THE REVIEW OF NATURAL PRODUCTS

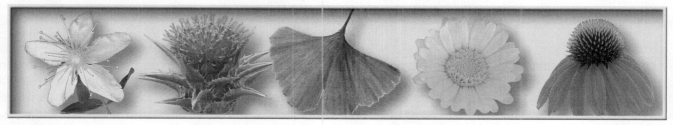

the most complete source of natural product information

2001

The Review of Natural Products®, First Edition, 2001

Adapted from *The Review of Natural Products* loose-leaf drug information service.
© 1996-2000 by Facts and Comparisons®
© 1989-1996 *The Lawrence Review of Natural Products* by Facts and Comparisons®

Cover photos © 2000 Steven Foster

ISBN 1-57439-100-3

Printed in the United States of America

Published by

Facts and Comparisons®
111 West Port Plaza, Suite 300
St. Louis, Missouri 63146-3098
www.factsandcomparisons.com
314/216-2100 • 800/223-0554

Facts and Comparisons®

Editor

Ara DerMarderosian, PhD
Professor of Pharmacognosy
University of the Sciences in Philadelphia

Facts and Comparisons® Publishing Group:

President and CEO — Steven K. Hebel, RPh

Senior Managing Editor — Teri H. Burnham

Managing Editor — Renée M. Short

Associate Editors — Wendy L. Bell
Kirsten K. Novak
Sara L. Schweain

Assistant Editor — Lindsay D. Harmon

Quality Control Editor — Susan H. Sunderman

SGML Specialist — Linda M. Jones

Senior Composition Specialist — Jennifer K. Walsh

Composition Specialist — Jennifer M. Reed

Director, Drug Information — Bernie R. Olin, PharmD

Cover Design — Mark L. Wickersham

Director, Sales and Marketing — Robert E. Brown

Marketing Manager — Laura V. Harter

Product and Market Analyst — Ann E. Burnett

Manufacturing Services Manager — Susan L. Polcyn

Consulting Editors:

Contributor

Lawrence Liberti, RPh, MS
President, Pharmaceutical Information Associates

Advisory Panel

John A. Beutler, PhD
Natural Products Chemist
National Cancer Institute

Michael Cirigliano, MD, FACP
Assistant Professor of Medicine
University of Pennsylvania
School of Medicine

Derrick DeSilva Jr., MD
President, American Nutraceutical Association

Constance Grauds, RPh
President, Association of Natural Medicine
 Pharmacists

Mary J. Ferrill, PharmD
Associate Professor
Drug Information Specialist
University of the Pacific
School of Pharmacy

David S. Tatro, PharmD
Drug Information Analyst

Facts and Comparisons® Editorial Advisory Panel

Table of Contents

Preface

As the premier publisher of drug information, Facts and Comparisons® provides a broad range of print, electronic, and on-line resources to fulfill the day-to-day needs of practicing health care professionals. The new bound edition of *The Review of Natural Products (RNP)* is being made available to continue our goal of fulfilling the various needs of our customers.

We acquired *The Lawrence Review of Natural Products* in 1989, and in 1996, we changed the name to *The Review of Natural Products,* established a reviewer panel, and added a patient information box to monographs. *RNP* provided objective information on herbal and other natural products at a time when the popularity of such products was just beginning to be noticed in the United States. Since that time, the natural product industry has exploded, and Facts and Comparisons® continues to stay on top of this ever-changing market.

Although the annual bound edition of *RNP* is one manner in which to access the primary source of natural product information, we provide *RNP* in many formats. The original version of RNP, a monthly updated monograph system, is intended to keep subscribers constantly up-to-date. A pocket-size, abridged version, *Guide to Popular Natural Products,* is a quick-reference publication. An electronic version is available on CD-ROM, which is updated monthly as part of the *CliniSphere*® library of drug reference resources and also as a stand-alone version *(Natural Products Explorer)*. We are also pleased to announce that the internet version of RNP became active in 2000 and can be accessed via www.drugfacts.com, your drug information destination.

All monographs in *RNP* are consistent and easy to follow. Each monograph lists scientific and common names and includes the following sections: Botany, History, Chemistry, Pharmacology, Toxicology, and a Summary. A patient information section discusses uses, side effects, drug interactions, and where appropriate, dosing. An appendix contains many other interesting sections, including Herbal Diuretics; a Mushroom Poisoning Decision Chart; Mushroom Societies; Poison Control Centers; Scientific and Trade Organizations that provide information on natural product research, evaluation, and education; and Herb/Drug Interaction Tables. A useful primary index as well as an in-depth therapeutic index rounds out this premier source of natural product information.

As this edition goes to press, we continue to update our database daily for use in future editions and formats of *RNP*. We also continue to expand our extensive library of drug information resources to remain the full service drug information provider that our customers have come to expect. However, this can only be accomplished with feedback from the loyal health care professionals who use our information daily. Comments, criticisms and suggestions are always welcome and encouraged. Please call or visit us at www.factsandcomparisons.com.

Steven K. Hebel, RPh
President and CEO

Introduction

The *Review of Natural Products*, is intended to provide a referenced guide to the numerous plant and dietary supplements now widely used in medicine. It contains more than 300 monographs on natural products alphabetically arranged and categorized by scientific name(s), common name(s), botany, chemistry, history, pharmacology, toxicology, patient information (a synopsis of uses, drug interactions, and side effects), and pertinent medical and scientific references.

This introduction provides an overview of historical and epidemiological data, the complimentary and alternative medicine (CAM) movement, the Dietary Supplement and Health Education Act (DSHEA) of 1994, and sufficient coverage of botany and pharmacology for the reader to appreciate and understand the details of proper use of natural products as medicinal agents.

Historical and epidemiological data: There is little doubt that herbal medicine or pharmacognosy is one of the oldest forms of health care. Almost every culture around the world has noted its individual contributions to pharmacognosy and use of foods as medicine. The oldest "prescriptions," found on Babylonian clay tablets and the hieratic writing of ancient Egyptians on papyrus, archive numerous ancient pharmaceutical and medical uses of hundreds of botanicals and foods (eg, olive oil, wine, turpentine, myrrh, opium, castor oil, garlic). This worldwide botanical cornucopia represents an eclectic collection of the most reliable early medicines that even today serve the ills of the world. The World Health Organization records the fact that 80% of the world's population still relies on botanical medicines. Several phytomedicines have advanced to widespread use in modern times and are familiar to all. These include morphine and related derivatives (from opium), colchicine (from Autumn crocus), cocaine (from Coca), digitoxin (from Foxglove), vincristine and vinblastine (from the Vinca plant), reserpine (from Indian Snakeroot), etoposide (from Mayapple), and taxol (from Yew). Many botanicals remain to be reevaluated as continued folkloric use around the world entices researchers to further scientific study.

History and science have shown repeatedly that almost all things are cyclical. Currently, we find ourselves in an era of resurgent interest in natural products as medicine. Ethnobotany, rain forest depletion of species, and certain limits in advancement using synthetic drugs continuously remind us that nature has and will always provide us with clues on how to develop new medicines. We have learned over and over the need to identify plants as to correct genus, species, variety, and even chemovar (chemical races) in order to obtain the same chemistry and medicinal properties desired for a particular botanical. Computers have helped us identify and categorize plants using the best of classical morphology and modern chemotaxonomy. Lessons from the complex phytochemistry of biologically active constituents have taught us that each plant is a unique chemical factory. We are trying to reach back to the old pharmacopoeias to update early attempts to standardize botanical medicines. Modern chemical procedures using chromatography, infrared spectroscopy, nuclear magnetic resonance spectroscopy, and mass spectrometry for molecular characterization of individual pharmacologically active principles have greatly facilitated the methodology. We now understand the complexity of standardization because of the innate biological variability of plant biochemistry. This allows us to fully appreciate all the complexities and variables that are introduced in plant collection, storage, transport, processing, and extraction to prepare uniform, stable dosage forms.

Natural product research has led to new physiological and pharmacological concepts, particularly when a new compound is found to have a specific biological effect. These have been referred to as "molecular keys" and include such examples as morphine (the chemical basis for natural and synthetic opioid analgesics), cocaine (the chemical basis for synthetic local anesthetics like procaine), and ephedra (the chemical basis for CNS stimulants like the amphetamines and the decongestants such as pseudoephedrine). Another recent resurrected plant drug is capsaicin from hot peppers. Previously used in topical analgesics as a "counterirritant," it is being reintroduced as a true analgesic because in low doses it depletes newly discovered substance P, which is involved in pain transmission.

Along similar lines, the ongoing competition with our new resistant pathogenic microbes has led us back into the race to find new antibiotics from soil microbes and fungi. New pandemic diseases like AIDS have taught us the importance of stimulating and protecting our immune system to fight such diseases. We are all living longer, and we need to help conquer cancer as well. Many promising agents are being developed from plants. New uses of certain supplements and vitamins have also focused our attention on food as medicine (nutraceuticals) and phytochemicals (eg, flavonoids, betacarbolenes, phytosterols) that may help prevent diseases.

Current epidemiological data and the current complimentary and alternative medicine movement: There are several factors that may be cited for the resurgence of interest in complementary and alternative medicine including the use of botanical medicines. These include consumer interest in perceived "natural" medicines, increased interest in fitness, health, and prevention directed toward longer and healthier lives, the general interest in improving the environment, and the increase in chronic diseases related to aging. Coupled with these factors has been the rise in cost of conventional medicines, an increased fear of potential adverse reactions to modern powerful drugs, and a desire to self-medicate to circumvent these difficulties. This has led to the movement toward complimentary and alternative medicines (CAM) (eg, acupuncture, biofeedback, chiropractic, diet, homeopathy, hypnosis, massage), particularly herbal medicine. A brief overview of the prevalence, costs, and patterns of use of CAM therapies in the US compiled by Dr. David Eisenberg at Peter Bent Brigham Hospital in Boston is quite revealing. The prevalence of CAM use increased from 33.8% in 1990 to 42.1% in 1997. The total number of visits to CAM providers increased by 47%, from 427 million in 1990 to 629 million in 1997. The total visits to CAM providers (629 million) exceeded total visits to all primary care physicians (386 million) in 1997. The estimated expenditures for alternative medicine professional services increased by 45% exclusive of inflation and in 1997 were estimated at $21.2 billion. An estimated 15 million adults in 1997 took prescription medications concurrently with herbal remedies or high-dose vitamins. It is obvious that there is a high risk for potential adverse drug-herb or drug-supplement interactions. The monographs provided herewith are intended to provide information that can preclude some of these difficulties. There is little doubt that even the current use of CAM services is underrepresented and that insurance coverage for holistic therapies will increase in the future. Health professionals and laity need reliable data to base decisions about which botanical supplements are possibly useful for various medical conditions.

The Dietary Supplement Health and Education Act (DSHEA): While several phytomedicinal agents have been used for a long time and thoroughly evaluated for safety and efficacy (eg, cascara, psyllium, digitalis, ipecac, belladonna), the majority of herbs have not been fully evaluated. For the most part, this rests with the problem of not being able to patent natural products in the US and the enormous costs (several hundred million dollars) and time (8 to 12 years) required to fully evaluate them. These reasons, coupled with the strong consumer movement to maintain the freedom of choice in self-medication, led to the DSHEA Act of 1994. For the first time, this law defined herbal products, vitamins, minerals, and amino acids as "dietary supplements." It also prohibited dietary supplements from being regulated as food additives, which normally require premarket approval. Further, it states that the burden of proof for safety and adulteration falls on the FDA. However, if a supplement poses an imminent health hazard, DSHEA allows the Secretary of Health and Human Services emergency powers to remove it from the market. The act permits general health claims regarding the activity of herbals but does not permit therapeutic claims. The herbal product manufacturer must be able to substantiate any health claim as being truthful and not misleading. The label must also include the following statement: "This statement has not been evaluated by the Food and Drug Administration. This product is not intended to diagnose, treat, cure, or prevent any disease." Finally, the label must include the designation "dietary supplement" and list each ingredient by name and quantity. Another provision allows for the distribution of information at the time of sale, giving a balanced view from scientific and related literature on the herbal products. The literature must not be misleading or false, cannot promote any specific brand, and should be displayed in an area physically separate from the product. It is up to the FDA to prove that any such information is misleading or false. Before this time, such literature was viewed as an extension of the label and any implied therapeutic claims could be considered in judging a product "misbranded."

On January 6, 2000 the FDA issued final regulations regarding types of structure/function claims that are allowed to be made under DSHEA. In general, claims that a product affects the normal structure/function of the human body are allowed. Any claim that explicitly or implicitly claims that the product can be used to "prevent, treat, cure, mitigate, or diagnose disease" are considered "disease claims" and would subject the product to the drug requirements under the

Act. The rule clarifies that such prohibited express or implied claims are made through the name of a product, through a statement about the formulation of a product (contains aspirin) or through the use of pictures, vignettes, or symbols (EKG tracings). The rule allows for claims that do not relate to disease, including health maintenance claims ("maintains a healthy circulatory system"), other nondisease claims ("for muscle enhancement," "helps you relax"), and claims for common, minor symptoms often associated with life stages ("for common symptoms of PMS," "for hot flashes").

DSHEA allowed for the establishment of a commission to conduct a 2-year study of the regulation of label claims and literature used in the sale of supplements. Finally, the bill also established the Office of Dietary Supplements (ODS) at the National Institutes of Health to coordinate research on dietary supplements. In order to keep up with the continuously evolving status, legal, and regulatory issues relating to the botanicals covered by ODS, refer to its web site: http://odp.od.nih.gov/ods

Another important web site for information on complementary and alternative medicine in general is http://nccam.nih.gov

Basic botany, pharmacognosy, and pharmacology: As it relates to herbals, basic botany, pharmacognosy, and pharmacology require the understanding that all plants have Latin binomial names (usually accurate and understood around the world) and numerous common names and synonyms. Therefore, botanical products should be identified with the proper Latin name and the most common synonym. Secondly, the active principles in a given plant may be found in one or more parts of the plant (eg, seeds, flowers, leaves). This is the reason that the plant part used should be indicated on the label of a commercial herbal product. For example, in ginkgo biloba, the active components are found in the leaves; in ginseng (*Panax* species), the roots contain the active constituents. Because the species or variety used may have differing concentrations of active principles, it is important to note this as well as geographic source, local environmental conditions of growth, and the processing procedures. All of these factors may influence the final product. Whichever plant part has shown the most active level of therapeutic effect and accompanying clinical evidence should be standardized and used. The proper extract or solvent should be specified by the manufacturer. Some require water soluble extraction while others may need a more non-polar or lipid extraction. Many of the commercial extracts do not follow official procedures, so it may be necessary to contact the manufacturer to determine how they produced the product. This may be difficult for proprietary reasons, and this is why particular extracts by particular manufacturers that have been clinically evaluated must be used for further studies verifying effects.

All solvents used to yield tinctures, extracts, etc. need to be fully defined for comparison studies and proper dosage determination. When advanced, concentrated, or standardized to active ingredients, the herb or dietary supplement comes closer to the definition of a drug. Yet many manufacturers do not bother to carry the quality control of their products to as high a level as traditional medicine dictates. It must be noted that pharmacologically active compounds in crude herbs are often present in lower concentrations than in conventional advanced, concentrated, or extracted products (eg, tablets, capsules, tinctures). This usually means that the toxicological risks associated with crude botanicals are minimal with moderate use. This may be true, particularly if there is data indicating safe use in many countries for centuries. Unfortunately, the US has always promoted the idea of "more is better," and this is where adverse reaction potential increases.

Another important factor about herbal products is that they often contain a wide variety of compounds from various classes. Often, therapeutic action is due to the combined action of several constituents. Some, like the primary metabolites (cellulose, starches, sugars, and fixed oils), are not particularly active pharmacologically. Others, like the secondary metabolites (alkaloids, cardiac glycosides, and steroids), are quite active pharmacologically. Content varies depending on genetics, environment (sunlight and rainfall), and fertilization. In fact, it is possible to see mixed activity depending on which compounds predominate. Selection at different times of the year also affects herb quality and clinical efficacy.

Potential toxicity, carcinogenicity, or liver toxicity: One must keep in mind dose levels and duration of use. In addition, there are growing concerns about plants such as comfrey *(Symphytum officinale)* that contain the externally useful drug allantoin (which promotes tissue regeneration) and rosmarinic acid (which acts as an anti-inflammatory). When taken internally, the content of pyrrolizidine alkaloids from comfrey is potentially hepatotoxic, mutagenic, and carcinogenic as seen in test animals. Many countries have banned or restricted its use. Unfortunately, because comfrey is regulated in the US as a dietary supplement and not a drug, it has remained on the market. The same story is seen with borage *(Borago officinalis)* and coltsfoot *(Tussilago farfara)* that also contain pyrrolizidine alkaloids. Fortunately, many products such as these have been withdrawn by reputable manufacturers and suppliers.

On occasion, there have been some unusual toxicities reported with commercial herbal products because of contamination with poisonous plants (eg, belladonna) or arsenic or mercury (imported products) and purposeful adulteration with synthetic drugs such as analgesics, anti-inflammatory agents, corticosteroids, and tranquilizers. These problems can be precluded by using products from reliable sources where rigorous good manufacturing practices (GMPs) are observed. Be aware that many imported products from underdeveloped countries may not adhere to good manufacturing practices.

While documented and published reports on herb-drug interactions are still minimal, there is the possibility that these can occur. The relatively few reports of herb-drug interactions probably is due to safety and a lack of professional surveillance. Because herbs have been classified as dietary supplements, there are no requirements for reporting acute or chronic toxicity. This is why the health professional should carefully monitor the use of herbal products by patients. There is a voluntary system for reporting suspected adverse effects (USP at 800-4USP-PRN and Medwatch at 800-FDA-1088).

Basic factors for the patient: The following general guidelines should be considered before advising patients about natural products: All products should be purchased from reliable sources. Even though GMPs are implicit in DSHEA guidelines for identity, cleanliness, and good quality control in manufacturing, there are significant differences in the purity, quality, and potency of products on the market. Further, many structure or function claims have not been evaluated by the FDA or by other independent and objective agencies. Generally, the more ambitious the claims, the more one should be suspicious of the quality of the product. One way to determine reliability of a manufacturer is to request professional health information from the company about the products, the nature of the company, testing, quality control standards, and the like. As with all legitimate and reliable pharmaceutical firms, such requests should elicit data on which decisions can be made about quality, return policies, and guarantees of structure and function claims in research and literature.

Most botanical products (particularly crude herbals) should be dry, appear fresh, and have appropriate colors (eg, bright yellows or reds for flowers, green for leaves, tan for roots). Moldy appearance or off odors are cause for return. Crude herbs, their extracts, or capsule forms should be stored in a cool, dry environment away from direct sunlight and out of the reach of children. Anyone handling crude botanicals should wear plastic gloves. Botanical dust should be kept at a minimum because of contamination concerns and potential allergy problems (eg, to molds, spores, pollen). All surfaces where herbs are handled should be wiped clean immediately. Botanicals should be dated. Discard it after one year.

Excessive dosages of phytomedicines should be avoided. Because many herbs are considered mild, the tendency is to use them for prolonged periods of time or to use too much at one time. Patients can delude themselves into thinking that they can avoid more potent and effective drugs by using "natural" herbs. All patients should be advised of risk/benefit ratios on all medical treatments and that serious illnesses can develop by assuming an herb will solve the problem over time. Also patients should be counseled about abuses seen with "diet teas" containing herbal laxatives that may lead to colonic impairments and excessive loss of potassium. Generally, natural products should not be used for serious health conditions without the advice and supervision of a qualified health practitioner. Most natural products are intended to treat mild, short-term disorders (eg, headaches, insomnia, dyspepsia, constipation). Any natural products causing undesirable side effects should be discontinued or the mode of administration changed. For example, while feverfew may be useful in preventing migraine headaches, aphthous mouth ulcers can result from chewing the leaves. Thus, capsules should be taken to avoid such local effects. Like many prescription and *otc* drugs, most natural products should be discontinued during pregnancy or lactation and not used in young children. Qualified health professionals should be consulted in these situations. Generally, avoid excessive combination products. Most research with prescription and *otc* medications has shown that more than two or three ingredients in one product is not always justifiable. Fixed combinations of active principles often result in excessive doses of one ingredient or use of an ingredient that may not be needed.

There is a good rationale for well-conceived combination products when appropriate, standardized dosages of a few synergistic herbals are coupled with vitamins and minerals. Herbal supplement users often start their nutritional regimen coupled with multivitamins. There is a growing market in higher quality, recognized brand-name products that feature concentrated, standardized botanical extracts in combination with appropriate dosages of vitamins and minerals. These offer convenience and simple once-daily dosing for patients. Examples of recent commercial products of this type have combined echinacea, vitamin C, and zinc for colds; echinacea polysaccharides and vitamin C may stimulate and improve the immune system, and zinc is an essential nutrient for immune system function. While not a cure, this combination may decrease the incidence and severity of the cold. Similar ideas have spawned combinations of B-vitamins, chromium, and ginseng for energy support, and combinations of St. John's wort and kava-kava for tension and mood control. Further research is needed to substantiate the efficacy of such combinations, but many companies have started to document the usefulness of such products. However, excessive use of more than a few botanicals in combination can be a potential problem because each botanical contains numerous active principles.

There is no doubt that efficacy becomes very difficult, if not impossible, to prove with excessive mixtures. Polypharmacy, an older pharmacy practice where small amounts of 10 to 15 ingredients were used in one combination product, is shunned today. Unfortunately, the practice of using many botanicals (often each in minute dosages) is still common in Asian and even in some American botanical products. It is highly unlikely that any of these are effective because there are often too many ingredients in ineffective amounts. Some patients feel that all of these botanicals work together, and therefore, such combinations are better, or that if one ingredient doesn't work another will. In reality, there is virtually no reliable clinical data on the efficacy of such complex mixtures.

Caution is advised not only in using combination herbal products but also in using single botanical products. *The Review of Natural Products* is intended to provide the reader with scientific data on both the benefits and the risks of various products.

Ara DerMarderosian, PhD
Editor
Philadelphia, Pennsylvania

MONOGRAPHS

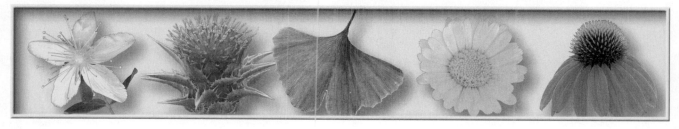

Acacia Gum

SCIENTIFIC NAME(S): *Acacia senegal* (L.) Willd. (syn. with *A. verek* Guill et Perr.). Other species of Acacia have been used in commerce. Family: Leguminosae or Fabaceae

COMMON NAME(S): Acacia gum, acacia vera.[1] Egyptian thorn,[1] gummi africanum,[2] gum Senegal, gummae mimosae, kher, Sudan gum arabic, Somali gum, yellow thorn

BOTANY: The acacia tree (*A. senegal*) is a thorny, scraggly tree that grows to heights of about 15 feet. It grows most prolifically in regions of Africa, in particular in the Republic of Sudan. During times of drought, the bark of the tree splits, exuding a sap that dries in small droplets or "tears."[3] In the past, these hardened sap tears served as the major source of acacia gum, but today commercial acacia gum is derived by tapping trees periodically and collecting the resin semi-mechanically. At least three grades of acacia gum are available commercially and their quality is distinguished by the color and character in the collected tears.[4] There is considerable variation in gum quality depending on whether it is obtained by natural flow secondary to extreme drought, obtained by tapping or induced by the boring of beetles at sites of branch injury.[5] Gums derived from *Combretum* are readily available at low prices in East and West Africa and are often offered for sale as "gum arabic." Because there is no toxicologic data supporting the safety of these gums, they are not recognized as food additives by most countries.[14] Similarly, trees of the genus *Albizia* are often confused with *Acacia* and should not be used as acacia substitutes.[15]

HISTORY: Acacia gum has long been used in traditional medicine and in everyday applications. The Egyptians used the material as a glue and as a pain-reliever base. Arabic physicians treated a wide variety of ailments with the gum, resulting in its current name.[3] Today, it is used widely in the pharmaceutical industry as a demulcent and in the cooking industry to give body and texture to processed food products. It also is used to stabilize emulsions. The fibers of the bark are used to make cordage.[6]

CHEMISTRY: Acacia gum is a brittle, odorless and generally tasteless material that contains a number of neutral sugars, acids, calcium and other electrolytes.[7] The main component of the gum is arabin, the calcium salt of arabic acid.[4] The structure of the gum is complex and has not yet been fully explained. A comprehensive analysis, including NMR spectra for 35 samples of gum arabic, has been published to serve as the basis for international standardization of acacia gum.[11] The gum is built upon a backbone of D-galactose units with side chains of D-glucuronic acid with L-rhamnose or L-arabinose terminal units. The molecular weight of the gum is large and estimates suggest the weight lies in the range of 200,000 to 600,000 daltons.[7] It is very soluble in water, but does not dissolve in alcohol.

PHARMACOLOGY: Acacia gum has no significant systemic effects when ingested. Although related gums have been shown to be hypocholesterolemic when ingested, there is no evidence for this effect with acacia. When administered to hypercholesterolemic patients for periods ranging from 4 to 12 weeks, acacia gum had no effect on the level of any plasma lipid evaluated.[9,12] Some studies suggest that ingestion of acacia gum may increase serum cholesterol levels in rats.[7] In the past, the gum has been administered intravenously to counteract low blood pressure following surgery and to treat edema associated with nephrosis, but this administration caused renal and liver damage and allergic reactions, and its use was abandoned.[5]

Acacia gum is a demulcent, and soothes irritated mucous membranes. Consequently, it is used widely in topical preparations to promote wound healing and as a component of cough and some gastrointestinal preparations. Whole gum mixtures of acacia have been shown to inhibit the growth of periodontic bacteria, including *Porphyromonas gingivalis* and *Prevotella intermedia* in vitro when added to culture medium in concentrations ranging from 0.5% to 1.0%.[8] At a concentration of 0.5%, acacia whole gum mixture also inhibited bacterial protease enzymes, suggesting acacia may be useful in limiting the development of periodontal disease. In addition, chewing an acacia-based gum for 7 days has been shown to reduce mean gingival and plaque scores compared to a sugar-free gum; the total differences in these scores was significant ($p < 0.05$) between groups suggesting that acacia gum primarily inhibits the early deposition of plaque.[13]

TOXICOLOGY: Acacia is essentially nontoxic when ingested. Allergic reactions to the gum and powdered forms of acacia have been reported and include respiratory problems and skin lesions.[7]

Acacia contains a peroxidase enzyme, which is typically destroyed by brief exposure to heat. If not inactivated, this enzyme forms colored complexes with certain amines and phenols and enhances the destruction of many pharmaceutical products including alkaloids and readily oxidizable compounds such as some vitamins.[5,7] Acacia gum reduces the antibacterial effectiveness of the preservative methyl-p-hydroxybenzoate against *Pseudomonas*

aeruginosa, presumably by offering physical barrier protection to the microbial cells from the action of the preservative.[10] A trypsin inhibitor also has been identified, but the clinical significance of the presence of this enzyme is not known.[6]

SUMMARY: Gum acacia has been used in commerce for millennia. Because of its soothing properties, it is included in cough and cold remedies and it is used topically in wound healing preparations. It is used as a stabilizer for foods. Although generally considered safe for internal use, some persons have developed severe allergic reactions following exposure to the gum.

PATIENT INFORMATION – Acacia Gum

Uses: Acacia gum has been used in food as a stabilizer and in pharmaceuticals as a demulcent. It is used topically for healing wounds and has been shown to inhibit the growth of periodontic bacteria and the early deposition of plaque.

Side Effects: Ingestion may raise serum cholesterol. Intravenous administration causes renal and liver damage. Various forms of acacia gum can cause allergic reactions, including respiratory problems and skin lesions.

---

[1] Meyer JE. *The Herbalist*. Hammond, IN: Hammond Book Co., 1934:13.

[2] Osol A, Farrar GE Jr. eds. *The Dispensatory of the United States of America*. 25th ed. Philadelphia: J.B. Lippincott, 1955:1.

[3] Dobelis IN, ed. *Magic and Medicine of Plants*. Pleasantville, NY: Reader's Digest Association, Inc., 1986.

[4] Evans WC. Trease and Evans' Pharmacognosy, 13th ed. London: Bailliere Tindall, 1989.

[5] Morton JF. Major medicinal plants. Springfield, IL: C.C. Thomas Publisher, 1977.

[6] Duke JA. Handbook of Medicinal Herbs. Boca Raton, FL: CRC Press, 1985.

[7] Leung AY. Encyclopedia of Common Natural Ingredients Used in Food, Drugs, and Cosmetics, New York, NY: J. Wiley and Sons, 1980.

[8] Clark DT, et al. The effects of Acacia arabica gum on the in vitro growth and protease activities of periodontopathic bacteria. *J Clin Periodontol* 1993;20:238.

[9] Jensen CD, et al. The effect of acacia gum and a water-soluble dietary fiber mixture on blood lipids in humans. *J Am Coll Nutr* 1993;12:147.

[10] Kurup TR, et al. Interaction of preservatives with macromolecules: Part I- natural hydrocolloids. *Pharm Acta Helv* 1992;67:301.

[11] Anderson DM, et al. Gum arabic (*Acacia senegal*); Unambiguous identification by 13C-NMR spectroscopy as an adjunct to the Revised JECFA Specification, and the application of 13C-NMR spectra for regulatory/legislative purposes. *Food Addit Contam* 1991;8:405.

[12] Haskell WL, et al. Role of water-soluble dietary fiber in the management of elevated plasma cholesterol in healthy subjects. *Am J Cardiol* 1992;69:433.

[13] Gazi MI. The finding of antiplaque features in Acacia arabica type of chewing gum. *J Clin Periodontol* 1991;18:75.

[14] Anderson DM, Morrison NA. The identification of Combretum gums which are not permitted food additives, II. *Food Addit Contam* 1990;7:181.

[15] Anderson DM, Morrison NA. Identification of Albizia gum exudates which are not permitted food additives. *Food Addit Contam* 1990;7:175.

Acerola

SCIENTIFIC NAME(S): *Malpighia glabra* L. and *M. punicifolia* L. Family: Malpighiaceae

COMMON NAME(S): Acerola, Barbados cherry, West Indian cherry, Puerto Rican cherry

BOTANY: The acerola is the fruit of a shrub that is native to the West Indies, but which is also found in northern South America, Central America, Texas and Florida.[1]

Because the fruit is small and bright red, it is said to resemble a cherry. Mature fruits are juicy with a pleasant tart flavor.[1]

HISTORY: Both species of *Malpighia* cited above have been reported to be excellent sources of vitamin C. More accurately, however, it is the fruit of *M. punicifolia* that is known as acerola and which is one of the richest sources of vitamin C known.

CHEMISTRY: Acerola contains from 1% to 4.5% vitamin C (1000 to 4500 mg/100 g) as ascorbic acid and dehydroascorbic acids in the edible portion of the fruit. This far exceeds the content of vitamin C in peeled oranges (about 0.05% or 50 mg/100 g).[1] The content of vitamin C in acerola varies with ripeness (highest in green and lowest in fully ripened fruit), season and climate.

In addition, acerola contains about the same amount of vitamin A as carrots, as well as thiamine, riboflavin and niacin.[1]

A number of other excellent natural sources of vitamin C have been identified including the fruits of *Terminalia ferdinandiana* (2767 mg/100 g), sea buckthorn (*Hippophae rhamnoides*, 450 mg/100 g), ambla (*Emblica officinalis*, 600 mg/100 g), and rose hips (*Rosa canina*, 1250 mg/100 g).[2]

PHARMACOLOGY: Vitamin C is an essential coenzyme that is required for normal metabolic function. While many animals can synthesize vitamin C from glucose, humans must obtain their vitamin totally from dietary sources. Deficiencies of this water-soluble vitamin result in scurvy, a potentially fatal disease with multisystem involvement. Dietary supplements have traditionally provided adequate protection against the development of this disease.

However, controversy has focused on whether vitamin C derived from "natural" sources is more physiologic than that produced synthetically or semisynthetically (as ascorbic acid). To date, there is no clear evidence that naturally-derived vitamin C is superior in its clinical effectiveness than synthetic ascorbic acid. A potential advantage to using acerola as a source of vitamin C is that one derives not only ascorbic acid, but also several other useful vitamins and minerals from the fruit. Whether this is superior to the use of a multiple vitamin preparation has not been determined.

TOXICOLOGY: No specific adverse events have been associated with the ingestion of acerola. Because vitamin C is a water-soluble compound, it is readily excreted by the body, and it is not typically associated with toxicity. However, the ingestion of large doses may induce gastrointestinal side effects, including diarrhea. Prolonged use of massive doses of ascorbic acid may predispose to the development of renal calculi.

SUMMARY: The acerola fruit is a natural source of vitamin C; it is among the most concentrated sources of the vitamin known. It is used as a nutritional supplement and foodstuff in the West Indies and portions of Central America, and today is widely used in the health food industry.

PATIENT INFORMATION – Acerola

Uses: Acerola provides natural vitamin C and other useful vitamins and minerals.

Side Effects: Large doses may produce gastrointestinal distress. Prolonged, massive dosage may predispose to formation of renal calculi.

---

[1] Leung AY. Encyclopedia of Common Natural Ingredients Used in Food, Drugs, and Cosmetics. New York, NY: J. Wiley and Sons, 1980.

[2] Brand JC, et al. An outstanding food source of vitamin C. *Lancet* 1982;2:873.

Acidophilus

HISTORY: For several decades, health and nutritional benefits have been claimed for products containing *Lactobacillus* cultures. The topical or intravaginal application of yogurt products has been reported to control yeast and bacterial infections, and the ingestion of these preparations has been recommended to reduce the symptoms of antibiotic-induced diarrhea or sore mouth due to candida infections.[1] Other reports have indicated that the ingestion of acidophilus-containing products can reduce serum cholesterol levels, improve lactose intolerance and slow the growth of experimental tumors.[2]

CLINICAL USES: Replenishment of normal bacterial flora: Products containing live cultures have been investigated for their ability to compete with pathogens in the microenvironment, thereby permitting the re-establishment of normal bacterial flora. Lactobacilli have been shown to inhibit the growth of other vaginal microorganisms including *Escherichia coli*, *Candida albicans* and *Gardnerella vaginalis*.[3] Several factors may contribute to the possible activity of *Lactobacillus*, including their ability to generate lactic acid, hydrogen peroxide and exogenous antibacterial compounds, to influence the production of interferon by target cells[4] and to alter the adherence of bacteria. Lactacin F, an antibacterial compound produced by *L. acidophilus*, has been isolated and partially characterized as a heat-stable protein with at least 56 amino acid residues.[5,6]

Lactobacillus has long been considered to be a component of the protective flora in the vagina. Recently, *Lactobacillus* species that produce hydrogen peroxide have been found in normal vaginal flora. Consequently, the therapeutic benefits of *Lactobacillus* products have been investigated in women with vaginal and urinary tract infections. Women who used either acetic acid jelly, an estrogen cream, a fermented lactobacillus-containing milk product or metronidazole (eg, *Flagyl*), were evaluated to determine the effects of intravaginal therapy on bacterial vaginosis. Clinical cures were obtained for 13 of 14 women receiving metronidazole but for only 1 of 14 using the fermented milk product. This latter intervention did not influence the predominance of lactobacilli in the vagina.[7] An evaluation of 16 commercially available products containing *Lactobacillus* in the form of capsules, powders and tablets (in addition to yogurt and milk) found that all 16 products contained lactobacilli, of which 10 strains produced hydrogen peroxide. At least one contaminant was detected in 11 of the products, including

Enterococcus faecium, *Clostridium sporogenes* and *Pseudomonas* species. Only 4 of the products contained *L. acidophilus* and therefore, the authors concluded that most commercially available products may not be appropriate for recolonization of the vagina.[3] The weekly instillation of *Lactobacillus* has been shown to reduce the recurrence rate of uncomplicated lower urinary tract infections in women, and the use of a strain that is resistant to nonoxynol-9, a spermicide that kills protective vaginal flora, may have potential for use in women with recurrent cystitis using this contraceptive agent.[8]

L. acidophilus is normally found in the human alimentary tract. Being acid-resistant, it persists in the stomach much longer than other bacteria do. Consequently, the oral administration of products containing *L. acidophilus* may be useful in the management of a variety of conditions associated with altered gastrointestinal flora. Their beneficial effects may be related to the ability to suppress the growth of pathogens. In vitro, *L. acidophilus* has been shown to suppress the growth of *Campylobacter pylori*, a pathogen implicated as a causative factor in acid-peptic disease, although the therapeutic implications of these findings are not clear.[9,10]

No consensus has been reached regarding the effectiveness of lactobacillus-containing products in ameliorating antibiotic-induced diarrhea. When *Lactinex* granules, a combination of *L. acidophilus* and *L. bulgaricus*, was given four times daily for 10 days to children concomitantly with amoxicillin (eg, *Amoxil*) therapy under double-blind conditions, 70% of the patients receiving placebo and 66% of those taking *Lactinex* experienced diarrhea. Closer analysis suggested that the incidence of diarrhea diminished during the last 4 days of therapy for the *Lactinex* patients, while it remained constant for those given placebo.[11] However, in a study of 40 children who received amoxicillin concomitantly with fermented lactobacillus milk products, the treated group showed a lower frequency of stool passages and more fully-formed feces compared with no treatment.[12]

The ingestion of these products has been associated with decreases in the concentration of several fecal enzymes that have the capacity to convert procarcinogens to carcinogens in the colon. This suggests that consumption of lactobacillus-containing products may have beneficial health effects, although no data are available to support this hypothesis.[13]

Effect on cholesterol levels: A mutant strain of *L. acidophilus* with unique metabolic characteristics, led to the isolation of mevalonic acid, an important intermediate of the isoprenoid compound pathwa.[14] and a precursor to cholesterol synthesis. It has been suggested that appropriately selected strains of *Lactobacillus* may be useful adjuncts for the control of hypercholesterolemia in humans, by virtue of the bacteria's ability to assimilate cholesterol and to grow well in the presence of bile.[15] The results of one study, in which 354 subjects took *Lactinex* tablets or placebo four times a day for 3 weeks in a crossover fashion, found no clinically significant changes in lipoprotein concentrations for either group.[16] Additional work is required to confirm the effects of *Lactobacillus* preparations on serum lipid levels.

TOXICOLOGY: No significant toxicity has been reported among users of *Lactobacillus* products.

SUMMARY: Preparations containing *Lactobacillus acidophilus* include yogurt, milk, tablets, capsules and granules. They are used most frequently to restore normal flora to the gastrointestinal tract and vagina. However, the data supporting the efficacy of these products for these uses are conflicting.

PATIENT INFORMATION – Acidophilus

Uses: Lactobacillus acidophilus has been used to restore normal oral, gastrointestinal, and vaginal flora in those affected by antibiotics, candida, and bacterial infections. Its value in treating all these, as well as lower urinary tract infections, remains unclear. In vitro, it suppresses growth of *Campylobacter pylori*, implicated in acid-peptic disease.

Side Effects: L. acidophilus is considered safe, being normally found in the human alimentary tract.

---

[1] Lewis WH. Medical Botany. New York, NY: J. Wiley and Sons, 1977.

[2] Gorbach SL. Lactic acid bacteria and human health. *Ann Med* 1990;22(1):37.

[3] Hughes VL, Hillier SL. Microbiologic characteristics of *Lactobacillus* products used for colonization of the vagina. *Obstet Gynecol* 1990;75(2):244.

[4] Mihal V, et al. Immunobiologic properties of lactobacilli. *Cesk Pediatr* 1990;45(10):587.

[5] Muriana PM, Klaenhammer TR. Purification and partial characterization of Lactacin F, a bacteriocin produced by *Lactobacillus acidophilus* 11088. *Appl Environ Microbiol* 1991;57(1):114.

[6] Muriana PM, Klaenhammer TR. Cloning, phenotypic expression and DNA sequence of the gene for Lactacin F, an antimicrobial peptide produced by *Lactobacillus* spp. *J Bacteriol* 1991;173(5):1779.

[7] Fredricsson B, et al. Bacterial vaginosis is not a simple ecological disorder. *Gynecol Obstet Invest* 1989;28(3):156.

[8] Reid G, et al. Is there a role for lactobacilli in prevention of urogenital and intestinal infections? *Clin Microbiol Rev* 1990;3(4):335.

[9] Bhatia SJ, et al. Lactobacillus acidophilus inhibits growth of *Campylobacter pylori* in vitro. *J Clin Microbiol* 1989;27:2328.

[10] Gismondc MR, et al. Competitive activity of a bacterial preparation of colonization and pathogenicity of *C. pylori*. A clinical study. *Clin Ter* 1990;134(1):41.

[11] Tankanow RM, et al. A double-blind, placebo-controlled study of the efficacy of *Lactinex* in the prophylaxis of amoxicillin-induced diarrhea. *DICP Ann Pharmacother* 1990;24(4):382.

[12] Contardi I. Oral bacteria therapy in prevention of antibiotic-induced diarrhea in childhood. *Clin Ter* 1991;136(6):409.

[13] Marteau P, et al. Effect of chronic ingestion of a fermented dairy product containing *Lactobacillus acidophilus* and *Bifidobacterium bifidum* on metabolic activities of the colonic flora in humans. *Am J Clin Nutr* 1990;52(4):685.

[14] Evans WC. Trease and Evans' Pharmacognosy, 13th ed. London, England: Bailliere Tindall, 1989.

[15] Gilliland SE, Walker DK. Factors to consider when selecting a culture of *Lactobacillus acidophilus* as a dietary adjunct to produce a hypocholesterolemic effect in humans. *J Dairy Sci* 1990;73(4):905.

[16] Lin SY, et al. *Lactobacillus* effects on cholesterol: In vitro and in vivo results. *J Dairy Sci* 1989;72(11):2885.

Ackee

SCIENTIFIC NAME(S): *Blighia sapida* K. Konig. Family: Sapindaceae

COMMON NAME(S): Ackee, akee, aki, arbre fricasse', seso vegetal

BOTANY: The ackee is found widely throughout the West Indies and has been naturalized to parts of Central America, Florida and Hawaii. The ackee tree grows to about 40 feet. Its oval, compound leaves have five pairs of leaflets, the longest of which is about 6 inches at the tip. The plant produces small greenish-white flowers. The red fruit pods split open at maturity, exposing three shiny black seeds embedded in a white waxy aril.[1]

HISTORY: The ackee tree was imported to Jamaica from West Africa in the late 1700s and is often grown as an ornamental.[2] Although the unripened walnut-like seeds are toxic, the ripe fruits are used in traditional island cooking.[1] In Jamaica, fresh ackee berries are available in season in markets and canned fruit is available throughout the year. Poisonings have long been associated with the use of the ackee, and published reports of Jamaican intoxications date back to 1904.[3] In South America, the fruit is used to treat colds, fever and diseases as varied as edema and epilepsy.[2]

CHEMISTRY: The primary compound of clinical interest is hypoglycin A, a cyclopropyl amino acid. This compound is found in the aril and the seeds of the unripe fruit.[4] In addition, other hypoglycemic compounds, including hypoglycin B and cyclopropanoid amino acids, are found in the seed.

PHARMACOLOGY/TOXICOLOGY: Hypoglycin A is a water-soluble liver toxin that induces hypoglycemia by inhibiting gluconeogenesis by limiting the activity of cofactors (CoA and carnitine) that are required for the oxidation of long-chain fatty acids.[3] The pink raphe (the portion of the seed that attaches to the ovary wall) and the aril in the immature plant are poisonous because of the presence of the hypoglycins. The arils become edible when the fruit ripens. Hypoglycin A appears to be approximately twice as toxic as hypoglycin B.[4] The powdered fruits are used in Africa as a fish poison.[2]

Large-scale poisonings appear to be limited to the island of Jamaica where they may reach epidemic proportions during the winter months under the name of "vomiting sickness."[1] More than 5000 people have died from ackee poisoning since 1886[4] and 271 cases have been reported since 1980. In a recent review of ackee poisonings in Jamaica, 28 patients who had symptoms of ackee poisoning were identified during the period of January 1989 through July 1991. Six of these patients died. The most common symptoms were vomiting, coma and seizures. Seven of the patients had confirmed hypoglycemia. Most of the cases occurred between January and March.[3]

Poisoning may be present in one of two distinct forms. In the first case, vomiting is followed by a remission period of 8 to 10 hours, followed by renewed vomiting, convulsions and coma. The second type is characterized by convulsions and coma at the onset. Diarrhea and fever are usually absent. Six hours or more may elapse between ingestion of the fruit and the onset of symptoms. Severe hypoglycemia develops[1] and blood glucose levels as low as 3 mg/dL are observed in many cases.[3]

Management of ackee intoxication consists of fluid therapy and the administration of glucose and electrolytes. Because patients with preexisting nutritional deficits and children may be more sensitive to the toxic effects of the fruit, vitamin and nutritional supplements should be administered.[1,3]

SUMMARY: The ripe ackee fruit is used traditionally in Jamaican cooking. However, the unripened fruit is toxic, causing severe hypoglycemia, often accompanied by convulsions and death.

PATIENT INFORMATION – Ackee

Uses: Ackee fruit is used in Jamaican cooking and in folk treatments for various diseases, including colds and fever.

Side Effects: The toxic unripe fruit causes hypoglycemia, convulsions, coma, and death. Symptoms may be delayed or intermittent.

---

[1] Lampe KF. AMA Handbook of Poisonous and Injurious Plants. Chicago, IL: Chicago Review Press, 1985.
[2] Duke JA. Handbook of Medicinal Herbs. Boca Raton, FL: CRC Press, 1985.
[3] Toxic Hypoglycemic Syndrome-Jamaica, 1989-1991. *MMWR* 1992;41(4):53.
[4] Farnsworth NR, Segelman AB. Hypoglycemic Plants. *Tile and Till* 1971;57(3):52.

Aconite

SCIENTIFIC NAME(S): *Aconitum napellus* L. *A. columbianum* also is described in cases of aconite toxicity. Family: Ranunculaceae

COMMON NAME(S): Aconite, monkshood, friar's cap, helmet flower, soldier's cap, wolfsbane[1]

BOTANY: These erect perennial plants grow to a height of 2 to 6 feet. In general, they resemble delphiniums. The characteristic helmet-shaped blue flowers grow in a raceme at the top of the stalk in summer or fall. Occasionally, the flowers may be white, pink or peach. The seed pods dry and contain numerous tiny seeds.[1] More than 100 species of *Aconitum* are distributed throughout the temperate zones of the United States and Canada. These plants also are found throughout many parts of Asia, Africa, Europe and Russia.

HISTORY: Aconite is well known because it is extremely toxic. The tuberous root has been used in traditional medicine although all parts of the plant are considered to be toxic. While the extracts of the plant are used rarely in medicine today in the United States, they continue to find use in liniments as rubifacients for external application. Extracts are used in homeopathic medicine as hypotensives, to decrease fever and to treat neuralgias.[2] Extracts of the plant have been used in traditional medicine as cardiac depressants and topically to treat neuralgias. In traditional Asian medicine, extracts of the roots are typically mixed with other ingredients (ie, licorice, ginger) for ailments ranging from sciatica to nephritis. Extracts have been used as arrow poisons.

CHEMISTRY: Alkaloids account for up to 1.5% of the plant. These consist primarily of the related alkaloids aconitine, picraconitine, aconine and napelline.[3] Aconitine is hydrolyzed to picraconitine, which hydrolyzes to aconine. A wide variety of minor alkaloids have been isolated from the various species of aconite.

PHARMACOLOGY: Aconite is a fast-acting toxin through the action of the active principles aconitine and related alkaloids. As little as 2 mg to 5 mg of aconitine (approximately one teaspoonful of the root) may cause death due to paralysis of the respiratory center or cardiac muscle.

Toxicity from the wild plant has resulted when the plant was confused for wild parsley or the roots for horseradish.[2]

Aconitine's toxicity is characterized by a burning sensation of the lips, tongue, mouth and throat almost immediately following ingestion. Numbness of the throat may ensue with difficulty in speaking. Salivation, nausea and emesis may occur along with visual blurring or yellow-green color vision distortion. A single dose of 0.6 mg/kg of aconitine administered intraperitoneally to rabbits has been shown to alter visual evoked potential and to cause histopathologic damage to the myelin sheath of the visual pathway, spinal cord and peripheral nerves.[4] Weakness, dizziness and incoordination may occur. Gastric lavage or emesis following the injection of atropine has been recommended.[5]

Cardiac arrhythmias of often unusual electrical characteristics have been observed following aconite poisoning.[6] These arrhythmias may not respond to procainamide and may worsen following verapamil administration. Putrescine, a compound used experimentally as a molecular probe, has been shown to attenuate aconitine-induced arrhythmias.[7] Death may ensue secondary to cardiac arrhythmias,[1] which may occur within minutes or days.[2]

Aconitine produces tingling and numbness when applied to the skin and significant toxicity may develop following percutaneous absorption.

Some *Aconitum* species have been reported to exert antitumor activity in vitro and in animals while others possess antibacterial and antifungal activity.[3] In animal models, aconitine and related compounds have been shown to possess anti-inflammatory and analgesic properties.[8]

There is some evidence to suggest that aconite may lose its potency after undergoing certain manufacturing procedures, and therefore processed aconite may not have a similar toxicity profile to crude plant material.[9]

SUMMARY: Aconite is recognized as a highly toxic plant. Its extracts find little use in medicine in the United States today, but continue to be used in traditional medicine throughout Europe and Asia. Severe toxicity, including death from cardiac arrhythmia, may ensue following ingestion of as little as one teaspoonful of the root.

PATIENT INFORMATION – Aconite

Uses: Aconite extracts have been used externally and homeopathically in Europe and Asia, but rarely in the United States. Research suggests a variety of possible applications.

Side Effects: Aconite is highly toxic, at times even through percutaneous absorption.

[1] Lampe KF. AMA Handbook of Poisonous and Injurious Plants. Chicago, IL: Chicago Review Press, 1985.

[2] Spoerke DG. Herbal Medications. Santa Barbara, CA: Woodbridge Press Publishing Company, 1980.

[3] Leung AY. Encyclopedia of Common Natural Ingredients Used in Food, Drugs and Cosmetics. New York, NY: J. Wiley and Sons, 1980.

[4] Kim SH, et al. Myelo-optic neuropathy caused by aconitine in rabbit model. *Jpn J Ophthalmol* 1991;35:417.

[5] Duke JA. Handbook of Medicinal Herbs. Boca Raton, FL: CRC Press, 1985.

[6] Tai YT, et al. Bidirectional tachycardia induced by herbal aconite poisoning. *PACE* 1992;15:831.

[7] Bozzani C, et al. Putrescine reverses aconitine-induced arrhythmia in rats. *J Pharm Pharmacol* 1989;41:651.

[8] Murayama M, et al. Studies on the constituents of *Aconitum* species. *J Ethnopharmacol* 1991;35:159.

[9] Thorat S, Dahanukar S. Can we dispense with Ayurvedic Samskaras? *J Postgrad Med* 1991;37:157.

Agrimony

SCIENTIFIC NAME(S): *Agrimonia eupatoria* L. Family: Rosaceae

COMMON NAME(S): Cocklebur, stickwort, liverwort

BOTANY: Agrimony (of British Herbal Pharmacopoeia) is a perennial herb with small, star-shaped yellow flowers. The plant possesses a short rhizome and is supported by a firm, hairy stem. The basal leaves are arrayed in a rosette and they, as well as the alternate sessile stem leaves, are pinnate, serrate and glabrous.[1] The flowers and fruit (achene) grow at the top of the stem in a long, terminal spike. Agrimony is common in grasslands throughout Europe. It is imported from Bulgaria, Hungary and the former Yugoslavia.[2]

HISTORY: The name Agrimonia may have its origin in the Greek "agremone" which refers to plants which supposedly healed cataracts of the eye. The species name *eupatoria* probably relates to Mithradates Eupator, King of Pontres, who is credited with introducing many herbal remedies. Its ancient uses include treatment for catarrh (mucous membrane inflammation with discharge), bleeding, tuberculosis and skin diseases.[1] In folk medicine, it has been reported, without verification, to be useful in gallbladder disorders. Numerous other reported uses include use as a dye, flavoring, gargle for performers and speakers, antitumor agent, astringent, cardiotonic, coagulant, diuretic, sedative, antiasthmatic and for corns or warts.[3]

CHEMISTRY: The aerial parts of the plant contain 4-10% condensed tannins, small amounts of ellagitannins and traces of gallotannins.[2,4] Also reported are some 20% polysaccharides.[4] A triterpenoid, urosolic acid, has been isolated. Silicic acid and traces of essential oil are listed as constituents. The flavonoids, luteolin and apigenin 7-0–β-D-glucosides, are present.[4] Organic acids, vitamin B$_1$, vitamin K and ascorbic acid are also listed as components. The fresh herb contains agrimoniolide, palmitic and stearic acids, ceryl alcohol and phytosterols. Seeds contain 35% oil which contains oleic, linoleic and linolenic acids.[2,3]

PHARMACOLOGY: Agrimony is used widely in Europe as a mild astringent (externally and internally), particularly against inflammation of the throat, gastroenteritis and intestinal catarrh. Studies of ethanolic extracts display the anti-viral properties. This plant is often included in phytomedicine mixtures for "liver and bile teas," again without true scientific verification. Agrimony extracts are often used in small amounts in prepared European cholagogues and stomach and bowel remedies (eg, Neo-Gallonorm®-Dragees) and urological products (eg, Rhoival©). Agrimony is also a component of the British product Potter's Piletabs®.[2,4,5,6]

TOXICOLOGY: Agrimony has been reported to produce photodermatitis in man.[3]

SUMMARY: Agrimony is used as a tea and gargle for sore throats, in compresses or poultices for skin rashes and cuts, and in various bath preparations. It does appear to have justifiable use as a mild antiseptic and topical astringent. Internal uses of this herb require further verification.

PATIENT INFORMATION – Agrimony

Uses: Agrimony is used as a tea and gargle for sore throat and externally as a mild antiseptic and astringent.

Side Effects: Agrimony reportedly can produce photodermatitis.

---

[1] Bunney S, ed. The Illustrated Encyclopedia of Herbs: Their Medicinal and Culinary Uses. New York: Dorset Press, 1984.
[2] Bisset NG, ed. Herbal Drugs and Phytopharmaceuticals. Stuttgart: Medpharm Scientific Publishers, 1994.
[3] Duke JA. Handbook of Medicinal Herbs. Boca Raton, FL: CRC Press 1985.
[4] von Gizycki F. *Pharmazie* 1949;4:276, 463.
[5] Hoppe HA. Drogenkunde, 8th ed., vol. 1. Berlin: Walter deGruyter, 1975.
[6] Drozd GA, et al. *Prir Soedin* 1983;1:106.
[7] Chon SC, et al. *Med Pharmacol Exp* 1987;16:407.

Agropyron

SCIENTIFIC NAME(S): *Agropyron repens*, *Elymus repens*, *Graminis rhizoma*, *Triticum repens*. Family: Gramineae

COMMON NAME(S): Couch-grass root, dog grass, quack grass

BOTANY: Agropyron is a weed that is widely distributed throughout the northern hemisphere. The grass grows up to 1.5 m tall with spikes up to 15 cm long containing many flowered spikelets.[1] The leaves alternate with sheaths; the blades are long and narrow, and the veins are parallel.[2] The grass also contains shiny, pale yellow, hollow pieces of rhizome and longitudinally grooved stems that are 2 to 3 mm thick. Thin roots and short fiber-like cataphylls are present at the unthickened nodes. It has an almost bland, but slightly sweet taste.[1] The rhizomes, roots and stems are used to formulate the drug.[1]

HISTORY: Based on folk medicine, agropyron has been used as a diuretic in cases of bladder catarrh and bladder/kidney stones, and as a cough medicine to alleviate bronchial irritation. Other uses in folk medicine include gout, rheumatic disorders and chronic skin disorders. The drug products are typically imported from Romania, Hungary, the former Yugoslavia and Albania.[1]

CHEMISTRY: The major constituent of agropyron is triticin (3% to 8%), a polysaccharide related to inulin. Upon hydrolysis, triticin releases: fructose; mucilage (10%); possible saponins; sugar alcohols (mannitol, inositol, 2% to 3%); essential oil with polyacetylenes or carvone (0.01% to 0.05%); small amounts of vanilloside (vanillin monoglucoside), vanillin and phenolcarboxylic acids; silicic acid; and silicates. Lectins found in the seedlings and leaves may also be present in the rhizome.[1] However, the lectin content of the leaves varies from season to season.[3]

PHARMACOLOGY: Couch grass leaf lectin exhibits specificity for N-acetylgalactosamine and agglutinates, preferentially blood-group-A erythrocytes.[3]

In addition to the folk uses of couch grass, it has also been indicated for irrigation therapy in inflammatory disorders of the urinary tract, in the prevention of renal gravel, as well as to supplement treatment in catarrh of the upper respiratory tract. The essential oil has shown antimicrobial effects, and extracts of the drug are used as a dietary component for diabetics.[1] Despite these indications, pharmacological and clinical studies are lacking.

TOXICOLOGY: There are no known side effects or drug interactions associated with the use of agropyron or couch grass.

SUMMARY: Agropyron has been used in folk medicine for a variety of diuretic ailments and as a cough remedy to alleviate bronchial irritation. Other uses include gout, various rheumatic disorders, chronic skin conditions and various urinary tract, bladder and kidney disorders. Extracts of the drug are used as a dietary component for diabetics. However, no large scale clinical studies have proven any of these indications for agropyron; further investigation is needed.

PATIENT INFORMATION – Agropyron

Uses: Agropyron has been used to treat gout, various rheumatic disorders, chronic skin conditions and various urinary tract, bladder and kidney disorders. Various extracts have been used as a dietary component for diabetics.

Side Effects: There are no known side effects.

---

[1] Bisset NG, ed. Herbal Drugs and Phytopharmaceuticals. Stuttgart: Medpharm Scientific Publishers, 1994.
[2] Trease GE. Pharmacognosy, ed. 12. London: Bailliére Tindall, 1983.
[3] Cammue B, et al. A new type of cereal lectin from leaves of couch grass (Agropyrum repens). *Eur J Biochem* 1985;148(2):315.

Alchemilla

SCIENTIFIC NAME(S): *Alchemilla xanthochlora* Rothm. (Syn. *Alchemilla vulgaris* auct. non L.). Family: Rosaceae

COMMON NAME(S): Lady's mantle

BOTANY: Lady's mantle is a perennial herb with a short rhizome carrying ascending or sprawling stems, and a rosette of basal leaves with dentate lobes of a circular or kidney-shaped outline. The inflorescence is a compound terminal cyme made up of dense clusters of small hellow-green flowers. Sepals are seen in two rings of four without petals. The fruit is of the achene type. Overall, the plant is softly pubescent. It is found throughout Europe in meadows, woodland clearings, pastures and in the lowland areas of the British Isles. Currently, it is distributed in Europe, North America and Asia.[1,2]

HISTORY: *Alchemilla* is one of an aggregate of species collectively referred to as lady's mantle, all possessing similar medicinal properties. Many are cultivated. Medieval alchemists collected rain water or dew collected in the leaf center and used it for its purported magical and medicinal powers. This custom derived from the plant's generic name, *alchemilla*, which is from the Arabic word, "alkimiya" (universal cure for diseas). In medieval tradition, it was used to treat wounds and female ailments. It has long been dedicated to the Virgin Mary, since the leaf lobes resemble the edges of a mantle. Among lady's mantle's historical uses are as a mild astringent, anti-inflammatory, diuretic, menstrual cycle regulator, treatment for digestive disorders and relaxant for muscular spasms. Externally, it was widely used in bath preparations, wound healing, skin bruises and as an herbal cosmetic.[1,2]

CHEMISTRY: Lady's mantle contains 6% to 8% tannins (elligiannins, such as pedunculagin and alchemillin) and flavonoids (quercetin 3–0–β-D-glucuronide).[2,3]

PHARMACOLOGY: The historical uses of lady's mantle as an astringent against bleeding and as a treatment for diarrhea seem justified on the bases of its tannin content.[2] Newer studies show that the water extract of *A. xanthochlora* possesses lipid peroxidation and superoxide anion scavenging activity.[4]

Several rosaceae species, including *A. xanthochlora*, have high tannin content and elastase inhibitin activity.[5] In a similar vein, flavonoids extracted from *Alchemilla* inhibit the activity of the proteolytic enzymes elastase, trypsin and alpha-chymotrypsin.[6] These results suggest a possible role by these inhibitors in the protection of conjunctive and elastic tissues.

A number of traditional plant treatments have been studied for diabetes in normal and streptozotocin diabetic mice, but no useful effects for lady's mantle have been found in this disorder.[7]

A study on the mutagenic potencies of several plant extracts (including Tinctura Alchemillae) containing quercetin in *Salmonella typhimurium* TA98 and TA100 found that the mutagenic potential of the plant extracts correlates well with their quercetin content.[8] The cytostatic activity of a lactone fraction from Alchemilla pastoralis has also been reported.[9]

TOXICOLOGY: No significant toxicological studies appear to have been carried out on lady's mantle and long use for various purposes (internal and external) seem to bear out the fact that it is safe in low doses. The warning in the Standard License about possible liver damage appears to be exaggerated.[2]

SUMMARY: The use of lady's mantle for its local astringent and anti-diarrheal properties are mildly justified by the known tannin content of the plant. Newer chemistry and pharmacological studies are sparse, revealing only possible usefulness for its anti-oxidant properties and vague protective effects as well as mutagenic potential and cytostatic activity. More human clinical data are needed to justify its use for its historical medical applications.

PATIENT INFORMATION – Alchemilla

Uses: Alchemilla has been used topically and internally, as a treatment for wounds, gastrointestinal complaints and female ailments. Its tannin content appears to justify astringent and antidiarrheal uses. It may protect conjunctive and elastic tissues and possibly be useful as an antioxidant.

Side Effects: None known for low doses, with the possible exception of liver damage.

---

[1] Bunney S, ed. The Illustrated Encyclopedia of Herbs. New York: Dorset Press, 1984.

[2] Bisset NG, ed. Herbal Drugs and Phytopharmaceuticals. Stuttgart: Medpharm Scientific Publishers, 1994.

[3] Lamaison JL, et al. [Quercetin-3–glucuronide, Main Flavonoid of *Alchemilla, Alchemilla xanthochlora* Rothm. (Rosaceae),] [French] *Ann Pharm Fr* 1991;49(4):186.

[4] Filipek J. Effect of *Alchemilla xanthochlora* Water Extracts on Lipid Peroxidation and Superoxide Anion Scavenging Activity. *Pharmazie* 1992;47:717.

[5] Lamaison JL, et al. [Tannin Content and Inhibiting Activity of Elastase in Rosaceae.] [Review] [French] *Ann Pharm Fr* 1990;48(6):335.

[6] Jonadet M, et al. [Flavonoids Extracted From *Ribes nigrum* L. and *Alchemilla vulgaris* L.: 1. In vitro inhibitory activities on elastase, trypsin and chymotrypsin. 2. Angioprotective activities compared in vivo.] [French] *J Pharmacologie* 1986;17(1):21.

[7] Swanston-Flatt SK, et al. Traditional Plant Treatments for Diabetes. Studies in normal and streptozotocin diabetic mice. *Diabetologia* 1990;33(8):462.

[8] Schimmer O, et al. The Mutagenic Potencies of Plant Extracts Containing Quercetin in *Salmonella typhimurium* TA98 and TA100. *Mutation Res* 1988;206(2):201.

[9] Sokolowska-Wozniak A. [Cytostatic Activity of the Lactone Fraction of *Alchemilla pastoralis* B u s.] [Polish] *Ann Univ Mariae Curie Sklodowska [Med]* 1985;40:107.

Aletris

SCIENTIFIC NAME(S): *Aletris farinosa* L. Family: Liliaceae

COMMON NAME(S): Unicorn root, stargrass, whitetube stargras, crow corn, Ague grass, Aloerot, Devil's-bit, colic root, ague root, starwort, blazing star.[1,4,5,6]

BOTANY: Aletris (of *NF* VII) is a perennial herb with grassy leaves that grow in a rosette. These leaves surround a slender stem that reaches about 3 feet in height. The plant is native to North America and is distributed widely throughout the continent.[1]

HISTORY: Aletris is an old American plant that has now been recognized worldwide in traditional folk medicine.[2] It had been used by Native American Indians in the Carolinas as an antidiarrheal tea and in Appalachia for the management of rheumatisms (known as ague in Colonial times), as a tonic and as a sedative.[1] Aletris is used in the preparation of herbal remedies designed to ameliorate female disorders including dysmenorrhea and menstrual discomfort. The fabled "Lydia Pinkham's Vegetable Compound," which was touted as a cure-all for female discomforts, contained aletris, among other plant derivatives.[3] It has been included in laxatives and has been used as an antiflatulent (hence the name "colic root")[4] and antispasmodic.

The roots and rhizomes are collected in the fall and dried for preservation.

CHEMISTRY: Little is known about the chemical composition of the plant. Diosgenin has been isolated, along with gentrogenin, from the related Japanese species *A. foliata* and *A. formosana*. An oil derived from the plant is reported to have pharmacologic activity, but this has not been well defined.[1] The plant also contains a resin and a saponin-like glycoside that is the likely source that yields diosgenin on hydrolysis.[1]

PHARMACOLOGY: Aletris has been reported to have estrogenic activity, although estrogenic compounds have not been isolated nor have detailed studies confirmed this activity. The potential estrogenic properties of aletris may be due to a diosgenin-derived steroid that has not yet been characterized.

TOXICOLOGY: No significant adverse events have been reported regarding the use of aletris. The plant has been reported to have narcotic properties, and in small doses can induce colic, stupefaction and vertigo.[2]

SUMMARY: Aletris is a common plant that has been used widely in folklore for the management of female discomforts. The pharmacologic activity of the plant has not been well defined, but steroidal compounds identified in the plant may form the basis of its purported estrogenic activity.

PATIENT INFORMATION – Aletris

Uses: Aletris has been used as a sedative, laxative, antiflatulent, antispasmodic and as a treatment for diarrhea and rheumatism. Its potential estrogenic properties may account for use treating female disorders.

Side Effects: None significant are known, but it reportedly has narcotic properties and can induce colic, stupor, and vertigo.

---

[1] Leung AY. Encyclopedia of Common Natural Ingredients Used in Food, Drugs and Cosmetics. New York, NY: J. Wiley and Sons, 1980.
[2] Duke JA. Handbook of Medicinal Herbs. Boca Raton, FL: CRC Press, 1985
[3] Tyler VE. The Honest Herbal: a sensible guide to the use of herbs and related remedies. Binghamton, NY: The Haworth Press, 1993.
[4] Osol A, Farrar GE Jr. The Dispensatory of the United States of America. 25th ed. Philadelphia: J.B. Lippincott, 1955:1535.
[5] Meyer JE. *The Herbalist.* Hammond, IN: Hammond Book Co, 1934:244.
[6] Dobelis IN, ed. Magic and Medicine of Plants. Pleasantville, NY: Readers Digest, 1986:144.

Alfalfa

SCIENTIFIC NAME(S): *Medicago sativa* L. Common cultivars include Weevelchek, Saranac, Team, Arc, Classic and Buffalo. Family: Leguminosae

COMMON NAME(S): Alfalfa

BOTANY: This legume grows throughout the world under widely varying conditions. A perennial herb, it has trifoliate dentate leaves with an underground stem that is often woody. Alfalfa grows to about 3 feet. Its blue-violet flowers bloom from July to September.

HISTORY: Alfalfa has played an important role as a livestock forage. Its use probably originated in Southeast Asia. The Arabs fed alfalfa to their horses claiming it made the animals swift and strong, naming the legume "Al-fal-fa" meaning "father of all foods." The medicinal uses of alfalfa stem from anecdotal reports that the leaves cause diuresis, and are useful in the treatment of kidney, bladder and prostate disorders. Leaf preparations have been touted for their antiarthritic and antidiabetic activity, for treatment of dyspepsia and as an antiasthmatic. Alfalfa extracts are used in baked goods, beverages and prepared foods, and the plant serves as a commercial source of chlorophyll and carotene.[1]

CHEMISTRY: Dried alfalfa leaves are ground and sold as tablets or powder for use as nutritional supplements. Leaf tablets are rich in protein, calcium and trace minerals, carotene, vitamins E and K and numerous water-soluble vitamins.[2] A steroidal saponin fraction (composed of soyasapogenols, medicagenic acid and others)[3,4] is believed to play a role in the hypocholesterolemic and hemolytic activity of the leaves and sprouts.[5] Alfalfa seeds contain the toxic amino acid L-canavanine, an analog of arginine. Sprouts of certain cultivars of alfalfa contain up to 13 g/kg canavanine (dry weight). Canavanine levels decrease as the plant matures. The alkaloids stachydrine and l–homo–stachydrine found in the seed possess emmenagogue and lactogenic activity.[6] Seeds contain up to 11% of a drying oil used in the preparation of paints and varnishes. The chemistry of alfalfa has been well characterized.[1]

PHARMACOLOGY: There are no studies to provide evidence that alfalfa leaves or sprouts possess effective diuretic, anti-inflammatory, antidiabetic or antiulcer activity in man. Alfalfa saponins are hemolytic in vitro.[7]

Several studies indicate that the ingestion of alfalfa reduces cholesterol absorption and atherosclerotic plaque formation in animals.[8,9,10] Alfalfa plant saponins and fibe.[11] bind significant quantities of cholesterol in vitro; sprout saponins interact to a lesser degree. In vitro bile acid adsorption is greatest for the whole alfalfa plant, and this activity is not reduced by the removal of saponins from the plant material. In one study, the ability of alfalfa to reduce liver cholesterol accumulation in cholesterol-fed rats was enhanced by the removal of saponins. Therefore, alfalfa plant saponins appear to play an important role in neutral steroid excretion, but are not essential for increasing bile acid excretion.[12] There is no evidence that canavanine or its metabolites affect cholesterol levels.

TOXICOLOGY: Significant changes in intestinal cellular morphology were noted in rats fed alfalfa; these effects were more extensive in animals fed whole plant material compared to sprouts. The interaction of saponins with cholesterol in cell membranes may only be in part responsible for these changes.[12] The significance of the changes in animal intestinal morphology is not clear; it is known that these changes, when observed concomitantly with changes in steroid excretion, may be related to an increased susceptibility to colon cancer.[13]

A disease similar to systemic lupus erythematosus (SLE) has been observed in monkeys fed alfalfa seeds.[14] The disease was characterized by hemolytic anemia, decreased serum complement levels, immunologic changes and deposition of immunoglobulins in the kidney and skin. Alfalfa ingestion has provoked pancytopenia and hypo-complementenemia in normal subjects.[15] L-canavanine has been implicated as the possible causative agent. The toxicity of L-canavanine is due in large part to its structural similarity to arginine. Canavanine binds to arginine-dependent enzymes interfering in their action. Arginine reduces the toxic effects of canavanine in vitro.[16] Further, canavanine may be metabolized to canaline, an analog of ornithine. Canaline may inhibit pyridoxal phosphate and enzymes that require the B_6 cofactor.[14] L-canavanine has also been shown to alter intercellular calcium levels[17] and the ability of certain B or T cell populations to regulate antibody synthesis.[18,19] Alfalfa tablets have been associated with the reactivation of SLE in at least two patients.[20]

A case of reversible asymptomatic pancytopenia with splenomegaly has been reported in a man who ingested up to 160 g of ground alfalfa seeds daily as part of a cholesterol-reducing diet. His plasma cholesterol fell from 218 mg/dl to 130-160 mg/dl.[15] Pancytopenia was believed to be due to canavanine.

A popular self-treatment for asthma and hay fever suggests the ingestion of alfalfa tablets. There is no scientific evidence that this treatment is effective.[21] Fortunately, the occurrence of cross-sensitization between alfalfa (a legume) and grass pollens appears unlikely, assuming the tablets are not contaminated with materials from grasses.[22] One patient died of listeriosis following the ingestion of contaminated alfalfa tablets.[23]

SUMMARY: Alfalfa is a nutritious legume of importance as animal forage. Leaf preparations have been used in the treatment of kidney and bladder disorders and as an antirheumatic agent. There is no evidence supporting these uses in humans. Evidence from animal studies suggests that alfalfa saponins may lower cholesterol levels. Ingestion of alfalfa preparations is generally without significant side effects, but these may reactivate latent SLE and have caused reversible pancytopenia.

PATIENT INFORMATION – Alfalfa

Uses: No study evidence currently supports use of various parts of the alfalfa plant for diuretic, anti-inflammatory, antidiabetic or antiulcer purposes. The plant appears to reduce cholesterol.

Side Effects: Alfalfa ingestion, especially of the seeds, has been associated in some instances with various deleterious effects, but alfalfa preparations are generally without significant side effects.

---

[1] Duke JA. Handbook of Medicinal Herbs. Boca Raton, FL: CRC Press, 1985.
[2] Worthinton-Roberts B, Breskin MA. Fads or Facts? A Pharmacist's guide to controversial nutrition products. Am Pharm 1983;23:421.
[3] Massiot G, et al. Reinvestigation of the sapogenins and prosapogenins from alfalfa (Medicago sativa). J Ag Food Chem 1988;36:902.
[4] Oleszek W. Solid-phase extraction-fractionation of alfalfa saponins. J Sci Food Ag 1988;44:43.
[5] Malinow MR, et al. Effect of alfalfa meal on shrinkage (regression) of atherosclerotic plaques during cholesterol feeding in monkeys. Atherosclerosis 1978;30:27.
[6] AHA Quarterly Newsletter 1984;3:4.
[7] Small E, et al. The Evolution of Hemolytic Saponin Content in Wild and Cultivated Alfalfa (Medicago sativa, Fabaceae). Economic Botany 1990;44:226.
[8] Malinow MR, et al. Effect of alfalfa saponins on intestinal cholesterol absorption in rats. Am J Clin Nutr 1977;30:2061.
[9] Malinow MR, et al. Cholesterol and Bile Acid Balance in Macaca Fascicularis Effects of alfalfa saponins. J Clin Invest 1981;67:156.
[10] Wilcox MR, Galloway LS. Serum and liver cholesterol, total lipids and lipid phosphorus levels of rats under various dietary regimes. Am J Clin Nutr 1961;9:236.
[11] Story JA, et al. Adsorption of bile acids by components of alfalfa and wheat bran in vitro. J Food Sci 1982;47:1276.
[12] Story JA, et al. Interactions of alfalfa plant and sprout saponins with cholesterol in vitro and in cholesterol-fed rats. Am J Clin Nutr 1984;39:917.
[13] Sprinz H. Factors influencing intestinal cell renewal. Cancer 1971;28:71.
[14] Malinow MR, et al. Systemic Lupus Erythematosus-Like Syndrome in Monkeys Fed Alfalfa Sprouts: Role of a Nonprotein Amino Acid. Science 1982;216:415.
[15] Malinow MR, et al. Pancytopenia During Ingestion of Alfalfa Seeds. Lancet 1981;i:615.
[16] Natelson S. Canavanine to Arginine Ratio in Alfalfa (Medicago sativa), Clover (Trifolium), and the Jack Bean (Canavalia ensiformis), J Ag Food Chem 1985;33:413.
[17] Morimoto I. A study on immunological effects of L-canavanine. Kobe J Med Sci 1989;35:287.
[18] Prete PE. The mechanism of action of L-canavanine in inducing autoimmune phenomena. Arthritis Rheum 1985;28:1198.
[19] Morimoto I, et al. L-canavanine acts on suppressor-inducer T cells to regulate antibody synthesis: Lymphocytes of systemic lupus erythematosus patients are specifically unresponsive to L-canavanine. Clin Immunol Immunopathol 1990;55:97.
[20] Roberts JL, Hayashi JA. Exacerbation of SLE associated with Alfalfa ingestion. N Engl J Med 1983;308:1361.
[21] Polk IJ. Alfalfa pill treatment of allergy may be hazardous. JAMA 1982;247:1493.
[22] Brandenburg DM. Alfalfa of the Family Leguminosae. JAMA 1983;249:3303.
[23] Farber JM, et al. Listeriosis traced to the consumption of alfalfa tablets and soft cheese. N Engl J Med 1990;322:338.

Alkanna Root

SCIENTIFIC NAME(S): *Alkanna tinctoria* (L.) Tausch Family: Boraginaceae

COMMON NAME(S): Alkanet, alkannawurzel (German), alkermeswurzel, (German) anchusa, Dyers's Bugloss, henna, orchanet (English), racine d'alcanna (French), racine d'orcanette(French), radix anchusea (tinctoriae) (Latin), rote ochsenzungenwurzel (German), schminkwurzel (German)

BOTANY: Alkanna is typically a biennial or perennial herbaceous plant growing from 1 to 2 feet in height with pubescent lanceolate leaves. It bears blue to purple trumpet-shaped flowers arranged in loose, one-sided scorpiorid racemes. The root is usually seen as a cylindrical, fissured rhizome with exfoliating, brittle and dark purple bark on the outside and remains of bristly leaf and stem pieces near the crown region.[1] While native to southern Europe, the plant is also grown in and imported from Albania, India and Turkey.[1]

Alkanna should not be confused with another plant also known as alkanet, but which is in the related genus *Anchusa officinalis* (L.) of the same family (Borage).[2] *A. officinalis* has had some use in the form of a decoction (tea) of the leaves and roots for coughs and chest disorders in older herbals.[2]

HISTORY: Alkanna and related plants have long been referred to as "henna" and used as a dye for cloth. Alkanna has also been used to impart a red color to fats, oils and waxes. It also has medicinal historical uses as an astringent. Currently, alkanna has no medicinal importance, and many countries have prohibited its use as a food dye.[1]

CHEMISTRY: Alkanna root contains a mixture of red pigments in the bark at levels up to 5%-6%. These consist mainly of fat soluble naphthazarin (5,8–dihydroxy-1, 4–naphthaquinone) components such as alkannin and related esters.[1,3] The red pigments are soluble in fatty oils which make them useful for the detection of oily materials in microscopic powders during histological examination. Like some of the other members of the Borage family, pyrrolizidine alkaloids have been found in *Alkanna tinctoria*, but levels have not been determined.[1] The alkannin esters of beta, beta=dimethylacrylic acid, beta-acetoxy-isovaleric acid, isovaleric acid and angelic acid have also been isolated from the root.[4]

PHARMACOLOGY: Currently, alkanna root has no recognized medical uses except for its older use as an astringent. Even its use as a pigment is minimal and many countries have prohibited its use as a food coloring. Today, it is used almost exclusively as a cosmetic dye.[1] The esteric pigments, however, displayed excellent antibiotic and wound-healing properties in a clinical study on 72 patients with ulcus cruris (indolent leg ulcers).[1,4]

TOXICOLOGY: No toxicological data on alkanna root are available in the current medical literature.

SUMMARY: Alkanna root has historically been used for its mild astringent properties and as a source of pigments for coloring purposes. However, except for little use as a red color in cosmetics, it is not a major pigment source or a particularly useful drug by today's standards. One study indicates some potential for its esteric pigments in wound healing in patients with ulcus cruris (indolent leg ulcers).[1]

PATIENT INFORMATION – Alkanna Root

Uses: Alkanna is an astringent and a source of red pigment used in cosmetics. It appears to have antibiotic and wound-healing properties.

Side Effects: Unknown.

---

[1] Bisset, NG, ed. Herbal Drugs and Phytopharmaceuticals. Stuttgart: Medpharm Scientific Publishers, 1994.
[2] Dobelis IN, ed. Magic and Medicine of Plants. Pleasantville, NY: Reader's Digest Association, Inc., 1986.
[3] Papageorgiou VP, Digenis GA. Isolation of 2 new alkannin esters from Alkanna tinctoria. *Planta Medica* 1980;39:81.
[4] Papageorgiou VP. Wound healing properties of naphthaquinone pigments from Alkanna tinctoria. *Experientia* 1978;34(11):1499.

Allspice

SCIENTIFIC NAME(S): *Pimenta dioica* (L.) Merr. synonymous with *P. officinalis* and *Eugenia pimenta*. Family: Myrtaceae

COMMON NAME(S): Allspice, pimenta, Jamaica pepper, clove pepper, pimento.[2,3]

BOTANY: Pimenta is a sturdy tree that grows to 13 meters. It has leathery, oblong leaves and is native to the West Indies, Central America and Mexico. The parts of the plant used medicinally are the dried, full-grown but unripe fruit and leaves.[2] Allspice powder available commercially consists of the whole ground dried fruit.[3]

HISTORY: The plant has been used as a carminative. Besides its use in cosmetics and toothpastes, it is used as a food flavoring. Its odor is reminiscent of a combination of cloves, cinnamon and nutmeg. Allspice has been used medicinally as a tonic, purgative, carminative and antidiarrheal[1] and for rheumatisms, neuralgia and stomachache.[3]

CHEMISTRY: Allspice berries contain from 1% to 4% of a volatile oil, which contains from 60% to 80% eugenol and eugenol methylether (40% to 45%).[1,2,3] The leaf oil contains more eugenol (up to 96%) and bears many similarities to the composition of clove leaf oil.[2] The oil is known as pimenta or allspice oil, and also contains cineole, levophellandrene, caryophyllene and palmitic acid.[1] Enzymes released after harvesting appear to be responsible for producing many of the volatile components from chemical precursors.[2] More than three dozen chemical constituents have been identified in the plant.[2] In addition, small amounts of resin, tannic acid and an acrid fixed oil are present.[1]

PHARMACOLOGY: Any pharmacologic activity associated with the plant is most likely due to the presence of eugenol. Eugenol has local antiseptic and anesthetic properties. Eugenol also has antioxidant properties and allspice may serve as a potential source of new natural antioxidants.[2,4] Furthermore, allspice appears to have in vitro activity against yeasts and fungi.[5,6]

Eugenol, aqueous extracts of allspice and allspice oil, has been shown to enhance trypsin activity and to have larvicidal properties.[2]

TOXICOLOGY: Allspice and extracts of the plant can be irritating to mucous membranes. Although allspice generally has not been associated with toxicity, eugenol can be toxic in high concentrations. Ingestion of more than 5 ml of allspice oil may induce nausea, vomiting, central nervous system depression and convulsions.[1]

When pimento oil and eugenol were applied to intact shaved abdominal skin of the mouse, no percutaneous absorption was observed.[2]

SUMMARY: Allspice is a popular spice and fragrance. The oil may induce topical irritation and ingestion of the oil may result in toxicity.

PATIENT INFORMATION – Allspice

Uses: Apart from use for spices and fragrance, allspice has been used for various gastrointestinal ills, rheumatism and neuralgia. Extracts have antiseptic, anesthetic, and antioxidant properties and efficacy in vitro against yeasts and fungi.

Side Effects: Allspice can irritate mucosa. Ingestion of extracts may produce toxicity and affect the CNS.

---

[1] Spoerke DG. Herbal Medications. Santa Barbara, CA: Woodbridge Press, Inc. 1980.
[2] Leung AY. Encyclopedia of Common Natural Ingredients Used in Food, Drugs and Cosmetics. New York, NY: J. Wiley and Sons, 1980.
[3] Duke JA. Handbook of Medicinal Herbs. Boca Raton, FL: CRC Press, 1985.
[4] Krishnakantha TP, Lokesh BR. Scavenging of superoxide anions by spice principles. *Indian J Biochem Biophys* 1993;30:133-4.
[5] Conner DE, Beuchat LR. Sensitivity of heat-stressed yeasts to essential oils of plants. *Appl Environ Microbiol* 1984;47:229-33.
[6] Hitokoto H, et al. Inhibitory effects of spices on growth and toxin production of toxigenic fungi. *Appl Environ Microbiol* 1980;39:818-22.

Aloe

SCIENTIFIC NAME(S): *Aloe vera* L., *A. perryi Baker* (Zanzibar or Socotrine aloe), *A. barbadensis Miller* (also called *A. vera* Tournefort ex Linne or *A. vulgaris* Lamark; Curacao or Barbados aloe), or *A. ferox* Miller (Cape aloe). *A. vera* Miller and *A. vera* L. may or may not be the same species. Family: Liliaceae

COMMON NAME(S): Cape, Zanzibar, Socotrine, Curacao, Barbados aloes, aloe vera

BOTANY: Aloes, of which there are some 500 species, belong to the family Liliaceae.[1] The name, meaning "bitter and shiny substance," derives from the Arabic "alloeh." Indigenous to the Cape of Good Hope, these perennial succulents grow throughout most of Africa, Southern Arabia and Madagascar, and are cultivated in the Caribbean, Mediterranean, Japan and America. They do not grow in rain forests or arid deserts. Often attractive ornamental plants, their fleshy leaves are stiff and spiny along the edges and grow in a rosette. Each plant has 15 to 30 tapering leaves, each up to 0.5 meters long and 8 to 10 cm wide. Beneath the thick cuticle of the epidermis lies the chlorenchyma. Between this layer and the colorless mucilaginous pulp containing the aloe gel are numerous vascular bundles and inner bundle sheath cells, from which a bitter yellow sap exudes when the leaves are cut.[2]

HISTORY: Drawings of aloe have been found in the wall carvings of Egyptian temples erected in the fourth millennium B.C. Called the "Plant of Immortality," it was a traditional funerary gift for the pharaohs. The Egyptian Book of Remedies (ca. 1500 B.C.) notes the use of aloe in curing infections, treating the skin and preparing drugs that were chiefly used as laxatives. *John* 19:39-40 says that Nicodemus brought a mixture of myrrh and aloes for the preparation of Christ's body. Alexander is said to have conquered the island of Socotra to obtain control of it. The Greek physician Dioscorides, in 74 A.D., recorded its use to heal wounds, stop hair loss, treat genital ulcers and eliminate hemorrhoids. In the 6th century A.D., Arab traders carried it to Asia. From the Mediterranean, it was carried to the New World in the 16th century by the Spaniards. In the modern era, its clinical use began in the 1930s as a treatment for roentgen dermatitis.[2]

CHEMISTRY: The aloe yields two commercially important products. "Aloe" is the solid residue obtained by evaporating the latex obtained from the pericyclic cells beneath the skin.[3] The bitter yellow latex contains the anthraquinone barbaloin (a glucoside of aloe-emodin) and iso-barbaloin in addition to a series of O-glycosides of barbaloin, called aloinosides, chrysophanic acid and up to 63% resin. Filtering out certain resins from the exudate and concentrating the remaining anthraglycoside material (which is up to 25% barbaloin) into crystalline form produces aloin. Aloin is a mixture of water-soluble glycosides obtained from aloe.

A second product, aloe gel, is a clear, thin, gelatinous material obtained by crushing the mucilaginous cells found in the inner tissue of the leaf. The gel is the product used most frequently in the cosmetic and health food industries. It is generally devoid of anthraquinone glycosides. The gel contains a polysaccharide glucomannan, similar to guar gum. It is this component that is believed to contribute mostly to the emollient effect of the gel. "Aloe vera gel extract" is not actually an extract, but rather the pulverized whole leaves of the plant.

Other compounds such as tannins, polysaccharides, organic acids, enzymes, vitamins and steroids have been identified.[4] Aloe contains bradykininase, a protease inhibitor, which relieves pain and decreases swelling and redness. Magnesium lactate, by blocking histamine production, may contribute to the antipruritic effect of aloe. An antiprostaglandin that reduces inflammation has also been isolated. The anthraquinones are local irritants in the gastrointestinal tract and have been used in treating certain skin diseases, eg, psoriasis.

Chemical composition differs among the species of aloe, eg, *A. barbadensis* Miller may contain 2.5 times the aloe-emodin of *A. ferox* Miller. The time of harvest is a further factor in composition.

PHARMACOLOGY: Aloe latex has been used for centuries as a drastic cathartic. The aloinosides exert strong purgative effects by irritating the large intestine. These should be used cautiously in children.

The most common use of the gel remains in the treatment of minor burns and skin irritation. Early studies of its use generally had been poorly controlled, and the data had been incomplete and conflicting. These reports described the use of aloe in the treatment of radiation-induced dermatitis.[5] Subsequent reports of the use of topical aloe in treating human and animal radiation burns suggested that although healing occurred, a clear advantage over aggressive wound care could not be established.

The activity of aloe in treating burns may stem from its moisturizing effect, which prevents air from drying the wound.[6] Its activity has also been ascribed to its chlorophyll content and that of other minor components, but this has not been adequately substantiated. Current theory suggests healing is stimulated by mucopolysaccharides in combination with sulfur derivatives and nitrogen compounds. Topical aloe treatment for burns has not been adequately documented. Two FDA advisory panels found insufficient evidence to show *A. vera* is useful in the treatment of minor burns and cuts or vaginal irritations.

More recent studies have generally found preparations containing aloe to accelerate wound healing. In patients who underwent dermabrasion, aloe accelerated skin healing by about 72 hours compared to polyethylene oxide gel dressing.[7] and aloe has been found to accelerate wound healing in patients with frostbite.[8] However, at least one study found that aloe applied as standard wound therapy delayed wound healing significantly (83 days vs 53 days).[9]

Studies of the antibacterial activity of aloe have yielded conflicting results. One study using *A. vera* gel[10] found no activity against *S. aureus* and *E. coli*. Other test.[11] found that *A. chinensis* inhibited growth of *S. aureus*, *E. coli* and *M. tuberculosis*, but that *A. vera* was inactive. Further, these extracts lost their in vitro activity when mixed with blood. The latex has shown some activity against pathogenic strains.[12] Two commercial preparations (*Aloe gel* and *Dermaide Aloe*) exerted antimicrobial activity against gram negative and positive bacteria as well as *Candida albicans* when used in concentrations greater than 90%.[13] Aloe has been found to be more effective than sulfadiazine and salicylic acid creams in promoting wound healing and as effective as sulfadiazine in reducing wound bacterial counts.[14]

Aloe-emodin is antileukemic in vitro;[15] other studies showed *A. vera* gel to be less cytotoxic[16] than indomethacin or prednisolone in tissue cultures. The National Cancer Institute concluded that *A. vera* latex was not worthy of further study as a cancer cure.

Other health claims are generally poorly documented. An emulsion of the gel was reported to cure 17 of 18 patients with peptic ulcers, but no control agent was used in this study.[17]

In one laboratory experiment, rats subcutaneously injected with 1, 10 or 100 mg/kg doses of *A. vera* (without anthraquinones) daily for 7 days showed improved circulation and wound healing.[18] Arthritic mice were subcutaneously injected with a 150 mg/kg suspension of anthraquinones once a day for 13 days. This aloe extract caused a 48% inhibition of inflammation, due to anthraquinone and cinnamic acid and a 72% inhibition of arthritis, due to anthranilic acid, which also had an anti-inflammatory effect. *A. vera* extracts have bradykininase activity in vitro.[19] Topical administration of aloe extracts reduced swelling in an animal model of inflammation by 29%.[20] Recent investigations have established that certain components of aloe inhibit the complementary system, thereby reducing inflammatory responses.[21,22]

A small study from China has found that parenteral administration of aloe extract protects the liver from chemical injury and has been shown to ameliorate SGPT levels dramatically in patients with chronic hepatitis.[23]

Only the dried latex is approved for internal use as a cathartic. In some cases, *A. vera* is sold as a food supplement, allegedly with FDA approval. FDA has only approved *A. perryi*, *A. vera*, *A. ferox* and certain hybrids for use as natural food flavorings.[24]

TOXICOLOGY: Since aloe is used extensively as a folk medicine, its adverse effects have been well documented. Except for the dried latex, aloe is not approved as an internal medication. Aloe-emodin and other anthraquinones may cause severe gastric cramping and its use is contraindicated in pregnant women and children.[25] The external use of aloe has not been generally associated with severe adverse reactions. Reports of burning skin following topical application of aloe gel to dermabraded skin have been described.[26] Contact dermatitis from the related *A. arborescens* has been reported.[1]

SUMMARY: Aloe products derived from the latex of the outer skin are drastic cathartics to be used with caution. Compounds derived from the inner gel intended for internal administration have not been shown to exert any consistent therapeutic effect. The effective topical use of the gel in the treatment of minor burns and wounds has not been established, although several human trials indicate a potential therapeutic benefit.

PATIENT INFORMATION – Aloe

Uses: Aloe appears to inhibit infection and promote healing of minor burns and wounds, and possibly of skin affected by diseases such as psoriasis. Dried aloe latex is used, with caution, as a drastic cathartic.

Side Effects: There has been one report that using the gel as standard wound therapy delayed healing. The gel may cause burning sensations in dermabraded skin.

---

[1] Nakamura T, Kotajima S. Contact dermatitis from *aloe arborescens. Contact Dermatitis* 1984;11(1):50.

[2] Grindlay D, Reynolds T. The *aloe vera* phenomenon: a review of the properties and modern uses of the leaf parenchyma gel. *J Ethnopharmacol* 1986;16:117.

[3] Leung AY. Encyclopedia of Common Natural Ingredients Used in Food, Drugs and Cosmetics. New York, NY: J Wiley and Sons, 1980.

[4] Henry R. An updated review of *aloe vera. Cosmetics and Toiletries* 1979;94:42.

[5] Row TD, et al. Further observations on the use of *aloe vera* leaf in the treatment of third degree x-ray reactions. *J Am Pharm Assn* 1941;30:266.

[6] Ship AG. Is topical *aloe vera* plant mucus helpful in burn treatment? *JAMA* 1977;238(16):1770.

[7] Fulton JE, Jr. The stimulation of postdermabrasion wound healing with stabilized *aloe vera* gel-polyethylene oxide dressing. *J Dermatol Surg Oncol* 1990;16(5):460.

[8] McCauley RL, et al. Frostbite-methods to minimize tissue loss. *Postgrad Med* 1990;88(8):67.

[9] Schmidt JM, Greenspoon JS. *Aloe vera* dermal wound gel is associated with a delay in wound healing. *Obstet Gynecol* 1991;78(1):115.

[10] Fly, Kiem. *Economic Bot* 1963;14:46.

[11] Gottshall, et al. *J Clin Invest* 1949;28:920.

[12] Lorenzetti LJ, et al. Bacteriostatic property of *aloe vera. J Pharm Sci* 1964;53:1287.

[13] Haggers JP, et al. *J Am Med Technol* 1979;41:293.

[14] Rodriguez-Bigasm, et al. Comparative evaluation of *aloe vera* in the management of burn wounds in guinea pigs. *Plast Reconstr Surg* 1988;81(3):386.

[15] Kupchan, Karmin. *J Nat Prod* 1976;39:223.

[16] Fischer JM. Medical use of aloe products. *US Pharmacist* 1982;7(8):37.

[17] Blitz JJ, et al. *J Am Osteopath Assoc*1963;62:731.

[18] Davis RH, et al. *Aloe vera* and wound healing. *J Am Podiatr Med Assoc* 1987;77(4):165.

[19] Yagi A, et al. Bradykinin-degrading glycoprotein in *aloe arborescens* var. *natalensis. Planta Med* 1987;X:19.

[20] Davis RH, et al. Isolation of a stimulatory system in an aloe extract. *J Am Podiatr Med Assoc* 1991;81(9):473.

[21] t'Hart LA, et al. An anti-complementary polysaccharide with immunological adjuvant activity from the leaf parenchyma gel of *aloe vera. Planta Med* 1989;55(6):509.

[22] t'Hart LA, et al. Effects of low molecular constituents from *aloe vera* gel on oxidative metabolism and cytotoxic and bactericidal activities of human neutrophils. *Int J Immunopharmacol* 1990;12(4):427.

[23] Fan YJ, et al. Protective effect of extracts from *aloe vera* L. var. Chinensis (Haw.) Berg. on experimental hepatic lesions and a primary clinical study on the injection of in patients with hepatitis. *Chung Kuo Chung Yao Tsa Chih* 1989;14(12):746.

[24] Hecht A. The overselling of *aloe vera. FDA Consumer* 1981;July-Aug:27.

[25] Spoerke DG, Ekins BR. *Aloe vera-* fact or quackery. *Vet Hum Toxicol* 1980;222:418.

[26] Hunter D, Frumkin A. Adverse reactions to vitamin E and *aloe vera* preparations after dermabrasion and chemical peel. *Cutis* 1991;47(3):193.

Alpha Lipoic Acid

SCIENTIFIC NAME(S): 1,2-dithiolane-3-pentanoic acid; 1,2-dithiolane-3-valeric acid; 6,8-thioctic acid; alpha-lipoic acid; 5-(1,2-dithiolan-3-yl) valeric acid.

COMMON NAME(S): Alpha-lipoic acid, lipoic acid, thioctic acid, acetate replacing factor, biletan, lipoicin, thioctacid, thioctan.

SOURCE: Lipoic acid is a fat-soluble, sulfur-containing, vitamin-like antioxidant. It is not a true vitamin because it can be synthesized in the body and is not necessary in the diet of animals. Lipoic acid functions in the same manner as many B-complex vitamins. Good sources of lipoic acid are yeast and liver.[1,2] Other sources include spinach, broccoli, potatoes, kidney, heart, and skeletal muscle.[3]

HISTORY: In the 1930s, it was found that a certain "potato growth factor" was necessary for growth of certain bacteria.[3] In 1951, a fat-soluble coenzyme factor was discovered from work done on lactic acid bacteria. Reed et al, isolated this naturally occurring d-form and found it to be an important growth factor for many bacteria and protozoa. This compound was isolated and identified as "alpha lipoic acid."[4]

CHEMISTRY: Alpha lipoic acid is a molecule with 2 sulfur high-energy bonds. It functions as a coenzyme with pyrophosphatase in carbohydrate metabolism to convert pyruvic acid to acetyl-coenzyme A (Kreb's cycle) to produce energy.[1]

PHARMACOLOGY: Pharmacokinetics and bioavailability of different enantiomers of alpha lipoic acid (ALA) have been performed in 12 subjects.[5] Pharmacology of ALA has been studied in the areas of **oxidation**, **diabetes**, **AIDS**, **cancer**, and **liver ailments**.

Oxidation: ALA's antioxidant properties have been demonstrated. It has the ability to chelate metals and to scavenge free radicals.[6] ALA is easily absorbed and transported across cell membranes; thus, free radical protection occurs both inside and outside of cells. It is also water- and fat-soluble, which makes it effective against a broader range of free radicals than vitamin C (water-soluble) and vitamin E (fat-soluble) alone.[2] ALA administration also increases intracellular levels of glutathione, an important antioxidant.[7] ALA regenerates or recycles antioxidant vitamins C and E[3] but in one report, had no effect on vitamin E tissue concentration in animals, contradicting this effect.[8]

The body routinely converts ALA to dihydrolipoic acid, an even more powerful antioxidant. Both forms "quench" the dangerous peroxynitrite radicals, which are responsible in part for heart, lung, and neurological disease and inflammation as well.[9] In oxidative stress models such as ischemia, reperfusion injury, and radiation injury, ALA has been shown to be beneficial.[10,11]

Diabetes: ALA has been shown to be beneficial in type 1 and type 2 diabetes. ALA has prevented various pathologies associated with this disease, such as reperfusion injury, macular degeneration, cataracts, and neuropathy.[2,3,10 12] ALA reduced diabetic neuropathy in rats, which was improved in a dose-dependent manner. In part, the mechanism was suggested to be caused by reduction of the effects of oxidative stress.[12] ALA is approved in Germany to treat diabetic neuropathy. High doses (600 mg/day) improve this condition.[2]

ALA also improves the diabetic condition by improving blood sugar metabolism. It facilitates better conversion of sugar into energy.[2] In 13 non-insulin-dependent diabetes mellitus patients, ALA increased insulin-stimulated glucose disposal. Metabolic clearance rate for glucose rose by 50% compared with the control group.[13]

ALA improves blood flow to peripheral nerves and stimulates regeneration of nerve fibers.[2] A German study evaluating 800 mg/day ALA in diabetics with damaged autonomic nervous systems was compared against placebo. After 4 months, sympathetic systems showed improvement and autonomic nerve disorder decreased in the ALA group.[14]

Antioxidants in general may lead to regression of diabetic complications. When ALA was compared with antioxidant vitamin E, results failed to justify the higher cost of ALA over less-expensive and equally effective nutritional antioxidants.[2]

AIDS: Patients with HIV have a compromised antioxidant defense system, which may benefit from ALA's role as an effective antioxidant.[2] A small pilot study was conducted administering 150 mg ALA 3 times daily to HIV patients. It increased glutathione in all 10 patients and increased vitamin C in most patients as well. In addition, it improved the T-helper lymphocyte to T-helper suppressor cell ratio in 6 of 10 patients.[2]

ALA significantly inhibits replication of HIV by reducing the activity of reverse transcriptase, the enzyme which makes virus from DNA of lymphocytes.[2] In another report, ALA was found to also inhibit activation of "nuclear factor kappa-B," a substance involved in AIDS progression.[15]

Cancer: There is limited information available concerning ALA's role in cancer. Its mechanism of action and anticarcinogenic and cytoprotective effects have been addressed.[16] ALA administration, in conjunction with cyclophosphamide, lowered the toxic effects of this anticancer drug when tested in animals.[17]

Liver ailments: ALA has been used as an antidote to *Amanita* mushroom poisoning.[4] A review on mushroom intoxications employing ALA and other antidotes is available.[18]

Various: Various reports on ALA pharmacology include the following: Suppression of T-4 metabolism, exerting a lipid-lowering effect in rats,[19] treatment in Wilson's disease,[4] and cardiovascular disease.[3]

TOXICOLOGY: No adverse effects from ALA supplementation have been reported in either animal or human studies, even with large doses or extended use.[2] Its use in diabetes may warrant a reduction in dose of insulin or other oral diabetic medications. Close monitoring of blood sugar levels must be performed. In addition, ALA use may spare vitamins C and E, as well as other antioxidants.[2]

SUMMARY: ALA is a vitamin-like, "universal antioxidant." It functions to produce energy and has been studied in a number of areas. Its ability to scavenge free radicals has been clearly demonstrated. Its use in diabetes, AIDS, cancer, and liver ailments offer promising results such as reduction of pathologies associated with these diseases. No adverse events from ALA supplementation have been reported.

PATIENT INFORMATION – Alpha Lipoic Acid

Uses: Alpha lipoic acid has been used as an antioxidant for the treatment of diabetes and HIV. It also has been used for cancer, liver ailments, and various other conditions.

Side effects: No adverse effects have been reported.

---

[1] Ensminger A, et al. Foods and Nutrition Encyclopedia, 2nd edition. Boca Raton, FL: CRC Press Inc. 1994:1318-19.
[2] Murray M. Encyclopedia of Nutritional Supplements. Rocklin, CA: Prima Publishing. 1996;343-46.
[3] Ley B. The Potato Antioxidant, Alpha Lipoic Acid. BL Publications. 1996.
[4] Budavari S, et al, eds. The Merck Index, 11th ed. Rahway: Merck and Co. 1989.
[5] Hermann R, et al. *European J Pharm Sci* 1996;4(3):167-74.
[6] Nichols T. *Alt Med Rev* 1997;2(3):177-83.
[7] Busse E, et al. *Arzneimittel-Forschung* 1992;42(6):829-31.
[8] Podda M, et al. *Biochem Biophys Res Commun* 1994;204:98-104.
[9] Whiteman M, et al. *Febs Letters* 1996;379:74-76.
[10] Schonheit K, et al. *Biochimica et Biophysica Acta* 1995;1271:335-42.
[11] Cao X, et al. *Free Radical Research* 1995;23:365-70.
[12] Nagamatsu M, et al. *Diabetes Care* 1995;18:1160-67.
[13] Jacob S, et al. *Arzneimittel-Forschung* 1995;45(8):872-74.
[14] Ziegler D, et al. *Diabetes Care* 1997;20:369-73.
[15] Suzuki Y, et al. *Biochemical and Biophysical Research Communications* 1992;189:1709-15.
[16] Dovinova I. *Ceska A Slovenska Farmacie* 1996;45(5):237-41.
[17] Berger M, et al. *Arzneimittel-Forschung* 1983;33(9):1286-88.
[18] Lampe K. *Clinical Toxicology* 1974;7(1):115-21.
[19] Segermann J, et al. *Arzneimittel-Forschung* 1991;41(12):1294-98.

Alpinia

SCIENTIFIC NAME(S): *Alpinia officinarum* Hance

COMMON NAME(S): China root, Chinese ginger, East Indian root, galangal, rhizoma galangae

BOTANY: Galangal is a reed-like perennial herb bearing stems that grow up to 3 feet high and that are covered by sheaths of narrow lanceolate leaves. Its inflorescence is a short raceme of white flowers which are veined and shaded in dull red. The plant has been cultivated for the rhizomes in the idland of Hainan off Southern China, and in coastal areas around Pak-hoi. Galangal rhizomes appear on the market as branched or simple rhizome fragments and show wavy annulations of the leaf bases. These are reddish-brown in color and have an aromatic, spicy and pungent odor and flavor.[1]

HISTORY: The rhizomes of galangal and its derivatives have long been used for its aromatic stimulant, carminative and condiment properties much like ginger (the dried rhizome of *Zingiber officinale*). Galangal oil is used to flavor French liqueurs and in some tobaccos.[1] The "ginger" of Thailand is obtained from *Alipinia galanga* Willd., a species related to galangal. Likewise, the large, ordinary, preserved ginger of China is also from *A. galanga*.[2] *A. galanga* (greater galangal), containing the volatile oil essence d'Amali, is used in China and northern India for various respiratory complaints in children, particularly bronchial catarrh (mucous membram inflammation).[3]

CHEMISTRY: Galanga contains a greenish-yellow volatile oil containing cineol, eugenol, sesquiterpenes, isomerides of cadinene, a resin containing galangol, kaempferide, galangin, as well as starch and other constituents.[1] Recent studies reveal sevel flavonoids,[4] acetoxychavicol acetate (*A. galanga*),[5] a cardiotonic principle (*A. oxyphylla*),[6] catecquic tannins, phenols, alkalokds and essential oils (*A. speciosa*),[7] nootkatone (*A. oxyphylla*),[8] dehydrokawain derivatives (*A. speciosa*),[9] diterpenes (*A. galanga*),[10] essential oils (*A. speciosa*),[11] nootkatol (*A. oxyphylla*),[12] starch (*A. galanga*),[13] monoterpenes (*A. galanga*),[14] the pungent principle 5–hydroxy-7–(4–hydroxy-3-methoxyphenyl)-1–phenyl-3-heptanone (*A. officinarum*).[15] The constituents in the essential oil of *A. khulanjan* M. Sheriff are 38.42% methylcinnamate, 20.21% cineol 1:8, 9.15% l-camphene, 8.75% l-borneol, 7.97% methylchavicol, 7.34% DELTA3–carene and 2.69% alpha-pinene.[16]

PHARMACOLOGY: Although the major uses of Alpinia involve its use as a carminative and condiment, there have been a number of recent interesting medical applications. Antifungals are found in *A. galanga*[5,10] and *A. officinarum*.[17] *A. speciosa* oils are also effective anitfungal agents, inhibiting 80% of the dermatophyte strains tested in a recent in vitro study.[18]

A. oxyphylla (bitter cardamon) significantly inhibits gastric lesions by 57% in rats; susquiterpenois nootkatone is suggested as the active principle.[8] Guaiacol, a cardiotonic principle, has been found in *A. oxphylla*.[6] Anti-ulcer activity is found in the seeds of *A. galanga*.[19]

A. speciosa extracts have shown diuretic and hypotensive properties.[7,20,21] The dehydrokawain derivatives from *A. speciosa*, 5,6–Dehydrokawain (DK) and dihydro-5,6–dehydrokawain (DDK), are antiplatelets due to their inhibition of thromboxane A2 formation.[9]

A. Galanga shows antitumor activity in mic.[22] and has been found to be moderately effective as an anthelmintic against the human *Ascaris lubricoides*.[23] Alpinia fructus (the fruit of *A. oxyphylla*) is effective as an anti-diuretic, anti-ulcerative and anti-dementia agent in rats.[24]

A. officinarum and ginger (*Zingiber officinalis*) roots contain potent inhibitors against prostaglandin biosynthesizing enzyme (PG synthetase). Gingerols and diarylheptanoids were identified as the active constituents. The structure of these components indicates that they might also be active again arachidonate 5–lipoxygenase, an enzyme of leukotriene (LT) biosynthesis.[25]

A. officinarum, used as an antirheumatic in Saudi traditional medicine, does not produce significant inhibition of carrageenan-induced inflammation.[26]

TOXICOLOGY: A hydroalcoholic extract of *A. speciosa*, injected intra-peritoneally (I.P.) in rats at a dose range of 100 to 1400 mg/kg, caused writhing, psychomotor excitation, hypokinesis and pruritus. The LD-50 by I.P. injection was 0.760 ± 0.126 g/kg, and 10.0 ± 2.5 g/kg by the oral route. Subacute toxicity studies in rats revealed an increase in transaminases and lactate dehydrogenase.

Blood glucose, urea and creatinine were normal; a histopathological study of the liver, spleen, gut, lung and heart showed no changes. The extract caused a prolongation of sleeping time and a dose-dependent fall in blood pressure in doses of 10 to 30 mg/kg.[7]

Another toxicity study on *A. galanga* found no significant mortality or weight gain in rats. However, the *A. galanga* treated animals showed a significant rise in red blood cell levels, weight gain of sexual organs and increased sperm motility and sperm counts. No spermatotoxic effects were noted.[27]

Cytotoxic diterpenes have been found in the seeds of *A. galanga*.[10]

SUMMARY: The rhizomes of *Alpinia officinarum* have had long use as aromatic, stimulant, carminative and condiment agents. Numerous recent studies reveal the presence of many pharmacologically active compounds in various species of the genus. Among the newer activities revealed for the various *Alpinia* species are anthelmintic effects, antifungal properties, anti-ulcer effects in seeds, a cardiotonic property, diuretic and hypotensive effects, inhibition of gastric lesions, antiplatelet action, antitumor principles and inhibition against prostaglandin synthetase. Toxicity is generally low in the *Alpinia* species. Because most of these investigations deal with animal studies, much more is needed to verify these effects and provide proof of true clinical usefulness.

PATIENT INFORMATION – Alpinia

Uses: Beyond common use as a flavoring, aromatic stimulant, carminative, and traditional use to treat children's respiratory complaints, Alpinia species show promise as antifungals, hypotensives, enhancers of sperm count and motility, etc. Antitumor and anti-dementia effects have been observed in rodents.

Side Effects: Toxicity is low; injections can produce psychomotor excitation and the like.

---

[1] Youngken HW. Textbook of Pharmacognosy, 6th ed. Philadelphia: Blakiston Co., 1950.

[2] Osol A. The Dispensatory of the United States of America, 25th ed. Philadelphia: J.B. Lippincott, 1955.

[3] Lewis WH. Elvin-Lewis MPF. Medical Botany: Plants affecting man's health. New York: John Wiley & Sons, 1977.

[4] Karlsen J, Beker F. Flavonoids of Rhizoma Galangae (*Alpinia officinarum* Hance). *Farm Aikak* 1971;80:95.

[5] Janssen A, Scheffer JJ. Acetoxychavicol Acetate, an Antifungal Component of *Alpinia galanga*. *Planta Med* 1985;51(6):507.

[6] Shoji, N, et al. Isolation of a Cardiotonic Principle from *Alpinia oxyphylla*. *Planta Med* 1984;50(2):186.

[7] Mendonca VL, et al. Pharmacological and Toxicological Evaluation of *Alpinia speciosa*. *Mem Inst Oswaldo Cruz* 1991;86(Suppl)2:93.

[8] Yamahara J, et al. Anti-ulcer Effect in Rats of Bitter Cardamon Constituents. *Chem Pharm Bull* 1990;38(11):3053.

[9] Teng CM, et al. Antiplatelet Action of Dehydrokawain Derivatives Isolated From *Alpinia speciosa* Rhizoma. *Chin J Physiol* 1990;33(1):41.

[10] Morita H, Itokawa H. Cytotoxic and Antifungal Diterpenes From the Seeds of *Alpinia galanga*. *Planta Med* 1988;54(2):117.

[11] Luz AIR, et al. Essential Oils of Some Amazonian *Zingiberaceae*. Part 3. Genera Alpinia and Rengalmia. *J Nat Prod* 1984;47:907.

[12] Shoji N, et al. Structural Determination of Nootkatol, New Sesquiterpene Isolated From *Alpinia oxyphylla* Miquel, Possessing Calcium Antagonistic Activity. *J Pharm Sci* 1984;73:843.

[13] Misra SJ, Dixit VK. Pharmaceutical Studies on Starches of Some *Zingiberaccous* Rhizomes. *Indian J Pharm Sci* 1983;45:216.

[14] Scheffer JJC, et al. Monoterpenes in the Essential Oil of *Alpinia galanga* (L.) Willd. *Scientia Pharmaceutica* 1981;49:337.

[15] Inque T, et al. Studies on the Pungent Principle of *Alpinia officinarum* Hance. *J Pharm Soc Jap* 1978;98:1255.

[16] Goutam MP, Purohit RM. Chemical Examination of Essential Oil Derived From Rhizomes of *Alpinia khulanjan*. *Parfuemeric Kosmetik* 1977;58:10.

[17] Ray PG, Majumdar SK. Antifungal Flavonoid From *Alpinia officinarum* Hance. *Indian J of Exp Biol* 1976;14(6):712.

[18] Lima EO, et al. In Vitro Antifungal Activity of Essential Oils Obtained From Official Plants Against Dermatophytes. *Mycoses* 1993;36(9–10):333.

[19] Mitsui S, et al. Constituents From Seeds of *Alpinia galanga* Wild, and Their Anti-Ulcer Activities. *Chem Pharm Bull* 1976;24(10):2377.

[20] Laranja SM, et al. Evaluation of Acute Administration of Natural Products with Potential Diuretic Effects in Humans. *Mem Inst Oswaldo Cruz* 1991;86(Suppl)2:237.

[21] Laranja SM, et al. [Evaluation of Three Plants with Potential Diuretic Effect.] [Portuguese] *Revis Assoc Med Brasil* 1992;38(1):13.

[22] Itokawa H, et al. Antitumor Principles from *Alpinia galanga*. *Planta Med* 1987;53(1):32.

[23] Kaleysa RR. Screening of Idigenous Plants for Anthelmintic Action Against Human *Ascaris lumbricoides*. Part 1. *Indian J Physiol Pharmacol* 1975;19:47.

[24] Kubo M, et al. [Study on Alpiniae Fructus. I. Pharmacological evidence of efficacy of Alpiniae Fructus on ancient herbal literature.] [Japanese] *Yakugaku Zasshi* 1995;115(10):852.

[25] Kiuchi F, et al. Inhibition of Prostaglandin and Leukotriene Biosynthesis by Gingerols and Diarylheptanoids. *Chem Pharm Bull* 1992;40(2):387.

[26] Ageel AM, et al. Experimental Studies on Antirheumatic Crude Drugs Used in Saudi Traditional Medicine. *Drugs Exp & Clin Res* 1989;15(8):369.

[27] Qureshi S, et al. Toxicity Studies on *Alpinia galanga* and *Curcuma longa*. *Planta Med* 1992;58(2):124.

Althea

SCIENTIFIC NAME(S): *Althaea officinalis* L. Family: Malvaceae

COMMON NAME(S): Altheae radix, althea, marshmallow

BOTANY: Althea is a perennial that grows to 5 feet in salt marshes and moist regions throughout Europe, western and northern Asia, and the eastern US. Its 3-lobed leaves are velvety, and the plant resembles hollyhock (*Althaea rosea*). The plant blooms from July to September. The family Malvaceae is known as the mallow family, and confusion may surround the common nomenclature and identification of the plants in this group. The root is collected in the fall, peeled of its brown corky layer, dried, and used in commerce. The leaves share many of the properties of the bark and have also been used in traditional medicine.[1,2]

HISTORY: Althea root has been recognized as a source of useful mucilage, which has been used for more than 2 millennia to treat topical wounds and as a remedy for sore throats, coughs, and stomach ailments. The mucilage is incorporated into ointments to soothe chapped skin and is added to foods in small quantities ($\approx$ 20 ppm) to provide bulk and texture.[1] One report discusses Althea-type plants in a Neanderthal gravesite in Iraq.[3]

CHEMISTRY: The root contains 25% to 35% of mucilage.[1,4] but the content of the individual, purified mucilaginous polysaccharides is much lower. The mucilage content varies considerably with the season, being highest in the winter. A purified mucilage has been shown to be composed of L-rhamnose:D-galactose:D-galacturonic acid:D-glucuronic acid in a molar ratio of 3:2:3:3.[1] Asparagine (2%), sugars, pectin, and a tannin have also been identified in the root.[2,4] Fatty oil of althea has been addressed.[5] Flavonoid compounds of the leaves, flowers, and roots have also been described, including glucosidoesters and monoglucosides.[6,7]

PHARMACOLOGY: The mucilaginous properties of the althea root yield a soothing effect on mucous membranes. Althea reduces the transport velocity of isolated ciliated epithelium cells of the frog esophagus in vitro and may be useful in the management of coughs and colds because of its ability to protect mucous layers in the hypopharynx along with its spasmolytic, antisecretory, and bactericidal activity.[8] Althea extract and polysaccharide were tested for antitussive activity in cats. Although the polysaccharide component was more effective, both possessed cough-suppressing capabilities.[9]

Combinations of althea extracts with steroids have been used in the management of dermatologic conditions.[10,11] and the plant appears to possess anti-inflammatory activity that potentiates the effect of topical steroids.[12]

TOXICOLOGY: Althea extracts have not been generally associated with toxicity.

SUMMARY: Althea root and extracts have demulcent properties that make them useful in the management of sore throats and coughs along with topical dermal irritations. The plant has a long history of use and is not associated with any important toxicity.

PATIENT INFORMATION – Althea

Uses : Althea mucilage has been used to soothe dermal irritations, sore throats, and coughs. It appears to have bactericidal and anti-inflammatory properties.

Side Effects: Long used as a food additive, althea has no observed toxicity.

---

[1] Evans WC. *Trease and Evans' Pharmacognosy*, 13th ed. London: Bailliere Tindall, 1989.

[2] Leung AY. *Encyclopedia of Common Natural Ingredients Used in Food, Drugs and Cosmetics*. New York: J. Wiley and Sons, 1980.

[3] Lietava, J. Medicinal plants in a Middle Paleolithic grave Shanidar IV? *J Ethnopharmacol* 1992;35(3):263-6.

[4] *Merck Index*, 10th ed. Rahway, NJ: Merck & Co., Inc., 1983.

[5] Mishina, A, et al. Fatty oil of *Althea officinalis*, stoloniferous valerian and golden wallflower. *Farm Zh* 1975;(5):92-3. Ukrainian.

[6] Gudej, J. Flavonoid compounds of leaves of *Althea officinalis* L. (Malvaceae). Part 1. Glucosidoesters and monoglucosides. *Acta Pol Pharm* 1985;42(2):192-8.

[7] Gudej, J. Determination of flavonoid in leaves, flowers, and roots of *Althea officinalis* L. *Farmacja Polska* 1990;46:153-5.

[8] Muller-Limmroth W, et al. Effect of various phytotherapeutic expectorants on mucociliary transport. *Fortschr Med* 1980;98(3):95–101. German.

[9] Nosal'ova, G, et al. Antitussive action of extracts and polysacchrides of marsh mallow. *Pharmazie* 1992;47(3):224-6. German.

[10] Piovano PB, et al.Mazzocchi S. Clinical trial of a steroid derivative (9-alpha-fluoro-prednisolone-21-acetate) in association with aqueous extract of althea in the dermatological field. *G Ital Dermatol Minerva Dermatol* 1970;45(4):279.

[11] Huriez C et al. On the association of althea and dexamethasone: Dexalta ointment. *Lille Med* 1968;13(2)(suppl):121.

[12] Beaune A, et al. Anti-inflammatory experimental properties of marshmallow: Its potentiating action on the local effects of corticoids. *Therapie* 1966;21(2):341.

Ambrette

SCIENTIFIC NAME(S): *Abelmoschus moschatus* Medic. Family: Malvaceae

COMMON NAME(S): Ambrette, musk okra, muskmallow

BOTANY: This plant is cultivated for its seeds, which have a characteristic musk-like odor. The seeds are the source of ambrette, an aromatic oil used in perfumery. The plant grows to about 3 feet with showy yellow flowers with crimson centers. The plant is indigenous to India and is cultivated throughout the tropics.[1]

HISTORY: Several parts of the plant have been used throughout history, most notably the seed oil, which is valued for its fragrant smell. The oil is used in cosmetics and has been used to flavor alcoholic beverages, especially bitters, and coffee.[2] The tender leaves and shoots are eaten as vegetables and the plant is often grown as an ornamental.

Philippine native have used decoctions of the plant to treat stomach cancer, and extracts of the plant have bene used to treat such diverse ailments as hysteria, gonorrhea and respiratory disorders.[2]

CHEMISTRY: Distillation of the plant yields farnesol and furfural. The volatile oil is high in fatty acids, including palmitic and myristic acids. The ketone ambrettolide (a lactone of ambrettolic acid) is responsible for the characteristic muck-like odor. A variety of other related compounds have also been identified in quantities of less than 1% of the oil.[1]

The bark yields a fiber that is used to produce tough cloths.[2]

PHARMACOLOGY: Little is known about the pharmacologic activity of this plant. The related species *A. manihot* has been shown to limit the development of renal injury in rabbits with immune complex-induced glomerulonephritis, and *A. ficulneus* may contain substances that inhibit the development of the fetal sheep brain and that may impair the health of the ewe.[3]

TOXICOLOGY: Although the seeds were once considered to be stimulants with antispasmodic activity, the plant has been classified as an "Herb of Undefined Safety" by the FDA.[2] However, the extracts are classified as GRAS (Generally Recognized as Safe) for use in baked goods, candies and alcoholic beverages. Ambrettolide is reported to be nontoxic.[1]

Ambrette and related "nitro musks" are highly lipophilic and have been shown to persist in human mother's milk, presumably following absorption through the skin from dermally-applied cosmetics.[4]

Musk ambrette and musk ketone, both found in cosmetics and aftershaves, have been shown to cause photosensitivity and dermatitis in sensitive individuals.[5,6]

SUMMARY: Ambrette is commonly used as a fragrance in perfumes and cosmetics. The safety of ingesting the oil and other extracts of the seeds has been questioned and extracts and components of the plant are known to cause dermal irritation. In small quantities, however, ambrette is safe for internal consumption as a flavor for foods and drinks.

PATIENT INFORMATION – Ambrette

Uses: Ambrette has been used as a stimulant and as treatment for a variety of ills, from stomach cancer to hysteria. It is commonly used to scent cosmetics and to flavor foods and drinks.

Side Effects: Ambrette has been eaten as a vegetable. With the possible exception of seed extracts, ingestion of small amounts is considered safe. Ingestion or application of ambrette derivatives produces photosensitivity and dermatitis in some individuals.

---

[1] Leung AY. Encyclopedia of Common Natural Ingredients Used in Food, Drugs and Cosmetics. New York, NY: J Wiley and Sons, 1980.

[2] Duke JA. Handbook of Medicinal Herbs. Boca Raton, FL: CRC Press, 1985.

[3] Walker D, et al. Some effects of feeding *Tribulus terrestris, Ipomoea, Lonchophylla* and the seed of *Abelmoschus ficulneus* on fetal development and the outcome of pregnancy in sheep. *Reprod Fertil Dev* 1992;4:135.

[4] Liebl B, Ehrenstorfer S. Nitro-musk compounds in breast milk. *Gesundheitswesen* 1993;55:527.

[5] Machet L, et al. Persistent photosensitivity: treatment with puvatherapy and prednisolone. *Ann Dermatol Venereol* 1992;119:737.

[6] Gardeazabal J, et al. Successful treatment of musk ketone-induced chronic actinic dermatitis with cyclosporine and PUVA. *J Am Acad Dermatol* 1992;27:838.

Ammi

SCIENTIFIC NAME(S): *Ammi majus* L. and *A. visnaga* Lam. Family: Umbelliferae

COMMON NAME(S): Ammi, visnaga, bishop's weed

BOTANY: These annual plants grow to ≈ 120 cm in height, primarily in Egypt, other regions of the Middle East, and the Mediterranean. *A. visnaga* has been naturalized to parts of the southeastern US. It has a slightly aromatic odor and a very bitter taste. The drug product of ammi consists of the dried ripe fruits, typically of *A. visnaga*.

HISTORY: The plant has been cultivated for hundreds of years and was known by the Assyrians. *A. majus* was cultivated for the cut-flower trade, and both species have been used medicinally. These plants have been used in traditional medicine for millennia, particularly for the management of angina and respiratory diseases. Portions of the plant are made into toothpicks.[1] The fruits have been used in Egyptian folk medicine as diuretics and for the treatment of kidney and bladder stones.[2] Ammi has also been used for the traditional management of diabetes in Israel.[3]

CHEMISTRY: *A. visnaga* contains coumarins and furocoumarins (psoralens), the most important of which are khellin and visnagin. Khellin is present in fruits in a concentration of ≈ 1% and visnagin in a concentration of ≈ 0.3%.[4] Biosynthesis of khellin, visnagin, furocoumarin, and visnadin have been investigated.[5] Two furocoumarins, xanthotoxin (methoxsalen) and ammidin (imperatorin), from ammi fruits have been discovered, as well.[6] Solubility and dissolution studies of khellin have also been described.[7]

Numerous reports regarding ammi constituents are available evaluating their concentrations at various stages of maturity,[2,8] their presence in certain plant parts,[9] and interactions with different plant extracts.[10]

Various methods for determination of ammi components have been performed including the following: Micro method (khellin and visnagin),[11] TLC separation (khellin and visnagin),[12] spectrometric determination (khellin and bergapten),[13] HPLC (khellin and visnagin),[4,14] and a polarographic method (khellinum in fruits).[15] Recent improved analyses to determine ammi components have also been performed.[16,17]

Dihydroseselins have been determined from ammi fruits and extracts.[18] Genetically transformed ammi cultures have been evaluated.[19] In addition, marmesin, ammoidin, and ammidin have been characterized.[20] The fruit contains a small amount (< 0.03%) of a volatile oil.

PHARMACOLOGY: Khellin is commercially available in several multi-ingredient European proprietary preparations for oral and parenteral administration as a vasodilator. It is used in the management of bronchial asthma and angina pectoris.[6] The structure of cromolyn sodium, used in the management of allergic respiratory illness, was based on components derived from *A. visnaga*.[21] Lipophilic extracts from the plant, including the active components visnadin, khellin, and visnagin exhibited calcium channel blocking actions, with visnadin being the most active.[22] Acting at multiple sites, visnagin inhibited induced contractile responses in rat vascular smooth muscle.[23] Similarly, visnadine demonstrated peripheral and coronary vasodilatory activities in isolated rat vascular smooth muscle.[24]

Ammi extract showed marked antimicrobial activity against gram-positive bacteria and *Candida* species.[25] Constituent khellin from ammi fruit parts inhibited the mutagenicity of certain promutagens in *Salmonella typhimurium*.[26]

An ethnobotanical survey including 130 respondants reported ammi to be one of 16 species of Israeli medicinal plants used for diabetes.[3] However, literature searches found no clinical trials to support this hypoglycemic action.

Extracts of *A. majus* seeds fed to rats with experimentally-induced kidney stones showed no beneficial effect in terms of stone passage or size reduction.[27]

A combination product containing ammi demonstrated spasmolytic activity on guinea pig ileum in one report.[28] Extracts of the plants have been used to treat vitiligo and psoriasis.[2] When given orally in a dose of 50 mg 4 times daily, khellin increases HDL-cholesterol levels without affecting total cholesterol or triglyceride concentrations.[7]

TOXICOLOGY: *A. majus* has been associated with the development of severe ophthalmologic changes, particularly pigmentary retinopathy in photosensitized fowl.[29,30] Therefore, patients receiving *ammi* or its extracts should be monitored for ophthalmologic changes.

The furocoumarins (psoralens) may cause photosensitization and dermatitis.[31] One study reports 4 irritant compounds from ammi seeds and evaluates potential for contact dermatitis.[32]

In patients who received khellin to reduce blood lipids, nausea and vomiting were observed frequently. Elevated AST and ALT were also observed during therapy.[33]

SUMMARY: Plants of the genus *Ammi* have been used for thousands of years for the treatment of urologic, dermatologic, and respiratory symptoms. Clinical evidence supports their vasodilatory actions. The plant also possesses antimicrobial activity and inhibits certain mutagens. The use of khellin, a major component of the plant, is limited by toxicity.

PATIENT INFORMATION – Ammi

Uses: Ammi has been used for the treatment of urologic, dermatologic, and respiratory symptoms. The plant also possesses antimicrobial activity and inhibits certain mutagens.

Side Effects: Monitor for ophthalmic changes. The use of khellin is limited by toxicity (eg, elevated liver enzymes, phototoxicity, dermatitis).

[1] Mabberley D. *The Plant-Book.* Cambridge: Cambridge University Press, 1987.
[2] Franchi G, et al. High performance liquid chromatography analysis of the furanochromones khellin and visnagin in various organs of *Ammi visnaga* (L.) Lam. at different developmental stages. *J Ethnopharmacol* 1985;14(2-3):203-12.
[3] Yaniv Z, et al. Plants used for the treatment of diabetes in Israel. *J Ethopharmacol* 1987;19(2):145-51.
[4] Martelli P, et al. Rapid separation and quantitative determination of khellin and visnagin in *Ammi visnaga* (L.) Lam. fruits by high-performance liquid chromatography. *J Chromatogr* 1984;301:297-302.
[5] Chen M, et al. The biosynthesis of radioactive khellin and visnagin from C14 - acetate by *Ammi visnaga* plants. *Planta Med* 1969;17:319-27.
[6] Le Quesne P, et al. Furocoumarins from the fruit of *Ammi visnaga. J Nat Prod* 1985;48:496.
[7] Fromming K, et al. Influence of biopharmaceutical properties of drugs by natural occurring compounds as exemplified with khellin in an *Ammi visnaga* dry extract. *Pharmazeutische Industrie* 1989;51(4):439-43.
[8] Balbaa S, et al. Study of the active constituent of *Ammi visnaga* fruits collected at different stages of maturity. *J Pharm Sci UAR* 1968;9:15-26.
[9] Franchi G, et al. *Ammi visnaga* (L.) Lam.: occurrence of khellin and visnagin in primary rib channels and endosperm, and emptiness of vittae, revealed by U.V. microscopy. *Intl J Crude Drug Research* 1987;25:137-44.
[10] Gharbo S, et al. Modified chromatographic method of assay of *Ammi visnaga* L. fruits and its galenicals. *J Pharm Sci* 1968;9:7-14.
[11] Karawya M, et al. Micro method for the estimation of khellin and visnagin in *Ammi visnaga* fruits and in formulations. *J Pharm Sci* 1969;10:189-96.
[12] Karawya M, et al. Simultaneous TLC separation of khellin and visnagin and their assay in *Ammi visnaga* fruits, extracts, and formulations. *J Pharm Sci* 1970;59:1025-27.
[13] Ibrahim S, et al. Use of acid-dye technique in the analysis of natural products. Part 3. Spectrophotometric microdetermination of khellin and bergapten. *loydia* 1979;42:366-73.
[14] Mesbah M. Determinatioin of khellin and visnagin in *Ammi visnaga* fruits and in renal teas by high-performance liquid chromatography. *Egyptian J Pharm Sci* 1992;33(5-6):897-904.
[15] Orlov Y, et al. Polarographic determination of khellinum in *Ammi visnaga* fruits. *Farmatsiia* 1989;38(5):47-50.
[16] El-Domiaty M. Improved high-performance liquid chromatographic determination of khellin and visnagin in *Ammi visnaga* fruits and pharmaceutical formulations. *J Pharm Sci* 1992;81:475-78.
[17] Zgorka G, et al. Determination of furanochromones and pyranocoumarins in drugs and *Ammi visnaga* fruits by combined solid-phase extraction-high-performance liquid chromatography and thin-layer chromatography-high-performance liquid chromatography. *J Chromatogr A* 1998;797(1-2):305-09.
[18] Karawya M, et al. Determination of dihydroseselins in fruits and extracts of *Ammi visnaga* L. *J Pharm Sci* 1969;58:1545-547.
[19] Kursinszki L, et al. Biologically active compounds of genetically transformed *Ammi visnaga* cultures. *Gyogyszereszet* 1997;41:84-87.
[20] Abu-Mustafa E, et al. Isolation of Marmesin from the Fruits of *Ammi majus* Linn. *Nature* 1958;182(4627):54.
[21] Evans W. *Trease and Evans' Pharmacognosy,* 13th ed. London: Bailliere Tindall, 1989.
[22] Rauwald H, et al. The involvement of a Ca2+ channel blocking mode of action in the pharmacology of *Ammi visnaga* fruits. *Planta Med* 1994;60(2):101-05.
[23] Duarte J, et al. Vasodilator effects of visnagin in isolated rat vascular smooth muscle. *Eur J Pharmacol* 1995;286(2):115-22.
[24] Duarte J, et al. Effects of visnadine on rat isolated vascular smooth muscles. *Planta Med* 1997;63(3):233-36.
[25] Jawad A, et al. Antimicrobial activity of sesquiterpene lactone and alkaloid fractions from Iraqi plants. *Int J Crude Drug Research* 1988;26:185-88.
[26] Schimmer O, et al. Inhibition of metabolic activation of the promutagens, benzo pyrene, 2-aminofluorene and 2-aminoanthracene by furanochromones in *Salmonella typhimurium. Mutagenesis* 1998;13(4):385–89.
[27] Ahsan S, et al. Effect of *Trigonella foenum-graecum* and *Ammi majus* on calcium oxalate urolithiasis in rats. *J Ethnopharmacol* 1989;26(3):249-54.
[28] Westendorf J, et al. Spasmolytic and contractile effects of a combination product from plants on the smooth muscle of the guinea pigs. *Arzneimittelforschung* 1981;31(1):40-43.
[29] Shlosberg A, et al. The comparative photosensitizing properties of *Ammi majus* and *Ammi visnaga* in goslings. *Avian Dis* 1974;18(4):544-50.
[30] Shlosberg A, et al. Examples of poisonous plants in Israel of importance to animals and man. *Arch Toxicol Suppl* 1983;6:194-96.
[31] Kavli G, et al. Phytophotodermatitis. *Photodermatol* 1984;1(2):65-75.
[32] Saeed M, et al. Studies on the contact dermatitic properties of indigenous Pakistani medicinal plants. Part 3. Irritant principles of *Ammi visnaga* L. seeds. *Gazi Universitesi Eczacilik Farultesi Dergisi* 1993;10(1):15-23.
[33] Harvengt C, et al. HDL-cholesterol increase in normolipaemic subjects on khellin: A pilot study. *Int J Clin Pharmacol Res* 1983;3(5):363-66.

Andrachne

SCIENTIFIC NAME(S): *Andrachne cordifolia* Muell. and related species viz. *A. aspera* Spreng. and *A. phyllanthoides* (Nutt.) Muell. Arg. Family: Euphorbiaceae

BOTANY: The Andrachne genus has about 20 tropical American species and a few species in North Africa, Europe and elsewhere.[1] These are generally seen as shrubs and undershrubs, possessing many ascending leafy branches, in tropical and warm regions. The leaves are oval or obovate, while the flowers are monoecious, pedicellate and usually solitary in the axils. The fruit is dry, splitting into three 2–valved carpels. *A. phyllanthoides* is found in the dry hills and rocky barrens from Montana to Texas in May through October.[2] *A. aspera* is widely distributed throughout the Middle East.

CHEMISTRY: Two bisbenzylisoquinoline alkaloids, cocsuline and pendulin, have been isolated from the roots of *A. cordifolia*.[3] Previously, the two alkaloids were reported only from the Menispermaceae family.

PHARMACOLOGY: The plants in the genus are marginally used as medicinal plants in some countries. *A. aspera* roots are used for treating eye inflammation in Yemen, where pieces of the crushed roots are placed on the eyelids.[4] Some species also have pest-control properties.

TOXICOLOGY: No toxicological data have been recorded for this genus.

SUMMARY: Andrachne species have marginal folkloric use for treating eye inflammation. Some are used for controlling pests.

PATIENT INFORMATION – Andrachne

Uses: One species has been used to treat eye inflammation in Yemen. Others act as pest controls.

Side Effects: No data available.

---

[1] Mabberley DJ. The Plant-Book. New York: Cambridge University press, 1987.
[2] Fernald ML. Gray's Manual of Botany, ed. 8. Portland, OR: Dioscorides Press. 1950.
[3] Khan MI, et al. Bisbenzylisoquinoline Alkaloids from *Andrachne cordifolia*. *Planta Med* 1983;47:191.
[4] Ghazanfur SA. Handbook of Arabian Medicinal Plants. Boca Raton, FL: CRC Press, 1994.

Angelica

SCIENTIFIC NAME(S): *Angelica* spp. Family: Umbelliferae

COMMON NAME(S): Angelica, wild angelica, garden angelica

BOTANY: Angelica is a tall, aromatic biennial plant of the parsley family. It possesses deeply indented, very large leaves and strong stems. The plant is commonly used as an attractive border for herb gardens and to shield other herbs from the wind. The stems, leaves and flowers are light green in color. The species *A. archangelica*, also referred to as *A. officinalis* (Moench) Hoffm., is native to shady places in Iceland, Lapland and other northern regions. The species *A. atropurpurea* is found in North America, and *A. sylvestris* L. is a small European species. Other species include *A. curtisi* and *A. rosaefolia*.[1] *A. atropurpurea* is also known in the United States by the common name alexanders, but this name is also used to identify another related plant, *Smyrnium olusatrum*. *A. pubescens* roots are used in Chinese herbal medicine for the treatment of arthritis, headaches and as a carminative.

HISTORY: According to legend, angelica was revealed to humans by an angel as a cure for the plague, hence its name. It was introduced to England during the 16th century. Angelica is best known today in the form of cadied or crystallized stems. Dried leaves have been used to make tisanes, which resemble Chinese tea, and as a scent in potpourri. Angelica has been used as a flavoring in gin because of its resemblance to the flavor of juniper berries. The candied leaves and stalks are used as decoration on cakes and pastries. When cooked with rhubarb, angelica reduces the tartness of the other plant. According to one source, angelica is responsible for the muscatel flavor of Rhine wines.[1] Teas made from the roots and leaves of *A. archangelica* have been used as expectorant, diuretic, diaphoretic, antiflatulent, and externally to treat rheumatic and skin disorders. Angelica has been used as a remedy for respiratory ailments, and in the Faeroe Islands the plant is used as a vegetable.[2]

CHEMISTRY: The roots and fruit of *A. archangelica* yield about 1% angelica oil, used as a flavoring and scent. Ether-pentane extracts contain volatile components including at least 16 monoterpene hydrocarbons, 13 sesquiterpene hydrocarbons, 12 monoterpene alcohols, 4 oxygenated sesquiterpenes, 11 esters, 3 lactones, 7 aliphatic carbonyls and 4 aromatic compounds. Alcohol extracts contain an additional 20 compounds.[3]

Experimental confirmation has shown that coumarin osthol and xanthotoxin, extracts from *A. pubescens*, have significant anti-inflammatory and analgesic properties.[4] The essential oil is known to contain alpha-phelandrene, alpha-pinene, osthenole, alpha-thujene and camphene.[5] Root oil is considered to be of superior quality to oils obtained from other parts of the plant.

PHARMACOLOGY: Angelica contains alpha-angelica lactone, which has been shown to augment calcium binding in canine cardiac microsomes in the presence of ATP. With or without ATP, the compound also augments calcium turnover. Its action may involve increasing the contract-dependent calcium pool to be released upon systolic depolarization.[6]

An attempt to identify non-viral inducers of interferon failed to find any active extracts of angelica.[7] Experimental confirmation has shown that osthole, a component of *A. pubescens*, has a non-specific relaxing effect on the trachaelis of guinea pigs.[8] Volatile oil from angelica has been shown to inhibit phasic contraction of ileal muscle fibers. In contrast to some other plant extracts, angelica oil has a greater effect on tracheal tissue than on ileal tissue.[9]

A mitogen consisting of 90% sugar and 10% protein has been found in *A. actiloba* (Kitagawa); the activity of this compound is reduced by at least half in the presence of acid or base.[10] An aqueous extract of *A. koreana* (radix) has shown wormicidal activity against *Clonorchis sinensis*.[11] Alpha-angelica lactone inhibits the formation of metabolites of the carcinogen benzo(alpha)pyrene in the mouse forestomach and liver, but not in lung tissue.[12] Volatile emissions of *A. archangelica* have demonstrated fungistatic activity against species of Aspergillus, Rhizopus, Mucor and Alternaria.[13]

A. archangelica L. has shown some antimutagenic properties in murine bone marrow cells.[14] Anti-tumor effects on mice with Ehrlich Ascites tumors have been demonstrated by *A. sinensis*. *In vitro* and *in vivo* immunostimulating effects were also produced.[15] *A. sinensis* given to healthy mice promoted clone stimulating factors (CSF) in

32

spleen conditioned medium (SCM).[16] Sodium ferolate, and active component of *A. sinensis* Diels, exhibited hepato-protective action in mice.[17] Ferulic acid, a phenolic compound in *A. sinesis* Diels, has inhibited uterine contractions in rats.[18]

TOXICOLOGY: Angelica is generally recognized as safe for consumption as a natural seasoning and flavoring. The coumarins and furocoumarins may induce photosensitivity if applied topically.[19] These compounds may also be photocarcinogenic and may be mutagenic in laboratory animals. It is possible to confuse this plant with water hemlock (*Cicuta maculata* L.), which is extremely toxic.

SUMMARY: The term angelica refers to a number of species of herbs of the genus *Angelica*. These plants have been used for flavorings and scents, as vegetables and herbs, and in folk remedies for respiratory illnesses and arthritis. Pharmacologically, angelica contains compounds with cardiac, smooth muscle and metabolic effects, and volatile components appear to control the growth of some fungi. Topical administration of the extract may induce photosensitity in sensitive persons.

PATIENT INFORMATION – Angelica

Uses: Angelica species are used as flavoring, scent and vegetable, It has been a folk remedy for respiratory and a range of other ailments, including arthritis. Evidence suggest it has immunostimulant, antimutagenic (but also possibly mutagenic), and anti-tumor effects. It inhibits muscle tissue.

Side Effects: Generally recognized as safe, angelica may be photocarcinogenic. Applied extract produces photosensitivity in some individuals.

---

[1] Lowenfeld C, Back P. The Complete Book of Herbs and Spices. London: David E. Charles, 1974.

[2] The New Encyclopedia Britannica, vo. 1. Chicago: Encyclopedia Britannica, Inc., 1985.

[3] Taskinen J, Nykanen L. Chemical composition of angelica root oil. *Acta Chem Scand* 1975;29(7):757.

[4] Chen YF, et al. Anti-inflammatory and analgesic activities from roots of Angelica pubescens. *Planta Med* 1995;61(1):2.

[5] Tagawa M, Murai F. New iridoid glucoside, nepetolglucosylester, from Nepeta cataria. *Planta Med* 1980;39:144.

[6] Entman ML, et al. The influence of ouabain and alpha angelica lactone on calcium metabolism of dog cardiac microsomes. *J Cin Invest* 1969;48(2):229.

[7] Zielinska-Jenczylik J, et al. Effect of plant extracts on the in vitro interferon synthesis. *Arch Immunol Ther Exp (Warsz)* 1984;32(5):577.

[8] Teng CM, et al. The relaxant action of osthole isolated from Angelica pubescens in guinea-pig trachea. *Naunyn-Schmiedebergs Arch Pharmacol* 1994;349(2):202.

[9] Reiter M, Brandt W. Relaxant effects on tracheal and ileal smooth muscles of the guinea pig. *Arzneimittelforschung* 1985;35(1A):408.

[10] Ohno N, et al. Biochemical and physiocochemical characterization of a mitogen obtained from an oriental crude drug, Tohki (Angelica actiloba Katagawa). *J Pharmacobiodyn* 1983;6(12):903.

[11] Rhee JK, et al. Screening of the wormicidal Chinese raw drugs on Clonorchis sinensis. *Am J Chin Med* 1981;9(4):227.

[12] Ioannou YM, et al. Effect of butylated hydroxyanisole, alpha-angelica lactone, and beta-naphthoflavoneo n benzo (alpha) pyrene: DNA adduct formation in vivo in the forestomach, lung, and liver of mice. *Cancer Res* 1982;42(4):1199.

[13] Saksena N, Tripathi HHS. Plant volatiles in relation to fungistasis. *Fitoterapia* 1985;56/4:243.

[14] Salikhova RA, Poroshenko GG. [Antimutagenic properties of Angelica archangelica L. (Russian).] *Vestn Akad Med Nauk SSSR* 1995;(1):58.

[15] Choy YM, et al. Immunopharmacological studies of low molecular weight polysaccharide from Angelica sinensis. *Am J Chin Med* 1994;22(2):137.

[16] Chen YC, Gao YQ [Research on the mechanism of blood-tonifying effect of danggui buxue decoction (Chinese).] *Chung-Kuo Chung Yao Tsa Chih - China J of Chin Materia Med* 1994;19(1):43.

[17] Wang H, Peng RX. [Sodium ferulate alleviated paracetamol-induced liver toxicity in mice (Chinese).] *Chung-Kuo Yao Li Hsueh Pao - Acta Pharamacologica Sinica* 1994;15(1):81.

[18] Ozaki Y, Ma JP. Inhibitory effects of tetramethylpyrazine and ferulic acid on spontaneous movement of rat uterus in situ. *Chem Pharm Bull* 1990;38(6):1620.

[19] Opdyke DL. Monographs on fragrance raw materials. *Food Cosmet Toxicol* 1975;13(suppl):683.

Anise

SCIENTIFIC NAME(S): *Pimpinella anisum* L. Family: Umbelliferae (Apiaceae). In some texts, anise is referred to as *Anisum vulgare* Gartner or *A. officinarum* Moench. Do not confuse with the "Chinese star anise" (*Illicium verum* Hook. filius. Family: Magnoliaceae).

COMMON NAME(S): Anise, aniseed, sweet cumin

BOTANY: Anise is an annual herb that grows 1 to 2 feet and is cultivated widely throughout the world.[1] The flowers are yellow, compound umbels. Its leaves are feather-shaped. The 2 mm long, greenish-brown, ridged seeds are used for the food or the drug. They are harvested when ripe in autumn.[2] Aniseed has an anethole-like odor and a sweet, aromatic taste,[3] described as "licorice-like," which has led to traditional use of anise oils in licorice candy.[1]

HISTORY: Anise has a history of use as a spice and a fragrance. It has been cultivated in Egypt for at least 4000 years. Recordings of its diuretic use and treatment of digestive problems and toothache are seen in medical texts from this era. In ancient Greek history, writings explain how anise helps breathing, relieves pain, provokes urine and eases thirst.[2] The oil has been used commercially since the 1800s. The fragrance is used in food, soap, creams and perfumes. Anise is often added to licorice candy or used as a "licorice" flavor substitute; it is a fragrant component of anisette.

CHEMISTRY: Anise oil (1% to 4%) is obtained by steam distillation of the dried fruits of the herb. The highest quality oils result from anise seeds of ripe umbels in the central location of the plant.[4] A major component of the oil is trans-anethole (75% to 90%), responsible for the characteristic taste and smell, as well as for its medicinal properties.[3,5,6] The cis-isomer is 15 to 38 times more toxic than the trans-isomer.[7] Spectrophotometric determination of anethole in anise oil has been performed.[8]

The volatile oil also has related compounds that include estragole (methyl chavicol, 1% to 2%), anise ketone (p-methoxyphenylacetone) and betacaryophyllene. In smaller amounts are anisaldehyde, anisic acid, limonene, alpha-pinene, acetaldehyde, p-cresol, cresol and myristicin (the psychomimetic compound previously isolated from nutmeg).[3,9,11] Oil of *Feronia limonia* has some similarity to anise oil and may be used as a substitute.[12]

Other constituents include coumarins such as umbelliferone, umbelliprenine, bergapten and scopoletin. Lipids (16%) include fatty acids, beta-amyrin, stigmasterol and its salts.[1,11] Flavonoids in aniseed include flavonol, flavone, glycosides, rutin, isoorientin and isovitexin,[11] protein (18%) and carbohydrate (50%). Terpene hydrocarbons in the plant have also been described.[13]

PHARMACOLOGY: Anise is widely used as a flavoring in all food categories including alcohols, liqueurs, dairy products, gelatins, puddings, meats and candies.[1] It is sold as a spice, and the seeds are used as a breath freshener.[7] The essential oil is used medicinally as well as in perfume, soaps and sachets.[1,5] The oil, when mixed with sassafras oil, is used against insects.[5] Applied externally, the oil has been used for lice and scabies.[2] As a skin penetration enhancer, anise oil has little activity compared with eucalyptus oil and others.[14] but topical application of the constituent bergapten, in combination with ultraviolet light has been used in psoriasis treatment.[11]

Pharmacological effects of anise are mainly caused by anethole, which has structural similarities to catecholamines (eg, adrenaline, noradrenaline, dopamine).[11] Sympathomimetic-type effects have been attributed to anethole in at least one report.[15]

Anise is well known as a **carminative** and an **expectorant**. Its ability to decrease bloating and settle the digestive tract is still used today, especially in pediatrics. In higher doses, anise is used as an antispasmodic and an antiseptic for cough, asthma and bronchitis.[2,3,5,11]

Anise has also been evaluated for its **antimicrobial** action against gram-negative and gram-positive organisms.[16] Constituent anethole also inhibits growth of mycotoxin producing *Aspergillus* in culture.[1] Anise is used in dentifrices as an antiseptic and in lozenges and cough preparations for its weak antibacterial effects.[1,7] A German report testing aromatic waters (including anise) on the growth and survival of *Pseudomonas aeruginosa* has been published.[17] Anise has been tested for odor preference in rats[18] and dietary preference in cows.[19] Anise has promoted iron absorption in rats, suggesting possible use as a preventative agent in iron deficiency anemia.[20]

TOXICOLOGY: Anise oil has GRAS status and is approved for food use. The acute oral LD-50 of the oil in rats is 2.25 g/kg. No percutaneous absorption of the oil occurred through mouse skin within 2 hours.[21] The oral LD-50 of anethole is 2090 mg/kg in rats; rats fed a diet containing 0.25% anethole for 1 year showed no ill effects, while those receiving 1% anethole for 15 weeks had microscopic changes in hepatocytes.[7]

The German commission E monograph lists side effects of anise as "occasional allergic reactions of the skin, respiratory tract and gastrointestinal tract."[3] When applied to human skin in a 2% concentration in petrolatum base, anise oil produced no topical reactions. The oil is not considered to be a primary irritant. However, anethole has been associated with sensitization and skin irritation and may cause erythema, scaling and vesiculation.[10] Anise oil in toothpaste has been reported to cause contact sensitivity, cheilitis and stomatitis.[7] The constituent bergapten may cause photosensitivity.[11] As mentioned, the cis-isomer of anethole is 15 to 38 times more toxic to animals than the trans-isomer, their relative content being depen-

dent on plant species.[1,7] Ingestion of the oil in doses as small as 1 ml may result in pulmonary edema, vomiting and seizures.[22] Large doses may interfere with anticoagulant and MAOI therapy. Anethole's (and its dimers') estrogenic activity may alter hormone therapy (eg, contraceptive pills). Aniseed is a reputed abortifacient. Excessive use is not recommended in pregnancy.[2,11]

The mycoflora of anise seed has been evaluated, making it possible to isolate 15 fungal genera, 78 species and six varieties, including *Aspergillus*, *Penicillium* and *Rhizopus*.[23] Naturally occurring mycotoxins are also present in TLC analysis of anise spice extract.[24] Gamma radiation has inhibited mold growth on anise in humid conditions.[25]

SUMMARY: Anise oil is a common fragrance, flavorant and spice. It has a history of uses in traditional medicine. It has carminative, antimicrobial and expectorant effects and may also be useful for psoriasis and iron deficiency anemia. Anise may cause occasional skin, respiratory and GI allergic reactions in sensitive individuals.

PATIENT INFORMATION – Anise

Uses: Anise has been used as a flavoring in alcohols, liqueurs, dairy products, gelatins, puddings, meats and candies and as a scent in perfumes, soaps and sachets. The oil has been used for lice, scabies and psoriasis. Anise is frequently used as a carminative and expectorant. Anise is also used to decrease bloating and settle the digestive tract in children. In high doses, it is used as an antispasmodic and an antiseptic and for the treatment of cough, asthma and bronchitis.

Side Effects: Anise may cause allergic reactions of the skin, respiratory and GI tract. Ingestion of the oil may result in pulmonary edema, vomiting and seizures. It is not recommended for use in pregnancy.

Drug Interactions : Anise may interfere with anticoagulant, MAOI therapy and hormone therapy.

---

[1] Leung AY. Encyclopedia of Common Natural Ingredients, 2nd ed. New York: J Wiley and Sons, 1996;36-38.
[2] Chevallier A. Encyclopedia of Medicinal Plants. New York: DK Publishing, 1996;246-47.
[3] Bisset N. Herbal Drugs and Phytopharmaceuticals. Stuttgart, Germany: CRC Press, 1994;73-75.
[4] Tsvetkov R. *Planta Medica* 1970 Aug;18:350-53.
[5] Chandler R, et al. *Can Pharm J* 1984 Jan;117:28-29.
[6] Tabacchi R, et al. *Helvet Chim Acta* 1974;57:849.
[7] Duke J. CRC Handbook of Medicinal Herbs. Boca Raton, FL: CRC Press, 1989;374-75.
[8] Mohamed Y, et al. *Indian J Pharm* 1976 Sep-Oct;38:117-19.
[9] Harborne JB, et al. *Phytochemistry* 1969;8:1729.
[10] *Food Cosmetic Toxicol* 1973;11:865.
[11] Newall C, et al. Herbal Medicines. London, England: Pharmaceutical Press, 1996;30-31.

[12] Shah N, et al. *Parfum Kosmetic* 1985 Mar;66:182-83.
[13] Burkhardt G, et al. *Pharm Weekb [Sci]* 1986 Jun 20;8: 190-93.
[14] Williams, A. et al. *Int J Pharmaceutics* 1989 Dec 22;57:R7-R9.
[15] Albert-Puleo M. *J Ethnopharmacol* 1980;2:337-44.
[16] Narasimha B, et al. *Flavor Ind* 1970 Oct;1:725-29.
[17] Ibrahim Y, et al. *Pharm Acta Helv* 1991;66(9–10):286-88.
[18] Lucas F. et al. *Behav Neurosci* 1995;109(3):446-54.
[19] Nombekela S, et al. *Journal of Dairy Science* 1994;77(8):2393-99.
[20] el-Shobaki F, et al. *Z Ernahrungswiss* 1990;29(4):264-69.
[21] Meyer F and Meyer E. *Arzneim Forsch* 1959;9:516.
[22] Spoerke DG. Herbal Medications. Santa Barbara, CA: Woodbridge Press, 1980.
[23] Moharram A, et al. *J Basic Microbiology* 1989;29(7):427-35.
[24] El-Kady I, et al. *Folia Microbiologica* 1995;40(3):297-300.
[25] Mahmoud M, et al. *Egyptian J Pharmaceutical Sciences* 1992;33(1–2):21-30.

Apple

SCIENTIFIC NAME(S): *Malus sylvestris* Mill. Family: Rosaceae

COMMON NAME(S): Apple

BOTANY: The apple is a deciduous tree with simple clusters of flowers. The fruit is termed a "pome." Apple trees are widely cultivated throughout the temperate climates of the world and the fruit is broadly available in commercial markets.[2] More than 1000 cultivars of apple have been identified.[3]

HISTORY: The apple has long been recognized as a valuable food. Its uses in traditional medicine have been varied, including the treatment of cancer, diabetes, dysentery, fever, heart ailmetns, scurvy and warts.[1] Apples are also said to be effective in cleaning the teeth. The fruit jice is drunk fresh, fermented as cider or as apple brandy. The wood of the apple tree is valued as a firewood.

CHEMISTRY: Apple leaves, bark and root contain an antibacterial substance (phloretin), which is active in vitro in low concentrations.[1] Hydrogen cyanide (HCN), present in the form of a cyanogenic glycoside (amygdalin), is found in the seeds.[1,2] In addition, the seeds contain a yellow semi-drying oil (Glucoside phlorizin with the odor of bitter almonds.

The fruit contains up to 17% pectin and pectic acids. A variety of other components, many of them with aromatic qualities, are found in apples, including tannins, quercetin, alpha-farnesene, shikimic acid and chlorogenic acid.[1]

PHARMACOLOGY: The apple is often eaten to alleviate contipation or to control diarrhea. Both therapeutic effects appear to be related to the fruit's pectin content. Pectin absorbs water in the gastrointestinal tract and swells to a gummy mass. As such, it can provide bulk and moisture to hardened stools, or aid in producing formed stools by adding bulk in the presence of diarrhea.

The antibacterial phloretin is active agains some gram-positive and gram-negative pathogens.[4] Extracts of the related *M. sativa* have been shown to be active against *Vibrio cholerae*.[5]

TOXICOLOGY: Because of their HCN content, apple seeds should not be ingested in large quantities. (A small number of seeds, however, may be ingested without symptoms.)[2] Large amounts of seeds have the potential for txicity. One recurring report cites the case of a man dying of cyanide poisoning after ingesting a cupful of apple seeds.[1] Because cyanogenic glycoside must be hydrolyzed in the stomach in order to release cyanide, several hours may elapse before symptoms of poisoning occur.[2]

SUMMARY: The apple is a widely cultivated fruit that has been used as a food for thousands of years. It has also been used in traditional medicine for a variety of applications; the most consistent pharmacologic effect appears to be related to the fruit's pectin content, which helps regulate bowel consistency.

PATIENT INFORMATION – Apple

Uses: Traditional uses include treatment for cancer, diabetes, fever, heart ailments, scurvy, and warts. Leaves, bark, and root contain antibacterials active in low concentrations. The large pectin content makes the fruit valuable for both constipation and diarrhea.

Side Effects: The seeds, which contain hydrogen cyanide, should not be consumed in large quantities.

---

[1] Duke JA. Handbook of Medicinal Herbs. Boca Raton, FL: CRC Press, 1985.
[2] Lampe KE, McCann MA. AMA Handbook of Poisonous and Injurious Plants. Chicago: American Medical Association, 1985.
[3] Mabberley DJ. The Plant-Book. Cambridge: Cambridge University Press, 1987.
[4] Lewis WH, Elvin-Lewis MPF. Medical Botany: Plants affecting man's health. New York: John Wiley & Sons, 1977.
[5] Guevara JM, et al. The in vitro action of plants on Vibrio cholorae. *Rev Gastroenterol Peru* 1994;14:27.

Apricot

SCIENTIFIC NAME(S): *Prunus armeniaca* L. (Rosaceae)

COMMON NAME(S): Apricot, Chinese almond

BOTANY: Apricots grow on trees up to 30 feet in height. The plant's leaves are oval and finely serrated. The five-petaled, white flowers grow together in clusters. Fruits vary in color from yellows and oranges to deep purples. They ripen in late summer.

The apricot is native to China and Japan but is also cultivated in warmer temperate areas of the world, mainly the regions including Turkey through Iran, Southern Europe, South Africa, Australia and California. There are many varieties and species of apricot, differing in flavor, color and size.[1,2,3,5]

HISTORY: In India and China, the apricot has been used for over 2000 years. During the 2nd century AD, a physician, Dong Feng, is said to have received his payment in apricot trees. There are also biblical references to the plant.[1,2]

The Greeks wrongly assumed the apricot to have originated in Armenia, hence its botanical name " *Prunus armeniaca*." The Romans termed the fruit "praecocium" meaning "precocious," referring to the fruit's early ripening. From this, the name "apricot" evolved.[5]

CHEMISTRY: Acids present in apricot fruits include malic, citric, tartaric, quinic, succinic, acetic, caffeic, p-coumaric and ferulic.[1,3]

The cyanogenic glycoside amygdalin also present in the plant has been determined from seeds, using gas chromatography.[6] Cyanide content in kernels varies from 2 to 200 mg/100 g.[3] Kernels contain up to 8% amygdalin, which yields laetrile and hydrocyanic acid.[2]

Sugars present in apricot include xylose, glucose, fructose and sorbitol.[1] Araginose and galactose have been detected by thin layer chromatography (TLC).[6] Vitamins include K, C, β-carotene, thiamine, niacin and iron.[1]

Other constituents in apricot include tannins (bark), volatile essences (myrcene, limonene, p-cymene, geranial and others), cholesterol, flavonols and pectin (fruits).[1,2,3]

The apricot gum has been studied in tablet and emulsion preparations.[7] Tablets prepared with apricot gum are comparable with those made with acacia gum.[8]

PHARMACOLOGY: Apricots are usually eaten as a fruit, either fresh or dried, made into jams and jellies or alcoholic beverages. The seeds are used like almonds by Chinese and Afghan cultures. The oil (apricot kernel oil) is also used. Its use in food, flavorings, confection, juices, jams, etc. is common. Some cultures use certain varieties of apricot kernels as almonds.[1,3]

In very small amounts, the toxic prussic acid (hydrogen cyanide) present in apricot kernels is prescribed in Chinese medicine for asthma treatment, cough and constipation.[2] Decoction of the plant's bark serves as an astringent to soothe irritated skin.[2] The oil is used in cosmetics or as a pharmaceutical vehicle.[1,2] Other folk medicine uses of apricot include treatment of hemorrhage, infertility, eye inflammation and spasm.[1] Apricot kernel paste may help eliminate vaginal infections.[2]

Laetrile, a semi-synthetic derivative of the naturally occuring "amygdalin," has been used (during late '70s, early '80s) in a highly controversial treatment for cancer.[2,3] A theory claimed that laetrile, when metabolized by the enzyme beta-glucosidase, released toxic cyanide. The enzyme was said to be most prevalent in tumor tissue (as opposed to normal tissue). As a result, this reaction was believed to destroy mainly cancer cells. It was later proven that both cancerous and normal cells contained only trace amounts of this enzyme. Although the treatment may have had slight activity in some cases, it was not as valuable as once thought.[4] A report in 1980 concluded laetrile to be ineffective in cancer treatment. Other proposed theories of laetrile in cancer treatment have not been substantiated by scientific evidence.[1,2,3]

TOXICOLOGY: Excess ingestion of apricot fruit may cause bone and muscle harm, blindness, hair loss and reduction in mental capacity.[1] Contact dermatitis has been reported from apricot kernels. Kernel ingestion may be teratogenic as well.[3]

Apricot kernel ingestion is a common source of cyanide poisoning, with over 20 deaths reported.[3] Deaths are reported from as little as ingesting two kernels.[1] Extract of amygdalin and water extract of apricot kernel produced sedation, convulsion, hyperventilation and death in mice.[8] Amygdalin content in apricot pits varies and can be up to 8%. Wild varieties may contain 20 times the amount of cultivated apricot varieties.[1] Hydrolysis of amygdalin yielding the toxic hydrogen cyanide (HCN) is more rapid in alkaline pH (than acidic, in the GI tract), which can delay symptoms of poisoning. Symptoms of cyanide toxicity include: Dizziness, headache, nausea/vomiting; and quickly progress to palpitations, hypotension, convulsion, paralysis, coma and death, from 1 to 15 minutes after ingestion. Antidotes to cyanide poisoning include nitrite, thiosulfate, hydroxocobalamin and aminophenol.[3]

SUMMARY: The apricot, native to China and Japan, has become a popular fruit. Apricots contain acids, sugars, tannins and the cyanogenic glycoside amygdalin. Prussic acid (hydrogen cyanide), present in the kernels, has been used in Chinese medicine. Apricot has also been used for asthma, inflammation and infection. In the late 1970s, laetrile (a synthetic derivative of amygdalin) had been used for cancer treatment but was later found to be ineffective. Excess ingestion of apricot kernels causes cyanide poisoning in both animals and humans. The apricot kernel oil is used in cosmetics.

PATIENT INFORMATION – Apricot

Uses: Apricots are usually eaten as fruit. Apricot kernel oil is used in cosmetics. In Chinese medicine, it has been used for asthma, cough and constipation.

Side Effects: Excess ingestion of apricot fruit may cause bone and muscle damage, blindness, hair loss and reduction in mental capacity. Ingestion of apricot kernels causes cyanide poisoning.

---

[1] Duke J. *CRC Handbook of Medicinal Herbs* Boca Raton, FL: CRC Press 1989;394-5.

[2] Chevallier A. *Encyclopedia of Medicinal Plants* New York, NY: DK Publishing 1996;254-5.

[3] Newall C, et al. *Herbal Medicines* London, England: Pharmaceutical Press 1996;32–33.

[4] Moertel, et al. *New Eng J Med* 306(4):201-6.

[5] Davidson A, et al. *Fruit, a Connoisseur's Guide and Cookbook* London, England: Mitchell Beazley Publishers 1991;26–7.

[6] Yao Q, et al. *Chung Yao Tung Pao Bulletin of Chinese Materia Medica* 1987;12(Apr):234–6.

[7] Farid D, et al. *Trav Soc Pharm Montpellier* 1980;40(1):61–6.

[8] Farid D, et al. *Trav Soc Pharm Montpellier* 1985;42(1–2):35–41.

[9] Yamashita M, et al. *Pharmaceuticals Monthly* 1987;29(Jun):1291–4.

Arnica

SCIENTIFIC NAME(S): *Arnica montana* L. In addition, other related species have been used medicinally including *A. sororia* Greene, *A. fulgens* Pursh., *A. cordifolia* Hook., *A. chamissonis* Less. subsp. *foliosa* (Nutt.) Family: Compositae or Asteraceae

COMMON NAME(S): Leopard's bane, mountain tobacco, mountain snuff, wolf's bane

BOTANY: Arnica is a perennial that grows from 1 to 2 feet.[1,2] Its oval, opposite leaves form a basal rosette close to the soil surface. It has bright yellow, daisy-like flowers.[1,2,3] The dried flower heads are the primary parts used from the plant. The rhizome is also used.[2,4] Arnica is native to the mountainous regions of Europe to southern Russia.[3,4] The unrelated plant, monkshood (*Aconitum* spp) is sometimes referred to as wolf's bane.

HISTORY: Internal and external preparations made from the flowering heads of arnica have been used medicinally for hundreds of years. Alcoholic tinctures were used by early settlers to treat sore throats, as a febrifuge, and to improve circulation. Homeopathic uses included the treatment of surgical or accidental trauma, as an analgesic, and in the treatment of postoperative thrombophlebitis and pulmonary emboli.[5] It has been used externally for acne, bruises, sprains and muscle aches, and as a general topical counterirritant.[6] Arnica has been used extensively in European folk medicine. German philosopher Johann Wolfgang von Goethe (1749–1832) was said to have drunk arnica tea to "ease" his angina.[2] Arnica's bactericidal properties were employed for abrasions and gunshot wounds.[7]

CHEMISTRY: A number of flavonoid glycosides have been identified in arnica.[8] Flavonoids (0.4% to 0.6%)[3] include betuletol, eupafolin, flavonol glucuronides hispidulin, isorhamnetin, luteolin, patuletin, spinacetin, tricin, 3,5,7,-trihydroxy-6,3',4'-trimethoxyflavone, kaempferol, quercetin,[9] and kaempferol and quercetin derivatives,[10] jaceosidin, and pectolin-arigenin.[4] Isomeric alcohols include arnidiol and foradiol.[7,8]

Terpenoids in arnica include arnifolin, arnicolide[2], sesquiterpenes (helenalin[9] and helenalin derivatives,[11] dihydrohelenalin,[9] etc). Pseudoguaianolide helenalinmethacrylate, a helenalin ester, has been isolated from the flowers.[12]

Amines present in the plant are betaine, choline, and trimethylamine. Coumarins include scopoletin and umbelliferone.[9]

Carbohydrates such as mucilage and polysaccharides (ie, inulin) are found in arnica.[2] Two homogeneous polysaccharides, for example, include an acidic arabino-3,6-galactan-protein, and a neutral fucogalactoxyloglucan.[13] Further polysaccharide isolation has been performed on a group of water-soluble acidic heteroglycaines.[14]

Volatile oils (0.3% to 1%) may be obtained from rhizomes and roots or from flower parts (used in perfumery).[7] Constituents in the oil include thymol, its derivatives,[2] and fatty acids (palmitic, linoleic, myristic, and linolenic).[4] The fatty acid content in arnica leaf essential oil has been evaluated, as well.[15]

Other components found in arnica include bitter compound arnicin, caffeic acid,[7,9] carotenoids (alpha- and beta-carotene, cryptoxanthin, lutein),[4,9,16] phytosterols, resin, tannins,[2,4] and anthoxanthine.[7]

PHARMACOLOGY: Not only is arnica employed in hair tonics, antidandruff preparations, perfumery, and cosmetics, it is used in herbal and homeopathic medicines as, well.[4,7] The plant possesses a slight **anti-inflammatory and mild analgesic effect**, most likely due to the sesquiterpene lactones. Helenalin and dihydrohelenalin exert mild anti-inflammatory and **antibacterial** activity.[6,9] They expressed anti-inflammatory activity in mice and rats,[4] and in humans, as well. Arnica improved feelings of stiffness associated with hard physical exertion (vs placebo) when tested in 36 marathon participants in a double-blinded, randomized trial.[17] However, in another report, contradictory results were seen.

Patients who had impacted wisdom teeth removed received either metronidazole, arnica, or placebo. Metronidazole was more effective than arnica in controlling postoperative pain, inflammation, and healing. Patients receiving arnica had greater pain and inflammation than those receiving placebo.[18]

Arnica contains a group of polysaccharides with 65% to 100% galacturonic acid that can inhibit the complement system, thereby modifying the immune system response.[19] This polysaccharide displays marked phagocytosis enhancement in vivo.[13] Yet another compound stimulates macrophages to excrete tumor necrosis factor.[20] Arnica, as well as other plant polysaccharides, possesses significant immunostimulatory activity.[14,21] Phenolic compounds of arnica improved toxic liver injury in rats.[22]

Extracts of arnica blossoms have been used in traditional medicine to improve blood flow. The sesquiterpene lactones helenalin and 11-alpha, 13-dihydrohelenalin have been shown to inhibit platelet aggregation by interacting with platelet sulfhydryl groups, suggesting therapeutic potential for these compounds.[23] Arnica increases the rate of reabsorption of internal bleeding.[2] However, in one report, it was not shown that arnica had any significant impact on certain blood coagulation parameters in a randomized, controlled trial.[24]

A report on arnica's use in facial injury is available.[25]

Arnica has been used traditionally as a topical agent to improve wound healing. It has been used externally (eg, ointment, compress) for acne, boils, bruises, rashes, sprains, pains, and other wounds.[3,7] Constituent helenalin and related esters have strong antimicrobial activity.[3] It has bactericidal (against salmonella, for example)[9] and fungicidal activity, as well.[4,7] The plant also possesses counterirritant properties[9] due to constituents arnidiol and foradiol, two isomeric alcohols.[26]

Arnica has been used for heart problems[2,3,7] (as it contains a cardiotonic substance[9]), to improve circulation,[3] to reduce cholesterol,[3,7] and to stimulate the CNS.[7]

TOXICOLOGY: The internal use of arnica and its extracts cannot be recommended. The plant is considered poisonous, and oral use should be avoided (or very strictly controlled).[2,3,9] Arnica irritates mucous membranes, causes stomach pain, diarrhea, and vomiting.[4,9] Gastroenteritis has occurred with high oral dosages; dyspnea and cardiac arrest may occur and result in death.[3] The flowers and roots of the plant have caused vomiting, drowsiness, and coma when eaten by children. Gastric lavage or emesis followed by supportive treatment is recommended.[27] A 1 oz tincture reportedly produced serious, but not fatal effects.[4]

The helenolide constituents of arnica are cardiotoxic, proven in animal experimentation.[39]

The plant's sesquiterpene lactones are responsible for its oxytocic activity. In folk medicine, arnica was used as an abortifacient because of these actions.[3]

Numerous cases of contact dermatitis related to arnica have been reported. Chemical and animal experimentation have proven the high sensitizing capacity of the plant. Sesquiterpene lactones helenalin, helenalin acetate, and methacrylate are the primary "culprits" in this type of allergy.[28] Another report is available identifying the allergans in arnica.[29] Three cases of patients with occupational contact dermatitis to arnica have been reported.[30] A case report of a 65-year-old male (a garden hobbyist) suffered from chronic eczema on his face and hands related to arnica's sesquiterpene lactones.[31] Cases such as these and others confirm arnica's prevalence in this allergy class.

SUMMARY: Although arnica and its extracts have a long history of use, few studies suggest its extracts are clinically useful. Its use as a topical counterirritant and wound-healing stimulant continues. Internal consumption of arnica is not recommended, because it is considered poisonous. Numerous cases of contact dermatitis have been reported from the plant.

PATIENT INFORMATION – Arnica

Uses: Arnica and its extracts have been widely used in folk medicine. It is used externally as a treatment for acne, boils, bruises, rashes, sprains, pains, and other wounds. It has also been used for heart and circulation problems, to reduce cholesterol, and to stimulate the CNS.

Side Effects: The plant is poisonous and ingestion can cause stomach pain, diarrhea and vomiting, dyspnea, cardiac arrest, and death. Contact dermatitis also has occurred.

1 Schauenberg P, Paris F. Guide to Medicinal Plants. New Canaan, CT: Keats Pub., 1977.
2 Chevallier A. Encyclopedia of Medicinal Plants. New York, NY: DK Publishing, 1996;170.
3 Bisset N. Herbal Drugs and Phytopharmaceuticals. Stuttgart, Germany: CRC Press, 1994:83–87.
4 Leung A. Encyclopedia of Common Natural Ingredients, 2nd ed. New York: John Wiley & Sons, 1996;40–41.
5 Ghosh A. Lancet 1983;8319:304.
6 DerMarderosian A. Natural Product Medicine. Philadelphia, PA: George F. Stickley Co, 1988;253–54.
7 Duke J. CRC Handbook of Medicinal Herbs. Boca Raton, FL: CRC Press 1989;64.
8 Merfort I. Planta Medica 1989;55:608.
9 Newall C, et al. Herbal medicines. London, England: Pharmaceutical Press, 1996;34–35.
10 Saner V, et al. Pharmaceutica Acta Helvetiae 1966;41:431–45.
11 List P, et al. Arzneimittelforschung 1974;24(2):148–51.
12 Herrmann H, et al. Planta Med 1978;34(3):299–304.
13 Puhlmann J. Phytochemistry 1991;30(4):1141–145.
14 Wagner V, et al. Arzheim-Forsch 1984;34(6):659–61.
15 Willuhn G. Z Naturforsch B 1972;27(6):728.
16 Vanhaelen M. Planta Med 1973;23(4):308–11.
17 Tveiten D, et al. Tidsskr Nor Laegeforen 1991;111(30):3630–631.
18 Kazirc G. Br J Oral Maxillofac Surg 1984;22(1):42–49.
19 Knaus U, Wagner H. Planta Med 1988;54:565.
20 Puhlmann J, Wagner H. Planta Medica 1989;55:99.
21 Wagner H, et al. Arzneimittelforschung 1985;35(7):1069–75.
22 Marchishin S. Farmakol Toksikol 1983;46(2):102–6.
23 Schroder H, et al. Thromb Res 1990;57:839.
24 Baillargeon L. Can Fam Physician 1993;39:2362–67.
25 Anon. Otolaryngol Chir Cervicofac 1977;94(1–2):65.
26 Tyler V. Herbs of Choice. New York: Pharmaceutical Products Press, Haworth Press, Inc. 1994:157.
27 Hardin JW, Arena JM. Human Poisoning from Native and Cultivated Plants. Duke University Press, 1974.
28 Hausen B. Hautarzt 1980;31(1):10–17.
29 Hausen B. Contact Dermatitis 1978;4(5):308.
30 Hausen B. Contact Dermatitis 1978;4(1):3–10.
31 Spettoli E, et al. Am J Contact Dermat 1998;9(1):49–50.

Artichoke

SCIENTIFIC NAME(S): *Cynara scolymus* L., *C. cardunculus*, Family: Compositae

COMMON NAME(S): Artichoke, globe artichoke

BOTANY: The artichoke is native to Mediterranean regions; 80% are grown in Italy, Spain, and France. In the US, most artichokes are grown in the vicinity of Castroville, California. The plant is a perennial herb, growing to approximately 150 cm in height. Its large leaves are thistle-like and are grayish-green on top and white underneath. The edible purple-green flower heads contain leaf-like scales that enclose the bud.[1,2] The vegetable heads are commonly available in supermarkets in the US and are considered a delicacy, being cooked and served in various ways.

HISTORY: The artichoke has been cultivated for thousands of years. In the first century AD, the plant's root was reputed to have been mashed and applied to the body to "sweeten" offensive odors. Artichokes were valued by the ancient Greeks and Romans. The plants were brought to America by French and Spanish explorers. The artichoke has been used for its diuretic, choleretic, and hepatostimulating properties.[1,2,3]

CHEMISTRY: Many polyphenolic substances, flavonoids (0.1% to 1%), and acids have been found in artichoke. Some of these include the following: Flavone glycosides (such as luteolin-7-beta-rutinoside, luteolin-4'-glucoside, luteolin-7-gentiobioside), luteolin, apigenin, scolimoside, cosmoside, quercetin, rutin, scopoletin, hesperitin, hesperidoside, and maritimein. Cynaroside, cynarine, cynaropicrin (very bitter), and cynarin (responsible for liver-protective qualities) have also been identified.[1,3,4,5] Flavonoids from Egyptian artichoke have been reviewed.[6] Organic acids, primarily acid-alcohols, have been evaluated from artichoke.[7] Examples include the following: Isochlorogenic, chlorogenic, quinic, glycolic, glyceric, and caffeic acids.[3,4,8] Its derivatives have been addressed in detail.[9]

Volatile oil constituents in artichoke include beta selinene, caryophyllene, eugenol, phenylacetaldehyde, and decanal. The aspartic proteases cardosin A and B have been isolated and identified from the flowers.[10,11] Molecular modeling and biochemical characterization of these proteases have been performed.[12,13]

Other constituents in artichoke include phytosterols, tannins, sugars, and inulin.[3]

Artichoke extract preparations have been evaluated in one report, comparing 11 marketed formulas.[14]

PHARMACOLOGY: Artichoke is reported to have diuretic and hypoglycemic effects.[1,2,3,15] However, additional research is needed to confirm any claims made by older reports and herbal uses of the plant.

Hypocholesterolemic, hypolipidemic, and choleretic effects from various artichoke preparations have been demonstrated. Some studies report decreases in serum cholesterol.[15] Artichoke extract may inhibit cholesterol synthesis indirectly but efficiently, as seen in one report in rat hepatocytes.[16] Artichoke had no effect; however, on cholesterol and triglyceride levels when administered orally to 17 (type IIa and IIb) familial hyperlipoproteinemic patients in a 3-month period.[17]

Constituent cynarine is listed in the *Martindale* text as a choleretic.[5] This increase of bile by the liver is essential in treatment of dyspeptic disorders. In a randomized, placebo-controlled, double-blind trial in 20 patients administered artichoke extract, marked increase in bile secretion was recorded. The authors concluded that artichoke can be recommended for dyspepsia treatment, especially in bile duct problems.[15] Artichoke's choleretic effects make the plant useful in abdominal and gallbladder problems, nausea, and indigestion.[1]

Both leaf extract of artichoke and the isolate, cynarine, demonstrated cytoprotective action in rat hepatocytes.[8,18] The leaf extract displayed marked antioxidative and protective effects in rat hepatocytes.[19] Artichoke's effects on regeneration of rat liver have also been reported.[20,21]

Other effects of artichoke include the following: Inhibitory actions against mouse skin tumor formation from phytosterol constituents taraxasterol and faradiol,[22] anti-inflammatory and analgesic effects,[23] and effects on sympatho-adrenal system activity in rats.[24]

TOXICOLOGY: No side effects were observed in 20 patients given standardized artichoke extract (1.92 g in

50 ml water) intraduodenally.[15] The LD $_{50}$ values in rats have been determined to be > 1000 mg/kg (total extract) and 265 mg/kg (purified extract).[3] No detrimental effects from artichoke have been found when studied in male rat gonads.[25]

Patients with an allergy to the Compositae family pollen may develop an allergic reaction to artichoke.[3] Contact dermatitis[26,27] and occupational contact urticaria syndrome have been reported.[28]

Nephrotoxic effects of artichoke mixtures and other Chinese herbal drugs have been reviewed.[29]

SUMMARY: The artichoke has been used for many centuries. It has diuretic and hypoglycemic effects. Its choleretic actions make the plant useful to treat dyspepsia and other digestive problems. Artichoke also demonstrates cytoprotective actions in the liver and hypocholesterolemic effects as well. The main toxicity of the plant is allergic dermatitis.

PATIENT INFORMATION – Artichoke

Uses: Artichoke has been used as a diuretic, in the treatment of dyspepsia and other digestive problems, and for its hypoglycemic effects. It also possesses cytoprotective actions in the liver and hypocholesterolemic effects.

Side Effects: Artichoke can cause allergic dermatitis.

---

1 Chevallier A. *Encyclopedia of Medicinal Plants.* New York, NY: DK Publishing, 1996;196-97.

2 Ensminger A, et al. *Foods and Nutrition Encyclopedia.* 2nd ed. Boca Raton, FL: CRC Press, 1994.

3 Newall C, et al. *Herbal Medicines.* London, England: Pharmaceutical Press, 1996;36-37.

4 Hinou J, et al. Polyphenolic substances of *Cynara scolymus* L. leaves. *Ann Pharm Fr* 1989;47(2):95-98.

5 Reynolds J, ed. *Martindale The Extra Pharmacopoeia.* 31st ed. London, England: Royal Pharmaceutical Society, 1996;1696.

6 Hammouda F, et al. Flavonoids of *Cynara scolymus* L. cultivated in Egypt. *Plant Foods Hum Nutr* 1993;44(2):163-69.

7 Bogaert J, et al. Organic acids, prinicipally acid-alcohols, in *Cynara scolymus* L. *Ann Pharm Fr* 1972;30(6):401-8.

8 Adzet T, et al. Hepatoprotective activity of polyphenolic compounds from *Cynara scolymus* against CC14 toxicity in isolated rat hepatocytes. *J Nat Prod* 1987;50(4):612-17.

9 Nichiforesco E. Variation of caffeic acid type o-dihydroxyphenolic derivatives of the artichoke (*Cynara scolymus* L.) during its period of vegetation. *Ann Pharm Fr* 1966;24(6):451-56.

10 Verissimo P, et al. Purification, characterization and partial amino acid sequencing of two new aspartic proteinases from fresh flowers of *Cynara cardunculus* L. *Eur J Biochem* 1996;235(3):762-68.

11 Ramalho-Santos M, et al. Identification and proteolytic processing of procardosin A. *Eur J Biochem* 1998;255(1):133-38.

12 Cordeiro M, et al. Substrate specificity and molecular modelling of aspartic proteinases (cyprosins) from flowers of *Cynara cardunculus* subsp. flavescens cv. cardoon. *Adv Exp Med Biol* 1998;436:473-79.

13 Brodelius P, et al. Aspartic proteinases (cyprosins) from *Cynara cardunculus* spp. Flavescens cv. cardoon; purification, characterisation, and tissue-specific expression. *Adv Exp Med Biol* 1995;362:255-66.

14 Brand N. Extract in artichoke preparations: pharmaceutical quality of a plant active principle. *Pharmazeutische Zeitung* 1997 Oct 9;142:60, 63-64, 66, 63, 70-72, 75-76.

15 Kirchhoff R, et al. Increase in choleresis by means of artichoke extract. *Phytomedicine* 1994;(1):107-15.

16 Gebhardt R. Inhibition of cholesterol biosynthesis in primary cultured rat hepatocytes by artichoke (*Cynara scolymus* L.) extracts. *J Pharmacol Exp Ther* 1998;286(3):1122-28.

17 Heckers H, et al. Inefficiency of cynarin as therapeutic regimen in familial type II hyperlipoproteinaemia. *Atherosclerosis* 1977;26(2):249-53.

18 Gebhardt R. Hepatoprotection with artichoke extract. *Pharmazeutische Zeitung* 1995 Oct 26;140:34-37.

19 Gebhardt R. Antioxidative and protective properties of extracts from leaves of the artichoke (*Cynara scolymus* L.) against hydroperoxide-induced oxidative stress in cultured rat hepatocytes. *Toxicol Appl Pharmacol* 1997;144(2):279-86.

20 Maros T, et al. Effects of *Cynara Scolymus* extracts on the regeneration of rat liver. 1. *Arzneimittelforschung* 1966;16(2):127-29.

21 Maros T, et al. Effects of *Cynara Scolymus* extracts on the regeneration of rat liver. 2. *Arzneimittelforschung* 1968;18(7):884-86.

22 Yasukawa K, et al. Inhibitory effect of taraxastane-type triterpenes on tumor promotion by 12-O-tetradecanoylphorbol-13-acetate in two-stage carcinogenesis in mouse skin. *Oncology* 1996;53(4):341-44.

23 Ruppelt B, et al. Pharmacological screening of plants recommended by folk medicine as anti-snake venom—I. Analgesic and anti-inflammatory activities. *Mem Inst Oswaldo Cruz* 1991;86 (Suppl 2): 203-5.

24 Khalkova Z, et al. An experimental study of the effect of an artichoke preparation on the activity of the sympathetic-adrenal system in carbon disulfide exposure. *Probl Khig* 1995;20:162-71.

25 Ilieva P, et al. The action of the artichoke (*Cynara scolymus*) on the male gonads in an experiment. *Probl Khig* 1994;19:105-11.

26 Turner T. Compositae dermatitis in South Australia: contact dermatitis from *Ixodia achillaeoides* and *Cynara cardunculus* or the tribulations of a dry flower arranger. *Contact Dermatitis* 1980;(6):444.

27 Meding B. Allergic contact dermatitis from artichoke, *Cynara scolymus.* *Contact Dermatitis* 1983;9(4):314.

28 Quirce S, et al. Occupational contact urticaria syndrome caused by globe artichoke (*Cynara scolymus*). *J Allergy Clin Immunol* 1996;97(2):710-11.

29 Violon C. Belgian (Chinese herb) nephropathy: why? *Farmaceutisch Tijdschrift voor Belgie* 1997 Apr;74:11-36.

Asparagus

SCIENTIFIC NAME(S): *Asparagus officinale* L. Family: Liliaceae

COMMON NAME(S): Garden asparagus

BOTANY: Asparagus is a dioecious perennial herb with scale-like leaves and an erect, much-branched stem that grows to a height of up to 3 meters. Asparagus is native to Europe and Asia and is widely cultivated. The part used as a vegetable consists of the aerial stems, or spears, arising from rhizomes. The fleshy roots and, to a lesser degree, the seeds have been used for medicinal purposes.

HISTORY: Asparagus spears are widely used as a vegetable and are frequently blanched before use. Extracts of the seeds and roots have been used in alcoholic beverages, with the maximum levels averaging 16 ppm. The seeds have been used in coffee substitutes, diuretic preparations, laxatives, remedies for neuritis and rheumatism, to relieve toothache, to stimulate hair growth and as cancer treatments. Chinese medicine has used them to treat parasitic diseases. Extracts are said to have served as contraceptives. Home remedies have employed the topical application of preparations containing the shoots and extracts to cleanse the face and dry acneiform lesions.

CHEMISTRY: Asparagus roots contain inulin and at least eight fructo-oligosaccharides. Two glycoside bitter principles, officinalisins I and II, were isolated from dried roots in yields of 0.12% and 0.075%, respectively. Other root components are beta-sitosterol, steroidal glycosides (asparagosides A to I, in order of increasing polarity) and asparagusic acid. The shoots have several sulfur-containing acids (asparagusic, dihydroasparagusic and S-acetyldihydroasparagusic); alpha-amino-dimethyl-gamma-butyrothetin, a glycoside bitter principle different from those in roots; flavonoids (rutin, quercetin and kaempferol); as well as asparagine, arginine, tyrosine, sarsasapogenin, beta-sitosterol, succinic acid and sugars. Asparagusic acid, and its derivatives, are plant growth inhibitors; they are also nematocidal (imparting resistance to several important plant parasite nematodes).[1]

Asparagus seeds contain large quantities of sodium hydroxide-soluble polysaccharides consisting of linear chains of beta-glucose and beta-mannose in a 1:1 ratio, 1 to 4 linked to alpha-galactose as a terminal group.[1] Seeds also contain three ribosome-inactivating proteins, in concentrations of 8 to 400 mg/100 g of starting material. These proteins, with molecular weights of about 30,000, have alkaline isoelectric points and inhibit protein synthesis by rabbit reticulocyte lysate.[2] Asparagus stalks contain folate and the folate conjugases asparagusate dehydrogenase I and II, as well as lipoyl dehydrogenase. Folate levels can be accurately measured only after inactivation of the conjugases.[3] Stalks may also contain residues of permethrin, an insecticide often applied to protect asparagus during growth. These residues peak about 3 days after insecticide treatment and then decline by about 85% by the seventh day.[4] Other herbicides applied during the growth of asparagus have been detected in commercial stock.[5]

PHARMACOLOGY: Asparagus roots have been used in diuretic preparations, but no data are available to substantiate this pharmacologic effect.

Ingestion of asparagus spears produces a characteristic pungent odor in the urine of some individuals within a few hours.[6] According to one report, the odor is produced by a combination of six sulfur-containing alkyl compounds: methanethiol, dimethyl sulfide, dimethyl disulfide, bis-(methylthio)methane, dimethyl sulfoxide and dimethyl sulfone. Possible precursors of these compounds are S-methylmethionine and asparagusic acid.[7] Other researchers attribute the urine odor to S-methylthioacrylate and S-methyl 3-(methylthio)thiopropionate.[8]

In one study, 43% of 800 volunteers had urine odor following asparagus ingestion. Production of the odor appears to be an autosomal dominant genetic trait that is evident throughout life.[9] A study of 307 volunteers found that 10% had the ability to smell high dilutions of urine from asparagus-fed individuals, suggesting that the ability to smell asparagus-tainted urine is also a specific trait.[10] A study of 19 volunteers confirmed that only some people have the ability to produce or detect the odor.[11] This may suggest a genetic composition to these traits.

Related species of Asparagus have demonstrated antiviral activity in vitro.[12] Asparagus juice has demonstrated in vitro antimutagenic activity[13] and cytotoxic saponins have been found in the plant.[14]

TOXICOLOGY: There are no reports of serious toxicity from the ingestion of asparagus or its extracts. There is one report of botulism poisoning following the ingestion of improperly home-preserved asparagus.[15]

SUMMARY: Asparagus is cultivated universally and used as a vegetable. The stalks are cooked and eaten. and extracts of the seeds and roots have been used as flavorings. Preparations of asparagus have been used in folk medicine of different nations, although there is little evidence to support any consistent pharmacologic effect. Asparagus is noted for its ability to produce a pungent odor in the urine of many persons consuming it.

PATIENT INFORMATION – Asparagus

Uses: The stalks are commonly eaten. Roots, seeds and extracts of these have been used as a treatment for various ills and as a diuretic.

Side Effects: None known except for pungent odor in urine of almost half those who eat it.

---

[1] Leung AY. Encyclopedia of Common Natural Ingredients Used in Food, Drugs and Cosmetics. New York, NY: J. Wiley and Sons, 1980.

[2] Stirpe F, et al. Ribosome-inactivating proteins from the seeds of Saponaria officinalis L. (soapwort), of Agrostemma githago L. (corn cockle) and of Asparagus officinalis L. (asparagus), and from the latex of Hura crepitans L. (sandbox tree). *Biochem J* 1983;216(3):617.

[3] Leichter J, et al. Folate conjugase activity in fresh vegetables and its effect on the determination of free folate content. *Am J Clin Nutr* 1979;32(1):92.

[4] George DA. Permethrin and its two metabolite residues in seven agriculture crops. *J Assoc Off Anal Chem* 1985;68(6):1160.

[5] Goewie CE, Hogendoorn EA. Liquid chromatographic determination of the herbicide diuron and its metabolite 3,4–dicholoraniline in asparagus. *Food Addit Contam* 1985;2(3):217.

[6] Richer C, et al. Odorous urine in man after asparagus [letter]. *Br J Clin Pharmacol* 1989;27(5):640.

[7] Waring RH, et al. The chemical nature of the urinary odour produced by man after asparagus ingestion. *Xenobiotica* 1987;17(11):1363.

[8] White RH. Occurrence of S-methyl thioesters in urines of humans after they have eaten asparagus. *Science* 1975;189:810.

[9] Mitchell SC, et al. Odorous urine following asparagus ingestion in man. *Experientia* 1987;43(4):382.

[10] Lison M. A polymorphism of the ability to smell urinary metabolites of asparagus. *Br Med J* 1980;281(6256):1676.

[11] Sugarman J, Neelon FA. You're in for a Treat: Asparagus. *NC Med J* 1985;46(5):332.

[12] Aquino F, et al. Antiviral activity of constituents of Tamus communis. *J Chemother* 1991;3(5):305.

[13] Edenharder R, et al. [Antimutagenic activity of vegetable and fruit extracts against in-vitro benzo(a)pyrene.] *Z Gesamte Hyg* 1990;36(3):144.

[14] Sati OP, et al. Cytotoxic saponins from Asparagus and Agave. *Pharmazie* 1985;40(3):586.

[15] Paterson DL, et al. Severe botulism after eating home-preserved asparagus. *Med J Aust* 1992;157(4):269.

Aspidium

SCIENTIFIC NAME(S): *Dryopteris filix-mas* (L.) Schott Family: Polypodiaceae

COMMON NAME(S): Aspidium, male fern, bear's paw, knotty brake, shield fern

BOTANY: *D. filix-mas* is a hardy ornamental fern.[1] It grows in dry terrain in rich woods and on rocky slopes. It is found throughout many areas of the United States.

HISTORY: The fern has been used in traditional medicine for the treatment of worm infections. The early physician Theophrastus recognized the value of the fern for treating tinea (ringworm) infections.[1] In Chinese medicine, extracts are used to treat recurrent bloody nose, heavy menstrual bleeding and wounds. The components of the plant have been used as veterinary vermifuges.

CHEMISTRY: The fern contains about 6% of an oleoresin. In addition, the plant is the source of albaspidin, filicic (filixic) acid, filicin, margaspidin, filmarone and more than two dozen additional chemically unique compounds.[1]

PHARMACOLOGY: Filicin and filmarone are active vermifuges and are particularly toxic to tapeworms.[1,2] Following ingestion of the drugs, tinea are expelled within hours; however, a purgative is typically ingested concomitantly with the vermifuge to aid expulsion.[3]

The oleoresin paralyzes intestinal voluntary muscle and the analogous muscles of the tapeworm, which is then readily eliminated by the action of the purgative.[1]

TOXICOLOGY: Large doses of the extracts are potentially toxic resulting in muscular weakness, coma and temporary or permanent blindness.[1] Even therapeutic doses are associated with adverse events.[2] Symptoms include headache, dyspnea, nausea, diarrhea, vertigo, tremors, convulsions and cardiac and respiratory failure.[1,2]

SUMMARY: Aspidium is no longer commonly used in the United States, although it had been listed in the US Pharmacopeia as late as 1965.[4] Some herbal enthusiasts may continue to find access to the extracts. While the evidence from traditional uses strongly indicates that extracts are potent vermifuges, their potential toxicity precludes any recommendation of their use.

PATIENT INFORMATION – Aspidium

Uses: A traditional vermifuge

Side Effects: Aspidium can produce adverse reactions, from headache to cardiac and respiratory failure.

---

[1] Duke JA. Handbook of Medicinal Herbs. Boca Raton, FL: CRC Press, 1985.

[2] Spoerke DG. Herbal Medications. Santa Barbara CA: Woodbridge Press, 1980.

[3] Schauenberg P, Paris F. Guide to Medicinal Plants. New Canaan, CT: Keats Publishing, 1977.

[4] Dobelis IN. Magic and Medicine of Plants. Pleasantville, NY: Reader's Digest Association, 1986.

Astragalus

SCIENTIFIC NAME(S): *Astragalus membranaceus* Bunge, and *Astragalus membranaceus* var. mongholicus (Bunge) P.K. Hsiao, Family: Fabaceae (Beans)

COMMON NAME(S): Huang chi, huang qi, astragalus

BOTANY: The genus *Astragalus* is an enormous group of more than 2000 species distributed worldwide, commonly known as milk vetches. The Chinese species *A. membranaceus* and the related *A. mongholicus* are now thought to be varieties of the same species.[1] Both are perennial herbs native to the northern provinces of China and are cultivated in China, Korea, and Japan. The dried root is used medicinally. Astragalus roots are sold as 15- to 20-cm long pieces, which have a tough, fibrous skin with a lighter interior. Some products are produced by frying the roots with honey, although the untreated root itself also has a sweetish, licorice-like taste.

HISTORY: Astragalus root is a very old and well-known drug in traditional Chinese medicine, and is currently official in the Chinese Pharmacopeia. It is used in China principally as a tonic and for treatment of diabetes and nephritis. It is an important component of Fu-Zheng therapy in China, where the goal is to restore immune system function. There is extensive Chinese language literature on the drug.

CHEMISTRY: A PCR method for measuring astragalus content in a polyherbal preparation has been published. Markers for each component were developed using decamer oligonucleotide primers.[2] Hairy root culture of Astragalus have been established and found to produce cycloartane saponins.[3,4,5]

Astragalus root contains a series of cycloartane triterpene glycosides denoted astragalosides I to VII, that are based on the genin cycloastragenol and contain from 1 to 3 sugars attached at the 3-, 6-, and 25-positions.[6,7,8,9] In the predominant astraglosides I to III the 3-glucose is acetylated. Several saponins based on the oleanene skeleton have also been reported.[10] The aboveground parts of astragalus contain similar but distinct saponins n the cycloartane series.[11,12] and many other species of astragalus contain cycloartane saponins.[13]

A variety of polysaccharides have been reported from astragalus root. Astragalan I is a neutral 36 kD heterosaccharide containing glucose, galactose, and arabinose, while astragalans II and III are 12 kD and 34 kD glucans, respectively.[1,14] Huang, et al., isolated 3 similar polysaccharides and an acidic polysaccharide, AG-2, as well.[1] Tomoda reported a complex 60 kD acidic polysaccharide, AMem-P with a high hexuroic acid content from *A. membranaceus*[15] and a similar but distinct 76 kD acidic polysaccharide, AMon-S from *A. mongholicus*.[16] Bombardelli and Pozzi patented polysaccharides known as astroglucans A-C from *A. membranaceus*.[17]

Isoflavan glycosides based on mucronulatol and isomucronulatol have been found in the roots of *A. membranaceus*.[9,18] Several products appear to use these compounds for standardization despite the lack of reported biological activity. In addition, the free isoflavones afrormosin, calycosin, formononetin, and odoratin have been isolated from the roots.[19,20]

A unique biphenyl was isolated from *A. membranaceus* var. mongholicus as an antihepatotoxic agent.[18]

PHARMACOLOGY: The most common use of astragalus root in herbal medicine in the US is as an immunostimulant to counteract the immune suppression associated with cancer chemotherapy. This use is based on several observations. The cycloartane saponins are capable of stimulating the growth of isolated human lymphocytes.[13] The polysaccharides astragalans I and II were found to potentiate immunological responses in mice following IP administration, though not after oral administration.[14] The glycans AMem-P and AMon-S increased phagocytic indices on IP injection into mice.[15,16]

Aqueous extract of astragalus root stimulated phagocytosis of murine macrophages, and augmented proliferation of human monocytes in response to phytohemagglutinin, concanavalin A, and pokeweed mitogen.[21,22] In cells from cancer patients, which were comparatively resistant to such stimulation, astragalus extract also stimulated mononuclear cells. Using a graft-vs-host model, astragalus extract restored the GVH reaction in vivo for healthy and immune-suppressed patients.[23]

These in vitro and in vivo effects justify further human trials of the immunostimulant activity of astragalus root extracts in patients whose immune system has been suppressed by cancer chemotherapeutic drug regimens.

A second use of astragalus root in the US is for HIV infection. Such use must depend on a host-mediated response because the aqueous extract of astragalus had no direct effect on viral infectivity,[24] and little effect on viral reverse transcriptase.[25] A pilot trial of a Chinese herbal formula containing astragalus root was found to improve subjective measures and symptomatology; however, the number of subjects was too small to detect statistically meaningful effects.[26]

A series of reports from China claim that treatment with herbal mixtures including astragalus can induce seronegative conversion in a small fraction of HIV patients.[27,28] These reports need to be verified.

In view of revised opinions on the population dynamics of the HIV virus in infected humans, an attempt to stimulate T-cell proliferation may not be a realistic therapeutic objective because the turnover rate is already quite rapid. Nevertheless, improvement in subjective symptoms in the above study[26] cannot be ignored, and a larger clinical trial might confirm these effects as significant.

Astragalus is often recommended for the prevention of the common cold; however, there are no published clinical trials that support this use.

The bipyhenyl compound 4,4′,5,5′,6,6′-hexahydroxy-2,2′-biphenyldicarboxylic acid 5,6:5′,6′-bis (methylene), 4,4′-dimethyl ether, dimethyl ester was isolated as the antihepatotoxic principle of astragalus root.[18] The isoflavones afrormosin, calycosin, and odoratin had antioxidant activity similar to butyl hydroxytoluene or alpha-tocopherol in several experimental models of air oxidation of lipids.[19,20]

Astragalus root saponins also have been found to have diuretic activity which was presumed to be caused by local irritation of the kidney epithelia.[29] Astragalus saponins showed anti-inflammatory and hypotensive effects in rats.[1]

TOXICOLOGY: An astragalus hot water extract that had been boiled for 90 minutes was mutagenic in the Ames test in *S. typhimurium* TA98 when activated by S9 rat liver fractions. The activity was dose-dependent. In addition, the mutagenic activity was not removed by XAD-2 resin treatment. The same preparations given by IP injection at 1 to 10 g/kg produced chromosomal abberations in the bone marrow of mice, and increased the incidence of micronucleated cells in bone marrow. No attempt was made to isolate the mutagenic compounds responsible for these effects.[30]

The pharmacology and toxicology of the genus *Astragalus* have been reviewed.[31]

SUMMARY: Astragalus root is a well-known Chinese traditional medicine that may have use in the restoration of immune function after cancer chemotherapy. The active principles are primarily cycloartane saponins and polysaccharides. The root appears to be safe; however, an observation of mutagenicity in the Ames test must be explored. Astragalus root is monographed by the World Health Organization, vol. 1.[32] An American Herbal Pharmacopeia monograph is nearing completion.

PATIENT INFORMATION – Astragalus

Uses: Astragalus root may have use in the restoration of immune function after cancer chemotherapy and for the treatment of HIV infection.

Side Effects: There is no known toxicity.

---

[1] Tang W, et al. *Chinese Drugs of Plant Origin*. Berlin: Springer-Verlag, 1992:191.

[2] Cheng K, et al. Determination of the components in a Chinese prescription, Yu-Ping-Feng San, by RAPD analysis. *Planta Med* 1998;64:563.

[3] Hirotani M, et al. Astragalosides from hairy root cultures of Astraglus membranaceus. *Phytochemistry* 1994;36:665.

[4] Hirotani M, et al. Cycloartane triterpene glycosides from hairy root cultures of Astragalus membranaceus. *Phytochemistry* 1994;37:1403.

[5] Zhou Y, et al. Two triglycosidic triterpene astragalosides from hairy root cultures of Astragalus membranaceus. *Phytochemistry* 1995;38:1407.

[6] Kitagawa I, et al. Chemical constituents of astragali radix, the root of Astragalus membranaceus Bunge. (1). Cycloastragenol, the 9,19-cyclolanostane-type aglycone astragalosides, and the artifact aglycone astragenol. *Chem Pharm Bull* 1983;31:689.

[7] Kitagawa I, et al. Chemical constituents of astragali radix, the root of Astragalus membranaceus Bunge. (2). Astragalosides, I, II, IV, acetylastragaloside I and isoastragalosides I and II. *Chem Pharm Bull* 1983;31:698.

[8] Kitagawa I, et al. Chemical constituents of astragali radix, the root of Astragalus membranaceus Bunge. (3). Astragalosides III, V, and VI. *Chem Pharm Bull* 1983;31:709.

[9] He Z, et al. Constituents of Astragalus membranaceus. *J Nat Prod* 1991;54:810.

[10] Kitagawa I, et al. Chemical constituents of astragali radix, the root of Astragalus membranaceus Bunge. (4). Astragalosides VII and VIII. *Chem Pharm Bull* 1983;31:716.

[11] Zhu Y, et al. Two new cycloartane-type glucosides, Mongholicoside I and II, from the aerial part of Astragalus mongholicus. *Chem Pharm Bull* 1992;40:2230.

[12] Ma Y, et al. Studies of the constituents of Astragalus membranaceus Bunge. III. Structures of triterpenoidal glycosides, huangqiyenins A and B, from the leaves. *Chem Pharm Bull* 1997;45:359.

[13] Calis I, et al. Cycloartane triterpene glycosides from the roots of Astragalus melanophrurius. *Planta Med* 1997;63:183.

[14] Liu X, et al. Isolation of astragalan and its immunological activities. *Tianran Chanwu Yanjiu Yu Kaifa* 1994;6:23.

[15] Tomoda M, et al. A reticuloendothelial system-activating glycan from the roots of Astragalus membranaceus. *Phytochemistry* 1991;31:63.

[16] Shimizu N, et al. An acidic polysaccharide having activity on the reticuloendothelial system from the root of Astragalus mongholicus. *Chem Pharm Bull* 1991;39:2969.

[17] Bombardelli E, et al. Polysaccharides with immunomodulating properties from Astragalus membranaceus. Eur Pat 441278 A1, 1994.

[18] He Z, et al. Isolation and identification of chemical constituents of Astragalus root. *Chem Abs* 1991;114:58918u.

[19] Shirataki Y, et al. Antioxidative components isolated from the roots of Astragalus membranaceus Bunge (Astragali Radix). *Phytother Res* 1997;11:603.

[20] Toda S, et al. Inhibitory effects of isoflavones in roots of Astragalus membranaceus Bunge (Astragali Radix) on lipid peroxidation by reactive oxygen species. *Phytother Res* 1998;12:59.

[21] Sun Y, et al. Preliminary observations on the effects of the Chinese medicinal herbs Astragalus membranaceus and Ligustrum lucidum on lymphocyte blastogenic responses. *J Biol Response Mod* 1983;2:227.

[22] Lau B, et al. Macrophage chemiluminescence modulated by Chinese medicinal herbs Astragalus membranaceus and Ligustrum lucidum. *Phytother Res* 1989;3:148.

[23] Sun Y, et al. Immune restoration and/or augmentation of local graft-vs-host reaction by traditional Chinese medicinal herbs. *Cancer* 1983;52:70.

[24] Yao X, et al. Mechanism of inhibition of HIV-1 infection in vitro by purified extract of Prunella vulgaris. *Virology* 1992;187:56.

[25] Ono K, et al. Differential inhibitory effects of various herb extracts on the activities of reverse transcriptase and various deoxyribonucleic acid (DNA) polymerases. *Chem Pharm Bull* 1989;37:1810.

[26] Burack J, et al. Pilot randomized controlled trial of Chinese herbal treatment for HIV-associated symptoms. *J Acquir Immune Defic Syndr and Hum Retrovirol* 1996;12:386.

[27] Lu, W. Prospect for study on treatment of AIDS with traditional Chinese medicine. *J Tradit Chin Med* 1995;15:3.

[28] Lu W, et al. A report on 8 seronegative converted HIV/AIDS patients with traditional Chinese medicine. *Chin Med J* 1995;108;634.

[29] Hostettmann K, et al. *Saponins.* Cambridge; England: Cambridge University Press, 1995;267.

[30] Yin X, et al. A study on the mutagenicity of 102 raw pharmaceuticals used in Chinese traditional medicine. *Mutat Res* 1991;260:73.

[31] Ríos J, et al. A review of the pharmacology and toxicology of Astragalus. *Phytother Res* 1997;11:411.

[32] World Health Organization. *WHO Monographs on Selected Medicinal Plant Materials*, vol 1. Geneva, Switzerland: WHO, 1999.

Autumn Crocus

SCIENTIFIC NAME(S): *Colchicum autumnale* L. Other species used medicinally have included *C. speciosum* Steven and *C. vernum* (L.) Ker-Gawl. Family: Liliaceae

COMMON NAME(S): Crocus, autumn crocus, fall crocus, meadow saffron, mysteria, vellorita, wonder bulb

BOTANY: These plants are members of the lily family and are often cultivated for their long, ornamental flowers. This perennial herb grows to about 1 foot in height and has a fleshy conical root (corm). The corm has a bitter, acrid taste and radish-like odor.[2] Low-lying leaves are found around the base of the plant, emanating from the bulb. The plant is native to grassy meadows and woods and riverbanks in Ireland, England and portions of Europe, and has been cultivated throughout much of the world.

HISTORY: The plant and its extracts have been used for centuries in the treatment of gout, rheumatism, dropsy, prostate enlargement and gonorrhea.[2] Extracts have been used to treat cancers. Today the plant serves as the primary source of colchicine, which is used therapeutically to treat gout and experimentally in cellular chromosomal studies. In addition to its FDA approved use (gout), colchicine has been used in the following conditions: Treatment of neurologic disability due to chronic progressive multiple sclerosis, familial Mediterranean fever, hepatic cirrhosis, primary biliary cirrhosis, adjunctive treatment of primary amyloidosis, Behcet's disease, pseudogout, skin manifestations of scleroderma, psoriasis, palmo-plantar pustulosis and dermatitis herpetiformis.[3]

CHEMISTRY: Colchicine is the main active principle and is present in a concentration of about 0.6% in the corm; concentrations can exceed 1% in the seeds.[2] A variety of other related alkaloids have been isolated from the plant including colchicerine and colchamine. Colchicine is not destroyed by heat or boiling and is highly soluble in water.[2]

PHARMACOLOGY: Colchicine inhibits normal cell division, specifically by interfering with microtubule growth and mitosis during cell division. It also may interfere with the normal function of cAMP or the cellular membrane.[3]

Because colchicine arrests mitosis during metaphase, it was hoped that it might be useful as an anticancer agent. Although it demonstrates antineoplastic activity in vitro and in some in vivo models, the toxicity of the drug has limited use in humans.[2]

Colchicine is now being investigated for its effectiveness in limiting the progression of chronic hepatitis and cirrhosis; it appears to decrease inflammation, inhibit collagen synthesis and increase collagen degradation, thereby slowing disease progression and fibrosis and perhaps extending survival time.[5,6,7,8,9]

TOXICOLOGY: The entire plant is toxic, due primarily to the colchicine content. Gastrointestinal disturbances are common following acute therapeutic use of colchicine.

After ingestion of the plant, immediate burning of the mouth and throat is followed by intense thirst, nausea and vomiting. Abdominal pain and persistent diarrhea develop. Fluid loss may lead to hypovolemic shock. Renal impairment with oliguria has been reported.[1] The intoxication follows a long course due to the slow elimination of colchicine from the body. Fluid replacement and supportive therapy is recommended.[1] No specific antidote is available for colchicine poisoning. Emesis followed by gastric lavage has been of value along with supportive therapy for shock.[10]

Veterinary poisonings have been associated with the autumn crocus, and these are often observed in grazing animals. Children, as well as calves, have been reported to have been intoxicated by drinking milk from cows that have ingested the plant. Human intoxications have occurred after corms were mistaken for onions and others have suffered overdosages from seed- or corm-derived natural medicinals.[2]

The volatiles emitted during the commercial slicing of the fresh corm can irritate the nostrils and throat and fingertips holding the corm may become numb.[2] Toxicity has been observed when colchicine accidentally was taken by nasal insufflation in place of methamphetamine.[10]

Prolonged therapeutic use of colchicine may cause agranulocytosis, aplastic anemia and peripheral neuritis. The lowest reported human lethal dose is 186 g in 4 days.[10] Although ingestion of 7 mg of colchicine has been reported to be lethal to man, the more typical lethal dose is 65 mg.[2]

SUMMARY: The autumn crocus is a pretty ornamental that has a long history of medicinal use. The main component, colchicine, is highly effective in the management of gout and related inflammatory disorders, but also is extremely toxic. Colchicine is now being investigated for the management of chronic inflammatory hepatic diseases.

PATIENT INFORMATION – Autumn Crocus

Uses: The plant and its extracts are used to treat gout and related inflammatory disorders. Autumn crocus may ameliorate hepatitis, cirrhosis and various other ills.

Side Effects: All parts are highly toxic. It can produce intoxication, severe gastric distress, shock, etc., and inhibit normal cell growth.

---

[1] Lampe KF. AMA Handbook of Poisonous and Injurious Plants. Chicago, Il: Chicago Review Press, 1985.

[2] Morton JF. Major Medicinal Plants. Springfield, IL: Thomas Books, 1977.

[3] Olin BR, Hebel SK, eds. *Drug Facts and Comparisons*, St. Louis: Facts and Comparisons, 1991.

[4] Levy M, et al. Colchicine: a state-of-the-art review. *Pharmacotherapy* 1991;11:196.

[5] Brenner DA, Alcorn JM. Therapy for hepatic fibrosis. *Semin Liver Dis* 1990;10:75.

[6] Groover JR. Alcoholic liver disease. *Emerg Med Clin North Am* 1990;8:887.

[7] Warnes TW. Colchicine in primary biliary cirrhosis. *Aliment Pharmacol Ther* 1991;5:321.

[8] Kershenobich D et al. *N Engl J Med* 1988;318:1709.

[9] Messner M, Brissot P. Traditional management of liver disorders. *Drugs* 1990;40(Suppl 3):45.

[10] Duke JA. Handbook of Medicinal Herbs. Boca Raton, FL: CRC Press, 1985.

[11] Baldwin L, et a. Accidental overdose of insufflated colchicine. *Drug Safety* 1990;5:305.

Avocado

SCIENTIFIC NAME(S): *Persea americana* Mill. Synonymous with *P. gratissima* Gaertn. Also referred to as *Laurus persea* L. Family: Lauraceae

COMMON NAME(S): Avocado, alligator pear, ahuacate, avocato

BOTANY: The avocado grows as a large tree to heights of 50 to 60 feet. It bears a large fleshy fruit that is oval or spherical in shape; the skin of the fruit can be thick and woody. Although the plant is native to tropical America (Mexico and Central America), numerous varieties are now widely distributed throughout the world.[1]

HISTORY: The avocado has been the subject of intense and varied use during the past, not only for food but also for medicinal purposes. The pulp has been used as a pomade to stimulate hair growth and to hasten the healing of wounds. The fruit also has been purported as an aphrodisiac and emmenagogue. Native Americans have used the seeds to treat dysentery and diarrhea. Today, the fruit is eaten widely throughout the world, and the oil is a component of numerous cosmetic formulations.

CHEMISTRY: The pulp of the avocado fruit is rich in a fatty oil, and this can account for up to 40% of its composition. In addition to sugars and carbohydrates, two bitter substances have been identified.[1]

Avocado oil is derived from the fruit pulp and is composed primarily of glycerides of oleic acid and approximately 10% unsaponifiable compounds, such as sterols and volatile acids. The vitamin D content of the oil exceeds that of butter or eggs.[1]

The large seed contains a wide variety of compounds, including fatty acids, alcohols and a number of unsaturated compounds with exceedingly bitter tastes.

The leaves of the Mexican avocado have been reported to contain approximately 3% of an essential oil composed primarily of estragole and anethole.

PHARMACOLOGY: Avocado oil has been used extensively for its purported ability to heal and soothe the skin. This use is based on the high hydrocarbon content of the pulp and oil, which is likely to be beneficial to dry skin.

A condensed flavonol isolated from the seed has been reported to have antitumor activity in mice and rats.[1]

Several of the unsaturated oxygenated aliphatic compounds in the pulp and seed have been shown to possess strong in vitro activity against gram-positive bacteria, including *Staphylococcus aureus*.

Avocados are frequently included in health diets, and recent evidence suggests that they are highly effective in modifying lipid profiles. In a randomized study, women chose either a diet high in monounsaturated fatty acids enriched with avocado or a high-complex-carbohydrate diet. After three weeks, the avocado diet resulted in a significant reduction in total cholesterol level from baseline (8.2%); a nonsignificant decrease (4.9%) occurred with the comparison diet. Low density lipoprotein cholesterol and apolipoprotein B levels decreased significantly only in the avocado group. The authors concluded that an avocado-supplemented diet rich in monounsaturates can benefit serum lipid levels.[2]

TOXICOLOGY: The poisoning of grazing animals that have ingested avocado has been reported, and this toxicity also has been observed in species as diverse as fish and birds.[1] Nevertheless, only a small number of reports of toxicity due to avocado have been published over the past 50 years. In a review of avocado toxicity, Craigmill et a.[3] reported that feeding dried avocado seed in a 1:1 ratio with normal food rations killed all mice tested. The amount of avocado ingested ranged from 10 to 14 g. Signs of toxicity became apparent after two to three days and the animals generally died within the next 24 hours. Gross findings included hemorrhage into the brain, lungs and liver.

In cattle and goats, acute toxicity has been characterized by a cessation of milk flow and nonbacterial mastitis. Fish have been killed as a result of avocado leaves falling into a backyard pond.[3] Although the specific mechanism of toxicity is not clear, leaves fed to goats reproducibly decreased milk production and increased SGOT and LDH enzyme levels.

A published case report suggests that the anticoagulant effects of warfarin may be antagonized by the avocado.[4]

SUMMARY: The fruit of the avocado is widely used as a food and as an ingredient in cosmetics and topical preparations. Ingestion of the fruit has been reported to reduce total cholesterol levels and to improve the overall lipid profile. No significant toxicity has been reported in humans, but toxicities have been observed in animals that have eaten large amounts of the seeds or leaves.

PATIENT INFORMATION – Avocado

Uses: The fruit is commonly eaten and the fruit oil is used for cosmetics. Studies indicate avocado reduces cholesterol and improves lipid profile. Seed derivatives reportedly have antitumor activity in rodents.

Side Effects: Large quantities of seeds or leaves appear to be toxic.

---

[1] Leung AY. Encyclopedia of Common Natural Ingredients Used in Food, Drugs, and Cosmetics. New York, NY: John Wiley and Sons, 1980.

[2] Colquhoun DM, et al. Comparison of the effects on lipoproteins and apolipo- proteins of a diet high in monounsaturated fatty acids, enriched with avocado, and a high-carbohydrate diet. *Am J Clin Nutr* 1992;56:671.

[3] Craigmill AL, et al. Toxicity of Avocado (*Persea americana* [Guatamalan Var]) Leaves: Review and Preliminary Report. *Vet Hum Toxicol* 1984;26:381.

[4] Blicksten D, et al. Warfarin antagonism by avocado. *Lancet* 1991;337:914.

Barberry

SCIENTIFIC NAME(S): *Berberis vulgaris* L. and *B. aquifolium* Pursh. However, more appropriately designated *Mahonia aquifolium* Nutt. Family: Berberidaceae

COMMON NAME(S): Barberry, Oregon grape, trailing mahonia, berberis, jaundice berry, woodsour, sowberry, pepperidge bush, sour-spine[1,2]

BOTANY: The barberry grows wild throughout Europe but has been naturalized to many regions of the eastern United States. *B. aquifolium* is an evergreen shrub native to the Rocky mountains. Barberry grows to more than 10 feet with branched, spiny holly-like leaves. Its yellow flowers bloom from May to June and develop into red to blue-black oblong berries.[3]

HISTORY: The plant has a long history of use, dating back to the Middle Ages. The extracts of the plant are used today in homeopathy for treatment of intestinal disorders and sciatica. A decoction of the plant has been used to treat gastrointestinal ailments and coughs.[3] The plant has been used as a bitter tonic and antipyretic. Duke[4] lists more than 3 dozen traditional uses for barberry, including cancer,[5] cholera and hypertension. The alkaloid berberine had been included as an astringent in eye drops, but its use has become rare. The fruits have been used to prepare jams and jellies. The medicinal use of the plant has been limited by the bitter taste of the bark and root.

CHEMISTRY: The root and wood are rich in isoquinoline alkaloids including palmatine, berbamine, oxyacanthine, jatrorrhizine, bervulcine, magnoflorine and columbamine.[2,3] However, the most important alkaloid is berberine. The root may contain as much as 3% alkaloids, which impart a yellow color to the wood. The edible berries are rich in vitamin C, sugars and pectin.

PHARMACOLOGY: Berberine is perhaps the best studied of the barberry alkaloids. Berberine and several related alkaloids have been shown to have bactericidal activity, which in one study exceeded that of chloramphenicol (eg, *Chloromycetin*) against *Staphylococcus epidermidis*, *Neisseria meningitidis*, *Escherichia coli* and other bacteria.[2]

Berberine (100 mg four times a day), given either alone or together with tetracycline (eg, *Achromycin V*), has been found to significantly improve acute watery diarrhea and excretion of vibrios after 24 hours, compared with placebo in patients with cholera-induced diarrhea. Berberine had no benefit over placebo in patients with non-cholera diarrhea.[6] Berberine does not appear to exert its antidiarrheal effect by astringency, and the mechanism of action has not been defined.[7]

Berberine has anticonvulsant, sedative and uterine stimulant properties. Local anesthesia can occur following subcutaneous injection of berberine.[4] Berbamine produces a hypotensive effect.[8]

TOXICOLOGY: Symptoms of poisoning are characterized by stupor and daze, diarrhea and nephritis.

SUMMARY: Although barberry has a long history of traditional use, today it plays a minor role in herbal and standard medicinal practice. Berberine, its best-studied alkaloid, has been shown to have significant pharmacologic activity, particularly in the management of bacterial-induced diarrheal conditions.

PATIENT INFORMATION – Barberry

Uses: The fruits have been used in jams and jellies. Plant alkaloids have been found to be bactericidal, antidiarrheal, anticonvulsant, hypotensive and sedative. Berberine is a uterine stimulant.

Side Effects: Barberry can produce stupor, daze, diarrhea and nephritis.

---

[1] Windholz M ed. *The Merck Index, 10th ed.* Rahway, NJ: Merck and Co., 1983.
[2] Leung AY. *Encyclopedia of Common Natural Ingredients Used in Food, Drugs and Cosmetics.* New York, NY: J Wiley and Sons, 1980.
[3] Schauenberg P, Paris F. *Guide to Medicinal Plants.* New Canaan, CT: Keats Publishing, Inc., 1977.
[4] Duke JA. *Handbook of Medicinal Herbs.* Boca Raton, FL: CRC Press, 1985.
[5] Hartwell JL. Plants Used Against Cancer: A Survey. *Lloydia* 1968;31(2):71.
[6] Maung KU, et al. Clinical trial of berberine in acute watery diarrhoea. *Br Med J* 1985;291:1601.
[7] Akhter MH, et al. Possible mechanism of antidiarrhoeal effect of berberine. *Indian J Med Res* 1979;70:233.
[8] Tyler VE. *The New Honest Herbal.* Philadelphia, PA: G.F. Stickley Co, 1987.

Barley

SCIENTIFIC NAME(S): *Hordeum vulgare* L. Family: Gramineae

COMMON NAME(S): Barley, Hordeum[1]

BOTANY: Barley is a well-known cereal grain that is cultivated throughout the world.

HISTORY: The use of barley for food and medicinal purposes dates to antiquity. The Roman physician Pliny noted that if a person affected with a boil took nine grains of barley, traced a circle around the boil three times with each grain, and then threw the barley into a fire with his left hand, the boil would be immediately cured.[2] The mucilage derived from the cereal (known as ptisane by the ancient Greeks) was used to treat gastrointestinal inflammation.[3] Barley has served as a food staple in most cultures. Gladiators ate barley for strength and stamina and were called *hordearii* from the Latin word for barley, *hordeum*.[4] Although supplanted by wheat and rye in the baking process, barley is now used extensively in soups, cereals, animal feeds, and beer making.[5] Roasted seeds are used in coffees and seeds are fermented into miso. "Covered" barley is used for animal feed and malting. For human consumption, the barley hull is removed by abrasions producing "pearl" barley.

CHEMISTRY: Barley contains β-glucan, a fiber also found in oat bran and reported to reduce cholesterol levels. It also contains the oil tocotrienol. Protein extracted from the leaves is said to be an adequate food supplement.[5]

Barley is the source of a natural sweetener known as malt sugar or barley jelly sugar, which is high in maltose.[5]

The root of the germinating grain contains the alkaloid hordenine, an aminophenol.[3]

"Pearling" removes essential amino acids and vitamins concentrated in the outer layers of the seed, although the grain retains its fiber content.

An oxalate oxidase that has commercial applications in monitoring oxalate levels in patients with hyperoxaluria, has been obtained from barley seedling plants.[8] Analogs of barley ribosomes and peptides are being used to enhance the potency and stability of in vitro immunoconjugate tests.[6,7]

PHARMACOLOGY: Hordenine is a sympathomimetic with a pharmacologic profile similar to that of epinephrine.[3] It stimulates peripheral blood circulation and has been used as a bronchodilator for bronchitis.

Barley's natural flavor may make it a more versatile grain for baking. In a taste test of muffins made with 100% barley flour, the barley muffins were rated more moist and flavorful than wheat bran muffins.[4]

The fiber content of barley suggests that it may be useful in reducing cholesterol levels and in controlling hyperglycemia in man. Ingestion by healthy subjects of barley-based breads resulted in lower glycemic and insulin indices than in subjects who ingested a control pumpernickel[9] or white bread.[10]

Of interest has been the finding of statistically significant reductions in total serum cholesterol and LDL-C in 79 hypercholesterolemic patients who supplemented their diet for 30 days with barley bran flour or barley oil. HDL-C also decreased significantly in the barley bran flour group, but not in the oil group.[11]

In a rat model of chemically-induced colon cancer, spent barley grain has been shown to protect against the risk of cancer, and this effect was greater than that observed with wheat bran and commercial barley bran.[12] This may be related in part to the ability of barley bran flour to decrease GI transit time. In 44 volunteers, barley bran significantly decreased transit time by 8.0 hours from baseline compared to 2.9 hours in the control group supplemented with cellulose.[13]

TOXICOLOGY: Because barley contains low levels of gluten, it should be ingested with caution by persons with celiac disease.[14] No other significant side effects have been associated with dietary ingestion of barley.

SUMMARY: Barley is a widely cultivated grain used as a food and in the brewing process. Interest has focused on the ability of components in the bran to reduce cholesterol levels and more extensive investigations into this effect are warranted.

PATIENT INFORMATION – Barley

Uses: Barley is a food staple also brewed to make beer, fermented to make miso, and processed to yield malt sugar. Studies indicate it may protect against colon cancer, reduce cholesterol and control hyperglycemia.

Side Effects: None of significant known, except that those with celiac disease should be cautioned about its low levels of gluten.

---

[1] Osol A, Farrar GE Jr, eds. *The Dispensatory of the United States of America, 25th ed*. Philadelphia: JB Lippincott, 1955:1713.

[2] Dobelis IN. *Magic and Medicine of Plants*. Pleasantville, NY: Reader's Digest Association, 1986.

[3] Schauenberg P, Paris F. *Guide to Medicinal Plants*. New Canaan, CT: Keats Publishing, 1977.

[4] Kreiter T. Beneficial barley. *Saturday Evening Post* 1993;Sept/Oct:22.

[5] Facciola S. *Cornucopia: source book of edible plants*. Vista, CA: Kampung Publications, 1990.

[6] Ellis HJ, et al. Demonstration of the presence of coeliac-activating gliadin-like epitopes in malted barley. *Int Arch Allergy Immunol* 1994;104:308.

[7] Bernhard SL, et al. Cysteine analogs of recombinant barley ribosome inactivating protein from anitbody conjugates with enhanced stability and potency in vitro. *Bioconjug Chem* 1994;5:126.

[8] Pundir CS, et al. Isolation, purification, immobilization of oxalate oxidase and its clinical applications. *Hindustan Antibiot Bull* 1993;35:173.

[9] Liljeberg H, et al. Bioavailability of starch in bread products. Postprandial glucose and insulin responses in healthy subjects and in vitro resultant startch content. *Eur J Clin Nutr* 1994;48:151.

[10] Granfeldt Y, et al. Glucose and insulin responses to barly produces: influence of food structure and amylose-amylopectin ratio. *Am J Clin Nutr* 1994;59:1075.

[11] Lupton JR, et al. Cholesterol-lowering effect of barley bran flour and oil. *J Am Diet Assoc* 1994;94:65

[12] McIntosh GH. Colon cancer: dietary modifications required for a balanced protective diet. *Prev Med* 1993;22:767.

[13] Lupton JR, et al. Barley bran flour accelerates gastrointestinal transit time. *J Am Diet Assoc* 1993;93:881.

[14] Ciclitira PG, et al. Determination of the gluten content of foods. *Panminerva Med* 1991;33:75.

Bayberry

SCIENTIFIC NAME(S): *Myrica cerifera* L. Family: Myricaceae

COMMON NAME(S): Bayberry, wax myrtle plant

BOTANY: The bayberry grows as a large evergreen shrub or small tree that is widely distributed throughout the southern and eastern US. It is known for its small bluish-white berries.[1]

HISTORY: The bayberry is best known for its berries, from which a wax is derived to make fragrant bayberry candles. In folk medicine, it has been used internally as a tea for its tonic and stimulant properties and has been used in the treatment of diarrhea. The dried root bark is often used medicinally.[2] The plant is astringent, which may account for this latter use along with its use for topical wound healing.[1]

CHEMISTRY: A number of compounds have been identified in the plant. Tannins account for the plant's astringency. The triterpenes myricadiol, taraxerol and taraxerone are present, along with the flavonoid glycoside myricitrin.[1]

PHARMACOLOGY: Myricadiol has been reported to have mineralocorticoid activity. Myricitrin has choleretic activity, stimulating the flow of bile.[1] The dried root is reported to have antipyretic properties.[2]

TOXICOLOGY: The elevated tannin concentration of the plant precludes its general internal use. The percutaneous injection of bark extracts in rats produced a significant number of malignant tumors following long-term (78-week) administration.[1,2] Ingestion of the plant may cause gastric irritation and vomiting.[3] The plant is said to be an irritant and sensitizer.[4]

SUMMARY: Bayberry is best known for its use in the production of a fragrance used in the preparation of scented Christmas candles. There is little evidence to support its use for the treatment of any disease and its high tannin content suggests that it should not be taken internally in any form.

PATIENT INFORMATION – Bayberry

Uses: Bayberry tea has been used as a tonic, stimulant and diarrhea treatment. Plant parts are also used to heal wounds, etc. Bayberry wax is used to make fragrant candles.

Side Effects: Bayberry probably should not be taken internally. Ingestion may cause GI distress. Long-term injection produced malignancies in rats.

---

[1] Tyler VE. *The New Honest Herbal.* Philadephia, PA: G.F. Stickley Co. 1987.
[2] Leung AY. *Encyclopedia of Common Natural Ingredients Used in Food, Drugs, and Cosmetics.* New York, NY: J. Wiley and Sons, 1980.
[3] Spoerke DG Jr. *Herbal Medications.* Santa Barbara, CA: Woodbridge Press, 1980.
[4] Duke JA. *Handbook of Medicinal Herbs.* Boca Raton, FL: CRC Press, 1985.

Bee Pollen

SOURCE: Bee pollen consists of plant pollens collected by worker bees, combined with plant nectar and bee saliva. These are packed by the insects into small dust pellets which are used as a food source for the male drones. commercially, the pollen is gathered at the entrance of the hive by forcing the bees to enter through a portal partially obstructed with wire mesh, thus brushing the material off the hind legs into a collection vessel. Because of the increasing popularity of this health food, this means of pollen collection has been supplemented by the direct collection of the material from within the hives. Alternately, pollen is collected directly from the wind-pollinated plants by automated means, and the pollen is compressed into tablets, with or without added nutritional supplements.[1] Claims have been made that machine-collected pollen is safer and less likely to cause allergic reactions because pollen collected by bees may contain fungal or bacterial contaminants. There is no adequate evidence to support this claim.

HISTORY: The use of bee pollen increased during the late 1970s following testimonials by athletes that supplementation with this product increased stamina and improved athletic ability.

CHEMISTRY: Bee pollen is a good nutritional source for drone bees. It contains approximately 30% protein, 55% carbohydrate, 1% to 2% fat, and 3% minerals and trace vitamins.[2] Vitamin C concentrations of 3.6% to 5.9% have also been found in some pollen samples.[3] Promotional literature lists almost 100 vitamins, minerals, enzymes, amino acids and other compounds identified in bee pollen. The physiologic importance of many of these components is poorly understood. Bee pollen preparations often contain mixtures of pollens from diverse types of plants, and these pollens vary with the geographic origin of the material.

PHARMACOLOGY: Articles in the lay press reported that athletes could enhance their performance by ingesting bee pollen; however, an investigation conducted by the National Athletic Trainer Association with Louisiana State University swim team members found no beneficial effect. The 2-year double-blind study found bee pollen "absolutely not a significant aid in the metabolism, workout training of performance" of these athletes.[4] The results of a study conducted in track runners suggested that athletes who took bee pollen recovered faster after exercise and that bee pollen would therefore be of value in relieving common tiredness and lack of energy. Critics of the study found the test group to be small, the blinding to be inadequate and the conclusions to be premature.[5]

Pregnant Sprague-Dawley rats fed bee pollen were experimentally found to have fetuses with higher birth weights and decreased death rates, suggesting bee pollen is an effective prenatal nutrient.[6] Bee pollen administered to rats was also experimentally found to possibly display anti-aging effects.[7] Bee pollen has been recommended to immunologically strengthen multiple sclerosis patients being treated with prednisolone and *Proper-Myl*.[8] Bee pollen may relieve or cure cerebral hemorrhage, bodily weakness, anemia, weight loss, enteritis, colitis and constipation.[3] However, all of these certainly bear clinical verification.

TOXICOLOGY: Reports of adverse reactions to bee pollen have been related to allergic reactions after ingestion by sensitive persons. There is a popular, but unadvisable, home practice of using bee pollen to treat allergic disorders. Despite the usually limited response to oral hyposensitization techniques and the potential for severe allergic reactions, this practice has spread considerably.

In one report of anaphylaxis, a 46-year-old man with a history of seasonal allergic rhinitis took a teaspoonful of bee pollen to treat his hay fever symptoms. Fifteen minutes later he developed paroxysm of sneezing and by 30 minutes experienced generalized angioedema, itching, dyspnea and lightheadedness. He recovered following treatment with epinephrine, corticosteroids and diphenhydramine.[1]

Other investigators have reported similar allergic reactions after single doses among patients with a history of allergic rhinitis. The dose required to precipitate an acute allergic reaction was less than one tablespoonful of bee pollen.[9] By contrast, the development of hypereosinophilia, neurologic and gastrointestinal symptoms in a woman who ingested bee pollen for more than 3 weeks was also reported.[10] These chronic allergic symptoms resolved upon discontinuation of the preparation. Although infrequent, some reports of severe allergic reactions to bee pollen have been observed. A 33-year-old man with no prior allergies had an acute anaphylactic reaction 15 minutes after ingesting bee pollen. He recovered fully after emergency medical treatment with epinephrine, lactated ringer's solution and methylprednisolone sodium succinate.[11]

Several reports suggested that bee pollen may have been used as a vehicle to carry the biochemical warfare toxin, T-2 mycotoxin, in Asia and Afghanistan, but this theory has come under considerable criticism.[12]

SUMMARY: Bee pollen is an expensive source of carbohydrates and trace nutrients. Although claims have been made that it may increase stamina and provide a source of instant energy, there is little supportive evidence for these claims. It should be taken with caution by persons with a history of pollen-sensitive allergies. Bee pollen is sold as loose granules, compressed tablets, and in capsules in combination with vitamin E and other nutritional supplements. A 100 tablet bottle (500 mg) retails for approximately $5, but imported products can retail for more than $15.00 for 30 pollen pods (a 30-day supply).

PATIENT INFORMATION – Bee Pollen

Uses: Although bee pollen is nutritionally rich, claims that it enhances athletic performance have not been reliably verified. Some evidence indicates it may benefit a range of conditions, from constipation to aging.

Side Effects: Ingestion produces allergic reactions in sensitive individuals. Attempts to hyposensitize by administering bee pollen may produce severe anaphylaxis and other acute or chronic responses.

---

[1] Mansfield LE, Goldstein GB. Anaphylactic Reaction After Ingestion of Local Bee Pollen. *Ann Allergy* 1981;47:154.

[2] Mirkin G. Can Bee Pollen Benefit Health? *JAMA* 1989;262(13):1854.

[3] Tyler VE. *The Honest Herbal: A Sensible Guide to the Use of Herbs and Related Remedies, ed. 3.* New York: Haworth Press, 1993.

[4] Montgomery PL. *New York Times* 1977;Feb. 6.

[5] Blustein P. *Wall Street Journal* 1981;Feb. 12.

[6] Xie Y, et al. [Effect of bee pollen on maternal nutrition and fetal growth (Chinese).] *Hua-Hsi I Ko Ta Hsueh Hsueh Pao [J West China Univ Med Sc]* 1994;25(4):434.

[7] Liu X, Li L. [Morphological observation of effect of bee pollen on intercellular lipofuscin in NIH mice (Chinese).] *Chung-Kuo Chung Yao Tsa Chich – China J of Chin Materia Medica* 1990;15(9):561.

[8] Iarosh AA, et al. [Changes in the immunological reactivity of patients with disseminated sclerosis treated by prednisolone and the preparation Proper-Myl (Russian).] *Vrach Delo* 1990;(2):83.

[9] Cohen, SH, et al. Acute allergic reaction after composite pollen ingestion. *J Allergy Clin Immunol* 1979;64(4):270.

[10] Lin FL, et al. Hypereosinophilia, neurologic, and gastrointestinal symptoms after bee-pollen ingestion. *J Allergy Clin Immunol* 1989;83(4):793.

[11] Geyman JP. Anaphylactic Reaction After Ingestion of Bee Pollen. *J Am Board Fam Pract* 1994;7(3):250.

[12] Marshall E. Bugs in the Yellow Rain Theory. *Science* 1983;220:1356.

Bee Venom

SCIENTIFIC NAME(S): Derived from *Apis Mellifera*

COMMON NAME(S): Bee venom, honeybee venom

SOURCE: Honeybee venom is obtained from *Apis Mellifera*, the common honeybee. Other venoms are derived from related members of the hymenoptera.

HISTORY: Anaphylaxis to insect stings is a relatively uncommon problem, believed to have affected only 0.4% of the general US population in the early 1990s. It is the cause of approximately 40 deaths per year in the United States.[1]

The allergic reactions are mediated by IgE antibodies directed at constituents of honeybee, yellow jacket, hornet and wasp venoms. In order to minimize the allergic reaction, hyposensitization immunotherapy techniques have been developed in which small doses of the venom are administered under controlled conditions over a period of months to years. Patients allergic to honeybee venom may be particularly sensitive to hymenoptera venoms in general and have been found to be at a significantly higher risk of developing systemic side effects to venom immunotherapy than patients who are sensitive to yellow jacket venom.[2]

More recently, it has been suggested that honeybee venom may alleviate the symptoms and slow the progression of immune-modulated diseases such as arthritis and multiple sclerosis.

CHEMISTRY: Bee venoms are complex mixtures of amino acids and polysaccharides. They are collected from the insects and diluted to standardized concentrations. Melittin, a phospholipase activating protein in bee venom, has been shown to induce neutrophil degranulation[3] and to both increase[3] and inhibit[4] the formation of superoxide. This difference in activity appears to be dependent upon the test method employed. Melittin induces neutrophil degranulation with subsequent superoxide formation;[3] however, melittin binds to calmodulin, and this effect is associated with an inhibition of the production of superoxide.[4]

The polypeptide adolapin isolated from bee venom inhibits inflammation in animals (carrageenan, prostaglandin and adjuvant rat paw edema models) and appears to inhibit the prostaglandin synthase systems.[5]

PHARMACOLOGY:

Immunotherapy: Hypersensitivity to honeybee venom is mediated by a number of antibodies and immunomodulators, the most important of which appears to be IgE. The infusion of beekeepers' plasma has been shown to protect patients against systemic reactions that can occur during active immunotherapy.[6] Following infusion of this plasma, a decrease in the sensitivity to honeybee venom has been noted; in one study, this was accompanied by increases in the levels of anti-idiotypic antibodies and decreases in specific antibodies to honeybee venom (IgG and IgE). (The study was conducted over a 76-week period of immunotherapy with the venom.) These findings suggest that several mechanisms play an interrelated role in the development of immunity to honeybee venom.

Arthritis Therapy: For some time it has been speculated that honeybee venom may prevent the development or improve the status of patients with rheumatoid arthritis. This conclusion was based largely on anecdotal observations of a general lack of arthritis among beekeepers stung routinely during their lifetimes. In one survey of a random sampling of the general population, 83% of respondents believed that bee venom could be an effective treatment for arthritis based on information they had read in the popular press.[7]

Honeybee venom administered to rats with adjuvant arthritis resulted in a significant suppression of the disease.[8] Melittin has been shown to block the production of superoxide and hydrogen peroxide in human neutrophils. Melittin and other agents that bind calmodulin have been shown to decrease superoxide production. An elevated superoxide level has been suggested as a possible cause of oxidative damage to synovial fluid and other joint membranes. Therefore, agents that decrease the production of the superoxide may prevent or halt the progression of inflammatory diseases such as arthritis. Also, honeybee venom has been found to decrease the production of the inflammatory mediator interleukin-1 (IL-1) in rat splenocytes.[9] Honeybee venom treatment of rats with adjuvant arthritis inhibits certain macrophage activities and, thus, indirectly inhibits the activation of T and B cells.[9]

Other Uses: Other uses for bee venom, though poorly substantiated, include the treatment of diseases of the locomotor system,[10] particularly multiple sclerosis (MS).

Despite widespread reports of true effectiveness of bee venom therapy for MS, there is no scientific consensus as to its safety and true effectiveness in the management of this disorder.

TOXICOLOGY: While single honeybee stings can cause anaphylaxis, the most severe reactions generally result from multiple stings. Signs and symptoms of multiple stings include urticaria (hives), nausea, vomiting, diarrhea, hypotension, confusion, seizures and renal failure. Treatment is supportive, with attention to blood pressure, renal function and maintaining an open airway. Stingers should be removed with gentle scraping to prevent further venom injection.[11] Because cardiac levels of noradrena-line have been found to increase dramatically in animals following injection with bee venom, it is suggested that all patients, regardless of sensitivity history, have cardiac monitoring if they are victims of multiple bee stings.[12] Rare cases of anuria and rhabdomyolysis/rhabdomyonecrosis have been reported.[13,14]

SUMMARY: Bee venom is used in hyposensitization immunotherapy for patients who are highly sensitive to the effects of bee stings. In addition, the venom finds use in the nontraditional treatment of arthritis and multiple sclerosis. The latter uses are based on observations of an anti-inflammatory and immunomodulating effect induced by bee venom.

PATIENT INFORMATION – Bee Venom

Uses: Bee venom is used to hyposensitize individuals highly sensitive to bee stings. There is some evidence it also helps inhibit or suppress arthritis and multiple sclerosis.

Side Effects: A single bee sting can produce anaphylaxis in sensitive individuals. Regardless of history, any patient with multiple stings should be monitored.

---

[1] Reisman RE. Stinging insect allergy. *Med Clin North Am* 1992;76:883.

[2] Muller U, et al. Immunotherapy with honeybee venom and yellow jacket venom is different regarding efficacy and safety. *J Allergy Clin Immuno* 1992;89:529.

[3] Bomalaski JS, et al. Rheumatoid arthritis synovial fluid phospholipase A2 activating protein (PLAP) stimulates human neutrophil degranulation and superoxide ion production. *Agents Actions* 1989;27:425.

[4] Somerfield SD, et al. Bee venom melittin blocks neutrophil O2–production. *Inflammation* 1986;10:175.

[5] Shkenderov S, Koburova K. Adolapin-a newly isolated analgetic and anti-inflammatory polypeptide from bee venom. *Toxicon* 1982;20:317.

[6] Boutin Y, et al. Possible dual role of anti-idiotypic antibodies in combined passive and active immunotherapy in honeybee sting allergy. *J Allergy Clin Immunol* 1994;93:1039.

[7] Price JH, et al. The public's perceptions and misperceptions of arthritis. *Arthritis Rheum* 1983;26:1023.

[8] Yiangou M, et al. Modulation of alpha 1-acid glycoprotein (AGP) gene induction following honey bee venom administration to adjuvant arthritic (AA) rats; possible role of AGP on AA development. *Clin Exp Immunol* 1993;94:156.

[9] Hadjipetrou-Kourounakis L, Yiangou M. Bee venom, adjuvant induced disease and interleukin production. *J Rheumatol* 1988;15:1126.

[10] Mund-Hoym WD. Bee venom containing forapin in the treatment of mesenchymal diseases of the locomotor system. Report on treatment results in 211 patients. *Med Welt* 1982;33:1174.

[11] Tunget CL, Clark RF. Invasion of the "killer" bees. Separating fact from fiction. *Postgrad Med* 1993;94:92.

[12] Ferreira DB, et al. Cardiac noradrenaline in experimental rat envenomation with Africanized bee venom. *Exp Toxicol Pathol* 1994;45:507.

[13] Azevedo-Marques MM, et al Rhabdomyonecrosis experimentally induced in Wistar rats by Africanized bee venom. *Toxicon* 1992;30:344.

[14] Beccari M, et al. Unusual case of anuria due to African bee stings. *Int J Artif Organs* 1992;15:281.

Bergamot Oil

SCIENTIFIC NAME(S): *Citrus bergamia* Risso et Poit. Synonymous with *C. aurantium* L. subspecies *bergamia*. Family: Rutaceae

COMMON NAME(S): Bergamot, oleum bergamotte. The plant should not be confused with *Monarda didyma* L. also known as scarlet bergamot or more commonly as oswego tea.[1]

BOTANY: The bergamot is a small tree native to tropical Asia, which is cultivated extensively on the southern coasts of Italy. The peel of the fresh, nearly ripe fruit is the source of bergamot oil. The oil is obtained by cold expression. Further purification by vacuum distillation solvent extraction or chromatography yields terpeneless (rectified) bergamot oil.[2] The oil is now used as a citrus flavor and is often added to perfumes and cosmetics.

CHEMISTRY: Bergamot oil is a complex mixture of more than 300 compounds. The most prevalent compounds are linalyl acetate (30% to 60%), linalool (11% to 22%) and other alcohols.[2] Furocoumarins include bergapten (approximately 0.4%), bergamottin,[3] citropten[4] and others. Rectified bergamot oil contains lower concentrations of terpenes and has no coumarins.[2]

PHARMACOLOGY:

Pharmacology/Toxicology: Some furocoumarins (such as bergapten and xanthotoxin, known as 5-5-methoxypsoralen and 8-methoxypsoralen, respectively) have been shown to be phototoxic in humans.[2] Bergamottin accounts for about two-thirds of the absorption of UVA and UVB light by bergamot oil.[5] Photosensitivity reaches its peak approximately two hours after topical administration of the oil.[6] Hyperpigmentation of the face and other areas exposed to the sun is thought to be due to the photosensitizing effects of cosmetics that contain these compounds.

The furocoumarins can induce genetic changes in cells exposed to UV light even in concentrations as low as 5 ppm.[7] These changes can be minimized by the application of a cinnamate-containing sunscreen,[8] but sunscreens in low concentrations (up to 1%) added to perfumes cannot suppress the phototoxicity of bergamot oil on human skin.[6] Studies suggest that many of the changes induced by bergamot oil and its components are malignant in nature.[7]

The furocoumarins have been used therapeutically in conjunction with long-wave ultraviolet light therapy for the management of psoriasis and vitiligo.

SUMMARY: Bergamot oil is a widely used material that imparts a citrus flavor to foods and beverages. Its odor has made it a component of perfumes and cosmetics. Unfortunately, bergamot oil contains photosensitizing compounds that can induce rashes and pathologic cellular changes when applied topically and exposed to sunlight or other sources of UV radiation.

PATIENT INFORMATION – Bergamot Oil

Uses: Bergamot oil is widely used as a flavoring and scenting agent. Some of its components are useful in therapy for psoriasis and vitiligo.

Side Effects: Photosensitizing components can induce rashes and pathologic cellular changes.

---

[1] Simon JE. *Herbs: an indexed bibliography, 1971-1980.* Hamden, CT: The Shoestring Press, 1984.

[2] Leung AY. *Encyclopedia of Common Natural Ingredients Used in Food, Drugs and Cosmetics.* New York, NY: John Wiley and Sons, 1980.

[3] Morliere P, et al. Photoreactivity of 5-geranoxypsoralen and lack of photoreaction with DNA. *Photochem Photobiol* 1991;53(1):13.

[4] Makki S, et al. High-performance liquid chromatographic determination of citropten and bergapten in suction blister fluid after solar product application in humans. *J Chromatogr* 1991;563(2):407.

[5] Morliere P, et al. In vitro photostability and photosensitizing properties of bergamot oil. Effects of a cinnamate sunscreen. *J Photochem Photobiol B* 1990;7(2-4):199.

[6] Dubertret L, et al. Phototoxic properties of perfumes containing bergamot oil on human skin: photoprotective effect of UVA and UVB sunscreens. *J Photochem Photobiol B* 1990;7(2-4):251.

[7] Young AR, et al. Phototumorigenesis studies of 5-methoxypsoralen in bergamot oil: evaluation and modification of risk of human use in an albino mouse skin model. *J Photochem Photobiol B* 1990;7(2-4):231.

[8] Averbeck D, et al. Genotoxicity of bergapten and bergamot oil in Saccharomyces cerevisiae. *J Photochem Photobiol B* 1990;7(2-4):209.

Beta Glycans

SCIENTIFIC NAME(S): Beta-1,3-glucan, beta-1,3/1,6-glycan

COMMON NAME(S): Beta glycans, beta glucans

SOURCE: Beta glycans are carbohydrates. They are natural substances that come from a variety of sources including mushrooms (eg, lentinan [see specific monograph]), oats, barley, baker's yeast, algae, and mannin.[1]

HISTORY: Beta-1,3/1,6-glycan has been studied for more than 30 years. It has immune system stimulant properties. In the 1980s, beta glycans were used to make salmon more disease resistant.[2]

CHEMISTRY: The chemistry of fungal beta-1,3-glucans has been reported. Structures were classified into triple helix, single helix, and random coil, which determined a variety of certain pharmacological characteristics.[3]

PHARMACOLOGY: In vitro testing demonstrated beta glycans induced non-specific macrophage-mediated tumor cell killing.[4] Beta glycans also increased hemagglutinin titers in certain cell lines.[5] Another report on soluble glycan demonstrates enhanced IL-1 and IL-2 production, which can be maintained 12 days post-glycan administration.[6] Beta glycans also cause a rapid decrease in tumor cells as shown in affected mice.[7] Fungal beta-1,3-glycan orally administered to mice inhibited tumor growth and potentiated immune response.[8] Another report confirms beta glycan's marked antitumor activity and enhanced ability of natural killer cell and macrophage activities in mice.[9] A review on mushroom beta glycans found differences in their effectiveness against certain tumors, primarily in cytokine expression and production.[10] Beta glycans were found to be immunostimulant in postsplenectomy sepsis in mice. Beta glycans increased survival by 75% in certain groups compared with 27% in the control group.[11] In mice with experimental colon and skin wounds, beta glycans increased tensile strength of the wounds by 42% and increased collagen biosynthesis as well.[12] Beta glycans obtained from oats were also found to possess immunostimulatory function in vitro and in vivo.[13] An overdose of a beta glycan preparation (sonifilan) failed to display antitumor activity in another report.[14]

Norwegian beta glycan is sold as an all-natural dietary supplement to boost the immune system and protect against colds and flu. It is claimed to strengthen the body's ability to fight disease-causing organisms. Because of its molecular shape, it binds specifically to macrophage surfaces, activating the immune system and increasing resistance.[2] In another product claim, beta glycans are said to be acid-resistant and pass through the stomach unchanged. Once in the intestine, macrophages attach to activate them.[1] Other product claims include beta glycans' ability to heal bed sores, nail fungus, and ear infections.[15]

Beta glycan's role in HIV appears promising in phase I and II human trials but needs confirmation.[16]

TOXICOLOGY: Baker's yeast beta-1,3/1,6-glycan has a "GRAS" rating by the FDA, meaning "generally recognized as safe."[1] A report on Norwegian beta glycans noted that if a patient with an existing disease takes beta glycans, symptoms may actually worsen for a couple of days.[2] In a clinical trial testing beta glycans use in AIDS patients, side effects severe enough to be reported to the FDA were anaphylactoid reaction, back pain, leg pain, depression, rigor, fever, chills, granulocytopenia, and elevated liver enzymes (1 case each); 4 of 98 patients discontinued therapy because of side effects.[16] Beta glycans may potentiate airway allergic responses.[17,18]

A preclinical safety evaluation of soluble glycan in mice, rats, guinea pigs, and rabbits is available. Data from this report indicate that "administration of soluble glycan over a wide dose range does not induce mortality or significant toxicity."[19]

SUMMARY: Beta glycans are carbohydrates that come from mushrooms, oats, baker's yeast, and other sources. Reports in animals and a few in humans have shown that beta glycans have immunostimulant effects and antitumor actions. Beta glycans have a "GRAS" rating by the FDA, but some reports of toxicity exist, including allergy.

PATIENT INFORMATION – Beta Glycans

Uses: Although few studies in humans are available (primarily in HIV patients), beta glycans are sold as supplements to boost the immune system and have also been studied in animals for their antitumor actions.

Side Effects: The FDA classifies baker's yeast beta-1,3/1,6-glycan as "GRAS" (generally recognized as safe), but reports show beta glycans may potentiate airway allergic responses and worsen symptoms in patients with existing disease.

[1] http://www.immunehealthsystems.com/questions.htm.

[2] Levy S. Echinacea, move over; Norwegian beta glucan is here. *Drug Topics* 2000 Apr 17:73.

[3] Yadomae T. Structure and biological activities of fungal beta-1,3-glucans. *Yakugaku Zasshi* 2000;120(5):413-31. [Japanese.]

[4] Artursson P, et al. Macrophage stimulation with some structurally related polysaccharides. *Scand J Immunol* 1987;25(3):245-54.

[5] Rios-Hernandez M, et al. Immunopharmacological studies of beta-1,3-glucan. *Arch Med Res* 1994;25(2):179-80.

[6] Sherwood E, et al. Enhancement of interleukin-1 and interleukin-2 production by soluble glucan. *Int J Immunopharmacol* 1987;9(3):261-67.

[7] Baba H, et al. Rapid tumor regression and induction of tumor-regressing activity in serum by various immune-modulating agents. *Int J Immunopharmacol* 1986;8(6):569-72.

[8] Suzuki I, et al. Immunomodulation by orally administered beta-glucan in mice. *Int J Immunopharmacol* 1989;11(7):761-69.

[9] Suzuki I, et al. Antitumor and immunomodulating activities of a beta-glucan obtained from liquid-cultured *Grifola frondosa*. *Chem Pharm Bull* 1989;37(2):410-13.

[10] Borchers A, et al. Mushrooms, tumors, and immunity. *Proc Soc Exp Biol Med* 1999;221(4):281-93.

[11] Browder W, et al. Protective effect of nonspecific immunostimulation in postsplenectomy sepsis. *J Surg Res* 1983;35(6):474-79.

[12] Portera C, et al. Effect of macrophage stimulation on collagen biosynthesis in the healing wound. *Am Surg* 1997;63(2):125-31.

[13] Estrada A, et al. Immunomodulatory activities of oat beta-glucan in vitro and in vivo. *Microbiol Immunol* 1997;41(12):991-98.

[14] Miura T, et al. Failure in antitumor activity by overdose of an immunomodulating beta-glucan preparation, sonifilan. *Biol Pharm Bull* 2000;23(2):249-53.

[15] http://www.immunehealthsystems.com/beta.htm.

[16] Gordon M, et al. A placebo-controlled trial of the immune modulator, lentinan, in HIV-positive patients: A phase I/II trial. *J Med* 1998;29(5-6):305-30.

[17] Wan G, et al. An airborne mold-derived product, beta-1,3-D-glucan, potentiates airway allergic responses. *Eur J Immunol* 1999;29(8):2491-97.

[18] Tarlo S. Workplace respiratory irritants and asthma. *Occup Med* 2000;15(2):471-84.

[19] Williams D, et al. Pre-clinical safety evaluation of soluble glucan. *Int J Immunopharmacol* 1988;10(4):405-14.

Betel Nut

SCIENTIFIC NAME(S): *Areca catechu* L. Family: Palmaceae

COMMON NAME(S): Betel nut, areca nut, pinlang, pinang

BOTANY: The areca tree is a feathery palm that grows to approximately 15 meters in height. It is cultivated in tropical India, Sri Lanka, south China, the East Indies, the Philippines and parts of Africa. The nut is about 2.5 cm in length and is very hard.[1]

HISTORY: The chewing of betel nut quids dates to antiquity. Betel nut is used in India and the Far East as a mild stimulant and digestive aid. The quid is generally composed of a mixture of tobacco, powdered or sliced areca nut and slaked lime often obtained from powdered snail shells. This mixture is wrapped in the leaf of the "betel" vine (*Piper betel* L. Family: Piperaceae). Users may chew from 4 to 15 quids a day with each quid being chewed for about 15 minutes.[2] Because of its CNS stimulating effects, betel nut is used in a manner similar to the Western use of tobacco or caffeine.[3] Chewing the nut stimulates salivary flow, thereby aiding digestion. The leaves have been used externally as a counterirritant and internally as an antitussive.

CHEMISTRY: The structurally-related pyridine alkaloids arecoline, arecaidine, arecaine, arecolidine, guvacine, isoguvacine and guvacoline are the pharmacologically active principles of betel nut.[4] The total alkaloid content can reach 0.45%.

The methyl esters of arecoline and guvacoline are hydrolyzed in the presence of alkali to the respective acids, arecaidine and guvacine. The hydrolysis is catalyzed by lime, which is added to the quid. Arecoline is most likely present in the nut as a salt of tannic acid, and the lime facilitates the release of the base from the salt.

The leaves of *P. betel* contain about 1% of a volatile oil and contain chaibetol, chavicol, cadinene and allylpyrocatechol.

PHARMACOLOGY: Arecoline is a basic oily liquid that has been used in veterinary medicine as a cathartic for horses and as a worm killer. These alkaloids have a cholinergic action similar to that of pilocarpine. The alkaloids of betel nut cause pupil dilation, vomiting, diarrhea, and in high doses, convulsions and death. The central stimulating activity of arecoline is greater than that of pilocarpine. Consequently, extracts of the nut have been used for the management of glaucoma in traditional medicine.[5] Betel nut chewing induces a number of physiologic changes including an increase in salivation,[6] gradual resorption of oral calcium induced by the lime, gingivitis, periodontitis and chronic osteomyelitis.[7]

TOXICOLOGY: As with chewing or smoking tobacco, the long-term use of betel nut is not without health consequences. Leukoplakia, which is considered to be a precancerous lesion, and squamous cell carcinoma of the oral mucosa have been found with unusually high frequency in long-term users of betel nut. Studies in New Guinea have also shown that chewing a betel nut-slaked lime mixture has been associated with oral leukoplakia that is precancerous in up to 10% of the cases.[8] By contrast, in persons chewing betel nut alone, such lesions are infrequent.

Experimental evidence indicates that arecaidine and arecoline have the greatest carcinogenic potential. When tested by an in vitro cell transformation assay, both alkaloids gave a positive response, implicating both as suspected human carcinogens.[9] Other compounds, in particular NMPA, are also highly active in decreasing mucosal cell viability, colony-forming efficiency and in causing DNA strand breaks and cross-links in buccal cells in vitro. These effects indicate that these compounds may contribute to the oral carcinogenicity associated with chewing betel nut quid.[10]

To confirm the carcinogenic potential of the plant, mice were fed daily doses of aqueous extracts of betel nut or betel leaf, the polyphenolic fraction of the nut or distilled water. Aqueous extracts of the nut induced tumors of the gastrointestinal tract, liver and lung in 58% of the treated mice. The polyphenolic fraction induced tumors in 17% of the mice. The aqueous extract of betel leaf and the water control did not induce tumors. Other studies by the same investigators indicate that betel *leaf* extract exerts an antineoplastic effect in mice when injected simultaneously with betel nut extract.[11]

The clinical implications of these animal data are poorly understood. The incidence of oral cancers increases among heavy long-term chewers of betel quids; whether this is due to the alkaloids or to the associated tannin (which accounts for 15% of the nut weight) or to carcinogens in the tobacco that is often added to the quid, is unknown. What "protective" value chewing betel leaf has is also unknown.

The results of one small study of Filipino betel chewers found that dietary supplementation with retinol (100,000 IU/week) and beta-carotene (300,000 IU/week) for 3 months was associated with a threefold decrease (from 4.2% to 1.4%) in the mean proportion of oral cells with nuclear alterations suggestive of precancerous lesions.[2]

Arecaine is poisonous and affects respiration, heart rate, increases intestinal peristalsis and can cause tetanic convulsions. Although doses of the seed in the range of 8 to 10 g have been reported to be fatal, others have suggested that doses up to 30 g may have a low toxicity potential.[4]

Betel nut chewing has been associated with an aggravation of asthma, and a dose-response relationship may exist between the use of this drug and the development of asthmatic symptoms.[12]

SUMMARY: Betel nut is used widely in many parts of the tropical world as a stimulant. In the United States, the nut is available through many Oriental grocery stores. Most chewers are middle- or older-aged women who spend several dollars per day on the product. Health professionals should suspect betel chewing as a cause of changes in the oral mucosa, particularly in persons of Asian descent, who may not readily discuss their use of the nut.

PATIENT INFORMATION – Betel Nut

Uses: Many Asians chew betel nut, usually along with other components in a quid. Betel nut is a CNS and salivary stimulant. The leaves may act as an antitussive and topically as a counterirritant.

Side Effects: Oral cancer and precancerous conditions are common among users, possibly due to other components of the quid. Betel may exacerbate asthma and bring other ill effects such as periodontitis.

---

[1] Evans WC. *Trease and Evans' Pharmacognosy*, ed. 13. London, England: Bailliere Tindall, 1989.

[2] Stich HF, et al. Reduction with vitamin A and beta-carotene administration of proportion of micronucleated buccal mucosal cells in Asian betel nut and tobacco chewers. *Lancet* 1984;8388(i):1204.

[3] Boyland E. The possible carcinogenic action of alkaloids of tobacco and betel nut. *Planta Med* 1968(suppl):13.

[4] Duke JA. Handbook of Medicinal Herbs. Boca Raton, FL: CRC Press, 1985.

[5] Morton JF. *Major Medicinal Plants*. Springfield, IL: CC Thomas, 1977.

[6] Reddy MS, et al. Effect of chronic tobacco-betel-lime "quid" chewing on human salivary secretions. *Am J Clin Nutr* 1980;33:77.

[7] Westermeyer J. Betel nut chewing. *JAMA* (letter) 1982;248:1835.

[8] McCallum CA. Hazards of betel nut chewing. *JAMA* (letter) 1982;247(19):2715.

[9] Ashby J, et al. Betel nuts, arecaidine and oral cancer. *Lancet* (letter) 1979;1(8107):112.

[10] Sundqvist K, et al. Areca-nut toxicity in cultured human buccal epithelial cells. *IARC Sci Publ* 1991;105:281.

[11] Bhide SV, et al. Carcinogenicity of betal quid ingredients: feeding mice with aqueous extract and the polyphenol fraction of betel nut. *Br J Cancer* 1979;40:922.

[12] Kiyingi KS. Betel-nut chewing may aggravate asthma. *PNG Med J* 1991;34(2):117.

Betony

SCIENTIFIC NAME(S): *Stachys officinalis* (L.) Trevisan, also referred to as *Betonica officinalis* L. in some older texts. Family: Labiatae

COMMON NAME(S): Betony, wood betony, and bishop wort. The genus is often collectively referred to as hedge-nettles.

BOTANY: Betony is a square-stemmed, mat-forming perennial of the mint family. It is distributed widely throughout western and southern Europe. It has a rosette of hairy leaves and a dense terminal spike of pink, white or purple flowers that bloom from June to September. The plant reaches a height of 1 meter, and the above-ground parts are dried and used medicinally. It is native to Europe and is often cultivated as a garden ornamental.[1,2]

HISTORY: Few plants have as widespread a history as betony. Its use has been known since the Roman Empire, where it was considered a panacea for practically every disease. During the Middle Ages, the plant was ascribed magical powers.[3]

Today the plant continues to be used in traditional medicine. A weak infusion is sometimes taken as a tea. It is used as an astringent to treat diarrhea and as a gargle or tea for irritations of the mouth and throat. It has been given to treat anxiety and has been given as a tincture or smoked for the treatment of headache.[4] The name "betony" may derive from the Celtic form of "bew" (a head) and "ton" (good).[5]

CHEMISTRY: Betony contains about 15% tannins, which account for its astringency. A mixture of flavonoid glycosides has been isolated and found to have hypotensive properties. In addition to tannins, betony contains stachydrine, which is a systolic depressant and active against rheumatism. The plant contains about 0.5% betaine along with small amounts of numerous other compounds, none of which contribute to the activity of the plant.[4] A report lists six new phenylethanoid glycosides from the aerial parts of the plant. Phenylethanoid glycosides formerly known include acetoside, campneosides, forsythoside B and leucosceptoside B.[6]

PHARMACOLOGY: The high tannin content of the plant most likely contributes to the **antidiarrheal** effect. In large doses, the plant may have a **purgative** and **emetic** action. A powder of the dried pulverized leaves has been used to induce sneezing.[7] Betony possesses **sedative** properties, relieving nervous stress and tension. It is still used as a remedy for headache and facial pain. In combination with herbs such as comfrey or linden, betony is effective for sinus headache and congestion.[2] Other uses for betony include: Treatment of nosebleeds; use as a gargle for its positive effect on gums, mouth and throat; and treatment of diarrhea and irritations of mucous membranes. Folk remedies of betony include treatment of tumors, spleen and liver sclerosis, colds, convulsions, kidney stones, palpitations, stomachache and toothaches.[4] Betony is known to stimulate the digestive system and the liver, which may support some of these claims.[2]

TOXICOLOGY: Although there is little documented evidence of betony toxicity, caution suggests that overdosage may cause gastrointestinal irritation because of the tannin content.[4] Betony polyphenols were found to be toxic in animals.[8] Betony should not be taken during pregnancy.[2]

SUMMARY: Betony is an ornamental plant that has been used in traditional medicine for centuries. It possesses sedative properties, which may relieve stress, headache, facial pain and congestion. Because of betony's high tannin content, its treatment for diarrhea can be useful. Betony also stimulates the digestive system, but additional studies are needed to establish efficacy. The plant is non-toxic in small doses, but it may cause gastrointestinal irritation if taken in excess.

PATIENT INFORMATION – Betony

Uses: Betony is used as an astringent to treat diarrhea and as a gargle or tea for mouth and throat irritations. It has been used to treat anxiety and headaches.

Side Effects: Overdosage can cause stomach irritation, and betony should not be taken during pregnancy.

---

[1] Bremness L. *The Complete Book of Herbs*. London, England: Dorling Kindersley Ltd., 1988;278.

[2] Chevallier A. *Encyclopedia of Medicinal Plants*. New York, NY: DK Publishing, 1996:270.

[3] Tyler VE. *The New Honest Herbal*. Philadelphia, PA: GF Stickley Co., 1987.

[4] Duke J. *CRC Handbook of Medicinal Herbs*. Boca Raton, FL: CRC Press Inc., 1989;457.

[5] http://www.botanical.com/botanical/mgmh/b/betowo35.html.

[6] Miyase T, et al. *Phytochemistry* 1996;43(2):475-79.

[7] Schauenberg P, Paris F. Guide to Medicinal Plants. New Canaan, CT: Keats Publishing Inc., 1977.

[8] Lipkan G, et al. *Farmatsevtychnyi Zhurnal* 1974;29(1):78–81.

Bilberry Fruit

SCIENTIFIC NAME(S): *Vaccinium Myrtillus,* Myrtilli fructus

COMMON NAME(S): Bilberries, bog bilberries,[1] blueberries (variety of),[2] whortleberries

BOTANY: Bilberry fruit originates from Northern and Central Europe and has been imported from parts of south-eastern Europe. These black, coarsely wrinkled berries contain many small, shiny brownish-red seeds. They have a somewhat caustic and sweet taste.[1]

HISTORY: The historical uses of dried bilberry fruit include being a supportive treatment of acute, non-specific diarrhea when administered as a tea and serving as a topical decoction for the inflammation of the mucous membranes of the mouth and throat.[1]

During World War II, British Royal Air Force pilots ate bilberry preserves before night missions in order to improve their vision. After the war, studies confirmed the folk beliefs that bilberry extracts could improve visual acuity and lead to faster visual adjustments between light (eg, glare) and darkness.[2] Some European physicians went on to recommend bilberry extracts for other eye complaints (eg, retinitis pigmentosa, diabetic retinopathy). Clinical studies, however, have not confirmed these therapeutic applications.

CHEMISTRY: According to older studies, bilberry consists of up to 10% tannins, most of which are catechol tannins. However, recent studies suggest that tannins constitute only 1.5%. In addition to tannins, bilberry contains anthocyans, flavonoids, plant acids, invert sugars and pectins. The fresh fruit does not have the antidiarrhetic effects; therefore, it must be dried to obtain the tannins which come about by the condensation of the monomeric tannin precursors during the drying process.[1]

PHARMACOLOGY: Dried bilberry fruit is used as an antidiarrhetic drug, especially in mild cases of enteritis. It is also used as a topical treatment for mild inflammation of the mucous membranes of the mouth and throat.[1]

Most clinical studies have concentrated on the fruit's anthocyanoside content. An experiment using a preparation of anthocyanosides from bilberry (equal to 25% of anthocyanidins) indicated vasoprotective and antiedema effects in experimental animals. Oral doses of 25–100 mg/kg increased the permeability of the skin capillary. Antiedema activity was discovered after intravenous or topical use.[3]

When vascular permeability is increased in rabbits by cholesterol-induced atheroma, a treatment of anthocyanosides from bilberry decreases vascular permeability. This is acheived when the drug interacts with collagen to increase its cross-links.[4] The administration of anthocyanosides before the induction of hypertension in rats maintains normal blood-barrier permeability and limits the increase in vascular permeability. This may also result from the interaction of the drug with collagens of the blood vessel walls to protect against the permeability-increasing action of hypertension.[5]

Vaccinium myrtillus anthocyanosides are effective in promoting and intensifying arteriolar rhythmic diameter changes which aid in the redistribution of microvascular blood flow and interstitial fluid formation.[6]

An investigation using an anthocyanidin pigment (IdB 1027) found in bilberries showed protective gastric effects without influencing acid secretion. The pigment was administered orally using 600 mg b.i.d. for 10 days in 10 laboratory animals. The results showed an increase in the gastric mucosal release of prostaglandin E2 which may explain the antiulcer and gastroprotective effects of IdB 1027.[7]

Anthocyans and vitamin E are natural antioxidants which produce a protective effect on liver cells damaged by injury.[8]

TOXICOLOGY: The effects of ingesting large doses of bilberry are not known. There are no known side effects or interactions with other drugs.

It is important that the fruit has not been attacked by insects and that it is free of mold. The berries should be as soft as possible or the long-stored drug will become hard and brittle.[1]

SUMMARY: The bilberry fruit is administered as a tea to treat acute, non-specific diarrhea. It may also be used topically for mild inflammation of the mucous membranes of the mouth and throat. Studies have shown various possible effects such as vasoprotectivity, antiedemic effects, decreasing vascular permeability, gastroprotectivity, hepatoprotectivity and intensifying arteriolar rhythmic diameter. However, further studies are need to prove these effects.

PATIENT INFORMATION – Bilberry Fruit

Uses: Dried bilberry tea is used internally to treat nonspecific diarrhea and topically to treat inflamed mouth and throat mucosa. Bilberry extracts demonstrably improve visual acuity and ability to adjust to changing light. Derivatives demonstrate vasoprotective, antiedema and gastroprotective effects.

Side Effects: None known.

---

[1] Bissett NG, ed. *Herbal Drugs and Phytopharmaceuticals.* Stuttgart: Medpharm Scientific Publishers, 1994.

[2] Murray MT. *The Healing Power of Foods.* Rocklin, CA: Prima Publishing, 1993.

[3] Lietti A. et al. Studies on Vaccinium myrtillus anthocyanosides. I. Vasoprotective and antiinflammatory activity. *Arzneimittel-Forschung* 1976;26(5):829.

[4] Kadar A, et al. Influence of anthocyanoside treatment on the cholesterol-induced atherosclerosis in the rabbit. *Paroi Arterielle* 1979;5(4):187.

[5] Detre Z, et al. Studies on vascular permeability in hypertension: action of anthocyanosides. *Clin Physiol Biochem* 1986;4(2):143.

[6] Colantuoni A, et al. Effects of Vaccinium Myrtillus anthocyanosides on arterial vasomotion. *Arzneimittel-Forshung* 1991;41(9):905.

[7] Mertz-Nielsen A, et al. A natural flavonoid, IdB 1027, increases gastric luminal release of prostaglandin E2 in healthy subjects. *Ital J Gastroenterol* 1990;22(5):288.

[8] Mitcheva M, et al. Biochemical and morphological studies on the effects of anthocyans and vitamin E on carbon tetrachloride induced liver injury. *Cell Microbiol* 1993;39(4):443.

Bitter Melon

SCIENTIFIC NAME(S): *Momordica charantia* L. Family: Cucurbitaceae

COMMON NAME(S): Bitter melon, balsam pear, bitter cucumber, balsam apple, "art pumpkin", cerasee, carilla cundeamor

BOTANY: Bitter melon is an annual plant growing to 6 feet tall. It is cultivated in Asia, Africa, South America, and India and is considered a tropical fruit. The plant has lobed leaves, yellow flowers, and edible (but bitter-tasting), orange-yellow fruit. The unripe fruit is green and is cucumber-shaped with bumps on its surface. The parts used include the fruit, leaves, seeds, and seed oil.[1,2,3]

HISTORY: Bitter melon has been used as a folk remedy for tumors, asthma, skin infections, GI problems, and hypertension.[4] The plant has been used as a traditional medicine in China, India, Africa, and southeastern US.[3] The plant has been used in the treatment of diabetes symptoms. In the 1980s, the seeds were investigated in China as a potential contraceptive.[1]

CHEMISTRY: Chemical constituents from whole plants, fruits, and seeds of bitter melon have been isolated and described.[5,6,7]

Specifically, bitter melon contains the glycosides mormordin and charantin. Charantin is a hypoglycemic agent composed of mixed steroids.[2,4] A pyrimidine glycoside has also been found.[8] The alkaloid mormordicine is also present, along with a fixed oil.[1] Leaves contain iron, sodium, and vitamins including thiamine, riboflavin, niacin, and ascorbic acid.[4]

An insulin-like, hypoglycemic peptide[1] "polypeptide-P"[2] is present in bitter melon. This has been isolated from the fruit, seeds, and tissue of the plant and has a molecular weight of 11,000 in 1 report.[9] An overview of specific antidiabetic constituents in bitter melon is available.[10]

Bitter melon seeds contain 32% oil, with stearic, linoleic, and oleic acids.[4] The seeds also contain the pyrimidine nucleoside vicine,[10] the glycoproteins alpha-momorcharin and beta-momorcharin (abortifacients) and lectins.[3] Amino acid composition in seeds is described as well.[11] Insulin-like molecules also have been found in the seeds.[12]

PHARMACOLOGY: Beneficial effects of bitter melon have been studied and reviewed.[3,13,14,15] These effects include **hypoglycemic**, **antimicrobial**, **antifertility**, and others.

The hypoglycemic effects of bitter melon have been clearly established in animal and human studies.[16,17] Constituents of the plant that contribute to its hypoglycemic properties include charantin, polypeptide P, and vicine.[2,10,18,19] Reduction of blood glucose and improvement of glucose tolerance are the mechanisms by which the plant exerts its actions.

Animal studies document the hypoglycemic effects and include reports in diabetic mice;[20,21,22] studies in rats,[23,24,25,26] including improvement in glucose tolerance,[27] sustained decrease in blood glucose levels even after 15 days of discontinuation of bitter melon treatment (as well as a decrease in serum cholesterol levels),[28] and a suggested oral hypoglycemic mechanism involving the presence of viable beta cells;[29] and a study in diabetic rabbits, which also confirmed the plant's consistent hypoglycemic effects.[30]

Other mechanisms for hypoglycemic effects include extrapancreatic actions such as increased glucose uptake by tissues, glycogen synthesis in liver and muscles, triglyceride production in adipose tissue, and gluconeogenesis.[31] Another report suggests the mechanism to be partly attributed to increased glucose use in the liver, rather than an insulin secretory effect.[32] Hepatic enzyme studies demonstrate bitter melon's hypoglycemic activity without glucose tolerance improvement in mice;[33] hypoglycemic activity by depression of blood glucose synthesis through depression of enzymes glucose-6-phosphatase and fructose-1,6-bisphosphatase, along with enhancement of glucose oxidation by enzyme G6PDH pathway;[34] and hypoglycemic actions involving hepatic cytochrome P450 and glutathione S-transferases in diabetic rats.[35] One report finds retardation of retinopathy (a diabetic complication) in diabetic rats administered a fruit extract of bitter melon.[36] At least 1 animal study finds no hypoglycemic effects in diabetic rats given a freeze-dried preparation of the plant for 6 weeks.[37]

Bitter melon improved glucose tolerance in humans.[27] Another study reported improved glucose tolerance in 18 type 2 diabetic patients with 73% success from a juice preparation of bitter melon.[38] Another report observed a

54% decrease in postprandial blood sugar, as well as a 17% reduction in glycosylated hemoglobin in 6 patients taking 15 g of aqueous bitter melon extract.[2] A trial is also available on patients taking a powder preparation of the plant.[39] Clinical trials using fresh fruit juice in 160 diabetic patients controlled diabetes. Bitter melon did not promote insulin secretion but did increase carbohydrate use.[4] A review describing the antidiabetic activity of bitter melon discusses in vitro, animal, and human studies, mechanisms of action, and the phytochemicals involved.[10]

Antimicrobial effects of bitter melon have been documented. Roots and leaf extracts have shown antibiotic activity.[3,4] One study reports 33.4% cytostatic activity from bitter melon aqueous extract,[40] as constituents momorcharins have antitumor properties and can inhibit protein synthesis.[41] Similarly, the plant also inhibits replication of viruses, including polio, herpes simplex 1, and HIV.[3,10] A study on antipseudomonal activity reports bitter melon to be effective, but not promising, in overall results.[42] Antiviral and other effects of bitter melon have been reviewed.[3]

Bitter melon exhibits genotoxic effects in *Aspergillus nidulans*.[43] It is cytotoxic in leukemia cells as a guanylate cyclase inhibitor.

Bitter melon's role in fertility has been reported. A protein found in the plant was found to show antifertility activity in male rats.[44] Oral administration of the fruit (1.7 g/day extract) to male dogs caused testicular lesions and atrophy of spermatogenic aspects. In female mice, the plant exhibited similar, but reversible, antifertility effects.[10] Momorcharins are capable of producing abortions.[41] Uterine bleeding has been induced in pregnant rats given the juice, as well as in rabbits, but not in nonpregnant females.[10] The ripe fruit has been said to induce menstruation.[1]

Other effects of bitter melon include the following: Dose-related analgesic activity in rats and mice,[45] anti-inflammatory actions,[10] and treatment for GI ailments, such as gas, ulcer, digestion, constipation, dysentery,[1,4] or hemorrhoids.[46] The plant has also been used for skin diseases (eg, boils, burns, infections, scabies, psoriasis),[4] and for its lipid effects[10] and hypotensive actions.[4,10] The plant has also been used as an insecticide.[3,4]

TOXICOLOGY: Bitter melon as an unripe fruit is commonly eaten as a vegetable.[2,3] Bitter melon extract is said to be nontoxic.[3] The plant is relatively safe at low doses and for a duration of $\leq$ 4 weeks.[1] There are no published reports of serious effects in adults given the "normal" oral dose of 50 ml. In general, bitter melon has low clinical toxicity, with some possible adverse GI effects.[10]

Because of the plant's ability to reduce blood sugar, some caution is warranted in susceptible patients who may experience hypoglycemia.[1] Two small children experienced hypoglycemic coma resulting from intake of a tea made from the plant. Both recovered upon medical treatment.[10] Another report concerning increased hypoglycemic effect noted an interaction in a 40-year-old diabetic woman between *M. charantia* (a curry ingredient) and chlorpropamide, which she was taking concurrently for her condition.[47]

The red arils around bitter melon seeds are toxic to children. The juice given to a child in 1 report caused vomiting, diarrhea, and death.[4]

Bitter melon's hepatotoxic effects have been demonstrated in animals, in which enzymes became elevated following plant administration. The momorcharin constituents may induce morphological changes in hepatocytes as well.[10]

The seed constituent, vicine, is a toxin said to induce "favism," an acute condition characterized by headache, fever, abdominal pain, and coma.[3,10]

Bitter melon is not recommended in pregnant women because of its reproductive system toxicities (see Pharmacology, antifertility section), including induction of uterine bleeding and contractions or abortion induction.[3,10,41]

SUMMARY: Bitter melon is an edible tropical fruit used mainly as a traditional medicine in China, India, and Africa. Its effects are well documented in the area of hypoglycemia but also include antimicrobial and antifertility actions. Human studies to substantiate the plant's use as an antidiabetic drug are promising. Its toxicity profile in adults is low but may cause problems in children. Bitter melon use is not recommended in pregnant women.

PATIENT INFORMATION – Bitter Melon

Uses: Bitter melon's effects include hypoglycemic, antimicrobial, antifertility, and others.

Side Effects: Use with caution in hypoglycemic patients. The red arils around bitter melon seeds are toxic to children. The plant is not recommended in pregnant women because it may cause uterine bleeding and contractions or may induce abortion.

Drug Interactions: Increased hypoglycemic effect when *M. charantia* and chlorpropamide are coadministered.

---

[1] Chevallier A. *Encyclopedia of Medicinal Plants*. New York, NY: DK Publishing, 1996:234.

[2] Murray M. *The Healing Power of Herbs, 2 ed*. Rocklin, CA: Prima Publishing, 1995;357-58.

[3] Cunnick J, et al. Bitter Melon (*Momordica charantia*). *J Nat Med* 1993;4(1):16-21.

[4] Duke J. *CRC Handbook of Medicinal Herbs*. Boca Raton, FL: CRC Press Inc., 1989;315-16.

[5] Visarata N, et al. Extracts from *Momordica charantia* L. *J Crude Drug Res* 1981 Oct;19:75-80.

[6] Zhu Z, et al. Studies on active constituents of *Momordica charantia* L. *Acta Pharmaceutica Sinica* 1990 Dec;25:898-903.

[7] Chang F. Studies on the chemical constituents of balsam pear (*Momordica charantia*). *Chin Traditional and Herb Drugs* 1995 Oct;26:507-10.

[8] El-Gengaihi S, et al. Novel pyrimidine glycoside from *Momordica charantia* L. *Pharmazie* 1995 May;50:361-62.

[9] Khanna P, et al. Hypoglycemic activity of polypeptide-p from a plant source. *J Nat Prod* 1981;44(6):648-55.

[10] Raman A, et al. Anti-diabetic properties and phytochemistry of *Momordica charantia* L. (Cucurbitaceae). *Phytomedicine* 1996;2(4):349-62.

[11] Barron D, et al. Comparative study of 2 medicinal Cucurbitaceae. *Planta Med* 1982 Nov;46:184-86.

[12] Ng T, et al. Insulin like molecules in *Momordica charantia* seeds. *J Ethnopharmacology* 1986 Jan;15:107-17.

[13] Sankaranaravanan J, et al. Phytochemical, antibacterial and pharmacological investigations on *Momordica charantia* Linn., *Emblica officinalis* Gaertn., and *Curcuma longa* Linn. *Indian J Pharm Sci* 1993;55(1):6-13.

[14] Platel K, et al. Plant foods in the management of diabetes mellitus: vegetables as potential hypoglycaemic agents. *Nahrung* 1997;41(2):68-74.

[15] Avedikian J. Herbs: what are they...and do they work? *California Pharmacist* 1994 Aug;42:15.

[16] Lei Q, et al. Influence of balsam pear on blood sugar level. *J Tradit Chin Med* 1985 Jun;5(2)99-106.

[17] Aslam M, et al. Hypoglycemic properties in traditional medicines with specific reference to karela. *Internat Pharm J* 1989 Nov-Dec;3:226-29.

[18] Wong C, et al. Screening of *Trichosanthes kirilowii*, *Momordica charantia* and *Cucurbita maxima* for compounds with antilipolytic activity. *J Ethnopharmacology* 1985 Jul;13:313-21.

[19] Handa G, et al. Hypoglycemic principle of *Momordica charantia* seeds. *Indian J Nat Prod* 1990;6(1):16-19.

[20] Bailey C, et al. Cerasee, a traditional treatment for diabetes. Studies in normal and streptozotocin diabetic mice. *Diabetes Res* 1985;2(2):81-84.

[21] Day C, et al. Hypoglycaemic effect of *Momordica charantia* extracts. *Planta Med* 1990 Oct;56(5):426-29.

[22] Cakici I, et al. Hypoglycemic effect of *Momordica charantia* extracts in normoglycemic or cyproheptadine-induced hyperglycemic mice. *J Ethnopharmacology* 1994;44(2):117-21.

[23] Karunanayake E, et al. Oral hypoglycemic activity of some medicinal plants of Sri Lanka. *J Ethnopharmacology* 1984 Jul;11:223-31.

[24] Chandrasekar B, et al. Blood sugar lowering potentiality of selected Cucurbitaceae plants of Indian origin. *Indian J Med Res* 1989;90:300-5.

[25] Higashino H, et al. Hypoglycemic effects of Siamese *Momordica charantia* and *Phyllanthus urinaria* extracts in streptozotocin-induced diabetic rats. *Nippon Yakurigaku Zasshi* 1992 Nov;100(5):415-21.

[26] Ali L, et al. Studies on hypoglycemic effects of fruit pulp, seed, and whole plant of *Momordica charantia* on normal and diabetic model rats. *Planta Med* 1993 Oct;59(5):408-12.

[27] Leatherdale B, et al. Improvement in glucose tolerance due to *Momordica charantia*. *Br Med J (Clin Res Ed)* 1981 Jun 6;282(6279):1823-24.

[28] Singh N, et al. Effects of long term feeding of acetone extract of *Momordica charantia* (whole fruit powder) on alloxan diabetic albino rats. *Indian J Physiol Pharmacol* 1989 Apr-Jun;33(2):97-100.

[29] Karunanayake E, et al. Effect of *Momordica charantia* fruit juice on streptozotocin-induced diabetes in rats. *J Ethnopharmacology* 1990;30(2):199-204.

[30] Akhtar M, et al. Effect of *Momordica charantia* on blood glucose level of normal and alloxan diabetic rabbits. *Planta Med* 1981;42(3):205-12.

[31] Welihinda J, et al. Extra-pancreatic effects of *Momordica charantia* in rats. *J Ethnopharmacology* 1986 Sep;17:247-55.

[32] Sarkar S, et al. Demonstration of the hypoglycemic action of *Momordica charantia* in a validated animal model of diabetes. *Pharmacol Res* 1996 Jan;33(1):1-4.

[33] Tennekoon K, et al. Effect of *Momordica charantia* on key hepatic enzymes. *J Ethnopharmacology* 1994;44(2):93-97.

[34] Shibib B, et al. Hypoglycaemic activity of *Coccinia indica* and *Momordica charantia* in diabetic rats. *Biochem J* 1993 May 15;292(Pt. 1):267-70.

[35] Raza H, et al. Effect of bitter melon fruit juice on the hepatic cytochrome P450-dependent monooxygenases and glutathione S-transferases in streptozotocin-induced diabetic rats. *Biochem Pharmacol* 1996 Nov 22;52(10):1639-42.

[36] Srivastava Y, et al. Retardation of retinopathy by *Momordica charantia* L. fruit extract in alloxan diabetic rats. *Indian J Exp Biol* 1987 Aug;25(8):571-72.

[37] Platel K, et al. Effect of dietary intake of freeze dried bitter gourd in streptozotocin induced diabetic rats. *Nahrung* 1995;39(4):262-68.

[38] Welihinda J, et al. Effect of *Momordica charantia* on the glucose tolerance in maturity onset diabetes. *J Ethnopharmacology* 1986 Sep;17:277-82.

[39] Akhtar M. Trial of *Momordica charantia* Linn. powder in patients with maturity-onset diabetes *JPMA J Pak Med Assoc* 1982 Apr;32(4):106-7.

[40] Rojas N, et al. Antitumoral potential of aqueous extracts of Cuban plants. Part 2. *Revista Cubana de Farmacia* 1980 May-Aug;14:219-25.

[41] Bruneton J. Pharmacognosy, PhytoChemistry, Medicinal Plants. Paris, France: Lavois er, 1995;192.

[42] Saraya A, et al. Antipseudomonal activity of *Momordica charantia*. *Mahidol Univ J Pharm Sci* 1985 Jul-Sep;12:69-73.

[43] Ramos R, et al. Screening of medicinal plants for induction of somatic segregation activity in *Aspergillus nidulans*. *J Ethnopharm* 1996;52(3):123-27.

[44] Chang F, et al. Studies on the antifertility chemical constituents of balsam pear. *Chin Traditional and Herbal Drugs* 1995 Jun;26:281-84.

[45] Biswas A, et al. Analgesic effect of *Momordica charantia* seed extract in mice and rats. *J Ethnopharmacology* 1991;31(1):115-18.

[46] Hocking G. A Dictionary of Natural Products. Medford, NJ: Plexus Publishing Inc., 1997;504-5.

[47] Aslam M, et al. Interaction between curry ingredient (karela) and drug (chlorpropamide). *Lancet* 1979 Mar 17;1:607.

Bittersweet Nightshade

SCIENTIFIC NAME(S): *Solanum dulcamara* L. Family: Solanaceae

COMMON NAME(S): Bittersweet nightshade, deadly nightshade, bittersweet, bitter nightshade, felonwort, violet-bloom, woody nightshade, fellen, scarlet berry, snake berry, mortal,[1] fever twig,[1] dulcamara[2]

BOTANY: The bittersweet is a member of the same family as the potato and tomato. A number of members of the genus have been identified. This plant is found throughout Eurasia, the United States and Canada. Bittersweet is a vine-like perennial that grows to heights of 10 feet. It has alternating heart-shaped oval leaves that usually have two small ear-like segments at their bases. Its star-shaped flowers bloom from April to September; the flowers are pinkish-purple with bright yellow stamens. The flowers produce green berries that turn bright red upon maturing.[3]

HISTORY: The Latin name "dulcamara" refers to the flavor of the berries, which are first bitter, then unpleasantly sweet.[3] Although the plant has long been recognized as being highly toxic, it has been used as an external remedy for skin abrasions. Its use to treat "felons" (inflammations around nail beds) may be the source of the name "felonwort." The plant has been investigated for possible antirheumatic, diuretic, narcotic and sedative activity, but these actions are linked to the toxicity of the plant and therefore have not been exploited.

CHEMISTRY: Chemical investigations into the composition of bittersweet have identified an ever-growing number of alkaloids and other organic compounds in the leaves and fruits. The most widely recognized of these compounds are solanine and the glucoside dulcamarin. Related compounds include gamma-soladulcine, soladulcidine, solasonine, solamargine and lycopene. Other compounds include soladulcosides A and B.[4] Green and yellowing fruits contain a higher percentage of the glycoalkaloids than ripe fruits.[5]

PHARMACOLOGY/TOXICOLOGY: The FDA classifies bittersweet as an unsafe poisonous herb because of the presence of the toxic compounds solanine, solanidine and dulcamarin.

Solanine is poorly absorbed from the gastrointestinal tract and is rapidly eliminated in the urine and feces of animals. Because of its structural similarity to cardiac glycosides, solanine has weak cardiotonic activity. Like saponin, solanine causes hemolytic and hemorrhagic damage to the gastrointestinal tract.[6] Although a 200 mg oral dose of solanine has not been associated with toxicity in man, the oral LD_{50} in rats is about 590 mg/kg.[6] Solanine poisoning is often confused with bacterial gastroenteritis, with symptoms appearing only after a latent period of several hours following ingestion. The most common source of solanine poisoning has been the tuber of the potato.[6] Symptoms of solanine poisoning include headache, convulsions, cyanosis, stomach ache, scratchy throat, subnormal temperature, paralysis, dilated pupils, vertigo, vomiting, diarrhea, speech difficulties, shock, circulatory and respiratory depression and death.

Adults appear to be relatively resistant to the toxicity of solanine, but fatal intoxications are more common in children.[7]

Emesis, fluid replacement and supportive care as for gastroenteritis should be given.[7] Despite this typically aggressive therapy, the results of one study in mice fed ripened fruit suggested that because no gastrointestinal or neurologic toxicity was observed, aggressive treatment of children who ingest ripened berries may not be necessary.[8] Nevertheless, these investigators found significant neurologic and pathologic gastrointestinal toxicity when mice were fed unripened fruits, indicating that poisoning with this plant should be considered a critical situation. Other investigators have confirmed the pathologic changes in the gastrointestinal tract (glandular mucosal necrosis and necrosis of the small intestine) in hamsters fed ground bittersweet.[9]

Concern has emerged linking the glycosides of certain solanum species (ie, potato) to fetal malformations in animals and humans. Extracts of bittersweet have been shown to cause an elevated incidence of craniofacial malformations in hamsters, which was statistically significant compared to controls.[10] The alkaloids solasodine, soladulcine and related compounds were linked to the malformations.

SUMMARY: Bittersweet is a toxic plant that grows wild throughout most of the United States. Although the plant has been used in traditional medicine, its use was generally limited to external application. Ingestion of the unripened berries, particularly by children, constitutes a medical emergency; other parts of the plant are also toxic. The toxicity is caused by solanine and related glycoalkaloids.

PATIENT INFORMATION – Bittersweet Nightshade

Uses: Bittersweet has been used as a traditional external remedy.

Side Effects: The plant is toxic. Ingestion of unripened berries should be considered a medical emergency. Toxic symptoms may be delayed for several hours.

---

[1] Meyer JE. *The Herbalist.* Hammond. IN: Hammond Book Co., 1934.

[2] Osol A, Farrar GE Jr., eds. *The Dispensatory of the United States of America, 25th ed.* Philadelphia, PA: J.B. Lippincott, 1955.

[3] Dobelis IN, ed. *Magic and Medicine of Plants.* Pleasantville, NY: Reader's Digest Association, 1986.

[4] Yamashita T, et al. Structures of two new steroidal glycosides, soladulcosides A and B from *Solanum dulcamara. Chem Pharm Bull* 1991;39(6):1626.

[5] Duke JA. Handbook of Medicinal Herbs. Boca Raton, FL: CRC Press, 1985.

[6] Dalvi RR, Bowie WC. Toxicology of solanine: An overview. *Vet Hum Toxicol.* 1983;25(1):13.

[7] Lampe KF. AMA Handbook of Poisonous and Injurious Plants. Chicago, IL: Chicago Review Press, 1985.

[8] Hornfeldt CS, Collins JE. Toxicity of nightshade berries (*Solanum dulcamara*) in mice. *J Toxicol Clin Toxicol* 1990;28(2):185.

[9] Baker DC, et al. Pathology in hamsters administered *Solanum* plant species that contain steroidal alkaloids. *Toxicon* 1989;27(12):1331.

[10] Keeler RF, et al. Spirosolane-containing *Solanum* species and induction of congenital craniofacial malformations. *Toxicon* 1990;28(8):873.

Black Cohosh

SCIENTIFIC NAME(S): *Cimicifuga racemosa* (L.) Nutt. Family: Ranunculaceae. Plants associated with the name include other *Cimicifuga* species, *Macrotys actaeoides* and *Actaea racemosa* L.

COMMON NAME(S): Black cohosh, baneberry, black snakeroot, bugbane, squawroot, rattle root[1]

BOTANY: Black cohosh grows in open woods at the edges of dense forests from Ontario to Tennessee and west to Missouri. This perennial grows to 8 feet and is topped by a long plume of white flowers that bloom from June to September. Its leaflets are shaped irregularly with toothed edges. The term "black" refers to the dark color of the rhizome. The name "cohosh" comes from an Algonquian word meaning "rough," referring to the feel of the rhizome.[2]

HISTORY: The roots and rhizomes of this herb are used medicinally. Traditional uses include the treatment of dysmenorrhea, dyspepsia and rheumatisms. A tea from the root has been recommended for sore throat. The Latin name cimicifuga means "bug-repellent" and the plant has been used for this purpose. American Indians used the plant to treat snakebites.

Old-time remedy "Lydia Pinkham's Vegetable Compound" (early 1900s) contained many natural ingredients, one of which was black cohosh.[3]

Remifemin, the brand-name of the standardized extract of the plant, has been used in Germany for menopausal management since the mid-1950s.[4]

CHEMISTRY: German reports from the late 1960s discussing the contents of black cohosh (eg, acetin) are available.[5,6,7]

Black cohosh contains alkaloids including N-methylcytisine and others, tannins and terpenoids. The terpenoid mixture consists of actein, 12-acetylactein and cimigoside. Other constituents found in the plant include acetic, butyric, formic, isoferulic, oleic, palmitic and salicylic acids, racemosin, formononetin (an isoflavone), phytosterols, acteina (resinous mixture) and volatile oil.[8]

An amorphous resinous substance called cimicifugin (macrotin) accounts for approximately 15% to 20% of the root. Cimigoside (cimifugoside) and 27–deoxyactein have also been isolated.[9,10]

PHARMACOLOGY: The purported estrogenic effects of the plant could not be reproduced in extensive tests in mice. In one study, there was no evidence of a direct or indirect influence on gonadal function.[11] However, other studies indicate that methanol extracts of *C. racemosa* contain substances that bind to estrogen receptors.[12] Intraperitoneal injection of the extract in ovariectomized rats caused a selective reduction in luteinizing hormone (LH) level with almost no effect on follicle-stimulating hormone (FSH) or prolactin levels.[13]

In women treated for 8 weeks with the commercial product *Remifemin* and luteinizing hormone but not follicle-stimulating hormone, levels were reduced significantly. This product is used for the management of menopausal hot flashes. Analysis of the commercial product identified at least three fractions that contribute synergistically to the suppression of LH and bind to estrogen receptors. These data suggest that black cohosh has a measurable effect on certain reproductive hormones.[14] The product may offer an alternative to conventional hormone replacement therapy (HRT). In patient populations with a history of estrogen-dependent cancer (although it possesses some estrogenic activity), *Remifemin* shows no stimulatory effects on established breast tumor cell lines dependent on estrogen's presence. Instead, inhibitory actions were seen. In addition, the product exerts no effect on endometrium, so there is no need to "oppose" therapy with progesterone as with conventional HRT. The plant extract's action proves to be more like estriol than estradiol, which is associated with higher risk for breast, ovarian and endometrial cancers. Estriol exerts its effects mainly on the vaginal lining rather than the uterine lining, as estradiol does. More studies are needed, however, to address osteoporosis and bone health with use of the product.[4]

One report finds no signs of uterine growth and vaginal cornification in ovariectomized rats given black cohosh extract. This helps to confirm that the plant's beneficial effects on menopausal discomfort cannot be explained as the traditional estrogenic type.[15]

A clinical and endocrinologic study has been performed in 60 patients under 40 years old who had hysterectomies.

Four randomized treatment groups included estriol, conjugated estrogens, estrogen-gestagen sequential therapy or black cohosh extract. Results of this report showed no significant differences between groups in success of therapy.[16]

Other actions of black cohosh include: Constituent actein (it has been shown to have a hypotensive effect in rabbits and cats and causes peripheral vasodilation in dogs);[17,18] antimicrobial activity (both by black cohosh[19] and related species *Cimicifuga dahurica*);[8] in vivo hypocholesteremic activity; and therapy for patients with peripheral arterial disease (by causing peripheral vasodilation and increase in blood flow from constituent acteina).[8]

TOXICOLOGY: Overdose of black cohosh may cause nausea, vomiting, dizziness, nervous system and visual disturbances, reduced pulse rate and increased perspiration. The constituent acteina does not possess toxicity in animal studies.[8]

Large doses of the plant may induce miscarriage.[2] Black cohosh is contraindicated in pregnancy and may cause premature birth in large doses.[8]

A case report describes a 45-year-old woman who experienced seizures, possibly related to consumption of an herbal preparation containing black cohosh.[20]

SUMMARY: Black cohosh has been used to control symptoms of menopause as an alternative to conventional HRT therapy. The plant seems to have no effect on estrogen-dependent cancers and may even exhibit inhibitory effects against the disease. Black cohosh may also be useful in other areas such as treatment for hypercholesteremia or peripheral arterial disease. Overdose of the plant reportedly causes nausea, dizziness and nervous system disturbances. It is contraindicated for use in pregnant women.

PATIENT INFORMATION – Black Cohosh

Uses: Black cohosh has been used to help manage some symptoms of menopause and as an alternative to HRT therapy. It may be useful for hypercholesteremia treatment or peripheral arterial disease.

Side Effects: Overdose causes nausea, dizziness, nervous system and visual disturbances, reduced pulse rate and increased perspiration.

---

[1] Meyer JE. *The Herbalist*. Hammond, IN: Hammond Book Co., 1934.
[2] Dobelis IN, ed. *Magic and Medicine of Plants*. Pleasantville, NY: Reader's Digest Association, 1986.
[3] Tyler V. *Pharmacy in History* 1995;37(1):24-28.
[4] Murray M. *Am J Nat Med* 1997;4(3):3-5.
[5] Linde H. *Archiv Der Pharmazie Und Berichte Der Deutschen Pharmazeutischen Gesellschaft* 1967;300(10):885-92.
[6] Linde H. *Arch Pharm Ber Disch Pharm Ges* 1967;300(12):982-92.
[7] Linde H. *Arch Pharm Ber Disch Pharm Ges* 1968;301(5):335-41.
[8] Newall C, et al. *Black Cohosh Herbal Medicines*. London, England: Pharmaceutical Press, 1996;80-81.
[9] Duke JA. Handbook of Medicinal Herbs. Boca Raton, FL: CRC Press, 1985.
[10] Berger S, et al. *Planta Med* 1988;54:579.
[11] Siess VM, et al. *Arzneimittelforschung* 1960;10:514.
[12] Jarry H, et al. *Planta Medica* 1985;(4):316-19.
[13] Jarry H, et al. *Planta Medica* 1985;(1):46-49.
[14] Duker E, et al. *Planta Medica* 1991;57(5):420-24.
[15] Einer-Jensen N, et al. *Maturitas* 1996;25(2):149-53.
[16] Lehmann-Willenbrock E, et al. *Zentralbl Gynakol* 1988;110(10):611-18.
[17] Genazzani E, et al. *Nature* 1962;194:544.
[18] Corsano S, et al. *Gazz Chimica Ital* 1969;99:915.
[19] Bukowiecki H, et al. *Acta Pol Pharm* 1972;29:432.
[20] Shuster J. *Hosp Pharm* 1996 Dec;31:1553-54.

Black Culver's Root

SCIENTIFIC NAME(S): *Veronica virginica = Veronicastrum virginicum* (L) Farw. (syn: *V. sibiricum* L. Pennell, *V. Sibirica* L.) *Leptandra virginica* (Nutt.)[1] Fam: Scrophulariaceae

COMMON NAME(S): Black Root, Culver's Root, Culveris Root, Culvers Physic, Physic Root, Bowman's Root, Brinton Root, Hini, Leptandra, Leptandra-Wurzel, Oxadody, Tall Speedwell, Tall Veronica Whorlywort[1,2,3]

BOTANY: Black culver's root is a tall, herbaceous perennial consisting of a simple, erect stem growing from approximately 0.9 to 2 m tall. Whorled leaves (from 4 to 7) terminate in spikes of white flowers approximately 8 to 25 cm long, which bloom in July through August. The purple flower variety is termed *Leptandra purpurea*. Native to North America, but growing elsewhere, black culver's root prefers meadows and rich woodlands. The medicinal parts of the plant include the dried rhizome with the roots.[2,3]

HISTORY: The first documented use of culver's root was when Puritan leader Cotton Mather requested it as a remedy for his daughter's tuberculosis in 1716. Culver's root was used by early physicians as a powerful laxative and emetic. Native American tribes also used the plant and drank tea preparations to induce vomiting and to help cleanse the blood. Herbalists have used culver's root for its ability to increase the flow of bile from the liver.[2]

CHEMISTRY: Chemical analysis studies report constituents from genus *Veronicastrum* and *Veronica*,[4] and the presence of aucubin from *Veronica* species.[5] Culver's root is known to contain volatile oil, cinnamic acid derivatives (such as 4-methoxy cinnamic acid, 3,4-dimethoxy-cinnamic acid and their esters), tannins, and bitter principle leptandrin.[1,3] Asian studies involving *Veronicastrum sibiricum* list the constituents mannitol, resin, gum, phytosterols, glycoside, and saponins as also being present in the plants.[6,7,8,9]

PHARMACOLOGY: Black culver's root has been used for years as a liver tonic, for liver or gallbladder disorders, and to promote bile flow. Culver's root is also a stomach tonic, aiding in digestion. It is used both for diarrhea and chronic constipation, and hemorrhoids as well.[1,2,3] Anti-ulcer activity in rats given related species *Veronica officinalis* L. has been demonstrated.[10]

TOXICOLOGY: No health hazards have been associated with proper administration of culver's root. Avoid using with bile duct obstruction, gallstones, internal hemorrhoids, menstruation, and pregnancy.[11]

SUMMARY: Black culver's root has been used for centuries as a liver tonic and to increase the flow of bile. It may also be useful for GI problems such as indigestion, diarrhea, or constipation. No major toxicity from the plant has been reported. More studies are needed to confirm the plant's uses. A taxonomic revision of the genus is needed.

PATIENT INFORMATION – Black Culver's Root

Uses: Black culver's root has been used as a liver tonic, for liver or gallbladder disorders, and to promote bile flow. It has also been used for various GI problems; however, no studies are available to confirm these uses.

Side Effects: No health hazards have been associated with proper administration. Avoid using with bile duct obstruction, gallstones, internal hemorrhoids, menstruation, and pregnancy.[11]

---

[1] Note: This plant was assigned by Linnaeus to the genus *Veronica*, but later was put in genus *Leptandra* by Nuttall, which is now used by present-day botanists. Different taxonomic names are confusing and a revision of the genus is needed.[1,2,3]

[1] Hocking G. *A Dictionary of Natural Products*. Medford, NJ: Plexus Publishing, Inc. 1997;438, 846.

[2] Dwyer J, Rattray D, eds. *Magic and Medicine of Plants*. Pleasantville, NY: The Reader's Digest Assoc., Inc. 1986;156.

[3] http://botanical.com/botanical/mgmh/b/blaroo53.html

[4] Swiatek L. Aucubin content in medicinal plants from *Veronica* species. *Acta Pol Pharm* 1968;25(6):597-600. [Polish.]

[5] Shimada H, et al. Studies on the constituent of plants of genus *Pedicularis*, *Veronicastrum*, and *Veronica*. *Yakugaku Zasshi* 1971;91(1):137-38. [Japanese.]

[6] Lee S, et al. Chemical components of the root of *Veronicastrum sibiricum* Pennell. *Saengyak Hakhoechi* 1987;18(3):168-76.

[7] Zhou B, et al. Chemical constituents of *Veronicastrum sibiricum* (L.) Pennell. *Zhongguo Zhongyao Zazhi* 1992;17(1):35-6, 64.

[8] Zhou B, et al. Determination of the active constituent in *Veronicastrum sibiricum* (L.) Pennell. *Zhongguo Zhongyao Zazhi* 1992;17(2):102-03, 127. [Chinese.]

[9] Lin W, et al. Structures of new cinnamoyl glucoside from the roots of *Veronicastrum sibiricum*. *Yaoxue Xuebao* 1995;30(10):752-56.

[10] Scarlat M, et al. Experimental anti-ulcer activity of *Veronica officinalis* L. extracts. *J Ethnopharmacol* 1985;13(2):157-63.

[11] Brinker F. Herb Contraindications and Drug Interactions. 2nd ed. Sandy, OR: Eclectic Medical Publications, 1998.

Bloodroot

SCIENTIFIC NAME(S): *Sanguinaria canadensis* L. Family: Papaveraceae

COMMON NAME(S): Bloodroot, red root, red puccoon, tetterwort, Indian red plant, Indian plant, sanguinaria

BOTANY: This perennial grows in rich woods from Ontario to Manitoba, Florida and Oklahoma. It grows close to the ground and produces a large white flower in April. The stout rhizome contains a red juice that oozes following damage to the root; hence the name, bloodroot. The root and rhizome are collected and dried for use.

HISTORY: Blood root has a long history of use, especially in Russia and North America. A root tea was used externally by American Indian tribes for the treatment of rheumatisms. Other folk uses included the treatment of warts, nasal polyps and skin cancers. During the mid-1800s, topical preparations containing bloodroot extracts were used as part of the "Fell Technique" for the treatment of breast tumors. Solutions of the root were also used as a dental analgesic. Extract of the root has been used as an emetic and expectorant[1] and in combination products as a cough remedy.[2] A number of these folk uses have spurred research into the pharmacology of this plant.

CHEMISTRY: Bloodroot contains a number of compounds, many of which are pharmacologically active. These include the related isoquinoline derivatives sanguinarine, chelerythrine, protopine, homochelidonine[3] and sanguidimerine,[4] berberine, coptisine and sanguirubine.[5] The chemical structure of many of these compounds is similar to that of alkaloids found in *Fagara zanthoxlyoides*, a plant used in Africa for chew sticks.[6]

PHARMACOLOGY: Sanguinarine and its related compounds can induce slight central nervous system depression and narcosis if ingested. These compounds have papaverine-like action on smooth and heart muscle. It inhibits sodium/potassium ATPase in the guinea pig brain and can react with nucleophiles in particular sulfhydryl enzymes thereby inhibiting oxidative decarboxylation of pyruvate.[7]

Because of its long folk history in the treatment of cancers, the root has been investigated in detail for its antineoplastic activity. The alkaloids sanguinarine and chelerythrine have long been known to exert a distinct antineoplastic effect on Ehrlich carcinoma in mice;[8] more recently, the compounds were found to be effective in controlling mouse sarcomas.[9] Carcinomas of the human nose and ear have responded to topical treatment with a preparation containing bloodroot extract.[10]

Bloodroot toothpastes are commercially available for use in the reduction of plaque. A large body of well-designed studies has found that toothpastes and oral rinses containing sanguinarine help reduce and limit the deposition of dental plaque in as little as 8 days.[6] Sanguinarine contains a negatively charged iminiun ion, which permits it to bind to dental plaque.[11] Sanguinarine is effective in vitro against a number of common oral bacteria, some of which are considered to play an important role in plaque formation.[12,13] Bloodroot extracts have also been shown to reduce glycolysis activity in saliva.[14]

TOXICOLOGY: Despite the general opinion that bloodroot is considered to have a low oral toxicity potential,[15] its ingestion has been discouraged because of safety concerns. Sanguinarine appears to be very poorly absorbed from the gastrointestinal tract.[7]

The LD^{50} of sanguinarine administered to rats is approximately 1.66 g/kg orally and 29 mg/kg IV.[7] When applied topically, the LD^{50} exceeded 200 mg/kg in the rabbit.

When ingested in large doses, extracts of the root produced nausea and vomiting. Sanguinarine may cause slight CNS depression. In large doses in animals it may result in hypotension, shock and coma. It has been used to produce experimental glaucoma in animals,[16] but the potential for inducing this disease in humans is unknown.

Sanguinarine is a mild irritant to the eye and dust of the root irritates mucous membranes.[17] Sanguinarine rinses in concentrations ranging from 0.03% to 0.045% generally did not induce mucosal irritation. No dermal sensitization or irritation has been noted in humans. Although the oral toxicity is low, it is suggested that reasonable precautions be used during processing of the crude drug to protect against inhalation exposure.[18] It is not mutagenic in the Ames mutagen assay.[7]

If ingested in large quantities, gastric lavage or emesis followed by symptomatic treatment has been suggested if tolerated by the patient.[19]

SUMMARY: Bloodroot is an old-time herbal remedy that continues to find use in modern society. While its oral toxicity is low, its ingestion is not recommended. However, its topical use as a mouthwash and toothpaste to fight plaque has been documented and products containing bloodroot extracts find use in modern dentistry.

PATIENT INFORMATION – Bloodroot

Uses: Used externally in folk remedies to treat rheumatism, warts, polyps and cancers. Evidence indicates derived compounds are antineoplastic. Derivatives in mouthwash and toothpaste limit dental plaque.

Side Effects: Because of low oral toxicity, ingestion is not recommended.

---

[1] Morton JF. *Major Medicinal Plants*. Springfield, IL: C.C. Thomas, 1977.

[2] Leung AY. *Encyclopedia of Common Natural Ingredients Used in Food, Drugs, and Cosmetics*. New York, NY: J. Wiley and Sons, 1990.

[3] Henry TA. *The Plant Alkaloids*. Philadelphia, PA: Blakiston Co., 1949.

[4] Tin-Wa M, et al. Structure of sanguidimerine, a new major alkaloid from *Sanguinaria canadensis* (Papaveraceae). *J Pharm Sci* 1972;61(11):1846.

[5] William JJ, Hui-lin Li. *Lloydia* 1957; 33(3A):1.

[6] Southgard GL, et al. *J Am Dent Assoc* 1984;108:338.

[7] Becci PJ, et al. Short-term toxicity studies of sanguinarine and of two alkaloid extracts of *Sanguinaria canadensis* L. *J Toxicol Environ Health* 1987;20:199.

[8] Stickl O. *Virchow's Arch [A]* 1929;270:801.

[9] Shear MJ, Hartwell JL. *Cancer Chemother Rep* 1960;July:19.

[10] Phelan JT, Juardo J. *Surgery* 1963;53:310.

[11] Bonesvoll P, Gjermo A. *Arch Oral Biol* 1978;23:289.

[12] Dzink JL, Socransky SS. *Antimicrob Agents Chemother* 1985;27:663.

[13] Eisenberg AD, et al. *J Dent Res* 1985;64:341.

[14] Boulware RT, et al. *J Dent Res* 1984;63:1274.

[15] Lewis WH, Elvin-Lewis MPF. *Medical Botany*. New York, NY: J. Wiley and Sons, 1977.

[16] Hakim, et al. *Nature* 1961;189:198.

[17] Duke JA. *Handbook of Medicinal Herbs*. Boca Raton, FL: CRC Press, 1985.

[18] Schwarts H, et al. *Toxicologist* 1985;5:702.

[19] Hardin JW, Arena JM. *Human Poisoning from Native and Cultivated Plants*, ed. 2. Durham, NC: Duke University, 1974.

[20] Meyer JE. *The Herbalist*. Hammond, IN: Hammond Book Co., 1934.

Blue Cohosh

SCIENTIFIC NAME(S): *Caulophyllum thalictroides* (L.) Michx. Family Berberidaceae (barberries)

COMMON NAME(S): Blue cohosh, squaw root, papoose root, blue ginseng, yellow ginseng

BOTANY: Blue cohosh is an early spring perennial herb whose yellowish-green flowers mature into bitter, bright blue seeds. It is found throughout woodlands of the eastern and midwestern United States, especially in the Allegheny Mountains. The matted, knotty rootstock, collected in the autumn, is used for medicinal purposes. The root of an Asian species, *C. robustum* Maxim., has also been used medicinally.

HISTORY: Blue cohosh was used by Native Americans; the name "cohosh" comes from the Algonquin name of the plant. It was used by Menomini, Meskawi, Ojibwe, and Potawatomi tribes for menstrual cramps, to suppress profuse menstruation, and to induce contractions in labor.[1] It was widely used in 19th century Eclectic medicine as an emmenagogue, parturient, and antispasmodic. It continues to be used for regulating the menstrual cycle and for inducing uterine contractions.

CHEMISTRY: The quinolizidine alkaloids anagyrine, baptifoline, and N-methylcytisine were isolated from blue cohosh rhizomes.[2] Other lupine alkaloids have been detected.[3] In addition to the quinolizidines, the aporphine alkaloid magnoflorine is found in substantial quantities.[2] Levels of the major quinolizidine alkaloids in herbal preparations have been determined by gas chromatography.[4] Blue cohosh root also contains triterpene saponins derived from hederagenin;[5] however, these saponins have not been purified or elucidated by modern chemical techniques. The saponins of the related species *C. robustum* have recently been more thoroughly characterized as a series of hederagenin bisdesmosides.[6]

PHARMACOLOGY: N-methylcytisine (caulophylline) was found to be a nicotinic agonist in animals[7] and to displace [3H]nicotine from nicotinic acetylcholine receptors with 50 nm potency.[8] It was essentially inactive at muscarinic receptors. Other quinolizidine alkaloids were considerably less potent nicotinic ligands, with anagyrine having IC50 values greater than 100 mcm in these test systems.[8]

Magnoflorine has its own pharmacological properties, decreasing arterial blood pressure in rabbits and inducing hypothermia in mice, as well as inducing contractions in the isolated pregnant rat uterus and stimulating isolated guinea pig ileal preparations in cell membranes.[9] The blue cohosh saponins have uterine stimulant effects, as well as cardiotoxicity presumably due to vasoconstriction of coronary blood vessels.[10] Extracts of *Caulophyllum* given to rats were found to inhibit ovulation and affect the uterus.[11] The saponins of the Siberian species *C. robustum* (caulosides) have antimicrobial activity.[12] A mechanism for cytotoxicity has been suggested for cauloside C involving formation of pH-dependent channels.[13]

TOXICOLOGY: Blue cohosh berries are poisonous to children when consumed raw although the roasted seeds have been used as a coffee substitute. The root can cause contact dermatitis.[14] The alkaloid anagyrine is a teratogen in ruminants,[15] causing "crooked calf syndrome." Another quinolizidine alkaloid in the plant, N-methylcytisine, was teratogenic in a rat embryo culture.[3] The skeletal malformations seen in calves have been postulated to be due to the action of the quinolizidine alkaloids on muscarinic and nicotinic receptors of the fetus, preventing normal fetal movements required for proper skeletal development.

A case was reported in which a newborn human infant, whose mother was administered blue cohosh to promote uterine contractions, was diagnosed with acute MI associated with CHF and shock. The infant eventually recovered after being critically ill for several weeks.[16] The FDA Special Nutritionals Adverse Event Monitoring System notes fetal toxicity cases of stroke and aplastic anemia following ingestion by the mother.

SUMMARY: Blue cohosh root is a dangerous product that can be toxic to humans. While it appears to be effective for inducing uterine contractions, its toxicity appears to outweigh any medical benefit.

PATIENT INFORMATION – Blue Cohosh

Uses: Blue cohosh has been used to induce uterine contractions. It is widely advertised on the internet but is dangerous (see Toxicology and Side Effects).

Side Effects: Blue cohosh root is a dangerous product. Its toxicity appears to outweigh any medical benefit.

[1] Erichsen-Brown C. *Medicinal and other uses of North American plants. A historical survey with special reference to the Eastern Indian tribes.* NY: Dover Press, 1980;355.

[2] Flom M, et al. Isolation and characterization of alkaloids from *Caulophyllum thalictroides. J Pharm Sci* 1967;56:1515-17.

[3] Kennelly E, et al. Detecting potential teratogenic alkaloids from blue cohosh rhizomes using an in vitro rat embryo culture. *J Nat Prod* 1999;62:1385-89.

[4] Betz J, et al. Gas chromatographic determination of toxic quinolizidine alkaloids in blue cohosh *Caulophyllum thalictroides* (L.) Michx. *Phytochem Anal* 1998;9:232.

[5] McShefferty J, et al. Caulospogenin and its identity with hederagenin. *J Chem Soc* 1956;449:2314.

[6] Strigina L, et al. Cauloside A, a new triterpenoid glycoside from *Caulophyllum robustum* Maxim.: Identification of cauloside A. *Phytochem* 1975;14:1583.

[7] Scott C, et al. The pharmacological action of N-methylcytisine. *J Pharmacol Exp Ther* 1943;79:334.

[8] Schmeller T, et al. Binding of quinolizidine alkaloids to nicotinic and muscarinic acetylcholine receptors. *J Nat Prod* 1994;57:1316-19.

[9] El-Tahir K. Pharmacological actions of magnoflorine and aristolochic acid-1 isolated from the seeds of *Aristolochia bracteata. Int J Pharmacognosy* 1991;29:101.

[10] Ferguson H, et al. A pharmacologic study of a crystalline glycoside of *Caulophyllum thalictroides. J Am Pharm Assoc (Sci Ed)* 1954;43:16.

[11] Chandrasekhar K, et al. Proceedings: Observation on the effect of low and high doses of Caulophyllum on the ovaries and the consequential changes in the uterus and thyroid in rats. *J Reprod Fertil* 1974;38:236-37.

[12] Anisimov M. [The antimicrobial activity of the triterpene glycosides of *Caulophyllum robustum* Maxim.] *Antibiotiki* 1972;17:834-37. Russian.

[13] Likhatskaya G, et al. The pH-dependent channels formed by cauloside C. *Adv Exp Med Biol* 1996;404:239-49.

[14] Hardin J, et al. *Human poisoning from native and cultivated plants* Durham, NC: Duke University Press,1974;60.

[15] Keeler R. Lupin alkaloids from teratogenic and nonteratogenic lupins. III. Identification of anagyrine as the probable teratogen by feeding trials. *J Toxicol Environ Health* 1976;1:887-98.

[16] Jones T, et al. Profound neonatal congestive heart failure caused by maternal consumption of blue cohosh herbal medication. *J Pediatr* 1998;132:550-52.

Boldo

SCIENTIFIC NAME(S): *Peumus boldus* Molina also referred to as *Boldu boldus* [Molina] Lyons and *Boldea fragrans* Gay. Family: Monimiaceae

COMMON NAME(S): Boldo, boldus, boldoa, boldea

BOTANY: An evergreen shrub or small tree native to central Chile, Peru and Morocco.

HISTORY: In Chile, the yellowish-green fruit is eaten, its bark used in tanning and its wood used for charcoal.[1] Boldo leaves have been used by South American natives against diseases of the liver and for the treatment of gallstones.[2] The plant is used in homeopathy in the treatment of digestive disorders, as a laxative, choleretic (a stimulant of bile secretion), diuretic[3] and for hepatic disturbances.[1] The leaves have also been used for worms, urogenital inflammations (eg, gonorrhea, syphilis), gout, rheumatism, head colds and earaches.[4] Boldo extract is used as a flavoring for alcoholic beverages.

CHEMISTRY: The alkaloid fraction has been reported to contain at least 17 alkaloids.[5] Dried boldo leaves contain a total alkaloid content of 0.25% to 0.5%.[6] The alkaloid boldine comprises approximately 0.1%.[7] The leaves also contain about 2% volatile oils[8] and the glycoside bolden or boldoglucin.[9]

PHARMACOLOGY: The choleretic activity of the plant is due to the alkaloid boldine[5] which also causes diuresis,

increasing urinary excretion by 50% in dogs.[10] The pharmacologic effects of the volatile oils are similar to those of boldine.[8] Boldo leaves, like the American wormseed fruit (*Chenopodium ambrosioides*), contain ascaridole, an anthelmintic, in its volatile oils.[11]

TOXICOLOGY: Oral doses of 0.5 mg/g were needed to kill mice, while doses of 15 g caused fatal intoxications in dogs.[2] Death was due to respiratory depression. Physiologically, boldus stimulates the central nervous system in particular, causing exaggerated reflexes, disturbed coordination and convulsions. In large doses, it causes paralysis of both the motor and sensory nerves and eventually the muscle fibers as well, causing death due to respiratory arrest.[1]

SUMMARY: Boldo leaves are included in herbal teas as a diuretic, "hepatic tonic" and laxative. The plant is used widely in Europe and Canada. Although no data are available comparing its effect to standard diuretic agents, boldo often causes clinically significant diuresis.

PATIENT INFORMATION – Boldo

Uses: The fruit is eaten and boldo extracts used to flavor alcoholic beverages. Leaves are widely used in teas, tonics, etc., as diuretic, laxative and treatment for liver, gallbladder and other conditions.

Side Effects: Boldo is a CNS stimulant. Large doses cause paralysis and death.

---

[1] Osol A, Farrar G, eds. *The Dispensatory of the U.S., 25th ed.* Philadelphia, PA: Lippincott, 1955.
[2] Genest K, Hughes DW. *Can J Pharm Sci* 1965;3:85.
[3] DaLegnano LP. The Medicinal Plants. *Edizione Mediterranea* 1968.
[4] Duke JA. *The Handbook of Medicinal Herbs.* Boca Raton, FL: CRC Press, 1985.
[5] Hughes DW, et al. Alkaloids of *Peumus boldus.* Isolation of (+) Reticuline and Isoboldine. *J Pharm Sci* 1968;57:1023.
[6] Rueggett A. *Helv Chim Acta* 1959;42:754.

[7] Windholz M, et al The Merck Index, 10th ed. Rahway, NJ: Merck & Co., 1983.
[8] Guici G. *Boll Soc Ital Biol Sper* 1932;7:992.
[9] Reynolds JE, et al. *Martindale – The Extra Pharmacopoeia, 29th ed.* London: The Pharmaceutical Press, 1989.
[10] Kreitmar H. *Pharmazie* 1952;7:507.
[11] Johnson MA, Croteau R. Biosynthesis of Ascaridole: Iodide Peroxidase-Catalyzed Synthesis of a Monoterpene Endoperoxide in Soluble Extracts of *Chenopodium ambrosioides* Fruit. *Arch Biochem Biophys* 1984;235(1):254.

Boneset

SCIENTIFIC NAME(S): *Eupatorium perfoliatum* L. Family: Asteraceae

COMMON NAME(S): Boneset, thoroughwort, vegetable antimony, feverwort, agueweed, Indian sage, sweating plant, eupatorium, crosswort

BOTANY: A ubiquitous plant found growing in swamps, marshes and shores from Canada to Florida and west to Texas and Nebraska. The plant is easily recognized by its long, narrow, tapering leaves that oppose each other around a single stout stem giving the impression of one long leaf pierced at the center by the stem. Hence its name "perfolia," meaning "through the leaves." The plant grows from July to October to a height of 3 to 4 feet, flowering in late summer with white blossoms. The entire plant is hairy and light green in color.

HISTORY: Boneset has been used as a charm and as a medicinal remedy for centuries by the North American Indians. As a charm, the root fibers were applied to hunting whistles, believing they would increase the whistle's ability to call deer.[1] As an herbal remedy, Indians used boneset as an antipyretic. The early settlers used the plant to treat rheumatisms, dropsy, dengue fever, pneumonia and influenza. The name "boneset" was derived from the plant's use in the treatment of break-bone fever, a term describing the high fever that often accompanies influenza.[2]

CHEMISTRY: The plant is known to contain a glucoside (eupatorin), volatile oil, tannin, resin, inulin and wax.[3] A number of sterols and triterpenes (including sitosterol and stigmasterol) have been isolated[4,5] along with more than eight sesquiterpene lactones.[6] The flavonoids quercetin, kaempferol and eupatorin have been identified in the plant.[7]

In an analysis of nine species of *Eupatorium*, which included *E. perfoliatum*, all species were found to contain alkaloids; boneset was found to contain pyrrolizidine alkaloids.[8] Other investigators have found pyrrolizidine alkaloids in the roots of the related *E. masculatum.*[9]

PHARMACOLOGY: Based on data from early medical compendia, boneset is believed to have diuretic and laxative properties in small doses; large doses may result in emesis and catharsis.[7] The "usual" dose of boneset was the equivalent of 2 to 4 grams of plant administered as a fluid extract. When used as a household remedy, the plant has been taken as a tea ranging in concentration from 2 teaspoonfuls to 2 tablespoonfuls of crushed dried leaves and flowering tops steeped in a cup to a pint of boiling water. Boneset had been used by physicians to treat fever, but its use was supplanted by safer and more effective antipyretics. It is not known which components of boneset reduce fever, or what the relative degree of effectiveness of these compounds is. An ethanolic extract of the whole plant has been found to exhibit weak anti-inflammatory activity in rats.[7]

A number of the sesquiterpene lactones isolated from the plant and related species (ie, eupatilin, eupafolin) and flavones (eupatorin) have been shown to possess cytotoxic or antineoplastic activity.[7,10]

An extract of *E. perfoliatum* combined with other herbs has been shown to stimulate phagocyte activity in vitro.[11] Compounds isolated from the related species *E. odoratum* have been found to enhance blood coagulation by accelerating clotting time through the activation of certain clotting factors.[12] Extracts of *E. cannabinum* exert choleretic and hepatoprotective effects in rat models.[13]

TOXICOLOGY: Although few reports of adverse effects have been reported with the use of boneset, the FDA has classified this plant as an "Herb of Undefined Safety." [14] Large amounts of teas or extracts result in severe diarrhea. The identification of pyrrolizidine alkaloids in *Eupatorium* species is disconcerting. This class of alkaloids is known to cause hepatic impairment after long-term ingestion. While direct evidence for a hepatotoxic effect from boneset does not exist, there is sufficient evidence to indicate that any plant containing pyrrolizidine alkaloids should not be ingested.

The sesquiterpene lactones of the related species *E. cannabinum* L. have been reported to induce contact dermatitis, although no documented cross-allergenicity to *E. perfoliatum* has been reported.[15]

A toxic unsaturated alcohol called tremetrol may cause hypoglycemia and may induce fatty degeneration of the liver and kidneys as well as gastrointestinal hemorrhage.[16]

Symptoms of toxicity are often observed in grazing animals and include weakness, nausea, loss of appetite, thirst and constipation. Animals may show muscle trembling and drooling progressing to muscle paralysis and death. Milk sickness in humans has been attributed to boneset poisoning from animals.[16] These symptoms also are seen after ingestion of the related *E. rugosum* (white snakeroot) and the activation of a toxic component by the cytochrome P450 system appears to be required for the toxic effect to occur.[17]

SUMMARY: Boneset is an old, popular remedy for the treatment of fever. There are no controlled studies evalu-

ating its safety or effectiveness in the treatment of fevers. Although its use was denounced by the editors of the 25th edition of the US Dispensatory who noted that boneset "is never prescribed by the medical profession,"[18] a variety of unique pharmacologic activities have been characterized suggesting that further studies are warranted to establish the clinical value of this plant and its extracts. Until the safety of the pyrrolizidine alkaloids present in boneset is better understood, the use of this plant should be discouraged.

PATIENT INFORMATION – Boneset

Uses: Boneset has chiefly been used to treat fevers.

Side Effects: Large amounts of teas or extracts can cause severe diarrhea. Because of liver damage and other toxic effects of its alkaloids, the use of boneset is discouraged.

[1] Densmore F. *How Indians Used Wild Plants.* NY: Dover Publications, 1974.
[2] Dobelis IN, ed. *Magic and Medicine of Plants.* Pleasantville, NY: Reader's Digest Association, Inc., 1986.
[3] Windholz M, et al. *The Merck Index. 9th ed.* Raway, NJ: Merck and Co., 1976.
[4] Dominguez XA, et al. *Phytochemistry* 1974;13:673.
[5] Bohlmann F, Grenz M. *Chem Berlin* 1977;110:1321.
[6] Herz W, et al. *J Org Chem* 1977;42:2264.
[7] Leung AY. *Encyclopedia of Common Natural Ingredients Used in Food, Drugs and Cosmetics.* New York, NY: J. Wiley and Sons, 1980.
[8] Locock. *Lloydia* 1966;29:201.
[9] Tsuda, Marion. *Canadian J Chem* 1963;8:1919.
[10] Woerdenbag HJ, et al. Enhanced cytostatic activity of the sesquiterpene lactone eupatoriopicrin by glutathione depletion. *Br J Cancer* 1989;59:63.
[11] Wagner H, Jurcic K. Immunologic studies of plant combination preparation. *Arznforsch* 1991;41:1072.
[12] Triratana T, et al. Effect of *Eupatorium odoratum* on blood coagulation. *J Med Assoc Thai* 1991;74:283.
[13] Lexa A, et al. Choleretic and hepatoprotective properties of *Eupatorium cannabinum* in the rat. *Planta Med* 1989;55:127.
[14] Duke JA. *Handbook of Medicinal Herbs.* Boca Raton, FL: CRC Press, 1985.
[15] Evans FJ, Schmidt RJ. *Planta Medica* 1980;38:289.
[16] Spoerke DG, Jr. *Herbal Medications.* Santa Barbara, CA: Woodbridge Press, 1980.
[17] Beier RC, Norman JO. The toxic factor in white snakeroot: identity, analysis and prevention. *Vet Hum Toxicol* 1990;32:81.
[18] Osol A, Farrar GE, Jr, eds. *The Dispensatory of the United States of America, 25th ed.* Philadelphia, PA: J.B. Lippincott Co., 1955.

Borage

SCIENTIFIC NAME(S): *Borago officinalis* L. Family: Boraginaceae

COMMON NAME(S): Borage, common borage, bee bread, common bugloss, starflower, ox's tongue, cool tankard[1,2,3]

BOTANY: A hardy annual that grows to about 2 feet. The entire plant is covered with coarse hairs. Borage has oval leaves and star-shaped bright blue flowers with black anthers. The flowers bloom from May to September. It is found throughout Europe and North America. The fresh plant has a salty flavor and a cucumber-like odor.[3]

HISTORY: Borage leaves have been a part of European herbal medicine for centuries. In the Middle Ages, the leaves and flowers were used, steeped in wine, to dispel melancholy. It has been suggested for the relief of symptoms of rheumatisms, colds and bronchitis and has been said to increase breast milk production.[3] Infusions of the leaves and stems were once used to induce sweating and diuresis. Although it is now only sold as an herbal remedy, borage has been an official drug in Germany, Spain, Portugal, Romania, Venezuela and Mexico.[3] The preserved leaves, soaked in vinegar, have been used as hors d'oeuvres and are eaten like spinach.[4] An infusion of borage flowers and dried stems is valued for its refreshing effect. It is often used to accent salads, pickles, and vegetables.[3]

CHEMISTRY: The plant is devoid of significant pharmacologically active components. It contains a mucilage, tannin and traces of an essential oil. While other members of the family Boraginaceae (*Symphytum* spp. and *Heliotropium* spp.) have been found to contain pyrrolizidine alkaloids that induce liver damage, there are no reports of similar compounds being noted in *Borago* spp.

PHARMACOLOGY: Borage has essentially no pharmacologic activity. In small amounts, it may have a slight constipating effect most likely due to the tannin content.[5]

The mucilage may contribute to the purported expectorant action. The mild diuretic effect has been attributed to the presence of malic acid and potassium nitrate.[6] Borage is often found in OTC herbal preparations designed for the relief of cold symptoms. While there is no direct evidence for its beneficial action, at least one of its components has the ability to act as an expectorant.

TOXICOLOGY: Borage has been used without significant adverse effects for hundreds of years. It can be eaten raw or cooked like spinach and has been used in jams, jellies and teas. The toxicologic importance of its chemotaxonomic association with toxic members of the family Boraginaceae is not known. Current research, however, suggests that it may be harmful in large doses.[2]

SUMMARY: Borage has a long history of use in herbal medicine. It has not been associated with significant toxicity, nor is it renown for its pharmacologic activity.

PATIENT INFORMATION – Borage

Uses: Leaves and flowers may be eaten, used for tea, or steeped in wine. Although credited with increasing lactation, dispelling melancholy, relieving cold symptoms, etc., borage exhibits little pharmacological significance.

Side Effects: None known.

---

[1] Tyler VE, et al. *Pharmacognosy, 9th ed.* Philadelphia, PA: Lea and Febiger, 1988.
[2] Dobelis IN, ed. *Magic and Medicine of Plants.* Pleasantville, NY: Reader's Digest Association, 1986.
[3] Awang DVC. Herbal Medicine Borage. *Can Pharm J* 1990;123:121.
[4] Schauenberg P, Paris F. *Guide to Medicinal Plants.* New Canaan, CT: Keats Publishing, 1977.
[5] Hannig E. *Die Pharmazie* 1950;5:35.
[6] Tyler VE. *The New Honest Herbal.* Philadelphia, PA: G.F. Stickley Co., 1987.

Boron

SCIENTIFIC NAME(S): Boron, an element

COMMON NAME(S): Boron

SOURCE: The element boron (B, atomic number 5) is found in deposits in the earth's crust at a concentration of about 0.001%. It is obtained in the form of its compounds and never in its elemental state.[1] Environmental boron is taken up by plants in trace amounts, thereby contributing to dietary boron intake. Boron was originally obtained in 1895 from the reduction of boric anhydride; today this remains a commercially important way to produce impure boron. Pure boron takes the form of clear red or black crystals, depending upon its crystalline shape.[1] The crystals can be as hard as diamonds. The chemistry of boron is extremely complex, with entire texts devoted solely to this topic.

HISTORY: Boron has been used in nuclear chemistry as a neutron absorber. It has also been added to other metals to form harder alloys. In medicine, boron is most commonly found in the form of boric acid, which is used as a topical astringent and anti-infective, as well as an ophthalmologic irrigant. Sodium borate is bacteriostatic and is commonly added to cold creams, eye washes and mouth rinses.

PHARMACOLOGY: Over-the-counter supplements containing boron compounds are purported to enhance mental power, sometimes citing poorly substantiated studies that found alterations in the electroencephalogram in the presence of a low-boron diet. These studies also reported a correlation between a low-boron diet and a decrease in mental alertness. There is no evidence, however, that diet supplementations of boron compounds, above the levels derived from a normal balanced diet, can enhance mental acuity or improve alertness.

Because of boron's ability to absorb electromagnetic radiation, boron-based compounds are used in conjunction with radiation therapy to enhance the selective killing of neoplastic cells, particularly those of resistant neoplasia such as glioblastoma.[2]

Boric acid solutions for topical use are generally used in diluted concentrations. A 2.2% solution of boric acid is isotonic with lacrimal fluid. Because boric acid has weak antifungal and antibacterial activity, it is employed as a mild disinfectant in concentrations ranging from 2% to 10%.[3]

Boric acid powder has been used as an insect and rodent repellent, being sprinkled in corners and along floor boards. This use, however, should be avoided because of the serious toxicity that can occur if ingested orally by small children or pets.

TOXICOLOGY: Boric acid and borates are toxic when ingested or absorbed through broken skin. An oral dose of 0.3 g/kg can be fatal, and serious toxicity can occur following the ingestion of as little as 5 g in infants and 15 to 20 g in adults.[4] Boric acid solutions should be labeled not to be used on broken skin or on severely irritated or inflamed mucous membranes in order to prevent toxicity as a result of its topical absorption.

Fatalities have been reported because of confusion between boric acid and similar-looking powders (ie, baking soda, dextrose). Stringent controls should be maintained in hospitals, nursing homes and other public facilities to prevent possible intoxications due to boron-containing products.

There is no effective antidote to boron poisoning, and treatment is symptomatic and supportive. Symptoms of toxicity include irritation and sloughing of skin, gastrointestinal irritation, restlessness, weakness, kidney and liver damage, convulsions, coma or death.

SUMMARY: The element boron is distributed throughout the earth's crust and found in trace quantities in normal diets. Compounds containing boron are used medicinally, but all pose a potential toxic hazard if ingested or absorbed through nonintact skin.

PATIENT INFORMATION – Boron

Uses: Boric acid is a topical astringent, mild disinfectant and eye wash. Sprinkled in crevices and corners, boric acid powder controls rodents and insects. Sodium borate is used in cold creams, eye washes and mouth rinses. Boron compounds are used to enhance the cell selectiveness of radiation therapy.

Side Effects: Boric acid and borates are toxic and potentially fatal when ingested or absorbed through broken skin. Solutions should not be used on broken skin or severely affected mucous membranes.

[1] Windholz M, ed. *The Merck Index, ed. 10.* Rahway, NJ: Merck & Co., 1983.
[2] Haselsberger K, et al. Subcellular boron-10 localization in glioblastoma for boron neutron capture therapy with Na2B12H11SH. *J Neurosurg.* 1994;81:741.

[3] Olin BR, Hebel SK, eds. *Drug Facts and Comparisons.* St. Louis: Facts and Comparisons, July 1992.
[4] Haddad LM, Winchester JF. *Clinical Management of Poisoning and Drug Overdose.* ed. 2. Philadelphia: Saunders, 1990:1447.

Bovine Colostrum

SCIENTIFIC NAME(S): Bovine colostrum

COMMON NAME(S): Cow milk colostrum

SOURCE: Colostrum is the premilk fluid produced from mammary glands during the first 2 to 4 days after birth. It is a rich natural source of nutrients, antibodies, and growth factors for the newborn.[1]

CHEMISTRY: Colostrum contains immune factors, immunoglobulins, antibodies, proline-rich polypeptides (PRP), lactoferrin, glycoproteins, lactalbumins, cytokines (eg, interleukin 1 and 6, interferon γ), growth factors, vitamins, and minerals.[1,2,3,4,5] Specific bovine colostrum growth factor has been purified, stimulating synthesis of certain cell lines, for example.[6] Colostrokinin is also a constituent isolated from bovine colostrum, responsible for uterine and intestinal contraction, and lowering of blood pressure.[7]

PHARMACOLOGY: Bovine colostrum, with its rich pool of nutrients, has successfully supported and maintained a variety of cell cultures.[8,9,10,11,12] Various concentrations of bovine colostral constituents, including certain immunoglobulins, have been studied in calves fed colostrum or colostral supplement products.[13,14,15,16,17] Certain immune factors and antibodies also fight a variety of organisms, allergens, or toxins including pneumonia, candida, and flu. Constituent lactoferrin prevents pathogens from getting the iron they need to flourish. Lactalbumins and cytokines (interleukin 1 and 6, interferon γ) are also important as antivirals and anticancer agents.[5]

Several studies show how bovine colostrum concentrates, including G immunoglobulin isolates, are highly successful alternative agents used to improve GI health and to treat diarrhea caused by a variety of pathogens. In > 50% of AIDS patients, diarrhea and subsequent weight loss pose a problem. The severity of symptoms in some cases and sometimes unidentifiable pathogens unaffected by antibiotics welcome alternative therapy with bovine colostrum.

In one study, 29 AIDS patients received a bovine colostrum preparation. The average stool per day decreased from 7.4 before therapy to 2.2 after treatment.[18] Another report finds similar results in animals, including high capacity for neutralization of bacterial toxins and high effectiveness in treating severe diarrhea, using a specialized colostrum preparation.[19] A 25- patient study of HIV subjects with chronic diarrhea administered bovine colostrum preparation also confirms therapeutic effectiveness, resulting in 64% of patients experiencing complete (40%) or partial (24%) remission of diarrhea.[20] *Cryptosporidium*, a human GI parasite, can also cause life-threatening diarrhea in immunodeficient patients when antibiotics or other anti-diarrheals may be ineffective. Bovine colostrum therapy has reduced significantly oocyst excretion of pathogen in stools vs placebo and relieved a previously untreatable AIDS patient of severe *cryptosporidium*-associated diarrhea.[21,22] *Lactobin*, a registed bovine colostral product, shows antibody reactivity and neutralization against certain *E. coli* strains and shiga-like toxins.[23] Immunoglobulin preparation supplementation was found to protect against *Shigellosis* (*S. flexneri*), and suggests its usefulness in high-risk groups including travelers and military personnel during *Shigella* outbreaks.[24] Bovine colostrum use against organisms *Yersinia enterocolitica* and *Campylobacter jejuni* has also been reported.[25] Bovine colostrum also inhibits *Helicobacter pylori* and *Helicobacter mustelae* by binding to certain lipid receptors, which may modulate the interaction of these pathogens to their target sites.[26] One report investigates the bovine colostral immunoglobulin proteins and how they are subject to degradation by gastric acid and intestinal enzymes under certain conditions.[27] Bovine colostrum supplementation, in another report, has been shown to prevent NSAID-induced gut injury in various in vivo and in vitro models, suggesting its possible usefulness for certain ulcerative bowel conditions.[1]

The immune-boosting properties of bovine colostrum have been greatly proclaimed as performance enhancers and anti-aging/healing supplements. Certain Web pages, for instance, promote significant fitness gains for athletes, noting its "anabolic effects" and claiming it can "promote muscle growth."[28] One clinical trial finds bovine colostrum supplement to increase serum IGF-1 concentration in athletes.[29] IGF-1 is a growth factor that speeds up protein synthesis and slows catabolism.[23]

TOXICOLOGY: A few symptoms, including mild nausea and flatulence, were seen in certain trials, but most have reported bovine colostrum to be well tolerated.[18,19,20] At least 2 allerginicity studies have been performed in humans.[30,31]

SUMMARY: Bovine colostrum is rich in nutrients, immune factors, immunoglobulins, antibodies, and other important constituents, all of which benefit the immune system. Many studies have been performed resulting in its successful use for severe diarrhea in certain populations such as the immunocompromised. Bovine colostrum also has other positive GI effects and may help rebuild muscle and other tissue. There is no major toxicity associated with bovine colostrum supplementation. Continued studies will further elucidate its true benefits.

PATIENT INFORMATION – Bovine Colostrum

Uses: Bovine colostrum has been used to treat diarrhea, to improve GI health, to boost the immune system.

Side effects: Bovine colostrum appears to be safe and effective.

---

[1] Playford R, et al. Bovine colostrum is a health food supplement which prevents NSAID induced gut damage. *Gut* 1999;44:653-58.

[2] Rumbo M, et al. Detection and characterization of antibodies specific to food antigens (gliadin, ovalbumin and beta-lactoglobulin) in human serum, saliva, colostrum and milk. *Clin Exp Immunol* 1998;112(3):453-58.

[3] Behrman R, et al. *Nelson Textbook of Pediatrics* 16th ed. Philadelphia, PA: W.B. Saunders Co. 2000;155-56.

[4] Joseph M, et al. Research shows colostrum to be one of nature's most potent, broad-spectrum substances. *Chiropract J* 1998 Mar;12(6):33,41,45.

[5] Fauci A, et al. *Harrison's Principles of Internal Medicine* 14th ed. New York, NY: McGraw Hill. 1998;1753,1760.

[6] Kishkawa Y, et al. Purification and characterization of cell growth factor in bovine colostrum. *J Vet Med Sci* 1996;58:1,47-53.

[7] Budavari S, et al, eds. *The Merck Index* 11th ed, Rahway, NJ: Merck and Co. 1989.

[8] Steimer KS, et al. Serum-free growth of normal and transformed fibroblasts in milk: differential requirements for fibronectin. *J Cell Biol* 1981;88(2):294-300.

[9] Steimer KS, et al. The serum-free growth of cultured cells in bovine colostrum and in milk obtained later in the lactation period. *J Cell Physiol* 1981;109(2):223-34.

[10] Tseng MT, et al. Selective maintenance of cultured epithelial cells from DMBA-induced mammary tumours by bovine colostrum supplement. *Cell Tissue Kinet* 1983;16(1):85–92.

[11] Pakkanen R, et al. Bovine colostrum ultrafiltrate: an effective supplement for the culture of mouse-mouse hybridoma cells. *J Immunol Methods* 1994;169(1):63-71.

[12] Viander B, et al. Viable AC-2, a new adult bovine serum- and colostrum-based supplement for the culture of mammalian cells. *Biotechniques* 1996;20(4):702-7.

[13] Garry FP, et al. Comparison of passive immunoglobulin transfer to dairy calves fed colostrum or commercially available colostral-supplement products. *J Am Vet Med Assoc* 1996;208(1):107-10.

[14] Mee JF, et al. Effect of a whey protein concentrate used as a colostrum substitute or supplement on calf immunity, weight gain, and health. *J Dairy Sci* 1996;79(5):886-94.

[15] Morin DE, et al. Effects of quality, quantity, and timing of colostrum feeding and addition of a dried colostrum supplement on immunoglobulin G1 absorption in Holstein bull calves. *J Dairy Sci* 1997;80(4):747-53.

[16] Hopkins BA, et al. Effects of method of colostrum feeding and colostrum supplementation on concentrations of immunoglobuln G in the serum of neonatal calves. *J Dairy Sci* 1997;80(5):979-83.

[17] Quigley J, III, et al. Effects of a colostrum replacement product derived from serum on immunoglobulin G absorption by calves. *J Dairy Sci* 1998;81(7):1936-39.

[18] Rump JA, et al. Treatment of diarrhoea in human immunodeficiency virus-infected patients with immunoglobulins from bovine colostrum. *Clin Investig* 1992;70(7):588-94.

[19] Stephan W, et al. Antibodies from colostrum in oral immunotherapy. *J Clin Chem Clin Biochem* 1990;28(1):19-23.

[20] Plettenberg A, et al. A preparation from bovine colostrum in the treatment of HIV-positive patients with chronic diarrhea. *Clin Investig* 1993;71:42-45.

[21] Okhuysen P, et al. Prophylactic effect of bovine anti-*Cryptosporidium* hyperimmune colostrum immunoglobulin in healthy volunteers challenged with *Cryptosporidium parvum*. *Clin Infect Dis* 1998;26:1324-29.

[22] Ungar B, et al. Cessation of *Cryptosporidium*-associated diarrhea in an acquired immunodeficiency syndrome patient after treatment with hyperimmune bovine colostrum. *Gastrenterology* 1990;98:486-89.

[23] Lissner R, et al. A standard immunoglobulin preparation produced from bovine colostra shows antibody reactivity and neutralization activity against *Shiga*–like toxins and EHEC-hemolysin of *Escherichia coli* O157:H7. *Infection* 1996;24(5):378-83.

[24] Tacket CO, et al. Efficacy of bovine milk immunoglobulin concentrate in preventing ilness after *Shigella flexneri* challenge. *Am J Trop Med Hyg* 1992;47:3,276-83.

[25] Lissner R, et al. Antibody reactivity and fecal recovery of bovine immunoglobulins following oral administration of a colostrum concentrate from cows (Lactobin) to healthy volunteers. *Int J Clin Pharmacol Ther* 1998;36(5):239-45.

[26] Bitzan M, et al. Inhibition of *Helicobacter pylori* and *Helicobacter mustelae* binding to lipid receptors by bovine colostrum. *J Infect Dis* 1998;177:955-61.

[27] Petschow BW, et al. Reduction in virus-neutralizing activity of a bovine colostrum immunoglobulin concentrate by gastric acid and digestive enzymes. *J Pediatr Gastroenterol Nutr* 1994;19:228-35.58.

[28] http://www.metafoods.com/athletic.htm.

[29] Mero A, et al. Effects of bovine colostrum supplementation on serum IGF-I, IgG, hormone, and saliva IgA during training. *J Appl Physiol* 1997;83(4):1144-51.

[30] Savilahti E, et al. Low colostral IgA associated with cow's milk allergy. *Acta Paediatr Scand* 1991;80(12):1207-13.

[31] Lefranc- Millot C, et al. Comparison of the IgE titers to bovine colostral G immunoglobulins and their F(ab')2 fragments in sera of patients allergic to milk. *Int Arch Allergy Immunol* 1996;110(21):56-62.

Brahmi

SCIENTIFIC NAME(S): *Bacopa monnieri* (L.) Wettst. family: Scrophulariaceae (figworts); also known as *Bacopa monniera*, *Herpestis monniera*, or *Moniera cuneifolia*

COMMON NAME(S): Brahmi, Jalnaveri, Jalanimba, Sambrani chettu, thyme-leaved gratiola

BOTANY: *Bacopa monnieri* is a creeping herb that grows in marshy places and is frequently planted in freshwater aquaria. It is native to India but has spread throughout the tropics. The name brahmi has also been applied to *Centella asiatica* (better known as *gotu kola*), as well as *Merremia gangetica*, however most authorities consider it most appropriate for *B. monnieri*.[1] A tissue culture method has been developed for the plant.[2]

HISTORY: Brahmi is a well-known drug in the Ayurvedic medical tradition in India, and is used in many Ayurvedic herbal preparations. It has been traditionally used to treat asthma, hoarseness, insanity, epilepsy, and as a nerve tonic, cardiotonic, and diuretic.[1] It was prominently mentioned in Indian texts as early as the 6th century A.D.[3]

CHEMISTRY: The principal constituents of *B. monnieri* are triterpene saponins of the dammarane class, which have been named bacosides[4] and bacopasaponins,[5,6] and which contain 2 or 3 sugars each. The saponins are considered to be primarily responsible for the bioactivity of the plant. Due to the proclivity of the sapogenins to rearrange on acid hydrolysis,[7] the correct structures of the saponins have been difficult to elucidate, despite many chemical investigations.[8,9,10,11,12] An analytical HPLC method for the quantitation of bacoside A3 has been published.[13] The structure of 4 saponins of *B. monnieri* have also been determined by HPLC coupled to 2-D NMR, mass spectrometry, and an anthelmintic bioassay.[14] While alkaloids were initially suspected to be the CNS-active agents in brahmi,[15] the very small amounts of nicotine and other simple alkaloids are no longer considered to be of pharmacologic importance.[16] A free triterpene, bacosine, has been reported from *B. monnieri*.[17] Other reported constituents include mannitol, common plant sterols, and betulinic acid,[4] as well as glutamic and aspartic acids.[18]

PHARMACOLOGY: In mice, the ethanolic extract of *B. monnieri* was found to increase cerebral levels of GABA 15 minutes after administration.[19] Oral treatment of rats with the extract of *B. monnieri* for 24 days facilitated their ability to learn mazes.[20] A saponin fraction of *B. monnieri* reduced spontaneous motor activity in rats, and lowered rectal temperatures in mice.[21] The same extract showed tranquilizing effects in rats but did not block the conditioned avoidance response. It also protected against audiogenic seizures.[22] More recently, the extract was found to improve the performance of rats in various behavioral models of learning.[3] Furthermore, the purified bacosides A and B showed dose-dependent effects in the same rat models, as well as in a taste aversion response test.[23] Bacosine, a free triterpene isolated from the aerial parts of *B. monnieri*, was found to have analgesic effects operating through opioidergic pathways.[17] The ethanolic extract of *B. monnieri* relaxed smooth muscle preparations of guinea pig and rabbit pulmonary arteries, rabbit aorta, and guinea pig trachea by a mechanism that was postulated to involve prostacyclins.[24] The same investigators found spasmolytic effects of the ethanol extract in guinea pig ileum and rabbit jejunum to be nonspecifically mediated through calcium channels.[25] The saponins were found to have anthelmintic activity using *C. elegans* as a test organism.[14] They are also reported to be hemolytic.[26]

TOXICOLOGY: Brahmi appears to be free of reported side effects. Its CNS actions do not include serious sedation, although the potentiation of chlorpromazine's effect on conditioned avoidance responses may indicate caution with phenothiazine coadministration.[22]

SUMMARY: Brahmi is an extract of *Bacopa monnieri* used in Ayurvedic medicine as a nerve tonic and aid to learning. Animal studies lend support to these indications, however no human trials have been reported to date. It is not monographed in any of the European or American compendia.

PATIENT INFORMATION – Brahmi

Uses: Brahmi is used as a nerve tonic and an aid to learning.

Side Effects: Brahmi has no reported side effects.

Drug Interactions: Use caution when coadministering with phenothiazine.

---

[1] *The Wealth of India.* Raw Materials. Vol.2:B, Publications & Information Directorate, CSIR, New Dehli, 2-3.

[2] Tiwari V, et al. Shoot regeneration and somatic embryogenesis from different explants of Brahmi (*Bacopa monniera*). *Plant Cell Rep* 1998;17:538.

[3] Singh H, et al. Effect of *Bacopa monniera* Linn. (brahmi) extract on avoidance responses in rat. *J Ethnopharmacol* 1982;5:205.

[4] Chatterji N, et al. Chemical examination of *Bacopa monniera* Wettst.: Part I - Isolation of chemical constituents. *Indian J Chem* 1963;1:212.

[5] Garai S, et al. Dammarane-type triterpenoid saponins from *Bacopa monniera*. *Phytochemistry* 1996;42:815.

[6] Garai S, et al. Bacopasaponin D--a pseudojujubogenin glycoside from *Bacopa monniera*. *Phytochemistry* 1996;43:447.

[7] Kulshreshtha D, et al. Identification of ebelin lactone from bacoside A and the nature of its genuine sapogenin. *Phytochemistry* 1973;12:2074.

[8] Chatterji N, et al. Chemical examination of *Bacopa monniera* Wettst.: Part II - The constitution of bacoside A. *Indian J Chem* 1965;3:24.

[9] Kawai K, et al. Crystal and molecular structure of bacogenin-A1 dibromoacetate. *Acta Crystallogr* 1973;B29:2947.

[10] Kulshreshtha D, et al. Bacogenin-A1. A novel dammarane triterpene sapogenin from *Bacopa monniera*. *Phytochemistry* 1973;12:887.

[11] Jain P, et al. Bacoside A1, a minor saponin from *Bacopa monniera*. *Phytochemistry* 1993;33:449.

[12] Rastogi S, et al. Bacoside A3--a triterpenoid saponin from *Bacopa monniera*. *Phytochemistry* 1994;36:133.

[13] Pal R, et al. Quantitative determination of bacoside by HPLC. *Indian J Pharm Sci* 1998;60:328.

[14] Renukappa T, et al. Application of high-performance liquid chromatography coupled to nuclear magnetic resonance spectrometry, mass spectrometry and bioassay for the determination of active saponins from *Bacopa monniera* Wettst. *J Chromatogr A* 1999;847:109.

[15] Brown I, et al. Constituents of *Bacopa monnieri* (L.) Pennell. *J Chem Soc* 1960;2783.

[16] Schulte K, et al. Components of medicinal plants. XXXVI. Nicotine and 3-formyl-4-hydroxy- 2H-pyran from *Herpestis monniera*. *Phytochemistry* 1972;11:2649.

[17] Vohora S, et al. Analgesic activity of bacosine, a new triterpene isolated from *Bacopa monnieri*. *Fitoterapia* 1997;68:361.

[18] Ahmad S, et al. Amino acid analysis of *Intellan*, a herbal product used in enhancing brain function. *Pak J Pharm Sci* 1994;7:17.

[19] Dey P, et al. Effect of psychotropic phytochemicals on cerebral amino acid levels in mice. *Indian J Exp Biol* 1966;4:216.

[20] Dey C, et al. Effect of some centrally active phyto products on maze-learning of albino rats. *Indian J Physiol Allied Sci* 1976;30:88

[21] Ganguly D, et al. Neuropharmacological and behavioral effects of an active fraction from *Herpestis monniera*. *Indian J Physiol Pharmacol* 1967;11:33.

[22] Ganguly D, et al. Some behavioral effects of an active fraction from *Herpestis monniera*. *Indian J Med Res* 1967;55:473.

[23] Singh H, et al. Effect of bacosides A and B on avoidance responses in rats. *Phytother Res* 1988;2:70.

[24] Dar A, et al. Relaxant effect of ethanol extract of *Bacopa monniera* on trachea, pulmonary artery and aorta from rabbit and guinea pig. *Phytother Res* 1997;11:323.

[25] Dar A, et al. Calcium antagonistic activity of *Bacopa monniera* on vascular and intestinal smooth muscles of rabbit and guinea-pig. *J Ethnopharmacol* 1999;66:167.

[26] Basu N, et al. Chemical examination of *Bacopa monniera*. III. Bacoside B. *Indian J Chem* 1967;5:84.

Broom

SCIENTIFIC NAME(S): *Cytisus scoparious* (L.) Link, sometimes referred to as *Sarothamnus scoparious* (L.) Wimm. Family: Fabaceae (Papilionaceae or Leguminosae)

COMMON NAME(S): Bannal, besenginaterkraut (German), broom, broom top, ginsterkraut (German), herbe de genet a balais (French), herba genistac scopariae, herba soartii scoparii, hog week, Irish broom top (English)[1], sarothamni herb, scoparii cacumina (Latin); scotch broom, Scotch broom top (English). Scotch broom should not be confused with Spanish broom (*Spartium junceum*), which also is pharmacologically active. The related *Cytisus laburnum* (golden chain) contains the toxic alkaloid cytisine.

BOTANY: Broom is native to central and southern Europe. It grows throughout the United States along the Eastern coastline and across the Pacific Northwest. The plant grows as a deciduous bush up to 6–feet tall and possesses 5–sided, greenish, rod-like twigs with small leaves. On flowering, it show yellow, butterfly-like flowers that bloom from May to June.[1] It is often used as an outdoor ornamental to hold steep, barren banks in place. The crude drug is made up mostly of short fragments (1–2 inches) of the woody twigs.[1]

HISTORY: In early American traditional medicine, a fluid extract of broom was used as a cathartic and diuretic. Large doses of the extract were used as an emetic.[2] An alkaloid derived from the plant (sparteine) was once used to induce labor and as an antiarrhythmic, but has now been abandoned for safer compounds.

The plant has been touted as a potential drug of abuse or "legal high." In describing the preparation of the drug, some counter-culture magazines suggest that the flowers be collected and aged for about 10 days in a closed jar.[2] The moldy, dried blossoms are then pulverized, rolled in cigarette paper and smoked like marijuana.

Before the advent of hops, the tender green tops were used to impart bitterness and to increase the intoxicating effects of beer. In homeopathy, extracts of the plant are used for the management of arrhythmias, congestion of the head and throat, and occasionally for diphtheria.[3]

CHEMISTRY: The main alkaloid in the plant is l-sparteine found in the floral parts of the plant in concentrations ranging up to 0.22%, but may exceed 1.5% in other parts of the plant. In addition, the alkaloids sarothamnine,[4] genisteine,[4] lupanine[5] and oxysparteine[6] have been identified. A number of minor alkaloids and other componenets have also been isolated.[7] The flavone glycoside scoparoside has also been isolated, primarily from the flowers. Apparently, the toxic alkaloid cytisine is not present in this species.[8]

The plant alkaloids are mainly found in the stem, but are also in the epidermis and sub-epidermis. Also present are flavonoids (spiraeoside, isoquercitin, genitoside, scoparoside) as well as other kaempferol and quercetin derivatives. Isoflavones such as sarothamnoside have also been reported. Broom also contains caffeic-acid derivatives and small amounts of essential oil. The seeds contain phytohaemagglutinins or lectins.[1] Fresh flower essential oils contain cis-3–hexan-l-ol, l-octen-3–ol, benzyl alcohol, phenethyl alcohol and various phenols and acids.[9]

PHARMACOLOGY: Sparteine is a powerful oxytocic drug once used to stimulate uterine contractions. Sparteine slows the cardiac rate and shares some pharmacologic similarities with quinidine[10] and nicotine.[3] It also has antiarrhythmic effects.[11]

Scoparoside is an active diuretic and may exert a pharmacologic effect if ingested in sufficient quantities.

A number of lectins have been isolated from broom seeds and these are being used as pharmacologic probes.[12]

Broom has long been used as a tea in Europe for improved regulation of the circulation. This activity is related to the alkaloidal content, particularly sparteine. It possesses an antiarrhythmic property, based on its ability to inhibit the transport of sodium ions across the cell membrane. The alkaloid reduces overstimulation of the system that conducts the nerve impulse. Hence, impulses arising in the auricle are normalized. Sparteine extends diastole, but does not show a positive inotropic effect. With low blood pressure, this property can lead to normalization.

TOXICOLOGY: Sparteine is an oily liquid that vaporizes readily when heated. Therefore, persons who smoke broom cigarettes may inhale significant amounts of the alkaloid. One such cigarette is said to produce a feeling of relaxation and euphoria lasting about 2 hours. However, some studies indicate that doses in excess of that which one would obtain by smoking the leaves would be needed to induce euphoria; the same studies concluded that "apparently this plant is not very toxic and the use of it as a 'legal high' probably would not precipitate a severe toxic episode."[8]

Smoking broom cigarettes may pose a number of health hazards. These include adverse cardiac effects such as headaches, uterine stimulant effects and residual effects. The inhalation of moldy plant material cannot be recommended as this may be associated with the development of pulmonary aspergillosis or similar fungal infections.

Broom tea is contraindicated during pregnancy because it can increase the tonus of the gravid uterus. For similar reasons (tonus increasing properties), it is not recommended with hypertensive individuals.[1]

The FDA considers broom an unsafe herb. Symptoms of toxicity suggest nicotine poisoning and are characterized by tachycardia with circulatory collapse, nausea, diarrhea, vertigo and stupor. The seeds have been used as a coffee substitute, a dangerous and unwarranted practice.[3]

SUMMARY: Broom is a traditional medicinal herb that is found throughout many regions of the United States and Europe. Broom contains the pharmacologically active alkaloid sparteine, which has oxytocic and antiarrhythmic properties. The plant has been touted as a "legal high," but the authenticity of these experiences has been doubted. The German Commission E monograph on this herb lists its uses as an effective agent for functional disorders of the heart and circulation.[1] Nevertheless, broom is considered an unsafe herb by the FDA and should not be used in modern therapeutics.

PATIENT INFORMATION – Broom

Uses: Extracts have been used for cathartic, diuretic, emetic, antiarrhythmic and labor-inducing effects. Tender plant tops have been used to flavor beer and increase its intoxicating effect. Leaves and aged flowers have been smoked to produce euphoria.

Side Effects: Although broom appears an effective agent for heart and circulatory disorders, the FDA has designated broom an unsafe herb.

[1] Bisset NG, ed. *Herbal Drugs and Phytopharmaceuticals.* Stuttgart: Medpharm Scientific Publishers, 1994.
[2] Tyler VE. *The New Honest Herbal.* Philadelphia: G.F. Stickley Co., 1987.
[3] Duke JA. *Handbook for Medicinal Herbs.* Boca Raton, FL: CRC Press, 1985.
[4] Henry TA. *The Plant Alkaloids.* Philadelphia: Blakiston Co., 1949.
[5] Wink M, et al. Accumulation of Quinolizidine Alkaloids in Plants and Cell Suspension Cultures: General Lupinus, Cytisus, Baptisia, Genista, Laburnum, and Sophora. *Planta Med* 1983;48:253.
[6] Jusiak L, et al. Analysis of Alkaloid Extract from the Herb of *Cytisus scoparious* by Chromatography on Moist Buffered Paper and Countercurrent Distribution. *Acta Pol Pharm* 1967;24(6):618.
[7] Murakoshi I, et al. (-)-3α, 13β -Dihydroxylupanine from *Cytisus scoparius.* *Phytochem* 1986;25(2):521.
[8] Brown JK, Malone MH. "Legal Highs" — Constituents, Activity, Toxicology, and Herbal Folklore. *Pacific Information Service on Street Drugs* 1977;5(3–6):21.
[9] Kurihara T, Kikuchi M. Studies on the Constituents of Flowers, XIII. On the Components of the Flower of *Cytisus scoparius* Link. *Yakugaku Zasshi* 1980;100(10):1054.
[10] Bowman WC, Rand MJ. *Textbook of Pharmacology.* Ondon: Bowman & Blackwell Scientific Publishers, 1980.
[11] Rashack VM. Wirkungen von Spartein und Sparteinderivaten auf Herz and Kreislauf. *Arzneim-Forsch* 1974;24(5):753.
[12] Young NM, et al. Structural differences between two lectins from Cytisus scoparius, both specific for D-galactose and N-acetyl-D-galactosamine. *Biochem J* 1984;222(1):41.

Buchu

SCIENTIFIC NAME(S): *Agathosma betulina* (Berg.) Pillans (syn. *Barosma betulina* [Berg.] Bartl. & Wendl.) (short buchu); *B. serratifolia* (Curt.) Willd. (long buchu); *B. crenulata* (L.) Hook. (ovate buchu). Family: Rutaceae. These plants should not be confused with "Indian buchu" (*Myrtus communis* L.), which is native to the Mediterranean regions.

COMMON NAME(S): Bookoo, buku, diosma, bucku, bucco.[1]

BOTANY: Buchu is harvested from the dried leaves obtained from three species of *Barosma*. The species derive their common names from the shape of the aromatic leaf.[2] The buchus grow up to 6 feet tall as low, bushy, drought-resistant shrubs with colorful blossoms. The leaves are described as yellowish green to brown, glossy and leathery, revealing oil-glandular dots on the underside. The three species produce oval, serrated leaves with the leaf of *B. serratifolia* being the longest and most slender. Harvesting of the leaves occurs in summer. Most commonly, *B. betulina* is used in commerce. Native to South Africa, buchu undergoes hillside cultivation. Odor and taste of the plants is described as spicy, resembling black currant but also reminiscent of a mixture between rosemary and peppermint.[3,4] Buchu oil is sometimes added as a component of black currant flavorings.

HISTORY: The Hottentots employed the leaves for the treatment of a great number of ailments. Early patent medicines sold in the United States hailed the virtues of the plant and its volatile oil for the management of diseases ranging from diabetes to nervousness. The drug had been included in the US National Formulary and was described as a diuretic and antiseptic. Its use has since been abandoned in favor of more effective diuretics and antibacterials. Buchu remains a popular ingredient in over-the-counter herbal diuretic preparations.[5]

Buchu was first exported to Britain in 1790. In 1821, it was listed in the *British Pharmacopoeia* as a medicine for "cystitis, urethritis, nephritis and catarrh of the bladder."[4]

CHEMISTRY: Buchu leaves contain from 1.5% to 3.5% volatile oil. Over 100 components exist in the oil,[1,5] including diosphenol (the main component in distilled oil, also called buchu camphor, barosma camphor or 1–pulegone), limonene, methone, pulegone, terpinen-4-ol and p-menthan-3-on-8-thiol (responsible for the aroma of the plant).[2,3,6]

Flavonoids include diosmetin, quercetin, diosmin, quercetin-3,7-diglucoside and rutin. Other constituents include mucilage, resin, thiamine and sulfur compounds. Coumarins have been reported from other *agathosma* species.[4,6]

PHARMACOLOGY: No scientific evidence is available to justify buchu's herbal uses, but its **diuretic** and **anti-inflammatory** effects may be attributed to the volatile oil and flavonoid's irritant nature.[6] Diosphenol, the flavonoids and terpinen-4-ol may contribute to the plant's diuretic activity but this action of buchu teas is probably no greater than that of the xanthine alkaloids in coffee or tea.[7] Buchu is listed in the German Commission E Monographs to treat inflammation, kidney and urinary tract infections and is also used as a diuretic, but the monograph explains that the plant's activity in these claimed uses has not been substantiated.[3]

Other reported uses of buchu include **carminative** action, treatment for **cystitis, urethritis, prostatitis, gout** and as a **stomach tonic**.[8]

An infusion of the leaves has been used gynecologically as a douche for **leukorrhea** and for **yeast infections**.[4] Diosphenol may be responsible for buchu's antibacterial effects.[3]

Despite the lack of evidence, buchu is still used today in western herbal medicine for urinary tract ailments, cystitis or urethritis prophylaxis and prostatitis. It is also used in combination with other herbs such as cornsilk, juniper and uva-ursi.[4]

TOXICOLOGY: There is little evidence to suggest that the casual intake of teas brewed from buchu are harmful.[9] Poisoning has not been reported.[3,6] Essential oil components diosmin and pulegone can cause GI and renal irritation.[3,6] Pulegone is known to be an abortifacient and to increase menstrual flow; therefore, use is not recommended during pregnancy. Pulegone is also a hepatotoxin, present in the plant "pennyroyal," in larger quantities.[4,5]

SUMMARY: Buchu leaves and extracts are recognized in herbal medicine as diuretics and weak antiseptics.

Their use is a popular treatment of kidney and urinary tract infections and prostatitis. More clinical trials are needed to substantiate these claims. There is little known toxicity associated with the plant, but because some of its components are associated with uterine stimulation, it is not recommended during pregnancy.

PATIENT INFORMATION – Buchu

Uses: Buchu has been used to treat inflammation and kidney and urinary tract infections; as a diuretic and as a stomach tonic. Other uses include carminative action and treatment of cystitis, urethritis, prostatitis and gout. It has also been used for leukorrhea and yeast infections.

Side Effects: Buchu can cause stomach and kidney irritation and can be an abortifacient. It can also induce increased menstrual flow.

---

[1] Leung AY. *Encyclopedia of Common Natural Ingredients Used in Food, Drugs, and Cosmetics*, NY: J Wiley and Sons, 1980.

[2] Gentry HS, *Economic Botany* 1961;15:326.

[3] Bisset N. *Herbal Drugs and Phytopharmaceuticals*. Stuttgart, Germany: CRC Press 1994;102-3.

[4] Chevallier A. *Encyclopedia of Medicinal Plants*. New York, NY: DK Publishing. 1996;67.

[5] Osol A, et al. *The Dispensatory of the USA, 25 ed.* Philadelphia, PA: J. B. Lippincott Co. 1960;196-97.

[6] Newall C, et al. *Herbal Medicines*. London, England: Pharmaceutical Press. 1996;51.

[7] *Medical Letter* 1979;21:29.

[8] Duke J. *CRC Handbook of Medicinal Herbs*. Boca Raton, FL: CRC Press Inc. 1989;77.

[9] DerMarderosian AH, Liberti LE. *Natural Product Medicine*. Philadelphia: G. F. Stickley Co, 1988.

Bupleurum

SCIENTIFIC NAME(S): *Bupleurum chinense* DC., related species include *B. falcatum* L., *B. scorzoneraefolium* , *B. fruticosum* L., *B. ginghausenii, B. rotundifolium* L., *B. stewartianum.* Family: Umbelliferae[1]

COMMON NAME(S): Thoroughwax, hare's ear root, chai hu (Chinese)

BOTANY: Bupleurum is a perennial herb that grows mainly in China, but also is cultivated in other areas. The plant grows to ≈ 1 m in height and requires plenty of sun to flourish. The leaves are long and sickle-shaped with parallel veining. Terminal clusters of small, yellow flowers appear in autumn.[2,3]

HISTORY: Bupleurum is a traditional Chinese herb dating back to the first century B.C. It is one of China's "harmony" herbs purported to organs and energy in the body. Bupleurum has been used as a liver tonic, with spleen and stomach toning properties as well. The plant has also been said to clear fevers and flu, promote perspiration, and alleviate female problems.[1,2,3]

CHEMISTRY: Bupleurum contains triterpene saponins or saikosides, also known as saikosaponins.[1,2] The highest levels of these saikosaponins are found in species *B. falcatum* (2% to 8%) and *B. chinense* (1.7%).[4] Saikosaponin content varies depending on certain growing periods and also between wild and cultivated species.[5] Root parts of bupleurum have been analyzed, resulting in the discovery of many saikosaponins.[6] Saponins, along with 8 flavonoid compounds, have also been found in the aerial parts of 6 species.[7] Saikogenins A, B, C, and D are also present in the plant. Spinasterol, stigmasterol, and rutin have also been found, as well as pectin-like polysaccharides (bupleurans).[1,4]

PHARMACOLOGY: Bupleurum's traditional role as a liver tonic has been substantiated by research. The saikosides are known liver protectants, and bupleurum has been found to be beneficial in both acute and chronic liver disease.[2,4] Doses of saikosaponins demonstrate marked hepatoprotective activity in several animal models.[8,9,10,11] IV injection of bupleurum provided beneficial therapeutic outcomes in 100 cases of infectious hepatitis in adults and children.[12] Saikosaponins increase hepatic protein synthesis both in vitro and in vivo.[4]

Bupleurum's effects on the immune system have been widely reported. Traditional use of the plant for acute infection, cold with chills and fever, headache, vomiting, and malaria treatment have been discussed.[3,4] Bupleurum was also found to possess antitussive effects.[13] The saikosides stimulate corticosteroid production, thus increasing the anti-inflammatory effects.[2] Bupleurum inactivated enveloped viruses including measles and herpes, but had no effect on naked viruses such as polio.[14] Bupleurum demonstrated cytotoxic effects in certain human cell lines in vitro.[4] Mitogenic activity has been shown from certain extracts of the plant.[15] Other immune problems may benefit from bupleurum including SLE, inflammatory disorders, and autoimmune disease.[4]

Improvement in certain GI conditions has also been seen with bupleurum. Constituents bupleurans and saikosaponins have been shown to decrease gastric ulcer development.[4] Bupleurum in combination has been reported to inhibit gastric secretion and acid output.[16] One study reports improved integrity of gastric mucosa in rats.[17]

A Chinese medicinal treatment including *B. chinense* was found to be comparable to methylphenidate (eg, *Ritalin*) in a 100-patient study of children 7 to 14 years of age with minimal brain dysfunction (MBD). The group that was administered the Chinese combination had far fewer side effects, as well as more improvement in parameters such as intelligence or enuresis than the methylphenidate group.[18]

Bupleurum is often used as part of the popular Japanese herbal remedy Sho-saiko-to (Tj-9, Xino-chai-hu-tang), which is used extensively for the treatment of various liver diseases. In one study, this product was found to reduce the incidence of hepatocellular carcinoma in patients.[19]

Other ailments for which bupleurum is used include irregular menstruation, PMS, hot flashes, prolapsed uterus,[1,3] kidney problems (protectant), high cholesterol (saponins decrease cholesterol by increasing excretion in bile),[4] and hemorrhoids.[2]

TOXICOLOGY: Limited pharmacokinetic information is available in humans, but in mice it was determined that certain saikosaponins are transformed into ≈ 30 compounds for potential absorption. Saikosaponin metabolites undergo enterohepatic recycling. Crude saikosaponins show medium toxicity after intraperitoneal administration and low toxicity if taken orally (LD_{50} = 4.7 g/kg in mice).[4] One report regarding bupleurum in combination finds no effects on CNS, respiratory, cardiovascular, or blood coagulation systems in mice, concluding that no important adverse events occur at pharmacologically effective doses.[16]

Bupleurum has produced sedative effects in some patients, along with increased flatulence and bowel movements in large doses. Some combinations with bupleurum may have certain undesirable effects such as induction of pneumonitis, or nausea and reflux in sensitive patients. Some reports are unclear as to whether or not the ill effects are due specifically to bupleurum.[4]

SUMMARY: Bupleurum has been used in China for over 2000 years as a liver tonic. Research finds bupleurum beneficial as a liver protectant. It also has positive effects on the immune system, including treatment for cold and flu, inflammatory disorders, and certain cancers. Bupleurum is also useful in GI ailments, certain brain disorders, and gynecological problems. The toxicity profile is low, with no important adverse effects being reported in animals.

PATIENT INFORMATION – Bupleurum

Uses: Bupleurum has been found beneficial as a liver protectant and possesses positive effects on the immune system, including treatment for cold and flu, inflammatory disorders, and certain cancers. It is also useful in GI ailments, certain brain disorders, and for gynecological problems.

Side Effects: Bupleurum has caused sedative effects in some patients, along with increased flatulence and bowel movements in large doses. Some combinations with bupleurum may have certain undesirable effects such as induction of pneumonitis, or nausea and reflux in sensitive patients.

---

[1] Hocking, G. *A Dictionary of Natural Products.* Plexus Publ. Inc.: Medford NJ, 1997;132-33.

[2] Chevallier, A. *Encyclopedia of Medicinal Plants.* DK Publishing: New York, NY, 1996;68.

[3] *A Barefoot Doctor's Manual* (American translation of official Chinese paramedical manual). Running Press: Philadelphia, PA, 1977;848.

[4] Bone, K. Bupleurum: a natural steroid effect. *Can J Herbalism* . 1996;22-25,41.

[5] Du X, et al. Dynamic variation of saikosaponin contents. *Chung Kuo Chung Yao Tsa Chih* 1991;16(11):652-55, 701.

[6] Jing H, et al. Chemical constituents of the roots of *Bupleurum longicaule* Wall. ex DC. var. franchetii de Boiss and *B. chaishoui* Shan et Sheh. *Chung Kuo Chung Yao Tsa Chih* 1996;21(12):739-41, 762.

[7] Luo S, et al. Chemical constituents of the aerial parts of six species of Bupleurum genus medicinally used in southwest region of China. *Chung Kuo Chung Yao Tsa Chih* 1991;16(6):353-56, 383.

[8] Chiu H, et al. The pharmacological and pathological studies on several hepatic protective crude drugs from Taiwan (I). *Am J Chin Med* 1988;16(3-4):127-37.

[9] Lin C, et al. The pharmacological and pathological studies on Taiwan folk medicine (III): the effects of *Bupleurum kaoi* and cultivated *Bupleurum falcatum* var. komarowi. *Am J Chin Med* 1990;18(3-4):105-12.

[10] Lin C, et al. The pharmacological and pathological studies on Taiwan folk medicine (IV): the effects of echinops grijisii and e. Latifolius. *Am J Chin Med* 1990;18(3-4):113-20.

[11] Yen M, et al. Evaluation of root quality of Bupleurum species by TLC scanner and the liver protective effects of "xiao-chai-hu-tang" prepared using three different Bupleurum species. *J Ethnopharmacol* 1991;34(2-3):155–65.

[12] Chang H, et al. *Pharmacology and Applications of Chinese Materia Medica.* World Scientific: Singapore, 1987.

[13] Takagi K, et al. Pharmacological studies on *Bupleurum falcatum* L. I. Acute toxicity and central depressant action of crude saikosides. *Yakugaku Zasshi* 1969;89(5):712-20.

[14] Ushio Y, et al. Inactivation of measles virus and herpes simplex virus by saikosaponin d. *Planta Med* 1992;58(2):171-73.

[15] Ohtsu S, et al. Analysis of mitogenic substances in *Bupleurum chinense* by ESR spectroscopy. *Biol Pharm Bull* 1997;20(1):97-100.

[16] Amagaya S, et al. General pharmacological properties of Tj-9 extract. *Phytomedicine* 1998;5(3):165-75.

[17] Hung C, et al. Comparison between the effects of crude saikosaponin and 16, 16-dimethyprostaglandin E2 on tannic acid-induced gastric mucosal damage in rats. *Chin J Physiol* 1993;36(4):211-17.

[18] Zhang H, et al. Preliminary study of traditional Chinese medicine treatment of minimal brain dysfunction: analysis of 100 cases. *Chung Hsi I Chieh Ho Tsa Chih* 1990;10(5):278-79, 260.

[19] Oka H, et al. Prospective study of chemoprevention of hepatocellular carcinoma with Sho-saiko-to (Tj-9). *Cancer* 1995;76(5):743-49.

Burdock

SCIENTIFIC NAME(S): *Arctium lappa* L. (Synonymous with A Majus Bernh, great burdock as well as A munus Bernh., lesser burdock.) Family: Asteraceae or Compositae.

COMMON NAME(S): Bardana, beggar's buttons, clotbur, edible burdock, great bur, great burdocks, lappa

BOTANY: Budock is considered to be native in Europe and Northern Asia; it is neutralized in the US. Burdock is widely cultivated in Eastern Europe especially former Yugoslavia, Poland, Bulgaria and Hungary. The plant is a perennial or biennial herb, growing up to 3 meters (about 9 feet), with large ovate, acuminate leaves, broad pinkish flowers made up of reddish-violate tubular florets, surrounded by many involucral bracts ending in a stiff spiny or hooked tip. Overall, these are rounded and spiny in appearance. The root pieces are used in teas and are very hard, minimally fibrous, longitudinally wrinkled and grayish brown to balck in color.[1,2]

HISTORY: In traditional medicine, the fruits (seeds), roots and leaves of burdock have been used as decoctions or teas for a wide range of ailments including colds, catarrh, gout, rheumatism, stomach ailments, cancers and as a diuretic, diaphoretic and laxative. It has even been promoted as an aphrodisiac. Externally, it has been used for various skin problems.

CHEMISTRY: Burdock root yields a wide variety of compounds on analysis that include inulin (up to 50%), tannins, polyphenolic acids (caffeic and chlorogenic), volatile acids (acetic, butyric, costic, 3–hexenoic, isovaleric, 3–octanoic, propionic, etc), polyacetylenes (0.001–0.002%, dry-weight basis), and a crystalline plant hormone, glamma-guanidino-n-butyric acid. Studies conducted have isolated and characterized a xyloglucan from the 24% KOH extract of edible burdock.[3] The seeds of burdock yield 15% to 30% fixed oils; a bitter glycoside (arctiin), two lignans (lappaols A and B), chlorogenic acid, a germacranolide and other materials. Other studies have isolated six compounds from burdock seeds including daucosterol, arctigenin, arctiin, matairesinol, lappaol and a new lignan named neoarctin.[4] The levels of arctiin and arctigen in the fruits of burdock that are used in Chinese medicine for the treatment of common colds have also been studied.[5] Others have also reported on the fruit

constituents,[6] and even the fruit pulp (pomace). The fruit pulp contains 11% proteins, 19% lipids and 34% inulin.

PHARMACOLOGY: Several researchers have reported on the various biological acitivites of burdock which include **antipyretic**, **antimicrobial**, **antitumor**, **diuretic**, and **diaphoretic** properties.[2] Beyond these effects are reported fruit extracts with hypoglycemic activity in rats and fresh root juices with antimutagenic effects probably due to a lignan.[2] Some cosmetic and toiletry type products used for skin-cleaning, antidandruff and hair tonic applications are given in the recent literature. It should be noted that burdock root is fairly commonly used as a food in Asia.[2] Occasionally, US health food stores carry fresh burdock root for sale as a food and nutraceutical (medical food). Among the more recent studies are the uses of burdock in the treatment of urolithiasis,[8] potential inhibition of HIV-1 infection in vitro,[9] metabolism of burdock lignans in rat gastrointestinal tract,[10] platelet activating factor (PAF) antagonism by burdock,[11] effects of burdock dietary fiber in digestion,[12] lack of effectiveness of burdock in treating streptozotocin diabetic mice,[13] potential antitumor activity of burdock extract[14] and a desmutagenic factor isolated from burdock.[15]

TOXICOLOGY: While burdock is generally considered a safe and edible food product, a few reports have appeared on burdock root tea poisoning[16] due to adulteration (subsequently shown to be extraneous atropine), and allergic contact dermatitis due to burdock.[17]

SUMMARY: Burdock root is generally considered an edible food product with some potential medical benefits as a mild diuretic, diaphoretic, antipyretic, antimicrobial and possible antitumor product. Many of the recent chemical and pharmacological studies verify some of these activities. Further investigations are warranted, particularly as a potential medical food or nutraceutical.

PATIENT INFORMATION – Burdock

Uses: Treatment of fever, infection, cancer, fluid retention and kidney stones. Effectiveness and safety for these have not been adequately evaluated. In addition, burdock has been used topically to cleanse the skin and treat dandruff.

Side Effects: Oral: Root tea poisoning due to extraneous atropine (blurred vision, headache, drowsiness, slurred speech, loss of coordination, incoherent speech, restlessness, hallucinations, hyperactivity, seizures, disorientation, flushing, dryness of mouth and nose, rash, lack of sweating, fever). Topical: Allergic skin irritation.

---

[1] Bisset G, ed. *Herbal Drugs and Phytopharmaceuticals.* Stuttgart: Medpharm Scientific Publishers, 1994.

[2] Leung A, et al. *Encyclopedia of Common Natural Ingredients, 2nd ed.* New York: John Wiley & Sons, 1996.

[3] Kato Y, et al. Isolation and Characterization of a Xyloglucan from Gobo (*Arctium lappa* L). *Bio Biotechnol Biochem* 1993;57(9):1591.

[4] Wang H, et al. Studies on the Chemical Constituents of (*Arctium lappa* L.) *Acta Pharma Sinica* 1993;28(12):911.

[5] Sun W. Determination of Arctiin and Arctigenin in Fructus Arctii by Reverse-phase HPLC. *Acta Pharm Sinica* 1992;27(7):549.

[6] Yamaguchi S. On the Constituents of the Fruit of Arctium lappa. *Yakugaku Zasshi* 1976;96(12):1492.

[7] Chalcarz W, et al. Evaluation of Technological Use of Pomaces Obtained at the Production of Juice from Burdock (Succus bardanae). *Herba Pol* 1984;30(2):109.

[8] Grases F, et al. Urolithiasis and Phytotherapy. *Int Urol Nephrol* 1994;26(5):507.

[9] Yao X, et al. Mechanism of Inhibition of HIV-1 Infection in vitro by Purified Extract of Prunella Vulgaris. *Virology* 1992;187(1):56.

[10] Nose M, et al. Structural Transformation of Lignan Compounds in Rat Gastrointestinal Tract. *Planta Med* 1992;58(6):520.

[11] Iwakami S, et al. Platelet Activating Factor (PAF) Antagonists Contained in Medicinal Plants: Lignans and sesquiterpenes. *Chem Pharm Bull* 1992;40(5):1196.

[12] Tadeda H, et al. Effect of Feeding Amaranth (Food Red No. 2) on the Jejunal Sucrase and Digestion-Absorption Capacity on the Jejunum in Rats. *J Nutr Sc Vit* 1991;37(6):611.

[13] Swanston-Flatt S, et al. Glycaemis Effects of Traditional European Plant Treatments for Diabetes. Studies in normal and streptozotocin diabetic mice. *Diabetes Res* 1989; 10(2):60.

[14] Donbradi C, et al. Screening Report on the Antitumor Activity of Purified Arctium lappa Extracts. *Tumori* 1966;53(3):173.

[15] Morita K, et al. A Desmutagenic Factor Isolated from Burdock (*Arctium lappa* Linne). *Mut Res* 1984;129(1):25.

[16] Bryson P, et al. Burdock Root Tea Poisoning: Case report involving a commercial preparation. *JAMA* 1978;239(May 19):2157.

[17] Rodriguez P, et al. Allergic Dermatitis due to Burdock (*Arctium lappa*). *Contact Dermatitis* 1995;33(3):134.

Butcher's Broom

SCIENTIFIC NAME(S): *Ruscus aculeatus* L. Family: Liliaceae. The nomenclature of this plant should not be confused with broom (*Cytisus scoparius* L.) or Spanish broom (*Spartium junceum* L.).

COMMON NAME(S): Butcher's broom, box holly, knee holly, pettigree

BOTANY: Butcher's broom is a low-growing common evergreen shrub. It is widely distributed, from Iran to the Mediterranean[1] and the southern US.[2] This plant develops shoots from rhizomes that in many ways are similar to asparagus in form.[3]

HISTORY: This plant has a long history of use. Almost 2000 years ago, this plant had been used as a laxative and diuretic. Extracts, decoctions and poultices have been used throughout the ages, but the medicinal use of this plant did not become common until this century. Early investigations during the 1950s indicated that extracts of the rhizomes of butcher's broom could induce vasoconstriction and therefore may have a clinical use in the treatment of certain circulatory diseases. Novel uses for this plant have included its use as an anti-inflammatory agent and to prevent atherosclerosis. The recent focus of research into butcher's broom has been in the elucidation of the pharmacologic activity of its components.

CHEMISTRY: A variety of compounds have been isolated from butcher's broom. A mixture of steroidal saponins had been identified during the preliminary investigations of the plant. The two primary saponin compounds are ruscogenin and neoruscogenin.[4] In addition, a variety of flavonoids, a fatty acid mixture composed primarily of tetracosanoic acid and related compounds, chrysophanic acid, sitosterol, campesterol and stigmasterol, have been isolated from the roots.[2] The benzofuran euparone has also been isolated.[5]

PHARMACOLOGY: Extracts of Ruscus have been included in commercial phytotherapeutic agents designed for the management of venous insufficiency.

In dogs, an extract of the root was shown to cause a dose-dependent increase in contraction of isolated veins. These contractions were inhibited by the alpha-adrenergic blocking agent phentolamine, suggesting that compounds in Ruscus activated both alpha-1 and alpha-2 receptors in smooth muscle. Ruscus had no influence on prostaglandin levels in these tests.[6] Prazosin also reduced the activity of Ruscus extract.[7]

In man, a drug containing Ruscus extract has been shown to be effective in improving the signs and symptoms of lower limb venous disease in patients with chronic phlebopathy.[8] Combined with hesperidin and ascorbic acid, this preparation was evaluated in a 2-month double-blind placebo-controlled crossover trial. A trend toward improvement was noted among treated patients, although statistical significance was not always noted. In particular, edema, itching and paresthesias improved greatly, as did a feeling of limb heaviness and cramping.

The combined action of the flavonoids, sterols and proteolytic enzymes found in the root has been shown to reduce dextran- and carrageenan-induced rat paw edema, indicating that the extract has the potential for providing some anti-inflammatory activity.[9] It should be noted that this mixture was administered intraduodenally, thereby reducing the possibility of inactivation by stomach acids. The effectiveness of orally administered butcher's broom preparations has not been firmly established.

TOXICOLOGY: Butcher's broom has not been associated with significant toxicity. The rhizomes had been eaten in a manner similar to asparagus in some early cultures. In the clinical trial conducted by Cappelli et al, no adverse events were attributable to therapy by the 40 patients evaluated.

SUMMARY: Butcher's broom has been used in traditional medicine and for culinary applications for centuries. Its popularity, however, has grown during this century with the observation that components of the plant may be useful in the management of circulatory disorders. There is little data to indicate that extracts of Ruscus are effective for the management of circulatory disorders, but these products are used popularly in Europe. The plant does not appear to be associated with significant toxicity concerns.

PATIENT INFORMATION – Butcher's Broom

Uses: Butcher's broom has been used in many forms to provide laxatives, diuretics and treatments for circulatory disease. Modern research has shown evidence of further medicinal potential. Rhizomes have been eaten as a vegetable.

Side Effects: Not known to be significantly toxic.

---

[1] Tyler VE. *The New Honest Herbal.* Philadelphia, PA: G.F. Stickley Co., 1987.

[2] ElSohly MA. Constituents of *Ruscus aculeatus. Lloydia* 1975;38(2):106.

[3] Mabberley DJ. *The Plant-book.* New York, NY: Cambridge University Press, 1987.

[4] Pourrat H, et al. Isolation and confirmation of the structure by C-NMR of the main prosapogenin from *Ruscus aculeatus* L. *Ann Pharm Fr* 1982;40:451.

[5] ElSohly MA, et al. Euparone, a New Benzofuran from *Ruscus aculeatus* L. *J Pharm Sci* 1974;63(10):1623.

[6] Marcelon G, et al. Effect of *Ruscus aculeatus* On Isolated Canine Cutaneous Veins. *Gen Pharmacol* 1983;14:103.

[7] Rubanyi G, et al. Effect of Temperature on the Responsiveness of Cutaneous Veins to the Extract of *Ruscus aculeatus. Gen Pharmacol* 1984;15(5):431.

[8] Capelli R, et al. Use of Extract of *Ruscus aculeatus* in Venous Disease In the Lower Limbs. *Drugs Exp Clin Res* 1988;14(4):277.

[9] Tarayre JP, Lauressergues H. The anti-edematous effect of an association of proteolytic enzymes, flavonoids, sterolic heterosides of *Ruscus aculeatus* and ascorbic acid. *Ann Pharm Fr* 1979;37:191.

Butterbur

SCIENTIFIC NAME(S): *Petasites Hybridus*

COMMON NAME(S): Butterbur, fuki

BOTANY: Butterbur is a perennial shrub, cultivated throughout Europe and North and West Asia, which can grow to 3 feet tall. It prefers damp areas, such as near rivers and streams. Its distinctive pink-lilac flowers grow on large spikes at the stem ends. The leaves are large and heart-shaped and used along with the root of the plant.[1,2] Microscopic analysis of butterbur's pollen grains has been reported[3,4] and examination of epidermal cells and stomata parts.[4] Anatomical and morphological features of the plant's leaves also have been described.[5]

HISTORY: Butterbur's genus name *Petasites* is derived from the Latin word *Petasus*, meaning "hat." Some were said to have worn the leaves in this manner. In 1652, herbalist Nicholas Culpeper documented the use of butterbur root to treat plague and fevers by inducing sweat.[2] Traditionally, the antispasmolytic actions of the plant have been used to treat asthma, cough, and GI disorders.[6]

CHEMISTRY: Butterbur contains pyrrolizidine alkaloids (primarily senecione) which are known to be liver toxins and to cause cancer in animals.[2,6,7] These pyrrolizidine alkaloids have been detected by gas chromatography (GC) and mass spectrophotometry (MS) methods and also include integerrimine and senkirkine.[8] Treatment of pyrrolizidine alkaloids to reduce their content in alcoholic extracts has been investigated.[9]

Sesquiterpene determination in butterbur has been reported,[10,11,12] including content in the plant according to season and location,[13] the sesquiterpene content in different plant parts,[14,15] and 6 sesquiterpene furanoeremophilanes.[16] Sesquiterpene lactones also found in butterbur include petasins (< 4%, such as isopetasin 0.15%, [antispasmolytic actions]), angelicoyleneopetasol, fukinone, and fukinanolide.[1,6,7]

The plant also contains volatile oil (0.1%), including dodecanal, pectin, mucilage, inulin (in the root), the flavonoids isoquercitrin and astragalin, and tannins.[1,2] Quantitative determination of active principles in butterbur in general has been reported.[17]

PHARMACOLOGY: Butterbur has been used for its antispasmodic and analgesic properties due in part to its petasin and isopetasin components.[1,2,6] The fact that its sesquiterpenes are reducers/inhibitors of peptido-leukotriene synthesis may also contribute to butterbur's antispasmodic and gastroprotective activity.[18,19]

Antispasmodic actions make butterbur useful for urinary tract disorders, mild kidney stone disease, obstruction of bile flow, and other liver, GI, or pancreas disorders.[1,2,3,6,7] For these disorders, 1 source suggests 5 to 7 grams of dried herb/day for short-term therapy only.[7] The plant also may be useful to treat dysmenorrhea and other cramp-like states such as pain or colic.[20] Bronchospasmolytic actions of the plant may be therapeutic for lung ailments, asthma, cough, and for its tonic and expectorant properties.[1,2]

Analgesic, anti-inflammatory, and sedative actions of butterbur are helpful in treating restlessness, back pain, and headache. Reports have concluded that migraine sufferers taking *Petasites* vs placebo had migraine attacks of shorter duration with no adverse effects. Overall, the treated group reported a 56% reduction in migraine attacks similar to results of conventional treatments currently available.[6]

Butterbur has also been used as a poultice with fresh leaves for wounds and skin eruptions.[1,2] A review on butterbur's actions and other highlights is available.[21]

TOXICOLOGY: Side effects have not been reported,[6,20] but butterbur's pyrrolizidine alkaloids are known to damage organs, primarily the liver, and cause cancer in animals.[2,20] Daily doses of these alkaloids should not exceed 1 mcg, and duration of use should not exceed 4 to 6 weeks per year.[20] Use of the plant root during pregnancy or breastfeeding is contraindicated.

Enzyme immunoassay for assessing toxic potential of the pyrrolizidine alkaloids from butterbur has been reported.[22]

SUMMARY: Butterbur has been used traditionally for its antispasmodic, analgesic, and anti-inflammatory actions.

These properties make the plant useful in treating urinary tract disorders, bronchial ailments, cramping, and migraine headaches. The plant's pyrrolizidine alkaloids are liver toxins and cause cancer in animals; therefore, limit butterbur's use.

PATIENT INFORMATION – Butterbur

Uses: Butterbur has traditionally been used for its antispasmodic and analgesic properties to aid in treatment of asthma, cough, and GI disorders. It has also been used for urinary tract disorders, bronchial ailments, cramping, and migraines.

Side Effects: Side effects have not been reported, but butterbur's pyrrolizidine alkaloids have damaged organs and caused cancer in animals; limit use. Do not use during pregnancy or breastfeeding.

---

[1] Bisset N. *Herbal Drugs and Phytopharmaceuticals*. CRC Press: Stuttgart, Germany, 1994; 366-68.

[2] Chevallier A. Encyclopedia of Medicinal Plants. DK Publishing: New York, NY, 1996;244.

[3] Lindauerova T. Palynomorphological investigation of the species *Petasites hybridus* and *Petasites albus*. *Farmaceuticky Obzor* 1981;50(11):569-74.

[4] Lindauerova T, et al. Study of the leaf epidermis of the species *Petasites hybridus* and *Petasites albus*. *Farmaceuticky Obzor* 1981;50(12):605-09.

[5] Saukel J. Pharmacobotanical investigations of plant drugs. *Scientia Pharmaceutica* 1991 Dec 31;59:307-19.

[6] Eaton J. Butterbur, herbal help for migraine. *Natural Pharmacy* 1998;2(10):1, 23-24.

[7] Schulz V, et al. *Rational Phytotherapy*. Springer-Verlag: Berlin, Germany, 1998;221-25.

[8] Luthy J, et al. Pyrrolizidine alkaloids in *Petasites hybridus* L. and *P. albus* L. *Pharm Acta Helv* 1983 Apr;58:98-100.

[9] Mauz C, et al. Method for the reduction of pyrrolizidine alkaloids from medicinal plant extracts. *Pharm Acta Helv* 1985;60(9-10):256-59.

[10] Steinegger E, et al. Investigation of the sesquiterpene fraction of *Petasites hybridus*. *Pharm Acta Helv* 1979;54(1):23-25.

[11] Steinegger E, et al. Investigation of the sesquiterpene fraction of *Petasites hybridus*. *Pharm Acta Helv* 1979;54(2):54-59.

[12] Predescu I, et al. Contributions to the chromatographic and spectral study of *Petasites hybridus* extract. *Farmacia* 1980 Oct-Dec;28:241-48.

[13] Debrunner B, et al. Sesquiterpenes of *Petasites hybridus* . *Pharm Acta Helv* 1995;70(4):315-23.

[14] Steinegger E, et al. Investigation of the sesquiterpene fraction from *Petasites hybridus*. *Pharm Acta Helv* 1979;54(2):57-59.

[15] Debrunner B, et al. Sesquiterpenes of *Petasites hybridus*. *Pharm Acta Helv* 1995;70(2):167–73.

[16] Siegenthaler P, et al. Sesquiterpenes of *Petasites hybridus*. *Pharm Acta Helv* 1997;72(2):57-67.

[17] Barza P, et al. New spectral method for quantitative determination of the active principles in *Petasites hydridus* extracts, based upon the ninhydrin reaction. *Farmacia* 1979 Apr-Jun;27:125-28.

[18] Brune K, et al. Gastro-protective effects by extracts of *Petasites hybridus*: the role of inhibition of peptido-leukotriene synthesis. *Planta Med* 1993;59(6):494-96.

[19] Bickel D, et al. Identification and characterization of inhibitors of peptido-leukotriene synthesis from *Petasites hybridus*. *Planta Med* 1994;60(4):318-22.

[20] Blumenthal M, ed. The Complete German Commission E Monographs. American Botanical Council: Austin, TX 1998:183, 365.

[21] Debrunner B, et al. *Petasites hydridus*: a tool for interdisciplinary research in phytotherapy. *Pharm Acta Helv* 1998;72(6):359-62.

[22] Langer T, et al. A competitive enzyme immunoassay for the pyrrolizidine alkaloids of the senecionine type. *Planta Med* 1996;62(3):267-71.

Calabar Bean

SCIENTIFIC NAME(S): *Physostigma venenosum*. Family: Leguminosae (Fabaceae).[1]

COMMON NAME(S): Calabar bean, physostigma, ordeal bean, chop nut, esere nut, faba calabarica.[2]

BOTANY: The calabar bean is the dried ripe seed of the *P. venenosum*, a perennial woody climbing plant found on the banks of streams in West Africa. Vines of the plant extend more than 50 feet in the air, climbing high among the trees.[3] The plant bears showy purple flowers and seed pods that grow to about 6 inches in length.[3] Each pod contains from 2 to 3 seeds.[4] The dark brown seeds are about 1 inch wide and thick and have an extremely hard shell.

HISTORY: This plant is native to an area of Africa around Nigeria once known as Calabar. The plant is widely known in Africa because the seeds had been used as an "ordeal poison" to determine if a person was a witch or possessed by evil spirits.[5] When used for this purpose, the victim was made to ingest several beans; if the person regurgitated the beans and survived the "ordeal," his innocence was proclaimed. Western settlers who were captured by native tribes and who underwent the "ordeal" soon learned not to chew the bean, but to swallow the kidney-shaped bean intact, thereby not permitting the release of the toxic constituents. The plant has been long recognized as a commercial source of the alkaloid physostigmine, first isolated in 1864.

CHEMISTRY: The seeds contain the alkaloid physostigmine (eserine) in a concentration of about 0.15%, along with the related alkaloids eseramine, physovenine, calabatine, and geneserine, among others. These alkaloids are derived from a tryptophan precursor. On exposure to air, physostigmine oxidizes to a reddish compound, rubreserine, and therefore should be protected from air and light.

PHARMACOLOGY: Physostigmine (usually as the stable salicylate salt) (*Antilirium*) is an acetylcholinesterase inhibitor, that prolongs the neuronal activity of acetylcholine. It is used clinically to contract the pupil of the eye, often to counter the dilating effects of mydriatic drugs, reverse the CNS toxicity of anticholinergic drugs, including tricyclic antidepressants, and to manage intraocular pressure in patients with glaucoma. Physostigmine and related drugs have been investigated for their ability to increase cognition, particularly in demented patients, but these therapies have met with minimal success. Physostigmine and the related synthetic agent neostigmine (eg, *Prostigmin*) have been used for the diagnosis and treatment of myasthenia gravis.[6]

Physostigmine is extremely toxic, with an oral LD50 of 4.5 mg/kg in mice. The maximum reported number of beans eaten followed by survival of a human is 35.[5] Physostigmine kills by affecting heart contractility and inducing respiratory paralysis.

SUMMARY: The use of the calabar bean as an "ordeal bean" has long been outlawed in Africa, although its use persists in tribal ritual. The bean is the source of physostigmine, a medically valuable drug that prolongs the activity of the neural transmitter acetylcholine. Physostigmine is highly toxic.

PATIENT INFORMATION – Calabar Bean

Uses: Originally consumed in African ritual ordeals which killed many subjects, the bean produces alkaloids clinically used to contract the pupil, manage ocular pressure in glaucoma, reverse toxicity of certain other drugs, and treat myasthenia gravis.

Side Effects: Toxic principle affects heart and induces respiratory paralysis.

---

[1] Lewis W, et al. *Medical Botany: Plants affecting man's health.* New York: John Wiley & Sons, 1977.

[2] Osol A, et al. *The Dispensatory of the United States of America,* 25th ed. Philadelphia: JB Lippincott, 1955:1054.

[3] Dobelis I. *Magic and Medicine of Plants.* Pleasantville, NY: Reader's Digest Association, 1986.

[4] Evans, W. *Trease and Evans' Pharmacognosy.* 13th ed. London: Balliere Tindall, 1989.

[5] Duke J. *Handbook of Medicinal Herbs.* Boca Raton, FL: CRC Press, 1985.

[6] Olin B, Hebel S, eds. *Drug Facts and Comparisons.* St. Louis: Facts and Comparisons, 1994.

Calamus

SCIENTIFIC NAME(S): *Acorus calamus* L. At least four subtypes have been identified and are differentiated by their content of the compound isoasarone. Family: Araceae

COMMON NAME(S): Calamus, rat root, sweet flag, sweet myrtle, sweet root, sweet sedge

BOTANY: Calamus is a perennial that is found in damp, swampy areas. It has sword-shaped leaves and grows to 6 feet tall. It is similar in appearance to the iris. It is found throughout North America, Europe, and Asia,[1] and is often imported from India and the former Yugoslavia and USSR.[2]

HISTORY: The fragrant underground portion (the rhizome) has been used medicinally since biblical times. Popular European books on medicinal plants touted calamus as a "wonder drug." It was commonly used in folk medicine as a "nervine," most likely linked to the tranquilizing effect of cis-isoasarone (the major component of the oil).[2] It has been used in traditional medicine for the treatment of digestive disorders and childhood colic. Infusions of the rhizome have been suggested for the treatment of fever, and chewing the rhizome has been said to relieve irritated throats and to remove the odor of tobacco.

The ground rhizome is used as a spice and commercial flavoring in drinks, cosmetics, and toothpastes. However, because of an association with isoasarone and the development of tumors in animals, the use of calamus and its extracts is prohibited in the US.[1]

CHEMISTRY: Calamus contains from 1.5% to 3.5% of a volatile oil responsible for the plant's characteristic odor and taste.[1] A major component of the oil (up to 75%) from some types of calamus is beta-asarone (also referred to as cis-isoasarone).[2] More than a dozen additional fragrant compounds have been identified in the oil.

Acorus calamus has recently been classified into four separate varieties which grow in different locations worldwide. The virtually isoasarone-free plant grows in North America (drug type I). Western Europe is home for yet another type of calamus, the oil of which contains less than 10% isoasarone (drug type II). The two other varieties, however, have been found to contain oils which are composed of up to 96% isoasarone (drug types III and IV).[1]

Calamerone, a bicyclic sesquiterpene, has been discovered in the roots of *A. calamus* Calamendiol and isocalamendiol, two known sesquiterpenes, were isolated from the same plant.[3] The essential oil consists of sesquiterpenes and phenylpropanes. The composition of the oil varies depending upon the degree of the ploidy of the plants. Other constituents are acorone, a sesquiterpene diketone, tannins, mucilage, and small startch grains.[2]

PHARMACOLOGY: A variety of studies have been conducted to evaluate the pharmacologic effects of calamus and its extracts. The crude drug has been found to possess sedative properties and to potentiate barbiturate and ethanol-induced sedation in mice; calamus potentiates the CNS effects of reserpine.[4] Doses of 10 to 100 mg/kg intraperitoneally of calamus oil to rats, mice, dogs, cats, and monkeys resulted in a dose-dependent reduction in spontaneous movement; at the 100 mg/kg dose, spontaneous motor activity was reduced by 95% compared to a control. No deaths occurred at any dose. The depressant effect did not induce hypnosis, but was characteristic of sedation induced by reserpine or chlorpromazine.[4]

In low doses, calamus oil has an acetylcholine-like action on smooth muscle; at high doses, it has an antispasmodic and relaxant effect.[4] It boasts stomachic, carminative, and (externally) rubefacient indications.[2] When tested *in vitro*, calamus oil abolished drug-induced contractions of isolated animal intestine, aorta, and uterus; its action was about 10 times less potent than that of papaverine.[5] The oil induced hypotension when administered parenterally to dogs.[1]

This sedative activity has been ascribed to asarone, which in part is chemically related to the reserpine molecule. The sedative effects of intraperitoneal doses of asarone in mice lasted 4 to 6 hours.[6]

Although calamus oil inhibits monoamine oxidase in vitro, this effect occurs primarily at doses higher than are required for usual pharmacologic activity. It has been suggested that the effects of the drug are mediated through 5–hydroxytryptamine[4] or norepinephrine; however, this mechanism has been disputed. Some experts suggest that asarone may mediate its effect through depression of hypothalamic function.[6]

When tested in vitro, it was found that isoasarone-free oil (type I) had a pronounced spasmolytic action comparable to that of a standard antihistamine. However, at a similar dose, isoasarone-rich oil (type IV) showed no spasmolytic action at all.[7] Researchers also noted that the oil decreased the mortality of guinea pigs caused by histamine.[5]

Such results suggest that the isoasarone-free oil from type I (North American) calamus plants can be an effective herbal remedy for dyspepsia and similar spasmodic gastrointestinal complaints.[1]

The essential oil of calamus has also been used as an insecticide. Several studies have found that the vapors of the oil are sufficient to control the hatching and molting of several types of common pests in doses of approximately 10 ml of a 100 ppm dilution.[8]

TOXICOLOGY: The primary toxicologic concern focuses on the carcinogenic effect of isoasarone, a major component of the volatile oil of calamus. Feeding studies conducted more than 20 years ago provided evidence for the mutagenic potential of this compound. Subsequently, all calamus-containing products were removed from the US marketplace.[1] However, a recent study found extracts of *A. calamus* to exhibit no mutagenic activity in the salmonella mutagenicity screen.[9] The plant and its extracts continue to find use throughout the world.

The LD_{50} of asarone in mice is 417 mg/kg (oral) and 310 mg/kg (IP).[10] Although *A. calamus* exhibited no mutagenic activity in the salmonella mutagenicity screen, recent experiences showed that calamus oil exhibited genotoxic effects on Swiss mice.[11] Another experiment showed that calamus oil was strongly mutagenic.[12]

SUMMARY: Calamus is a fragrant plant that grows throughout many parts of the world and has been used in traditional medicine since biblical times. Although used in many countries as a flavoring, the oil contains asarone, a compound which has been considered to be mutagenic. Hence, calamus and its derivatives are not used in foods in the US. The oil has a strong sedative and antispasmodic action that appears to resemble the activity of the phenothiazine tranquilizers.

PATIENT INFORMATION – Calamus

Uses: Traditionally used as a tranquilizer and general "wonder drug," calamus also is used as a flavoring. The oil is a sedative, hypotensive, and muscle relaxant.

Side Effects: Because of mutagenic properties, calamus derivatives are not used in foods in the US.

---

[1] Tyler V. *The New Honest Herbal.* Philadelphia: G.F. Stickley, 1987.
[2] Bisset N. *Herbal Drugs and Phytopharmaceuticals*, Stuttgart: MedPharm Scientific Publishers, 1994.
[3] Wu L, et al. *Yakugaku Zasshi* 1994;114(3):182.
[4] Dhalla N, et al. *Arch Int Pharmacodyn Ther* 1968;172(2):356.
[5] Maj T, et al. *Acta Poloniae Pharma* 1966;23(5):477.
[6] Menon M, et al. *J Pharm Pharmacol* 1967;19(3):170.
[7] Keller K, et al. *Planta Med* 1985;1:6.
[8] Saxena B, et al. *Experientia* 1974;30(11):1298.
[9] Riazuddin S, et al. *Environ Mol Mutagen* 1987;10(2):141.
[10] Belova L, et al. *Farmakol Toksikol* 1985;48(6):17.
[11] Balachandran B, et al. *Ind J Med Res* 1991;94:378.
[12] Sivaswamy S, et al. *Indian J Exp Biol* 1991;29(8):730.

Calanolide A

SCIENTIFIC NAME(S): Originally isolated from species *Calophyllum lanigerum* var. *austrocoriaceum*

COMMON NAME(S): Calanolide A

BOTANY: Calanolide A is a compound isolated from the latex of the tree, *Calophyllum lanigerum* var. *austrocoriaceum*, that grows in the rain forest of the Malaysian state of Sarawak on the island of Borneo. There are at least 200 species in the genus *Calophyllum*.[1,2]

HISTORY: Rain forests are a very promising source of natural medicines because of its vast diversity. It has been estimated that more than half of the world's 250,000 plant species exist in tropical rain forests. Searching for natural drugs in these areas, the National Cancer Institute (NCI) contracts scientists to gather specimens for analysis. In 1987, an Illinois team obtained samples from many trees, one of which was *Calophyllum lanigerum*. Four years later, the NCI discovered that a preparation from this gum tree was very effective against the human immunodeficiency virus type 1 (HIV-1).[1,3] Confirmation of species was performed by comparison to Arnold Arboretum species and samples from the Singapore Botanic Garden.[3]

CHEMISTRY: Plants from the genus *Calophyllum* have been shown to contain xanthones, steroids, triterpenes, coumarins, and benzopyrans. Calanolide A falls into the category of a dipyranocoumarin.[2] It is classified as a nonnucleoside HIV-1 specific reverse transcriptase (RT) inhibitor.[2,4] Many studies in this area discuss findings from the genus *Calophyllum*, and offer structural representations, related compounds and their derivatives, modifications of the molecule, etc.[2,4,5,6,7,8,9] Calanolide A has been synthesized in the lab and was found to have similar actions to the natural product.[10]

PHARMACOLOGY:

HIV: This recently discovered natural product has been found to specifically inhibit the DNA polymerase activity of HIV-1 RT, but not HIV-2 RT.[11] This information warrants further investigation in human clinical trials. Calanolide A has been found to inhibit a wide variety of HIV-1 strains, drug-resistant strains, and HIV disease in various stages. Calanolide A appears to act early in the infection process similar to dideoxycytidine.[12] Calanolide A's complex biochemical mechanism of inhibition has suggested the presence of 2 binding sites, 1 competitive, 1 noncompetitive. Calanolide A binds near the active site of the enzyme and interferes with deoxynucleotide triphosphate binding.[13] Many RT inhibitors bind to a common site on HIV-1 RT; whereas calanolide A may bind to a different site or sites on the enzyme.[14] Changes in the nonnucleoside inhibitor binding site itself may also alter effects. One report discusses cross-resistance of certain viral strains. Single mutations at certain amino acids can yield virus with either higher or lower resistance.[15]

In vivo, calanolide A has suppressed (HIV) viral replication in both IP and SC compartments in the hollow fiber mouse model. When combined with zidovudine, calanolide A had a synergistic effect.[16]

Other related compounds from the genus *Calophyllum* possess HIV-inhibitory actions. Examples include costatolide,[17,18] dihydrocalanolide,[18] and certain cordatolides.[19] Calanolides, their derivatives and/or structural analogs from *C. lanigerum* and other *Calophyllum* species, and their anti-HIV activities have been reported.[5,6,7,8,9,20,21] HIV RT inhibitors of natural origin, including calanolide A, have been reviewed.[22]

TOXICOLOGY: It has been mentioned that substance from *C. lanigerum* destroys the HIV virus without killing healthy cells,[1] but toxicology information is limited because of its recent discovery.

SUMMARY: Calanolide A offers promising treatment for HIV-1, although most studies have been performed in vitro. Clinical investigation and human trials are underway to further evaluate the effects of *Calophyllum*, a natural substance found in the tropical rain forest.

PATIENT INFORMATION – Calanolide A

Use: Initial studies show promise for treating HIV-1.

Side effects: Because this product is a relatively new discovery, no data are available.

---

1 Sheron P. Hunt in forests of Borneo aims to track down natural drugs. *New York Times* 1994 Dec 6.

2 McKee T, et al. Pyranocoumarins from tropical species of the genus *Calophyllum*: A chemotaxonomic study of extracts in the National Cancer Institute Collection. *J Nat Prod* 1998;61:1252-56.

3 Anonymous. Arnold Arboretum launches $8.2M capital campaign. *The Harvard University Gazette*. 1996 Jul 3.

4 McKee T, et al. New pyranocoumarins isolated from *Calophyllum enigerum* and *Calophyllum teysmannii. J Nat Prod* 1996;59:754–58.

5 Kashman Y, et al. The calanolides, a novel HIV-inhibitory class of coumarin derivatives from the tropical rainforest tree, *Calophyllum lanigerum. J Med Chem* 1992;35(15):2735-43.

6 Galinis D, et al. Structure-activity modifications of the HIV-1 inhibitors (+)- calanolide A and (-)-calanolide B. *J Med Chem* 1996;39(22):4507-10.

7 Boyd M, et al. Extraction of calanolide antiviral compounds from *Calophyllum*. US Pat Appl 1993 #Pat-appl-7-861 249, 1993.

8 Boyd M, et al. Calanolide and related antiretroviral compounds isolated from *Calophyllum*. 30 pp cont-in-part of US Patent Ser No. 861, 249, 1997.

9 Zembower D, et al. Structural analogues of the calanolide anti-HIV agents. Modification of the trans-10,11-dimethyldihydropyran-12-0l ring (ring C). *J Med Chem* 1997;40(6):1005-17.

10 Flavin M, et al. Synthesis, chromatographic resolution, and anti-human immunodeficiency virus activity of (+/-)-calanolide A and its enantiomers *J Med Chem* 1996;39(6):1303-13.

11 Hizi A, et al. Specific inhibition of the reverse transcriptase of human immunodeficiency virus type 1 and the chimeric enzymes of human immunodeficiency virus type 1 and type 2 by nonnucleoside inhibitors. *Antimicrob Agents Chemother* 1993;37(5):1037-42.

12 Currens M, et al. Antiviral activity and mechanism of action of calanolide A against the human immunodeficiency virus type-1. *J Pharmacol Exp Ther* 1996;279(2):645-51.

13 Currens M, et al. Kinetic analysis of inhibition of human immunodeficiency virus type-1 reverse transcriptase by calanolide A. *J Pharmacol Exp Ther* 1996;279(2):652-61.

14 Boyer P, et al. Analysis of nonnucleoside drug-resistant variants of human immunodeficiency virus type 1 reverse transcriptase. *J Virol* 1993;67(4):2412-20.

15 Buckheit R Jr, et al. Resistance to 1–[(2–hydroxyethoxy) methyl]-6-(phenylthio) thymine derivatives is generated by mutations at multiple sites in the HIV-1 reverse transcriptase. *Virology* 1995;210(1):186-93.

16 Xu Z, et al. In vivo anti-HIV activity of (+)-calanolide A in the hollow fiber mouse model. *Bioorg Med Chem Lett* 1999;9(2):133-38.

17 Fuller R, et al. HIV-inhibitory natural products. 16. HIV-inhibitory coumarins from latex of the tropical rain forest tree *Calophyllum teysmannii* var. inophylloide. *Bioorg Med Chem Lett* 1994;4(16):1961-64.

18 Buckheit R Jr, et al. Unique anti-human immunodeficiency virus activities of the nonnucleoside reverse transcriptase inhibitors calanolide A, costatolide, and dihydrocostatolide. *Antimicrob Agents Chemother* 1999;43(8):1827-34.

19 Dharmaratne H, et al. Inhibition of human immunodeficiency virus type 1 reverse transcriptase activity by cordatolides isolated from *Calophyllum cordato-oblongum. Planta Med* 1998;64(5):460-61.

20 Xu Z, et al. In vitro anti-human immunodeficiency virus (HIV) activity of the chromanone derivative, 12-oxocalanolide A, a novel NNRTI. *Bioorg Med Chem Lett* 1998;8(16):2179-84.

21 Newman R, et al. Pharmaceutical properties of related calanolide compounds with activity against human immunodeficiency virus. *J Pharm Sci* 1998;87(9):1077-80.

22 Matthee G, et al. HIV reverse transcriptase inhibitors of natural origin. *Planta Med* 1999;65(6):493-506.

Calendula

SCIENTIFIC NAME(S): *Calendula officinalis* L. Family: Compositae

COMMON NAME(S): Calendula, garden marigold, gold bloom, holligold, marygold, pot marigold, marybud[1]

BOTANY: Believed to have originated in Egypt, this plant has almost world wide distribution. There are numerous varieties of this species, each one varying primarily in flower shape and color. Calendula grows to about two feet in height and the wild form has small, bright yellow-orange flowers that bloom from May to October. It is the ligulate florets, mistakenly called the flower petals, that have been used medicinally. This plant should not be confused with several other members of the family that also carry the "marigold" name.

HISTORY: The plant has been grown in European gardens since the 12th century and its folkloric uses are almost as old. Tinctures and extracts of the florets had been used topically to promote wound healing and to reduce inflammation; systemically, they have been used to reduce fever, to control dysmenorrhea and to treat cancer. The dried petals have been used like saffron as a seasoning and have been used to adulterate saffron.[2]

The pungent odor of the marigold has been used as an effective pesticide. Marigolds are often interspersed among vegetable plants to repel insects.[3]

CHEMISTRY: A number of studies have been reported describing the chemistry of calendula. Almost all of the investigations regarding this plant have been conducted in Eastern Europe. The plant contains a number of oleanolic acid glycosides.[4] Flavonol-2-O–glycosides have been recovered from *C. officinalis* via high pressure chromatography.[5] Calendulin (also known as bassorin) has been identified in the plant.[1] Sterols and fatty acids, such as calendic acid, are present in the plant.[6,7,8] In addition, the plant contains triterpenoids,[9] tocopherols,[10] mucilage and a volatile oil. The carotenoid pigments have been used as coloring agents in cosmetics and the volatile oil has been used in perfumes.[11]

PHARMACOLOGY: Despite the history of use of calendula and the rather detailed studies of its chemistry, there are almost no studies regarding its efficacy in the treatment of human disorders.

Calendula extracts have been used topically to promote wound healing, and experiments in rats have shown that this effect is measurable. An ointment containing 5% flower extract in combination with allantoin was found to "markedly stimulate" epithelialization in surgically-induced wounds. On the basis of histological examination of the wound tissue, the authors concluded that the ointment increased glycoprotein, nucleoprotein and collagen metabolism at the site.[12]

Russian investigators found that sterile preparations of calendula extracts alleviated signs of chronic conjunctivitis and other chronic ocular inflammatory conditions in rats;[13] the extracts also had a systemic anti-inflammatory effect. Other Russian investigators have used plant extract mixtures containing calendula for the treatment of chronic hyposecretory gastritis. Extracts of the florets are uterotonic in the isolated rabbit and guinea pig uterus.

Calendula extracts have in vitro antibacterial, antiviral[14,15] and immunostimulating properties.[16] Published reports of small clinical trials conducted in Poland and Bulgaria suggest that extracts of the plant may be useful in the management of duodenal ulcers, gastroduodenitis and periodontopathies.

TOXICOLOGY: Despite its widespread use, there have been no reports in the Western literature describing serious reactions to the use of calendula preparations. A report of anaphylactic shock in a patient who gargled with a calendula infusion has been reported in Russia.

Allergies to members of the family Compositae (chamomile, feverfew, dandelion) have been reported, in particular to the pollens of these plants. Users of calendula preparations should consider the potential for allergic reactions to occur.

In animals, doses of up to 50 mg/kg of extract had essentially no pharmacologic effect and induced no histopathologic changes following either acute or chronic administration.[17] Saponin extracts of *C. officinalis* have not been found to be mutagenic.[18]

SUMMARY: Calendula is one of the many plants used persistently despite no clear evidence that its components exert any consistent pharmacologic effect. Some support in the form of animal studies exists for its topical wound healing and anti-inflammatory uses, and these properties should be investigated further. The plant ap-

pears to have a low potential for toxicity, but nevertheless, cannot be recommended at this time for the systemic treatment of any disease.

PATIENT INFORMATION – Calendula

Uses: Calendula has been used in folk medicine topically to treat wounds and internally to reduce fever, treat cancer and control dysmenorrhea. Extracts have proved antibacterial, antiviral and immunostimulating in vitro. Petals are consumed as a seasoning. The plant has been used to repel insects.

Side Effects: Allergic reactions to the botanical family and one case of anaphylaxis have been reported.

---

[1] Meyer JE. *The Herbalist.* Hammond, IN: Hammond Book Co, 1934.

[2] Duke JA. *Handbook of Medicinal Herbs.* Boca Raton, FL: CRC Press, 1985.

[3] Lewis WH, Elvin-Lewis MPF. *Medical Botany: Plants affecting man's health.* New York: John Wiley & Sons, 1977.

[4] Kasprzky Z, et al. Metabolism of triterpenoids in the seeds of *Calendula Officinalis* germinating. *Acta Biochim Pol* 1973;20:231.

[5] Pietta P, et al. Separation of flavonol-2-O-glycosides from Calendula officinalis and Sambucus nigra by high-performance liquid and micellar electrokeinetic capillary chromatography. *J Chromatogr* 1992;593(1–2):165.

[6] Chisholm MJ, Hopkins CY. *Can J Biochem* 1967;45:251.

[7] Badami RC, Morris LJ. *J Am Oil Chem Soc* 1965;42:1119.

[8] Szakiel A, Kasprzyk Z. Distribution of oleanolic acid glycosides in vacuoles and cell walls isolated from protoplasts and cells of *Calendula officinalis* leaves. *Steroids* 1989;53(3–5):501.

[9] Auguscinska E, Kasprzyk K. *Acta Biochim Pol* 1982;29:7.

[10] Janiszowska W, Jasinska R. *Acta Biochim Pol* 1982;29:37.

[11] Tyler VE. *The New Honest Herbal.* Philadelphia, PA: G.F. Stickley Co., 1987.

[12] Klouchek-Popava E, et al. *Acta Physiol Pharmacol Bulg* 1982;8:63.

[13] Marinchev VN, et al. *Oftalmol Zh* (USSR) 1971;26:196.

[14] Dumenil G, et al. *Ann Pharm Fr* 1980;38:493.

[15] De Tommasi N, et al. Structure and in vitro antiviral activity of sesquiterpene glycosides from *Calendula arvensis*. *J Nat Prod* 1990;53(4):830.

[16] Wagner H, et al. *Arzneimittelforschung* 1985;35:1069.

[17] Iatsyno AI, et al. *Farmakol Toksikol* 1978;41:556.

[18] Elias R, et al. Antimutagenic activity of some saponins isolated from *Calendula officinalis* L., *C. arvensis* L. and *Hedera helix* L. *Mutagenesis* 1990;5(4):327.

Canaigre

SCIENTIFIC NAME(S): *Rumex hymenosepalus* Torr. Family: Polygonaceae.

COMMON NAME(S): Canaigre, ganagra, tanner's dock, wild rhubarb[1,2]

BOTANY: Canaigre is native to the deserts of the southwestern United States and Mexico. It is a member of the dock (sorrel) family, and can attain a height of 3 feet.

HISTORY: Canaigre has long been known as a practical source of tannin. The common name derived from the Spanish "Cana Agria" or "sour cane"[2] and extracts of the plant were used in the tanning industry. The plant was also the source of a mustard-colored dye. However, canaigre does not have an extensive history of use in herbal medicine. Instead, it became popular during the latter half of this century and today is promoted for the treatment of a variety of ailments. More recent promotions suggest that canaigre may be used as an inexpensive alternative to ginseng because of its ability to manage disease states. Canaigre is not related botanically to ginseng and there is no evidence of any beneficial effects associated with the use of canaigre.

CHEMISTRY: The root of canaigre contains up to 25% of tannin.[2] The plant contains small amounts of anthroquinones (about 1%) as well as starch and resin.[3] There is no evidence that the plant contains any of the panaxoside-like saponin glycosides responsible for the pharmacologic activity of ginseng.

PHARMACOLOGY: There are no reports of any significant pharmacologic activity associated with canaigre. The high tannin content may provide an astringent effect when applied topically. The leucoanthocyanin fraction of the plant may have antitumor activity.[4]

TOXICOLOGY: Although the petioles are edible like rhubarb, this practice is not widespread and no significant reports of toxicity have been associated with canaigre. Tyler[3] notes that the high tannin concentration may pose a considerable carcinogenic risk. Consequently, the ingestion of canaigre should be avoided.

SUMMARY: Canaigre is being actively promoted for the treatment of a variety of disease states. The plant contains high concentrations of tannin but appears to be otherwise devoid of significant pharmacologic activity. There is no evidence that canaigre contains the same pharmacologically active compounds as ginseng. Its high tannin content may pose a toxicologic risk and the ingestion of the plant should generally be avoided.

PATIENT INFORMATION – Canaigre

Uses: Roots contain up to 25% tannin. The plant yields dye. It has in recent times been promoted as an alternative to ginseng.

Side Effects: High tannin may pose carcinogenic risk. Ingestion should be avoided.

---

[1] Mabberly DJ. *The Plant-Book*. New York, NY: Cambridge University Press, 1987.
[2] Balls EK. *Early Uses of California Plants*. Berkeley, CA: University of California Press, 1962.
[3] Tyler VE. *The New Honest Herbal*. Philadelphia, PA: G.F. Stickley Co, 1987.
[4] Duke JA. *Handbook of Medicinal Herbs*. Boca Raton, FL: CRC Press, 1985.

Capers

SCIENTIFIC NAME(S): *Capparis spinosa* L. Family: Capparidaceae

COMMON NAME(S): Caper, cappero

BOTANY: *C. spinosa* is a shrub native to the Mediterranean region. It is a tender perennial plant with deep roots and a long stem that grows to approximately 5 feet. Two forms of the caper can be found, a spiny and a nonspiny variety. Capers thrive best in dry soil.

HISTORY: The caper has a long history of use as a culinary spice and remains widely used as a spice today. In commercial operations, the unopened flower buds are collected by hand and pickled to produce the characteristic pungent taste and smell.[1] Leaves of related species are used as rubifacients and to treat skin disorders.

CHEMISTRY: No detailed investigations have been carried out regarding the chemical constituents of capers, although a number of aromatic volatile compounds are present in the unripe buds.

PHARMACOLOGY: Preliminary investigations have found that extracts of capers may be an effective treatment for improving the function of enlarged capillaries and for improving dry skin.[1]

TOXICOLOGY: The topical application of wet compresses soaked in fluid containing capers has been associated with the development of contact dermatitis. Therefore, patients with sensitive skin should be aware of the irritating potential of this plant when used topically.[2] The related species *C. fasicularis* and *C. tumentosa* are reported to be poisonous.[1]

SUMMARY: Capers are best known as spices used in Mediterranean cooking. Although they have not been used widely in herbal medicine, extracts of the buds and plant have been used for the treatment of some topical skin disorders. Unfortunately, capers may induce dermatitis.

PATIENT INFORMATION – Capers

Uses: Pickled flower buds are used as a condiment. Extracts of this or related species may improve dry skin and the function of enlarged capillaries.

Side Effects: Capers may cause contact dermatitis in sensitive individuals.

---

[1] Simon JE. *Herbs: An Indexed Bibliography, 1971-1980*. Hamden, CT: Shoe String Press, 1984.

[2] Angelini G, et al. Allergic contact dermatitis from *Capparis spinosa* L. applied as wet compresses. *Contact Dermatitis* 1991;24(5):382.

Capsicum Peppers

SCIENTIFIC NAME(S): *Capsicum frutescens* L., *Capsicum annuum* L., or a large number of hybrids or varieties of the species. Family: Solanaceae

COMMON NAME(S): *C. frutescens*: capsicum, cayenne pepper, red pepper, African chillies; *C. annuum*, var. conoides: tabasco pepper, paprika, pimiento, Mexican chilies; *C. annuum*, var. longum: Louisiana long pepper or hybridized to the Louisiana sport pepper.

BOTANY: *C. frutescens* is a small spreading annual shrub that is indigenous to tropical America. It yields an oblong, pungent fruit, while *Capsicum annum* (the common green pepper) yields paprika. At one time, it was believed that all peppers derived from *C. frutescens* or *C. annuum* or their hybrids. However, it is now recognized that approximately five species and their hybrids contribute as sources of "peppers."[1] Capsicum peppers should not be confused with the black and white pepper spices derived from the unripened fruit of *Piper nigrum*.

HISTORY: Capsicum was first described in the mid-1400s by a physician who accompanied Columbus to the West Indies. The plants derive their names from the Latin "capsa," meaning box, referring to the partially hollow, box-like fruit. Capsicum has been highly desired as a spice and has been cultivated in some form in almost every society. Peppers are among the most widely consumed spices in the world with an average daily per capita consumption in some South East Asian countries approaching 5 g of red pepper (approximately 50 mg of capsaicin).[2] Preparations of capsicum have been used use as topical rubifacients, and extracts have been ingested as a stomachic, carminative and gastrointestinal stimulant.

CHEMISTRY: Capsicum contains about 1.5% of an irritating oleoresin. The major component of the oil is capsaicin (0.02%), a very pungent phenolic chemical. Along with several closely related compounds, it is responsible for the pungency of the fruit.[3] The structure of capsaicin is similar to that of eugenol, the active principle in oil of cloves, which can also induce long-lasting local analgesia.[4] The pungency appears to be related to the presence of a 4-hydroxy-3-methoxyphenyl substituent.[5] It has been noted that the more tropical the climate, the more pungent the fruit.[5] The characteristic flavor of capsaicin can be detected in concentrations as low as 1 part in 11 million in aqueous solutions.

PHARMACOLOGY: Capsicum is a powerful irritant due to the effect of the oleoresin and capsaicin. Solutions of capsaicin applied topically can produce sensations varying from warmth to burning, depending on the concentration; with repeated applications, an apparent desensitization to the burning occurs. This effect has been studied in detail and has resulted in the elucidation of the mechanism of action of capsaicin.

In one study, four applications of a 0.1% solution of capsaicin were applied topically to the skin of healthy subjects and compared to untreated skin. Histamine was injected intradermally at the application site to test for chemical responsiveness. As expected, injection at the untreated area evoked a wheal, flare and itching. Interestingly, the capsaicin-treated areas developed a wheal but no flare. The flare response, also called axon reflex vasodilation, is believed to be mediated by the release of the vasoactive compound, substance P. This compound is involved in the transmission of painful stimuli from the periphery to the spinal cord. Following an initial application, substance P is released, causing the sensation of pain. However, upon repeated administration, the compound is depleted and a lack of pain sensation ensues. This effect usually occurs within 3 days of regular application. Pretreatment with capsaicin also abolishes airway edema and bronchoconstriction induced by cigarette smoke and other irritants.[4]

Capsaicin has become a valuable "pharmacologic probe" for the evaluation of nociception. Of more practical importance has been the use of capsaicin ointments for the treatment of pain due to herpes zoster (shingles). In patients affected with shingles, often excrutiating pain may persist around the infected nerve tracts for months to years after the initial flare. *Zostrix* cream (GenDerm Corp.), containing either 0.025% or 0.075% capsaicin, has been found to be effective when applied topically in the management of post-herpetic neuralgia.[6,7] It also has been found to be effective in the management of trigeminal and diabetic neuralgia, causalgia and post-mastectomy and post-surgical neuralgias.

The inhalation of a capsaicin solution can desensitize nasal nerves that cause running, sneezing and congestion. In a small study at Johns Hopkins Asthma & Allergy Center, such symptoms were alleviated in eight volunteers who received repeated nose sprays of capsaicin.[8]

One commercial product (*WarmFeet*, Divajex Inc, Tustin CA) contains powdered capsicum mixed with several other herbs. The powder is sprinkled into socks or massaged on the feet to stimulate a sensation of warmth during cold weather.

TOXICOLOGY: The most well-known adverse effect of peppers is the often intolerable burning sensation that occurs following contact with moist mucous membranes. For this reason, it is a common component of many self-defense sprays. When sprayed into an attacker's eyes, *Pepper Defense* (Security Barn, New Port Richey, FL) causes immediate blindness and irritation for up to 30 minutes, with no permanent damage. If capsicum comes in contact with mucous membranes, it should be flushed with water. Anecdotal reports suggest that flushing the area with milk may be beneficial.

Topical irritation is common, in particular with the use of commercial creams. One clinical study in patients with post-herpetic lesion was terminated early because approximately one-third of the patients experienced "unbearable" burning.[9]

The toxicity of *Tabasco* brand red pepper sauce was evaluated in rats.[10] The acute oral LD_{50} was 24 ml/kg. After 90 days of diet supplementation with the sauce, no signs of toxicity were noted. Mild eye irritation was observed when instilled, but vinegar, an ingredient in the sauce, was shown to contribute significantly to this effect.[11]

The intense gastrointestinal burning that often accompanies the ingestion of peppers may be reduced by removing the seeds from the pepper pods before ingestion[12] or by ingesting bananas along with the peppers.[13] One study found no difference in the healing rate of duodenal ulcers among patients who ingested 3 g of capsicum daily compared to untreated controls,[14] disproving a commonly held idea that peppers always exacerbate gastrointestinal problems.

SUMMARY: Peppers are one of the most common spices known, and their distribution is worldwide. Pungent peppers contain the highest concentration of the active principle capsaicin, a compound known to deplete neuronal stores of the pain transmitter, substance P. Capsaicin is applied topically in the management of topical neuritis syndromes.

PATIENT INFORMATION – Capsicum Peppers

Uses: Many varieties are eaten as vegetables and spices. The component capsaicin is both an irritant and analgesic, used in self-defense sprays and pain treatments for post-surgical neuralgia, shingles, etc.

Side Effects: Topical, mucosal and GI irritation are common.

---

[1] Leung AY. *Encyclopedia of Common Natural Ingredients Used in Food*, Drugs and Cosmetics. New York, NY: John Wiley and Sons, 1980.

[2] Buck SH and Burks TF. Capsaicin: hot new pharmacological tool. *Tips* 1983;4:84.

[3] Tyler VE. *The Honest Herbal*. Philadelphia, PA: G.F. Stickley Co., 1987.

[4] Editorial. Hot peppers and substance p. *Lancet* 1983;B335:1198.

[5] Tyler VE, et al. *Pharmacognosy*, 8th ed. Philadelphia, PA: Lea & Febiger, 1981.

[6] Bernstein JE, et al. Total capsaicin relieves chronic post herpetic neuralgia. *J Am Acad Dermatol* 1987;17:93.

[7] Olin BR, Hebel SK, eds. *Drug Facts and Comparisons*. St. Louis, MO: Facts and Comparisons, Jul 1992:632.

[8] Snyder M. Chili peppers heat up a cure for runny noses. *USA Today* 1992; Mar 18.

[9] GenDerm capsaicin for shingles pain relief. *F-D-C Reports* 1989;Feb 27.

[10] Winek CL, et al. Pepper sauce toxicity. *Drug Chem Toxicol* 1982;5(2):89.

[11] Monseraenuscrn Y. Subchronic toxicity studies of capsaicin and capsicum in rats. *Res Commun Chem Pathol Pharmacol* 1983;41(1):95.

[12] Prevost RJ. Preventing capsicum colon. *Lancet* 1982;8277(1):917.

[13] Roberts RM. Trouble with chillies. *Lancet* 1982;8270(1):519.

[14] Kumar N, et al. Do chillies influence healing of duodenal ulcer? *Brit Med J* 1984;288:1803.

Carrot Oil

SCIENTIFIC NAME(S): *Daucus carota* L. Subsp. *carota*. Fam: Umbelliferae or Apiaceae

COMMON NAME(S): Oil of carrot, Queen Anne's lace, wild carrot

BOTANY: The carrot is an annual or biennial herb, having an erect multi-branched stem, growing up to 1.5 m (4 ft) in height. The wild carrot is commonly seen in fields and roadsides throughout most of temperate North America and is seen with an intricately patterned flat flower cluster (Queen Anne's lace). The main cluster is made up of some 500 flowers, each showing at the center a single, small red-to-purplish flower. The wild carrot has an inedible tough white root. It is native to Asia and Europe, having been brought to America from England. The common cultivated carrot [*Daucus carota* L. subspecies *sativus* (Hoffm.) Arcang.] possesses an edible, fleshy, orange taproot. The parts that are used pharmaceutically are the dried fruit which yields carrot seed oil upon steam distillation and the orange carrot root which yields root oil by solvent extraction.[1,2]

CHEMISTRY: Carrot seed oil is made up of α-pinene (up to 13.3%), β-pinene, carotol (up to 18.29%), daucol, limonene, β-bisabolene, β-elemene, *cis*-β-bergamotene, γ-decalactone, β-farnesene, geraniol, geranyl acetate (up to 10.39%), caryophyllene, caryophyllene oxide, methyl eugenol, nerolidol, eugenol, *trans*-asarone, vanillin, asarone, α-terpineol, terpinene–4–ol, γ-decanolactone, coumarin, β-selinene, palmitic acid, butyric acid and other constituents. The seed oil varies in content from 0.005% to 7.15% of the plant.[2]

The chemical composition of the edible carrot root is 86% water, 0.9% protein, 0.1% fat, 10.7% carbohydrate, 1.2% fiber, trace elements and vitamin A (2,000 to 4300 I.U. in 100 grams).[1] Several tissue culture studies on *D. carota* identify new ingredients in the vegetative tissue (eg, enthocyanins,[3,5] chlorogenic acid,[3] flavonoids,[4] apigenin[6] and a soluble β-fructofuranosidase[7]).

PHARMACOLOGY: Carrot seed oil exhibits both smooth-muscle relaxant and vasodilatory action in isolated animal organ studies. It depresses cardiac activity in both frog and dog hearts.[2]

The cultivated fleshy taproot of the edible carrot is widely eaten as a raw or cooked vegetable; even wine has been brewed from the plant.[1] A wide array of older references lists the uses of carrot seed oil as an aromatic, carminative, diuretic, emmenagogue, aphrodisiac, nerve tonic and as a treatment for dysentery, worms, uterine pain, cancer, diabetes, gout, heart disease, indigestion and various kidney ailments.[1] Of course, many of these areas have not yet been fully studied. The continued use of carrot seed oil is primarily as a fragrance in detergents, soaps, creams, lotions and perfumes (which contain 0.4%, the highest level) and as a flavoring in many food products (eg, liqueurs, nonalcoholic beverages, frozen dairy desserts, candy, baked goods, gelatins, puddings, meat products, condiments, relishes and soups), usually in levels below 0.003%.[2] The root oil is used in sunscreen preparations, as a yellow food color (because of its high carotene content) and as a good source of β-carotene and vitamin A.[2]

Extracts of *D. carota* show only limited antifungal activity.[8] An ethanol extract (10 to 100 mg/kg dose) produced a dose-dependent decrease in systolic and diastolic blood pressure in anesthetized normotensive rats. Further experiments using beating guinea pig paired atria showed that the cardiovascular effects are independent of adrenergic or cholinergic receptors, and the extract induced a concentration-dependent (0.3 to 5 mg/ml) decrease in force and rate of atrial contractions. The same preparation applied to rabbit thoracic aorta produced inhibition of potassium-induced contractions. These results suggest that *D. carota* extract may exhibit calcium channel blocking-like direct relaxant action on cardiac and smooth muscle, and may explain its hypotensive action.[9] An extract of *D. carota* has also demonstrated hepatoprotective activity against carbon tetrachloride-induced intoxication in mouse liver.[10] Obviously, both these hypotensive and hepatoprotective properties need verification in humans.

TOXICOLOGY: Because myristicin (a known psychoactive agent) occurs in carrot seed, it has been proposed that ingestion of large amounts of *D. carota* may cause neurological effects. Some individuals have shown sensitivity (irritation, vesication) to carrot leaf when they handle it excessively, especially after exposure to sunlight.[1] Most data indicate that the vegetable and the seed oil are nontoxic.[2]

SUMMARY: The commonly cultivated edible carrot root is widely consumed as a vegetable because of its flavor and high vitamin A content. The seed and root oils of the wild and cultivated carrot are used pharmaceutically as a flavoring and fragrance, and the roots as sources of β-carotene and vitamin A. More recent pharmacological studies indicate its potential usefulness as cardiovascular and hepatoprotective agents. These still need further verification and human clinical studies.

PATIENT INFORMATION – Carrot Oil

Uses: Lab studies show that carrot seed oil, which had a wide range of applications in folk medicine, acts as a muscle relaxant and vasodilator. It is now most commonly used as fragrance, flavoring and a source of food color, beta-carotene and vitamin A. Hypotensive and hepatoprotective properties have yet to be confirmed in humans.

Side Effects: Ingestion of large amounts may have neurological effects.

---

[1] Duke JA. *Handbook of Medicinal Herbs*. Boca Raton, FL: CRC Press, 1989.

[2] Leung AY. *Encyclopedia of Common Natural Ingredients*, ed. 2. New York: John Wiley & Sons, 1996.

[3] Stark D, et al. Phenylalanine Ammonia Lyase Activity and Biosynthesis of Anthocyanins and Chlorogenic Acid in Tissue Cultures of *Daucus carota*. *Planta Med* 1976;30:104.

[4] El-Moghazi AM, et al. Flavonoids of *Daucus carota*. *Planta Med* 1980;40:382.

[5] Hemingson JC, Collins RP. Anthrocyanins Present in Cell Cultures of *Daucus carota*. *J Nat Prod* 1982;45:385.

[6] Gupta KR, Niranjan GS. New Flavone Glycoside From Seeds of *Daucus carota*. *Planta Med* 1982;46:240.

[7] Unger C, et al. Purification and Characterization of a Soluble Beta-Fructofuranosidase From *Daucus carota*. *Eur J Biochem* 1992;204(2):915.

[8] Guerin JC, Reveillere HP. Antifungal Activity of Plant Extracts Used in Therapy. Part 2. Study of 40 plant extracts against 9 fungal species. *Ann Pharma Fr* 1985;43(1):77.

[9] Gilani AH, et al. Cardiovascular Actions of *Daucus carota*. *Arch Pharmacal Res* 1994;17(3):150.

[10] Bishayee A, et al. Hepatoprotective Activity of Carrot (*Daucus carota* L.) Against Carbon Tetrachloride Intoxication in Mouse Liver. *J Ethnopharm* 1995;47(2):69.

Cascara

SCIENTIFIC NAME(S): *Rhamnus pushiana* DC. (Syn. *Frangula purshiana* (D.C.) A. Gray ex J.C. Cooper) Family: Rhamnaceae

COMMON NAME(S): Buckthorn, cascara sagrada, chittem bark, sacred bark

BOTANY: The official cascara sagrada is the dried bark of *Rhamnus pushiana* collected from small to medium-sized wild deciduous trees. They usually range from 20 to 40 feet high and possess thin, elliptic to ovate-oblong, acutely pointed leaves. The greenish flowers are arranged in umbellate cymes and the fruit is purplish-black and broadly obovoid (8 mm long). The commercial bark is flattened or transversely curved, longitudinally ridged with a brownish to red-brown color. It has gray or white lichen patches and occasional moss attachments. Cascara trees are found in North America in California, Oregon, Washington, Idaho, Montana and as far north as Southeast British Columbia.[1,2]

HISTORY: The American cascara is a folkloric medicine of relatively recent origin, having been introduced as a tree bark laxative by early Mexican and Spanish priests of California (probably *Rhamnus Californica*). *R. purshiana* itself was not described officially until 1805 and the bark was not brought into regular medicinal use until 1877. The European counterpart (European buckthorn, *Rhamnus frangula*) was described much earlier by the Anglo-Saxons. In fact, the berries were official in the 1650 London Pharmacopoeia.[3]

CHEMISTRY: The active laxative principles of cascara include at least 6% to 9% anthracene derivatives which exist as normal O-glycosides and C-glycosides. The four primary glycosides or cascaroside A, B, C and D, contain both O- and C-glycosidin linkages. Chemically these are designated as the C-10 isomers of the 8–O–β-D-glucopyranosides of aloin and chrysophanol. The probable breakdown products of the C-glycosides are the two aloins: Barbaloin which is derived from aloe-emodin anthrone and chrysaloin which is derived from chrysophanol anthrone. Other glycosides isolated include a number of O-glycosides derived from emodin, emodin oxanthrone, aloe-emodin and chrysophanol. A number of dianthrones are also present including emodin, aloe-emodin, chrysophanol and the heterodianthrones, palmidin A, B and C. Compounds found in the free state include aloe-emodin, emodin and chrysophanol.

The free anthraquinones are likely formed in the leaves and stored in the bark largely as C-glycosides. The older bark contains the most C-glycosides. Although uneconomical for commercial exploitation, *R. purshiana* cell suspension cultures produce anthracene derivatives.[2,3]

Cascara juice also contains other non-laxative compounds eg, rhamnol (cinchol, cupreol, quebrachol); linoleic, myristic and syringic-acids; resins, fat, starch and glucose; malic and tannic acid. The dried seeds contain 6.7% to 25.4% protein, 13.4% to 56.9% oil and 1.3% to 2.3% ash.[4] The presence in the bark of bitter substance and methylhydrocotoin is disputed.[5]

A variety of extraction methods have been examined for cascara. Boiling water prevents the losses and changes to the compound that occur in cold water extraction.[6] Active fractions of anthraquinone glucosides have been isolated from *R. pushiana* and *R. frangula* by high pressure liquid chromatography.[7] Hydrophilic anthraquinone glycosides have been separated from lesser hydrophilic anthraquinone aglycones by XAD-2 column chromatography.[8] The quantitative analysis of anthraquinones and anthranol in 16 species of *Rhamnus* from South and East Anatolia have been examined.[9] Likewise, a new naphthalene compound, nakahalene and known anthraquinones, including physcion and frangulin B, have been isolated from *Rhamnus* species.[10]

PHARMACOLOGY: As in other laxatives (aloe, senna, etc), the anthraglycosides are responsible for the cathartic properties in cascara. Cascarosides A and B are the major active principles which act on the large intestine to induce peristalsis and evacuation.[2] More specifically, the anthraglycosides produce an active secretion of water and electrolytes within the lumen of the small intestine and inhibit the absorption of these from the large intestine. This causes an increase in the volume of the bowel contents and strengthens the dilatation pressure in the intestine to stimulate peristalsis. They exert this action with a minimum of side effects.[5] In general, the cascarosides are more active than their hydrolyzed by-products.[2] Furthermore, these cascarosides possess a sweet and more pleasant taste than the aloins and hence should be extracted separately, if possible.[3] Cascara is largely used in the form of a liquid extract or elixir or as tablets made from a standardized dry extract.[2]

The daily dose ranges from 20 to 160 mg of the cascara derivatives for the treatment of constipation.[5] The average dose range of total hydroxyanthracene derivatives is 20 to 70 mg daily.[11] The laxative action is seen within 6 to 8 hours after administration. Basically, cascara can be used in most conditions where easy defecation with a soft stool is desired (eg, constipation, hemorrhoids, anal fissures and post rectal-anal surgery). It is contraindicated in ileus of any origin and during pregnancy and lactation.[5]

No major side effects are known; however, chronic use or abuse (eg, for weight loss) can result in electrolyte loss, especially potassium. Chronic use can also lead to pigmentation of the intestinal mucosa (melanosis coli). No direct interactions are known with cascara except where chronic use leads to a potassium deficiency which can potentiate the effects of cardiotonic glycosides (eg, digitalis). The anthraquinone glycosides should not be used for long periods of time because they can cause the above problems or lead to laxative dependence.[5]

Because the freshly prepared cascara products contain anthrones, it can lead to severe vomiting and intestinal cramping. Therefore, the bark should be stored for at least a year before use or artificially changed by heating (in air) to preclude the presence of anthrones.

Recent studies have shown that aloe-emodin has antileukemic activity against the P-388 lymphocytic leukemia in mice,[2] that *Rhamnus* anthraquinones can act as sunscreens in cosmetics,[12] that cascarosides are not readily metabolized in animal model gut microflora,[13] that a Formosan *Rhamnus* species contains physcion and frangulin B which exhibited a high activity against human hepatoma PLC/PRF/5 and KB cell lines,[10] that *R. purshiana* extracts are capable of inactivating herpes simplex virus,[14] that anthranoids are transformed to their corresponding glucuronide and sulfate derivatives and appear in the urine and bile,[15] and that a mixture of *Curcuma amara* and *R. purshiana* roots have choleretic and serum cholesterol lowering effects in rats.[16]

TOXICOLOGY: Extended or habitual use of cascara is to be avoided because it can cause chronic diarrhea and weakness, due to excessive potassium loss. Chronic use can cause melanin pigmentation of the mucous membranes of the colon.[4,5] Emodin can produce dermatitis.[4]

SUMMARY: Cascara bark is an anthraquinone-containing stimulant laxative commonly used for managing simple constipation in doses ranging from about 20 to 70 mg daily of total hydroxyanthracene derivatives. A laxative effect occurs 6 to 8 hours after administration.

Some commercial products containing cascara are Concentrated Milk of Magnesia-Cascara, Herbal Laxative and *Kondremul* with Cascara or Veracolate.

PATIENT INFORMATION – Cascara

Uses: Cascara extracts are used in laxatives.

Side Effects: Cascara should not be used during pregnancy and lactation, or in ileus of any origin. Extended use may cause chronic diarrhea and attendant ills.

---

[1] Osol A, Farrar GE, eds. *The Dispensatory of the United States of America* 25th ed. Philadelphia: JB Lippincott, 1955.

[2] Leung AY. *Encyclopedia of Common Natural Ingredients Used in Food, Drugs, and Cosmetics.* New York: J Wiley Interscience, 1980.

[3] Evans WC. *Trease and Evans' Pharmacognosy*, 13th ed. New York: Bailliere Tindall, 1989.

[4] Duke JA. *Handbook of Medicinal Herbs.* Boca Raton, FL: CRC Press, 1985.

[5] Bisset NG, ed. *Herbal Drugs and Phytopharmaceuticals.* Stuttgart: Medpharm Scientific Publishers, 1994.

[6] Fairbairn JW, Simic S. New dry extract of cascara (*Rhamnus pushiana* DC bark). *J Pharm Pharmacol* 1970;22:778.

[7] Terracciano M, et al. Analysis of the principle constituents in extracts of cascara and frangula by high pressure liquid chromatography. *Boll Chim Farm* 1977;116:402.

[8] Denee R, Huizing HJ. Purification and separation of anthracene derivatives on the polystyrene divinylbenzene copolymer. *J Nat Prod* 1981;44:257.

[9] Coskun M. Quantitative determination of anthraderivatives in *Rhamnus* species growing in South and East Anatolia (Turkey). Part 2. *Int J Crude Drug Res* 1989;27:167.

[10] Wei BL, et al. Nakahalene and cytotoxic principles of Formosan *Rhamnus* species. *J Nat Prod* 1992;55:967.

[11] Reynolds JEF ed. *Martindale: The Extra Pharmacopoeia*, 31st ed. London: Royal Pharmaceutical Society, 1996.

[12] Bader S, et al. Natural hydroxyanthracenic polyglycosides as sunscreens. *Cosmetics and Toiletries* 1981;96:67.

[13] Dreessen M, Lemli J. Studies in the field of drugs containing anthraquinone derivatives. Part 36. Metabolism of cascarosides by intestinal bacteria. *Pharm Acta Helv* 1988;63(9–10):287.

[14] Sydiskis RJ, et al. Inactivation of enveloped viruses by anthraquinones extracted from plants. *Antimicrob Agents Chemother* 1991;35(12):2463.

[15] de Witte P, Lemli L. The metabolism of anthranoid laxatives. [Review] *Hepato Gastroenterology* 1990;37(6):601.

[16] Beynen AC. Lowering of serum cholesterol by Temoe Lawak Singer, a Curcuma mixture. *Artery* 1987;14(4):190.

Castor

SCIENTIFIC NAME(S): *Ricinus communis* L. and *R. sanguines* L. Family: Euphorbiaceae

COMMON NAME(S): Castor, Palma Christi, Tangantangan oil plant, African coffee tree, Mexico weed, wonder tree, Bofareira.[16]

BOTANY: A common annual ornamental whose native habitat is in the West Indies, the castor grows to heights of 40 feet, bearing broad, deeply lobed leaves on broad stalks. The flowers develop into spiny capsules each containing three seeds. As the capsules dry, they explode, scattering the beans.[1] The castor has been naturalized to temperate regions of the contiguous United States and Hawaii.

HISTORY: The name "ricinus" is derived from the Latin word meaning insect, because the seeds resemble some beetles in shape and markings. The plant has been used as an ornamental since antiquity. Castor beans are used as art objects and ornaments.[2] The Egyptians used castor oil as a lamp oil and unguent[1] and ingested the oil with beer as a purgative. The fast-drying, non-yellowing oil is used in industry to coat fabrics, in the manufacture of high-grade lubricants and in dyes and inks. The plant and oil have been used medicinally for an innumerable variety of diseases, rarely with any true clinical benefit.[3]

CHEMISTRY: Castor oil is obtained by cold expression of the kernels, which contain 45% to 50% oil.[17] The oil is a mixture of triglycerides, of which 75% to 90% is ricinoleic acid.[4] This mixture is hydrolyzed by duodenal lipases to release ricinoleic acid, which exerts a cathartic effect.[5] The cake left after the expression of the oil is the castor pomace.[17]

The phytotoxins ricin and ricinine are present in the seed cake and oil. Ricin is a glycoprotein of approximate molecular weight 65,000, consisting of a neutral A chain and an acidic B chain connected by S-S bonds. The A chain inhibits protein synthesis, which causes cell death, and the B chain serves as a carrier that binds the protein to the cell surface.[6] Other designations indicate that ricin can be separated into the highly toxic ricin D, acidic ricin and basic ricin.[7] The alkaloid ricinine is found in the seeds and leaves. Commercially, the oils and cakes are obtained by cold expression or are steam treated to denature the toxins.

In addition the seeds contain a lipase and an allergen designated CBA.[7]

PHARMACOLOGY: Ricin is a protoplasmic poison. It binds with normal cells and disrupts DNA synthesis and protein metabolism resulting in cell death.[8] In vitro studies have shown that 10 molecules of ricin bound to HeLa cells in culture are sufficient to cause cell death. Ricin is engulfed within 30 seconds, rapidly inhibiting peptide elongation.[8]

Ingestion, inhalation or intravenous (IV) administration of ricin results in rapid organismal death, and the toxin has been explored as a chemical warfare agent.

Ricin has been evaluated in the treatment of cancers[10] and was found to be active in mice inoculated with L1210 leukemia cells. When given intraperitoneally (IP), its effect was superior to that of 5-fluorouracil, but less than that of adriamycin. It was ineffective when given IV.[11] Ricin has been used with some clinical success as an analgesic.[12]

TOXICOLOGY: The castor is a commonly cultivated plant. Ornamental use of the seeds increases the likelihood of toxicities since the beans usually have been drilled, rupturing the seed coat and exposing the contents. If the seeds are swallowed without chewing, poisoning is unlikely because the impermeable seed coat remains intact.

The minimal lethal dose (given IP) in mice is 0.028 mcg crude ricin/g of body weight. As few as one or two chewed beans are lethal to humans. Although the seeds are most toxic, the leaves also may induce poisoning. Toxicity is characterized by burning of the mouth and throat, severe stomach pains, dull vision, renal failure, uremia and death.[13] Treatment is similar to that of other phytotoxin poisonings and generally consists of supportive therapy. Ricinine causes nausea, vomiting, hemorrhagic gastroenteritis, hepatic and renal damage, convulsions and death.

It should be noted that more recent analyses of clinical data from confirmed castor poisonings suggest that ingestion of castor seeds may not always result in severe toxicity. In one event, more than nine school children ingested the seeds without any signs of toxicity. In another more dramatic case, a 38-year-old woman ingested not less than 24 beans that had been cut and chopped to insure absorption. She was treated with induced emesis and remained completely asymptomatic.[14] Regardless of these more recent successful experiences, castor poisoning always should be treated as a serious medical emergency.

The castor has been implicated as an inhalant allergen. Burlap sacks used in the shipment of coffee beans may be contaminated with castor beans or residual castor pomace; this often occurs in the holds of ships or freight cars that have held castor beans.[15] Repeated exposure to castor dust is an occupational hazard to coffee industry workers who handle these sacks.

SUMMARY: Ricin is one of the most potent plant toxins. The widespread cultivation of castor plants represents a potential hazard to small children who ingest and chew the seeds. More recent clinical data suggest, however, that the ingestion of castor seeds by man may not always result in severe toxicity.

PATIENT INFORMATION – Castor

Uses: The oil has long been used for laxative effect.

Side Effects: Ingestion of leaves or seeds is often fatal. Inhalation of residual dust is a hazard to those who handle sacks of castor beans or who work in enclosures where these have been stored.

---

[1] Dobelis IN, eds. *Magic and Medicine of Plants.* Pleasantville, NY: Reader's Digest Association, 1986.
[2] Gunn CR. *Science* 1969;164:245.
[3] Duke JA. *Handbook of Medicinal Herbs.* Boca Raton, FL: CRC Press, 1985.
[4] Leung AY. *Encyclopedia of Common Natural Ingredients Used in Food, Drugs and Cosmetics* New York, NY: John Wiley and Sons, 1980.
[5] Tyler VE, et al. *Pharmacognosy.* Philadelphia, PA: Lea and Febiger, 1981.
[6] Olsnes S, et al. *Nature* 1974;249:627.
[7] Morton JF. *Major Medicinal Plants.* Springfield, IL: CC Thomas, 1977.
[8] Lampe KE. *AMA Handbook of Poisonous and Injurious Plants.* Chicago, IL: Chicago Review Press, 1985.
[9] Snodgrass WR. *Law Rev Nat Prod* 1982;3:32.
[10] Lin J, et al. *Nature* 1970;227:292.
[11] Fodstad O, et al. *Int J Cancer* 1978;22:558.
[12] Chen CC, et al. *J Formosan Med Assn* 1976;75:239.
[13] Kinamore PA, et al. *Clinical Toxicol* 1980;17:401.
[14] Rauber A, Heard J. *Vet Hum Toxicol* 1985;27:498.
[15] Bernton HS. *JAMA* 1973;223:1146.
[16] Meyer JE. *The Herbalist.* Hammond, IN: Hamond Book Co, 1934:60.
[17] Osol A, Farrar GE Jr., eds. 25th ed. *The Dispensatory of the United States of America* Philadelphia, PA: J.B. Lippincott, 1955:261.

Catnip

SCIENTIFIC NAME(S): *Nepeta cataria* L. Family: Labiatae (Lamiaceae)

COMMON NAME(S): Catnip, catnep, catmint, catswort, field balm

BOTANY: Catnip is a native of Eurasia, now established throughout the northeastern US and Canada. It is an aromatic perennial with dark green, oval-toothed leaves growing as a branched bush to about 1 meter. The plant's dried leaves, along with its white flowering tops gathered in summer and autumn, are used medicinally.[1,2,3,4]

HISTORY: Catnip was documented in K'eogh's *Irish Herbal* in 1735. Historically, it had been promoted to induce urination, open lung and womb obstruction, and expel worms from the body.[2] However, catnip is widely recognized for its ability to elicit "euphoria" in some cats. In Appalachia, catnip tea is used by humans to treat colds, nervous conditions, stomach ailments, and hives. The dried leaves have been smoked to relieve respiratory ailments, and a poultice has been used externally to reduce swelling. In the early 1900s, the flowering tops and leaves were used to bring on delayed menses, a practice that continues today in Appalachia. During the 1960s, catnip was used by humans as an hallucinogen. A tea can be brewed from the leaves.[5]

CHEMISTRY: Catnip contains between 0.2% and 1% volatile oil, of which the major component is nepetalactone (alpha and betaforms) ranging from 80% to 95%.[2,3,6] Congeners of nepetalactone are also present and include epinepetalactone, dihydronepetalactone, neonepetalactone, and isodihydronepetalactone.[6] The minor isomer trans-cis-nepetalactone possesses the cat-attractant activity of the isomeric mixture.[7] Also contained in the volatile oil are citronellol and geraniol.[2,6] Beta-caryophyllene (14%), camphor, thymol, carvacrol, and nerol are also in the plant,[3] as are nepetalic acid,[8] nepetaside,[9] tannins,[2,6] and numerous other components.[10] Iridoids[2,11] in catnip include epideoxyloganic and 7-deoxyloganic acid.[6] One report discusses (1R,5R,8S,9S)-deoxyloganic acid from catnip.[12]

PHARMACOLOGY: Catnip is available in the wild or commercially in pet stores as the leaf or liquid extract. Best known for its appeal to felines, catnip transforms some cats into a "euphoric" state. Domestic cats and large cats, such as tigers and jaguars, respond to catnip by sniffing, licking, head shaking, rolling, and body rubbing.[6] This "catnip response" has been described in detail, consisting of 6 distinct phases, each lasting ≈ 10 minutes and ranging from stretching and animation to euphoria and sexual stimulation.[13] The response is observed in essentially all species of cats, but not all individuals respond to the plant. Furthermore, the response does not appear to develop until 3 months of age. In Siamese cats, the response is inherited as an autosomal dominant gene. In a random sampling of 84 cats from the Boston area, one-third of the animals did not respond to catnip.[14]

Similar reactions to catnip in other animals have been reported. Amphetamine-like effects and other behavioral changes in mice due to catnip have been discussed.[15] Catnip oil and nepetalic acid increased (induced) sleeping time in mice. Other studies showed decreased performance in rats using the Sidman avoidance schedule, following intraperitoneal injections of both constituents.[16] In another report, high levels of catnip alcohol extract caused fewer chicks to sleep, while low-to-moderate dosing caused more chicks to sleep.[17]

Catnip also contains iridoids and has been used as an herbicide and insecticide.[6,11] Iridoids, which are named after a certain ant species, *Iridomirmex*, are involved in the insect's defense mechanisms.

In humans, catnip tea has been used as a calmative and sleep aid. The essential oil component, nepetalactone, is similar to the sedative compounds in valerian, another calming herb.[4] This calming effect makes catnip useful for migraine headaches, nervous disorders, and digestive complaints. It purportedly helps indigestion, colic, cramping, and flatulence.[2,3,4] Catnip has also increased gallbladder activity and been used for its diuretic effects.[3] Because catnip exhibits antipyretic and diaphoretic actions, it has been promoted for the treatment of flu, colds, and fever.[2,3]

Topically, catnip has been applied for arthritis treatment as a tincture and for hemorrhoids as an ointment.[2]

INTERACTIONS: Catnip may interact with other sedatives. Use with caution in patients taking standard sedative medications or alcohol.

TOXICOLOGY: Reports by human users describe a happy intoxication similar to the experience one might subjectively observe in an intoxicated cat. Four cases of catnip abuse have been reported,[18] with 2 modes of use being described. The first is similar to marijuana smoking in that the dried leaves are smoked as a "joint" or in a pipe, with catnip burning more rapidly than marijuana. An alternate method involves spraying or soaking tobacco in the volatile oil or extract and then smoking it. The latter method is purported to yield a stronger "high." These users consistently reported mood elevation and euphoria. Effects were of variable intensity ranging from "giddy" to a "feeling of unreality." The experiences were generally short-lived, lasting only a few hours, and could be reactivated for up to 3 days after smoking by some subjects. However, the validity of these case reports has been subjected to skepticism.[19,20]

The intraperitoneal LD$_{50}$ for catnip oil is 1300 mg/kg.[10] Severe physical effects after catnip abuse are usually absent; however, users report some symptoms, generally consisting of headache and malaise. Large amounts of tea induce emesis. The ingestion of cupful quantities of catnip tea has not been associated with any important toxicity.[4] No health hazards or side effects have been associated with proper administration of catnip in designated dosages.[3] Catnip was once listed in the FDA's "Herbs of Undefined Safety" listing in the mid 1970s.[21]

Catnip is contraindicated during pregnancy because of its uterine stimulant activities. Because catnip may lead to excessive menstrual bleeding, it may be contraindicated in certain gynecological conditions.

SUMMARY: Catnip is mostly recognized for its euphoric effect in cats but may be useful in humans for certain minor ailments. It has been used as a sedative, and its calming effects are also useful for migraine, nervous disorders, or digestive problems. Catnip also reduces fever and may be beneficial for colds and flu. No major side effects have been associated with catnip ingestion when administered properly in the correct dosages.

PATIENT INFORMATION – Catnip

Uses: Catnip has been used as a sleep aid and calmative, in migraines, GI problems, colds, flu, fevers, and topically for arthritis and hemorrhoids.

Side Effects: Excessive ingestion may result in headache and malaise. Catnip is contraindicated in pregnancy because of its uterine stimulant activities and may be contraindicated in certain other gynecological conditions because it could lead to excessive menstrual bleeding.

Interactions: Catnip may interact with other sedatives. Use with caution in patients taking standard sedative medications or alcohol.

---

[1] Gleason H, et al. *Manual of Vascular Plants of the Northeastern United States and Adjacent Canada.* New York: D. VanNostrand and Co. 1963.

[2] Chevallier A. *Encyclopedia of Medicinal Plants.* New York, NY: DK Publishing, 1996;237.

[3] Fleming T, et al. *PDR for Herbal Medicines.* Montvale, NJ: Medical Economics Co., Inc., 1998.

[4] Peirce A. *Practical Guide to Natural Medicines.* New York, NY: William Morrow and Co., Inc. The Stonesong Press, Inc., 1999; 147-48.

[5] Boyd E, et al. *Home Remedies and the Black Elderly.* Ann Arbor, MI: University of Michigan, 1984.

[6] Leung A. *Encyclopedia of Common Natural Products.* New York, NY: John Wiley and Sons, Inc., 1996;137-38.

[7] Bates R, et al. Terpenoids. *Cis-trans-* and *Trans-cis* -nepetalactones. *Experientia* 1963;19:564.

[8] McElvain S, et al. The consitutients of the volatile oil of catnip. III. The structure of nepetalic acid and related compounds. *J Am Chem Soc* 1955;77:1599.

[9] Xie S, et al. Absolute structure of nepetaside, a new iridoid glucoside from *Nepeta cataria. Phytochemistry* 1988;27:469.

[10] Duke J. *Handbook of Medicinal Herbs.* Boca Raton, FL: CRC Press, 1985.

[11] Bruneton J. *Pharmacognosy, Phytochemistry, Medicinal Plants.* Paris, France: Lavoisier Publishing, 1995;475-76.

[12] Mura F, et al. (1R,5R,8S,9S)-Deoxyloganic acid from *Nepeta cataria. Chem Pharm Bull* 1984;32(7):2809-14.

[13] Tucker A, et al. Catnip and the catnip response. *Economic Botany* 1988;42:214.

[14] Todd N. Inheritance of the catnip response in domestic cats. *J Heredity* 1962;53:54.

[15] Massoco C, et al. Behavioral effects of acute and long-term administration of catnip (*Nepeta cataria*) in mice. *Vet Hum Toxicol* 1995;37(6):530-33.

[16] Harney J, et al. Behavioral and toxicological studies of cyclopentanoid monoterpenes from *Nepeta cataria. Lloydia* 1978;41(4):367-74.

[17] Sherry C, et al. The effect of an ethanol extract of catnip (*Nepeta cataria*) on the behavior of the young chick. *Experientia* 1979;35(2):237-38.

[18] Jackson B, et al. Catnip and the alteration of consciousness. *JAMA* 1969;207:1349-50.

[19] Poundstone J. *JAMA* 1969;208:360.

[20] Tyler V. *The New Honest Herbal.* Philadelphia, PA: G.F. Stickley Co., 1987.

[21] Miller L, et al, eds. *Herbal Medicinal — Clinician's guide.* Binghamton, NY: Pharmaceutical Products Press, 1998;334-35.

Cat's Claw (Uña De Gato)

SCIENTIFIC NAME(S): *Uncaria tomentosa* (Willd.) DC and *Uncaria guianensis* (Aubl.) (Gmel.) Family: Rubiaceae

COMMON NAME(S): Cat's claw, life-giving vine of Peru, samento, uña de gato

BOTANY: Cat's claw, or uña de gato (Spanish), is a tropical vine of the madder family (Rubiaceae). The name describes the small curved-back spines on the stem at the leaf juncture. The genus *Uncaria* is found throughout the tropics, mainly in Southeast Asia, the Asian continent and South America. The two species of current interest, *Uncaria tomentosa* (Willd.) DC and *Uncaria guianensis* (Aubl.) (Gmel.), are found in South America. These species are lianas or high climbing, twining woody vines.[1,2] Both species are known in Peru as uña de gato.

There are 34 reported species of *Uncaria*. One Asian species, known as gambir or pole catechu (*Uncaria gambir*) (Hunter) Roxb., is a widely used tanning agent which also has long medicinal use as an astringent and anti-diarrheal.[3]

HISTORY: *U. guianensis* has long folkloric use in South America as a wound healer and for treating intestinal ailments.[2] Large amounts of *U. guianensis* are collected in South America for the European market, while American sources prefer *U. tomentosa*.[1]

The bark decoction of *U. guianensis* is used in Peru as an anti-inflammatory, antirheumatic and contraceptive, as well as in treating gastric ulcers and tumors, gonorrhea (by the Bora tribe), dysentery (by the Indian groups of Columbia and Guiana) and cancers of the urinary tract in women.[2]

The center of the *U. tomentosa* range is in Peru and its uses are similar to those of *U. guianensis*: Treatment of arthritis, gastric ulcers, intestinal disorders, and some skin problems and tumors.[2]

The Ashanica Indians believe that samento (also *U. tomentosa*) has "life-giving" properties and use a cup of the decoction each week or two to ward off disease, treat bone pains and cleanse the kidneys.[4] Recent interest in uña de gato stems from a reference to the plant in a popular book: *Witch Doctor's Apprentice, Hunting for Medicinal Plants in the Amazonian* (3rd ed., New York: Citadel Press, 1990) by Nicole Maxwell.

Reviews and scientific studies by the National Cancer Institute in the last decade have led to verification of some of the anticancer and immunostimulant properties.[2] Some of the demand for the bark has been attributed to European reports on its clinical use with AZT in AIDS treatment. The demand for the bark in the US is based on the purported usefulness of its tea in treating diverticulitis, hemorrhoids, peptic ulcers, colitis, gastritis, parasites and leaky bowel syndrome.[4]

CHEMISTRY: Several studies on the chemistry of the genus *Uncaria* have been undertaken during the last 20 years. Research on Asian (Thai) species includes the isolation and identification of four pentacyclic oxindole alkaloids, isopteropodine, pteropodine, speciophylline and uncarine F from the leaves of *U. homomalla*,[5] as well as the alkaloids 3–isoajmalicine, 19–epi-3–isoajmalicine, mitraphylline and uncarine B from the leaves of *U. attenuata*.[6]

Of recent interest are the studies on Cat's claw (*U. guianensis*) oxindole alkaloids;[7] three indole alkaloidal glucosides (cadambine, 3–α-dihydrocadambine and 3–β-isodihydrocadambine) from the Oriental crude drug chotoko (*Uncaria* hooks);[8] alkaloids of *U. ferrea*;[9] three new quinovic acid glycosides from *U. tomentosa*;[10] the isolation and structure of six quinovic acid glycosides from the bark of *U. tomentosa*;[11] alkaloids of *U. rhynchophylla*;[12] three new polyhydroxylated triterpenes from *U. tomentosa*;[13] and the alkaloid gambirine from *U. callphylla*.[14] The major alkaloids (rhynchophylline and isorhynchophyllin) occur in the roots, stem bark and leaves of uña de gato, but show great seasonal variation in concentration.[4] Several of these constituents have verified some of the pharmacological activities reported for the crude extract of the bark used in folkloric preparations.

PHARMACOLOGY: Both species, *U. tomentosa* and *U. guianensis*, have been used folklorically in the form of a bark decoction for a wide range of disorders, including gastric ulcers, inflammation, rheumatism, tumors and as a contraceptive. Specifically, *U. guianensis* has been employed to treat dysentery, gonorrhea and cancer of the urinary tract in women.[1]

Recent reports have demonstrated *Uncaria's* role in improving immunity in cancer patients,[4] as well as its anti-mutagenic properties.[15] All the individual alkaloids of *U. tomentosa*, with the exception of hynchophylline and mitraphyllin, have immunostimulant properties[16] and the ability to enhance phagocytosis in vitro. Other researchers have shown pteropodine and isopteropodine to have immune-stimulating effects.[4]

The major alkaloid rhynchophylline has been shown to be anti-hypertensive, to relax the blood vessels of endothelial cells, dilate peripheral blood vessels, inhibit sympathetic nervous system activities, lower the heart rate and lower blood cholesterol.[4,17] The alkaloid mytraphylline has diuretic properties,[4] while the alkaloid hirsutine inhibits urinary bladder contractions and possesses local anesthetic properties.[4,18] At higher dosages, hirsutine showed a "curare-like" ability on neuromuscular transmission.[4,19] The Oriental crude drug "chotoko" (the dried climbing hooks of *Uncaria* species) has hypotensive properties.[8] Six quinovic acid glycosides in *U. tomentosa* have antiviral activity in vitro,[11,13] as well as anti-inflammatory activity in rats. The alkaloid gambirine isolated from *U. callophylla* has cardiovascular properties.[14] An intravenous injection of this alkaloid (dose range: 0.2 — 10.0 mg/kg) in normotensive rats produced a dose-related fall in both systolic and diastolic blood pressure. Plant extracts and fractions of *U. tomentosa* exhibit no mutagenic effects, but show a protective antimutagenic property in vitro and decreased the mutagenicity in a smoker who had ingested a decoction of the plant for 15 days.[15]

TOXICOLOGY: While there is little published data on the toxicology of uña de gato, there is an international patent (1982) and a German dissertation (1984) which indicate low toxicity for this material.[4] The scattered pharmacological studies also seem to indicate little hazard in ingesting the plant decoction.

SUMMARY: Cat's claw, or uña de gato, has folkloric use in Peru and elsewhere in South America for a variety of conditions, mostly gastrointestinal problems, tumors, cancers and as a contraceptive. No major toxicity problems appear in the world literature. Several chemical and pharmacological investigations have verified that the alkaloids have immune-stimulating effects (pteropodine and isopteropodine), anti-hypertensive properties (rhynchophylline), diuretic effects (mytraphylline) and smooth muscle relaxant and local anesthetic properties (hirsutine). Early reports indicate the clinical usefulness of uña de gato and AZT in AIDS treatment. This, and other uses, have prompted sporadic demand for the crude botanical in the United States. At least one company advertises its availability through the Worldwide Web under the title, "Peruvian Cat's Claw: A Gift from Nature."[20] More research is needed to determine the true efficacy of the crude material and its numerous constituents.

PATIENT INFORMATION – Cat's Claw (Uña De Gato)

Uses: Various species have been used as astringent, anti-inflammatory, GI and cancer treatment, contraceptive, general tonic, etc. Studies have verified some anticancer and immunostimulant properties. The major alkaloid is hypotensive.

Side Effects: Little known hazard ingesting the decoction.

---

[1] Duke J, Vasquez R. *Amazonian Etnobotanical Dictionary*. Boca Raton, FL: CRC Press, 1994.

[2] Foster S. Cat's Claw. *Health Food Bus* 1995;Jun:24.

[3] Duke JA. *Handbook of Medicinal Herbs*. Boca Raton, FL: CRC Press, 1985.

[4] Jones K. The Herb Report: Uña De Gato, Life-Giving Vine of Peru *Am Herb Assoc* 1994;10(3):4.

[5] Ponglux D, et al. Alkaloids from the leaves of *Uncaria homomalla*. *Planta Med* 1977;31:26.

[6] Tantivatana P, et al. Alkaloids of Uncaria. Part 7. Alkaloids of U. attenuata (U. salaccensis) from N.E. Thailand. *Planta Med* 1980;40:299.

[7] Lavault M, et al. [Alkaloids of Uncaria guianensis.] [French] *Planta Med* 1983;47:244.

[8] Endo K, et al. Hypotensive principles of Uncaria Hooks. *Planta Med* 1983;49:188.

[9] Holdsworth D, Mahana P. Traditional medicinal plants of the Huon Peninsula Morobe Province, Papua New Guinea. *Int J Crude Drug Res* 1983;21:121.

[10] Cerri R, et al. New quinovic acid glycosides from *Uncaria tomentosa*. *J Nat Prod* 1988;51(2):257.

[11] Aquino R, et al. Plant metabolites: Structure and in vitro antiviral activity of quinovic acid glycosides from *Uncaria tomentosa* and *Guettarda platypoda*. *J Nat Prod* 1989;52(4):679.

[12] Want Z. Quantitative determination of the alkaloids of *Uncaria rhynchophylla* by calcium chromatography-UV Spectrophotometry. *Chin Tradit Herbal Drugs* 1989;20 11.

[13] Aquino R, et al. New polyhydroxylated triterpenes from Uncaria tomentosa. *J Nat Prod* 1990;53(3):559.

[14] Mok JS, et al. Cardiovascular response in the normotensive rat produced by intravenous injection of gambirine isolated from *Uncaria callophylla* Bl. ex Korth. *J Ethnopharmacol* 1992;36(3):219.

[15] Rizzi R, et al. Mutagenic and antimutagenic activities of Uncaria tomentosa and its extracts. *J Ethnopharmacol* 1993;38(1):63.

[16] Wagner H, et al. Die Alkaloide von *Uncaria tomentosa* und ihre Phagozytose-steigernde Wirkung. *Planta Med* 1985:419.

[17] Hemingway SR, Phillipson JD. Alkaloids from S. American species of *Uncaria* (Rubiaceae). *J Pharm Pharmacol* 1974;26(Suppl):113P.

[18] Harada M, et al. Effects of Indole Alkaloids from *Gardneria nutans* Sieb. et Zucc. and *Uncaria rhynochophylla* Miq. on a Guinea Pig Urinary Bladder Preparation in Situ. *Chem Pharm Bull* 1979;27(5):1069.

[19] Harada M, Ozaki Y. Effect of Indole Alkaloids from *Gardneria* Genus and *Uncaria* Genus on Neuromuscular Transmission in the Rat Limb [in Situ.] *Chem Pharm Bull* 1976;24(2):211.

[20] Anonymous. Peruvian Cat's Claw: A Gift from Nature. Gilroy, CA: Bour-Man Medical.

Celery

SCIENTIFIC NAME(S): *Apium graveolens* L. var *dulce* (Mill.) Pers. Family: Umbelliferae

COMMON NAME(S): Celery, celery seed, celery seed oil

BOTANY: This biennial plant is native to Europe,[1] yet grown and consumed worldwide. A number of varieties of celery exist, many developed to meet commercial demands for particular colors, tastes and stalk sizes. Celery generally grows between 1 to 2 feet tall. They have tough ribbed green stems and segmented dark green leaves containing toothed leaflets. During June and July, small white flowers bloom which later bear the smooth gray fruits of seeds. Wet and salty soils, swamps and marshes are the preferred environment for celery.[1] Celery is blanced to generate the edible white stem during cultivation.[1] Celery seeds have a spicy odor and a spicy, yet slightly bitter taste.[2]

The generic name pascal applies to any green celery. In Europe, the term celery is frequently used to refer to a related root vegetable, *Apium graveolens* L. var *rapaceum, DC.* Wild celery can refer to *Vallisneria spiralis* L., an aquatic perennial.

Celery seed oil is obtained by the steam distillation of the seed. According to the US Department of Agriculture, US growers in 1983 produced 914 tons of celery on 35,000 acres of farmland. The crop was valued at $235 million.

HISTORY: Celery originated as a wild plant growing in salt marshes around the Mediterranean Sea. About 450 B.C., the Greeks used it to make a type of wine called selinites. It served as an award at early athletic games, much as laurel leaves or olive branches. By the Middle Ages, Europeans were cultivating celery. Since that time, the plant has been used widely both as a food and as a medicine.

Late in the 19th century, various celery tonics and elixirs appeared commercially. These generally contained the juice of crushed celery seeds, often with a significant amount of alcohol. Celery seed is mainly used as a diuretic for bladder and kidney complaints and for arthritis and rheumatism. Sedative effects have been produced from the essential oil.[2]

Celery continues to be used as a food flavor, in soaps and in gum. One product that is still available is a celery-flavored soda, Dr. Brown's Cel-Ray. Celery has become increasingly popular with dieters. This particular attraction stems from celery's high fiber content and the (mistaken) belief that chewing and digesting the stalks uses more calories than celery contains.[3]

CHEMISTRY: Celery is high in minerals (including sodium and chlorine) and is a poor source of vitamins.[4] The major constituents of celery seed oil are d-limonene (60%), selinene (10%) and a number of related phthalides (3%) which include 3–n–butylphthalide, sedanenolide and sedanonic anhydride. Celery contains a pheromone steroid previously identified in boars and parsnips.[5]

The furocoumarin, bergapten, has been found in celery.[6] UV spectographic studies have indicated the presence of a compound similar or identical to 8–methoxypsoralen. Infrared spectography has confirmed yet another compound with a furocoumarin glucoside, isoquercitrin, and the coumarin glucoside apiumoside also have been identified.[8]

Other organic components include isovalerianic aldehyde, propionic aldehyde and acetaldehyde.[9] Oil of celery seed is sometimes adulterated with celery chaff oil or d-limonene from less expensive sources.

PHARMACOLOGY: Herbalists recommend celery for treatment of arthritis, nervousness and hysteria. Oriental medicine uses the seeds to treat headaches and as a diuretic, digestive aid and emmenagogue. Celery has also been prescribed as an antiflatulent, antilactogen and aphrodisiac.

The phthalides have been reported to have sedative[10] and anticonvulsive[2] activity in mice. An extract of celery (var dulce) has been reported to have hypotensive properties in rabbits and dogs when administered intravenously. In man, the juice has been shown to have effectively lowered blood pressure in 14 of 16 hypertensive patients.[11]

The essential oil has in vitro fungicidal effects.[12] The oil has hypoglycemic activity.[13] Essential oils from celery may also possess potential anticarcinogenic properties.[14] Two component of celery, 3–n-butylphthalide and sedanolide were experimentally found to reduce tumors in mice.[15]

TOXICOLOGY: Celery allergies in patients have led to urticaria and angioedema, respiratory complaints and anaphylaxis.[16] IgE antibodies have been experimentally associated with mediating celery allergies.[17] Since 1926, a number of sources have reported the occurrence of dermatitis in workers who cultivate or process celery. The dermatitis had been attributed to an allergic reaction to the volatile oil.[18]

Some celery workers, primarily Caucasian, develop phototoxic bullous lesions. Workers in greenhouses are less susceptible to lesions than those who work outside. Once healed, the lesions often leave areas of depigmentation or hyperpigmentation. Significantly, the bullae develop only after contact with celery affected by "pink-rot" a condition caused by the fungus *Sclerotinia sclerotiorum*.

Skin reactions probably result from exposure to a furocoumarin followed by exposure to sunlight (UVA light). The pink-rot apparently increases the availability of the furocoumarin. Use of a sunscreen can prevent this reaction.[7] Furocoumarins may be carcinogenic, and their concentration increases 100–fold in celery that is injured or diseased.[19] Large doses of the oil may induce CNS depression, although the specific toxic syndrome has not been well characterized.

SUMMARY: Celery is a widely cultivated plant that remains popular, especially among dieters. It is a relatively poor source of vitamins and is relatively high in sodium. Contact with the plants by farmworkers or food processors may cause a phytophototoxic reaction that may be incapacitating. Ingestion of large amounts of celery oil may cause toxicity; however, the toxicity has not been well characterized in man. The medicinal uses for celery are beginning to be more thoroughly explored, particularly for potential anticancer properties.

PATIENT INFORMATION – Celery

Uses: The seed is used as a diuretic and as a treatment for arthritis and rheumatism. The seed oil has produced sedative effects. Celery has been used in herbal medicine to treat arthritis, nervousness, hysteria and various other conditions. The juice lowered blood pressure in several tested patients. Two components reduced tumors in mice.

Side Effects: Some patients have experienced allergic responses, including anaphylaxis. There are many reports of dermatitis among those cultivating and processing celery. Some develop phototoxic lesions, often followed by disturbed pigmentation in the same areas. Certain compounds in diseased or damaged plants may be carcinogenic. Large doses of the oil may produce CNS depression.

---

[1] Dobelis IN, ed. *Magic and Medicine of Plants.* Pleasantville, NY: Reader's Digest Assoc., Inc., 1986.

[2] Bisset N, ed. *Herbal Drugs and Phytopharmaceuticals.* Stuttgart: Scientific Publishers, 1994.

[3] Garfield E. From Tonic to Psoriasis — Stalking Celery's Secrets. *Current Contents* 1985;16(8):3.

[4] Blish J. *Dictionary of Health Foods.* Los Angeles: Nash Publishing, 1972.

[5] Claus R, Hoppen HO. The Boar-Pheromone Steroid Identified in Vegetables. *Experentia* 1979;35(12):1674.

[6] Musajo L, et al. *Gass Chim Ital* 1954;84:870.

[7] Birmingham DJ, et al. Phytotoxic Bullae Among Celery Harvesters. *Arch Dermatcl* 1961;83:73.

[8] Garg SK, et al. Glucosides of Apium graveolens. *Planta Medica* 1980;38(4):363.

[9] Madjarova D, et al. The biochemical nature of forms obtained by the remote hybridization between genera- Apium, Petroselinum. II. Essential oils. *Herba Hungarica* 1979;18(3):185.

[10] Bjeldanes LF, Kim IS. Phthalide Components of Celery Essential Oil. *J Org Chem* 1977;42(13):2333.

[11] Leung AY. *Encyclopedia of Common Natural Ingredients.* New York: John Wiley, 1980.

[12] Jain SR, Jain MR. Effect of some common essential oils on pathogenic fungi. *Planta Medica* 1973;24(2):127.

[13] Farnsworth NR, Segelman AB. Hypoglycemic Plants. *Tile and Till* (Eli Lilly and Company) 1971;57(3):52.

[14] Hashim S, et al. Modulatory effects of essential oils from spices on the formation of DNA adduct by aflatoxin B1 in vitro. *Nutr Cancer* 1994;21(2):169.

[15] Zheng GQ, et al. Chemoprevention of benzopyrene-induced forestomach cancer in mice by natural phthalides from celery seed oil. *Nutr Cancer* 1993;19(1):77.

[16] Pauli G, et al. Celery sensitivity: clinical and immunological correlations with pollen allergy. *Clin Allergy* 1995;15(3):273.

[17] Pauli G, et al. Celery allergy: clinical and biological study of 20 cases. *Ann Allergy* 1988;60(3):243.

[18] Palumbo JF, Lynn EV. Dermatitis from Celery. *J Am Pharm Assn* 1953;42(1):57

[19] Ames BN. Dietary carcinogens and anticarcinogens. Oxygen radicals and degenerative diseases. *Science* 1983;221(4617):1256.

Chamomile

SCIENTIFIC NAME(S): *Matricaria chamomilla* L. and *Anthemis nobilis* L. Sometimes referred to as *Chamaemelum nobile* (L.) All. L. Family: Compositae (Asteraceae).

COMMON NAME(S): *M. chamomilla*, is known as German, Hungarian, wild, or genuine chamomile and *A. nobilis* is called English, Roman, Scotch, garden, lawn, sweet, and true chamomile (common chamomile).[1]

BOTANY: *M. chamomilla* grows as an erect annual and *A. nobilis* is a slow-growing perennial. The fragrant flowering heads of both plants are collected and dried for use as teas and extracts.

HISTORY: Known since Roman times for their medicinal properties, the plants have been used as antispasmodics and sedatives in the folk treatment of digestive and rheumatic disorders. Teas have been used to treat parasitic worm infections and as hair tints and conditioners. The volatile oil has been used to flavor cigarette tobacco.

Chamomile has been utilized as a skin wash to cleanse wounds and ulcers, and has been used to increase the sloughing of necrotic tissue and promote granulation and epithelialization. It has also been reported to have anti-inflammatory, antibacterial, astringent, and deodorant properties. Various formulations of chamomile have been used to treat vomiting, colic, fever, flatulence, and cystitis.[1]

CHEMISTRY: Both plants contain related chemical constituents. The anti-inflammatory and antispasmodic effects of *M. chamomilla* are due to compounds contained in the light-blue essential oil, which constitutes about 0.5% of the flower head.[2] Chamazulene, an artifact formed during heating while preparing teas and extracts, comprises about 5% of the essential oil. Up to 50% of the essential oil consists of alpha-bisabolol, an unsaturated monocyclic sesquiterpene alcohol,[3] whose concentration can vary according to geographic origin and chemotype. Other minor components include apigenin and angelic acid.[4]

PHARMACOLOGY: Bisabolol exerts numerous pharmacologic effects, which may account for the many traditional uses of chamomile. The compound effectively reduces inflammation of carageenan-induced rat paw swelling and adjuvant-induced arthritis in rats, as well as inflammation induced by the cotton pellet granuloma test.[5] Bisabolol is antipyretic in yeast-induced fever in rats. It significantly shortens the healing time of cutaneous burns in guinea pigs.[3] In rats, the compound also inhibits the development of gastric ulcers induced by indomethacin, stress, and ethanol, and shortens the healing time of acetic acid-induced ulcers.[6]

Chamomile infusions have been used traditionally as GI antispasmodics. Alcohol extracts of *M. chamomilla* showed significant antispasmodic effects in vitro.[7] Bisabolol and the lipophilic compounds bisabolol oxides A and B, as well as the essential oil, have a papaverine-like antispasmodic effect. Bisabolol is about as potent as papaverine and twice as potent as the oxides.[8] The cis-en-in-ether and the flavones apigenin, luteolin, patuletin, and quercetin also have marked antispasmodic effects as do the coumarins umbelliferone and herniarin.

Chamazulene exerts anti-inflammatory and antiallergic activity in animal models.[9] The hydrophilic components of chamomile, principally the flavonoids, also contribute to the anti-inflammatory process. The most active flavonoids are apigenin and luteolin, with potencies comparable to those of indomethacin.[10] Because of the low water solubility of the essential oil, teas prepared from chamomile flowers contain only about 10% to 15% of the oil present in the plant. Despite the relatively low concentration of lipophilic components in water infusions, chamomile teas are generally used over long periods of time, during which a cumulative therapeutic effect may result.[11]

German chamomile flower is approved by the German Commission E for use as an inhalation in skin and mucous membrane inflammations, bacterial skin diseases (including those of the oral cavity and gums), and respiratory tract inflammations and irritations; for use in baths and irrigation for anogenital inflammation; and internally for GI spasms and inflammatory diseases.

Sedation and mood: A blinded, crossover, placebo-controlled study evaluating the effect of chamomile on both sedation and mood was conducted in 22 patients. Aromatized chamomile oil proved to have a sedative effect, as well as a positive effect on mood. Negative mood rating was also less pronounced when patients were using chamomile oil.[12]

Mucositis: The theory that chamomile could decrease 5-fluorouracil-induced mucositis was evaluated in 164 patients receiving chemotherapy. In this double-blind, placebo-controlled trial, 82 patients were randomized to receive chamomile mouthwash 3 times daily for 14 days starting on the first day of chemotherapy. An equal number of patients were randomized to a matching placebo regimen. At the end of the study, stomatitis scores between the 2 treatment groups did not differ. A limitation of this study may be the short, 2-week study period.[13]

Another study evaluating the efficacy of chamomile for both the prophylaxis and treatment of mucositis was conducted in 98 patients. Twenty patients were scheduled to receive a chamomile-derived oral rinse 3 times daily for the prophylaxis of radiation-induced mucositis. Additionally, 78 patients treated with chemotherapy were enrolled. In the group receiving chemotherapy, 46 patients received the rinse for prophylaxis and 32 patients received the rinse for treatment. Prophylactic use of the rinse prevented the occurrence of mucositis in 78% of the patients receiving chemotherapy, and delayed the onset and reduced the intensity of radiation-induced mucositis.[14]

Wound healing: Chamomile cream was tested against almond ointment to determine if it could decrease adverse skin reactions induced by radiation. Forty-eight women were included in this study for breast cancer surgery. Chamomile cream or almond ointment was randomly assigned to the area above and below the scar; therefore, each patient served as her own control. This study failed to show a difference in adverse skin reactions between the 2 groups.[15]

Diarrhea: A prospective, double-blinded, randomized trial assessed the efficacy of a chamomile preparation (n = 39) to that of placebo (n = 40) in children with acute, noncomplicated diarrhea. The patients ranged in age from 6 months to 5.5 years of age and all 79 subjects received rehydration and a realimentation diet. At the end of 3 days, more patients in the chamomile group had resolution of diarrhea. The treatment group also had a significant reduction in the duration of diarrhea.[16]

INTERACTIONS: Based on the actions of chamomile, potential drug interactions involving increased sedation, delayed gastric absorption, and altered anticoagulant activity have been proposed. Because chamomile is reported to have sedative effects, this action may be additive with other sedatives (eg, benzodiazepines) a patient is taking. Because chamomile has antispasmotic activity in the GI tract, the absorption of concomitantly administered drugs may be delayed. Chamomile contains coumarin derivatives. Thus, if patients take anticoagulants (especially warfarin), it would be prudent to closely monitor anticoagulant parameters. The clinical importance of these parameters has not been established.

TOXICOLOGY: The toxicity of bisabolol is low following oral administration in animals. The acute LD_{50} is $\approx$ 15 ml/kg in rats and mice. In a 4-week subacute toxicity study, the administration of bisabolol (1 to 2 ml/kg body weight) to rats did not cause significant toxicity. No teratogenic or developmental abnormalities were noted in rats and rabbits after chronic administration of 1 ml/kg bisabolol.[17]

The pollen in the *Matricaria chamomilla* flowers may cause hypersensitivity leading to sneezing, runny nose, anaphylaxis, dermatitis, and GI upset. The dried flowering heads can be emetogenic if ingested in large amounts. English chamomile is reported to be an abortifacient and to affect the menstrual cycle.

The use of chamomile is not without potential adverse effects. The tea prepared from the pollen-laden flower heads has resulted in contact dermatitis,[18] anaphylaxis,[19] and other severe hypersensitivity reactions in people allergic to ragweed, asters, chrysanthemums, and other members of the family Compositae.[20] People with allergies to ragweed pollens should refrain from ingesting chamomile. A previously healthy female in labor developed an anaphylactic reaction after receiving a chamomile enema. After an emergency cesarean section, the newborn died shortly, thereafter due to inutero asphyxiation.[21] The dried flowering heads are emetic when ingested in large quantities.[22]

SUMMARY: The chamomiles are used widely. They exert significant antispasmodic activity in the GI tract and the potential for delaying concomitant drug absorption from the gut should be considered. Chamomile should not be used by people taking anticoagulants. There is evidence from animal models that some components of chamomile exert anti-inflammatory activity, but the extent to which this is observed in humans has not been established. The toxicity and teratogenicity potential appear to be low, but hypersensitivity has been reported.

PATIENT INFORMATION – Chamomile

Uses: Chamomile has been used as an antispasmodic and sedative. Teas have been used to treat parasitic worm infections and as hair tints and conditioners. It has been used as a skin wash to increase the sloughing of necrotic tissue, promote granulation and epithelialization, as an anti-inflammatory, antibacterial, astringent, and for its deodorant properties. Various formulations have been used to treat vomiting, colic, fever, flatulence, and cystitis.

Side Effects: The tea has resulted in contact dermatitis, anaphylaxis, and other severe hypersensitivity reactions in people allergic to ragweed, asters, chrysanthemums, and other members of the family Compositae. Do not use if currently taking anticoagulants or are allergic to ragweed pollens.

[1] Craker, L. *Herb, Spices, and Medicinal Plants: Recent Advances in Botany Horticulture, and Pharmacology.* Vol 1. Phoenix, AZ: Oryx Press, 1986.

[2] Padula L, et al. Quantitative determination of essential oil, total azulenes and chamazulene in German chamomile (*Matricaria chamomilla*) cultivated in Argentina. *Planta Med* 1976;30:273-80.

[3] Isaac, O. Pharmacological investigations with compounds of chamomile 1. On the pharmacology of (-)-a-bisabolol and bisabolol oxides. *Planta Medica* 1979;35:118-24. German.

[4] Morton, J. *Major Medicinal Plants.* Springfield, IL: C.C. Thomas, 1977.

[5] Jakovlev V, et al. Pharmacological investigations with compounds of chamomile 11. New investigations on the antiphlogistic effects of (-)-a-bisabolol and bisabolol oxides. *Planta Medica* 1979;35:125-40. German.

[6] Szelenyi I, et al. Pharmacological experiments with compounds of chamomile 111. Experimental studies of the ulcer protective effect of chamomile. *Planta Medica* 1979;35:218-27. German.

[7] Forster H, et al. Antispasmodic effects of some medicinal plants. *Planta Medica* 1980;40:309-19.

[8] Achterrath-Tuckerman U, et al. V. Investigations on the spasmolytic effect of compounds of chamomile and kamillosant on the isolated guinea pig ileum. *Planta Medica* 1980;39:38-50. German.

[9] Stern P, et al. Die antiallergische und antiphlogistische Wirkung der Azulene. *Arzn Forsch* 1956;6:445.

[10] Hamon, N. Herbal Medicine. The Chamomiles. *Can Pharm J* 1989;Nov:612.

[11] Farnsworth N, et al. Herb drinks: Chamomile tea. *JAMA* 1972;221:410-11.

[12] Roberts A, et al. The effect of olfactory stimulation on fluency, vividness of imagery and associated mood: a preliminary study. *Br J Med Psychol* 1992;65:197-99.

[13] Fidler P, et al. Prospective evaluation of a chamomile mouthwash for prevention of 5-FU-induced oral mucositis. *Cancer* 1996;77:522-25.

[14] Carl W, et al. Management of oral mucositis during local radiation and sytemic chemotherapy: a study of 98 patients. *J Prosthet Dent* 1991;66:361-69.

[15] Maiche A, et al. Effect of chamomile cream and almond ointment on acute radiation skin reaction. *Acta Oncol* 1991;30(3):395-96.

[16] de la Motte S, et al. Doppelblind-Vergleich zwischen einem Apfelpektin/Kamillenextrakt-Praparat und Plazebo bei mit Diarrhoe. *Arzneim-Forsch Drug Res* 1997;47(II):1247-49.

[17] Habersang S, et al. Pharmacological studies with compounds of chamomile. IV. Studies on toxicity of (-)-a-bisabolol. *Planta Medica* 1979;37:115-23. German.

[18] Rowe, A. Chamomile (*Anthemis cotula*) as a skin irritant. *J Allergy* 1934;5:383.

[19] Benner M, et al. Anaphylactic reaction to camomile tea. *J Allergy Clin Immunol* 1973;52:307-08.

[20] Toxic reactions to plant products sold in health food stores. *Med Lett Drugs Ther* 1979;21:29-32.

[21] Jensen-Jarolim E, et al. Fatal outcome of anaphylaxis to camomile-containing enema during labor: a case study. *J Allergy Clin Immunol* 1998;102:1041-42.

[22] Lewis W, et al. *Medical Botany.* New York, NY: J. Wiley and Sons, 1977.

Chaparral

SCIENTIFIC NAME(S): *Larrea divaricata* Cav. [synon. with L. *tridentata* (DC) Coville], also referred to as *L. glutinosa* Engelm. Family: Zygophyllacea.

COMMON NAME(S): Chaparral, creosote bush, greasewood, hediondilla[1]

BOTANY: The chaparrals are a group of closely related wild shrubs found in the arid regions of the Southwestern United States and Mexico. Chaparral found in health food stores usually consists of leaflets and twigs. This branched bush grows to 9 feet. Its leaves are bilobed and have a resinous feel and strong smell.

HISTORY: Chaparral tea was used as a remedy by Native Americans and has been suggested for the treatment of bronchitis and the common cold, to alleviate rheumatic pain, stomach pain, chicken pox and snake bite pain. A strong tea from the leaves has been mixed with oil as a burn salve.[2] It is an ingredient in some over-the-counter weight loss teas.

In 1959, the National Cancer Institute (NCI) was informed through lay correspondence that several cancer patients claimed beneficial effects on their cancers from drinking chaparral tea. Years later, a similar treatment was brought to the attention of physicians at the University of Utah, when an 85-year-old man with a proven malignant melanoma of the right cheek with a large cervical metastasis refused surgery and treated himself with chaparral tea. Eight months later he returned with marked regression of the tumor.[3] Additional cases observed by the physicians at the University of Utah included four patients who responded to some degree to treatment with the tea, including two with melanoma, one with metastatic choriocarcinoma, and one with widespread lymphosarcoma. After two days of treatment, the patient with lymphosarcoma discontinued chaparral treatment, despite the disappearance of 75% of his disease. The choriocarcinoma patient, who had not responded well to other therapies, responded well to chaparral tea for two months after which the disease became progressive. Of the melanoma patients, one experienced a 95% regression and the remaining disease was excised; the other, after remaining in remission for four months, subsequently developed a new lesion.[4]

Reports subsequently appeared in the lay literature describing the virtues of chaparral tea as an antineoplastic treatment.

CHEMISTRY: Phytochemical investigations of *L. divaricata* resulted in the isolation of nor-dihydroguaiaretic acid (NDGA) and the related lignans nor-isoguaiasin, dihydroguaiaretic acid, partially demethylated dihydroguaiaretic acid, and 3'-demethoxyisoguaiasin. The total phenolics together with the small amounts of lipids produced by the plant range from 16% in older plants to 21% in younger growing plants.[4]

PHARMACOLOGY: NDGA is believed to be responsible for the biological activity of chaparral. Up until 1967, when more effective antioxidants were introduced, NDGA was used in the food industry as a food additive to prevent fermentation and decomposition. It is theorized that any anticancer effect of chaparral tea is due to the ability of NDGA to block cellular respiration. NDGA and its related compounds inhibit the beef heart mitochondrial NADH oxidase system and succinoxidase system, and therefore, exert some antioxidant activity at the cellular level.[5] NDGA inhibits the induction of the lipogenase inhibitor ornithine decarboxylase in mice.[6,7] DGA also inhibits collagen- and ADP-induced platelet aggregation and platelet adhesiveness in aspirin-treated patients.[8]

Studies conducted by the NCI found that in vitro, NDGA was an effective anticancer agent, being described as "the penicillin of the hydroquinones and the most potent antimetabolite in vitro."[9] This activity, however, is almost completely abolished in vivo. Chaparral failed to show any significant anticancer activity in two separate NCI chemotherapy screening tests in mice.[4] There is some evidence that when combined with ascorbic acid, NDGA shows some inhibitory effect against small Ehrlich ascites tumors in mice.

Other disconcerting data from 34 cancer patients treated for varying periods of time with chaparral suggest that a majority of malignancies are stimulated by NDGA, while some go on to regress.[4]

TOXICOLOGY: The creosote bush can induce contact dermatitis.[10] NDGA has been found to induce mesenteric lymph node and renal lesions in rats;[11] because of these problems, it was removed from the Generally Recognized as Safe (GRAS) list in 1970.[12]

Several recent reports have linked the ingestion of chaparral tea with the development of liver damage.[11,13] In all three cases, the patients took chaparral tablets or capsules for 6 weeks to 3 months. They developed signs of hepatic damage as evidenced by liver enzyme abnormalities; these resolved following discontinuation of the plant material. These reports indicate that chronic ingestion of chaparral may be associated with liver damage.

SUMMARY: Miracle cancer cures have an enormous public appeal. Like laetrile and taheebo, chaparral tea has gained attention as a natural cancer treatment, albeit with only inconclusive evidence to justify its safety or effectiveness. The results of in vivo and in vitro tests indicate that chaparral contains potent antioxidants that exert some biologic activity; however, the antineoplastic activity of chaparral is weak and inconsistent in vivo.

The numerous anecdotal reports of its efficacy suggest that further in vivo testing may be warranted. Because its use may stimulate the growth of certain tumors, however, chaparral cannot be recommended as an antineoplastic agent at this time.

PATIENT INFORMATION – Chaparral

Uses: Chaparral tea has been widely used in folk medicine to treat conditions ranging from the common cold to snake bite pain. A derivative was formerly used as a food preservative. Anecdotal and in vitro evidence suggests antineoplastic effects.

Side Effects: No longer classified safe. Chaparral may cause liver damage, stimulate most malignancies and cause contact dermatitis.

---

[1] Dobelis IN, ed. *Magic and Medicine of Plants*. Pleasantville, NY: Reader's Digest Association, Inc., 1986.

[2] Sweet M. *Common Edible and Useful Plants of the West*. Healdsburg, CA: Naturegraph Publications 1976.

[3] Smart CR, et al. *Cancer Chemother Reports* 1969;53:147.

[4] Unproven Methods of Cancer Management. American Cancer Society, 1970.

[5] Gisvold O, Thaker E. *J Pharm Sci* 1974;63:1905.

[6] Nakadate T, et al. *Cancer Res* 1982;42:2841.

[7] Bracco MM, et al. *Clin Exp Immunol* 1984;55:405.

[8] Gimeno MF, et al. *Prostaglandin Leukotrein Med* 1983;111:109.

[9] Burk D, Woods M. *Radiation Res Supp* 1963;3:212.

[10] Lampe KF, McCann MA. *AMA Handbook of poisonous and Injurious Plants*. Chicago, IL: AMA, 1985.

[11] *MMWR*. Chaparral-induced toxic hepatitis-California and Texas 1992. 1992;43:812.

[12] Tyler VE. *The Honest Herbal*. Philadelphia, PA: G.F. Stickley Co., 1981.

[13] Katz M, et al. Herbal hepatitis: subacute hepatic necrosis secondary to chaparral leaf. *J Clin Gastroenterol* 1990;12:203.

Charcoal

COMMON NAME(S): Activated charcoal, animal charcoal, charcoal, gas black, lamp black

SOURCE: Charcoal is produced by pyrolysis and high temperature oxidation of organic materials. Animal charcoal is obtained from charred bones, meat, blood, etc. "Activated" charcoal is obtained from charred wood or vegetable matter and treated with various substances to increase its adsorptive power. Amorphous carbons (or charcoals) are obtained from the incomplete combustion of natural gas, fats, oils or resins.

CHEMISTRY: The chemistry of charcoals is complex. Although the purest forms of charcoal are essentially all carbon, the small amounts of impurities that remain following combustion of the source material have been difficult to characterize. Medicinal charcoals have been developed with a high surface area-to-weight ratio in order to maximize the adsorption capacity.

The adsorptive properties of charcoal may be significantly increased by treating it with such substance as carbon dioxide, oxygen, air, steam, sulfuric acid, zinc chloride or phosphoric acid (or combinations of these) at high temperatures (500°-900°C). These matreials help remove impurities and reduce the particle size of carbon, allowing charcoal to be more adsorptive due to an increased surface area. One ml of finely subdivided and activated medicinal charcoal has a total surface area of about 1000 m^2. Medicinal or activated charcoal is a fluffy, fine, black, odorless and tasteless powder without any gritty material. It is insoluble in water or other common solvents, but may be suspended for a short time after vigorous shaking.[1]

PHARMACOLOGY: Activated charcoal has been used in the management of acute toxicity for almost a century. Its large surface area permits the absorption of a variety of complex chemicals, thereby rendering the toxic material unavailable for systemic absorption. In addition, charcoal may interrupt the enterohepatic circulation of compounds that are excreted into the bile. It is usually coadministered with a laxative and the combination may hasten the elimination of toxins from the gastrointestinal tract due to the resultant diarrhea and more rapid gastrointestinal transit time.[2]

Activated charcoal is used for the acute management of a wide variety of poisons, but is particularly used as an emergency antidote. It is commonly accepted by medical personnel as the antidote of choice for almost all drugs and chemicals (except mineral acids, alkalines and substances insoluble in aqueous acid solution, eg, tolbutamide).[1] Capsules of powdered medicinal charcoal are also used to relieve the discomfort of abdominal gas and flatulence. The capsules should be taken 2 hours before or 1 hour after any oral medication.

Charcoal is often underutilized or given in insufficient dosages. On average, it should be administered at least in a 10:1 proportion (charcoal-to-estimated poison dose). Caution should be used with the simultaneous administration of charcoal and the emetic ipecac, since charcoal may adsorb the ipecac and render it ineffective. The dosage range for medicinal charcoal (as an antidote) is 5 - 50 g. The usual adult dose is 50 g; children, 25 g. It is administered as an aqueous slurry and may be flavored, though the flavoring may reduce its effectiveness. As an antiflatulent, the dose range is 520–975 mg, taken after meals or at the first sign of discomfort. This may be repeated as needed, up to 4.16 g daily.[1]

It has long been known that uremic patients treated with charcoal hemoperfusion often have significant reductions in blood lipid levels. Repeated oral doses of activated charcoal have also been found to be effective in reducing blood lipid concentrations in uremic[3] and diabetic patients.[4] In a study of hypercholesterolemic patients given 8 g of activated charcoal three times a day for 4 weeks, the total cholesterol and low density lipoproteincholesterol (LDL) levels decreased by a mean of 25% and 41%, respectively. The high density lipoproteincholesterol (HDL) and the ratio of HDL:LDL increased.[5] Mention of this study in lay literature has resulted in an increased interest in the use of oral charcoal for the reduction of blood lipid levels. At present, however, there is insufficient evidence to confirm the effect of charcoal on lipid parameters or to determine an appropriate dose.

Numerous articles continue to appear in the medical literature on the usefulness of activated charcoal as an antidote in all kinds of poisoning and as a gastrointestinal decontaminant. Researchers discuss the controversy of whether activated charcoal should be used alone or if gastric lavage or ipecac syrup should be given before activated charcoal in treating poisonings.[6] Multiple studies indicate that a relatively small amount of gastric content is removed by ipecac syrup or gastric lavage. They argue that there are still no universal standards for the lavage method, the diameter of the orogastric tube or the size of the aliquot fluid. Furthermore, there is still a need for studies of lavage fluid temperatures, abdominal massage and even the positioning of patients during these procedures. Some studies, however, caution against the use of activated charcoal alone, since it does not adsorb all materials.

A later study comments on the gastric decontamination controversy and focuses on acute poisoning emergencies.[7] The researchers promote good supportive care in acute poisoning: Aggressive support of the cardiovascular, respiratory and central nervous systems and appropriate gastric decontamination. They contend that ipecac should be reserved for home use following ingestion of certain toxins and that activated charcoal should replace ipecac for the treatment of mild to moderate poisonings in the emergency room setting. Both gastric lavage and the proper dosage of activated charcoal (adults, 50-100 g; children, 25-50 g; infants 1 g/kg) should be considered in life-threatening cases. A cathartic should be considered after the administration of activated charcoal.

TOXICOLOGY: Activated charcoal is used in hemoperfusion for the removal of toxins from the blood following acute overdose. In general, there is little toxicity associated with the charcoal component of hemoperfusion.

The oral use of charcoal has been associated with unwanted side effects. Gastrointestinal obstruction, in the form of "briquettes," has been observed in patients who have received repeated doses of charcoal.[2,8,9] Other problems following the ingestion of charcoal preparations (in the form of a charcoal-sorbitol suspension) include hypernatremic dehydration[10] and aspiration pneumonia.[11] One drawback to the emergency use of oral charcoal is that adsorbed toxins may have the opportunity to dissociate from the charcoal and re-enter the systemic circulation before the charcoal is excreted. Although charcoal given alone may slow gastric transit time, it is often coadministered with a laxative to hasten its evacuation. It is not clear what effect the long-term ingestion of charcoal preparations may have on vitamin levels. At least one pediatric report has focused on the pulmonary aspiration of activated charcoal as a complication of its misuse in overdose management.[12]

SUMMARY: Charcoal has been used in the treatment of toxic events for almost 100 years with a remarkable record of safety. It adsorbs a wide variety of toxic compounds and facilitates their gastrointestinal removal. Charcoal is also used in hemoperfusion to remove toxic material from the systemic circulation. Recent reports indicating that blood lipid levels may be beneficially altered following the use of charcoal cannot be extrapolated to clinically useful therapeutic regimens until more is known about these effects.

PATIENT INFORMATION – Charcoal

Uses: Activated charcoal is used as an antidote to poisoning, as an antiflatulent and potentially as a treatment for reducing blood lipid concentrations in uremic and diabetic patients.

Side Effects: GI obstruction can develop in those receiving repeated doses.

---

[1] Gennaro AR, ed. *Remington: The Science and Practice of Pharmacy*, 19th ed. Easton, PA: Mack Printing Co., 1995.
[2] Pond SM. Role of repeated oral doses of activated charcoal in clinical toxicology. *Med Toxicol* 1986;1(1):3.
[3] Friedman EA. Oral sorbents in uremia: charcoal-induced reduction in plasma lipids. *Am J Med* 1977;62(4):541.
[4] Manis T, et al. *Am J Clin Nutr* 1980;33:1485.
[5] Kuusisto P, et al. Effect of activated charcoal on hypercholesterolaemia. *Lancet* 1986;2(8503):366.
[6] Harris CR, Kingston R. Gastrointestinal decontamination: Which method is best? *Postgrad Med* 1992;92(2):116.
[7] Krenzelok EP, Dunmire SM. Acute poisoning emergencies: Resolving the gastric decontaminiation controversy. *Postgrad Med* 1992;91(2):179.
[8] Watson WA, et al. Gastrointestinal obstruction associated with multiple-dose activated charcoal. *J Emerg Med* 1986;4(5):401.
[9] Anderson IM, Ware C. Syrup of ipecacuanha. *Br Med J* 1987;294:578.
[10] Farley TA. Severe hypernatremic dehydration after use of an activated charcoal-sorbitol suspension. *J Pediatr* 1986;109(4):719.
[11] Harsch HH. Aspiration of activated charcoal [letter]. *N Engl J Med* 1986;314(5):318.
[12] Givens T, et al. Pulmonary aspiration of activated charcoal: A complication of its misuse in overdose management. *Pediatr Emerg Care* 1992;8(3):137.

Chaste Tree

SCIENTIFIC NAME(S): Vitex agnus-castus L. Family: Verbenaceae

COMMON NAME(S): Chaste tree, chasteberry, monk's pepper

BOTANY: The chaste tree is a shrub that grows in moist river banks in southern Europe and in the Mediterranean region.[1] It can grow to 22 feet in height. The plant blooms in summer, developing light purple flowers and palm-shaped leaves. The dark brown to black fruits are the size of a pepper corn; these fruits have a pepperish aroma and flavor and are collected in autumn.[2,3]

HISTORY: The dried ripe fruit is used in traditional medicine. The plant has been recognized since antiquity and has been described in works by Hippocrates, Dioscorides, and Theophrastus.[2] In Homer's epic, *The Iliad*, the plant was featured as a "symbol of chastity, capable of warding off evil."[3] Early physicians recognized its effect on the female reproductive system, suggesting its use in controlling hemorrhages and expelling the placenta after birth. The English name "chaste tree" derives from the belief that the plant reduces unwanted libido. Monks have chewed its parts to decrease sexual desire.[2,3] At least one report is available discussing the chaste tree's use in ancient medicine to the present.[4]

CHEMISTRY: The chaste tree contains iridoids, flavonoids, progestins and essential oils.[5] Two iridoid glycosides have been isolated: Agnuside (0.6%) and aucubin (0.3%).[6,7] Another report confirms iridoid presence from the leaves of the plant using TLC and spectral data.[8]

Flavonoid content has been determined in chaste tree leaves (0.99% to 2.7%), flowers (1.01% to 1.47%) and fruits (0.45% to 0.97%).[9] Components of flavonoids include flavonol derivatives kaempferol and quercetagetin, the major constituent being casticin.[7] An earlier report isolates and identifies additional flavonols from the fruits including 6-hydroxykaempferol-3,6,7,4'-tetramethyl ether (penduletin 4'-methyl ether), penduletin and chrysosplenol.[10] Other flavonoids present in the plant include orientin and isovitexin.[2]

Progesterone and hydroxyprogesterone, in the free and conjugated forms, have been found in chaste tree leaves and flowers. Progesterone, testosterone and epitestosterone were detected from flower parts. Androstenedione was found in the leaves.[11]

Essential oils present in chaste tree include mainly the monoterpenoids, cineol and pinene (alpha and beta), along with limonene, sabinene, castine, eucalptol, myrcene, linalool, citronellol, cymene and camphene. Sesquiterpenoids such as caryophyllene, farnesene, cardinene and ledol are also present.[5,7,12]

The alkaloid vitricine is also present in the plant.[7] An overview of chaste tree is available, including chemical composition, pharmacology and side effects.[13]

PHARMACOLOGY: Chaste tree berries are thought to be **antiandrogenic**, inhibiting these male hormonal actions. In females, the berries exert **progesterogenic** effects, **balancing progesterone and estrogen production** from the ovaries and **regulating menstrual cycles**.[3] A preparation of chaste tree (0.2% w/w) has been available in Germany since the 1950s and is used in treatment of **breast pain, ovarian insufficiency** (some cases resulting in pregnancy) and **uterine bleeding**.[7] Crude herb or alcoholic or aqueous extracts of pulverized fruit are used in commercial preparations.[14]

Chaste tree preparations inhibit basal and TRH-stimulated prolactin secretion of rat pituitary cells in vitro, suggesting its possible use in treatment of **hyperprolactinemia**.[15] In addition, animal studies have found an increase in lactation and mammary enlargement, indicating an effect on prolactin release.[2]

When studied in 52 women with luteal phase defects caused by latent hyperprolactinemia, a chaste tree preparation reduced prolactin release, normalized luteal phases and eliminated deficits in luteal progesterone without side effects.[16] Chaste tree extract contains an active principle that binds to dopamine (D_2) receptor sites, inhibiting prolactin release. This suggests therapeutic usefulness of the plant for treatment of **premenstrual breast pain** associated with prolactin hypersecretion.[17]

A case report in a female patient evaluated chaste tree therapy in **multiple follicular development**. Hormone levels after administration of the herb became "disordered;" thus, the authors concluded not to use chaste tree to promote normal ovarian function.[18]

Chaste tree is reportedly effective in treating **endocrine abnormalities** such as **menstrual neuroses and dermatoses**. It has also been used to treat **acne**.[7]

In lactating women, extracts of the plant have also been used to **increase milk production**.[2] When analyzed chemically, the breast milk revealed no compositional changes after chaste tree use.[7]

TOXICOLOGY: Chaste tree administration has not been associated with significant adverse events. In one large German market surveillance study, 17 of 1542 women discontinued treatment because of an adverse event.[2] Minor side effects include gastrointestinal reactions, aller-gic reactions (eg, itching and rash), headaches and menstrual flow increase.[2,7] The safety of the plant has not been determined in children.

SUMMARY: The chaste tree is a popular European plant that is used in traditional medicine for the management of disorders of the female reproductive tract. Chemical analysis indicates the presence of components that can affect the function of these systems, and the results of preliminary human investigations indicate that extracts of the plant have measurable pharmacologic activity. This plant should be further investigated for its potential medicinal effects.

PATIENT INFORMATION – Chaste Tree

Uses: Chaste tree has been used in females to balance progesterone and estrogen production and regulate menstruation. It has been used for breast pain, ovarian insufficiency and uterine bleeding and to increase breast milk production.

Side Effects: Minor side effects include GI reactions, itching, rash, headaches and increased menstrual flow.

---

[1] Mabberley DJ. *The plant-book: A portable dictionary of the higher plants.* Cambridge: Cambridge University Press, 1987.
[2] Brown DJ. *Quarterly Rev Nat Med* 1994;Summer:111.
[3] Chevallier A. Encyclopedia of Medicinal Plants. New York, NY: DK Publishing 1996;149.
[4] Hobbs C. *Pharmacy in History.* 1991;33(1):19-24.
[5] Kustrak D, et al. *Farmaceutski Glasnik* 1992 May;48:149-58.
[6] Gomaa CS. *Planta Medica* 1978;33:277.
[7] Newall C, et al. Herbal Medicines. London, England: Pharmaceutical Press 1996;19-20.
[8] Kustrak D, et al. *Farmaceutski Glasnik* 1992 Nov;48:305-10.
[9] Kustrak D, et al. *Farmaceutski Glasnik* 1993 Nov;49:299-303.
[10] Wollenweber E, et al. *Planta Med* 1983 Jun;48:126-27.
[11] Saden-Krehula M, et al. *Acta Pharm Jugosl* 1991;41(3):237-41.
[12] Kustrak, Kuftinec J, et al. *Planta Med* 1992:58(Suppl 1):A681.
[13] Houghton P. *Pharm J* 1994 Nov 19;253:720-21.
[14] Leung, AY. *Encyclopedia of Common Natural Ingredients.* New York, NY: John J. Wiley & Sons 1996;151.
[15] Sliutz G, et al. *Horm Metab Res* 1993;25(5):253-55.
[16] Milewicz A, et al. *Arzneimittelforschung* 1993;43(7):752-56.
[17] Jarry H, et al. *Exp Clin Endocrinol* 1994;102(6):448-54.
[18] Cahill D, et al. *Hum Reprod* 1994;9(8):1469-70.

Chicken Soup

SOURCE: Chicken soup is obtained from a hot water infusion of selected parts of the common chicken *Gallus domesticus*.

HISTORY: Chicken soup has long been recognized as an important part of the physician's armamentarium. Therapeutic observations were recorded as far back as 60 A.D. by Pedacius Dioscorides, an army surgeon under the emperor Nero. He was responsible for the book "De Materia Medica," which, among other natural science knowledge, discusses chicken soup. Aretaeus the Cappadocian (2nd to 3rd century), an author of causes, symptoms and treatments of diseases, is credited with describing how boiled chicken can treat respiratory tract disorders.[1]

As early as the 12th century, the theologian and physician Moses Maimonides wrote "Chicken soup...is recommended as an excellent food as well as medication."[2] He further specified that "One should not use the too large, that is of more than 2 years of age; nor the too small, that is those in whom the mucus still prevails; neither too lean, nor those who through feeding becomes obese; but those that are fat by nature without being stuffed."[3]

Chicken soup was used in Europe for centuries, but disappeared from commercial production after the inquisition. It remained popular in European tradition, and its use has grown steadily over the last 300 years.

CHEMISTRY: While details of the chemistry of chicken soup are poorly understood, it is recognized that the composition of this material can vary considerably, generally being related to the production technique. Some investigators have expressed concern about the cholesterol content of chicken soup, but there appears to be little evidence of a hypercholesterolemic effect when ingested in moderation.

Circa 1990, Dr. Irwin Zimet (University of California, Los Angeles) found that chicken, a protein, contains the amino acid cysteine. This is chemically similar to the drug acetylcysteine, which is prescribed for respiratory infections because it thins the mucus in the lungs.[4]

A study has been performed proving increased calcium content with duration of cooking soup with bones. Chicken soup prepared this way may be of use in patients who require calcium, but cannot tolerate dairy products.[5]

PHARMACOLOGY: In 1975, the editor of the journal *Chest* published the scientific spoof on uncontrolled studies entitled "Chicken Soup Rebound and Relapse of Pneumonia: Report of a Case." The patients suffered severe pneumonia requiring a thoracotomy and treatment with penicillin after he discontinued a course of self-treatment with chicken soup.[2]

The result of this report was a flood of correspondence over the next 5 years expounding the virtues of chicken soup. Readers reported the isolation of the "active ingredient"[6] that was claimed to have antibacterial activity[7] and could be useful in the treatment of impotence,[8] frustration, anxiety and backache.[9] It was also suggested that appropriate blends of chicken soup could be used as substitutes for aircraft fuel.[10]

Despite these barbs, a serious investigation was conducted comparing the effects of drinking hot water, cold water and chicken soup on nasal mucus velocity and airflow resistance. Drinking 200 ml of hot water, by sipping, increased nasal mucus velocity, but not when the cup was covered and a straw used for drinking. The latter procedure prevented hot water vapor from penetrating the nares. Drinking chicken soup by sipping and by straw caused a response similar to that of drinking hot water. It is believed that the additional effect seen when drinking chicken soup by straw may be related to an aromatic compound acting on the nasal pharynx or through a mechanism related to taste. The authors recommend hot rather than cold liquids for fluid intake in patients with upper respiratory tract infections.[11]

While the aroma of this agent precludes double-blind investigations, it is encouraging to know that one of the properties of chicken soup is to hasten the removal of pathogens from the nose.[12] Chicken soup has also been reported as therapy for facial pain[13] and for asthma.[14]

A detailed letter discussed the therapeutic efficacy of chicken and other fowl. Conditions in areas such as neurological, respiratory, urinary tract, antibacterial and gastrointestinal are relieved by chicken parts, soup or other fowl (eg, leprosy, sexual potential, snake bite antidote and memory enhancement).[15] The use of prednisone vs chicken soup for treatment of lymphocytic thyroiditis with spontaneously resolving hyperthyroidism has also been reported.[16]

The ability of chicken soup to inhibit neutrophil chemotaxis (and therefore reduce inflammation) has been presented at the 1993 International Conference of the American Lung Association and the American Thoracic Society. It was proven that chemotaxis was markedly reduced, even when the soup was diluted 200 times. The soup included onions, sweet potatoes, carrots, turnips and parsnips, all of which may have contributed to the beneficial effects.[4]

A Japanese trial demonstrated chicken cartilage soup to have therapeutic efficacy in 38 rheumatoid arthritis patients.[17]

TOXICOLOGY: The ingestion of chicken soup is not without danger. One case of pneumonia secondary to the aspiration of a bone from a dose of chicken soup has been reported. The authors concluded that "only bone-free chicken soup" should be used.[18] Another report describes severe respiratory distress in a 6-month-old infant from a hollow chicken bone in the left main bronchus after the child was spoon-fed chicken soup.[19] Information on the dangers of chicken soup in pediatrics is available.[20]

Hypernatremia was reported in a 75-year-old Chinese woman who ingested one or two bowls of three different kinds of high-salt soups to correct hydrochlorothiazide-induced hyponatremia. She became delirious but was treated uneventfully with hypotonic solutions.[21] Similarly, a 17-month-old child, who was given six packets of HERB-OX chicken broth (prepared as directed in 6 oz of water), was hospitalized due to hypernatremic dehydration. She recovered uneventfully with rehydration.[20] Hypernatremia following high-salt supplements is a complication sometimes seen in children, in particular those with acute diarrheal disease. Large amounts of hypertonic solutions, such as chicken soup, should not be given to young children. In addition, commercial soup bouillons may contain trace amounts of mutagens.[22]

There is at least one case report of anaphylaxis to chicken soup.[23] Also of concern may be migration of mineral hydrocarbons from polystyrene containers from which hot beverages, including chicken soup, are served.[24]

SUMMARY: Chicken soup has a historical legacy that spans hundreds of generations. It appears to be an effective adjunct in the treatment of mild upper respiratory tract infections. Toxicity involves mainly hypernatremia and physical obstruction by bone fragments present in the soup.

PATIENT INFORMATION – Chicken Soup

Uses: Chicken soup has been used to treat respiratory tract disorders, asthma and facial pain among other ailments.

Side effects: Adverse events include severe respiratory distress from aspirating chicken bone fragments.

---

[1] Cohen S. *Allergy Proc* 1991;(12):47–59.
[2] Caroline NL, et al. *Chest* 1975;67:215.
[3] Rosner F, et al. *The Medical Writings of Moses Maimonides*. Philadelphia: Lippincott, 1969.
[4] Winter R. *A Consumer's Guide to Medicines in Food*. New York, NY: Crown Trade Paperbacks 1995;167-68.
[5] Rosen H. *Calcif Tissue Int* 1994;54(6):486-88.
[6] Levin S. *J Irresproducible Results* 1968;17:42.
[7] Dorna RJ, et al. *Chest* 1975;68:604.
[8] Greene LF. *Chest* 1975;68:605.
[9] Lindsey O. *Chest* 1976;70:2.
[10] Lawrence DS. *Chest* 1975;68:606.
[11] Saketkhoo K, et al. 1978;74(4):408-10.
[12] Weiss WM. *Chest* 1978;74:487.
[13] Marbach J. *NY State Dent J* 1979;45(5):232-33.
[14] Rosner F. *Lancet* 1979;2(8151):1079.
[15] Rosner F. *Chest* 1980;78(4):672-74.
[16] Dorfman S, et al. *Arch Intern Med* 1982;142(13):2261.
[17] Toda Y, et al. *Nihon Rinsho Meneki Gakkai Kaishi* 1997;20(1):44-51.
[18] Leiberman A, et al. *Chest* 1980;77:1.
[19] Avital A, et al. *Respiration* 1992;59(1):62-63.
[20] Chu E. *Pediatrics* 1986;77(5):785-86.
[21] Fujiwara P, et al. *N Engl J Med* 1985;313(18):1161-62.
[22] Stavric B, et al. *Food Chem Toxicol* 1993;31(12):981-87.
[23] Saff R, et al. *J Allergy Clin Immunol* 1992;89(5):1061-62.
[24] Castle L, et al. *Food Addit Contam* 1991;8(6):693-99.

Chickweed

SCIENTIFIC NAME(S): *Stellaria media* (L.) Villars. Family: Caryophyllaceae

COMMON NAME(S): Chickweed, Mouse-ear, Satinflower, Starweed, Starwort, Tongue Grass, White Bird's-Eye, Winterweed

BOTANY: Chickweed is a common plant, particularly throughout Europe and North America. This low-growing annual has a thin hairy stem with pointed oval leaves. It produces small white star-shaped flowers throughout much of the year.[1,5,6]

HISTORY: The whole dried plant has been used in the preparation of infusions. Chickweed extract has been used internally as a demulcent, but is more typically used externally for the treatment of rashes and sores. The young shoots are edible and have been used as salad greens.[2] In homeopathy, the plant is used to relieve rheumatic pains and psoriasis.[1]

CHEMISTRY: Nitrate salts, a saponin and vitamin C (375 mg/100 g) have been identified in the plant.[2,3]

PHARMACOLOGY: Although there is an extensive base of scientific literature describing chickweed, this literature focuses largely on its control as an unwanted weed. There is no indication that any of the plant's constituents possess significant therapeutic activity and its vitamin content is too low to be of therapeutic value.[4]

TOXICOLOGY: Grazing animals have experienced nitrate poisoning secondary to chickweed.[3] Although poorly documented, human cases of paralysis have been reported from large amounts of the infusion. However, there is no overwhelming evidence to suggest that chickweed possesses a significant toxic potential.[2]

SUMMARY: Although chickweed is ubiquitous and has been used in traditional medicine for centuries, there is no evidence that it offers any significant therapeutic activity. It is generally well tolerated, although the ingestions of large amounts of the plant may be associated with nitrate toxicity.

PATIENT INFORMATION – Chickweed

Uses: Chickweed infusions and extracts have been used internally as a demulcent and topically as treatment for rashes and sores. Young shoots are edible.

Side Effects: Ingestion of large amounts may be toxic.

---

[1] Schauenberg P, Paris F. *Guide to Medicinal Plants*. New Canaan, CT: Keats Publishing Inc., 1977.
[2] Spoerke DG, Jr. *Herbal Medications*. Santa Barbara, CA: Woodbridge Press 1980.
[3] Duke JA. *Handbook of Medicinal Herbs*. Boca Raton, FL: CRC Press, Inc., 1985.
[4] Tyler VE. *The New Honest Herbal*. Philadelphia, PA: G.F. Stickley Co., 1987.
[5] *The Herbalist*. Hammond, IN: Hammond Book Co, 1934.
[6] *Magic and Medicine of Plants*. Pleasantville, NY: Reader's Digest, 1986.

Chicory

SCIENTIFIC NAME(S): *Chicorium intybus* L. Family: Compositae or Asteraceae

COMMON NAME(S): Blue sailor's succory, chicory, wild succory

BOTANY: Chicory is a perennial plant indigenous to Europe, India, and Egypt. It was introduced to the US in the late 19th century. It grows as a weed in temperate climates and is widely cultivated in northern Europe. There are 2 principal types: The Brunswick variety has deeply cut leaves and generally spreads horizontally; the Magdeburg variety has undivided leaves and grows erect. Chicory has bright blue flowers that bloom from July to September. The dried root is the primary part of the plant used.

HISTORY: In cultivation, chicory roots are "forced" during the fall and winter to produce 2 types of leaves used as greens: Barbe de capucin and witloof (or French endive). The leaves of young plants are used as potherbs, in which case they are cooked like spinach. Leaves of older plants, when blanched, are used like celery. Chicory roots are boiled and eaten with butter. They are also roasted and used to add a bitter, mellow taste to coffee and tea or used as a substitute for coffee. Chicory is on the FDA Generally Recognized as Safe (GRAS) list.

CHEMISTRY: Chicory flowers contain cichoriin, which is 6,7-glucohydroxycoumarin. The roots contain up to 8% inulin (a polysaccharide), a bitter principle consisting of 1 part protocatechuic aldehyde to 3 parts inulin, as well as lactucin and lactucopicrin.[1] Constituents of the greens include chicoric acid (dicaffeoyl tartaric acid), flavonoids, catechol tannins, glycosides, carbohydrates, unsaturated sterols and triterpenoids, sesquiterpene lactones, and tartaric acid.[2,3] Leaf proteins from chicory greens have also been reported.[4]

The root contains a large number of steam-distillable aromatic compounds. Acetophenone provides the characteristic chicory aroma. Upon roasting, inulin is converted to oxymethylfurfural, a compound with a coffee-like smell.[3] Fructan:fructan 6G-fructosyltransferase (6G-FFT) was found to be an important enzyme in the formation of inulin. According to 1 report, introduction of 6G-FFT from 1 plant into chicory resulted in inulin synthesis.[5] Chicory is the source of the taste-modifier maltol, which is known to intensify the flavor of sugar.

The caffeine content of beverages containing chicory was determined using high pressure liquid chromatography (HPLC). A coffee/chicory mixture substitute contains 3.18 mg/fl oz of caffeine, whereas instant coffee contains 12.61 mg/fl oz of caffeine.[6]

In identifying closely related chicory varieties, the use of polyacrylamide gel electrophoresis followed by leucine aminopeptidase and esterase staining of bulked seed sample extracts has been developed.[7]

PHARMACOLOGY: The water-soluble fraction of chicory has a sedative effect and antagonizes the stimulating effects of coffee and tea via a CNS mechanism. Lactucin and related compounds may be in part responsible for the plant's sedative effects.

The naturally occurring oligosaccharides in chicory are considered "probiotics" entering the large intestine and are substrates for intestinal fermentation. This maintenance of microbial composition in the colon is important for GI tract health. Because of certain bond configurations, these oligosaccharides resist hydrolysis by salivary and intestinal enzymes. In the colon they are fermented by anaerobic bacteria. The most well-known effects of nondigestible oligosaccharides is the selective stimulation of bifidobacteria, reducing the growth of other pathogenic bacteria.[8,9,10,11,12]

Studies conducted on rats show that inulin from chicory seems very effective in promoting proprionic fermentation and enhances the calcium content of the large intestines.[13] A reduction in intestinal absorption of glucose was observed in another report in rats administered chicory extract.[14] Improved lipid metabolism was demonstrated in rats fed inulin-containing chicory extract, as well. This effect possibly was due to changes in absorption or synthesis of cholesterol.[15] Chicory's inulin type fructans may have potential to benefit many conditions or disease states including constipation, infectious diarrhea, cancer, cardiovascular disease, and non-insulin-dependent diabetes.[16,17] Long- vs short-chain fructans from chicory have also been compared in the intestine. Absorption, transit time, fermentation factors, and abdominal symptoms have been studied in a 10-patient, single-blind trial.[18] More human trials are needed.

Chicory fructans oligofructose and inulin have also been found to inhibit colon carcinogenesis in rats.[19,20] Another study reports weak-to-moderate comutagenic effects using an extract of chicory greens against induced mutagenicity in vitro.[21] Other fruits and vegetables have been studied with respect to induced mutagenic activities. Chicory was shown to have strong-to-moderate antimutagenic activities that remained heat stable.[22] Root callus extract of chicory demonstrated liver protectant effects against carbon tetrachloride-induced hepatocellular damage.[23] Alcoholic extracts of the root also have anti-inflammatory activity.[24]

Experiments with the isolated toad heart show that chicory extracts reduce cardiac rate in a manner similar to quinidine. Although variable from one preparation to another, this effect is evident before and after ganglionic blockade and atropinization. Its potency is increased by heating the extract. These findings suggest chicory constituents may be effective in treatment of disorders involving tachycardia, arrhythmias, and fibrillation.[1]

Contraceptive activity was observed in female rats orally administered (days 1 to 10 postcoitum) seed extracts of chicory, as well as certain other plant fractions.[25] Chicory has also been noted as an appetite stimulant and for dyspepsia.[26]

TOXICOLOGY: Handling of chicory has been reported to cause occupational contact dermatitis. This effect may be caused by the presence of sesquiterpene lactones.[27,28] Other allergies to chicory include case reports or letters of occupational asthma in a chicory grower,[29] occupational and ingestive allergy to the plant,[30] food allergy,[31] and other allergies.[32,33] A recent report investigates chicory

extract on mast cell-mediated immediate type allergic reactions. It was demonstrated that the extract inhibits this type of reaction in vivo and in vitro.[34]

A study of contamination showed that chicory absorbs the fungicide quintozene through the roots, which may present a toxic hazard.[35] In a study of 64 vegetable samples, 92.5% of the 654 bacterial lines isolated were Enterobacteriaceae, with the more contaminated being celery, fennel, onion, and chicory. These vegetables are a source of contamination and colonization of Enterobacteriaceae, especially in hospitals.[36]

Chicory sold commercially has, in some instances, been contaminated with crushed cashew shells that can cause an allergic toxicity similar to that observed with poison ivy.[37] High levels of inulin (greater than 10%) from chicory in the diet may affect growth in rats and lead to acidic (pH 5.65) cecal fermentation.[13]

In case of gallstones, consult with a physician before taking chicory.[26]

SUMMARY: Chicory is common to Europe, India, Egypt, and North America and is widely cultivated. The leaves are used as salad greens in cooked form; the roots are boiled and eaten or roasted for use as an additive or replacement for coffee or tea. Chicory's oligosaccharides are probiotic and are beneficial in maintaining healthy GI flora. Inulin type fractions of the plant may help certain conditions including constipation, diarrhea, cancer, and cardiovascular disease. Chicory has also been noted as an appetite stimulant and for dyspepsia. The principal toxicity related to chicory is contact dermatitis. In case of gallstones, consult with a physician before taking chicory.

PATIENT INFORMATION – Chicory

Uses: Chicory leaves and roots are used as a vegetable. Roasted roots are ground and brewed. Chicory is a sedative with potential cardioactive properties. Chicory's oligosaccharides are probiotic and are beneficial in maintaining healthy GI flora. Inulin type fractions of the plant may help certain conditions including constipation, diarrhea, cancer, and cardiovascular disease. Chicory has also been noted as an appetite stimulant and for dyspepsia.

Side Effects: Known toxicity includes contact dermatitis, contamination with foreign substances or bacteria, and various allergies. Significant contraceptive activity was observed in female rats orally administered seed extracts and other fractions of chicory. In case of gallstones, consult with a physician before taking chicory.

---

[1] Balbaa S, et al. Preliminary phytochemical and pharmacological investigations of the roots of different varieties of *Chicorium intybus*. *Pianta Med* 1973;24(2):133-44.

[2] Proliac A, et al. [Isolation and identification of the two beta-carbolins in roasted chicory root.] [French] *Helv Chim Acta* 1976;59(7):2503-05.

[3] Ruhl I, et al. [Organic acids in vegetables. I. Brassica, leaf and bulb vegetables as well as carrots and celery.] [German] *Z Lebensm Unters Forsch* 1985;180(3):215-20.

[4] Mahadeviah S, et al. Leaf protein from the green tops of *Chichorium intybus* L. (chicory). *Indian J Exp Biol* 1968;6(3):193-94.

[5] Vijn I, et al. Fructan of the inulin neoseries is synthesized in transgenic chicory plants (*Chicorium intybus* L.) harbouring onion (Allium cepa L.) fructan:fructan 6G-fructosyltransferase. *Plant J* 1997;11(3):387-98.

[6] Galasko G, et al. The caffeine contents of nonalcoholic beverages. *Food Chem Toxicol* 1989;27(1):49-51.

[7] Baes P, et al. Chicory seed lot variety identification by leucine-aminopeptidase and esterase zymogram analysis. *Electrophoresis* 1992;Nov 13(11):885-86.

[8] Roberfroid, M. Functional effects of food components and the gastrointestinal system: chicory fructooligosaccharides. *Nutr Rev* 1996;54(11 Pt. 2):S38-42. Review.

[9] Roberfroid, M. Health benefits of non-digestible oligosaccharides. *Adv Exp Med Biol* 1997;427:211-19. Review.

[10] Roberfroid M, et al. The bifidogenic nature of chicory inulin and its hydrolysis products. *J Nutr* 1998;128(1):11-19. Review.

[11] Gibson, G. Dietary modulation of the human gut microflora using prebiotics. *Br J Nutr* 1998;80(4):S209-12. Review

[12] Roberfroid, M. Caloric value of inulin and oligofructose. *J Nutr* 1999;129(7 Suppl):1436S-437S. Review.

[13] Levrat M, et al. High proprionic acid fermentations and mineral accumulation in the cecum of rats adapted to different levels of inulin. *J Nutr* 1991;121(11):1730-37.

[14] Kim M, et al. The water-soluble extract of chicory reduces glucose uptake from the perfused jejunum in rats. *J Nutr* 1996;126(9):2236-242.

[15] Kim M, et al. The water-soluble extract of chicory influences serum and liver lipid concentrations, cecal short-chain fatty acid concentrations and fecal lipid excretion in rats. *J Nutr* 1998;128(10):1731-736.

[16] Roberfroid M, et al. Dietary fructans. *Annu Rev Nutr* 1998;18:117-43. Review.

[17] Roberfroid, M. Concepts in functional foods: the case of inulin and oligofructose. *J Nutr* 1999;129(7 Suppl):1398S-401S.

[18] Rumessen J, et al. Fructans of chicory: intestinal transport and fermentation of different chain lengths and relation to fructose and sorbitol malabsorption. *Am J Clin Nutr* 1998;68(2):357-64.

[19] Reddy B, et al. Effect of dietary oligofructose and inulin on colonic preneoplastic aberrant crypt foci inhibition. *Carcinogenesis* 1997;18(7):1371-374.

[20] Reddy, B. Prevention of colon cancer by pre- and probiotics: evidence from laboratory studies. *Br J Nutr* 1998;80(4):S219-23.

[21] Tang X, et al. Inhibition of the mutagenicity of 2-nitrofluorene, 3-nitrofluoranthene and 1-nitropyrene by vitamins, porphyrins and related compounds, and vegetable and fruit juices and solvent extracts. *Food Chem Toxicol* 1997;35(3-4):373-78.

[22] Edenharder R, et al. In vitro effect of vegetable and fruit juices on the mutagenicity of 2-amino-methylimidazo-quinoline, 2-amino-3,4-dimethylimidazo-quinoline and 2-amino-3,8-dimethlimidazoquinoxaline. *Food Chem Toxicol* 1994;32(5):443-59.

[23] Zafar R, et al. Anti-hepatotoxic effects of root and root callus extracts of *Chicorium intybus* L. *J Ethnopharmacol* 1998;63(3):227-31.

[24] Benoit P, et al. Biological and phytochemical evaluation of plants. 14. Anti-inflammatory evaluation of 163 species of plants. *Lloydia* 1976;39:160-71.

[25] Keshri G, et al. Postcoital contraceptive activity of some indigenous plants in rats. *Contraception* 1998;57(5):357-60.

[26] Blumenthal, M, ed. *The Complete German Commission E Monographs.* Boston: American Botanical Council, 1998.

[27] Friis B, et al. Occupational contact dermatitis from Chicorium (chicory, endive) and Lactuca (lettuce). *Contact Dermatitis* 1975;1(5):311-13.

[28] Malten K. Chicory dermatitis from September to April. *Contact Dermatitis* 1983;9(3):232.

[29] Nemery B, et al. Occupational asthma in a chicory grower. *Lancet* 1989;1(8639):672-73.

[30] Cadot P, et al. Inhalative occupational and ingestive immediate-type allergy caused by chicory (Chichorium intybus). *Clin Exp Allergy* 1996;26(8):940-44.

[31] Helbling A, et al. Food allergy to Belgian endive (chicory). *J Allergy Clin Immunol* 1997;99(6 Pt. 1):854-56.

[32] Symons, M. Strange allergy to chicory. *Lancet* 1988;2(8618):1027.

[33] Escudero A, et al. Lettuce and chicory sensitization. *Allergy* 1999;54(2):183-84.

[34] Kim H, et al. Inhibitory effect of mast cell-mediated immediate-type allergic reactions by *Chicorium intybus*. *Pharmacol Res* 1999;40(1):61-65.

[35] Dejonckheere W, et al. Residues of quintozene, its contaminants and metabolites in soil, lettuce and witloof-chicory, Belgium-1969-74. *Pestic Monit J* 1976;10(2):68-73.

[36] Cavazzini G, et al [Gram-negative flora of horticultural produce destined for consumption mainly in the raw state.] [Italian] *Ann Ig* 1989;1(5):1279.

[37] Sengupta P, et al. Detection of cashew nut shells in coffee, tea, and chicory. *J Assoc Off Anal Chem* 1974;57(3):761-62.

Chinese Cucumber

SCIENTIFIC NAME(S): *Trichosanthes kirilowii* Maxim. Family: Cucurbitaceae

COMMON NAME(S): Chinese cucumber, Chinese snake gourd, gua-lou, tian-hua-fen, compound Q

BOTANY: The chinese cucumber is one of more than 40 recognized species of *Trichosanthes*. It is a member of the gourd family, and the root, fruit, seeds, stems and peel are used medicinally. While *T. kirilowii* is the plant most often referred to in Chinese materia medica, a number of related species are often used as adulterants.

HISTORY: *T. kirilowii* has a long history in traditional Chinese medicine where it is used to reduce fevers, swelling and coughing. A starch extracted from the root is used for abscesses, amenorrhea, jaundice and polyuria. Modern Chinese medicinal uses include the management of diabetes and use as an abortifacient.[1] The plant has been used for centuries in the treatment of tumors.

CHEMISTRY: The most studied component of *T. kirilowii* is the protein trichosanthin.[2,3] Two trichosanthins have been identified: Alpha from *T. kirilowii* and beta from *T. cucumeroides*. Alpha-trichosanthin is synonymous with Chinese cucumber. A highly purified form of trichosanthin has been investigated under the name GLQ-223. A second protein, trichokirin, was isolated and found to possess ribosome-inactivating activity.[4] A later study reports that a peptide trypsin inhibitor isolated from *T. kirilowii* roots may be the smallest naturally occurring protein inhibitor.[5]

An abortifacient protein, karasurin, has been isolated from fresh root tubers of the plant. It was found to express protein polymorphism separated by ion-exchange chromatography.[6,7] Three Japanese studies report structure and anti-inflammatory effects of five hydroxylated sterols from Chinese cucumber seeds.[8,9,10]

PHARMACOLOGY: The Chinese cucumber has gained enormous popularity because trichosanthin may be effective in the management of **acquired immunodeficiency syndrome (AIDS)** infections. A report by McGrath, et al described the ability of GLQ-223 to block HIV replication in infected T-cells and to kill HIV-infected macrophages. In vitro, this compound appears to selectively kill infected cells without damaging uninfected cells. Trichosanthin also appears to prevent the HIV virus from replicating in T-4 cells (immune cells that are killed by the virus). When freshly drawn blood samples from HIV-infected patients were treated with a single 3-hour exposure to GLQ-223, HIV replication was blocked for at least 5 days in subsequently cultured monocytes and macrophages.[11] Human clinical trials have been initiated in the United States to determine the drug's potential in man.

A report studied anti-HIV activity in trichosanthin purified from *T. kirilowii* root tubers.[12] A protein ("TAP 29"), distinct from trichosanthin, may offer a broader safe dose range compared with trichosanthin in AIDS treatment. The two proteins exhibit similar anti-HIV activity.[13]

Extracts of the plant have been known for centuries to be potent **abortifacients**. Trichosanthin inhibits ribosome activity and cellular replication.[14] One report says that trichosanthin inactivates ribosomes by cleaving the N-C glycosidic bond of adenylic acid at (position) 4324 of 28S rRNA in a hydrolytic fashion.[15] Another report discusses the importance of lysine and arginine to trichosanthin's activity.[16] Another ribosome-inactivating protein, beta-kirilowin, has recently been isolated from *T. kirilowii* seeds and exhibits strong abortifacient activity.[17] Studies on another abortifacient and antitumor protein, karasurin, report induction of mid-term abortion in pregnant mice.[6,7] Other proteins present in the plant have been reported to express similar abortive effects.[18]

Chinese cucumber juice, applied to a sponge inserted vaginally, can induce abortions. Trichosanthin has been used to abort ectopic pregnancies in place of management via salpingectomy.[19] The drug is also effective in inducing first-trimester abortion when administered intramuscularly or extra-amniotically.[19]

Trichosanthin possesses **antitumor activity** and has been used to treat invasive moles.[1,20] Selective killing of choriocarcinoma cells has occurred.[21] It also shows specificity as an antihepatoma agent.[22] Trichosanthin is a reported potent immunosuppressive protein, which could affect immunity and various cell-mediated processes.[23] The plant's other components, karounidiol and bryonolic acid, have been evaluated for their cytotoxic activity.[24,25,26]

Other immunological effects of trichosanthin include: Initiation of the alternative complement activation pathway in mice;[27] viability of human immunocytes, lymphocyte proliferation and cytotoxicity to lymphoma and leukemia cell lines;[28] and inhibitory effects on "IL-8 induction in lipopolysaccharide-activated rat macrophages."[29] Other effects of Chinese cucumber in animals include: Anti-inflammation,[8] anti-ulceration[30] and hypoglycemia.[31]

TOXICOLOGY: Extracts of the Chinese cucumber are extremely toxic, particularly if administered parenterally. Subacute LD-50 studies in mice resulted in deaths in 10 days. The LD-50 of intravenously administered freeze-dried root extract was 2.26 mg/mouse. Crystalline trichosanthin had an LD-50 of 0.236 mg/mouse.

Patients who receive injections of trichosanthin for abortion often develop strong sensitization to the compound. The risk of anaphylactic reaction secondary to a single exposure to trichosanthin may last longer than a decade.[1]

Other severe reactions produced by trichosanthin include pulmonary and cerebral edema, cerebral hemorrhage and myocardial damage. One report describes six patients with AIDS who purchased a cucumber root extract while in China. Following parenteral administration, the patients developed seizures and fever and were hospitalized.[20] The FDA has received a report of a patient who died following trichosanthin injections.[1] The crude mixture of plant proteins and lectins may have resulted in damage to blood cells. Clinical trials in the United States are confined to the use of highly purified trichosanthin.

Chinese cucumber use is contraindicated in pregnant women. Abortifacient effects have been well documented.[6,7,14,17] In vivo and in vitro teratogenic effects were evaluated in mice, resulting in aphysical abnormalities.[32] An additional study reported increased incidence of follicular atresia, ovulation changes and decreased hormone levels in mice given trichosanthin injections.[33]

SUMMARY: The Chinese cucumber has been recognized in oriental medicine for several thousand years. Extracts of the plant have been used to induce abortions. The primary component of the plant, trichosanthin, inhibits replication of the HIV virus in vitro. The plant also exhibits antitumor properties and other immunological effects. Extracts of the plant are extremely toxic and should never be ingested without supervision by a physician. The plant and its compounds are contraindicated in pregnant women or those of childbearing potential.

PATIENT INFORMATION – Chinese Cucumber

Uses: Chinese cucumber has been used to induce abortion. It possesses antitumor activity and has been used to treat invasive moles. Chinese cucumber is being studied as a treatment for the management of AIDS infections.

Side Effects: Side effects include allergic reaction, fluid in the lungs or brain, bleeding in the brain, heart damage, seizures, fever and death.

---

[1] Duke JA and Foster S. *Herbalgram* 1989;20:20.
[2] Yeung HW, et al. *Planta Med* 1987;53:164.
[3] Ke YP, et al. *Immunopharmacol Immunotoxicol* 1988;10:131.
[4] Casellas P, et al. *Eur J Biochem* 1988;176:581.
[5] Qian Y, et al. *Sci China* 1990;33(5):599-605.
[6] Toyokawa S, et al. *Chem Pharm Bull* 1991;39(3):716-19.
[7] Toyokawa S, et al. *Chem Pharm Bull* 1991;39(8):2132-34.
[8] Akihisa T, et al. *Chem Pharm Bull* 1994;42(5):1101-1105.
[9] Kimura Y, et al. *Chem Pharm Bull* 1995 Oct ;43:1813-17.
[10] Akihisa T, et al. *Chem Pharm Bull* 1992;40(5):1199-1202.
[11] McGrath, et al. *Proc Natl Acad Sci* 1989;86:2844-48.
[12] Ferrari P, et al. *AIDS* 1991;5(7):865-70.
[13] Lee-Huang S, et al. *Proc Natl Acad Sci U S A* 1991;88(15):6570-74.
[14] Yeung HW, et al. *Int J Pept Protein Res* 1988;31:265.
[15] Zhang J, et al. *Nucleic Acids Res* 1992;20(6):1271-75.
[16] Keung W, et al. *Int J Pept Protein Res* 1993;42(6):504-8.
[17] Dong T, et al. *Biochem Biophys Res Commun* 1994;199(1):387-93.

[18] Yeung H, et al. *Immunopharmacol Immunotoxicol* 1987;9(1):25-46.
[19] Lu PX and Jin YC. *Chinese Med J* 1989;102:365.
[20] Chang and But. *Pharmacology and Applications of Chinese Materia Medica.* World Scientific Publishing Co, Singapore 1986;1.
[21] Tsao S, et al. *Toxicon* 1986;24(8):831-40.
[22] Wang Q, et al. *Cancer Res* 1991;51(13):3353-55.
[23] Leung K, et al. *Asian Pac J Allergy Immunol* 1986;4(2):111-20.
[24] Yasukawa K, et al. *Biological Pharm Bull* 1994;17(3):460-62.
[25] Takeda T, et al. *Chem Pharm Bull* 1994;42(3):730-32.
[26] Kondo T, et al. *Biological Pharm Bull* 1995;18(5):726-29.
[27] Chen X, et al. *Clin Exp Immunol* 1993;93(2):248-52.
[28] Zheng Y, et al. *Immunopharmacol Immunotoxicol* 1995;17(1):69-79.
[29] Lee G, et al. *Planta Med* 1995;61(1):26-30.
[30] Takano F, et al. *Chem Pharm Bull* 1990;38(5):1313-16.
[31] Hikino H, et al. *Planta Med* 1989;55(4):349-50.
[32] Chan W, et al. *Teratogenesis Carcinog Mutagen* 1993;13(2):47-57.
[33] Ng T, et al. *Gen Pharmacol* 1991;22(5):847-49.

Chitosan

SCIENTIFIC NAME(S): Chitosan

COMMON NAME(S): Chitosan

SOURCE: Chitin is a cellulose-like biopolymer found mainly in exoskeletons of marine invertebrates and arthropods, such as shrimp, crabs or lobsters. Chitin can also be found in fungi and yeasts. Deacylated chitin is called chitosan.[1] Chitosan is unique in that, unlike plant cellulose that is negatively charged, it possesses positively charged amino groups. These bind to the negatively charged lipid and bile components, preventing absorption by the body.[2] "Squid pens" (waste by-product of New Zealand squid processing) are a renewable and inexpensive source of chitosan.[3]

HISTORY: Chitosan has been used in the past 30 years in water purification plants to absorb greases, oils, metals and toxic substances. It can absorb four to six times its weight, and ascorbic acid can potentiate this action even further.[4]

CHEMISTRY: Chitin consists mainly of unbranched chains of beta-(1 → 4)-2-acetamido-2-deoxy-D-glucose (=N-acetyl-d-glucosamine). It is similar to cellulose, where the C-2 hydroxyl groups are replaced by acetamido residue. Chitin is practically insoluble in water, dilute acids and alcohol. However, this varies depending on product origin.[1]

Chitosan, the partially deacetylated polymer of N-acetyl-D-glucosamine, is water-soluble.[3]

Rheology, flocculation and film formation testing have been performed with chitosan, demonstrating its usefulness in medical and analytical applications.[3] Biodegradable and biocompatible properties of chitosan films have been studied with good outcomes.[5] In vitro and in vivo degradation tests of chitin and chitosan have been evaluated,[6] as well as chitosan film chemistry on electrically charged metal plates.[7]

N-carboxymethylchitosan solubility and structure have been reported,[8] along with its ability to chelate metal ions and to enhance binding of dyes.[9]

Other chemical aspects involving chitin or chitosan include: Optical isomer separation,[10] mass-spectrometric analysis,[11] polyelectrolyte and sulfation studies,[12] adherence to liposomes[13] and properties of chitosan microspheres.[14]

PHARMACOLOGY: Chitosan is used in many areas, including the cosmetic and pharmaceutical industries, for medical use as a **hyperlipidemic** and in **hypercholesterolemia** therapy and for **biomaterials**. It is also used for **antimicrobial** and other effects.

Application of chitosan in the pharmaceutical industry is documented. Its ability to **mask bitter tastes** in oral pharmaceuticals has been reported.[15] There are reports employing chitosan in drug delivery systems of many types. Some of these reports include:

1.) *Peptide/Diabetic use:* Peptide drug delivery enhancement using chitosan,[16] colon-specific drug delivery of insulin using chitosan capsules,[17] mucoadhesion of chitosan-coated liposomes affecting insulin absorption in rats,[18] chitosan microcapsules to control insulin release,[19] and diabetic drugs in chitosan matrix tablets;[20]

2.) *Nasal route studies:* For insulin,[21,22] effects of chitosan on intranasal mucociliary clearance[23] and transport rates.[24] Pharmacokinetics on nasal administration on morphine-6–glucuronide in sheep;[25]

3.) *Transdermal delivery* using chitosan composite membranes;[26]

4.) *Various drug release evaluations on:* Chitosan hydrogels for organ specific antibiotic delivery in the stomach,[27] sustained release deoxytetracycline from chitosan microspheres,[28] biophosphonate-containing chitosan microspheres,[29] chitosan-indomethacin conjugates,[30] aspirin and heparin embedded in a chitosan matrix,[31] preparation and drug-release properties of chitosan-drug microspheres,[32] suitability of chitosan as a carrier, using indomethacin papaverine[33] and lidocaine,[34,35] cancer drug delivery,[36] buccal and vaginal tablets containing mycotic drugs and chitosan,[37] nifedipine release with chitosan microspheres,[38] chitosan beads to deliver salmon calcitonin;[39]

5.) *Chitosan to enhance absorption:* For poorly absorbable drugs[40] and across mucosal surfaces.[41]

Chitosan's role in the cosmetic industry has been reported.[42,43,44] Chitosan use as a natural product may substitute for the synthetic polymer elements in film-forming resins.[45]

Chitosan's characteristic as a film-forming and protective polysaccharide suggests its potential use as a biomaterial. Its applications in this area have been reported.[46] Safety and hemostatic potential have been evaluated, concluding low toxicity and tensile strength retention in many circumstances.[47] N,O-carboxymethyl chitosan gel and solution delivered postoperatively were effective in preventing peritoneal adhesions in rats.[48] A Russian article discusses chitosan's role in **reparative skin regeneration**.[49] Heparin-chitosan gel application has stimulated **wound healing** in human skin, hypothesized to possibly be caused by stabilization and activation of growth factors that bind to heparin.[50] In burn patients, where standard of care involves application of silver sulfadiazine cream, silver toxicity is a concern (because of reduced skin barriers). Membranes, including chitosan, reduce this toxicity caused by the entrapment of silver ions in the matrix.[51] Adsorption of lead ions on chitosan has also been evaluated.[52] Chitin's involvement with human enzymatic activity seems to be activation of macrophages and stimulation of fibroblasts, promoting normal tissue production.[53]

Fiber products such as bran, resins, pectins, etc. have been used in the past for cholesterol and weight reduction. Cross-linked O-carboxymethyl chitosan beads are capable of absorbing LDL-cholesterol in vitro.[54] Extensive animal studies have been reported on these topics. Chitosan decreases lipid concentrations in affected rats, decreasing VLDL and increasing HDL levels.[55] Chitosan also has hypocholesterolemic actions in rats,[56,57,58] and

has shown to lower cholesterol triglycerides.[59,60] Chitosan alters metabolism of bile in the intestines, affecting lipid and cholesterol levels.[61] One report relates many enzyme-involvements to oral administration of chitosan but proposes physical chitosan-lipid aggregate adsorption to be the mechanism of lipid adsorption.[53] **Hypocholesterolemic** effect in humans has been reported.[62,63]

Chitosan has been reported to exert some antimicrobial actions, exhibiting **bactericidal** actions against several pathogens in the field of dentistry,[64] inhibiting adhesion of *Candida albicans* to human vaginal epithelial cells[65] and inhibiting chlamydial infection by interfering with adsorption.[66]

One report suggests chitosan to be effective treatment for **renal failure** patients.[67]

Chitosan's use includes photographic emulsions and improving dyeability of synthetic fibers in the fabric industry.[1]

TOXICOLOGY: Chitosan's toxicity profile is relatively low. Dietary chitosan reportedly affects calcium metabolism in animals.[68] Toxic effects of chitosans are dependent mainly on their chemical composition.[40]

SUMMARY: Chitosan is deacylated chitin, which is a polymer found mainly in shellfish exoskeletons. It has been used in water treatment to soak up grease and other undesirable substances. Chitosan is used in many areas, including the pharmaceutical and cosmetic industries, in medicine as treatment of hyperlipidemias and as biomaterials. It has antimicrobial effects and other actions. Most studies report low toxicity profiles, but individuals with shellfish allergy or pregnant women should consult with their doctors before use. Chitosan may affect mineral metabolism. The chemical composition of chitosans may affect its toxicity.

PATIENT INFORMATION – Chitosan

Uses: Chitosan has been used in various drug delivery systems. It has antimicrobial and other effects and can be used for kidney failure and to lower cholesterol.

Side Effects: Consult your physician if you are allergic to shellfish or if you are pregnant or breastfeeding.

---

[1] Budavari, ed. *The Merck Index.* Rahway, NJ: Merck & Co., Inc., 1989.
[2] Furda I, et al. *New Developments in Dietary Fiber.* Plenum Press: New York. 1990;67-82.
[3] Shepherd R, et al. *Glycoconj J* 1997;14(4):535-42.
[4] Nauss J, et al. *Lipids* 1983;18(10):714-19.
[5] Cao Z, et al. *Chin J Pharm* 1996 Jan; 27:14–16.
[6] Tomihata K, et al. *Biomaterials* 1997;18(7):567-75.
[7] Ikeda H, et al. *Chem Pharm Bull* 1996 Jul;44:1372-75.
[8] Muzzarelli R, et al. *Int J Biol Macromol* 1994;16(4):177-80.
[9] Muzzarelli R, et al. *Chimicaoggi* 1993 Oct;11:31-35.
[10] Malinowska I, et al. *Biomed Chromatogr* 1997;11(5):272-75.
[11] Lopatin S, et al. *Anal Biochem* 1995;227(2):285-88.

[12] Holme K, et al. *Carbohydr Res* 1997;302(1-2):7-12.
[13] Henriksen I, et al. *Int J Pharm* 1994 Jan 25;101:227-36.
[14] Berthold A, et al. *S.T.P. Pharma Sci* 1996;6(5):358-64.
[15] Roy G. *Pharmaceut Tech* 1994 Apr;18:84,86,88,92,94,96–99.
[16] Luessen H, et al. *J Cont Rel* 1994 Mar;29:329-38.
[17] Tozaki H, et al. *J Pharm Sci* 1997;86(9):1016-21.
[18] Takeuchi H, et al. *Pharm Res* 1996 Jun;13:896-901.
[19] Aiedeh K, et al. *J Microencapsul* 1997;14(5):567-76.
[20] Ilango R, et al. *Indian Drugs* 1995 Dec;32:578-82.
[21] Aspden T, et al. *Eur J Pharm Sci* 1996;4(1):23-31.
[22] Illum L, et al. *Pharm Res* 1994 Aug;11:1186-89.
[23] Zhou M, et al. *Int J Pharm* 1996 Jun 17;135:115-25.
[24] Aspden T, et al. *J Pharm Sci* 1997;86(4):509-13.
[25] Illum L, et al. *Biopharm Drug Dispos* 1996 Nov;17:717-24.
[26] Thacharodi D, et al. *Int J Pharm* 1996 May 28;134:239-41.
[27] Patel V, et al. *Pharm Res* 1996 Apr;13:588-93.
[28] Mi F, et al. *J Microencapsul* 1997;14(5):577-91.
[29] Patashnik S, et al. *J Drug Target* 1997;4(6):371-80.
[30] Orienti I, et al. *Archiv Der Pharmazie* 1996 May;329:245-50.
[31] Vasudev S, et al. *Biomaterials* 1997;18(5):375-81.
[32] Onishi H, et al. *Drug Develop Ind Pharm* 1996;22(5):457-63.
[33] Miyazaki S, et al. *Chem Pharm Bull* 1981 Oct;29:3067-69.
[34] Kristl J, et al. *Farmaceutski Vestnik* 1991 Sep;42:207-13.
[35] Kristl J, et al. *Int J Pharm* 1993 Sep 1;99:13-19.
[36] Liu L, et al. *J Cont Rel* 1997 Jan;43:65-74.
[37] Knapczyk J, *Int J Pharm* 1992 Dec 8;88:9-14.
[38] Filipovic-Grcic J, et al. *Int J Pharm* 1996 Jun 17;135:183-90.
[39] Ayoin Z, et al. *Int J Pharm* 1996 Apr 5;131:101-3.
[40] Schipper N, et al. *Pharm Res* 1997;14(7):923-29.
[41] Kotze A, et al. *Pharm Res* 1997;14(9):1197-1202.
[42] Skaugrud O. *Manufactur Chem* 1989 Oct; 60:31,33,35.
[43] Onsoyen E, et al. *Seifen, Oele, Fette, Wachse* 1991 Oct 24;117:633-37.
[44] Naidoo N. *S Afr Pharm J* 1992 Jun;59:131-32.
[45] Gross P, et al. *Parfuem Kosmet* 1983 Jul;64:367-71.
[46] Shigemasa Y, et al. *Biotechnol Genet Eng Rev* 1996;13:383-420.
[47] Rao S, et al. *J Biomed Mater Res* 1997;34(1):21-28.
[48] Costain D, et al. *Surgery* 1997;121(3):314-19.
[49] Tolstikova T, et al. *Dokl Akad Nauk* 1996;350(4):557-59.
[50] Kratz G, et al. *Scand J Plast Reconstr Hand Surg* 1997;31(2):119-23.
[51] Tsipouras N, et al. *Clin Chem* 1997;43(2):290-301.
[52] Zheng F, et al. *J China Pharmaceut University* 1995 Oct;26:318-20.
[53] Muzzarelli R. *Cell Mol Life Sci* 1997;53(2):131-40.
[54] Yihua Y, et al. *Artif Cells Blood Substit Immobil Biotechnol* 1997;25(5):445-50.
[55] Ryzhenkov V, et al. *Vopr Med Khim* 1996;42(2):115–19.
[56] Sugano M, et al. *Nutr Rep Intl* 1978;18(5):531-37.
[57] Sugano M, et al. *Am J Clin Nutr* 1980;33:787-93.
[58] Michihiro S, et al. *Lab Nutr* 1988.
[59] Birketvedt G. *Clinical Report* 1991 May.
[60] Chobot V, et al. *Ceska A Slovenska Farmacie* 1995;44(4):190-95.
[61] Vahouny G, et al. *Am J Clin Nutr* 1983;38:278-84.
[62] Takaai, et al. *Nutritional Rep Int* 1979;19(3)327-34.
[63] Kestin M, et al. *Am J Clin Nutr* 1990;52(4):661-66.
[64] Tarsi R, et al. *J Dent Res* 1997;76(2):665-72.
[65] Knapczyk J, et al. *Int J Pharm* 1992 Feb 10;80:33-38.
[66] Petronio M, et al. *Chemotherapy* 1997;43(3):211-17.
[67] Jing S, et al. *J Pharm Pharmacol* 1997;49(7):721-23.
[68] Wada M, et al. *Biosci Biotechnol Biochem* 1997;61(7):1206-8.

Chondroitin

SCIENTIFIC NAME(S): Chondroitin sulfate, chondroitin sulfuric acid, chonsurid, structum

COMMON NAME(S): Chondroitin

SOURCE: Chondroitin is a biological polymer that acts as the flexible connecting matrix between the protein filaments in cartilage.[1] Chondroitin can come from natural sources, such as shark or bovine cartilage or can be manufactured in the lab, using different methods.[2] Danaparoid sodium, a mixture of heparan sulfate, dermatan sulfate and chondroitin sulfate (21:3:1), is derived from porcine intestinal mucosa.[3]

HISTORY: Chondroitin sulfates were first extracted and purified in 1960. Studies suggested that if enough chondroitin sulfate was available to cells manufacturing proteoglycan (one of the substances that forms the cartilage matrix), stimulation of matrix synthesis could occur, leading to an accelerated healing process.[4] This idea of natural regeneration of cartilage has been popularized with the publication of the J. Theodosakis Book, "The Arthritis Cure."[5]

CHEMISTRY: Chondroitin sulfate is a high-viscosity mucopolysaccharide (glycosaminoglycan) with N-acetylchondrosine as a repeating unit and one sulfate group per disaccharide unit. Its molecular weight is about 50,000, depending on product source or preparation.[1] Danaparoid sodium (a mixture containing chondroitin) has a low molecular weight (5500 to 6000).[3] Analytical determination including HPLC, spectrophotometric analysis, chemical methods, ultraviolet spectrometry, and IR spectroscopy has been performed on chondroitin and its related structures.[6,7,8,9,10] A method for potentiometric titration of chondroitin sulfate has also been reported.[11]

PHARMACOLOGY: The pharmacokinetics of chondroitin sulfate have been determined in rats and dogs.[12] Another pharmacokinetic study, involving eight healthy volunteers, reports similar results in metabolism to those in animals. Other parameters evaluated included half-lives of distribution and elimination, volumes of distribution, excretion values, urine and blood levels and bioavailablity.[13] Another report concludes oral chondroitin sulfate B (dermatan sulfate) to reach significant plasma levels, with 7% bioavailability.[14] In 22 patients with renal failure, chondroitin sulfate half-life was prolonged, but it could be administered for clot prevention during hemodialysis in this population.[15]

Chondroitin's role in treating **arthritis** has gained popularity. Ongoing research continues with some controversial outcomes.

Articular cartilage is found between joints (eg, finger, knee, hip) allowing for easy, painless movement. It contains 65% to 80% water, collagen and proteoglycans. Chondrocytes are also found within this matrix, to produce new collagen and proteoglycans from building blocks, including chondroitin sulfate, a glycosaminoglycan (GAG). Chondroitin helps attract essential fluid into the proteoglycan molecules, "water magnet," which not only acts as a shock absorber but "sweeps" nutrients into the cartilage as well.[4] Chondrocytes must derive nutrition from this synovial fluid as there is no vasculature to nourish them.[16] Glucosamine, another of the beneficial substances in this area, stimulates chondrocyte activity. It is also the critical building block of proteoglycans and other matrix components.[4] Both chondroitin and glucosamine play vital roles in joint maintenance, which is the reason the combination of the two are found in many arthritic nutritional supplements (eg, "chondroitin complex" by Nature's Bounty, Bohemia, NY; 11716).

In inflammation and repeated wear of the joint, chondrocyte function is disturbed, altering the matrix and causing breakdown.[16] Proper supplementation with glycosaminoglycans (eg, chondroitin sulfate) may enable chondrocytes to replace proteoglycans, offering "chondroprotection."[17] Cartilage contains the biological resources to enhance repair of degenerative injuries and inflammation. It has been proposed that a certain chondroitin sulfate sequence, released from cartilage proteoglycans, can inhibit elastase, regulating the matrix.[18]

Results of a multicenter study of chondroitin sulfate in finger, knee and hip joint therapy are comparable with other international, double-blind, placebo controlled studies, all indicating beneficial results in osteoarthritis treatment.[19] An overview of chondroitin sulfate in another report, however, concluded the product has no clear value in osteoarthritis treatment.[20]

There is considerable controversy regarding absorption of chondroitin. Absorption of glucosamine is 90% to 98%, but chondroitin absorption is only 0% to 13% because of molecule size. Chondroitin is 50 to 300 times larger than glucosamine. (Note in chemistry section "MW") Chondroitin may be too large to be delivered to cartilage cells. In addition, there also may be purification and identification problems with some chondroitin products, some of which have tested subpotent.[4]

The American College of Rheumatology has stated that although chondroitin sulfate is readily available in health food stores, the supplements are not regulated by the Food and Drug Administration. Longer-term clinical trials, with larger groups of people are warranted to determine whether or not it is safe and effective. They also warn against discontinuaton of conventional therapy without consulting a physician and stress the importance of maintaining proper body weight and exercising.[21]

Chondroitin sulfate has been used as a **drug delivery** system for diclofenac and flurbiprofen.[22] Additionally, the polymer has been used as a **stabilization agent** for iron injection hyperalimentation.[23]

Chondroitin sulfate B (dermatan sulfate) has potential as an **antithrombolytic** agent, as it inhibits venous thrombi, with less effect upon bleeding than heparin. It is an effective anticoagulant in hemodialysis.[24] Another study found dermatan sulfate to have no direct, observable relation to heparin aggregation.[25] Dermatan sulfate's efficacy, compared with heparin, has been determined in acute leukemia patients.[26]

Chondroitin sulfate has been used to treat **extravasation** after ifosfamide therapy, decreasing pain and inflammation.[27] It has also been used to treat extravasation from vindesine,[28] doxorubicin and vincristine[29] and an etoposide needlestick injury in a healthcare worker.[30]

Levels of chondroitin sulfate increase 10 to 100 times in tumors compared with normal tissue. In one report, all 44 cancer patients analyzed showed the structural anomaly of the urinary chondroitin sulfate. This may provide a potential new marker for diagnosis and follow-up of cancer therapy.[31]

General reviews are available on chondroitin sulfate and chondroitin sulfate B.[32,33]

TOXICOLOGY: Little information about long-term toxic effects of chondroitin sulfate is available. Most reports conclude that it is not harmful compared with other arthritis therapies, such as NSAIDs. Because the drug is concentrated in cartilage, the theory is that it produces no toxic or teratogenic effects.[19] Long-term clinical trials with larger populations are needed to fully determine toxicity.[21]

SUMMARY: Chondroitin sulfate is a biological polymer important in the formation of cartilage. Its role in treatment for arthritis has gained in popularity but is controversial. It seems to help arthritis sufferers in some clinical trials. Chondroitin sulfate has also been studied in drug delivery, antithrombotic therapy and extravasation treatment.

PATIENT INFORMATION – Chondroitin

Uses: Chondroitin has been used to treat arthritis. It has also been studied for use in drug delivery, antithrombotic and extravasation therapy.

Side Effects: There is little information on chondroitin's long-term effects. Most reports conclude that it is not harmful.

---

[1] Budavari S, et al, eds. *The Merck Index*, 11th ed. Rahway: Merck and Co., 1989.
[2] Ma S, et al. *Chin Pharm J* 1993 Dec 28;741-43.
[3] Reynolds J, ed. *Martindale, the Extra Pharmacopoeia*, 13th ed. London: Royal Pharmaceutial Society, 1996.
[4] Benedikt H. *Nat Pharm* 1997;1(8):1,22.
[5] Theodosakis J. The Arthritis Cure. New York, NY: St. Martin's Press, 1997.
[6] Murata K, et al. *J Biochem Biophys Methods* 1987;15(1):23-32.
[7] Fabregas, et al. *Pharm Acta Helvetiae* 1981;56(9-10):265-67.
[8] Volpi N, et al. *Farmaco* 1992 May;47 Suppl:841–53.
[9] Brizzi V. *Farmacia e Clinica* 1990;29(1):3-8.
[10] Ovsepyan A, et al. *Pharm Chem J* 1979 Sep;13:986-90.
[11] Mascellani G, et al. *Farmaco Ed Prat* 1988 May;43:165-75.
[12] Conte A, et al. *Arzneimittel-Forschung* 1995;45(8):918-25.
[13] Conte A, et al. *Arzneimittel-Forschung* 1991;41(7):768-72.
[14] Dawes J, et al. *Br J Clin Pharm* 1991 Sep;32:361-6.
[15] Gianese F, et al. *Br J Clin Pharm* 1993 Mar;35:335-39.
[16] Krane S, et al. *Eur J Rheumatol Inflamm* 1990;10(1):4-9.
[17] Pipitone V. *Drugs Exp Clin Res* 1991;17(1):3-7.
[18] Paroli E. *Int J Clin Pharmacol Res* 1993;13 Suppl:1-9.
[19] Leeb B, et al. *Wien Med Wochenschr* 1996;146(24):609-14.
[20] Anonymous. *Prescrire Int* 1995;4(20):165-67.
[21] American College of Rheumatology Patient Information WEB page (60 Executive Park S. Ste. 150, Atlanta, GA 30329), 1997. http://www.rheumatology.org/patient/970127.htm.
[22] Murata Y, et al. *J Controlled Release* 1996 Feb;38:101-8.
[23] Yamaji A, et al. *J Nippon Hosp Pharm Assoc* 1979 Jan;5:30-35.
[24] Lane D, et al. *Lancet* 1992 Feb 8;339:334-5.
[25] Racey T, et al. *J Pharm Sci* 1989 Mar;78:214-18.
[25] Cofrancesco E. *Lancet* 1992 May 9;339:1177-78.
[27] Mateu J, et al. *Ann Pharmacother* 1994 Nov;28:1243-44.
[28] Mateu J, et al. *Ann Pharmacother* 1994 Jul-Aug;28:967-68.
[29] Comas D, et al. *Ann Pharmacother* 1996 Mar;30:244-46.
[30] Mateu J, et al. *Am J Health-System Pharm* 1996 May 1;53:1068,1071.
[31] Dietrich C, et al. *Lab Invest* 1993;68(4):439-45.
[32] Dosa E, et al. *Acta Pharm Hungarica* 1977 May;47:102-12.
[33] Tamagnone G, et al. *Drugs of the Future* 1994 Jul;19:638-40.

Chromium

SOURCE: Chromium is abundant in the earth's crust and is found in concentrations ranging from 100 to 300 ppm.[1] Commercially, it is obtained from chrome ore among other sources. The organic form of chromium exists in a dinicotino-glutathionine complex in natural foods, and appears to be absorbed better than the inorganic form. Good dietary sources of chromium include brewer's yeast, liver, potatoes with skin, beef, fresh vegetables and cheese.[2]

HISTORY: Chromium is important as an additive in the manufacture of steel alloys (chrome-steel, chrome-nickel-steel, stainless steel) and greatly increases the durability and resistance of these metals. Synthetically-produced $_{51}Cr$ is used as a tracer in various hematologic disorders and in the determination of blood volume.[3] Because chromium is a recognized element required for the normal glucose metabolism, a number of over-the-counter products promote the use of chromium, alone or in combination with "glucose tolerance factor" (GTF), to improve carbohydrate utilization. The effectiveness of these products has not been established although they represent nutritionally sound sources of chromium.

CHEMISTRY: Chromium (Cr) has an atomic weight of 51.996. The element has four valences. A number of naturally-occurring isotopes have been identified, the most common of which is $_{52}Cr$ (approximately 84% of the isotopes). $_{51}Cr$ has a half-life of approximately 28 days. Chromium is a steel-gray lustrous metal. Many of the salts of chromium (ie, chromic acid) are industrial hazards.

PHARMACOLOGY: The recommended daily allowance for chromium in healthy adults is 50 to 200 mcg.[4]

Trivalent chromium plays a role in a cofactor complex for insulin, and is involved in normal glucose utilization.[5] Chromium forms part of the glucose tolerance factor (GTF) which may facilitate binding of insulin to insulin receptors, thereby amplifying its effects on lipid and carbohydrate metabolism.[6]

Chromium deficiency is rare in the general population but may play a role in the development of adult diabetes mellitus and atherosclerosis.[6] Persons who have a high intake of highly refined foods may be at risk for developing chromium deficiency, as are patients receiving total parenteral nutrition. Trace metal solution for intravenous administration are available containing chromium alone or in combination with other metals.[7] These patients may experience peripheral neuropathy or encephalopathy that could be alleviated by administration of chromium. Marginal levels of chromium have been associated with decreased glucose utilization during pregnancy and in the elderly. Administration of chromium has improved glucose tolerance in these patients. It should be noted that supplemental amounts of dietary chromium do not have a hypoglycemic effect in normal individuals.[5] Most absorbed chromium is eliminated through the kidneys (3 to 50 mcg/day).[6,7]

TOXICOLOGY: Acute oral ingestion of chromate salts may lead to irritation of the gastrointestinal tract (nausea, vomiting, ulcers), circulatory shock or hepatitis.[7] Renal damage (including acute tubular necrosis) has been observed following occupational exposure to chromium.[8] Trivalent chromium compounds (the kind found in foods) show little or no toxicity.

Exposure to occupational dust contaminated with hexavalent chromium and CrO_3 or CrF_2 (which are used as corrosion inhibitor pigments, and in metallurgy and electroplating) has been associated with the development of mucous hypersecretion and respiratory (lung) cancers.[9] The incidence of lung cancer is increased up to 15 times normal in workers exposed to chromite, chromic oxide or chromium ores.[10] The hexavalent species of chromium appears to be most highly associated with the development of cancers.[11]

Topical effects following exposure to chromium and chromates may lead to incapacitating eczematous dermatitis and ulceration. Ulceration and perforation of the nasal septum have also occurred.[10] About 1% to 4% of a topically applied dose of hexavalent and trivalent chromium penetrate guinea pig skin in 24 hours. Only 2 mcg of hexavalent chromium are required to induce a topical reaction in sensitive individuals.[12] Chromium may be chelated by the systemic administration of dimercaprol.[10]

SUMMARY: Chromium is a trace element that is required for normal metabolic function. Although dietary requirements may generally be met by a balanced diet, supplements are available. Certain forms of chromium are associated with the development of topical skin irritation and the induction of renal disease and cancers.

PATIENT INFORMATION – Chromium

Uses: Chromium is a necessary nutrient. Deficiencies, though rare, may contribute to adult diabetes and atherosclerosis and may complicate aging and pregnancy.

Side Effects: Ingestion or exposure to certain forms of chromium may cause or contribute to GI irritation and ulcers, cancer, dermatitis, circulatory shock, and hepatitis.

---

[1] Windholz M, ed. *The Merck Index,* 10th ed. Rahway, NJ: Merck & Co., 1983.

[2] Faelten S. *The Complete Book of Minerals for Health.* Emmaus, PA: Rodale Press, Inc., 1981.

[3] Davey RJ. The uses of radiolabeled red cells in trasfusion medicine. *Transfus Med Rev* 1988;2(3):151.

[4] The National Research Council: Recommended Dietary Allowances, 10th ed. Washington, D.C.: National Academy of Sciences, 1989.

[5] *AMA Drug Evaluations Annual 1991.* American Medical Association, 1990.

[6] Dubois F, Belleville F. Chromium: physiologic role and implications in human pathology: *Pathol Biol* (Paris) 1991;39(8):801.

[7] Olin BR, Hebel SK, eds. *Drug Facts and Comparisons.* St. Louis: Facts and Comparisons, 1992.

[8] Wedeen RP, Qian LF. Chromium-induced kidney disease. *Environ Health Perspect* 1991;92:71.

[9] Wilson JD, et al, eds. *Harrison's Principles of Internal Medicine,* 12th ed. New York, NY: McGraw-Hill, 1991.

[10] Meyers FH, et al, eds. *Review of Medical Pharmacology,* 5th ed. Los Altos, CA: Large Medical Publications, 1976.

[11] Lees PS. Chromium and disease: review of epidemiologic studies with particular reference to etiologic information provided by measures of exposure. *Environ Health Perspect* 1991;92:93.

[12] Bagdon RE, Hazen RE. Skin permeation and cutaneous hypersensitivity as a basis for making risk assessments of chromium as a soil contaminant. *Environ Health Perspect* 1991;92:111.

Ciguatera

CIGUATERA POISONING: Vertebrate fish containing toxins capable of causing human illness can be divided into three major groups based on the location of the toxin. Ichthyosarcotoxic fish (hagfish, lamprey, puffer, snapper, barracuda) contain toxin in their musculature, viscera, skin or mucus, and are responsible for most fish poisonings. Ichthyo-ootoxic fish contain toxins in their gonads, and ichthyohemotoxic species contain toxins in their blood. The most frequently implicated ichthyosarcotoxism is ciguatera.[1] Ciguatera poisoning is on the increase because of a recurrence of it in normally edible fish, the sporadic and unpredictable nature of the toxicity and the increased demand for seafood worldwide.[2]

HISTORY: Ciguatera (from "cigua," a poisonous tuban snail of the Spanish Antilles) is primarily a tropical disease but is also seen in the southern coastal United States. It is caused by the ingestion of a wide variety of normally safe, bottom-feeding coral-reef fish that contain toxins accumulated via the marine food chain. Ciguatera outbreaks are usually localized and often follow major disturbances of reefs, as in construction of wharves.[3] Over 400 species of fish and several invertebrates are known to contain ciguatera toxin (ciguatoxin). Ciguatoxic fish are restricted to species feeding on organisms around tropical reefs and include the sturgeon fish, reef sharks, moray eels, parrotfish, jacks, snappers, sea bass and barracuda.[4] The red snapper and barracuda are the most frequently implicated species, although, in Miami, grouper has been implicated in 60% of cases. The sale of barracuda is now prohibited there.[2]

CHEMISTRY: Ciguatera poisoning is caused by ciguatoxin, which fish are believed to acquire through the food chain. Other compounds that may also be involved include maitotoxin, lysophosphatidylcholine, scaritoxin and ciguatoxin-associated ATPase inhibitor.[5] The marine reef dinoflagellate *Gambierdiscus toxicus* (formerly misidentified as *Diplopsalis* spp.) is the most likely source of the toxin.[6] Reef disruptions release unusually large numbers of the organisms into surrounding waters. These organisms are eaten by reef herbivores, which are then eaten by successively larger carnivores, which store the toxin in their organs (muscle, liver, brain, intestines, gonads). For this reason, large fish are more likely to be toxic and have a higher concentration of toxin. In a study of Pacific red snapper, 69% of the fish weighing more than 2.8 kg were toxic, compared with 18% of smaller fish.[7]

Ciguatoxin has been difficult to characterize because it is present only in minute quantities. About 1000 kg of toxic eel liver yields approximately 1 mg of purified toxin. Ciguatoxin is a crystalline, colorless, heat-stable solid with a molecular weight of about 1100 (because it is heat-stable, it cannot be deactivated by freezing or cooking).[2] Only general functional groups (quaternary nitrogen, hydroxyl) have been identified. Certain features of ciguatera are thought to be caused by polycyclic ethers.[5]

PHARMACOLOGY: Ciguatoxin is one of the most potent marine toxins known, with an LD-50 of 0.45 mcg/kg (mouse IP). In an outbreak involving 14 members of an Italian freighter crew who ate portions of a 25–pound barracuda caught near Freeport, Bahamas, the CDC determined from remaining fish parts that the fish had an LD-50 (mouse IP) equivalent to 2 g to 5 g of original fish flesh.[8]

All persons known to have eaten at least one bite of fish associated with a documented outbreak developed symptoms of ciguatera.[9]

The main pharmacologic action of ciguatoxin is an increase in cell permeability to sodium, causing sustained depolarization. This change can be antagonized by large doses of calcium. The toxin has been shown to inhibit red cell cholinesterase in vitro.[10] Its mechanism of action in man is not only dependent on anticholinesterase activity, but also in part to a transmitter-like cholinomimetic action.[11]

Ciguatera poisoning is endemic in islands of the Pacific where a 43% annual incidence was found during one household study.[12] Florida and Hawaii are the states with the highest incidence. In an analysis of 129 cases reported to the Dade County (Miami) Department of Public Health from 1974 to 1976,[9] the estimated incidence of the disease was 5 cases per 10,000 residents. Ciguatera poisoning accounts for more than half of all foodborne outbreaks related to fish in the United States.[13] More than 600 people in the Hawaiian islands have reported contracting ciguatera during the years 1900 to 1980.[14] Although mortality rates as high as 20% have been reported,[15] no deaths occurred in the 184 cases reported to the Centers for Disease Control between 1970 and 1974[16] or among 129 cases reported in Dade County, Florida between 1974 and 1976. Isolated outbreaks in non-endemic areas, such as Maryland, North Carolina and Vermont, have been reported. These are usually attributed to importation of fish, recent travel to endemic areas or by migration of fish from endemic areas.[17]

The symptoms of ciguatera are various and complex, with over 175 manifestations.[5] Diagnosis is based largely on the clinical manifestations. Poisoning is usually characterized by gastrointestinal symptoms (abdominal cramps, nausea, vomiting, diarrhea) appearing within one to 6 hours after ingestion. Numbness of the lips, tongue and throat, paresthesias, blurred vision, hypotension, bradycardia and itching have been reported; reversal of hot and cold sensations (the feeling of heat when in contact with cold, or vice versa) is often diagnostic. Coma is unusual, but has been reported, which suggests possible confounding factors such as co-ingestion of alcohol or non-seafood related toxins, or genetic susceptibility to a more severe response to ciguatera toxin.[17] In severe cases shock, muscular paralysis and death may occur. Recovery is often prolonged. The gastrointestinal symptoms usually subside within 24 hours, but muscular weakness and numbness may persist for weeks to months. Repeated episodes may be more severe.[2]

Several case reports of ciguatera poisoning during pregnancy have been published reporting fetal symptoms beginning simultaneously with the mother's symptoms. These consisted of tumultuous fetal movements and an intermittent, peculiar fetal shivering. None of the liveborn infants appeared to have lasting effects from exposure ot the toxin (one fetus was aborted during the acute phase of the poisoning), although, this could not be ruled out in one infant exposed shortly before birth. Ciguatera is also, apparently, excreted in breast milk, and gastrointestinal problems and pruritic symptoms have been reported in infants whose mothers continue to nurse during their illness. Cessation of breastfeeding appears to resolve the problem.[18]

There is no antidote for ciguatera poisoning, and therapy is symptomatic. Although emesis and gastric lavage have been recommended if vomiting has not occurred,[16] up to 30 hours may have elapsed before the first signs of intoxication appear, and these maneuvers may be fruitless. A cathartic may be used to remove toxin from the lower gastrointestinal tract. Since calcium is a competitive inhibitor of ciguatoxin, infusions of calcium salts have been reported to be beneficial.[19] Other therapeutic agents have included atropine, neostigmine (*Prostigmin*), steroids, *Protopam* (pralidoxime Cl), vitamins B_{12} and C, antihistamines, amitriptyline (eg, *Elavil*), morphine and mannitol (*Osmitrol*).[20,21,22]

Immune sensitization is a major feature of ciguatera and can lead to substantial hypotension; sensitization can make responses to subsequent ingestions more serious. Hypotension can be a particular problem for patients who have been treated with opiates, which are cyclic ether histamine releasers. A "ciguatera diet" has been proposed that is high in protein, carbohydrates and vitamins and allows no fish or fish products, shellfish or shellfish products, seeds, nuts, mayonnaise or alcohol. The diet also specifies avoidance of marijuana, opiates, barbiturates, solvents, herbicides, cosmetics and other substances, as a means of reducing the potential effects of sensitization.[5]

DETECTION: Ciguatoxic fish appear normal in all ways including the smell and taste of the flesh. The detection of ciguatoxic fish has been based largely on unsubstantiated and erroneous rules of thumb such as: A lone fish separated from the rest of the school should not be touched; if ants are repelled by a fish, or a turtle refuses to eat it, it is probably unsafe for humans; if a thin slice of the fish does not show a "rainbow effect" when held up to the sunlight, it is inedible; a silver spoon will tarnish if placed in the cooking pot with a toxic fish.[23] There are no distinguishing routine laboratory features of ciguatera toxin, however, testing of the toxin source is available in some endemic areas. The stick enzyme immunoassay provides promise as a simple widespread test for clinical laboratories and the fishing industry. Other tests include the mouse intraperitoneal injection and radioimmunoassay (RIA) and guinea pig atrium assay.[17,24] RIA has been used to screen amberjack in Hawaii,[25] but this method is time consuming. An electrophoretic technique to evaluate potentially toxic fish has been described but requires further evaluation.[26]

SUMMARY: Although a common source of fish-induced poisoning, ciguatera is little known by the general public and poorly understood by health practitioners. The ingestion of large reef fish, especially snappers, jacks, parrotfish and barracuda, is associated with this illness, and consumption of these fish by natives and tourists in areas of recent reef disturbances should be avoided.

PATIENT INFORMATION – Ciguatera

Uses: None.

Side Effects: Ciguatera is a toxin which sometimes contaminates reef fish. Symptoms may be delayed up to 30 hours. Sensitization can render subsequent ingestion far more dangerous.

---

[1] Halstead BW, Courville DA. *Poisonous and Venomous Marine Animals of the World*, Vol 2. Washington DC: Government Printing Office, 1967.

[2] Haddad LM, Winchester JF, eds. *Clinical Management of Poisoning and Drug Overdose*. Philadelphia, PA: WB Saunders Co., 1983.

[3] Ciguatera (editorial). *Med J Aust* 1977;1:647.

[4] Withers NW. Ciguatera fish poisoning. *Annu Rev Med* 1982;33:97.

[5] Sims JK, A theoretical discourse on the pharmacology of toxic marine ingestions. *Ann Emerg Med* 1987;16:1006.

[6] Johnson R, Jong E. Ciguatera: Caribbean and Indo-Pacific fish poisoning. *Western J Med* 1983;138:872.

[7] Hessel DW, et al. *Ann NY Acad Sci* 1960;90:788.

[8] Ciguatera Fish Poisoning – Bahamas, Miami. *MMWR* 1982;31:391.

[9] Lawrence DN, et al. Ciguatera fish poisoning in Miami. *JAMA* 1980;244:254.

[10] Li KM. Ciguatera fish poison: A cholinesterase inhibitor. *Science* 1965;147:1580.

[11] Rayner MD, et al. Ciguatoxin: More than an anticholinesterase. *Science* 1968;160:70.

[12] Lewis N, Ciguaters, Health and Human Adaptation in the Pacific. PhD Thesis, University of California, Berkeley, 1981.

[13] Engleberg NC, et al. Ciguatera fish poisoning: A major common-source outbreak in the US Virgin Islands. *Ann Intern Med* 1983;98:336.

[14] Helfrich P. *Hawaii Med J* 1964;22:361.

[15] Craig CP. It's always the big ones that should get away (editorial). *JAMA* 1980;244:272.

[16] Hughes JM, Merson MH. Current concepts fish and shellfish poisoning. *NEJM* 1976;295:1117.

[17] DeFusco DJ, et al. Coma due to ciguatera poisoning in Rhode Island. *AM J Med* 1993;95:240.

[18] Briggs GG, Freeman RK, Yaffe SJ. Drugs in Pregnancy and Lactation, 4th ed. Baltimore, MD: Williams & Wilkins, 1994.

[19] Dawson J. *Hawaii Med J* 1977;36:239.

[20] Moon AJ. Ciguatera poisoning. *Practitioner* 1981;225:1176.

[21] Olin BR, Hebel SK, eds. *Drug Facts and Comparisons*. St. Louis, MO: Facts and Comparisons, 1994.

[22] Wilson L. Ciguatera fish poisoning in California. *Medical Sciences Bulletin* 1992;2:5.

[23] Heimbecker RO. Ciguatera poisoning-snowbirds beware (editorial). *Can Med Assoc J* 1979;120:637.

[24] Hokama, et al. *Toxicon* 1977;15:317.

[25] Morris JG Jr. Ciguatera fish poisoning (editorial). *JAMA* 1980;244:273.

[26] Emerson DL, et al. *JAMA* 1983;143:931.

Cinnamon

SCIENTIFIC NAME(S): *Cinnamomum* spp.

COMMON NAME(S): Cinnamon, cinnamomon, ceylon

BOTANY: The plant form of cinnamon consists of short, oval-lanceolate, rough-textured leaves up to 20 cm in length. The food additive form is a brown bark that forms quills and longitudinal striations. Cinnamon bark is also found in ground form as a spice.[1] The plant is native to Sri Lanka, southeastern India, Indonesia, South America and the West Indies.[2]

HISTORY: Cinnamon is primarily used as a spice, taste enhancer or aromatic. Historically, its drop-like oil ("Cinnamon drops") has been used to treat gastrointestinal upset and dysmenorrhea. The essential oil derived from the plant has also been used for its antagonist activities against various microorganisms and fungi.[1]

CHEMISTRY: The primary constituents of the essential oil are 65–80% cinnamaldehyde and lesser percentages of various other phenols and terpenes,[2] including eugenol, *trans*-cinnamic acid, hydroxycinnamaldehyde, o-methoxycinnamaldehyde, cinnamyl alcohol and its acetate, limonene, α-terpineol, tannins, mucilage, oligomeric procyanidins and trace amounts of coumarin.[1]

PHARMACOLOGY: Water and ether extract of *Cinnamomum cassia* have shown antidiarrheic effects in laboratory mice. Choleretic and analgesic effects have been seen in anesthetized laboratory rats. These effects are possibly due to the "warming" and analgesic effects of the stomach and spleen.[3] *Cinnamomum cassia* has also been shown to increase the levels of atrial natriuretic factor (ANF) in the plasma of mice during an experiment studying the action of pharmaceutically (with Wu Lin powder, WLP) increased urination.[4]

The essential oils of cinnamon were shown to halt mycelial growth and aflatoxin synthesis in Aspergillus parasiticus at a concentration of only 0.1%. The essential oils also displayed high activity against aflatoxino-genesis.[5]

TOXICOLOGY: Human consumption of large quantities of cinnamon bark or moderate quantities of cinnamon oil has been shown to increase heart rate, intestinal movement, breathing and perspiration via a chemical stimulation of the vasomotor center. This state of accelerated body function is followed by a period of centralized sedation which includes sleepiness or depression.[1]

Skin irritation and pruritus have been found after repeated contact with cinnamon powder. (Most of these outbreaks being observed at spice factoreis where contact is exceptionally high.)[6] Further skin cell irritation has been observed in oral leukoplakic lesions caused by allergic reactions to the cinnamon component of chewing gum.[7]

SUMMARY: Cinnamon has been in use for centuries, with references in ancient Greek and Latin writings, both as a spice and as a "folk medicine" for gastrointestinal disorders. The essential oil has displayed antidiarrheic, analgesic and germicidal properties. High contact with cinnamon powder has caused dermatitis.

PATIENT INFORMATION – Cinnamon

Uses: Cinnamon is used as a spice and aromatic. The bark or oil has been used to combat microorganisms, diarrhea and other GI disorders, dysmennorhea, etc.

Side Effects: Heavy exposure may cause skin irritation and allergic reactions. Ingestion of larger than usual amounts may accelerate and then depress body function.

---

[1] Bisset NG, ed. *Herbal Drugs and Phytopharmaceuticals*. Stuttgart: Medpharm Scientific Publishers, 1994.
[2] Evans WC. *Pharmacognosy*, ed. 13. London: Bailliere Tindall, 1989.
[3] Zhu ZP, et al. [Pharmacological study on spleen-stomach warming and analgesic action of Cinnamomum cassia Presl.] [Chinese] *Chung-Kuo Chung Yao Tsa Chih – China J Chinese Materia Medica* 1993;18(9):553.
[4] Zhou L, et al. [Effect of wu lin powder and its ingredients on atrial natriuretic factor level in mice.] [Chinese] *Chung-Kuo Chung Hsi i Chieh Ho Tsa Chih* 1995;15(1):36.

Citronella Oil

SCIENTIFIC NAME(S): *Cymbopogon nardus* (L.) Rendle and *C. winterianus* Jowitt. Sometimes referred to as *Andropogon nardus* L. Family: Gramineae

COMMON NAME(S): Citronella oil, Ceylon oil, citronella

BOTANY: *C. nardus* (Ceylon citronella) and *C. winterianus* (Java citronella) are both perennial grasses. The essential oils are obtained by steam distillation of the fresh or dried grass. The Java-type oil is generally considered to be of superior quality to the Ceylon oil.[1]

HISTORY: Citronella oil has been used as a flavoring for foods and beverages in very low quantities (approximately 45 ppm).[1] In traditional medicine, the oil has been used as an aromatic tea, as a vermifuge, diuretic and antispasmodic.[1] Perhaps the most widely recognized use for the oil is as an insect repellent. It is sometimes incorporated into perfumes and soaps.[2]

CHEMISTRY: Citronella oil contains a number of fragrant fractions of which citronellal, geraniol and citronellol are the major components.[1,3] The Java-type citronella oil appears to have a higher concentration of these compounds (about 35% citronellol, 21% geraniol) than does the Ceylon type (about 10% citronellol, 18% geraniol).[4] In addition, the oil contains esters, sesquiterpene hydrocarbons, alcohols and phenols.

PHARMACOLOGY: Citronella oil has been found to have in vitro antibacterial activity equivalent to that of penicillin, particularly against gram-positive organisms.[1]

TOXICOLOGY: Animal toxicity studies have shown that citronella oil has an LD_{50} in mice of 4600 mg/kg and in rats of 7200 mg/kg. A dose of 1 to 4 ml/kg given by stomach tube in rabbits caused paralysis, coma and death. At least one case of death has been reported in a child who ingested an unknown quantity of citronella oil. A review of five cases of childhood citronella oil poisoning suggests that dilution of the oil following ingestion may be sufficient to treat most cases of ingestion, and that emesis may be induced with a relatively low risk of major pulmonary complications. If spontaneous vomiting has occurred, observation for respiratory symptoms is required.[4]

Citronella oil has been reported to cause contact dermatitis in humans.[1]

SUMMARY: Citronella oil is commonly used as an insect repellent and has also found use in foods, cosmetics and toiletries. As with any volatile oil, ingestion of the product poses a toxicologic problem, which in rare cases may lead to severe toxicity and death.

PATIENT INFORMATION – Citronella Oil

Uses: Citronella oil is used in small amounts to flavor foods, scent cosmetics and repel insects. It has been used in aromatic tea as a vermifuge, diuretic and antispasmodic.

Side Effects: Citronella oil may cause contact dermatitis. Ingestion may be fatal in some cases.

---

[1] Leung AY. *Encyclopedia of Common Natural Ingredients Used in Food, Drugs, and Cosmetics.* New York, NY: J Wiley and Sons, 1980.
[2] Evans WC. *Trease and Evans' Pharmacognosy*, 13th ed. Bailliere Tindall, 1989.
[3] Windholz M, ed. *Merck Index*, 10th ed. Rahway, NJ: Merck and Co., Inc., 1983.
[4] Temple WA, et al. Management of oil of citronella poisoning. *Clin Toxicol* 1991;29(2):257.

Clematis

SCIENTIFIC NAME(S): *Clematis virginiana* L. Family: Ranunculaceae

COMMON NAME(S): Clematis, devil's-darning-needle, old-man's beard, traveler's-joy, vine bower, virgin's bower, woodbine

BOTANY: Clematis is a genus of mostly climbing perennial shrubs in the buttercup family and has over 200 species worldwide, mainly in North America and Asia. Several species are cultivated in North America for their beautiful flowers. The common species include: Woodbine (*C. virginiana*), virgin's bower (*C. cirrhosa*), old-man's beard (*C. vitalba*) and vine bower (*C. viticella*).

C. virginiana is a trailing vine which can grow up to 50 feet higher than other botanicals, often resulting in a bower or shaded shelter. The long, feathery, beard-like tail on the fruit led to the synonym, old-man's beard. This species is a North American native plant which was once in the continental pharmacopeia as a medicine.

Its habitat is in thickets, roadsides, woods and stream banks. It may be found from Manitoba to Quebec, as far south as Alabama and Louisiana, and west all the way to Kansas. The vine has leaves which are divided into three oval and toothed leaflets, each of which are on a long stalk. These stalks are like tendrils which aid in its climbing habit. From July to September, it displays creamy white flowers which bloom into large clusters; these become fruit heads with long plume-like tails.[1,2]

Other related species in the genus include: *C. dioica* from tropical America,[3] *C. recta* (*C. erecta*) of Southern Europe,[4] *C. vitalba* of Eurasian and North African origin,[4] *C. chinensis* (Wei Ling Xian) of Chinese origin[5] and *C. thunbergii* from Senegal.[3]

HISTORY: The popular use of *C. virginiana* in pioneer medicine was probably learned from the Native Americans. It was a common remedy for skin disorders (sores, cuts), itching and venereal eruptions.[1] Throughout history, the leaf of the plant was used in folk remedies for treating cancers and tumors, as well as for itching, fever, renosis, nephrosis, ulcers and scrofula.[2] Past uses also report diuretic, poisonous, rubefacient, sudorific, purgative and vesicant properties. Clematis has long been cultivated as a woody climbing or trailing vine for growing over a fence or wherever dense foliage is desired. Others have mentioned using the fuzzy seed mass for smoking and utilizing the young shoots of a Eurasian variety (*C. taurica*) in cooking.

CHEMISTRY: Early literature reports extraction of alkaloidal, glycosidal and saponic fractions from certain species.[6] Members of Ranunculaceae contain protoanemonin, an irritant compound found mostly in the fresh leaves and sap; this is derived from a precursor glycoside known as ranunculin.[7] Some report the same principles for *C. vialba*, as well as: Anemonin; caulosaponin; caulosapogenin; stigmasterol glycoside; ceryl alcohol; myricylalcohol; beta-siterosterol; trimethylamine; beheinc-, caffeic-, choregenic- and melissic-acid; n-triacontane; n-nonacosane; ginnone; ginnol; and campesterol.[2] The dried seeds contain about 15% protein and 14% fat.

More recent reports identified anemonin (the dilactone of cyclobutane-1,2–diol-1,2 diacrylic acid derived from the cyclodimerization of protoanemonin) in *C. hirsutissima*,[8] a new oleanic saponin named clemontanoside B from *C. montana* leaves,[9] two saponins named hushangoside and hederagenin glycoside from the stems of *C. montana*,[10] other saponins from *Clematis* species,[11] clemontanoside F from the roots of *C. montana*,[12] and two triterpenoid saponins named clematichineno-side A and B from the roots of *C. chinensis*.[13] The major components of the essential oil of *C. hexapetala* are palmitic acid and 3–hydroxy-4–methoxyl benzaldehyde.[14]

PHARMACOLOGY: Modern herbalists cite the older uses of *C. virginiana* as a treatment for **skin disorders**, but caution that the juice is a powerful irritant.[1] Generally, all of the historic uses stated above have not been verified in modern studies. Among the more recent verified pharmacological effects are: the **CNS stimulant** properties of anemonin in horses;[8] the CNS activity of clemontanoside B from *C. montana* in mice;[9] the **androgenic effects** (in mice) of *C. fusca* Turcz. preparations;[15] **the anti-inflammatory activity** of the Chinese medicine "Wei Ling Xian" (*C. chinensis* and related species);[16] and the **cardiovascular and hypotensive action**,[17] the **hepatic protective**[18] and the biliary tract effects of *C. chinensis*.[19]

TOXICOLOGY: A recent poisonous plant reference focused on those buttercup species which contained protoanemonin in the fresh leaves and sap (including Clematis). When the plants were handled or eaten, protoanemonin irritated and blistered the skin. Intense inflammation and burning around the mouth and digestive tract followed oral ingestion. Other side effects associated with oral intake included: Profuse salivation, blistering, inflamed eyes, abdominal cramping, vomiting of blood, weakness and bloody diarrhea.[7] Kidneys may also be irritated, resulting in painful and excessive urination and bloody urine, ultimately leading to diminished urinary output. Poisoning symptoms also include: Dizziness, confusion, possible fainting and convulsions.

Fatalities are not common, probably due to the rapid and intense acrid taste and irritation resulting from oral contact. If a large amount has been ingested accidentally, gastric lavage is recommended, followed by demulcents to soothe irritated membranes. Fortunately, the protoanemonin is present mainly in fresh plant material and cooking or drying should result in its decomposition.

SUMMARY: While there is considerable older literature on the use of Clematis for a wide variety of skin and other disorders, the human and animal toxicological experiences preclude recommending it for any of these purposes. Recent Asian studies hint at the presence of numerous active principles possessing CNS activity, anti-inflammatory effects, cardiovascular and hypotensive properties; however, none of these have been developed to the point where they have proven clinical value. Currently, the Chinese are clinically evaluating *Clematis chinensis* as one of their traditional medicines.

PATIENT INFORMATION – Clematis

Uses: Primarily used for skin disorders. In animals, it has caused CNS stimulant, androgenic, anti-inflammatory, cardiovascular, hypotensive and hepatic effects.

Side Effects: *Topical*: Can cause skin irritation. *Oral*: Notify physician if painful or bloody urine occurs. Profuse salivation, blistering, inflamed eyes, abdominal cramping, vomiting of blood, weakness, bloody diarrhea, and painful, excessive or bloody urine.

---

[1] Dobelis IN, ed. *The Magic and Medicine of Plants*. Pleasantville, NY: Reader's Digest Assoc., 1986.

[2] Duke JA. *Handbook of Medicinal Herbs*. Boca Raton, FL: CRC Press, Inc., 1985.

[3] Lewis WH, et al. *Medical Botany - Plants Affecting Man's Health*. New York: Wiley and Sons, 1977.

[4] Delaveau P. *Secrets et vertus des plantes médicinales*, 2nd ed. Paris: Reader's Digest, 1985.

[5] Ody P. *The Complete Medicinal Herbal*. New York: Dorling Kindersley, 1993.

[6] Kingsbury J. *Poisonous Plants of the United States and Canada*. Englewood Cliffs, NJ: Prentice-Hall, 1964.

[7] Turner NJ, et al. *Common Poisonous Plants and Mushrooms of North America*. Portland: Timber Press, 1991.

[8] Kern JR, et al. *J Ethnopharm* 1983:8:121.

[9] Jangwan JS, et al. *Int J Crude Drug Res* 1990;28:39.

[10] Bahuguna RP, et al. *Int J Crude Drug Res* 1990;28:125.

[11] Fujita M, et al. *Yagugaku Zasshi-J Pharma Soc Japan* 1974;94(2):194.

[12] Thapliyal RP, et al. *Phytochem* 1993;34(3):861.

[13] Shao B, et al. *Phytochem* 1995;38(6):1473.

[14] Jiang B, et al. *Chin J Materia Med* 1990;15(8):488.

[15] Moiseeva RK. *Buill Eksp Biol Med* 1975;80(7):60.

[16] Wei MJ, et al. *Acta Pharma Sinica* 1991;26(10):772.

[17] Ho CS, et al. *Am J Chin Med* 1989;17(3–4):189.

[18] Chin HF, et al. *Am J Chin Med* 1988;16(3–4):127.

[19] Geng BQ, et al. *Chung Yao Tung Pao Bull Chin Materia Med* 1985;10 (9):37.

Clove

SCIENTIFIC NAME(S): *Eugenia caryophyllata* Thunb. also described as *Caryophyllus aromaticus* L. and *Syzygium aromaticum* L. Merr. and Perry. Family: Myrtaceae

COMMON NAME(S): Clove, caryophyllus

BOTANY: The clove plant grows in warm climates and is cultivated commercially in Tanzania, Sumatra, the Molucca Islands and South America. The plant, a tall evergreen, grows up to 20 meters tall and has leathery leaves. The clove spice is the dried flower bud. Essential oils are obtained from the buds, stems and leaves. The dark brown buds are 12 to 22 mm in length with four projecting calyx lobes. The four petals above the lobes fold over to form a hood, which hides numerous stamens. The cloves are strongly aromatic.[1]

HISTORY: Cloves have a long history of culinary and medicinal use. The oil was used as an expectorant and antiemetic with inconsistent clinical results. Clove tea was used to relieve nausea. The use of the oil in dentistry as an analgesic and local antiseptic continues today. The oil has been used topically as a counterirritant.

CHEMISTRY: Clove buds yield approximately 15% to 20% of a volatile oil that is responsible for the characteristic smell and flavor. The stems yield about 5% of the oil and the leaves about 2%. In addition, the bud contains a tannin complex, a gum and resin and a number of glucosides of sterols. The principal constituent of distilled clove bud oil (60% to 90%) is eugenol (4–allyl-2–methoxyphenol). The oil also contains about 10% acetyleugenol and small quantities of gallic acid,[2] sesquiterpenes,[3] furfural, vanillin and methyl-n-amyl ketone.[4] Other constituents include flavonoids,[1] carbohydrates, lipids, oleanolic acid, rhamnetin and vitamins.[5]

PHARMACOLOGY: Clove oil has **antihistaminic** and **spasmolytic** properties, most likely because of the presence of eugenyl acetate.[6] Cloves have a positive effect on healing stomach ulcers.[1] A 15% tincture of cloves has been shown to be effective in treating topical ringworm infections. As with many other volatile oils, clove oil has been found to inhibit gram-positive and gram-negative bacteria. Its **fungistatic** action has been documented, suggesting use as an antidermatophytic drug.[7] Clove oil also has **anthelmintic** and **larvicidal** properties. Another report suggests clove oil suppresses aflatoxin production.[8] Sesquiterpenes from cloves show potential as anticarcinogenic agents.[9] Similarly, eugenol present in clove oil may ameliorate effects of environmental food mutagens.[10] Whole cloves were chemoprotective against liver and bone marrow toxicity in mice.[11] Eugenol in high concentrations can inhibit reactive oxygen species generated by macrophages during inflammation.[12] Eugenol has also been found to possess marked antipyretic activity in animals, similar to the activity of acetaminophen.[13]

Aqueous extracts of clove increase trypsin activity. Eugenol inhibits prostaglandin biosynthesis, the formation of thromboxane B2, and arachidonic acid-induced platelet aggregation in vitro. This effect has been postulated to contribute to the antidiarrheal effect of other oils that contain eugenol (such as nutmeg oil).[14] Other reports also confirm inhibition of platelet aggregation and antithrombotic activity of clove oil.[15,16]

Clove oil is applied for the symptomatic treatment of toothaches and is used for the treatment of dry socket (post-extraction alveolitis). Recent studies indicate that newer techniques, such as the application of collagen paste, may be more effective than clove oil/zinc oxide preparations in the management of alveolitis.[17]

TOXICOLOGY: Cloves and clove oils are used safely in foods, beverages and toothpastes. In general, the level of clove used in foods does not exceed 0.236%; the oil is not used in amounts greater than 0.06%. Toxicity has been observed following ingestion of the oil, but this type of poisoning is rare and poorly documented. In rats, the oral LD-50 of eugenol is 2680 mg/kg; however, the toxicity of the compound increases almost 200–fold when administered by the intratracheal route (LD-50 11 mg/kg).[18] This increase in toxicity by the pulmonary route has become more important in light of the toxicity reported among persons who have smoked clove cigarettes. Clove cigarettes, called "kreteks," generally contain about 60% tobacco and 40% ground cloves. More than a dozen brands of kreteks exist, and they enjoy some popularity in Asian countries. This popularity is growing in the US and Europe.

More than a dozen cases of pulmonary toxicity have been reported in people who have smoked clove cigarettes.[19,20] There is evidence that clove cigarettes may anesthetize the throat, leading to deeper and more prolonged inhalation of the smoke. Blood-tinged sputum and hemoptysis have been noted in smokers and may be related to eugenol's antiplatelet effects.[14] The American Lung Association has issued a warning against clove cigarette use, noting that they can have a higher tar content than ordinary cigarettes. One study, however, found no carcinogenic effect of hot aqueous clove extracts in the *Drosophila* mutagenicity assay, although metabolites and pyrolysis products of eugenol are carcinogenic.[21]

Clove oil can be a skin and mucous membrane irritant and sensitizer.[5] A case of a 24–year-old woman reports permanent local anesthesia and anhidrosis following clove oil spillage into the facial area.[22] Other case reports exist, including treatment of a 2–year-old child suffering from disseminated intravascular coagulation and liver failure following clove oil ingestion,[23] and development of depression and electrolyte imbalance in a 7–month-old child after accidental oral ingestion of clove oil.[24]

There has been no documentation of toxicity in the bud, leaf or stem of the plant.[5]

SUMMARY: Cloves are used as a common condiment and have found favor in most regional cuisines. Clove extracts and oil have been used medicinally for their antiseptic and analgesic effects. Cloves have also been studied for use in platelet aggregation inhibition, antithrombotic activity and chemoprotective and antipyretic effects. Toxicity from clove oil can occur by inhalation of smoke from clove cigarettes or by ingestion of large amounts of the oil.

PATIENT INFORMATION – Clove

Uses: Cloves have been used for their antiseptic and analgesic effects and have been studied for use in platelet aggregation inhibition, antithrombotic activity and chemoprotective and antipyretic effects.

Side Effects: Blood-tinged sputum and hemoptysis have been noted in clove cigarette smokers. Clove oil can irritate skin and mucous membranes.

---

[1] Bisset N. *Herbal Drugs and Phytopharmaceuticals.* Stuttgart, Germany: CRC Press, 1994;130–31.
[2] Kramer RE. *J Am Oil Chem Soc* 1985;62:111.
[3] Narayanan CS, et al. *Indian Perfum* 1985;29:15.
[4] Windholz M, et al, eds. *The Merck Index*, 10th ed. Rahway: Merck and Co., 1983.
[5] Newall C, et al. *Herbal Medicines.* London: The Pharmaceutical Press, 1996;79.
[6] Leung AY. *Encyclopedia of Common Natural Ingredients Used in Food, Drugs and Cosmetics.* NY: John Wiley and Sons, 1980.
[7] El-Naghy M, et al. *Zentralb Mikrobiol* 1992;147(3–4):214–20.
[8] Hasan H, et al. *Zentralb Mikrobiol* 1993;148(8):543–48.
[9] Zheng G, et al. *J Nat Prod* 1992;55(7):999–1003.
[10] Soudamini K, et al. *Indian J Physiol Pharmacol* 1995;39(4):347–53.
[11] Kumari M. *Cancer Lett* 1991;60(1):67–73.
[12] Joe B, et al. *Biochim Biophys Acta* 1994;1224(2):255–63.
[13] Feng J, et al. *Neuropharmacology* 1987;26(12):1775–78.
[14] Rasheed A, et al. *NEJM* 1984;310:50.
[15] Srivastava K. *Prostaglandins Leukot Essent Fatty Acids* 1993;48(5):363–72.
[16] Saeed S, et al. *J Pakistan Med Assoc* 1994;44(5):112–15.
[17] Mitchell R. *Int J Oral Maxillofac Surg* 1986;15:127.
[18] LaVoie EJ, et al. *Arch Toxicol* 1986;59:78.
[19] *MMWR* 1985;34:297.
[20] Hackett PH, et al. *JAMA* 1985;253:3551.
[21] Abraham SK, et al. *Ind J Exp Biol* 1978;16:518.
[22] Isaacs G. *Lancet* 1983 Apr 16;1(Apr. 16):882.
[23] Brown S, et al. *Blood Coagulation and Fibrinolysis* 1992;3(5):665-68.
[24] Lane B, et al. *Hum Exp Toxicol* 1991;10(4):291–94.

Cocoa

SCIENTIFIC NAME(S): *Theobroma cacao* L. subspecies *cacao*. Family: Sterculiaceaea or Byttneriaceae

COMMON NAME(S): Theobroma, cacao. Compounds derived from this product include cocoa, chocolate and cocoa butter.

BOTANY: The cocoa tree grows to heights exceeding 25 feet. The fruits are berry-like and are borne on branches with the seeds imbedded in a sticky pulp. The seeds, referred to as cocoa beans, are used in commerce. Cacao is often used to describe the crude material, while cocoa is used to describe the processed products. Although several varieties of cacao exist, the forastero variety from West Africa accounts for more than 90% of world production.[1]

HISTORY: Cortez described the use of a beverage called chocalatl, based on the seeds of *T. cacao*, among the members of the Aztec court. The words "theo broma" are Greek for "food of the Gods." The three main commercial products obtained from cacao seeds are cocoa powder, cocoa butter and cocoa extracts. Following curing and fermentation, the beans are dried and roasted to yield the desired flavor, color and aroma.

CHEMISTRY: The nib, which contains about 55% cocoa butter, is ground to a liquid mass called chocolate liquor, from which the butter is removed by hydraulic pressing. The remaining cocoa cake is dried and ground to a fine powder to yield cocoa powder with a fat content of 22% or more. Specially treated cocoa powder, called alkalinized cocoa, is considered to have improved color, flavor and dispersability over unalkalinized powder. Cocoa butter (also known as theobroma oil) may have a faint chocolate odor, which may be removed following further purification. Cocoa contains more than 300 volatile compounds. The important flavor components are aliphatic esters, polyphenols, aromatic carbonyls and theobromine.[1]

Cocoa contains the alkaloids theobromine (0.5% to 2.7%), caffeine (about 0.25% in cocoa), trigonelline and others.[1,2] The characteristic bitter taste of cocoa is due to the reaction of diketopiperazines with theobromine during roasting. Theobromine is produced commercially from cocoa husks.[1]

Cocoa butter contains triglycerides consisting mainly of oleic, stearic and palmitic acids. About three-quarters of the fats are present as monounsaturates.[1]

PHARMACOLOGY: Theobromine, the primary alkaloid in cocoa, has activity similar to that of caffeine. It is a weak CNS stimulant, but is a more potent diuretic, cardiac stimulant and coronary dilator than caffeine.[1,3]

The ingestion of high levels of theobromine in the form of dark chocolate for a one-week period did not alter the pharmacokinetics of theobromine administered concomitantly in healthy individuals.[4]

Cocoa products find extensive use in the food and pharmaceutical industries. Cocoa power and syrup are used as flavorings, while cocoa butter is used widely as a suppository and ointment base, as an emollient and as an ingredient in various topical cosmetic preparations.[5]

Cocoa powder and butter are important components of chocolate, where they are mixed with chocolate liquor (ground cacao nibs) sugar, milk and other flavors.

Cocoa butter has been reported to be a source of natural antioxidants.[1]

TOXICOLOGY: Although cacao is not considered to be toxic in typical confectionery doses, at least one report of animal toxicity has been published. A dog that had eaten 2 pounds of chocolate chips suffered hyperexcitability, convulsions and collapsed and died, most likely due to acute circulatory failure secondary to theobromine/caffeine toxicity.[6] Cocoa butter may be allergenic and have comedogenic properties in animals. The plant has been reported to contain small amounts of safrole, a carcinogen banned by the FDA.[7]

Chocolate and cocoa-containing products should be omitted from the diets of people with conditions such as irritable bowel syndrome.[8]

SUMMARY: Products derived from *T. cacao* are used in a variety of food and cosmetic applications including flavorings and pharmaceutical bases. Although toxicity has been reported, probably from the theobromine and caffeine components, it is generally nontoxic.

PATIENT INFORMATION – Cocoa

Uses: Cocoa products are used in foods and cosmetics. The primary alkaloid is a diuretic, cardiac stimulant and coronary dilator.

Side Effects: Those with irritable bowel syndrome should omit cocoa products from their diet. Cocoa butter may be topically allergenic and comedogenic. Large amounts of cocoa products may be fatal to pets.

---

[1] Leung AY. *Encyclopedia of Common Natural Ingredients Used in Food, Drugs and Cosmetics*. New York, NY: J. Wiley and Sons, 1980.

[2] Tyler VE. *The New Honest Herbal*. Philadelphia, PA: G.F. Stickley Co., 1987.

[3] Evans WC. *Trease and Evans' Pharmacognosy*, 13th ed. London, England: Bailliere Tindall, 1989.

[4] Shively CA, et al. High levels of methylxanthines in chocolate do not alter theobromine disposition. *Clin Pharmacol Ther* 1985;37(4):415.

[5] Morton JF. *Major Medicinal Plants*. Springfield, IL: CC Thomas, 1977.

[6] *Medical Sciences Bulletin* 1985;7(11):4.

[7] Duke JA. *Handbook of Medicinal Herbs*. Boca Raton, FL: CRC Press, 1985.

[8] Friedman G. Diet and the irritable bowel syndrome. *Gastroenterol Clin North Am* 1991;20(2):313.

Coltsfoot

SCIENTIFIC NAME(S): *Tussilago farfara* (L. Family: Compositae)

COMMON NAME(S): Coltsfoot, coughwort, feuilles de tussilage (Fr.), horse-hoof, huflattichblätter (Ger.), kuandong hua

BOTANY: Coltsfoot is a low-growing perennial (up to 30 cm high) with fleshy, woolly leaves. In early spring, the plant produces a stem with a single golden-yellow, narrow, ligulate flower head that blooms from April to June. As the stem dies, the hoof-shaped leaves appear. The plant is native to Europe, but also grows widely in sandy places throughout the United States and Canada.[1] Coltsfoot is collected widely from wild plants in the Balkans, Eastern Europe (Bulgaria, Czechoslovakia, Hungary, Poland, the former Yugoslavia), and Italy.[2] It has also been a part of Chinese folk medicine for centuries. The morphology and anatomy of coltsfoot have been described in detail, including the plant's underground parts.[3] A later report on leaf differentiation is also available.[4]

HISTORY: As part of its Latin name *Tussilago* implies, coltsfoot is reputed as an antitussive.[5] The buds, flowers, and leaves of coltsfoot have long been used in traditional medicine for dry cough and throat irritation. The plant has found particular use in Chinese herbal medicine for the treatment of respiratory diseases, including cough, asthma, and acute and chronic bronchitis. It is also a component of numerous European commercial herbal preparations for the treatment of respiratory disorders. A mixture containing coltsfoot has been smoked for the management of coughs and wheezes, but the smoke is potentially irritating. Its silky seeds were once used as a stuffing for mattresses and pillows.[6] Extracts of coltsfoot had once been used as flavorings for candies. All early references emphasize the usefulness of coltsfoot's mucilage for soothing throat and mouth irritation.[2]

CHEMISTRY: Coltsfoot contains a number of diverse components including tannins, a mucilage, terpene alcohols, carotenoids, and flavonoids.[7] The mucilage is present in a concentration of about 8%. It yields sugars following hydrolysis including arabinose, fructose, galactose, glucose, and others.[3] Water-soluble polysaccharides from coltsfoot leaves have been reported.[9,10] Mucilaginous polysacchrides have been investigated in another report.[11] Tussilagone, a sesquiterpene, has been isolated from ether extracts of the plant. It is a potent cardiovascular and respiratory stimulant.[12]

Acids found in coltsfoot include caffeic, caffeoyltartaric, ferulic, gallic, p-hydroxybenzoic, tannic, malic, and tartaric.[8]

Farfaratin, a novel sesquiterpenoid compound, has been isolated from flower buds collected from the Shaanxi Province in China.[13] At least 7 pyrrolizidine alkaloids,[14] including tussilagin,[15] senkirkine,[16] and senecionine[6] have been identified in coltsfoot. Coltsfoot leaves contain 2.8 to 4.1 ppm and the flowers 2.4 ppm senkirkine.[17] Quantitative gas chromatographical analyses of pyrrolizidine alkaloids have been performed for various commercial coltsfoot preparations.[18]

Other constituents in coltsfoot include choline, paraffin, phytosterols, amyrin, and volatile oil.[6,8] A recent report reviews chemistry and other aspects of the plant.[19]

PHARMACOLOGY: Coltsfoot preparations have long been used to soothe sore throats. The mucilage is most likely responsible for the demulcent effect of the plant. The mucilage is destroyed by burning; smoking the plant or inhaling vapors of the leaves steeped in water would not be expected to provide any degree of symptomatic relief. Instead, the smoke may exacerbate existing respiratory conditions. However, one source mentions coltsfoot in the form of a medicinal cigarette to help relieve asthma.[20] Coltsfoot components have been found to increase the cilia activity in the frog esophagus, and this action may contribute to the plant's expectorant effect.[21] Related conditions for which coltsfoot has been used include bronchitis, laryngitis, pertussis, influenza, and lung congestion.[5,6,8] It is one of the most popular European remedies to treat chest ailments.[20] Coltsfoot, in a mixture of Chinese herbs, has been evaluated in 66 cases of convalescent asthmatics and found useful in decreasing airway obstruction.[22]

Coltsfoot polysaccharides and flavonoids have anti-inflammatory actions.[20] This effect was similar to that of indomethacin in one report.[23] Weak anti-inflammatory actions have also been observed when tested against induced rat paw edema.[8]

A compound designated L-652,469, was isolated from coltsfoot buds. This compound has been found to be a platelet-activating factor (PAF) inhibitor and a calcium channel blocker. PAF is known to be an integral component of the complex cascade mechanism involved in both acute and chronic asthma, and a number of naturally occurring PAF antagonists are being clinically evaluated for the treatment of this and other inflammatory diseases. The isolation of PAF antagonists from coltsfoot indicates that the traditional uses of the plant in the management of certain inflammatory respiratory diseases may be verifiable.[24]

L-652,469 is also a competitive inhibitor of the calcium channel in the rat aorta, but the clinical importance of this finding has not been explored.

Tussilagone is a potent cardiovascular stimulant. When administered intravenously (0.02 to 0.3 mg/kg), it produced a rapid and dose-dependent pressor effect in dogs. This increase in blood pressure was similar to that observed following the administration of the cardiac stimulant dopamine. The increase in blood pressure was short-lived, lasting about 5 minutes. Tussilagone also increased the rate of respiration. The cardiovascular effects appear to be peripherally mediated, while the site of respiratory stimulation is central.[12]

Aqueous leaf extracts and phenolic components have been found to have in vitro antibacterial activity generally limited to gram-negative bacteria.[25] Some of these organisms include *Staphylococcus aureus*, *Bordetella pertussis*, *Pseudomonas aeruginosa*, and *Proteus vulgaris*.[8]

A report discusses coltsfoot's historical, traditional, and modern medical uses, along with the plant's pharmacology and toxicity.[26]

TOXICOLOGY: The use of teas prepared from coltsfoot has not generally been associated with acute toxicity. Several members of this family of plants (eg, chamomile, ragweed) cause common allergies, and some people may exhibit a cross-sensitivity to coltsfoot.[27] While coltsfoot is only a weak topical sensitizer in guinea pigs, other members of the family are strong sensitizers (blessed thistle, dwarf sunflower), and cross-sensitivity may exist.[28]

Several reports have noted the presence of hepatotoxic pyrrolizidine alkaloids in coltsfoot. Pre-blooming flowers have been reported to contain the highest concentration of these alkaloids, although considerable loss of both senkirkine and senecionine occurs upon prolonged storage of the plant.[8] In one long-term safety study, the alkaloid senkirkine (0.015% by weight in dried flowers) was incorporated into rat diets in concentrations of up to 8% of the diet for 2 years. Among the rats fed the 8% meal, two-thirds developed cancerous tumors of the liver characteristic of pyrrolizidine toxicity.[15] This alkaloid is also present in the leaves.[29] The acute intravenous LD-50 of tussilagone is 28.9 mg/kg.[12] These pyrrolizidine alkaloids have well documented toxicities in humans as well, presenting as anorexia, lethargy, abdominal pain and swelling, and liver changes. The alkaloids destroy the liver's hepatocytes and damage small branches of the hepatic vein. In Germany, consumption of > 1 mg of pyrrolizidine alkaloids per day is prohibited.[30]

Of interest is a case of reversible hepatic veno-occlusive disease in an infant after consumption of coltsfoot, later found to be *Adenostyles alliariae* (these two plants can be easily confused, especially after the time of flowering.) Seneciphylline and related hepatotoxins were identified via thin-layer chromatography, mass spectrometry, and NMR spectroscopy.[31]

Coltsfoot has been classified by the FDA as an herb of "undefined safety." [32] However, although the pyrrolizidine alkaloids of coltsfoot are hepatotoxic, mutagenic, and carcinogenic, there is little danger of acute poisoning when it is used as prescribed (as an occasional tea or cough preparation).[2] The German Commission E Monographs recommend a limit of 10 micrograms per day of pyrrolizidine alkaloids with the 1,2–unsaturated necine structure, including their N-oxides.[33]

Excessive consumption of coltsfoot may interfere with preexisting antihypertensive or cardiovascular therapy. Prolonged ingestion of the plant should be avoided. Duration of administration should not exceed 4 to 6 weeks per year.[33] Because the plant may be an abortifacient, it should not be taken during pregnancy or lactation.[8] The flowers of coltsfoot should not be used. The plant is subject to legal restrictions in some countries.[20]

SUMMARY: Coltsfoot has been used for centuries in the treatment of respiratory diseases. The plant contains a mucilage, which may provide some therapeutic effect in relieving sore throats, asthma and related conditions. It also has some anti-inflammatory and antibacterial activities. A PAF antagonist and cardiac and respiratory stimulant have been identified in the plant. The use of coltsfoot is not generally associated with acute toxicity, but users should be warned that the plant has the potential to cause allergic reactions, to increase blood pressure, and to pose a risk of carcinogenicity if used chronically. Its pyrrolizidine alkaloids are known hepatotoxins. Prolonged use of the plant should be avoided.

PATIENT INFORMATION – Coltsfoot

Uses: Coltsfoot has been used to treat sore throats, asthma, and some related conditions such as bronchitis, laryngitis, pertussis, influenza, and lung congestion.

Side Effects: Allergic reactions may occur. Coltsfoot has an "undefined safety" classification by the FDA. Avoid prolonged use of the plant; it may increase blood pressure and pose a risk of carcinogenicity, hepatotoxicity, or mutagenicity.

---

[1] Tyler, VE. *The New Honest Herbal.* Philadelphia: GF Stickley Co., 1987.

[2] Bisset NG. *Herbal Drugs and Phytopharmaceuticals.* Stuttgart: Medpharm Scientific Publishers, 1994.

[3] Engalycheva E, et al. *Farmatsiia* 1981;30(3):21-26.

[4] Saukel J. *Scientia Pharmaceutica* 1991(Dec 31);59:307-19.

[5] Bruneton J. *Pharmacognosy, Phytochemistry, Medicinal Plants, Technique and Documentation.* Paris, France, 1995.

[6] Duke J. *CRC Handbook or Medicinal Herbs.* Boca Raton, FL: CRC Press Inc. 1989;493-4.

[7] Didry N. *Annales Pharmaceutiques Francaises* 1980;38(3):237-41.

[8] Newall C, et al. *Herbal Medicines.* London, England: Pharmaceutical Press, 1996;85–86.

[9] Haaland E. *Acta Chem Scand* 1969;23(7):2546-48.

[10] Engalycheva E, et al. *Farmatsiia* 1984;33(3):13-16.

[11] Franz G. *Planta Medica* 1969(Aug);17:217-20.

[12] Li Y, et al. *Gen Pharmacol* 1988;19(2):261-63.

[13] Wang C, et al. *Yao Hsueh Hsueh Pao* 1989;24(12):913-16.

[14] Sener B, et al. *Gazi Universitesi Eczacilik Fakultesi Dergisi* 1993;10(2):137-41.

[15] Roder E, et al. *Planta Medica* 1981(Sep);43:99-102.

[16] Hirono I, et al. *Gann* 1976;67(1):125-9.

[17] Steinbach R, et al. *Pharmazeutische Zeitung* 1989(Jun 5);134:25-26, 28-29.

[18] Wiedenfeld H, et al. *Deutsche Apotheker Zeitung* 1995(Mar 23);135; 17-18, 21-22, 25-26.

[19] Berry M. *Pharmaceutical Journal* 1996(Feb 17);256:234-5.

[20] Chevallier A. *Encyclopedia of Medicinal Plants.* New York: DK Publishing, 1996;277.

[21] Muller-Limmroth W, et al. *Fortshr Med* 1980;98(3):95-101.

[22] Fu JX. *Chung Hsi I Chieh Ho Tsa Chih* 1989;9(11):658.

[23] Engalycheva E, et al. *Farmatsiia* 1982;31:37-40.

[24] Hwang S, et al. *Eur J Pharmacol* 1987;141(2):269-81.

[25] Didry N, et al. *Annales Pharmaceutiques Francaises* 1982;40(1):75-80.

[26] Salvador R. *Canadian Pharmaceutical Journal* 1996(Jul-Aug);129:48-50.

[27] Anonymous. Toxic Reactions to Plant Products Sold in Health Food Stores. *Med Lett* 1979;21(7):29.

[28] Zeller W, et al. *Arch Dermatol Res* 1985;227(1):28.

[29] Smith LW, et al. *J Nat Prod* 1981;44:129.

[30] Schulz V, et al. *Rational Phytotherapy — A Physician's Guide to Herbal Medicine,* 3rd ed. Berlin, Germany: Springer-Verlag, 1998;34.

[31] Sperl W, et al. *Eur J Pediatr* 1995;154(2):112-16.

[32] DerMarderosian AH, Liberti LE. *Natural Products Medicine.* Philadelphia: GF Stickley Co., 1988.

[33] Blumenthal M, ed. *The Complete German Commission E Monographs.* Austin, TX: American Botanical Council; Boston: Integrative Medicine Communications, 1998.

Comfrey

SCIENTIFIC NAME(S): *Symphytum officinale* L., *S. asperum* Lepechin, *S. tuberosum*, *Symphytum + uplandicum* Nyman (Russian comfrey) is a hybrid of *S. officinale* and *S. asperum*. Family: Boraginaceae

COMMON NAME(S): Comfrey, Russian comfrey, knitbone, bruisewort, blackwort, slippery root

BOTANY: A perennial that grows to about 3 feet. It has lanceolate leaves and bell-shaped purple or yellow-white flowers. It grows in moist grasslands.

HISTORY: Comfrey has been cultivated in Japan as a green vegetable and has been used in American herbal medicine.[1] Its old name, knitbone, derives from the external use of poultices of the leaves and roots to heal burns, sprains, swelling and bruises. Comfrey has been claimed to heal gastric ulcers, hemorrhoids and to suppress bronchial congestion and inflammation.[1] Its use has spanned over 2000 years.[2]

CHEMISTRY: The healing action of the poultices of the roots and leaves may be related to the presence of allantoin, an agent which promotes cell proliferation. The underground parts contain 0.6%-0.7% allantoin and 4%-6.5% tannin. The leaves are poorer in allantoin, but richer in tannin.[3] It has been recently found that the roots contain about 100 times the alkaloid content as compared to the aerial portions.[4] Large amounts of mucilage are found in both leaves and roots.[3] Rosmarinic acid,[5] lithospermic acid[5] and a pentacyclic triterpene glycoside of oleonolic acid[6] have been identified in the root. The alkaloid content of *S. asperum* ranges from 0.14% to 0.4%.[7] Numerous pyrrolizidine alkaloids have also been isolated from comfrey.

PHARMACOLOGY: Ointments containing comfrey have been found to possess an anti-inflammatory activity, which appears to be related to the presence of allantoin and rosmarinic acid[8] or to another hydrocolloid polysaccharide.[9] Lithospermic acid, isolated from the root, appears to have antigonadotropic activity.[5]

TOXICOLOGY: Despite its common use, the long-term ingestion of comfrey may pose a health hazard. Several members of the family Boraginaceae (*Senecio, Heliotropium*) contain related alkaloids reported to cause liver toxicity in animals and humans. Some of these compounds predispose hepatic tumor development.

The carcinogenic potential of *S. officinale* was tested in rats fed 0.5% to 8% comfrey root or leaves for 600 days.[10]

Signs of liver toxicity were seen within 180 days and hepatocellular adenomas were induced in all groups. Urinary bladder tumors were also induced at the lowest comfrey levels. The incidence of liver tumors was higher in groups fed a diet of roots rather than leaves.

The pyrrolizidine alkaloids symphytine, echimidine[11] and lasiocarpine have been found in *S. officinale*. Of these, lasiocarpine[12] and symphytine have been shown to be carcinogenic in rats.[13] In a recent experiment, rats were given doses of 50 mg/kg of comfrey-derived alkaloids. Subsequent liver analysis showed vascular congestion, necrosis and hepatocyte cellular membrane damage.[14] This liver damage was evident and was dose dependent.[15]

Similarly, the alkaloids of Russian comfrey caused chronic liver damage and pancreatic islet cell tumors after 2 years of use in animal models. Eight alkaloids have been isolated from *Symphytum + uplandicum*.[16] Alkaloid levels range from 0.003% to 0.115% with highest concentrations in small young leaves.[17] Of the 7200 inhabitants observed, 23% had severe liver impairment. An indirect estimate of alkaloid ingestion determined the consumption of toxic alkaloids to be 2 mg/700 g of flour. Based on this value, Roitman's calculation of 8 to 26 mg of toxic alkaloids per cup of comfrey root tea (4 to 13 times as great as the episode above) suggests that comfrey ingestion poses a significant health risk.[18] Herbal teas and similar preparations of *Symphytum* contain the pyrrolizidine alkaloid which has shown to cause blockage of hepatic veins and lead to hepatonecrosis.[19] Venoocclusive disease has been reported in a woman who ingested a comfrey-pepsin preparation for 4 months;[18] one woman died following the ingestion of large quantities of yerba mate tea (*Ilex paraguariensis*) which also contains pyrrolizidine alkaloids.[20] A woman who consumed large amounts of comfrey preparations developed ascites-caused veno-occlusive disease,[21] and four Chinese women who self-medicated with an herbal preparation that contained pyrrolizidine alkaloids from an unknown plant source also developed the disease.[22] One man presented portal hypertension with hepatic veno-occlusive disease and later died of liver failure. It was discovered that he used comfrey in his vegetarian diet.[23] Oral ingestion of pyrrolizidine-containing plants such as comfrey poses the greatest risk since the alkaloids are converted to toxic pyrrole-like derivatives following ingestion;[24] however, the alkaloids of comfrey applied to the skin of rats were detected in the urine, and lactating rats excrete pyrrolizidine alkaloids into breast milk.[25] If animals consume plants containing pyrrolizidine alkaloids, they could pass these alkaloids on to humans via milk.[26]

SUMMARY: The Henry Doubleday Research Assoc. (United Kingdom) issued a public statement which con-

cluded that until further research clarifies the long-term health hazard of comfrey ingestion, "no human being or animal should eat, drink, or take comfrey in any form."[27] Comfrey is widely used in the US. Chronic ingestion of its roots and leaves poses the potential for hepatic damage. The possibility of carcinogenicity should be kept in mind by the user. Based on a lack of scientific evidence of a therapeutic effect, the consumption or use of comfrey and its teas cannot be recommended until further evidence of its safety and efficacy is obtained.

PATIENT INFORMATION – Comfrey

Uses: Comfrey has been used as a vegetable, as topical treatment for bruises, burns and sprains and as internal medicine.

Side Effects: Evidence indicates that comfrey is unsafe in any form and potentially fatal.

---

[1] Bianchi F, Corbetta F. *Health plants of the world.* New York: Newsweek Books 1975.
[2] Castlemen M. Comfrey: Friend or Foe? *Herb Quarterly* 1989;44:18.
[3] Tyler VE. *The Honest Herbal,* ed. 3. New York: Haworth Press, 1993.
[4] Mutterlein R, Arnorld CG. Investigations concerning the content and the pattern of pyrrolizidine alkaloids in *Symphytum official L. (comfrey). Pharm Ztg Wiss* 1993;138(5–6):119.
[5] Wagner H, et al. [Lithospermic acid, the antihormonally active principle of Lycopus europaeus L. and Symphytum officinale.] *Arzneimittel-Forschung* 1970;20(5):705.
[6] Ahmad VU, et al. A new triterpene glycoside from the roots of Symphytum officinale. *J Nat Prod* 1993;56(3):329.
[7] Roitman JN. Comfrey and liver damage. *Lancet* 1981;1:944.
[8] Andres R, et al. Relating antiphlogistic efficacy of dermatics containing extracts of symphytum officinale to chemical profiles. *Pianta Med* 1989;55:643.
[9] Franz G. Polysaccharides in Pharmacy: Current Applications and Future Concepts. *Planta Med* 1989;55:493.
[10] Hirono, et al. Carcinogenic activity of symphytum officinale. *J Nat Cancer Inst* 1978;61(5):865.
[11] Furuya T, et al. Alkaloids and triterpenoids of Symphytum officinale. *Phytochem* 1971;10:2217.
[12] Svoboda DJ, Reddy JK. Malignant tumors in rats given lasiocarpine. *Cancer Res* 1972;32:980.
[13] Hirono I, et al. Induction of hepatic tumors in rats by senkirkine and symphytine. *J Nat Cancer Inst* 1979;63:469.
[14] Yeong ML. Hepatocyte membrane injury and bleb information following low dose comfrey toxicity in rats. *Inter J of Exp Pathol* 1993;74:211.
[15] Yeong ML. The effects of comfrey derived pyrrolizidine alkaloid on rat liver. *Path* 1991;23:35.
[16] Culvenor CCJ, et al. Structure and toxicity of the alkaloids of Russian comfrey (Symphytum X uplandicum Nyman) a medicinal herb and item of human diet. *Experientia* 1980;36:377.
[17] mattocks AR. Toxic pyrrolizidine alkaloids in comfrey. *Lancet* 1980;2:1136.
[18] Ridker PM, et al. Hepatic veno-occlusive disease associated with the consumption of pyrrolizidine-containing dietary supplements. *Gastroenterol* 1985;88:1050.
[19] Larrey D. [Liver involvement in the course of phytotherapy (editorial)]. [Review, French] *Presse Med* 1994;23(15):691.
[20] McGee J, et al. A case of veno-occlusive disease of the liver in Britain associated with herbal tea consumption. *J Clin Pathol* 1976;29:799.
[21] Bach N, et al. Comfrey Herb Tea-Induced Hepatic Veno-Occlusive Disease. *JAMA* 1989;87:97.
[22] Kumana CR, et al. Hepatic veno-occlusive disease due to toxic alkaloid in herbal tea. *Lancet* 1983;ii:1360.
[23] Yeong ML, et al. Hepatic veno-occlusive disease associated with comfrey ingestion. *J of Gastroent Hepatol* 1990;5(2):211.
[24] Mattocks AR. Toxicity of pyrrolizidine alkaloids. *Nature* 1986;217:724.
[25] Schoenta R. Health hazards of pyrrolizidine alkaloids: a short review. *Toxicol Lett* 1982;10:323.
[26] Panter KE, James LF. Natural plant toxicants in milk: a review. *J Animal Sci* 1990;68(3):892.
[27] Dunea G. Medical crises. *Brit Med J* 1979;6163:596.

Coral

SOURCE: Coral is harvested from a wide region of the Pacific and other tropical oceans. A number of coral genera have been collected for medicinal use, including *Goniopora* and *Porites*.

HISTORY: While coral has been used by the inhabitants of Pacific regions for cutting tools and as the basis of jewelry and amulets, it was not until the mid 1980s that its value in surgery was fully recognized. The natural material derived from the matrix of sea coral has been found to serve as an effective substrate for the growth of new bone in areas damaged by trauma or requiring reconstruction. Coral may be more durable than bone and appears to eliminate some of the complications inherent in traditional bone graft surgery.[1]

Today, coral-based material is used to aesthetically enhance the facial skeleton in cosmetic surgery and is used as a surgical aid in maxillofacial reconstructive surgery.[7]

CHEMISTRY: Although the structural and mineral composition of coral is very similar to that of bone, coral is not implanted in its natural state. Following its harvest, the coral is treated chemically together with heat and high pressure to convert the calcium carbonate matrix to hydroxyapatite (calcium phosphate hydroxide). Hydroxyapatite is the normal mineral portion of bone.

The pores of the processed coral exoskeletal matrix range from 150 to 600 microns in diameter, with interconnecting pore sizes averaging approximately 260 microns in diameter.[2,3] These dimensions are in the range for normal bone and, therefore, make the coral an excellent base for the spread of new bone growth.

SURGICAL USES: During surgery, the processed coral is shaped to fit the patient's facial structure. Sea coral has several advantages over human bone. Unlike traditional procedures that require the surgical removal of bone matrix from elsewhere in the patient's body (ie, hip) for grafting, coral implant requires only facial incision; it retains its shape well, and it provides a long-lasting matrix that closely resembles natural bone.[1,4]

In baboon studies, surgically made bone defects that were grafted with coral demonstrated substantial bone growth (p < 0.01) compared to bone grafts as early as 3 months after surgery, culminating with complete penetration of bone into the tridimensional porous spaces of the coral.[2] Similar good results were observed when the material was implanted in the mandibles of rabbits.[3] In dogs, bone regrowth in experimentally created proximal tibia defects demonstrated that the stereological distribution of regenerated bone in the porous hydroxyapatite was the same as in normal tibial bone; after 12 months, 66% of the surface of the coral was covered with new bone ingrowth.[6]

Although experience is somewhat limited, published results suggest that in man, the use of coral in maxillofacial surgery results in good bone conduction into the surgical site.[3] Bone defects in man have been shown to heal rapidly following reconstruction with coral microgranules. Biopsies at 8 and 18 months showed good bone formation around the coral particles.[5]

TOXICOLOGY: Follow-up of patients for 6 to 24 months found no deleterious host responses and good tolerability to coral implants.[3] To date, insufficient experience has been gained with the use of coral products to confirm their benefit in assisting bone growth in severely damaged weight-bearing bones.

SUMMARY: Coral is now under investigation for its use in facial reconstructive surgery. The chemically modified coral exoskeleton provides a strong matrix for bone regeneration. The product does not appear to be associated with adverse effects or tissue rejection.

PATIENT INFORMATION – Coral

Uses: Coral is used in cosmetic and reconstructive surgery and as a substrate for new bone growth.

Side Effects: Coral does not appear to be rejected or produce adverse effects.

---

[1] Smith V. Gift from the sea: coral finds place in facial surgery. *Quill* Winter 1989.
[2] Ripamonti U. Calvarial reconstruction in baboons with porous hydroxyapatite. *J Craniofac Surg* 1992;3:149.
[3] Zeng RS. The use of coral as a substitute for maxillofacial bone reconstruction. *Ching Hua Kou Chiang Hsueh Tsa Chih* 1991;26:345, 389.
[4] Hippolyte MP, Fabre D, Peyrol S. Coral and guided tissue regeneration. Histological aspects. *J Parodontol* 1991;10:279.
[5] Issahakian S, Ouhayoun JP. Clinical and histological evaluation of a new filling material: natural coral. *J Parodontol* 1989;8:251.
[6] Holmes RE, Bucholz RW, Mooney V. Porous hydroxyapatite as a bone-graft substitute in metaphyseal defects. A histometric study. *J Bone Joint Surg* 1986;68:904.
[7] Servera C, Souyris F, Payrot C, Jammet P. Coral in infra-osseous lesions. Evaluation after 7 years' use. *Rev Stomatol Chir Maxillofac* 1987;88:326.

Corkwood Tree

SCIENTIFIC NAME(S): *Duboisia myoporoides* Family: Solanaceae

COMMON NAME(S): Corkwood tree, pituri

BOTANY: The plant is found throughout most of Australia[1,2] and has also been cited in botanical texts from South America.[3]

HISTORY: The leaves of the corkwood plant are cured and rolled into a quid. These are chewed by the natives to ward off hunger, pain and tiredness.[1] Because the leaves contain anticholinergic stimulants, it has been reported that Australian aborigines taint waterholes in order to stun and capture animals. The alkaloids derived from the plant are sometimes used as a therapeutic substitute for atropine and the plant had once been an import source of Australia's scopolamine.[1] The plant has been used in homeopathy to treat eye disorders. The corkwood is used for carving.[2]

CHEMISTRY: The plant is rich in alkaloids, yielding more than 2% alkaloids. These consist primarily of hyoscyamine and hyoscine. Also isolated are the alkaloids scopolamine, atropine, butropine and more than a dozen additional related compounds. Nicotine and nornicotine have been reported to exist in the leaves.[1]

PHARMACOLOGY: The tropane alkaloids (atropine, scopolamine, etc) are potent anticholinergic agents. Even therapeutic doses may cause central nervous system disturbances. The alkaloid tigloidine has been found to have an antiparkinson effect, which is not unexpected from an anticholinergic compound.[1]

TOXICOLOGY: Scopolamine and related alkaloids can be fatal in large doses. This plant demonstrates stimulant and hallucinogenic properties by virtue of the anticholinergic effects of its major constituents.

SUMMARY: The corkwood tree is used as a central nervous system stimulant and hallucinogen by native Australians. There is little medicinal use of the plant, and other sources of scopolamine and atropine have become more commercially viable.

PATIENT INFORMATION – Corkwood Tree

Uses: Corkwood tree leaves have been used as a CNS stimulant and hallucinogen.

Side Effects: Even small doses may cause CNS disturbances. Large doses may be fatal.

---

[1] Duke JA. *Handbook of Medicinal Herbs*. Boca Raton, FL: CRC Press, 1985.
[2] Mabberley DJ. *The Plant-Book*. New York: Cambridge University Press, 1987.
[3] Penso G. *Inventory of Medicinal Plants Used in the Different Countries*. World Health Organization, 1982.

Corn Cockle

SCIENTIFIC NAME(S): *Agrostemma githago* L:, Family: Caryophyllaceae

COMMON NAME(S): Cockle, corn campion, corn cockle, corn rose, crown-of-the-field, purple cockle

BOTANY: *Agrostemma githago* is an annual herb showing a few erect branches which are heavily pubescent overall. The leaves are linear lanceolate and the flowers red growing up to 2 inches broad. It was originally native to Europe but has long been naturalized in the US to the extent that it is a troublesome weed in winter wheat fields.[1]

HISTORY: Though corn cockle has an attractive red flower, it is not usually cultivated horticulturally and is generally considered a weed. In fact, its seeds have long been considered poisonous; it causes problems when gathered together with cereal grains with which it grows as a weed. In European folklore, its seeds have been used for treating cancers, hard tumors, warts and apostemes (hard swellings in the uterus). Seeds have also been put into the conjunctival sac to induce keratoconjunctivitis. Its saponins are irritating and have been claimed to have local anesthetic effects.[2]

CHEMISTRY: At least two saponins, githagin and agrostemmic acid, are contained in corn cockle.[1] The saponin, sapotoxin A, with the prosapogenin githagin ($C_{35}H_{54}O_{11}$), the aglycone githagenin ($C_{30}H_{46}O_4$), and agrostemmic acid ($C_{35}H_{54}O_{10}$) have also been reported.[2] The ripe seeds contain a number of aromatic amino acids, including 2,4–dihydroxy-6–methylphenylalanine, L(+)-citrullin ($C_6H_{13}N_3O_3$), sugar, oil, fat and starch. The seedlings, like others, possess allantoin and allantoic acid. The roots are reported to contain up to 2.02% starch labeled "lactosin." The oil contains 41.4% unsaturated fatty acids and a high portion (3.42%) of unsaponifiable lipids.[3] These, in turn yield 8.3% mixed alkanes from C19 to C33. The unsaponifiable lipids were found to have 44.7%

crystalline alpha-spinasterol as well as small quantities of a triterpene ester and a di- or tri-terpene-like unsaturated acyclic ketone.

PHARMACOLOGY: Corn cockle has been used historically as a diuretic, emmenagogue, expectorant, poison and vermifuge. It has been used to treat cancer, dropsy (edema) and jaundice. Corn cockle roots have been used for exanthemata and hemorrhoids. The seeds have been used homeopathically in treating gastritis and paralysis.[2]

TOXICOLOGY: The sapoinins githagin and agrostemmic acid are reported to be absorbable from the alimentary canal and may produce systemic poisoning, including gastrointestinal irritation, severe muscle pain and twitching, followed by depression and coma. In veterinary experiences, poultry and livestock have been poisoned by the seeds of corn cockle. As a seed, it commonly contaminates wheat seed. Hogs that have ingested the roots have died. Consumption of 0.2% to 0.5% of the body weight of seed is lethal to young birds. Cows have also died from this seed. The repeated ingestion and chronic poisoning by small doses of corn cockle is referred to as githagism. Acute poisoning by large doses is manifested by vertigo, respiratory depression, vomiting, diarrhea, salivation and paralysis. Gastric lavage or emesis are recommended for poison treatment.[2]

SUMMARY: Since there are few, if any, modern acceptable medical uses for corn cockle, its record of toxicity relegates it to the category of a poisonous plant. It cannot be recommended for any of the reported folklore uses. The seeds and roots of *A. githago* are the most toxic parts of the plant, probably due to the numerous saponins reported.

PATIENT INFORMATION – Corn Cockle

Uses: Corn cockle has been used in folk medicine to treat a range of ills, from parasites to cancer.

Side Effects: Corn cockle may produce chronic or acute, potentially fatal poisoning.

---

[1] Osol A, Farrar GE Jr., eds. The Dispensatory of the United States of America, ed. 25. Philadelphia: Lippincott, 1955.
[2] Duke JA. *Handbook of Medicinal Herbs*. Boca Raton, FL: CRC Press, 1985.
[3] Jankov LK, Ivanov TP. Constituents of Agrostemma githago L. *Planta Medica* 1970;18(May):232.

Cranberry

SCIENTIFIC NAME(S): *Vaccinium macrocarpon* Ait. (cranberry, trailing swamp cranberry), *V. oxycoccos* L. (small cranberry), *V. erythrocarpum* Michx. (Southern mountain cranberry, *V. vitis* (lowbush cranberry), *V. edule* (highbush cranberry). Family: Ericaceae. Not to be confused with another highbush cranberry, *Viburnum opulus* L. Family: Caprifoliaceae[1]

COMMON NAME(S): See above.

BOTANY: A number of related cranberries are found in areas ranging from damp bogs to mountain forests. These plants grow from Alaska to Tennessee. Cranberry plants grow as small trailing evergreen shrubs. Their flowers vary from pink to purple and bloom from May to August depending on the species. The *Vaccinium* genus also includes the blueberry (*V. angustifolium* Ait.), deerberry (*V. stamineum* L.) and the cowberry (*V. vitis-idaea* L.).

HISTORY: During the mid-1800s, German physicians observed that the urinary excretion of hippuric acid increased after the ingestion of cranberries. It was believed that cranberries, prunes and plums contained benzoic acid or some other compound that the body metabolized and excreted as hippuric acid (a bacteriostatic agent in high concentrations. This hypothesis has always been disputed because the amounts of benzoic acid present in these fruits (about 0.1% by weight) could not account for the excretion of the larger amounts of hippuric acid.

Despite a general lack of scientific evidence to indicate that cranberries or their juice were effective urinary acid-fiers, interest persists among the public in the medical use of cranberries. Cranberries are used in eastern European cultures because of their folkloric role in the treatment of cancers and to reduce fever. Cranberries make flavorful jams and preserves.

CHEMISTRY: Natural, unprocessed cranberry juice contains a variety of constituents, few of which have shown significant pharmacologic activity. The berries contain about 88% water.[2] The juice contains anthocyanin dyes, catechin, triterpenoids, about 10% carbohydrates and small amounts of protein, fiber and ascorbic acid (2 to 10 mg %).[3] The major organic acids are citric, malic[4] and quinic acids, with small amounts of benzoic and glucuronic acids. The glycoside leptosine and several related compounds have been isolated[5] along with small amounts of alkaloids.[6]

Anthocyanin dyes obtained from cranberry pulp are used in commercial coloring applications.[7]

PHARMACOLOGY: The ability of cranberries to acidify urine was based on an early experiment with two healthy subjects.[8] Following a basal diet, one subject was given 305 g of cooked cranberries and the other an unspecified amount of prunes. In the first subject, urinary pH decreased from 6.4 to 5.3 with a concomitant increase in the excretion of total acids. Hippuric acid excretion increased from 0.77 g to 4.74 g. Presumably, urinary hippurate came from the slow biotransformation of quinic and benzoic acids or from a glucoside that hydrolyzes to quinic acid. Since mammalian tissues cannot convert quinic to hippuric acid, intestinal bacteria may play a role in this conversion.[9]

Despite these early observations, it appears that the value of cranberries in treating urinary tract infections continues to be controversial. In one study, three of four subjects given 1.5 to 4 L per day of cranberry cocktail (1/3 juice mixed with water and sugar) showed only transient changes in urinary pH.[10] The maximum tolerated amounts of cranberry juice (about 4 L per day) rarely result in enough hippuric acid excretion to achieve urinary concentrations that are bacteriostatic at the optimum activity level of pH 5. The antibiotic activity of hippuric acid decreases about five-fold at pH 5.6.[11] When five subjects were given 1.2 to 4 L per day of cranberry juice, urinary pH decreased only 0.2 to 0.5 units after 4 days of treatment; no urinary pH was ever lowered to pH 5.[11] A recent placebo controlled study assessed the value of drinking 300 ml per day of cranberry juice on bacteria and white blood cell counts in the urine of 153 elderly women.[2] The odds of having bacteria or white blood cells in the urine were significantly lower in the group of women that ingested the real cranberry juice and their odds of remaining bacteria-free from one month to the next were only 27% of the controls (p = 0.006). This is one of the largest and best designed studies of its kind and suggests that there may be a microbiologic basis for cranberry's activity.

It is therefore likely that the juice does not exert a direct antibacterial effect via a compound such as hippuric acid, but that an alternate mechanism accounts for the anti-infective activity.[13] This is supported by the observation that cranberry and blueberry juices contain a high molecular weight compound that inhibits the common urinary pathogen *Escherichia coli* from adhering to infection sites within the urinary tract, thereby limiting the ability of the bacteria to initiate and spread infections.[14]

One promising use for the juice is as a "urinary deodorant." The malodor of fermenting urine from incontinent patients is a persistent, demoralizing problem in hospitals and long-term care facilities. Cranberry juice appears to lower urinary pH sufficiently to retard the degradation of urine by *E. coli*, limiting the generation of the pungent ammoniacal odor.[15,16,17]

Using the juice in combination with antibiotics has been suggested for the long-term suppressive therapy of urinary tract infections.[18,19] Anecdotal reports have described the benefits of drinking 6 oz of juice twice daily to relieve symptoms of chronic pyelonephritis and to decrease the recurrence of urinary stones.[18] The juice shows slight antiviral activity in vitro.[20]

TOXICOLOGY: There have been no reports of significant toxicity with the use of cranberries or their juice. The ingestion of large amounts (more than 3 to 4 L per day) of the juice often results in diarrhea and other gastrointestinal symptoms.

SUMMARY: Based on more than 100 years of clinical experience, the data are still conflicting about whether cranberries and their juice can be expected to reliably decrease urinary pH to a level that would permit bacteriostasis. Hippuric acid excretion alone does not exert a reliable clinical effect and it is more likely that the effects of cranberries on urinary tract infections are related to their ability to interfere with bacterial adhesion. The juice has been given to decrease the rate of urine degradation and odor formation in incontinent patients.

PATIENT INFORMATION – Cranberry

Uses: Cranberries and cranberry juice appear to combat urinary tract infections. The acids lower urine pH levels enough to slow urine degradation and odor in incontinent patients.

Side Effects: Extremely large doses can produce GI symptoms such as diarrhea.

---

[1] Dobelis IN. *Magic and Medicine of Plants*. Pleasantville, NY: Reader's Digest Association, 1986.

[2] Geigy Scientific Tables, 7th ed. New York: Geigy Pharmaceutical.

[3] Melgalve I. Quantity of vitamin C in cranberries. *Latv Lauksaimn Akad Raksti* 1976;107:28. *Chem Abs* 86:154212.

[4] Borukh IF, Senchuk GV. Antimicrobial properties of cranberries. *Vopr Pitan* 1972;31:82. *Chem Abs* 80:35101.

[5] Jankowski K, Pare JRJ. Trace glycoside from cranberries (*Vaccinium oxicoccos*). *J Nat Prod* 1983;46:190.

[6] Jankowski K. Alkaloids of cranberries V. *Experientia* 1973;29:1334.

[7] Woo AH, et al. Anthocyanin recovery from cranberry pulp wastes by membrane technology. *J Food Sci* 1980;45:875.

[8] Blatherwick NR, Long ML. Studies of urinary acidity II: The increased acidity produced by eating prunes and cranberries. *J Biol Chem* 1923;57:815.

[9] DerMarderosian AH. Cranberry juice. *Drug Therapy* 1977;7:151.

[10] Kahn DH, et al. Effect of cranberry juice on urine. *J Am Dietetic Assn* 1967;51:251.

[11] Bodel PT, et al. Cranberry juice and the antibacterial action of hippuric acid. *J Lab Clin Med* 1959;54:881.

[12] Avorn J, et al. Reduction of bacteriuria and pyuria after ingestion of cranberry juice. *JAMA* 1994;271:751.

[13] Tyler V. The Honest Herbal: A sensible guide to the use of herbs and related remedies. Binghamtom, NY: The Haworth Press, 1993.

[14] Ofek I, et al. Anti-Escherichia coli adhesin activity of cranberry and blueberry juices. *N Engl J Med* 1991;324:1599.

[15] Kraemer RJ. Cranberry juice and the reduction of ammoniacal odor of urine. *Southwestern Med* 1964;45:211.

[16] Dugan C, Cardaciotto PS. Reduction of ammoniacal urinary odors by the sustained feeding of cranberry juice. *J Psychiatric Nurs* 1966;8:467.

[17] Walsh BA. Urostomy and urinary pH. *J ET Nurs* 1992;19:110.

[18] Zinsser HH, et al. Management of infected stones with acidifying agents. *NY State J Med* 1968;68:3001.

[19] Papas PN, et al. Cranberry juice in the treatment of urinary tract infections. *Southwestern Med* 1966;47:17.

[20] Konowalchuk J, Speirs JI. Antiviral effect of commercial juices and beverages. *Appl Envir Microbiol* 1978;35:1219.

Cucurbita

SCIENTIFIC NAME(S): *Cucurbita pepo* L. (pumpkin or pepo), *C. maxima Duchesne* (autumn squash), *C. moschata* Poir. (crookneck squash). Family: Cucurbitaceae.

BOTANY: The members of this genus are plants that develop long vine-like stems that produce large edible fruits. The large, yellow flowers are eaten in some Mediterranean cultures; whereas, the fruits are eaten world-wide. Many cultivated varieties can be found throughout the world.

HISTORY: The seeds of several species of cucurbita have been used in traditional medicine for centuries. They have been used to immobilize and aid in the expulsion of intestinal worms and parasites. Traditionally, the seeds of *Cucurbita* species are ingested after grinding or as a tea. The amount of seeds that can exert a pharmacologic effect appears to vary by species, from as few as 50 g to more than 500 g. These are usually taken in several divided doses. Some cultures suggest eating small amounts of the seeds on a daily basis as a prophylactic against worm infections. The seeds also have been used in the treatment of prostate gland disorders.[1]

CHEMISTRY: The pharmacologically active anthelmintic component of cucurbita seeds appears to be cucurbitin, a carboxypyrrolidine. The distribution of this compound is limited to seeds of this genus. The concentration of cucurbitin can vary from 0.53% to 1.94% in *C. maxima*, from 0.4% to 0.84% in *C. moschata*, and from 0.18% to 0.66% in *C. pepo*. A 1-dose pumpkin seed extract prepared from a Lebanese variety of cucurbita contained about 1.5 g of cucurbitin.[2]

Cucurbita is rich in carotenoids. Pressed seeds of *C. pepo* contain lutein, carotene, and beta-carotene.[3] *C. moschata* contains 19 carotenoids, with beta-carotene accounting for 74% of total carotenoid content. This "Baianinha" squash is one of the richest sources of provitamin A.[4] The species *C. maxima* is also high in carotenoid content containing 11 carotenoids, which include lutein and beta-carotene.[4,5]

C. pepo has a high fatty acid content containing mainly palmitic, stearic, oleic, and linoleic acids. The oil content of the seed is 50%. Vitamin E content, primarily gamma-tocopherol, is very high, making certain pumpkin varieties desirable.[6,7] Long chain hydrocarbons and fatty acids have been reported in fruits of *C. maxima*.[8]

Amino acid content in cucurbita has been reported. Amino acid patterns and certain protein isolates have been studied in the species *C. moschata*, evaluating nutritional characteristics.[9] Computer analysis of amino acids in *C. pepo* has been performed to find properties of phytochromes in the plant.[10]

Flavonol content from *C. pepo* has been discussed[11] and sterols in *C. moschata* seed oil have been reported.[12] *C. maxima* flowers contain spinasterol.[13] Sterols and triterpenoids in *C. maxima* tissue cultures also have been evaluated.[14]

Other reports concerning cucurbita chemistry include *C. pepo* male flower constituents,[15] lectins from related species of *C. ficifolia* seedlings,[16] and root starches from *C. foetidissima* and *C. digitata*.[17]

PHARMACOLOGY: Cucurbitin inhibits the growth of immature *Schistosoma japonicum* in vivo, and a patent has been granted for an effective aqueous extract of the seeds for use as a human anthelmintic.[2] Anthelmintic activity has been demonstrated in mice.[18] In certain species of parasites, cucurbita had no effect. A dried-seeds diet of *C. maxima* given to mice infected with *Vampirolepis nana* tapeworm had no anthelmintic actions.[19] Because cucurbitin varies widely among plants of the same species, it has often been difficult to replicate the efficacy of the crude preparations. Cucurbitin has been generally supplanted by more effective single-dose vermifuges.[2] In one report, *C. maxima* in an oral preparation displayed strong antimalarial activity in mice, reducing the parasites by 50%.[20] In another report, an extract of *C. maxima* demonstrated antitumor potential against *Neurospora crassa*.[21]

Characteristics[22] and nutritional aspects[23] of cucurbita have been addressed. Studies on antilipolytic activity of *C. maxima* also have been performed.[24]

The influence of *C. maxima* on age-associated impairments has been reported.[25]

In a randomized, 3-month, double-blind study, a preparation of *C. pepo* (curbicin) improved certain parameters of benign prostatic hyperplasia including urinary flow, micturition time, residual urine, and urinary frequency vs placebo.[26]

Related species *C. ficifolia* exhibits hypoglycemic actions in rabbits.[27,28]

TOXICOLOGY: Severe toxicity has not been reported with the use of cucurbita extracts. In a 53-patient, randomized, double-blind trial, no side effects from *C. pepo* were noted.[26] Ingestion of *C. maxima* seeds by rats and pigs over a 4-week period resulted in no changes in glucose, urea, creatinine, liver enzymes, blood counts, etc.[29] One report on *C. moschata* describes dermatitis.[30]

SUMMARY: Seeds of *Cucurbita* species have been used throughout the world for centuries as a vermifuge. The active component, cucurbitin, is an effective vermifuge agent in vitro and may also be effective in humans. Cucurbita also demonstrates antimalarial and antitumor activities. The plant improved symptoms of BPH in one trial. It may be useful in diabetes, but more human research is warranted. Preparations of this plant have not been generally associated with toxicity.

PATIENT INFORMATION – Cucurbita

Uses: Squashes, pumpkins, and other fruits of this family are consumed throughout the world. Flowers and seeds of some species are eaten. Seeds of some species are a traditional vermifuge. Also, components of some seeds may be useful in treating prostatic disorders.

Side Effects: Severe toxicity has not been reported with the use of cucurbita extracts.

---

[1] Tyler V. *The New Honest Herbal.* 2nd ed. Philadelphia: G.F. Stickley Co., 1987.

[2] Mihranian V, et al. Extraction, detection, and estimation of cucurbitin in Cucurbita seeds. *Lloydia* 1968;31:23.

[3] Matus Z, et al. Main carotenoids in pressed seeds (Cucurbitae semen) of oil pumpkin (*Cucurbita pepo* convar. pepo var. styriaca). *Acta Pharma* 1993;63(5):247-56. Hungarian.

[4] Arima HK, et al. Carotenoid composition and vitamin A value of a squash and a pumpkin from northeastern Brazil. *Arch Latinoam Nutr* 1990;40(2):284-92. Portuguese.

[5] Barua S, et al. Studies on dark green leafy vegetables and yellow vegetables. Part 5. Availability of carotene as a source of vitamin A. *Bangladesh Pharm J* 1977;6:8-12.

[6] Murkovic M, et al. Variability of vitamin E content in pumpkin seeds (Cucurbita pepo L.). *Z Lebensm Unters Forsch* 1996;202(4):275-8.

[7] Murkovic M, et al. Variability of fatty acid content in pumpkin seeds (*Cucurbita pepo* L.). *Z Lebensm Unters Forsch* 1996;203(3):216-9.

[8] Stoianova-Ivanova B, et al. Long chain hydrocarbons and fatty acids in different parts of the fruits of *Cucurbita maxima* linnaeus. *Rivista Italiana Essenze Profumi Piante Officinali Aromi Saponi Cosmetici Aerosol* 1975;57:377-82.

[9] Salgado J, et al. Chemical and biological characterization of meal and protein isolates from pumpkin seed (*Cucurbita moschata*). *Arch Latinoam Nutr* 1992;42(4):443-50. Portuguese.

[10] Partis M, et al. Computer analysis of phytochrome sequences from five species: implications for the mechanism of action. *Z Naturforsch [C]* 1990;45(9-10):987-98.

[11] Krauze-Baranowska M, et al. Flavonols from *Cucurbita pepo* L. herb. *Acta Pol Pharm* 1996;53(1):53-6.

[12] Rodriguez J, et al. The sterols of *Cucurbita moschata* ("calabacita") seed oil. *Lipids* 1996;31(11):1205-8.

[13] Villasenor I, et al. Antigenotoxic spinasterol from *Cucurbita maxima* flowers. *Muta Res* 1996;360(2):89-93.

[14] Caputo O, et al. Biosynthesis of sterols and triterpenoids in tissue cultures of *Cucurbita maxima*. *Planta Med* 1983;49:176-80.

[15] Itokawa H, et al. Studies on the constituents of the male flowers of *Cucurbita pepo* L. *Yakugaku Zasshi J Pharm Soc Japan* 1982;102(4):318-21. Japanese.

[16] Lorenc-Kubis I, et al. Lectins from squash (*Cucurbita ficifolia*) seedlings. *Acta Biochim Pol* 1993;40(1):103-5.

[17] Berry J, et al. Cucurbit root starches: isolation and some properties of starches from *Cucurbita foetidissima* HBK and *Curcurbita digitata* Gray. *J Agric Food Chem* 1975;23(4):825-6.

[18] Elisha E, et al. Anthelmintic activity of some Iraqi plants of the Cucurbitaceae. *Int J Crude Drug Res* 1987;25:153-57.

[19] De Amorim A, et al. Anthelmintic action of plants. Part 6. Influence of pumpkin seeds in the removal of *Vampirolepis nana* from mice. *Revista Brasileira de Farmacia* 1992;73:81-82.

[20] Amorim CZ, et al. Screening of the antimalarial activity of plants of the Cucurbitaceae. *Mem Inst Oswaldo Cruz* 1991;86(Suppl 2):177-80.

[21] Rojas N, et al. Antitumoral potential of aqueous extracts of Cuban plants. Part 2. *Revista Cubana de Farmacia* 1980:14:219-225.

[22] Basaran A, et al. Characteristics of Turkish *Cucurbita maxima* Duch seed oil. *Acta Pharmaceutica Turcica* 1998;40(1):17-19.

[23] Jaroniewska D, et al. Vegetables in diet and treatment: pumpkin. *Farmacja Polska* 1997;53(3):134-5.

[24] Wong C, et al. Screening of *Trichosanthes kirilowii, Momordica charantia* and *Cucurbita maxima* (family Cucurbitaceae) for compounds with antilipolytic activity. *J Ethnopharmacol* 1985;13:313-21.

[25] Wichtl M. Geriatrics of plant origin. *Dtsch Apoth Ztg* 1992;132:1569-76.

[26] Carbin B, et al. Treatment of benign prostatic hyperplasia with phytosterols. *Brit J Urol* 1990;66(6):639-41.

[27] Roman-Ramos R, et al. Hypoglycemic activity of some antidiabetic plants. *Arch Med Res* 1992;23(3):105-9.

[28] Roman-Ramos R, et al. Anti-hyperglycemic effect of some edible plants. *J Ethnopharmacol* 1995;48(1):25-32.

[29] Dequeiroz-Neto A, et al. Toxicologic evaluation of acute and subacute oral administration of *Cucurbita maxima* seed extracts to rats and swine. *J Ethnopharmacol* 1994;43(1):45-51.

[30] Potter T, et al. Butternut squash (*Cucurbita moschata*) dermatitis. *Contact Dermatitis* 1994;30(2):123.

Cumin

SCIENTIFIC NAME(S): *Cuminum cyminum* L. also referred to as *C. odorum* Salisb. Family: Apiaceae (Umbelliferae)

COMMON NAME(S): Cumin, cummin

BOTANY: This small annual plant is native to the Mediterranean region where it is cultivated extensively. The cumin seed is widely used in cooking. The dried seeds resemble those of caraway, but are straighter in form and have a coarser taste and odor than caraway seeds.[2] Major cumin seed producers include Egypt, Iran, India and Morocco.[1] The United States is among the largest producers of cumin oil. This spice should not be confused with sweet cumin, which is a common name for anise (*Pimpinella anisum*).[3] Black cumin (*Bunium persicum*) has smaller and sweeter seeds than *C. cyminum*, but is not commercially important. Another black cumin (*Nigella sativa*) is not related to cumin.[4]

HISTORY: Cumin is a major component of curry and chilir powders[1] and has been used to flavor a variety of commercial food products. The oil, which is derived by steam distillation,[4] is used to flavor alcoholic beverages, desserts and condiments, and has been used as a fragrant component of creams, lotions and perfumes.[1]

CHEMISTRY: Cumin seeds contain up to 5% of a volatile oil. In addition, the seeds yield about 22% fats, numerous free amino acids and a variety of flavonoid glycosides, including derivatives of apigenin and luteolin.[1]

The volatile oil is composed primarily of aldehydes (up to 60%) and the cuminaldehyde content varies considerably depending on the source of the oil (ie, fresh versus ground seeds). Fine grinding of the seed can result in the loss of up to 50% of the volatile oil,[1] with the greatest loss occurring within one hour of milling. Other major components of the oil include monoterpene hydrocarbons, and sesquiterpenes constitute minor constituents of the oil. The chief components of the characteristic aroma of unheated whole seeds are 3–p-menthen-7–al and cuminaldehyde in combination with other related aldehydes.

PHARMACOLOGY: The petroleum ether soluble fraction of cumin has been reported to have antioxidant activity when mixed with lard.[1] No in vivo inhibition of hepatic peroxidation has been observed, even with high concentrations of cuminaldehyde.[5] However, cuminaldehyde scavenges the superoxide anion.[6]

The spice appears to have and anticancer effect as demonstrated by the ability of cumin seeds to inhibit the induction of gastric squamous cell carcniomas in mice.[7] Furthermore, cumin seeds were not carcinogenic when tested by the reverse mutation *Salmonella typhimurium* test.[8]

Cumin, given at a level 5–fold higher than the normal human intake level, did not reduce serum or liver cholesterol levels in rats fed a hypercholesterolemic diet.[9]

Cumin oil and cuminaldehyde have been reported to exhibit strong larvicidal and antibacterial activity. At in vitro concentrations of 300 or 600 ppm, cumin oil inhibited the growth of *Lactobacillus plantarum*.[10]

TOXICOLOGY: Cumin is generally recognized as safe for human consumption as a spice and flavoring.[4] Cumin oil components appear to be absorbed rapidly through shaved intact abdominal mouse skin and undiluted cumin oil has phototoxic effects that are not related to cuminaldehyde, but to another photosensitizing component.[1]

SUMMARY: Cumin, a widely used spice, is a major ingredient in curry and chilies. Its aromatic fragrance makes it valuable in cooking and perfumery.

PATIENT INFORMATION – Cumin

Uses: The seeds are used in cooking. The oil flavors food and scents cosmetics. Components may have antioxidant, anticancer, larvicidal and antibacterial effects.

Side Effects: The oil may have photosensitizing effects.

[1] Leung AY. *Encyclopedia of Common Natural Ingredients Used in Food, Drugs and Cosmetics.* New York, NY: J. Wiley and Sons, 1980.

[2] Evans WC. *Trease and Evans' Pharmacognosy.* 13th ed. London: Balliere Tindall, 1989.

[3] Dobelis IN. *Magic and Medicine of Plants.* Pleasantville, NY: Reader's Digest Association, 1986.

[4] Simon JE. *Herbs: an indexed bibliography, 1971–1980.* Hamden, CT: The ShoeString Press, 1984.

[5] Reddy AC, Lokesh BR. Studies on spice principles as antioxidants in the inhibition of lipid peroxidation of rat liver microsomes. *Mol Cell Biochem* 1992;111:117.

[6] Krishnakantha TP, Lokesh BR. Scavenging of superoxide anions by spice principles. *Indian J Biochem Biophys* 1993;30:133.

[7] Aruna K, Sivaramakrishnan VM. Anticarcinogenic effects of some Indian plant products. *Food Chem Toxicol* 1992;30:953.

[8] Sivaswamy SN, et al. Mutagenic activity of south Indian food items. *Indian J Exp* Biol 1991;29:730.

[9] Sambaiah K, Srinivasan K. Effect of cumin, cinnamon, ginger, mustard and tamarind in induced hypercholesterolemic rats. *Nahrung* 1991;35:47.

[10] Kivanc M, et al. Inhibitory and stimulatory effects of cumin, oregano and their essential oils on growth and acid production of *Lactobacillus plantarum* and *Leuconostoc mesenteroides. Int J Food Microbiol* 1991;13:81.

Damiana

SCIENTIFIC NAME(S): *Turnera diffusa* Willdenow et Schultes var. *aphrodisiaca* Urban. Also known as *T. aphrodisiaca* Ward. and *T. microphylla* Desv. Family: Turneraceae

COMMON NAME(S): Damiana, herba de la pastora, Mexican damiana, old woman's broom, rosemary (not to be confused with the spice *Rosmarinus officinalis* L.)

BOTANY: Damiana is a Mexican shrub also found throughout the southern US and many parts of South America. It has small, yellow-brown aromatic leaves. The leaves are broadly lanceolate, 10 to 25 mm long with three to six teeth along the margins. The red-brown twigs are often found mixed in the crude drug along with the spherical fruits.

HISTORY: The scientific literature on the plant dates back more than 100 years when reports described its aphrodisiac effects.[1] Damiana history began with its early use by the Maya (under the name mizibcoc) in the treatment of giddiness and loss of balance. Its primary use in the last century has been as an aphrodisiac.[2] Father Juan Maria de Salvatierra, a Spanish missionary, first reported that the Mexican Indians made a drink from the damiana leaves, added sugar and drank it for its love-enhancing properties. In the 1970s, it was imported into the US as a tincture and advertised as a powerful aphrodisiac, to improve the sexual ability of the enfeebled and the aged and to provide increased activity to all the pelvic secretions. Suffice to say that in this patent medicine era, it enjoyed some success.

Damiana was admitted into the first edition of the National Formulary (NF) in 1888 as an elixir and fluid extract. However, it never made it into the US Pharmacopeia and the elixir was finally dropped from the NF in 1916. The fluid extract and the crude drug (leaves) were listed in the NF until 1947. Although some commercial companies continued to sell it to the American market, damiana had almost disappeared until the 1960s "hippy" movement brought it back into popularity.

Today, damiana has found its way into a number of herbal OTC products, in particular those claiming to induce a legal herbal "high." In the Caribbean, damiana leaves are boiled in water and the vapors inhaled for the relief of headaches. Teas are said to aid in the control of bed wetting.[3]

CHEMISTRY: Damiana contains from 0.5% to 1% of a complex volatile oil that gives the plant its characteristic odor and taste. Analysis of the oil has identified a low-boiling fraction composed mainly of 1,8–cineol and pinenes, but their consistent presence in all forms of the plant has been disputed.[4] A fraction with a higher boiling point is believed to contain thymol and a number of sesquiterpenes. In addition, the plant contains gonzalitosin, a cyanogenic glycoside and a brown amorphous, bitter substance (damianin) among other components.[5]

PHARMACOLOGY: No substantive data is available to support the aphrodisiac effects of damiana. Although it has been postulated that the plant may contain the central nervous system stimulant caffeine, the aphrodisiac effect has not been attributed to any specific components. The volatile oil in damiana might be sufficiently irritating to the urethral mucous membranes to account for its so-called aphrodisiac effects.[2] Despite containing a complex mixture of components, there is no evidence to support claims for an aphrodisiac or hallucinogenic effect.

TOXICOLOGY: No significant adverse effects have been reported in the literature. However, persons claiming to experience damiana-induced hallucinations should be monitored closely and the possibility of ingestion of other drugs should be considered.

SUMMARY: Damiana is a plant that has received considerable attention for its purported aphrodisiac and hallucinogenic effects. Although there are anecdotal reports of these effects, the plant lacks any verifiable pharmacologic activity. No new significant chemical or pharmacological studies could be found in the scientific literature up to mid-1996.

PATIENT INFORMATION – Damiana

Uses: Damiana is reportedly an aphrodisiac and hallucinogen.

Side Effects: Significant adverse effects have not been reported.

---

[1] Anonymous. New York Alumni Association of the Philadelphia College of Pharmacy: Meeting Minutes – August 3, 1875. *Am J Pharm* 1875;47:426.

[2] Tyler VE. Damiana: History of an Herbal Hoax. *Pharmacy in History* 1983;25(2):55.

[3] Eldridge J. Bush Medicine in the Exumas and Long Island Bahamas: A field study. *Econ Bot* 1975;29(4):307.

[4] Dominquez XA, Hinojosa M. Mexican medicinal plants. 28. Isolation of 5–hydroxy-7,3′4′-trimethoxyflavone from Turnera diffusa. *Planta Med* 1976;30:68.

[5] Leung AY. Encyclopedia of Common Natural Ingredients Used in Food, Drugs, and Cosmetics. New York: J. Wiley Interscience, 1980.

Dandelion

SCIENTIFIC NAME(S): *Taraxacum officinale* Weber, also referred to as *Leontodon taraxacum* L. Family: Compositae

COMMON NAME(S): Dandelion, lion's tooth

BOTANY: The dandelion is a weedy composite plant with a rosette of leaves radiating from its base. The stem is smooth and hollow and bears a solitary yellow head consisting solely of ray flowers, which produces a cluster of numerous tiny, tufted, single-seed fruits. The plant has a deep taproot. The leaves may be nearly smooth-edged, toothed or deeply cut; the toothed appearance gives rise to the plant's name (dent-de-lion means "lion's tooth" in French).[1] This perennial plant can reach 20 inches in height. It grows wild in most parts of the world and is cultivated in France and Germany.[2]

HISTORY: The dandelion is mentioned as early as the 10th century by Arab physicians, who used it for medicinal purposes.[3] The plant was also recommended in an herbal written in the 13th century by the physicians of Myddfai in Wales.[2] It is native to Europe and Asia, but was naturalized in North America and now grows widely as a weed in nearly all temperate climates. It is cultivated by some European growers, and more than 100 specialized varieties have been developed. The bitter greens are used raw in salads, in wine making or cooked like spinach. The root is roasted and used to brew a coffee-like beverage said to lack the stimulant properties of coffee. Dandelions have long been used in herbal remedies for diabetes and disorders of the liver (the sugars in the plant are said not to aggravate this disease) and as a laxative and tonic. The juice of the leaves has been used to treat skin diseases, loss of appetite and to stimulate the flow of bile.[3]

CHEMISTRY: Dandelions are one of nature's richest green vegetable source of beta-carotene, from which vitamin A is created (14,000 IU/100 g leaf vs. 11,000 IU/100 g in carrots). They are also a very good source of fiber, potassium (297 mg or 7.6 mEq/100 mg leaf), iron, calcium, magnesium, phosphorus, thiamine and riboflavin. Sodium and vitamins C and D are also present.[4]

Dandelions contain acids including caffeic, p-hydroxyphenyl-acetic, chlorogenic, oleic, palmitic and the fatty acids linoleic and linolenic. Other acids found are gallic and ascorbic acids.

The plant also contains terpenoids, sesquiterpenes (responsible for the bitter taste), triterpenes (beta-amyrin, taraxol and taraxerol), luteolin and the glycoside apigenin. Other reported constituents in dandelion include choline, inulin, pectin, glutin, gum, resin, sterols (β-sitosterol, stigmasterol, taraxasterol, homotaraxasterol) coumestrol and sugars (fructose, sucrose, glucose).[2,5,6]

Reports are available evaluating fructofuranosidases from dandelion roots,[7] taraxinic acid 1'-O-beta-D-glucopyranoside[8] and furan fatty acid content.[9]

PHARMACOLOGY: Dandelion has been classified as a **hepatic mild laxative, cholegogue, diaphoretic, analgesic, stimulant, tonic** and a **regulator of blood glucose.**[5,6 10,12-15] The roots have been used as a laxative, diuretic, tonic, hepatic and for spleen ailments.[6,12,14] Root and leaves have been used for heartburn, bruises, chronic rheumatism, gout, diabetes, eczema and other skin problems as well as for cancers.[12,14]

Diuretic effects of dandelion extracts have been documented in mice.[5] One reported animal study indicated a greater diuretic effect achieved from herbal extracts than root extracts and compared the effects of a 50 ml/kg body weight dose (2 g dried herb/kg) to the effects achieved with 80 mg/kg of furosemide.[5] This study also reported the effects of dandelion to be greater than other plant diuretics, including Equisetum and Juniper berry.[5,10] This diuretic effect, likely a result of sesquiterpene lactone activity and high potassium content,[10] has been used to treat high blood pressure.[2,10] A later report observed no significant diuretic activity from the plant.[11] These same sesquiterpene lactones may contribute to dandelion's mild anti-inflammatory activity demonstrated.[5,12]

It is effective as a detoxifying herb, working primarily on the liver and gallbladder to remove waste. It may aid gallbladder ailments and help "dissolve" gallstones.[2] However, dandelion should only be used for gallstones under a physician's direction; it is generally contraindicated in bile duct obstruction, empyema or ileus.[5,10,12,13] Increases of bile secretion in rats (≥ 40%) have been attributed to activity of bitter sesquiterpene lactones in the root.[12] These lactones also increase gastric secretions that can cause gastric discomfort.[10,12] Use for dyspeptic disorders may be attributed to the anti-ulcer and gastric antisecretory activity of taraxerol, one of the terpenoid alcohols also found in the root.[4] Dandelion is also considered an appetite-stimulating bitter.[4,10] The bitter principles, previously known as taraxacin which have recently been identified as eudesmanolides, are contained in the leaves and appear to be unique to dandelion.[10]

Hypoglycemic effects have been demonstrated in healthy, non-diabetic rabbits with a maximum decrease in blood glucose achieved at a dose of 2 g/kg.[5] The maximum effect of dandelion was reported to be 65% of the effect produced by tolbutamide 500 mg/kg.[5] Another report found no effect on glucose homeostasis in mice.[16] Inulin, reported to have antidiabetic activity, may contribute to dandelion's glucose regulating properties.[14,17]

In vitro antitumor activity with a mechanism similar to that of lentinan (a tumor polysaccharide) has been reported.[5], *Taraxacum* species have been used in China for over 1100 years in treating breast cancer and other breast ailments.[12] Clinical studies using Chinese *Taraxacum* species also support the use of dandelion to treat hepatitis as well as various respiratory infections.[12]

TOXICOLOGY: Like many plants in this family, dandelions are known to cause contact dermatitis in sensitive individuals.[18,19] A case report of a 9-year-old boy describes positive patch test reactions to dandelion and other compositae-plant oleo resins.[20] Two out of seven patients, each with histories of dandelion dermatitis, reacted not only to dandelion extracts, but to a sesquiterpene mix.[21] These sesquiterpene lactones are believed to be the allergenic principles in dandelion.[2] Taraxinic acid 1'-O-beta-D-glucopyranoside has also been identified as an allergenic component.[22]

Acute toxicity of dandelion is low. LD_{50} values in mice for the root are 36.8 g/kg and for herb are 28.8 g/kg.[2] A case report describes toxicity in a patient taking an herbal combination tablet that included dandelion. It was unclear as to which constituents were responsible.[23] Dandelion may be potentially toxic because of the high content of potassium, magnesium and other minerals.[24]

SUMMARY: The dandelion is a common weed that has been collected and used as a salad green, an ingredient for wine and an herbal medicine. It has limited documented pharmacological activity, but its use persists in herbal medicine for minor medicinal and nutritional purposes. The principal hazard appears to be contact dermatitis.

PATIENT INFORMATION – Dandelion

Uses: Dandelion has been used for its nutritional value in addition to other uses including diuresis, regulation of blood glucose; liver and gall bladder disorders; an appetite stimulant; and for dyspeptic complaints.

Side effects: Contact dermatitis and gastric discomfort have been reported.

---

[1] Seymour ELD. The Garden Encyclopedia. 1936.
[2] Chevallier A. Encyclopedia of Medicinal Plants. New York, NY: DK Publishing, 1996;140.
[3] Loewenfeld C, Back P. The Complete Book of Herbs and Spices. David E. Charles. London: Seymour, 1974.
[4] Brooks S. *Prot J Bot Med* 1996;1(4):231.
[5] Newall C, et al. Herbal Medicines. London, England: Pharmaceutical Press, 1996;96-97.
[6] Duke J. CRC Handbook of Medicinal Herbs. Boca Raton, FL: CRC Press Inc., 1989;476-77.
[7] Rutherford P, et al. *Biochem J* 1972;126(3):569-73.
[8] Hausen B. *Derm Beruf Umwelt* 1982;30(2):51-53.
[9] Hannemann K, et al. *Lipids* 1989;24(4):296-98.
[10] Bisset Ng, ed. Max Wichtl. Herbal Drugs and Phytopharmaceuticals. Boca Raton, FL: CRC Prss Inc., 1994;486-89.
[11] Hook I, et al. *Int J Pharmacognosy* 1993;31(1):29-34.

[12] Leung AY; Fosters. Encyclopedia of Common Natural Ingredients. New York: John Wiley and Sons, Inc., 1996;205-7.
[13] Brooks S. *Prot J Bot Med* 1998;2(3):268.
[14] Brooks S. *Prot J Bot Med* 1996;1(3):163.
[15] Brooks S. *Prot J Bot Med* 1995:1(1):70.
[16] Swanston-Flatt S, et al. *Diabetes Res* 1989;10(2):69-73.
[17] Duke JA. Handbook of Biologically Active Phytochemicals and Their Activities. Boca Raton, FL: CRC Press, Inc., 1992;86.
[18] Larregue M, et al. *Ann Dermatol Venerol* 1978;105:547.
[19] Hausen BM, Schulz KH. *Derm Beruf Umwelt* 1978;26:198.
[20] Guin J, et al. *Arch Dermatol* 1987;123(4):500-2.
[21] Lovell C, et al. *Contact Dermatitis* 1991;25(3):135-88.
[22] Hausen BM. *Derm Beruf Umwelt* 1982;30:51.
[23] DeSmet P, et al. *BMJ* 1996 Jul 13;313:92.
[24] Hamlin T. *Can J Hosp Pharm* 1991;44(1):39-40.

Danshen

SCIENTIFIC NAME(S): *Salvia miltiorrhiza* Bunge Family: Labiatae

COMMON NAME(S): Danshen, Tan-Shen, Tzu Tan-Ken (roots of purple sage), Hung Ken (red roots), Shu-Wei Ts'ao (rat-tail grass), Ch'ih Shen (scarlet sage), Pin-Ma Ts'ao (horse-racing grass)

BOTANY: Danshen is a perennial herb found mainly on sunny hillsides and stream edges. Violet-blue flowers bloom in the summer. The leaves are oval, with finely serrated edges. The fruit is an oval brown nut. Danshen's roots, from which many of the common names are derived, are a vivid scarlet red.[1] Danshen is related to common sage (of the same genus *Salvia*), the culinary herb.

HISTORY: Used in ancient Chinese medicine for generations, danshen joins many other of these remedies that must be evaluated scientifically to separate fact from myth in the therapeutic claims. In the mid-1980s, danshen (among other Chinese medicinal herbs similar in structure) was presented at the Chinese University of Hong Kong for discussion of its vasoactive properties.[2] The herb has also been used for menstrual irregularity, to "invigorate" the blood and for other ailments such as abdominal pain and insomnia.[1]

CHEMISTRY: Derivatives isolated from danshen include protocatechualdehyde and 3,4-dihydroxyphenyl-lactic acid, both of which are derived from a 4-substituted catechol structure. Structures of this type play a role as vasoactive agents.[2] Twenty-eight compounds, including tanshinones and related terpenoids, have been identified, using both HPTLC and mass spectrometric analysis.[3] Miltirone, an "active central benzodiazepine receptor ligand," has been isolated from the plant, from which twenty–one 0-quinonoid-type compounds and one coumarin-type compound have been synthesized.[4] Another report discusses the structure of "dihydroisotanshinone I" from danshen.[5] Salvianolic and rosmarinic acids have also been isolated from the plant.[6,7,8]

PHARMACOLOGY: Circulation improvement from danshen's use has long been practiced. Its ability to "invigorate" the blood is now being proven in many Chinese studies. Danshen has been used for **menstrual problems, to relieve bruising** and **to aid in granulation**.[1]

Pharmacokinetic studies of constituent 3,4-dihydroxyphenyl-lactic acid have been performed in rabbits.[9]

In animal studies, a mixture of danshen with chuanxiong excelled in preventing capillary contraction, thus improving circulation in a hypoxic, high-altitude environment.[10] However, this same mixture was not satisfactory to prevent cardiopulmonary changes caused by high altitudes in humans.[11]

Another danshen mixture, this time with foshousan, may offer protection to erythrocytes, improving blood flow to the placenta and increasing fetal birth weight in pregnant rats exposed to cigarette smoke.[12]

Danshen use in **ischemic stroke** has been reported.[13]

Danshen has been studied for its effects on mechanical activity and coronary flow rate in isolated rat hearts. After 30 minutes of ischemia, reperfusion was then allowed for 30 minutes. Although danshen exerted a negative inotropic effect, it caused an increase in coronary flow rate, suggesting some protective actions of the drug in ischemic situations.[14]

Antithrombotic actions of danshen have also been reported. A proposed mechanism of this effect may be related to a semisynthetic analog of plant constituent "salvianolic acid A." This "acetylsalvianolic acid A" reduced cerebral infarction and lessened neurological deficits in ischemic rats with cerebral artery thrombosis.[7] In another report, acetylsalvionolic acid A was also found to exert suppressive effects on collagen-induced platelet 5-HT release while inhibiting aggregation in vitro.[6] The rosmarinic acid isolate from danshen also displayed antithrombotic effects when injected into rats. This was because of platelet aggregation and promotion of fibrinolytic activity as well.[8]

Danshen use results in possible dilation of blood vessels, increase in portal blood flow and prevention of coagulation to improve tissue ischemia. This accelerates repair and enhances nutrition in hepatic cells.[2]

More than 70% of **chronic hepatitis** patients responded to danshen therapy in areas such as LFTY improvement and relief of symptoms such as nausea, malaise, liver pain and abdominal distention.[2] Another report confirms danshen therapeutic effects in chronic active hepatitis as well.[15]

Other effects of danshen include: **Cytotoxic activities** (of tanshinone analogs) against certain carcinoma cell lines, many of which were effective at concentrations less than 1 mcg per ml;[16] marked protective action against **gastric ulceration**;[17] and CNS effects[18] including **neurasthenia** and **insomnia** treatments.[1]

TOXICOLOGY: Coadministration of danshen and warfarin result in exaggerated warfarin adverse effects. Both pharmacodynamic and pharmacokinetic parameters were affected when studied in rats. Observed interactions such as increased warfarin bioavailability, decreased warfarin clearance and prolonged prothrombin times are all indicative of clinically important interactions if danshen and warfarin are taken together.[19,20] Severe clotting abnormalities have been reported in a case where danshen induces overcoagulation in a patient with rheumatic heart disease.[21] Another case report is available describing an interaction between danshen and methylsalicylate medicated oil.[22]

SUMMARY: Danshen has been used in ancient Chinese medicine for circulatory and related disorders. Some of its constituents are derived from a 4-substituted catechol structure responsible for the drug's vasoactive characteristics. Studies on dashen's effects on circulation improvement, protective actions against ischemia, antithrombotic effects and hepatitis are ongoing. Clinically important adverse interactions between warfarin and danshen have been reported more than once.

PATIENT INFORMATION – Danshen

Uses: Danshen's effects on circulation improvement have long been utilized. Danshen has also been used to alleviate menstrual irregularity, abdominal pains and insomnia.

Drug Interactions: Adverse effects of warfarin are exaggerated when danshen and warfarin are coadministered.

Side Effects: The most prominent side effect of danshen seems to be blood clotting disorders. Danshen can also cause difficulties when taken with warfarin or methylsalicylate medicated oil.

---

[1] A Barefoot Doctor's Manual (The American Translation of the Official Chinese Paramedical Manual). Running Press: Philadelphia, PA, 1997;657.
[2] Chang H, et al, ed. Advances in Chinese Medical Materials Research Symposium, 1984;217,559–80.
[3] Luo H, et al. Yao Hsueh Hsueh Pao 1989;24(5):341–47.
[4] Chang H, et al. J Med Chem 1991;43(5):1675–92.
[5] Kong D, et al. Yao Hsueh Hsueh Pao 1984;19(10):755–59.
[6] Yu W, et al. Yao Hsueh Hsueh Pao 1994;29(6):412–16.
[7] Dong J, et al. Yao Hsueh Hsueh Pao 1996;31(1):6–9.
[8] Zou Z, et al. Yao Hsueh Hsueh Pao 1993;28(4):241–45.
[9] Zhao F, et al. Biol Pharm Bull 1997;20(3):285–87.
[10] Zhang Z, et al. Chung Kuo Chung Yao Tsa Chih 1990;15(3):177–81.
[11] Feng S, et al. Chung Hsi I Chieh Ho Tsa Chih 1989;9(11):650–52.
[12] Han Q, et al. J Tongji Med Univ 1995;15(2):120–24.
[13] Anon. Chin Med J 1977;3(4):224–26.
[14] Zhou W, et al. Am J Chin Med 1990;18(1–2):19–24.
[15] Bai Y. Chung Hsi I Chieh Ho Tsa Chih 1984;4(2):86–87.
[16] Wu W, et al. Am J Chin Med 1991;19(3–4):207–16.
[17] Gu J. Chung Hua I Hsueh Tsa Chih (Taipei) 1991;71(6):630–32.
[18] Liao J, et al. Proc Natl Sci Counc Repub China B 1995;19(3):151–58.
[19] Lo A, et al. Eur J Drug Metab Pharmacokinet 1992;17(4):257–62.
[20] Chan K, et al. J Pharm Pharmacol 1995;47(5):402–6.
[21] Yu C, et al. J Intern Med 1997;241(4):337–39.
[22] Tam L, et al. Aust N Z J Med 1995;25(3):258.

Devil's Claw

SCIENTIFIC NAME(S): *Harpagophytum procumbens* DeCandolle. Family: Pediliaceae

COMMON NAME(S): Devils' claw, grapple plant

BOTANY: Devil's claw grows naturally in the Kalahari desert and Namibian steppes of southwest Africa. The secondary roots are used in decoctions and teas.

HISTORY: Devil's claw has been used by native Africans as a folk remedy for diseases ranging from liver and kidney disorders to allergies, headaches and, most commonly, rheumatisms. This drug, however, is more widely used in South Africa, expecially by Bushmen, Hottentots and Bantu.[1] Devil's claw is marketed in Canada and Europe as a home remedy for the relief of arthritic disease.[2]

CHEMISTRY: The major chemical component, which has been thought to be responsible for the anti-inflammatory activity of devil's claw, is harpagoside, a monoterpenic glucoside. Harpagide has also been shown to be one of the active principles of devil's claw.[3] Harpagoside is found primarily in the roots; secondary tubers contain twice as much glucoside as the primary roots. Flowers, stems and ripe fruits are essentially devoid of the compound while traces have been isolated from the leaves.[4] Harpagoside can be progressively hydrolyzed to harpagid and harpagogenin.[5] Commercial sources of devil's claw extract contain 1.4% to 2% harpagoside.[6]

The plant also contains procombide, a diasterio-isomer of antirrhinoside[7,8] and a variety of other glycosides, the pharmacologic significance of which is unknown.[9]

PHARMACOLOGY: Studies of the crude methanolic extract of the secondary roots of *Harpagophytum procumbens* indicate that its effect on smooth muscles is due to a complex interaction of the different active principles of the drug at the cholinergic receptors.[3] The dried crude methanolic extract, harpagoside, causes significant dose-dependent reduction in blood pressure, decreased heart rate and anti-arrhythmic activity on isolated rabbit heart and on intact rats.[10] The extract has shown that harpagoside interferes with the mechanisms that regulate the influx of calcium in cells of smooth muscles.[3] The methanolic extract also causes a mild decrease in the heart rate with a concomitant and positive inotropic effect at higher doses. The coronary flow decreases at higher doses only.

The negative chronotropic and positive inotropic effects of harpagoside are comparatively higher with respect to that of the extract, whereas harpagide has only a slight negative chronotropic effect and a considerable negative inotropic one.[11] In experiments on intact rats and on isolated rabbit heart, the *H. procumbens* extract has demonstrated a protective action with regard to arrhythmias induced by aconitine, and particularly to those provoked by calcium chloride and epinephrine chloroform.[11]

Aqueous extract of *H. procumbens* significantly reduces the carrageenan-induced edema at 400 and 800 mg/kg 4 hours after carrageenan injection. Orally administered extracts are inefficient, which could be attributed to the time in transition in the stomach, where the pH is acidic, causing a decrease in activity of the extract.[11]

The results of a German clinical study indicate that devil's claw has anti-inflammatory activity comparable to that of phenylbutazone. Analgesia was observed, along with a reduction in abnormally high uric acid and cholesterol levels.[12]

The suggestion that devil's claw possesses oxytocic or abortive properties has been largely disproved.

TOXICOLOGY: Harpagoside has been found to be of low toxicity with an LD$_{50}$ of greater than 13.5 g/kg in mice. Although no chronic toxicity studies have been reported, rats given oral doses of 7.5 g/kg/day harpagoside showed no clinical, hematologic or gross pathologic changes.[13] Adverse effects in human trials have been rare, generally consisting of headache, tinnitus or anorexia.

SUMMARY: Devil's claw extracts contain harpagoside and harpagide which possess anti-inflammatory activity, the ability to reduce blood pressure, decrease heart rate and slow anti-arrhythmic activities in animal studies. These extracts appear to be free of significant toxicities when given for short periods of time to animals and humans; little is known about their long-term toxicity or potential for interactions with other commonly used anti-inflammatory agents. Additional human clinical studies need to be conducted before the true efficacy of devil's claw can be stated.

PATIENT INFORMATION – Devil's Claw

Uses: Devil's claw is a folk remedy for an extensive range of diseases, including arthritis and rheumatism. Research suggests it may be useful as a hypotensive, anti-arrhythmic, anti-inflammatory, and analgesic.

Side Effects: Significant toxicity has not been observed in limited use.

---

[1] Ragusa S, et al. A drug used in traditional medicine. Harpagophytum procumbens D.C. Part I. Scanning electron microscope observations. *J Ethnopharmacol* 1984;11(3):245.

[2] Moussard C, et al. A drug used in traditional medicine, harpagophytum procumbens: no evidence for NSAID-like effect on whole blood eicosanoid production in human. *Prostaglandins Leuko Essent Fatty Acids* 2993;46(4):283.

[3] Occhiuto F, et al. A drug used in traditional medicine: *Harpagophytum procumbens* D.C. Part IV. Effects on some isolated muscle preparations. *J Ethnopharmacol* 1985;13(2):201.

[4] Czygan FC, Krueger A. *Planta Med* 1977;31:305.

[5] Vahaelen M, et al. Biological activity of Harpagophytum procumbens D.C. Part I. Preparation and structure of harpagogenin. *J Pharm Belg* 1981;36:38.

[6] Caprasse M. [Description, identification and therapeutic uses of the 'Devil's claw:' Harpagophytum procumbens D.C.] [French] *J Pharm Belg* 1980;35(2):143.

[7] Biancho A, et al. *Gazz Chim Ital* 1971;101:764.

[8] Bendall M, et al. The structure of procumbide. *Aust J Chem* 1979;32(9):2085.

[9] Tunmann P, Bauersfeld HJ. [Further components from radix Harpagophytum procumbens D.C.] [German] *Arch Pharm* 1975;308(8):655.

[10] Circosta C, et al. Drug used in traditional medicine: Harpagophytum procumbens D.C. Part 2. Cardiovascular activity. *J Ethnopharmacol* 1984;11:259.

[11] Soulimani R, et al. The role of stomachal digestion on the pharmacological activity of plant extracts, using as an example extracts of *Harpagophytum procumbens*. *Can J Physiol Pharmacol* 1994;72:1532.

[12] Kampf R. *Schweitz Apothek Zeitung* 1976;114:337.

[13] Whitehouse LW, et al. Devil's Claw (Harpagophytum procumbens): no evidence for anti-inflammatory activity in the treatment of arthritic disease. *Can Med Assoc J* 1983;129(3):249.

Devil's Club

SCIENTIFIC NAME(S): *Oplopanax horridus* (Sm.) Miq. Also referred to as *Panax horridum* Sm., *Echinopanax horridum* (Sm.) Decne. & Planch., *Fatsia horrida* (Sm.) Benth. & Hook. Family: Araliaceae (the ginseng family)

COMMON NAME(S): Devil's club, cukilanarpak (native Alaskan for "large plant with needles")[1]

BOTANY: This hardy plant grows in moist ravines and well-drained soils along much of the Alaskan coast and adjacent regions of Canada and northwestern United States; it can be found up to 100 miles inland, forming nearly impenetrable thickets.[2] The plants attain heights of 5 m, and the densely thorned stem can reach 3 cm in diameter.[2] Greenish-white flowers appear in June, producing scarlet berries in late summer.

HISTORY: This plant has a long tradition of use, particularly among native Alaskans and other populations in the Northwestern regions of the United States and Canada. The prickly outer bark sometimes is scraped from the stem, leaving the cambium for use in the preparation of decoctions and poultices; others, however, use both the cambium and stem together.[1] The cambium sometimes is softened by chewing prior to being placed on a cut or burn. In many cultures, the plant is believed to possess "magical" powers that impart great strength.[2] Traditional uses of extracts of the plant have included the treatment of arthritis, as a purgative and emetic, for the treatment of body pain, to promote wound healing, to control fever, tuberculosis, stomach trouble, coughs and colds and pneumonia.[1,2] The berries are not eaten and are considered useless or toxic by some.

CHEMISTRY: Preliminary chemical investigations into the constituents of devil's club reported the absence of alkaloids and gallic acid, and the presence of oleic and unsaturated fatty acids, saponins, glycerides and tannins.[3] An ether extract of the root yielded two oils, equinopanacene (a sesquiterpene) and equinopanacol (a sesquiterpene alcohol).[4]

PHARMACOLOGY: Several animal investigations were conducted in the 1930s and 1940s in an attempt to characterize the pharmacologic activity associated with the traditional uses of devil's club. Following reports that patients with diabetes could be managed successfully using water extracts of the root bark, animal-based investigations suggested that the extract had hypoglycemic activity in the hare and that the plant was not associated with toxicity.[5] Further investigations were unable to verify the hypoglycemic effect in rabbits.[3,6] No pharmacologically active component could be identified in the plant.[3] A report of a case study of two patients given extracts of the plant in conjunction with a glucose tolerance test found no hypoglycemic effects that could be attributed to devil's club.[2]

The dried roots and stalk have been reported to inhibit the effects of pregnant mare serum on the growth of the ovaries of the white rat. The ovaries of control rats weighed more than eight times those of test animals that received the serum together with 40 mg of dried plant per dose.[7]

TOXICOLOGY: Although no cases of significant toxicity have been reported, several points should be kept in mind regarding devil's club. The spiny covering of the stem can cause painful irritation and scratches upon contact. The use of devil's club extract as an emetic and purgative are reflective of potential toxicity from use of the plant. Although the hypoglycemic effect has not been confirmed, the continued traditional use of this plant for the management of diabetes suggests that some persons may be sensitive to the hypoglycemic effects of devil's club and should use the plant with caution.

SUMMARY: The use of devil's club is steeped in tradition, particularly among native Alaskans. Although the plant has been reported to have hypoglycemic activity, no strong evidence supports this effect.

PATIENT INFORMATION – Devil's Club

Uses: Devil's club has been traditionally made into decoctions and poultices for diabetes, arthritis, wounds, fever, pain, and as a purgative and emetic.

Side Effects: Traditional use as a hypoglycemic, purgative, and emetic suggests potential toxicity.

[1] Russell PN. English Bay and Port Graham Alutiq Plantlore. Homer, AK: Pratt Museum, 1991.

[2] Smith GW. Arctic pharmacognosia II. Devil's club, *Oplopanax horridus. J Ethnopharmacol* 1983;7:313.

[3] Stuhr ET, Henry FB. An investigation of the root bark of *Fatsia horrida. Pharmaceutical Arch* 1944;15:9.

[4] Kariyone T, Morotomi SJ. The essential oil of *Echinopanax horridus. J Pharm Soc Japan* 1927;546:671.

[5] Large RG, Brocklesby HN. A hypoglycemic substance from the roots of devil's club. *Can Med J Assoc* 1938;39:32.

[6] Piccoli LJ, Spinapolice BS, Hecht M. A pharmacologic study of devil's club root. *J Am Pharm Assoc* 1940;29:11.

[7] Graham RCB, Noble RL. Comparison of in vitro activity of various species of Lithospermum and other plants to inactivate gonadotrophin. *Endocrinology* 1955;56:239.

Devil's Dung

SCIENTIFIC NAME(S): *Ferula assafoetida* L., *F. foetida* Regel, *F. rubricaulis* Boissier and possibly other sp. Family: Umbelliferae

COMMON NAME(S): Asafetida, asafoetida, devil's dung, gum asafetida

BOTANY: Indigenous to eastern Iran and western Afghanistan, asafetida is the gum resin obtained from the dried roots and rhizomes of this plant. This perennial herb branches up to 9 feet and appears as a soft, almost semiliquid mass of tears, as irregular masses of agglutinated tears or as separate egg-shaped tears. This tear-like part of the plant undergoes a gradual change from a shimmering yellowish white to a violet-streaked pink and finally to reddish brown.[1]

HISTORY: The resin has been used as an expectorant, carminative and intestinal spasmodic, and was administered rectally to control colic. A suspension of the product has been used as a repellent against dogs, cats and other wildlife. Its use continues especially within African-American communities.[1] Asafetida has been used for tumors in the abdomen, corns and calluses, as an aphrodisiac, diuretic, sedative and stimulant. In folk remedies, it is used for amenorrhea, asthma, convulsions, croup, insanity and sarcomas.[2] However, its main use is as a fragrance component in perfumes.

With a taste stronger than onion or garlic, the product continues to be available as the gum resin or as a solution. It is found in pharmacies and ethnic and health food stores where it is sold as a food preservative and spice. At very low levels, it is sometimes used in candies, beverages, relishes and sauces.[2]

CHEMISTRY: Despite its popularity, asafetida gum has a major drawback — a putrid, almost nauseating odor and bitter, acrid taste — which serves as the basis for its common name, devil's dung. Asafetida contains a number of terpenes and lipid-soluble substances, which have not been well characterized. It is composed of up to 20% volatile oil, 65% resin and 25% gum. Isobutylpropanyld-isulfide, pinene, cadinene and vanillin are found in the oil. Umbelliferone, asaresinotannol and ferulic acid have been found in the resin.

PHARMACOLOGY: There are no animal or clinical studies evaluating the efficacy of devil's dung in any disorder. In a study in rats, asafetida did not reduce serum cholesterol levels.[3] In vitro, an alcoholic extract of asafetida showed some cytotoxicity against lymphoma ascites, tumor cells and human lymphocytes.[4]

TOXICOLOGY: The topical use of asafetida may result in skin irritation. Ingestion of the product has not been associated with severe toxicity in adults. However, one report described the case of a 5-week-old child who developed severe methemoglobinemia after being given an undetermined amount of glycerated asafetida solution (a mixture of asafetida, glycerol, propylene glycol and calcium carbonate, available over the counter).[5] In vitro testing found gum asafetida to exert a strong oxidative effect on purified fetal hemoglobin, leading to the recommendation that this folk remedy should be considered potentially life threatening if given to infants.

SUMMARY: Asafetida persists as a folk remedy, especially among the African-American population in the United States. There is no evidence that the material exerts any therapeutic effect, and its use should be discouraged in children because of a potential to induce methemoglobinemia. The resin is used safely in small quantities as a spice.

PATIENT INFORMATION – Devil's Dung

Uses: The gum resin, asafetida, is used as a flavoring, food preservative, and fragrance. It is used as a folk remedy for a wide variety of ills and as an aphrodisiac, diuretic, sedative, and stimulant.

Side Effects: It should be considered potentially life threatening to infants, although ingestion has not been associated with severe toxicity in adults. It may cause topical irritation.

[1] Tyler VE, et al. Pharmacognosy. Philadelphia, PA: Lea & Febiger, 1988.

[2] Duke JA. Handbook of Medicinal Herbs. Boca Raton, FL: CRC Press, 1985.

[3] Kamanna VS, Chandrasekhara N. Effects of garlic (*Allium sativum* Linn) on serum lipoproteins and lipoprotein cholesterol levels in albino rats rendered hypercholesteremic by feeding cholesterol. *Lipids* 1982;17:483.

[4] Unnikrishnan MC, Kuttan R. Cytotoxicity of extracts of spices to cultured cells. *Nutr Cancer* 1988;11:251.

[5] Kelly KJ, et al. Experience and reason. *Pediatrics* 1984;73:717.

Dichroa Root

SCIENTIFIC NAME(S): *Dichroa febrifuga Lour.* Family: Saxifragaceae.

COMMON NAME(S): Dichroa root, ch'ang shan (Chinese), huang ch'ang-shan (yellow alum root), t'u ch'ang-shan (native alum root), chi-ku feng, chi-ku ch'ang-shan (chicken-bone alum root), pai ch'ang-shan (white alum root), ta chin-tao (big golden sword), chi-fen ts'ao (chicken-droppings grass).

BOTANY: Dichroa root comes from a deciduous shrub that prefers damp areas such as wooded valleys or stream edges. The roots and leaves are used medicinally. The plant bears light-blue flowers and blue-colored berries.[1,2]

HISTORY: For many centuries in China, dichroa root was used to treat malaria.[3,4] One of the earliest recorded uses of "plants as medicine" include dichroa root.[5] Chinese scholar/emperor Shen Nung (c. 2735 BC) recorded the plant's effectiveness in treating fevers caused by malaria parasites.[6]

CHEMISTRY: Alkaloid febrifugine and its isomer isofebrifugine were isolated during World War II in order to study their effects against malaria.[3,4] Febrifugine is the main alkaloidal constituent present.[7]

PHARMACOLOGY: With drug resistance from medications such as chloroquine and quinine becoming prevalent, researchers sought other possible antimalarial sources. Isolates of *D. febrifuga*, febrifugine, and isofebrifugine were found to be the active principles against malaria. However, chemists could not separate adverse effects such as nausea, vomiting, and diarrhea from its beneficial actions.[6,8,9] Febrifugine and isofebrifugine in certain preparations (eg, acetone extract) demonstrated high antimalarial activity against *Plasmodium falciparum* and *P. berghei*.[4] Aqueous extract of dichroa studied in mice against *P. berghei* demonstrated an inhibition of infection rate and an increase in mean survival time.[10] Two reports suggest that dichroa extracts alter nitric oxide (NO) concentrations. It was found that infected mice administered febrifugine at 1 mg/kg/day orally increased NO production, thus contributing to host defense against

malaria infection. Febrifugine reduced mortality and parasitemia, as well as increased plasma NO concentrations.[7] Febrifugine had the same NO increasing effects in mice peritoneal macrophages with dose-dependent activations.[11] However, another report demonstrates aqueous extract of dichroa decreasing NO production as well as tumor necrosis factor, which plays a role in endotoxin-mediated shock and inflammation. In mouse macrophages, NO synthase and NO serum levels were decreased by the extract, suggesting a suppression of inflammatory response and possible use as an anti-inflammatory drug.[12]

Changrolin, a Chinese antiarrhythmic drug derived from dichroa, has been studied for its antiarrhythmic effects in small mammal cardiac cells.[13]

Other claims from animal studies for dichroa root include its use for bronchitis to remove sputum, as an emetic, and as an antipyretic.[1,3]

TOXICOLOGY: Little information concerning toxicity of dichroa root is available, except for the previously mentioned nausea, vomiting, and diarrhea.[6,14]

SUMMARY: Dichroa root has been used for many centuries in China, and its effectiveness in treating malaria has been noted as far back as 2735 BC. The active alkaloids are febrifugine and isofebrifugine. Modern studies in animals have shown febrifugine and isofebrifugine are active against malaria parasites, involving possible alteration of NO, which is important in host defense. Nausea, vomiting, and diarrhea are some adverse effects observed in animal studies.

PATIENT INFORMATION – Dichroa Root

Uses: Dichroa root has been used to treat malaria for centuries in China.

Side Effects: Possible adverse effects include nausea, vomiting, and diarrhea.

---

[1] A Barefoot Doctor's Manual: Practical Chinese Medicine and Health. Bethesda, MD: US Department of Health, Education & Welfare; 1977;878.

[2] http://www.gardenbed.com/D/4564.cfm.

[3] Hocking, G. A Dictionary of Natural Products. Medford, NJ: Plexus Publishing, Inc.; 1977;253.

[4] Takaya Y, et al. New type of febrifugine analogues, bearing a quinolizidine moiety, show potent antimalarial activity against *Plasmodium* malaria parasite. *J Med Chem* 1999;42:3163-66.

[5] Taylor J. Introductory Medicinal Chemistry. Chichester, UK: Ellis Horwood Ltd.; 1981.

[6] Burger, A. Understanding Medications. What the Label Doesn't Tell You. Washington, DC: American Chemical Society Publication; 1999.

[7] Murata K, et al. Potentiation by febrifugine of host defense in mice against *Plasmodium berghei* NK65. *Biochem Pharmacol* 1999;58(10):1593-601.

[8] Zhao C. Effect of *Dichroa febrifuga* L. on chloroquinsensible and chloroquin-resistant malaria parasites. [German]. *J Tongji Med Univ* 1986;6(2):112-15.

[9] Zeng, Y. Development of plant derived drugs in China. *Pharm Weekbl* 1982;117:1037-43.

[10] Gopal H, et al. Effect of *Dichroa febrifuga* on *Plasmodium berghei. Indian J Pathol Microbiol* 1982;25(4):269-72.

[11] Murata K, et al. Enhancement of NO production in activated macrophages in vivo by an antimalarial crude drug, *Dichroa febrifuga. J Nat Prod* 1998;61(6):729-33.

[12] Kim Y, et al. The production of nitric oxide and TNF-alpha in peritoneal macrophages is inhibited by *Dichroa febrifuga* Lour. *J Ethnopharmacol* 2000;69(1):35-43.

[13] Lu L, et al. Electrophysiological effects of changrolin, an antiarrhythmic agent derived from *Dichroa febrifuga*, on guinea pig and rabbit heart cells. *Clin Exp Pharmacol Physiol* 1995;22(5):337-41.

[14] http://ascaris.med.tmd.ac.jp/JSP/68meeting/program2.html.

Digitalis

SCIENTIFIC NAME(S): *Digitalis purpurea* L.; *D. lanata* Ehrh. Family: Scrophulariaceae, the figwort family. Related species that have found some use in traditional medicine include *D. lutea* (straw foxglove), *D. grandiflora* and D. ambigua (yellow foxglove), and *D. ferriginea* (rusty foxglove).[1]

COMMON NAME(S): Foxglove, purple foxglove, throatwort, fairy finger, fairy cap, lady's thimble, scotch mercury, lion's mouth, witch's bells, dead man's bells, wolly foxglove, digitalis.[1,2,7,8]

BOTANY: The foxglove is typically a biennial plant (but may be annual or perennial depending on the species) characterized by a thick, cylindrical downy stem that reaches a height of up to 6 feet. The leaves form a thick rosette during the first year of growth. The leaves, which are wooly and veined and covered with whitish hairs on the underside, have a very bitter taste. The flowers grow in the first or second year, depending on the species, and are tubular and bell-shaped, growing to 3 inches in length. Although many colors of flowers have been bred from digitalis, the flowers are rarely white. The plant is native to the British Isles, Western Europe and parts of Africa, but today is found as an ornamental throughout the world.

HISTORY: Although the use of foxglove has been traced back to 10th century Europe, it was not until its scientific investigation by William Withering in the late 1700s that the plant became widely used as a diuretic for the treatment of dropsy.[1] In South America, preparations of the powdered leaves are used to relieve asthma, as sedatives and as diuretic/cardiotonics. In India, an ointment containing digitalis glycosides is used to treat wounds and burns.[1] Today, digitalis glycosides are widely used in the treatment of congestive heart failure; however, because of their narrow therapeutic margin and high potential for severe side effects, the use of these products is beginning to be supplanted by newer agents including the angiotensin converting enzyme inhibitors and the calcium channel blocking agents.

CHEMISTRY: Ornamental strains of *D. purpurea* typically have low concentrations of active compounds. Leaves of wild varieties that have been used for medicinal purposes contain at least 30 different glycosides in total quantities ranging from 0.1% to 0.6%; these consist primarily of purpurea glycoside A (yielding digitoxin) and glycoside B, the precursor of gitoxin. Upon hydrolysis, digitoxin and gitoxin loose sugar molecules producing their respective aglycones, digitoxigenin and gitoxigenin. Seeds also contain digitalis glycosides.[1]

The main glycosides of *D. lanata* are the lanatosides, designated A through E. Removal of acetyl groups and sugars results in formation of digitoxin, gitoxin, digoxin, digitalin and gitaloxin.[1,3] *D. lanata* is not typically used in powder form in the United States, but serves as a major source of lanatoside C and digoxin.

PHARMACOLOGY: Digitoxin is 1000 times more potent than the powdered leaves and is completely and rapidly absorbed from the gastrointestinal tract.[1] Digoxin is 300 times more potent than the powder prepared from *D. purpurea*. All cardiac glycosides share the characteristic of improving cardiac conduction, thereby improving the strength of cardiac contractility. These drugs also possess some antiarrhythmic activity, but will induce arrhythmias at higher dose levels.

Digitoxin has shown antitumor activity in the KB tumor system.[2] Some investigators have suggested that the incidence of cancers is lower among patients receiving digitalis glycosides[4] and that these compounds may offer some protection by virtue of their structural similarity to estrogens. Tumors from patients receiving these glycosides were found to be smaller in size, less prone to distant metastasis, more uniform in morphology and their small nuclei had lower RNA and DNA contents than did those of breast cancer patients not taking digitalis glycosides.[5]

The pharmacology and pharmacokinetics of the digitalis glycosides have been extensively studied. For a concise review on the medicinal use of commercial products, please refer to a standard reference book.[9]

TOXICOLOGY: All parts of the plant are toxic. Animal toxicity occurs during grazing. Children have been made ill by sucking the flowers or ingesting seeds or parts of the leaves. The toxic doses of fresh leaves are reported as 6 to 7 ounces for an ox, 4 to 5 ounces for a horse, and 0.5 to 0.75 ounces for a pig.[1] Deaths have been reported among persons who drank tea made from foxglove mistakenly identified for comfrey.[2]

Digitalis glycosides are excreted slowly and accumulate; therefore, intoxications during therapy are common. The incidence of digitalis toxicity had been estimated to range from 5% to 23%. More stringent dosing guidelines and monitoring techniques have dramatically reduced the incidence of therapeutic overdose.

Signs of poisoning by the plant or purified drug include contracted pupils, blurred vision, strong but slowed pulse, nausea, vomiting, dizziness, excessive urination, fatigue, muscle weekness and tremors; in severe cases, stupor, confusion, convulsions and death occur.[1,10] Cardiac signs include atrial arrhythmias and atrioventricular block.[1] Chronic digitalis intoxication is characterized by visual halos, yellow-green vision and gastrointestinal upset.

Gastric lavage or emesis together with supportive measures such as electrolyte replacements, antiarrhythmias, such as lidocaine and phenytoin, atropine and other agents that can antagonize the cardiovascular effects of the glycosides, have been used to manage acute poisonings.[2,10] Digoxin-specific Fab antibody fragments (Digibind) are effective in managing acute intoxications caused by digitalis and related cardioactive glycosides.[6,9,10] This therapy is revolutionary for the severely poisoned patient.

SUMMARY: Foxglove and its derivatives are critically important in the management of congestive heart failure and related cardiac disorders. Their uses continue to be strong in underdeveloped countries where they can be used cost effectively. The plants are grown ornamentally throughout much of the world, and vigilance must be used if children or animals can come in contact with the potentially lethal plants.

PATIENT INFORMATION – Digitalis

Uses: In addition to a range of other traditional uses, digitalis has long been used as a recognized treatment for heart failure. The plant is cultivated as an ornamental.

Side Effects: Ingestion of extremely small amounts of the plant may be fatal to humans, especially children and to animals. Toxicity is cumulative.

---

[1] Morton JF. Major Medicinal Plants. Springfield, IL: Charles C. Thomas, 1977.
[2] Duke JA. Handbook of Medicinal Herbs. Boca Raton, FL: CRC Press, 1985.
[3] Evans WC. Trease and Evans' Pharmacognosy, 13th ed. London: Balliere Tindall, 1989.
[4] Goldin AG, Safa AR. Digitalis and cancer. *Lancet* 1984;8386:1134.
[5] Stenkvist B, Bengtsson E, Eklund G, et al. Evidence of a modifying influence of heart glycoside on the development of breast cancer. *Anal Quant Cytol* 1980;2:49.
[6] Shumaik GM, Wu AW, Ping AC. Oleander poisoning: treatment with digoxin-specific Fab antibody fragments. *Ann Emerg Med* 1988;17:732.

[7] Dobelis IN, ed. Magic and Medicine of Plants. Pleasantville, NY: Readers Digest, 1986:188.
[8] Meyer JE. The Herbalist. Hammond, IN: Hammond Book Co, 1934:96.
[9] Olin BR, Hebel SK, eds. Drug Facts and Comparisons. St. Louis: Facts and Comparisons, 1988:141,712b
[10] Dick M, Curwin J, Tepper D. Digitalis intoxication recognition and management. *J Clin Pharmacol* 1991;31:444.

Dolomite

COMMON NAME(S): Dolomite, dolomitic limestone

HISTORY: Dolomite has long been used as a source of calcium and magnesium for animal feeds. Dolomite is now available in a number of dosage forms including tablets and chewable wafers, to be taken as dietary supplements.

CHEMISTRY: Dolomite is a form of limestone rich in approximately equal parts of magnesium carbonate and calcium carbonate. It is found widely throughout the world. Dolomitic limestone contains about five times as much magnesium and five eighths as much calcium as ordinary limestone. Dolomite also contains small amounts of chlorine, phosphorus, and potassium,[1] in addition to more than 20 other trace minerals.[2]

PHARMACOLOGY: Dolomite appears to be a good source of magnesium and calcium supplementation. In animal models, minerals from dolomite are well absorbed.[3]

TOXICOLOGY: Although the use of pure dolomite supplements has not been associated with toxicity, concern has arisen over the use of dolomite preparations contaminated with heavy metals.

Dolomite mined from a location near a lead mine was found to contain up to 2,700 ppm (after addition to animal feed), a level that would have induced lead toxicity in the cattle that ingested it; milk and meat products from these animals would have been unsafe for human consumption.[4]

Of similar concern has been the detection of elevated levels of heavy metals in dolomite preparations intended for human consumption. One product, for example, that was used as a mineral supplement was contaminated with aluminum (187 ppm), lead (35 ppm), nickel (13 ppm), arsenic (24 ppm) and mercury (12 ppm), among other trace elements.[5]

Contaminated dolomite products have been reported to precipitate psychomotor seizures in otherwise controlled epileptics.[2]

SUMMARY: Dolomitic limestone preparations are good sources of calcium and magnesium for dietary supplementation. In general, they may be taken with little concern about toxicity or side effects. Some products, however, have been shown to be contaminated with often significant levels of heavy metals, which may pose a toxicologic hazard.

PATIENT INFORMATION – Dolomite

Uses: Dolomitic limestone is a supplementary source of magnesium and calcium.

Side Effects: Products contaminated with heavy metals are considered hazardous.

---

[1] Worthinton-Roberts B, Breskin MA. *Am Pharm* 1983;8:421.
[2] Roberts HJ. Potential toxicity due to dolomite and bonemeal. *South Med J* 1983;76(5):556.
[3] Greger JL, et al. Interactions of lactose with calcium, magnesium and zinc in rats. *J Nutr* 1989;119(11):1691.
[4] *FDA Consumer.* 1981;15(9):35.
[5] Roberts HJ. *N Engl J Med* 1981;304(7):423.

Dong Quai

SCIENTIFIC NAME(S): *Angelica sinensis* (Oliv.) Diels, synonymous with *A. polymorpha* var. *sinensis* Oliv. Family: Apiaceae (carrot family)

COMMON NAME(S): Dong quai, danggui, tang-kuei, Chinese angelica

BOTANY: Three species of *Angelica* are monographed separately in the Chinese pharmacopeia: Dong quai, the root of *Angelica sinensis*; Bai zi, the root of *Angelica dahurica* (Fisch.) Benth. et. Hook. f. or *A. dahurica* var. *formosana* (Boiss.) Shan et Yuan; and Du huo, the root of *A. pubescens* Maxim. *f. biserrata* Shan et Yuan.[1] In Korea, *A. gigas* Nakai is used medicinally, while in Japan, *A. acutiloba* Kitagawa is used. The European *A. archangelic* L. is used to flavor liqueurs and confections. While botanically related, do not confuse the various species of *Angelica*, which differ in chemistry, pharmacology, and toxicology. A molecular biology study of *A. acutiloba* may lead to efficient methods for distinguishing raw materials.[2]

HISTORY: Dong quai is widely used in traditional Chinese medicine and continues to be popular in China and elsewhere. It is used to treat menstrual disorders, as an analgesic in rheumatism, and used in suppressing allergy symptoms. It is promoted for similar uses in the American herb market.

CHEMISTRY: The chemistry of *A. sinensis* is distinct from the other species. While coumarins have been reported from this species,[3] a recent comparative study of commercial dong quai products and related species[4] found coumarins to be lacking, while the lactone Z-ligustilide was a major constituent. In fact, in this study, *A. sinensis* more closely resembled *Levisticum officinale* in chemical composition than it did the other species of *Angelica*. Thus, there is good justification for terming the latter plant "European dong quai." Several other lactones related to ligustilide have been found in *A. sinensis*.[5,6,7] Ferulic acid and its esters were also found in *A. sinensis*. A capillary electrophoresis method for measuring ferulic acid in *A. sinensis* has been published.[8]

In contrast, the roots of *A. dahurica* have been found to contain an abundance of coumarins. Imperatorin and isoimperatorin are the major constituents, with many other related compounds (eg, bergapten, phellopterin, scopoletin) reported.[9] Ferulic acid was also detected in this species.[10]

The root of *A. pubescens* contains coumarins, but with some differences from *A. dahurica*. The simple prenylcou-marin, osthole, and the linear furocoumarins, columbianadin and columbianetin acetate, are the major constituents while the coumarins, angelols A-H, are characteristic of the species.[11,12]

The common polyacetylene falcarindiol has been isolated from various species of *Angelica*.[4] Polysaccharides have been isolated from different species of *Angelica*; however, they have not been characterized sufficiently to permit comparison.[13] Simple plant sterols and lipids have also been found.[14]

PHARMACOLOGY:

Antiallergy effects: A water extract of *A. sinensis* inhibited IgE-antibody production in a mouse model of atopic allergy. The extract was active orally and the activity was retained on dialysis, indicating that it was caused by high molecular weight components of the extract.[15]

Antispasmodic effects: The simple lactone ligustilide is thought to be a major bioactive principle of dong quai. Its antiasthmatic action was studied in guinea pigs.[16] Ligustilide and the related butylidenephthalide and butylphthalide were found to have antispasmodic activity against rat uterine contractions and in other smooth muscle systems. The compounds were characterized as nonspecific antispasmodics with a mechanism different from papaverine.[17] The ligustilide and butylidenephthalide constituents of Japanese angelica root were found to reverse the decrease in pentobarbital sleep induced by either isolation stress or yohimbine, implicating central noradrenergic or GABA systems in their actions.[18]

Anticoagulant effects: The coumarins of *Angelica* species have been associated with both bioactivity and toxicity of the plants; however, the low coumarin content of *A. sinensis* minimizes its importance in dong quai pharmacology. In other species of *Angelica*, coumarins clearly play an important role. Simple coumarins often have anticoagulant effects, while the linear furocoumarins are well known as photosensitizing agents.[19]

Anti-inflammatory effects: The simple prenylcoumarin, osthole, is a major constituent of *A. pubescens* (Du huo).[20] Osthole showed anti-inflammatory activity in carageenan-induced rat paw edema and acetic acid-induced writhing in mice.[20] Osthole also caused relaxation of rat thoracic aorta preparations[21] and inhibited proliferation of rat vascular smooth muscle cells.[22] Another study found that osthole inhibited the second phase of edema caused by formalin in the rat.[23] An inhibitory effect was also seen for osthole on 5-lipoxygenase and cyclooxygenase.[24] The related prenylcoumarin angelols were shown to inhibit platelet aggregation.[25]

The linear furocoumarin phellopterin was found to bind with high affinity to benzodiazepine receptors in vitro; however, other closely related furocoumarins were weaker or inactive.[26] Phellopterin was characterized as a competitive partial agonist of central benzodiazepine receptors by GABA and TBPS shift assays.[27] No in vivo experiments were reported. Other furocoumarins from *A. dahurica* inhibited histamine release in a mouse peritoneal cavity assay,[28] while isoimperatorin was analgesic; columbianadin, columbianetin acetate, and bergapten were anti-inflammatory and analgesic.[23] Finally, the action of various coumarins from *A. dahurica* on lipolysis in fat cells of rats were examined, with some coumarins activating lipolysis and other coumarins inhibiting lipolysis.[29]

Menopause: Dong quai is widely used in the US to treat hot flashes and other symptoms of menopause. A randomized, double-blind, placebo-controlled trial of *A. sinensis* as a single agent found no effect on vasomotor flushes, endometrial thickness, or on the level of estradiol or estrone. The study material was standardized for ferulic acid content.[30] A polyherbal preparation including dong quai was shown to reduce menopausal symptoms in a much smaller clinical trial.[31]

INTERACTIONS: The possibility of herb-drug interactions between *Angelica* coumarins and warfarin has been postulated[32] and is supported by one case report,[33] a patient stabilized on warfarin therapy experienced more than a 2-fold increase in prothrombin time and international normalized ratio 4 weeks after starting dong quai.[33] The values returned to the therapeutic range 4 weeks after discontinuing dong quai. Monitor patients receiving warfarin.

TOXICOLOGY: Coumarins are the focus of toxicology in *Angelica*. Furanocoumarins such as bergapten and psoralen have been widely studied for their photoactivated toxicity; however, only *A. gigas* (Korean angelica) has been demonstrated to cause photodermatitis.[34] Clearly the risk of phototoxicity should be correlated with the content of specific toxic furocoumarins. In the case of A. sinensis, there appears to be little risk, but with *A. gigas*, *A. dahurica*, and *A. pubescens*, there is a very reasonable cause for caution. Possible synergism with calcium channel blockers may occur. *Angelica archangelica* L. is reported to be an abortifacient and to affect the menstrual cycle. *A. sinensis* has uterine stimulant activity.

SUMMARY: Dong quai is monographed in the Chinese Pharmacopeia, the British Herbal Pharmacopeia (vol. 2), and by WHO (vol. 2). An American Herbal Pharmacopeia monograph is in progress.

Dong quai is a Chinese medicine used widely to treat menopause symptoms; however, convincing proof of efficacy in humans is lacking. Animal studies support anti-inflammatory, antiasthmatic, and antiallergy effects, but these observations require clinical study. Monitor the potential interaction with warfarin and other anticoagulants. Phototoxicity appears to be a problem with related species of *Angelica*, but not with authentic dong quai.

PATIENT INFORMATION – Dong Quai

Uses: Traditionally used as an analgesic for rheumatism, an allergy suppressant, and in the treatment of menstrual disorders, dong quai has been shown to possess antiasthmatic, antispasmodic, anti-inflammatory, and anticoagulant properties. It has also been used to flavor liqueurs and confections.

Drug Interactions: The possibility of dong quai interactions with warfarin has been postulated and is supported by at least one report. Possible synergism with calcium channel blockers may occur.

Side Effects: No reported side effects have occurred with authentic dong quai, but with *A. gigas*, *A. dahurica*, and *A. pubescens*, there is a very reasonable risk of phototoxicity. *Angelica archangelica* L. is reported to be an abortifacient and to affect the menstrual cycle. *A. sinensis* has uterine stimulant activity.

1 Tang W, et al. Chinese Drugs of Plant Origin: Chemistry, Pharmacology, and Use in Traditional and Modern Medicine. Berlin: Springer-Verlag,1992:113-125.

2 Mizukami H. Amplification and sequence of a 5s-rRNA gene spacer region from the crude drug "angelica root". *Biol Pharm Bull* 1995;18:1299-301.

3 Hata K, et al. [On the coumarins of the roots of *Angelica polymorpha* Maxim.] *Yakugaku Zasshi* 1967;87:464-65. Japanese.

4 Zschocke S, et al. Comparative study of roots of *Angelica sinensis* and related Umbelliferous drugs by thin layer chromatography, high-performance liquid chromatography, and liquid chromatography-mass spectrometry. *Phytochem Anal* 1998;9:283.

5 Sheu S, et al. Analysis and processing of Chinese herbal drugs; VI. The study of *Angelicae radix*. *Planta Med* 1986;53:377.

6 Hon P, et al. A ligustilide dimer from *Angelica sinensis*. *Phytochemistry* 1990;29:1189.

7 Chen Y, et al. Analysis of the composition of *Angelica sinensis* –determination of the essential oil composition by capillary column GC/MS. *Gaodeng Xuexiao Huaxue Xuebao* 1984;5:125.

8 Ji S, et al. Determination of ferulic acid in *Angelica sinensis* and Chuanxiong by capillary zone electrophoresis. *Biomed Chromatogr* 1999;13:333-34.

9 Okuyama T, et al. Studies on the antitumor-promoting activity of naturally occurring substances. II. Inhibition of tumor-promoter-enhanced phospholipid metabolism by umbelliferous materials. *Chem Pharm Bull* 1990;38:1084-86.

10 Kwon Y, et al. Antimicrobial constituents of *Angelica dahurica* roots. *Phytochemistry* 1997;44:887-89.

11 Kozawa M, et al. Studies on coumarins from the root of *Angelica pubescens* Maxim. III. Structures of various coumarins including angelin, a new prenyl-coumarin. *Chem Pharm Bull* 1980;28:1782.

12 Baba K, et al. Studies on coumarins from the root of *Angelica pubescens* Maxim. IV. Structures of angelol-type prenylcoumarins. *Chem Pharm Bull* 1982;30:2025.

13 Choy Y, et al. Immunopharmacological studies of low molecular weight polysaccharide from *Angelica sinensis*. *Am J Chin Med* 1994;22:137-45.

14 Tani S, et al. Studies on constituents of *Angelica dahurica*. II. Identification of gamma-nonalactone and gamma-decalactone by GC and GC/MS as a part of the odor components. *J Nat Prod* 1980;47:734.

15 Sung C, et al. Effect of extracts of *Angelica polymorpha* on reaginic antibody production. *J Nat Prod* 1982;45:398-406.

16 Tao J, et al. [Studies on the antiasthmatic action of ligustilide of dang-gui, *Angelica sinensis* (Oliv.) Diels.] *Yao Hsueh Hsueh Pao* 1984;19:561-65. Chinese.

17 Ko W. A newly isolated antispasmodic - butylidenephthalide. *Jpn J Pharmacol* 1980;30:85-91.

18 Matsumoto K, et al. Effects of methylenechloride-soluble fraction of Japanese angelica root extract, ligustilide and butylidenephthalide, on pentobarbital sleep in group-housed and socially isolated mice. *Life Sci* 1998;62:2073-82.

19 Hoult J, et al. Pharmacological and biochemical actions of simple coumarins: natural products with therapeutic potential. *Gen Pharmacol* 1996;27:713-22. Review.

20 Kosuge T, et al. Studies on bioactive substances in crude drugs used for arthritic diseases in traditional Chinese medicine. II. Isolation and identification of an anti-inflammatory and analgesic principle from the root of *Angelica pubescens* Maxim. *Chem Pharm Bull* 1985;33:5351-54.

21 Ko F, et al. Vasorelaxation of rat thoracic aorta caused by osthole isolated from *Angelica pubescens*. *Eur J Pharmacol* 1992;219:29-34.

22 Guh J, et al. Antiproliferative effect in rat vascular smooth muscle cells by osthole, isolated from *Angelica pubescens*. *Eur J Pharmacol* 1996;298:191-97.

23 Chen Y, et al. Anti-inflammatory and analgesic activities from roots of *Angelica pubescens*. *Planta Med* 1995;61:2-8.

24 Liu J, et al. Inhibitory effects of *Angelica pubescens f. biserrata* on 5-lipoxygenase and cyclooxygenase. *Planta Med* 1998;64:525-29.

25 Liu J, et al. Angelol-type coumarins from *Angelica pubescens f. biserrata* and their inhibitory effect on platelet aggregation. *Phytochemistry* 1989;39:1099.

26 Bergendorff O, et al. Furanocoumarins with affinity to brain benzodiazepine receptors in vitro. *Phytochemistry* 1997;44:1121-24.

27 Dekermendjian K, et al. Characterisation of the furanocoumarin phellopterin as a rat brain benzodiazepine receptor partial agonist in vitro. *Neurosci Lett* 1996;219:151.

28 Kimura Y, et al. Histamine-release effectors from *Angelica dahurica* var. dahurica root. *J Nat Prod* 1997;60:249-51.

29 Kimura Y, et al. Effects of various coumarins from roots of *Angelica dahurica* on actions of adrenaline, ACTH and insulin in fat cells. *Planta Med* 1982;45:183-87.

30 Hirata J, et al. Does dong quai have estrogenic effects in postmenopausal women? A double-blind, placebo-controlled trial. *Fertil Steril* 1997;68:981-86.

31 Hudson T, et al. Clinical and endocrinological effects of a menopausal botanical formula. *J Naturopathic Med* 1998;7:73.

32 Fugh-Berman A. Herb-drug interactions. *Lancet* 2000;355:134-38. Review.

33 Page R, et al. Potentiation of warfarin by dong quai. *Pharmacotherapy* 1999;19:870-76.

34 Hann S, et al. Angelica-induced phytophotodermatitis. *Photodermatol Photoimmunol Photomed* 1991;8:84-85.

Echinacea

SCIENTIFIC NAME(S): *Echinacea angustifolia* DC. The related species *E. purpurea* (L.) Moench and *E. pallida* (Nutt.) Britton have also been used in traditional medicine. Family: Compositae

COMMON NAME(S): American coneflower, black susans, comb flower, echinacea, hedgehog, Indian head, Kansas snakeroot, narrow-leaved purple coneflower, purple coneflower, scurvy root, snakeroot

BOTANY: There are at least 9 species of echinacea. The ones most commonly studied are *E. purpura*, *E. pallida*, and *E. angustifolia*.[1]

Echinacea is native to Kansas, Nebraska, and Missouri. There has been confusion regarding the identification of echinacea. Because of this confusion, it should be recognized that much of the early research conducted on this plant (in particular with European *E. angustifolia*) was probably conducted on *E. pallida*.[2] At least 6 synonyms have been documented for these plants.

E. angustifolia is a perennial herb with narrow leaves and a stout stem that grows to 90 cm in height. The plant terminates in a single, colorful flower head. The plant imparts a pungent, acrid taste when chewed and causes tingling of the lips and tongue.

Echinacea products have been found to be adulterated with another member of the family Compositae, *Parthenium integrifolium* L. This plant has no pharmacologic activity.

HISTORY: Echinacea is a popular herbal remedy in the central US, an area to which it is indigenous. The plant was used in traditional medicine by the American Indians and quickly adopted by the settlers. During the 1800s, claims for the curative properties of the plant ranged from a blood purifier to a treatment for dizziness and rattlesnake bites.[3] During the early part of the 20th century, extracts of the plant were used as anti-infectives; however, the use of these products fell out of favor after the discovery of modern antibiotics.

The plant and its extracts continue to be used topically for wound-healing action and internally to stimulate the immune system. Most of the research during the past 10 years has focused on the immunostimulant properties of this plant.

CHEMISTRY: Echinacea contains about 0.1% echinacoside, a caffeic acid glycoside. The pungent component of the plant is echinacein, a isobutylamide.[4] This compound is toxic to adult houseflies. The plant also contains a complex mixture of components that are now being elucidated. Depending on the species, the essential oil obtained from the root may be high in unsaturated alkyl ketones or isobutylamides.[2] Fresh aerial portions of echinacea contain a highly volatile germacrene alcohol that is not usually identified in dried plant material.[5] In addition, a number of alkamides have been found in the lipophilic fraction of *E. angustifolia* and *E. purpurea* roots.[6]

PHARMACOLOGY: A small but growing body of evidence is developing to support the traditional uses of echinacea as a wound-healing agent and immunostimulant.

Most studies have indicated that the lipophilic fraction of the root and leaves contains the most potent immunostimulating components. Although a number of pharmacologically active components have been isolated, no single compound appears to be responsible for the plant's activity. Polyunsaturated alkamides from *E. angustifolia* have been shown to inhibit in vitro the activity of sheep cyclooxygenase and porcine 5-lipoxygenase assays.[7]

Treatment of the common cold: Nineteen German controlled clinical trials examined the efficacy of 7 different echinacea preparations, alone or in combination, for the prevention or treatment of upper respiratory tract infections (URIs) including the common cold. The authors rated the overall quality of the studies, with a median score of 37% and a range of 7% to 70%.[8] These results correspond to the average scores (38.5%) found for other clinical trials in journals from 1990.[9] The authors of this review determined that the studies available as of 1993 revealed that echinacea may have an effect on the immune system, but that there is insufficient evidence to provide specific recommendations.[8]

Barrett and colleagues published an evidence-based clinical review of echinacea in 1999. They examined 13 trials, 9 of which were reviewed by Melchart in 1994, and 4 additional studies (1 unpublished report). Barrett et al, found conclusions similar to those of Melchart in that there is some evidence that echinacea is effective for treatment, not for the prevention of URIs, but there is still a lack of definitive information to provide specific recommendations.[10] Brinkeborn and colleagues reported that patients receiving a commercially available echinacea product in Germany with 6.78 mg, 95% herb, and 5% root or a concentrate with 48.27 mg of the same crude extract, had a 50% reduction in 12 cold symptoms as judged by the patient and 60% as judged by physicians compared with placebo (see Table 1 for description of clinical trials). In addition, approximately 70% of physicians and 80% of patients judged the treatment to be effective. There was no information on whether echinacea decreased the duration of a cold. The authors did not speculate as to why it was effective while the fresh plant preparation was not.[11] Degenring provided information concerning an open-label, "adjunctive treatment" (term not described) trial in 77 patients receiving echinacea. Results showed that 72% of patients became symptom-free within 14 days. However, without a placebo-control, it is impossible to determine if patients would have improved without treatment.[12] Dorn and colleagues used an unidentified *E. pallida radix* extract 900 mg/day in an unspecified divided dose regimen for 8 to 10 days to determine its effect on both viral and bacterial infections compared with a placebo. *E. pallida* decreased the length of the illness from 13 to 9.8 days compared with placebo for bacterial infections and 12.9 days to 9.1 days for viral infections ($p < 0.0001$).[13]

Another study used a commercially available echinacea product in Germany. Results showed a direct correlation to time of administration with patients taking the medication during the early phase ("...identified by the course of an indicator symptom during the first three days of observation") showing faster improvement than those who started echinacea later. In the treatment group, 55.3% had greater than or equal to 50% improvement in global score compared with 27.3% in the placebo group.[14] Hoheisel and colleagues demonstrated that another commercially available product in Germany was more effective in shortening the duration of a cold and required treatment of a cold than placebo using subjective measures such as "Did you have a 'real cold'?" (fully expressed symptoms of acute respiratory tract infection). Although more patients experienced a "real cold" with placebo than echinacea, the severity of symptoms were similar in the 2 groups.[15] Thom and colleagues used a commercially available *E. pallida* root extract combination product (Kanjang mixture) in Scandinavia. Compared to placebo, the Kanjang mixture caused a decrease in subjective symptoms such as degree and frequency of cough, quality of sleep, efficacy of mucus discharge, nasal congestion, and global evaluation compared with placebo. These improvements were noted as early as 2 days after initiation of treatment and were more prominent at day 4. Patients took the echinacea treatment for an average of 5.2 days vs 9.2 days for placebo. No side effects were reported in either group; however, 2 patients discontinued the active treatment because they could not tolerate the taste of the medication.[16]

There were several limitations of the studies listed in Table 1. Only 2 studies measured patient compliance and 3 studies addressed concomitant medication use that might affect cold symptoms.[11,14,16] Inclusion and exclusion criteria were not always provided, and if provided, they were poorly defined. Four studies mentioned that the placebo product was similar to the echinacea preparation to help ensure blinding. However, one of these studies reported that the treatments "...could almost not be distinguished from one other by their smell or taste." However, Melchart mentioned that "because of the characteristic taste of echinacea extracts it is almost impossible to prepare a completely indistinguishable placebo."[11,14,17] None of the studies asked patients if they had tried an echinacea product before. If so, what kind was it and did it work? The methods for randomization and verification were not provided. The studies used subjective measures of a cold that can be highly variable from patient to patient, and the methods for measuring these subjective outcomes varied greatly. Some of the studies used plant parts (*purpurea* root) that are not approved by The German Commission E because they lack documentation pertaining to efficacy. There were 6 different preparations (extract vs. tab vs squeezed sap vs combination product), 2 different species (*E. purpurea* or *pallida*), and 6 different doses used in the 6 studies. None of the studies tested the products for quality high-pressure (performance) liquid chromatography (HPLC) testing procedures currently available or standardized the products prior to initiation of the study.[18] Two of the studies used patients who were more prone to the common cold.[11,15] One of the studies lacked a placebo control, which makes it virtually impossible to reach a conclusion regarding efficacy.[12] The exact time of initiation of echinacea treatment was not well defined in the studies. Some mentioned echinacea was taken at the first sign of a cold, others did not mention when therapy was initiated.

Prevention of the common cold: Three clinical trials, 2 were randomized, double-blind, placebo-controlled English-language trials, and 1 placebo-controlled have been conducted that examined the effectiveness of echinacea in the prevention of the common cold and other URIs (see

Table 2). None of the studies found echinacea to be effective. However, 1 study did not calculate power (ie, the ability of a study to find a significant difference, if in fact, one exists). One calculated the study power at only 20% and the other 75%, suggesting that neither study probably enrolled enough subjects.[17,19,36] Melchart and colleagues commented that echinacea may cause a 10% to 20% relative risk reduction for the occurrence of a cold; however, larger sample sizes than those used would be required to prove this theory.[17] As with the treatment trials, 2 of the studies determined whether the placebo was a true placebo.[17,19] The other study questioned whether patients thought they were receiving a placebo, and the investigators found no significant difference be-

tween groups. However, the dosage form used in this study was not described. Only 1 of the studies tested the products for quality.[36] However, the study did not list the species they used or if the product contained the desired components. None of the studies standardized their products prior to initiation of the study.[18] Melchart and colleagues reported that 45% of the subjects had tried echinacea before, which could have affected the results. This study also used an echinacea species (*angustifolio*) and plant parts (*purpurea* root) that are not approved by The German Commission E because they lack documentation of efficacy.[17]

Table 1: English–Language Studies of Echinacea for the Treatment of the Common Cold							
Study & country	N	Study design	Species	Formulation	Dose	Outcome	Side effects
Brinkeborn (1999) Sweden	246	R, D-B, P-C, intent-to-treat, healthy volunteers "prone to common cold"	*E. purpurea*	(1) *Echinaforce* (6.78 mg, 95% herb, and 5% root) or (2) *Echinaforce* concentrate (48.27 mg of the same crude extract) or (3) special *E. purpurea* extract preparation (29.6 mg crude extract based on root only).	2 tabs tid at the first sign of a cold for ≤ 7 days or until pt felt better	*Echinaforce* and the concentrate were more effective at relieving 12 symptoms[1] of the common cold compared with special *Echinacea* extract and placebo.	Similar to placebo. Most common was GI upset.
Degenring (1995) Austria	77	Open-label, 4-week observation	*E. purpurea*	*Echinaforce* (6.78 mg, 95% herb, and 5% root) "made from stems and leaves, together with the root." Alcohol content, 57%.	30 drops tid × 14 days at the first sign of a cold; ≤ 3 days after	88.2% of pts and 86.8% of physicians rated echinacea to have clinically relevant efficacy (very good, good, or satisfactory).	76 pts and physicians rated tolerability as good. One pt dc'd therapy due to SEs.
Dorn (1997) Germany	160	R, D-B, P-C, single-center	*E. pallida*	Liquid form of *E. pallida radix* extract.	90 drops (900 mg) in divided doses for 8 to 10 days	Length of illness, overall symptom scores, and whole clinical scores were decreased compared with placebo.	None mentioned.

Table 1: English–Language Studies of Echinacea for the Treatment of the Common Cold							
Study & country	N	Study design	Species	Formulation	Dose	Outcome	Side effects
Henneicke-von Zepelin (1999) Germany	259	R, D-B, P-C, multi-center, intent-to-treat	*E. purpurea*, *E. pallida*	*Esberitox N* tablets (ethanolic-aqueous extracts of 2 mg of *herba thujae occi-dentalis*, 7.5 mg of *radix echinaceae* [*purpureae + pal-lidae = 1+1*], 10 mg *radix baptiaiae tinc-torae*, plus other ingredients).	"3 tabs tid for 7 to 9 days, and at least until the final visit to the investigator"	*Esberitox N* was more effective in relieving 18 cold symptoms than pla-cebo. Mean time to response was 4.8 days in the echina-cea group vs 7 days in the placebo group.	Similar to placebo.
Hoheisel (1997) Sweden	120	R, D-B, P-C, intent-to-treat, healthy vol-unteers with history of recurrent URIs.	*E. purpurea*	*Echinagard* ("squeezed sap of the herb").	20 drops q2hrs for the first day, at the first sign of URI then tid for ≤ 10 days	60% of placebo and 40% of echinacea pts experienced a "real" cold, with faster improvement time by 4 to 5 days. Pts stopped treat-ment median 6 days on echinacea vs 10 on placebo.	None reported.
Thom (1997) Norway	60	R, D-B, P-C pts with the common cold	*E. pallida*	Kanjang mixture with *E. pallidia radix* 10 g/100 ml mixed with 4 other "active ingredients."	15 ml tid for 5 to 10 days	Kanjang mixture improved symptoms compared with pla-cebo on days 2 and 4.	None reported.

[1] Severity of illness, runny nose and sneezing, tearing/burning eyes, sore throat, headache, dizziness, weakness, drowsiness, muscle pain, limb pain, fever, cough, blocked nose, earache, or any other complaint most probably related to the cold. R = randomized; D-B = double-blind; P-C = placebo-controlled; pt = patients.

Table 2: English-Language Studies of Echinacea for Prevention of the Common Cold							
Study & country	N	Study design	Species	Formulation	Dose	Outcome	Side effects
Grimm (1999) Germany	108	R, D-B, P-C, pts with a his-tory of cold > 3x/yr	*E. purpurea*	Echinacin-Liquidum made from fresh expressed juice of whole flowering plants of *Echinacea purpurea* (verum) harvested without its roots with 22% alco-hol.	4 ml bid for 8 weeks	No difference in occurrence, sever-ity, or duration.	Similar to placebo.

Table 2: English-Language Studies of Echinacea for Prevention of the Common Cold

Study & country	N	Study design	Species	Formulation	Dose	Outcome	Side effects
Melchart (1998) Germany	289	R, D-B, P-C	*E. purpurea, E. angustifolia*	Ethanolic extracts (plant ratio 1:11 in 30% alcohol) from the roots of *E. angustifolia* or *E. purpurea.*	50 drops bid, M-F × 12 weeks	Not an effective preventative.	Similar to placebo.
Turner (2000) USA	92	P-C, experimental rhinovirus	*Possibly E. pallida, E. angustifolia* but not directly stated	0.16% cichoric acid with a most no echinacosices or alkamides.	300 mg tid × 14 days prior to virus challenge	Not an effective preventative.	Similar to placebo.

[1] R = randomized; D-B = double-blind; P-C = placebo-controlled; pt = patients.

When injected IV in mice or rats, echinacea extract almost completely inhibited carrageenan-induced mice or rat paw edema. Similarly, when the extract was applied topically, it inhibited almost completely the inflammation induced by croton oil applied to the mice or rats' ear.[20] Its activity was slightly less than that of topical indomethacin. The most active anti-inflammatory compound(s) has a molecular weight of between 30,000 and 100,000.[21]

Several caffeoyl conjugates have been isolated from *E. angustifolia* that demonstrate antihyaluronidase activity; these include chicoric acid, cynarine, chlorogenic acid, and caftaric acid.[22] The inhibition of this enzyme is believed to limit the progression of certain degenerative inflammatory diseases.

Perhaps the most intriguing activity of this plant rests in the ability of its extracts to enhance the immune response. A number of in vitro and animal studies have documented the activation of immunologic activity. These extracts appear to exert their effects by stimulating phagocytosis, increasing cellular respiratory activity, and increasing the mobility of leucocytes. When ethanolic extracts were administered orally to rats, phagocytosis was enhanced. The lipophilic fraction was more active than the polar fraction.[23]

The purified polysaccharide arabinogalactan, isolated from *E. purpurea*, was effective in activating macrophages to cytotoxicity against tumor cells and microorganisms following intraperitoneal injection in mice.[24] Arabinogalactan induces macrophages to produce tumor necrosis factor, interleukin-1, and interferon beta-2. Polysaccharides derived from *E. purpurea* enhance the cytotoxic activity of treated macrophages against tumor cells and the intracellular parasite *Leishmania enrietti*.[25] The research suggests that this activity may be of clinical value in the defense against tumors and infectious diseases, particularly in immunocompromised patients. However, a study involving 23 patients with tumors showed that an echinacea complex made with *E. angustifolia* had no effect on cytokine or leukocytes.[26]

Dietary supplementation with *E. purpurea* to rats who were undergoing experimental irradiation resulted in the mobilization and enhancement of vitamin E-mediated oxidation/reduction pathways, suggesting that echinacea could have potential as a radioprotector.[27]

One study found the administration of echinacea extracts to humans stimulated cell-mediated immunity following a single dose, but that repeated daily doses suppressed the immune response.[28] In a more recent German study conducted in a small number of patients (15) with advanced metastasized colorectal cancer, echinacin (a component of the plant) was added to treatment consisting of cyclophosphamide and thymostimulin; the mean survival time was 4 months, and two patients survived for more than 8 months, suggesting that this form of immunotherapy may have some value in treating these ill patients.[29]

Although the results are encouraging, they are too preliminary to draw conclusions about the appropriate therapeutic uses of echinacea extracts. Similarly, there are no well-controlled studies that have evaluated the effects of OTC echinacea supplements. Consequently, dosages are not well defined.

Photodamage prevention/treatment: An in vitro study demonstrated that typical constituents of echinacea species applied topically were effective in prevention/treatment of photodamage of the skin caused by UV/UVB radiation.[30]

TOXICOLOGY: Little is known about the toxicity of echinacea despite its widespread use in many countries. It has been documented in American traditional medicine for more than a century and generally has not been associated with acute or chronic toxicity. Purified echinacea polysaccharide is relatively nontoxic. Acute toxicity studies found that doses of arabinogalactan as high as 4 g/kg injected intraperitoneally or IV were essentially devoid of toxic effects.[24]

High-dose oral and IV administration (ie, several times the normal human therapeutic dose) of the expressed juice of E. purpurea to rodents for 4 weeks demonstrated no acute, subacute, genotoxic, carcinogenic, mutagenic, or other toxic reactions.[31]

Side effects: Exclusion criteria from clinical trials provide information regarding patients who should not receive echinacea. Some of the exclusion criteria were the following: Childhood, chronic diseases such as diabetes, bronchial asthma, allergy, or autoimmune deficiency, tuberculosis, leukemia, collagenous disease, multiple sclerosis, polyarthritis, HIV infection, organ transplantation, pneumonia, or fungal infections, other infections not involving the respiratory tract, known inflammatory GI disease or impairment of resorption, acute influenza, chronic diseases of the respiratory tract; patients taking any immunosuppressants including corticosteroids, antibiotics, or cytostatic therapy; pregnancy or lactation; fever; hypersensitivity to plants of the Asteraceae/Compositae family; and any type of acute infection.[11,12,13,14,15,16,17,19] Some of the exclusion criteria were taken from parenteral echinacea product information. Most of the contraindications and some of the possible side effects are theoretical and are not derived from actual case reports or studies of oral echinacea. According to The German Commission E, Echinacea purpurea and pallida, when taken orally, do not cause any side effects.[32] Parnham and colleagues reported results from an unpublished practice study to determine adverse effects and safety of the squeezed sap of E. purpurea. A total of 1231 patients with relapsing respiratory and urinary infections given echinacea for 4 to 6 weeks demonstrated the following side effects: Unpleasant taste (1.7%); nausea or vomiting (0.48%); abdominal pain, diarrhea, sore throat (0.24%). The authors reported that 90% of patients took the medication as directed. Parenteral administration was associated with immunostimulating-type reactions such as shivering, fever, and muscle weakness.[33] Degenring reported that 1 out of 77 patients who received the 6.78 mg, 95% herb, and 5% root formulation experienced nausea, restlessness, and aggravation of cold symptoms 4 days after starting the medication.[12] The symptoms were severe enough to require discontinuation of therapy. Other side effects reported in clinical trials were primarily GI in nature, such as mild nausea.[11,12,14,19] At the American Academy of Allergy, Asthma and Immunology 2000 annual meeting, 23 unpublished cases (2 "certain," 10 "probable," and 11 "possible") of allergic reaction to echinacea consistent with IgE-mediated hypersensitivity were reported. Of the 23 cases, 34% were atopic, 13% were nonatopic, and 44% did not provide this information. Of another 100 atopic patients who had never taken echinacea, 20% had positive skin test reactions to echinacea, indicating a hypersensitivity without prior exposure to echinacea.[34] There was also a case of anaphylaxis caused by a combination echinacea product (E. angustifolia and E. purpurea) with other dietary supplements. The amount of echinacea product consumed was approximately double that recommended by the manufacturer. The patient had a high incidence of allergies to other substances. Of an additional 84 patients with asthma or allergic rhinitis, 16 subjects (19%) reacted to an echinacea skin prick. Only 2 patients had prior exposure to echinacea.[35]

SUMMARY: Echinacea is a native American plant that has been documented in traditional herbal medicine for more than a century. Its uses have included topical application to stimulate wound healing and ingestion to improve immune function. Studies have indicated that the plant does possess pharmacologic activity that supports some of these traditional uses.

Echinacea has been shown to have some beneficial effects on the symptoms of the common cold. A few studies have shown echinacea (E. purpurea and E. pallida) to be effective for the treatment, but not prevention, of the common cold. However, the variation in products used in clinical trials (some products are not available in the US), including part of the plant used, variable dosing, treatment duration, and different extraction methods (eg, alcoholic extraction, pressed juice) makes specific dosing recommendations difficult to determine (see Table 1). There are 9 species of echinacea found in the US and south central Canada.[19] Many different parts of the plants can be used in formulations, such as the root, upper parts, sap, or the whole plant.

There is a lack of large clinical trial information. However, The German Commission E gives a positive rating to 2 echinacea monographs, *E. pallida* root (not herb or leaf) and *E. purpurea* herb or leaf (not root).[32] Some of the studies listed in the pharmacology section used parts of the herb that are not approved by The German Commission E.

PATIENT INFORMATION – Echinacea

Uses: There is some evidence that echinacea (*purpurea* and *pallida* species) is effective in shortening the duration of symptoms of URIs, including the common cold, but it has not been shown to be effective as a preventative. The variation in available products makes specific recommendations difficult to determine.

Side Effects: Side effects are rare. Patients with allergies, specifically allergies to daisy-type plants (Asteraceae/Compositae family) might be more susceptible to reactions. Nausea and other mild GI effects have been reported in clinical trials. Because of the potential immune stimulating property of echinacea, patients who are immunocompromised should not take echinacea. Many patients were excluded from clinical trials (see Pharmacology, Clinical Trials, Toxicology).

Dose: Variable doses and preparations were used in the studies that make specific dosing recommendations difficult. The dosing range for *E. pallida* root is 6 to 9 ml/day and *E. purpurea* leaf is approximately 900 mg/day. Because echinacea may be an immunostimulant, it should not be taken for more than 8 consecutive weeks. Usually 7 to 14 days is sufficient. However, there is no data to support or refute this theory.

---

[1] Chavez M, et al. Echinacea. *Hosp Pharm* 1998;33:180-88.

[2] Bauer R, et al. TLC and HPLC analysis of *Echinacea pallida* and *E. angustifolia* roots. *Planta Med* 1988;54:426.

[3] Tyler V. The New Honest Herbal. Philadelphia: GF Stickley Co., 1987.

[4] Jacobson M. The structure of echinacein, the insecticidal component of American coneflower roots. *J Org Chem* 1967;32:1646-47.

[5] Bauer R, et al. A germacrene alcohol from fresh aerial parts of *Echinacea purpurea*. *Planta Med* 1988;54:478.

[6] Bauer R. et al. New alkamides from *Echinacea angustifolia* and *E. purpurea* Roots. *Planta Med* 1988;54:563.

[7] Muller-Jakic B, et al. In vitro inhibition of cyclooxygenase and 5–lipoxygenase by alkamides from echinacea and achillea species. *Planta Med* 1994;60(1):37-40.

[8] Melchart D, et al. Immunomodulation with echinacea-a systematic review of controlled clinical trials. *Phytomedicine* 1994;1:245-54.

[9] Rochon P, et al. Evaluating the quality of articles published in journal supplements compared with the quality of those published in the parent journal. *JAMA* 1994;272:108-13.

[10] Barrett B, et al. Echinacea for upper respiratory infection. *J Fam Pract* 1999;48:628-35. Review.

[11] Brinkeborn R, et al. *Echinaforce* and other echinacea fresh plant preparations in the treatment of the common cold. A randomized, placebo-controlled, double-blind clinical trial. *Phytomedicine* 1999;6:1-5.

[12] Degenring F. Studies on the therapeutic efficacy of *Echinaforce*. Phytotherapy for adjunctive treatment for recurrent infections of the respiratory tract. *Schweiz Zschr Ganzheits Medizin* 1995;2:88-94.

[13] Dorn M. Placebo-controlled, double-blind study of *Echinacea pallidae* radix in upper respiratory tract infections. *Complement Ther Med* 1997;5:40-42.

[14] Henneicke-von Zepelin H, et al. Efficacy and safety of a fixed combination phytomedicine in the treatment of the common cold (acute viral respiratory tract infection): Results of a randomized, double blind, placebo controlled, multicentre study. *Curr Med Res Opin* 1999;15(3):214-27.

[15] Hoheisel O, et al. Echinagard treatment shortens the course of the common cold: A double-blind, placebo-controlled clinical trial. *Eur J Clin Res* 1997;9:261-68.

[16] Thom E, et al. A controlled clinical study of Kanjang mixture in the treatment of uncontrolled upper respiratory tract infections. *Phytother Res* 1997;11:207-10.

[17] Melchart D, et al. Echinacea root extracts for the prevention of upper respiratory tract infections: a double-blind, placebo-controlled randomized trial. *Arch Fam Med* 1998;7:541-45.

[18] Awang D, et al. Echinacea. *Can Pharm J* 1991;124:512-16.

[19] Grimm W, et al. A randomized controlled trial of the effect of fluid extract *Echinacea purpurea* on the incidence and severity of colds and respiratory infections. *Am J Med* 1999;106:138-43.

[20] Tubaro A, et al. Anti-inflammatory activity of a polysaccharidic fraction of *Echinacea angustifolia*. *J Pharm Pharmacol* 1987;39(7):567-69.

[21] Tragni E, et al. Anti-inflammatory activity of *Echinacea angustifolia* fractions separated on the basis of molecular weight. *Pharmacol Res Commun* 1988;20(Suppl 5):87-90.

[22] Facino R, et al. Direct characterization of caffeoyl esters with antihyaluronidase activity in crude extracts from *Echinacea angustifolia* roots by fast atom bombardment tandem mass spectrometry. *Farmaco* 1993;48(10):1447-61.

[23] Bauer V, et al. [Immunologic in vivo and in vitro studies on echinacea extracts.] *Arzneimittelforschung* 1988;38(2):276-81. German.

[24] Luettig B, et al. Macrophage activation by the polysaccharide arabinogalactan isolated from plant cell cultures of *Echinacea purpurea*. *J Nat Cancer Inst* 1989;81(9):669-75.

[25] Steinmuller C, et al. Polysaccharides isolated from plant cell cultures of *Echinacea purpurea* enhance the resistance of immunosuppressed mice against systemic infections with *Candida albicans* and *Listeria monocytogenes*. *Int J Immunopharmacol* 1993;15(5):605-14.

[26] Elsässer-Beile U, et al. Cytokine production in leukocyte cultures during therapy with echinacea extract. *J Clin Lab Anal* 1996;10:441-45.

[27] Peranich A, et al. [Effect of supposed radioprotectors on oxidation-reduction of vitamin E in the tissues of irradiated rats.] *Radiats Biol Radioecol* 1993;33(5):653-57. Russian.

[28] Coeugniet E, et al. Immunomodulation with *Viscum album* and *Echinacea purpurea* extracts. *Onkologie* 1987;10(Suppl 3):27-33.

[29] Lersch C, et al. Nonspecific immunostimulation with low doses of cyclophosphamide (LDCY), thymostimulin, and *Echinacea purpurea* extracts (echinacin) in patients with far advanced colorectal cancers: preliminary results. *Cancer Invest* 1992;10(5):343–48.

[30] Facino R, et al. Echinacoside and caffeoyl conjugates protect collagen from free radical-induced degradation: a potential use of echinacea extracts in the prevention of skin photodamage. *Planta Med* 1995;61:510-14.

[31] Mengs V, et al. Toxicity of *Echinacea purpurea*. Acute, subacute, and genotoxicity studies. *Arzneimittelforschung* 1991;41:1076-81.

[32] Blumenthal M, et al. (ed.) The Complete German Commission E Monographs: Therapeutic Guide to Herbal Medicines. S. Klein. Boston: American Botanical Council, 1998.

[33] Parnham M. Benefit-risk assessment of the squeezed sap of the purple coneflower (*Echinacea purpura*) for long-term oral immunostimulation. *Phytomedicine* 1996;3:95-102.

[34] Today's findings from the AAAAI Annual Meeting unveil new research on alternative therapies and food allergy: Echinacea can cause allergic reactions. American Academy of Allergy, Asthma, and Immunology, URL: www.aaaai.org/media/pressreleases/2000/03/000307.html.

[35] Mullins R. Echinacea-associated anaphylaxis. *Med J Aust* 1998;168:170-71.

[36] Turner R, et al. Ineffectiveness of echinacea for prevention of experimental rhinovirus colds. *Antimicrob Agents and Chemother* 2000;44(6):1708-09.

Elderberry

SCIENTIFIC NAME(S): The American elder (*Sambucus canadensis* L.) and the European Elder (*Sambucus nigra* L.). Family: Caprifoliaceae

COMMON NAME(S): Sweet elder, common elder, elderberry, sambucus[1]

BOTANY: The American elder is a tall shrub that grows to 12 feet. It is native to North America. The European elder grows to about 30 feet and while native to Europe, has been naturalized to the United States.

HISTORY: Elder flowers and berries have been used in traditional medicine and as flavorings for centuries. In folk medicine, the flowers have been used for their diuretic and laxative properties and as an astringent. Various parts of the elder have been used to treat cancer and a host of other unrelated disorders.[2] Distilled elder flower water has been used as a scented vehicle for topical preparations and extracts are used to flavor foods, including alcoholic beverages. The fruits have been used to prepare elderberry wine.

CHEMISTRY: European elder flowers contain about 0.3% of an essential oil composed of free fatty acids and alkanes. Triterpenes (alpha- and beta-amyrin), ursolic acid, oleanic acid, betulin, betulic acid and a variety of other minor components have been identified.[1,3] The elder leaf contains sambunigrin, a cyanogenic glucoside (0.042% by weight).[1]

The *Sambucus* species are now undergoing significant scrutiny because they contain a number of plant lectins that have hemagglutinin characteristics. These compounds are useful in blood typing and defining other hematologic characteristics.[4,5]

PHARMACOLOGY: Elder flowers are considered to have diuretic and laxative properties; however, the specific compounds responsible for these activities have not been well established. The compound sambuculin A and a mixture of alpha- and beta-amyrin palmitate have been found to exhibit strong antihepatotoxic activity against liver damage induced experimentally by carbon tetrachloride.[6]

TOXICOLOGY: Because of the cyanogenic potential of the leaves, extracts of the plant may be used in foods, provided HCN levels do not exceed 25 ppm in the flavor. Toxicity in children who used pea shooters made from elderberry stems has been reported.[2]

One report of severe illness following the ingestion of juice prepared from elderberries has been recorded by the Centers for Disease Control.[7] Persons attending a picnic who ingested several glasses of juice made from berries picked the day before reported nausea, vomiting, weakness, dizziness, numbness and stupor. One person who consumed five glasses of juice was hospitalized for stupor. All recovered. Although cyanide levels were not reported, there remains the possibility of cyanide-induced toxicity in these patients. While elderberries are safe to consume, particularly when cooked (uncooked berries may produce nausea), leaves and stems should not be crushed when making elderberry juice.

SUMMARY: Elderberries are edible berries (particularly when cooked) from the elder bush. They have been used medicinally although they are not typically associated with strong medicinal characteristics. One report of toxicity following the ingestion of elderberry juice has been recorded, but this appears to have been an isolated incident.

PATIENT INFORMATION – Elderberry

Uses: Elder flowers and berries have been used in flavorings and in traditional medicines.

Side Effects: There have been reports of toxicity, particularly involving the stems and leaves.

---

[1] Leung AY. Encyclopedia of Common Natural Ingredients Used in Food, Drugs, and Cosmetics. New York, NY: J. Wiley and Sons, 1980.

[2] Duke JA. Handbook of Medicinal Herbs. Boca Raton, FL: CRC Press, 1985.

[3] Inoue T, Sato K. Triterpenoids of *Sambucus nigra* and *S. canadensis*. Phytochemistry 1975;14:1871.

[4] Mach L, et al. Purification and partial characterization of a novel lectin from elder (*Sambucus nigra* L.) fruit. *Biochem J* 1991;278:667.

[5] Kaku H, et al. Isolation and characterization of a second lectin (SNA- II) present in elderberry (*Sambucus nigra* L.) bark. *Arch Biochem Biophys* 1990;277(2):255.

[6] Lin C-N, Tome W-P. Antihepatotoxic principles of *Sambucus formosana*. Planta Medica 1988;54(3):223.

[7] Anonymous. Poisoning from elderberry juice - California. *Morbidity & Mortality Weekly Report* 1984;33(13):173.

Eleutherococcus

SCIENTIFIC NAME(S): *Eleutherococcus senticosus* Maxim. *Acanthopanax senticosus* Rupr. et Maxim. *Hedera senticosa.* Family: Araliaceae

COMMON NAME(S): Devil's shrub, eleutheroccoc, shigoka, Siberian ginseng, touch-me-not, wild pepper

BOTANY: *E. senticosus* belongs to the same family as (Araliceae) *Panax ginseng*. The geographical distribution of eleutherococcus coincides with the borders of the distribution of *P. ginseng*. Eleutherococcus is found in forests of broadleaf trees, broadleafs with spruce, and broadleafs with cedar. It grows at elevations of up to 800 m or more above sea level. The plant is a shrub, commonly attaining a height of 2 to 3 m or, less commonly, 5 to 7 m. It possesses gray or grayish-brown bark and numerous thin thorns. The leaves are long-stalked and palmate. Eleutherococcus has male and female forms with globular umbrella-shaped flowers. Male plants produce violet flowers, while female plants have yellowish flowers; the fruit takes the form of black, oval berries. Most commonly, the root is used in herbal medicine; however, it was found that leaves and berries also produce pharmacologically active metabolites. Because it grows abundantly in areas such as Russia and China, it has become a popular substitute for ginseng.[1]

HISTORY: Eleutherococcus has been studied extensively in Russia. It is used as a health food in China, but Asian folk medicine has largely ignored eleutherococcus in favor of its relative, ginseng. As with ginseng, root extracts of the plant have been promoted as "adaptogens" that aid the body in responding to external (eg, environmental) and internal (eg, a disease) stress. The plant extracts have been used to normalize high or low blood pressure, to stimulate the immune system, and to increase work capacity. Reputed effects include increasing body energy levels, protection from motion sickness and against toxins, control of alloxan-induced diabetes, reduction of tumors, and control of atherosclerosis.[1,2]

CHEMISTRY: The chemical composition of the roots and leaves varies with season. It was observed that the roots contain the maximum active ingredient in October and drops sharply in July.[1,2] Methanolic extracts of eleutherococcus roots have been found to contain a glycoside fraction that includes different eleutherosides (isofraxidin, sesamin, syringin) as well as glucose, sucrose, betulinic acid, vitamin E, β-carotene, caffeic acid, and β-sitosterol. The eleutherosides found in the root, leaves, and berries are designated as A through M and have different structures belonging to different groups of chemical compounds.[1,3]

Several studies have differentiated between the botany, chemistry, and pharmacology of common ginseng (*P. ginseng* and *P. quinquefolium*) and Siberian ginseng (*E. senticosus*).[4] Only eleutheroside A has similar saponins structure (ginsenosides/panaxosides) to ginseng.[5] While some eleutherosides share common properties with panaxosides, others exhibit very different effects. Seven glycans (eleutherans A, B, C, D, E, F, G) have been isolated from aqueous extract of the crude drug shigoka (Siberian ginseng) roots.[6] New lignans have been isolated from the root of eleutherococcus: 7SR,8RS-dihydrodrodiconiferyl alcohol, dehydrodiconiferyl alcohol, 7,8-trans-dihydrodehydrodiconiferyl alcohol-4-O-β-D-glucopyranoside, meso-secoisolariciresinol, and (-)-syringoresinol-4-O-β-D-glucopyranoside.[7] The antiplatelet compound 3,4-dihydroxybenzoic acid has also been isolated from this species.[8] Eleutherosides have been isolated, identified, and measured in the rhizomes, roots, and liquid extracts of eleutherococcus.[9] Other relatively new compounds that have been isolated include phenylpropanes and polysaccharides, ciwujianosides C1 and D1,[10] and at least 10 phenolic compounds such as isofraxidin.[11] Chemical analysis is still in progress on eleutherococcus and indicates that there have been improvements in the procedures of isolation and analysis methods (such as reverse-phase HPLC) of the plant.[12,13,14]

PHARMACOLOGY: An animal study examined the effect of acute (4 to 320 mg/kg) or 4- to 5-day treatment (80 to 320 mg/kg/day) via intraperitoneal injection of eleutherococcus extract on the response of mice to hexobarbital. Both single dose and 4- to 5-day treatments increased sleep latency and duration. This may have drug-drug interaction implications if these 2 agents are taken together. Findings support the contention that the extract acts by inhibiting an enzyme system of hexobarbital metabolism.[15]

In another study with mice, intraperitoneal injection of an aqueous extract of eleutherococcus root reduced plasma sugar levels. Fractionation studies of the extract identified 7 eleutherosides, designated A through G, that produced synergistic hypoglycemic effects in normal mice and in mice with alloxane-induced diabetes.[6] Water-soluble, branched-chain heteroglycans isolated from polysaccharide fractions of extracts have been shown to have such properties in granulocyte and carbon-clearance tests.[16] However, in rats, oral administration of extracts did not affect plasma lactic acid, glucagon, insulin, or liver glycogen, nor did they increase swimming times in endurance tests. Thus, this study did not confirm an endurance-boosting effect of eleutherococcus. Decreased plasma glucose levels were found in resting rats.[17] Another study compared the effects of various orally administered infusions of P. ginseng and eleutherococcus for endurance effects in mice. Treatments lasting up to 96 days failed to show any increases in swimming endurance or longevity with any of the infusions. However, eleutherococcus was associated with increased aggressive behavior.[18] There is evidence that the adaptation effect of eleutherococcus may act through the pituitary-adrenocortical system.[19]

In vitro experiments have shown some activity of eleutherococcus against L1210 murine leukemia cells. When root extract was added to cytarabine or N-6-(delta-2-isopentenyl)-adenosine, the extract had an additive effect with conventional antimetabolite drugs, with an ED50 of about 75 mcg/ml. This suggests that addition of the extract to anticancer regimens might make it possible to reduce the doses of toxic drugs.[20] P. ginseng has been shown to protect cell cultures from the effects of gamma radiation. The mechanism seems to involve alteration of cellular metabolism rather than DNA repair. Eleutherococcus extract has a similar action, but only to a slight degree.[21]

The eleutherosides have 36 to 143 times the physiologic activity of the roots from which they are extracted.[2] Eleutherococcus extracts, like those of P. ginseng, bind to progestin, mineralocorticoid, and glucocorticoid receptors. In addition, eleutherococcus extracts bind to estrogen receptors. This may explain the observed glucocorticoid-like activity of the extracts.[22]

There is evidence of therapeutic benefits of eleutherococcus in humans. In 1 study of 36 healthy volunteers, a 3-times-daily injection of an ethanolic extract for 4 weeks produced increases in the absolute numbers of immunocompetent cells, particularly T-cells. The increase was most marked for helper/inducer cells, although cytotoxic and natural killer cells also increased in number. A general enhancement of the activation state of T cells was evident.[23]

In hypotensive children between 7 and 10 years of age, an eleutherococcus extract improved subjective signs, significantly raised systolic and diastolic blood pressures, and increased total peripheral resistance.[24]

Other studies have described the wide range of eleutherococcus properties, including the effects on the human physical working capacity,[25] the immune systems of cancer patients,[26] the heart structure in MI,[27] malignant arrhythmias,[28] myocarditis and other coronary heart diseases,[29] radiation recovery,[30] diabetes,[31] hyperlipemia,[32] its antimicrobial actions,[33] prenatal prevention of congenital developmental anomalies in rats,[34] and enhanced proliferation of human lymphocytes.[35] Although preparations from E. senticosus have been found to be effective against a variety of somatic disorders, the labels on otc preparations do not supply adequate directions for taking the product or clarify the ingredients.[36,37,38]

INTERACTIONS: Possible assay interference with digoxin may occur; concomitant therapy increased digoxin level to greater than 5 mg/ml without symptoms of toxicity.[39]

TOXICOLOGY: There are possible estrogenic effects in females. Side effects, toxicity, contraindications, and warnings similar to those for Panax species (see ginseng) apply. Experience suggests that this product should not be used for people under the age of 40 and that only low doses be taken on a daily basis. Patients are advised to abstain from alcohol, sexual activity, bitter substances, and spicy foods. Avoid use during pregnancy and lactation. High doses of eleutherococcus are associated with irritability, insomnia, and anxiety. Other adverse effects include skin eruptions, headache, diarrhea, hypertension, and pericardial pain in rheumatic heart patients. Use of eleutherococcus extract has been associated with little or no toxicity. No pathologic, cytotoxic, or histologic changes were noted in mice that ingested infusions of the plant for up to 96 days.[18] In 1 human study, there were no side effects during the 6 months of follow-up.[23] However, use is not recommended for patients in febrile states, hypertensive crisis, or those with MI. Use is contraindicated in hypertensive patients. Rare reported side effects have included slight languor or drowsiness immediately after administration; this may be the result of a hypoglycemic effect of the extract.[2]

Most of the reviewed literature on eleutherococcus suggests that the plant preparations bear minimal toxicity and are fairly safe to use. There was a case in which an eleutherococcus preparation caused severe side effects, but it was later discovered that the preparation did not include eleutherococcus but rather another related species.[1,4,5]

SUMMARY: Eleutherococcus is a plant botanically related to the more familiar *P. ginseng*. Eleutherococcus has a different chemical composition but has been named Siberian ginseng because of purported similar activities. Ethanol and water extracts of the roots of eleutherococcus have been used for a wide variety of therapeutic purposes in which they are said to have an adaptogenic effect. Among the studied properties of eleutherococcus are adaptogenic, hemodynamic, immunoboosting, car-dioprotective; usefulness in treatment of hyper- and hypotonia, inhibitory effects on platelet aggregation, potentiation of radioprotective agents, hypoglycemic properties, cytotoxicity against various cancer cells, usefulness in the treatment of hyperlipemia, potential histamine-inhibiting effects, and potential prevention of congenital defects. Continued studies on standardized extracts or isolated active constituents are needed to verify all of eleutherococcus' purported activities.

PATIENT INFORMATION – Eleutherococcus

Uses: Eleutherococcus is similar to ginseng in its properties and alleged effects. It has been used as a hypotensive, immunostimulant, energy enhancer, and aphrodisiac. Extracts of the roots have been used for a wide variety of therapeutic purposes in which they are said to have an adaptogenic effect. Although preparations from *E. senticosus* have been found to be effective against a variety of somatic disorders, the labels on *otc* preparations do not supply adequate directions for taking the product or clarify the ingredients. In addition, standardization of the active ingredients is not clear.[36,37,38] The German Commission E recommends limiting use to 3 months.[40]

Side Effects: Although side effects appear to be rare, eleutherococcus should not be used by patients in febrile states, hypertensive crisis, or those with MI. Use is contraindicated in hypertensive patients. In some individuals it may produce drowsiness or nervousness.

---

[1] Brekhman I, et al. Man and Biologically Active Substances: The Effects of Drugs, Diet, and Pollution on Health. Oxford: Pergamon Press, 1980.

[2] Brekhman I, et al. Comparative study of eleutherococcus preparations made from raw material of various origin. *Farmatsiia* 1991;40(1):39.

[3] Farnsworth N, et al. Siberian ginseng (*E. senticosus*): Current status as an adaptogen. *Economic and Medicinal Plant Research* 1985;1:155-215.

[4] Wagner H, et al. Plant adaptogens. *Phytomedicine* 1994;1:63-76.

[5] Wagner H, et al. Chemistry, pharmacology and TLC of ginseng and eleutherococcus drugs. *Dtsch Apoth Ztg* 1977;117:743.

[6] Hikino H, et al. Isolation and hypoglycemic activity of eleutherans A, B, C, D, E, F, and G: Glycans of *E. senticosus* roots. *J Nat Prod* 1986;49:293-297.

[7] Makarieva T, et al. Lignans from *E. senticosus* (Siberian ginseng). *Pharm Sci* 1997;3(10):525-27.

[8] Yun-Choi HS, et al. Potential inhibitors of platelet aggregation from plant sources. Part 3. *J Nat Prod* 1987;50(6):1059.

[9] Solovyeva AG, et al. Anaylsis and standardization of eleutherococcus roots and rhizomes and its liquid extract by the amount of biologically active compounds. *Farmatsiia* 1989;38(1):25.

[10] Umeyama A, et al. Ciwujianosides D1 and C1; Powerful inhibitors of histamine release induced by anti-immunoglobulin E from rat peritoneal mast cells. *J Pharm Sci* 1992;81(7):661.

[11] Nishibe S, et al. Phenolic compounds from stem bark of *Acanthopanax senticosus* and their pharmacological effect in chronic swimming and stressed rats. *Chem Pharma Bull* 1990;38(6):1763.

[12] Chen G, et al. Determination of syringin in slices of radix *Acanthopanax senticosi* by RP-HPLC. *Zhongguo Zhongyao Zazhi* 1999;24(8):472-73.

[13] Yat P, et al. An improved extraction procedure for the rapid, quantitative high-performance liquid chromatographic estimation of the main eleutherosides (B and E) in *E. senticosus* (Eluthero). *Phytochem Anal* 1998;9(6):291-95.

[14] Anetai M, et al. Determination of some constituents in *Acanthopanax senticosus* Harms. III. Differences among part, diameter, age, and harvest time. *Hokkaidoritsu Eisei Kenkyusho* 1995;45 63-65.

[15] Medon P, et al. Effects of *E. senticosus* extracts on hexobarbital metabolism in vivo and in vitro. *J Ethnopharmacol* 1984;10(2) 235-41.

[16] Wanger Von H, et al. Immunostimulierend wirkende polysaccharide (heteroglycane) aus Hoheren pflanzen. *Arzneimittelforschung* 1984;34:659-61.

[17] Martinez B, et al. The physiological effects of aralia, panax and eleutherococcus on exercised rats. *Jpn J Pharmacol* 1984;35(2):79.

[18] Lewis W, et al. No adaptogen response of mice to ginseng and eleutherococcus infusions. *J Ethnopharmacol* 1983;8(2):209.

[19] Filaretov A, et al. [Effect on adaptogens on the activity of the pituitary-adrenocortical system in rats.] [Russian] *Bull Eksper Bio Med* 1986;101(5):573.

[20] Hacker B, et al. Cytotoxic effects of *E. senticosus* aqueous extracts in combination with N6-(DELTA 2-isopentenyl)-adenosine and 1–beta-D-arabinofuranosylcytosine against L-1210 leukemia cells. *J Pharm Sci* 1984;73(2):270.

[21] Ben-Hur E, et al. Effect of panax ginseng saponins and *E. senticosus* on survival of cultured mammalian cells after ionizing radiation. *Am J Chin Med* 1981;9(1):48.

[22] Pearce P, et al. *P. ginseng* and *E. senticosus* extracts - in vitro studies on binding to steroid receptors. *Endocrinol Jpn* 1982;29(5):567-73.

[23] Bohn B, et al. Flow-cytometric studies with *E. senticosus* extract as an immunomodulatory agent. *Arzneimittelforschung* 1987;37(10):1193.

[24] Kaloeva, Z. [Effect of the glycosides of *E. senticosus* on the hemodynamic indices of children with hypotensive states.] [Russian] *Farmakol Toksikol* 1986;49(5):73.

[25] Asano K, et al. Effect of *E. senticosus* extract on human physical working capacity. *Planta Med* 1986;48(3):175.

[26] Kupin V, et al. [Stimulation of the immunological reactivity of cancer patients by eleutherococcus extract.] [Russian] *Vopr Onkol* 1986;32(7):21.

[27] Afanas'eva T, et al. [Effect of eleutherococcus on the subcellular structures of the heart in experimental myocardial infarct.] *Bull Eksper Bio Med* 1987;103(2):212.

[28] Tian B, et al. [Effects of ciwujia (*A. senticosus* harms) on reperfusion-induced arrhythmia and action potential alterations in the isolated rat heart.] [Chinese] *Chung Kuo Chun Yao Tsa Chih* 1989;14(8):493-95.

[29] Shang Y, et al. [Effect of eleutherosides on ventricular late potential with coronary heart disease and myocarditis.] [Chinese] *Chung Hsi i Chih Ho Tsa Chih* 1991;11(5):280.

[30] Minkova M, et al. Effect of eleutherococcus extract on the radioprotective action of adeturone. *Acta Physiol Pharmacol Bulg* 1987;13(4):66-70.

[31] Molokovskii D, et al. [The action of adaptogenic plant preparations in experimental alloxan diabetes.] [Russian] *Probl Endokrinol* 1989;35(6):82.

[32] Shi Z, et al. [Effect of a mixture of *A. senticosus* and *Elsholtzia splendens* on serum-lipids in patients with hyperlipemia.] [Chinese] *Chung Hsi i Chieh Ho Tsa Chih* 1990;10(3):155.

[33] Tarle D, et al. *E. senticosus* maxim - investigation of saponins and antimicrobial acitivity. *Farma Glasnik* 1993;49:161.

[34] Godeichuk T, et al [The prevention of congenital development anomalies in rats.] [Russian] *Ontogenez* 1993;24(1):48.

[35] Borchers A, et al. Comparative effects of three species of ginseng on human peripheral blood lymphocyte proliferative responses. *Int J Immunother* 1998;14(3):143-52.

[36] http://www.19nordiol.com/nutrionline/ginseng51.html

[37] http://www.enrich.com/us/prod_cat_eng/preprint_0251.html

[38] http://www.tfnutrition.com/sportsnutrition/sibgin60.html

[39] McRae S. Elevated serum digoxin levels in a patient taking digoxin and Siberian ginseng. *Can Med Assoc J* 1996;155(3):293.

[40] Blumenthal M, et al. The Complete German Commission E Monographs. Austin, TX: American Botanical Council. 1998;124-25.

Emblica

SCIENTIFIC NAME(S): *Emblica officinalis* Gaertin. Family: Euphorbiaceae

COMMON NAME(S): Indian gooseberry, Amla (Hindi), Amalaki (Sanskrit), Emblic Myrobalan (English).

BOTANY: Emblica is a deciduous tree native to India and the Middle East. The round greenish-yellow fruits are commonly used in the Indian diet. Its leaves are feather-like with pale green flowers.[1]

HISTORY: Emblica is mentioned in an Ayurvedia text dating back to the 7th Century.[1]

CHEMISTRY: A fixed oil, volatile oil, and tannins are also present in the plant.[1]

PHARMACOLOGY: Emblica has documented effects on cholesterol levels. Various reports from the 1980s demonstrated reduced serum, aortic, and hepatic cholesterol in rabbit experimentation.[2,3,4,5] A later report confirms the earlier studies reducing lipids and exhibiting atherosclerotic effects in rabbits. Parameters that decreased were serum cholesterol (82%), triglycerides (66%), phospholipids (77%), and LDL (90%).[6] In a human clinical trial, normal and hypercholesterolemic men (35 to 55 years of age) given emblica supplementation experienced a decrease in serum cholesterol levels, which was reversible upon discontinuation of the drug.[7] The plant also has inhibited lipid peroxidation in biological membranes[8] and has displayed a protective effect in myocardial necrosis in rats.[9]

Ancient Ayurvedic medicine also employs emblica, in the form of fruit juice, as therapy for diabetic patients to strengthen the pancreas.[1] Current investigation in this area was studied in dogs with acute pancreatitis. The treated group showed less cell damage and marked inflammatory score decreases confirmed by microscopic examination.[10]

Emblica has also been studied for its anticancer and antimicrobial effects. It has inhibited induced mutagenesis in *Salmonella* strains.[11] In another study, the plant significantly inhibited dose-dependent hepatocarcinogenesis as measured by parameters such as tumor incidence, enzyme measurements, and other liver injury markers.[12] Emblica has reduced cytotoxic effects in mice given carcinogens.[13] However, in 1 report emblica had no significant effect in reducing lung cancer parameters in mice.[14] Alcoholic extracts of emblica showed activity against a number of test bacteria in another report.[15] In addition, the plant was effective against certain dermatophytes in another study.[16]

Other reported effects of emblica include the following: Anti-inflammatory (in water fraction of methanol leaf extract),[17] dyspepsia treatment,[18] organ restoration, and treatment for eye problems, joint pain, diarrhea, and dysentery.[1]

TOXICOLOGY: No major reported toxicities have been associated with the fruit.

SUMMARY: Emblica, or Indian gooseberry, has been used in Ayurvedic medicine for thousands of years. Emblica has cholesterol-lowering effects, and other positive effects in certain heart diseases. The plant has also exhibited antimicrobial, anticancer, and anti-inflammatory actions. Little information on toxicity is available.

PATIENT INFORMATION – Emblica

Uses: Emblica has cholesterol-lowering, antimicrobial, anticancer, and anti-inflammatory effects.

Side Effects: No major toxicities have been reported.

---

[1] Chevallier A. Encyclopedia of Medicinal Plants. New York, NY: DK Publishing 1996;202.

[2] Mishra M, et al. Emblica officinalis Gaertn. and serum cholesterol level in experimental rabbits. *Br J Exp Pathol* 1981;62(5):526-28.

[3] Thakur C, et al. Effect of Emblica officinalis on cholesterol-induced atherosclerosis in rabbits. *Indian J Med Res* 1984;79:142-46.

[4] Thakur C, et al. Emblica officinalis reduces serum, aortic, and hepatic cholesterol in rabbits. *Experientia* 1985;41(3):423-24.

[5] Thakur C, et al. The Ayurvedic medicines Haritaki, Amala, and Bahira reduce cholesterol-induced atherosclerosis in rabbits. *Int J Cardiol* 1988;21(2):167-75.

[6] Mathur R, et al. Hypolipidaemic effect of fruit juice of Emblica officinalis in cholesterol-fed rabbits. *J Ethnopharmacol* 1996;50(2):61-68.

[7] Jacob A, et al. Effect of the Indian gooseberry (amla) on serum cholesterol levels in men aged 35-55 years. *Eur J Clin Nutr* 1988;42(11):939-44.

[8] Kumar K, et al. Medicinal plants from Nepal; II. Evaluation as inhibitors of lipid peroxidation in biological membranes. *J Ethnopharmacol* 1999;64(2):135-39.

[9] Tariq M, et al. Protective effect of fruit extracts of Emblica officinalis (Gaertn.) and Terminalia belerica (Roxb.) in experimental myocardial necrosis in rats. *Indian J Exp Biol* 1977;15(6):485-86.

[10] Thorat S, et al. Emblica officinalis: a novel therapy for acute pancreatitis—an experimental study. *HPB Surg* 1995;9(1):25-30.

[11] Grover I, et al. Effect of Emblica officinalis Gaertn. (Indian gooseberry) fruit extract on sodium azide and 4-nitro-o-phenylenediamine induced mutagenesis in *Salmonella typhimurium*. *Indian J Exp Biol* 1989;27(3):207-09.

[12] Jeena K, et al. Effect of Emblica officinalis, Phyllanthus amarus, and Picrorrhiza kurroa on N-nitrosodiethylamine induced hepatocarcinogenesis. *Cancer Lett* 1999;136(1):11-16.

[13] Nandi P, et al. Dietary chemoprevention of clastogenic effects of 3,4-benzo(a)pyrene by Emblica officinalis Gaertn. fruit extract. *Br J Cancer* 1997;76(10):1279-83.

[14] Menon L, et al. Effect of rasayanas in the inhibition of lung metastasis induced by B16F-10 melanoma cells. *J Exp Clin Cancer Res* 1997;16(4):365-68.

[15] Ahmad I, et al. Screening of some Indian medicinal plants for their antimicrobial properties. *J Ethnopharmacol* 1998;62(2):183-93.

[16] Dutta B, et al. Antifungal activity of Indian plant extracts. *Mycoses* 1998;41(11-12):535-36.

[17] Asmawi M, et al. Anti-inflammatory activities of Emblica officinalis Gaertn. leaf extracts. *J Pharm Pharmacol* 1993;45(6):581-84.

[18] Chawla Y, et al. Treatment of dyspepsia with Amalaki (Emblica officinalis Linn.)—an Ayurvedic drug. *Indian J Med Res* 1982;76 Suppl:95-98.

The Ephedras

SCIENTIFIC NAME(S): Many members of the genus Ephedra have been used medicinally. The most common of these include *E. major* Host., *E. vulgaris*, *E. altissima*, *E. distachya*, *E. sinica* Stapf., *E. helvetica*, C.A. Meyer, *E. intermedia* Schrenk and Meyer and *E. nevadensis* Watson. Family: Ephedraceae (Gnetaceae)

COMMON NAME(S): Sea grape, ma-huang, yellow horse, yellow astringent, joint fir, squaw tea, Mormon tea, popotillo, teamster's tea.

BOTANY: Ephedra species have a worldwide distribution. They are generally erect evergreen plants, often resembling small shrubs. The name yellow horse derives from the traditional name for its horse-shaped flowers. The plants resemble a bunch of jointed branches covered with minute leaves. These plants generally have a strong pine odor and astringent taste. They have been suggested as an economic cash crop for the southwestern United States.[1]

HISTORY: The Ephedras have a long history of use as stimulants and for the management of bronchial disorders. It is believed that these plants were used more than 5,000 years ago by the Chinese to treat asthma.[2] Ephedra has been used in Oriental medicine to treat colds and flu, fevers, chills, headaches, edema, lack of perspiration, nasal congestion, aching joints and bones, coughing and wheezing.[3] Today, Ephedra continues to find a place in herbal preparations designed to relieve cold symptoms and to improve respiratory function. The use of standardized ephedrine/pseudoephedrine preparations, however, has supplanted the use of the crude drug in most developed countries.

North American species which are alkaloid-free have been made into refreshing, non-stimulating beverages and used to treat venereal diseases. The fruits of some species are eaten, while ashes of *E. intermedia* are mixed with chewing tobacco in Pakistan.[4]

CHEMISTRY: Comprehensive pharmacologic studies of *E. sinica* at the turn of the 20th century led to the isolation of the alkaloid ephedrine. The natural form is levorotatory, while the synthetic compound is generally a racemic mixture. Members of this genus that contain the alkaloid yield from 0.5% to 2.5% alkaloids, 30% to 90% of which is ephedrine, depending on the species. Pseudoephedrine (isoephedrine) is also found in some members of the genus.[5] In trade, dried Ephedra should contain no less than 1.25% ephedrine.[4] The woody basal stems are low in alkaloids and the roots and fruits are nearly alkaloid-free. Ephedrine is highly stable, even in solution. These plants generally contain large amounts of tannin,[6] which contribute to their astringent taste.

Most North American species do not appear to contain any pharmacologically active alkaloids. *E. nevadensis* (Mormon tea) is one species that has been shown repeatedly to be devoid of ephedrine-like alkaloids. These plants are consumed under local names such as squaw tea and desert tea.[4] There has been considerable controversy about the alkaloid content of this plant, but the weight of evidence indicates that it is alkaloid free.[7,8]

PHARMACOLOGY: Ephedrine and its related alkaloids are central nervous system stimulants. Ephedrine is active when given orally, parenterally or ophthalmically. It stimulates the heart, causing increased blood pressure and heart rate and is an effective bronchodilator. It can stimulate contraction of the uterus and has diuretic properties. Because it constricts peripheral blood vessels, it can relieve congestion in mucous tissues. Pseudoephedrine has a weaker cardiac effect but a greater diuretic activity.[4] Strong diuretic activity has been reported experimentally for dogs and rabbits.[3] Administration of the fluid extract and decoction of Mormon tea has resulted in diuresis, most likely due to compounds other than ephedrine. Teas of these plants can cause constipation due to their tannin content.

Crude aerial parts of Ephedra (known in Chinese as mao) cause hyperglycemia, most likely induced by the ephedrine alkaloids. However, investigations into the crude drug found a fraction that exhibited repeated hypoglycemic effects.[9] At least five related glycans (ephedrans) reduce blood sugar levels in normal mice and these were also effective in alloxan-induced diabetes,[10] indicating that intact pancreatic cells are not required for the pharmacologic effect.

Although crude Ephedra aerial parts (mao) can induce hypertension, crude ephedra root (mao-kon) causes hypotension. This effect is due to several related macrocyclic spermine alkaloids designated ephedradines.[11] These exerted a hypotensive effect in rats at a dose of 1 mg/kg IV and appear to act as ganglionic blocking agents.

Others studying the hypotensive effect of the root preparation have isolated L-tyrosine betaine (maokonine) a compound that induces hypertension, suggesting that, depending on the species, a variable effect on bloodpressure may be observed.[12]

Crude aerial parts have been shown to exert anti-inflammatory activity in animal models; this effect was related to (+)-pseudoephedrine and ephedroxane (a minor component).[13]

Dry extract and tannin of Herba Ephedra have been experimentally linked to improving renal function in adenine-induced chronic renal failure in rats, correcting calcium and phosphorous disorders, and inhibiting production of methylguanidine.[14]

TOXICOLOGY: In large doses, ephedrine causes nervousness, headache, insomnia, dizziness, palpitations, skin flushing, tingling, vomiting, anxiety and restlessness. Toxic psychosis could be induced by ephedrine. Skin reactions have been observed in sensitive patients.[4,15] Patients with high blood pressure and diabetes should exercise caution when using these plants.

E. altissima yields several mutagenic n-nitrosamines under simulated gastric conditions. For example, N-nitrosephedrine causes metastasizing liver-cell carcinomas, as well as cancer of the lung and forestomach in animals. However, the investigators noted that the potential for endogenous formation of these compounds following ingestion of the tea is extremely small.[16]

SUMMARY: The Ephedras are a large genus of plants that have been used medicinally throughout the world. Most of the species contain ephedrine or pseudoephedrine, the major active components responsible for the stimulating and vasoactive effects of the plant. Most North American species, however, are devoid of alkaloids and are used to produce non-stimulating teas.

PATIENT INFORMATION – The Ephedras

Uses: Ephedra preparations are traditionally used to relieve colds, improve respiratory function and treat a range of ills from headaches to venereal disease. Evidence shows that plant parts of various species exert hypoglycemic, hypo- and hypertensive, diuretic, anti-inflammatory and other effects.

Side Effects: Large doses may cause a variety of ill effects from skin reactions to toxic psychosis and mutagenic effects. Those with high blood pressure and diabetes should exercise caution using ephedra.

---

[1] McLaughlin SP. Economic Prospects for New Crops in the Southwestern United States. *Economic Botany* 1985;39(4):473.

[2] Weiss RF. Herbal Medicine. Gothenburg, Sweden: AB Arcanum, 1988.

[3] Blumenthal M, King P. Ma Huang: Ancient Herb, Modern Medicine, Regulatory Dilemma. *Herbal Gram* 1995;34:22.

[4] Morton JF. Major Medicinal Plants: Botany, Culture and Uses. Springfield, IL: Charles C. Thomas, 1977.

[5] DerMarderosian AH, Liberti LE. Natural Product Medicine. Philadelphia: GF Stickley Co., 1988.

[6] Friedrich VH, Wiedemeyer H. [Quantitative Determination of the Tannin-Precursors and the Tannins in Ephedra helvetica.] [German] *Planta Medica* 1976;303(3):223.

[7] Tyler VE. The New Honest Herbal. Philadelphia: GF Stickley Co., 1987.

[8] Terry RE. Scientific Section: A Study for Ephedra Nevadensis. *J APHA* 1927;16:397.

[9] Shabana MM, et al. Study into wild Egyptian plants of potential medicinal activity. Ninth communication: hypoglycaemic activity of some selected plants in normal fasting and alloxanised rats. *Arch Exp Veterinarmed* 1990;44(3):389.

[10] Konno C, et al. Isolation and Hypoglycemic Activity of Ephedrans A, B, C, D and E, Glycans of *Ephedra distachya* Herbs. *Planta Medica* 1985;50(2):162.

[11] Hikino H, et al. Hypotensive Actions of Ephedradines, Macrocyclic Spermine Alkaloids of Ephedra Roots. *Planta Med* 1983;48(4):290.

[12] Tamada M, et al. Maokonine, Hypertensive Principle of Ephedra Roots. *Planta Medica* 1978;34(3):291.

[13] Hikino H, et al. Antiinflammatory Principle of *Ephedra* Herbs. *Chem Pharm Bull* 1980;28(10):2900.

[14] Wang GZ, Hikokichi O. [Experimental study in treating chronic renal failure with dry extract and tannins of herba ephedra.] [Chinese] *Chung-Kuo Chung Hsi i Chieh Ho Tsa Chih [Chinese Journal of Stomatology]* 1994;14(8):485.

[15] Kalix P. The pharmacology of psychoactive alkaloids from ephedra and catha. [Review] *J Ethnopharmacol* 1991;32(1-3):201.

[16] Tricker AR, et al. 2-(N-nitroso-N-methylamino) propiophenone, a direct acting bacterial mutagen found in nitrosated *ephedra altissima* tea. *Toxicol Lett* 1987;38(1-2):45.

Evening Primrose Oil

SCIENTIFIC NAME(S): *Oenothera biennis* L. Family: Onagraceae

COMMON NAME(S): Evening primrose

BOTANY: The evening primrose is a large, delicate wildflower native to North America and is not a true primrose. The blooms usually last only 1 evening. Primrose is an annual or biennial and can grow in height from 1 to 3 meters. The flowers are yellow in color and the fruit is a dry pod about 5 cm long that contains many small seeds.[3] The small seeds contain an oil characterized by its high content of gamma-linolenic acid (GLA).[1] Wild varieties of *O. biennis* contain highly variable amounts of linoleic acid and GLA; however, extensive cross-breeding has produced a commercial variety that consistently yields an oil with 72% cis-linoleic acid and 9% GLA. This is perhaps the richest plant source of GLA. A commercially grown mold has been reported to produce an oil containing 20% GLA, and newer strains may produce even greater yields.[2]

The oil from evening primrose (OEP) seeds is cultivated in at least 15 countries and is available in more than 30 countries as a nutritional supplement or as a constituent in specialty foods. US and Canadian production total more than 300 to 400 tons of seeds yearly. US production centers are in California, North Carolina, South Carolina, Oregon and Texas.[4]

CHEMISTRY: Seeds from *O. biennis* L. contain 14% of a fixed oil known as OEP. This oil can contain from 50% to 70% cis-linoleic acid and from 7% to 10% cis-GLA.[3] Plants of varying age and location have been studied for different GLA content.[5] Also found is cis-6,9,12–octadecatrienoic acid; small amounts of oleic, palmitic and stearic acids; steroids; campesterol; and beta-sitosterol.[3] Mucilage and tannin presence in plant parts of evening primrose has also been analyzed.[6]

PHARMACOLOGY: Essential fatty acids (EFAs) are important as cellular structural elements and as precursors of prostaglandins. Prostaglandins help regulate metabolic functions.[3] EFAs are the biologically active parts of polyunsaturated fats. Ingestion of EFAs is believed to help reduce the incidence of cardiovascular disease and obesity. EFAs cannot be manufactured by the body and must be provided by the diet in relatively large amounts. It has been recommended that 1% to 3% of total daily caloric intake should be in the form of EFAs.[7] The World Health Organization recommends 5% for children and pregnant or lactating women.[8]

Animal studies have shown that dietary EFA deprivation can lead to eczema-like lesions and hair loss, a generalized defect in connective tissue synthesis with poor wound healing, failure to respond normally to infection with poor immune function, infertility (especially in males), fatty degeneration of the liver, renal lesions with a lack of normal water balance and atrophy of exocrine glands (lacrimal, salivary). This suggests that a variety of human illnesses with similar symptoms may result from poor EFA metabolism or insufficient dietary EFA. Because OEP represents a rich source of EFAs, particularly GLA, its use has been suggested in the treatment of these deficiency syndromes. Theoretically, the GLA provided by EPO can be converted directly to the prostaglandin precursor dl-homo-GLA (DGLA) and might be beneficial to persons unable to metabolize cis-linoleic acid to GLA or with low dietary intake of cis-linoleic acid.

It has been postulated that GLA, DGLA and arachidonic acid are present in human milk for a very important and specific purpose.[9,10] It is believed that the conversion of linoleic acid to GLA in humans is a rate-limiting metabolic step,[11] with only a relatively small amount of dietary linoleic acid (LA) being converted to GLA and to other metabolites.[12] The delta-6-desaturase enzyme is required for this conversion. Factors interfering with this GLA production include aging, diabetes, high alcohol intake, high fat diets, certain vitamin deficiencies, hormones, high cholesterol levels and viral infections.[8] The essential fatty acids beyond this rate-limiting step are crucial for proper development of many body tissues, especially in the brain. The brain contains about 20% of 6-desaturated EFAs by weight. Infants cannot form an adequate amount of EFAs if linoleic acid is the only dietary source of n-6-EFA; this may be why preformed GLA, DGLA and arachidonic acid are present in human milk. Studies have compared fatty acids in the phospholipids of red blood cells from infants fed human milk with those from infants fed artificial milk formulas. Infants fed artificial formulas showed phospholipids containing higher levels of linoleic acid and significantly lower levels of DGLA and arachidonic acid. Dietary supplementation to pregnant women with OEP results in an increase of total fat and EFA content in breast milk.[13] The presence of linoleic acid metabolites in human milk can affect the composition of red blood cell membranes.[14]

Taking large amounts (30 g/day to 40 g/day) of linoleic acid has little effect on DGLA or arachidonic acid blood levels.[15,16,17] However, taking less than 500 mg GLA/day can produce a significant increase in DGLA concentration and a smaller increase in arachidonic acid in plasma phospholipids.[12] These elevated levels do not exceed normal amounts found in the American population.[18] Therefore, GLA, not linoleic acid, is capable of elevating the levels of linoleic acid metabolites in human blood. Below-normal plasma or adipose-tissue concentrations of GLA, DGLA or arachidonic acid may occur in: Healthy middle-aged men who will later develop heart disease;[19,20,21,22] healthy middle-aged people who will later suffer stroke;[23] diabetics;[24,25] patients with atopic dermatitis;[25,26,27] heavy drinkers;[28,29] females with premenstrual syndrome;[30] older people.[31,32]

The commercial product *Efamol* (Efamol Research Institute, Nova Scotia, Canada) is a standardized dosage form of EPO and has been tested clinically in a variety of illnesses. A large number of independently conducted studies and clinical trials, mainly sponsored by Efamol, Ltd., provide preliminary evidence that GLA in the form of EPO can be beneficial in certain conditions.

The effects of OEP can be categorized as follows:

Cardiovascular disease: Linoleic acid can reduce elevated serum cholesterol levels, but GLA has cholesterol-lowering activity about 170 times greater than the parent compound.[33] In 79 patients who took 4 g *Efamol*/day in a placebo controlled study, a significant ($p < 0.001$) decrease of 31.5% in serum cholesterol was noted after 3 months of treatment. A nonsignificant (NS) decrease was observed in the placebo group.[34] Preliminary unpublished data from double-blind trials suggest that EPO given to overweight patients with a family history of obesity results in a significant weight loss and a reduction in skin-fold thickness and systolic and diastolic blood pressures after 6 weeks of therapy. There is evidence that the oil inhibits ADP-induced platelet aggregation in treated guinea pigs, suggesting that an increase in the formation of the antithrombotic-1-series prostaglandins may inhibit in vivo thrombosis.[35] In some studies, GLA has lowered plasma cholesterol and triglycerides and inhibited in vivo platelet aggregation.[36] Elevated plasma lipids and in vivo platelet

aggregation are risk factors for heart disease and stroke, and GLA lowers both of these.[37] In a later report in 20 hyperlipidemic patients, 2.4 to 7.4 ml/day of *Pre-Glandin* I (containing 9% GLA) was administered. There were no changes in serum cholesterol, HDL cholesterol or triglyceride levels.[38]

Breast cancer and related disorders: Animal studies indicate that subcutaneous OEP injections (25 to 200 mcL/day) produced statistically significant reductions in transplanted mammary tumors from baseline size, while an olive oil control did not.[39] An in vitro experiment found a dose-related inhibition of the growth rate in the malignant BL6 tumor system.[40]

Improvement in serum fatty acid levels by OEP supplementation in women with benign breast disorders has not been associated with a clinical response.[41] In women with proven recurrent breast cysts, OEP treatment for 1 year resulted in a slightly lower (NS) recurrence rate compared with placebo.[42]

Premenstrual syndrome (PMS) and mastalgia: Clinical studies investigating OEP use in these conditions have had positive results. PMS involves a variety of symptoms, the most common being cyclical mood changes, fluid retention or redistribution, breast tenderness and discomfort and tension headaches. A variety of pharmacologic therapies have been suggested with variable results, including the use of progestogens, oral contraceptives, pyridoxine (vitamin B_6), bromocriptine, danazol, mineral supplements, opioid antagonists, diuretics, antidepressants, mefenamic acid, clonidine, lithium carbonate, ibuprofen and GLA.[43,44,45]

It has been suggested that an abnormal sensitivity to prolactin or a deficiency of PGE1 (thought to attenuate the biologic activity of prolactin) may contribute to PMS. Levels of GLA and subsequent metabolites were lower in women with PMS than in controls, indicating a possible defect in the conversion of linoleic acid to GLA. This may result in an exceptional sensitivity to normal changes in prolactin levels.[46] In 19 PMS patients receiving evening primrose oil each morning and evening during the last 14 days before menstruation for five consecutive cycles, PMS symptoms were decreased. OEP was most effective during the fifth cycle.[47]

PMS and breast pain are common with high fat intake. Women with breast pain may be unable to convert LA to GLA.[8] In some studies, PMS and premenstrual breast pain (cyclic mastalgia) have been relieved by GLA to a significantly greater degree than with placebo.[48] However, a placebo controlled evaluation of OEP found the oil to have no effect and that the effects observed in women with moderate PMS were solely due to a placebo effect.[49]

A number of clinical studies have evaluated the effect of OEP in women with nodular or polycystic breast disease. Treatments such as bromocriptine, danazol or OEP have been associated with improvement in breast pain in up to 77% of patients with cyclical mastalgia and 44% of those with noncyclical mastalgia.[50]

Further etiology and assessment of breast pain has been reported, along with OEP treatment in this condition.[51] PMS assessment and recommendations to affected patients can also be referenced.[52]

A recent report on the use of OEP to treat menopausal flushing concluded that there were no benefits over placebo in this condition.[53]

Rheumatoid arthritis: A double-blind, placebo controlled study investigated the effects of altering dietary EFAs on requirements for nonsteroidal anti-inflammatory drugs (NSAIDs) in patients with rheumatoid arthritis. The major aim was to determine whether OEP or OEP/fish oil could replace NSAIDs. An initial 1 year treatment period was followed by 3 months of placebo. At 1 year, OEP and OEP/fish oil produced significant subjective improvement compared with placebo. Furthermore, by 1 year, the patients taking OEP or EPO/fish oil had significantly reduced their use of NSAIDs. Following 3 months of placebo, those receiving initial NSAID treatment had relapsed. Despite decreased NSAID use, measures of disease activity did not worsen. However, there was no evidence that OEP and OEP/fish oil acted as disease-modifying agents.[54] OEP therapy for rheumatoid arthritis requires longer than 3 months for any beneficial effects.[8] A study of OEP vs olive oil found that OEP use resulted in a significant reduction in morning stiffness after 3 months.[55]

Properties, adverse effects, mechanism of action and clinical study overview of evening primrose oil for rheumatoid arthritis are further discussed.[56,57]

Multiple Sclerosis: In MS there is evidence of abnormality in both EFA metabolism and lymphocytic function. Several studies have shown slight but variable improvement in patients fed diets high in linoleic acid. In an open trial of OEP, three of eight patients with MS showed improvement in the manual dexterity test, but no improvement was noted in grip strength. When the oil was given with colchicine, four of six patients improved in their general physical tone.[58] Others have noted similar improvement with GLA therapy.[59,60,61]

Atopic dermatitis and dermatologic disorders: In atopic dermatitis, GLA was significantly more effective than placebo in improving skin condition, providing relief from pruritus and allowing reduced reliance on corticosteroid medication.[62,63] Other reports exist (most double-blind, crossover, randomized or placebo controlled) that evaluate OEP in atopic dermatitis treatment. These studies include: 15 adults and 17 children given 500 mg OEP (*Efamol*) orally twice daily for 3 weeks;[64] 60 adults and 39 children given higher EPO doses compared with lower doses;[63] 20 adults;[62] 24 children for a 4-week period, then 12 children for a long-term 20-week follow-up period;[65,66] 52 patients, age 16 to 64 years, given 500 mg OEP frequently for 4 months.[67] All reports suggest improvement in atopic eczema, regarding factors such as itch, scaling, disease severity, grade of inflammation, percent of body surface area involvement, dryness,[62,63] erythema and surface damage. Women with "premenstrual flare" of eczema reported improvement in their condition.[67] A meta-analysis involving 311 patients (age 1 to 60) in nine randomized, double-blind, placebo controlled studies determined OEP to be more effective than placebo.[68]

A defect in the function of delta-6-desaturase, the enzyme responsible for the conversion of linoleic acid to GLA, has been found in patients with atopic dermatitis.[69] Forty-eight children (age 2 to 8 years) administered 0.5 g/kg/day of *Epogam* showed significant improvement in disease severity independent of whether the patients had IgE-mediated allergy manifestations. OEP also increased percent content of n-6 fatty acids in red blood cell membranes, without affecting membrane microviscosity.[70] OEP doses of 6 g/day in a double-blind, placebo controlled study of 102 patients improved the lipid profile of the epidermis in patients with atopic dermatitis[71] but it was not effective in treatment of the disease itself.[72]

A recent report discusses OEP and fish oil in the treatment of atopic dermatitis and psoriasis.[73]

Other diseases: In diabetic patients, GLA has been shown to reverse neurological damage.[74] GLA supplementation to children with IDDM (insulin-dependent diabetes mellitus) indicated that favorable and statistically significant increases in serum essential fatty acid levels and decreases in PGE2 levels occurred, which may provide a therapeutic benefit.[75] One study demonstrated that GLA accelerated recovery of liver function in alcoholics and reduced the severity of withdrawal symptoms.[28]

OEP has been tested for use in diagnosis and symptom relief of myalgic encephalomyelitis (Tapanui flu).[76] OEP may be of use to prevent or slow the development of hypertension in pregnancy by its pressor response to angiotensin II.[77] In combination therapy, three patients with Crohn's disease remained in relapse-free remission after OEP administration.[78]

The value of a drug that is effective in a wide variety of EFA-deficiency disorders cannot be overstated. The treatment of several unique medical conditions with OEP has been undertaken, often with excellent results. Many of the published studies have been open trials that require confirmation through double-blind testing; however, these studies generally have been well designed and their results adequately analyzed. The disorders treated include autoimmune diseases, childhood hyperactivity, chronic inflammation, ethanol-induced toxicity and acute alcohol withdrawal syndrome, icthyosis vulgaris, scleroderma, Sjogren's syndrome and Sicca syndrome, brittle nails, mastalgia, psychiatric syndromes, tardive dyskinesia, ulcerative colitis and migraine headaches. GLA has shown in vitro antitumor activity against primary liver cancer cells, but this effect was not demonstrated in a clinical trial.[79] Reviews of evening primrose oil are listed in the bibliography.[80,81,82,83,84,85,86,87,88,89,90]

TOXICOLOGY: As a nutritional supplement, the maximum label-recommended daily dose of OEP is approximately 4 g. This dose contains 300 to 360 mg GLA, which contributes: (1) 6 to 7 mg GLA/kg/day likely to be produced from linoleic acid in the normal adult female, (2) 23 to 65 mg GLA/kg/day consumed by a breastfed baby or (3) 70 to 400 mg/kg/day of all the metabolites of linoleic acid consumed by a breastfed infant. According to these estimates, the amounts of GLA in the recommended doses of OEP are in the same range as the amounts of GLA and other related EFAs present in widely consumed foods. Thus, there is little concern about the safety of OEP as a dietary supplement in the recommended dosage range. There are considerable data on the safety of OEP from Efamol, Ltd., a major commercial supplier of oil derived from specially selected and hybridized forms of *Oenothera* species. In toxicological studies carried out for 1 year, OEP at doses up to 2.5 ml/kg/day in rats and 5 ml/kg/day in dogs was found to possess no toxic properties. Similar results were obtained in 2-year carcinogenicity and teratological investigations. With approximately 1000 tons of OEP sold in several countries as a nutritional supplement since the 1970s, there have been no complaints concerning the safety of the product.[91]

SUMMARY: The oil obtained from the seeds of inbred strains of evening primrose is a rich natural source of essential fatty acids, especially cis-linoleic acid and GLA. The biologic importance of these fatty acids in maintaining normal physiologic function is well documented. The use of GLA supplementation by the ingestion of OEP has been shown effective in a variety of medical disorders due to EFA deficiency or problems in EFA metabolism. Some of these illnesses include: Cardiovascular disease, female disorders, rheumatoid arthritis, multiple sclerosis and atopic dermatitis.

Evening primrose oil appears to be devoid of significant adverse effects. A small number of patients in published studies have discontinued therapy for reasons related to OEP, but the symptoms have been variable and usually mild. The use of OEP for periods of up to 18 months did not result in any adverse effects.

PATIENT INFORMATION – Evening Primrose Oil

Uses: OEP has been used to treat cardiovascular disease, breast disorders, premenstrual syndrome, mastalgia, rheumatoid arthritis, multiple sclerosis, atopic eczema dermatological disorders and other illnesses.

Side effects: There have been no adverse effects attributed to oil of evening primrose.

---

[1] DerMarderosian A, et al. *Natural Product Medicine*. Philadelphia, PA: George F. Stickley Co., 1988.
[2] *Market Letter* 1986;Aug 4:21.
[3] Leung A. *Encyclopedia of Common Natural Ingredients*, 2nd ed. New York, NY: John Wiley, 1996.
[4] Carter JP. *Food Technol* 1988;(6):7282.
[5] Koblicova Z, et al. *Cesk Farme* 1990;39(Jul):315–19.
[6] Runjaic-Antic D, et al. *Pharmazie* 1988;43(Aug):563–4.
[7] Horrobin DF. *Holistic Med* 1981;3:118.
[8] Winther M. *Nat Pharm* 1996;(Oct/Nov):8–9,27.
[9] Clandinin M, et al. *Lipid Res* 1982;20:901.
[10] Crawford MA. *Progr Food Nutr Sci* 1980;4:755.
[11] Brenner RR. *Progr Lipid Res* 1982;20:41.
[12] Manku MS, et al. *Eur J Clin Nutr* 1988;42:55.
[13] Cant A, et al. *J Nutr Sci Vitaminol* 1991;37:573.

[14] Putnam JC, et al. *Am J Clin Nutr* 1982;36:106.
[15] Dayton S, et al. *J Lipid Res* 1966;7:103.
[16] Lasserre M, et al. *Lipids* 1983;20:227.
[17] Singer P, et al. *Prostaglandins Leukotr Med* 1984;15(2):159.
[18] Holman RT. *Am J Clin Nutr* 1979;32:2390.
[19] Horrobin DF, Huang YR. *Intl J Cardiol* 1987;17:241.
[20] Miettinen TA, et al. *Br Med J* 1982;285:993.
[21] Salonen JT, et al. *Am J Cardiol* 1985;58:226.
[22] Wood DA, et al. *Lancet* 1984;2:117.
[23] Miettinen TA. *Monogr Atheroscler* 1986;4:19.
[24] Jones DB, et al. *Br Med J* 1983;286:178.
[25] Mercuri C, et al. *Biochem Biophys Acta* 1988;116:407.
[26] Manku MS, et al. *Br J Dermatol* 1984;110:643.
[27] Strannegard IL, et al. *Intl Arch Allergy Appl Immunol* 1987;82:423.
[28] Glen L, et al. *Clin Exp Res* 1987;11:37.

[29] Nervi AM, et al. *Lipids* 1980;15:263.
[30] Bruch MG, et al. *Am J Obstet Gynecol* 1984;150:363.
[31] Darcet P, et al. *Ann Nutr Alim* 1980;34:277.
[32] Horrobin DF. *Rev Pure Appl Pharmacol Sci* 1983;4:339.
[33] Horrobin DF, Manku MS. *Lipids* 1983;18:558.
[34] Horrobin DF, Manku MS. Intern conference on oils, fats and waxes 1983, Auckland, New Zealand.
[35] Fisher J, et al. *Prog Lipid Res* 1982;20:799.
[36] van Doormal JJ, et al. *Diabetologia* 1986;29:A603.
[37] Puolaka J, et al. *J Reprod Med* 1985;30:149.
[38] Viikari J, et al. *Int J Clin Pharmacol Ther Toxicol* 1986;24(Dec):668–70.
[39] Ghayor T, Horrobin DF. *IRCS Med Sci* 1981;9:582.
[40] Dippemaar N. *S Afr Med J* 1982;62:505.
[41] Gateley CA, et al. *Br J Surg* 1992;79:407.
[42] Mansel RE, et al. *Ann NY Acad Sci* 1990;586:288.
[43] Brush MG. *J Psychosomatic Obst Gyn* 1983;2:35.
[44] Van Tyle J, et al. *Pharm Times* 1987;53(Sep):110–20,122–3.
[45] Choy G, et al. *CA Pharm* 1992;40(Jul):30–4,37.
[46] Horrobin DF. Abstract, Int. Symposium on Premenstrual Tension and Dysmenorrhea (1983), Charleston, SC.
[47] Larsson B, et al. *Curr Ther Res* 1989;46(Jul):58–63.
[48] Pye J, et al. *Lancet* 1985;2(Aug 17):373–7.
[49] Khoo S, et al. *Med J Aust* 1990;153(Aug 20):189–92.
[50] Gateley CA, Mansel RE. *Br Med Bull* 1991;47:284.
[51] Mansel R. *Br Med J* 1994;309(Oct 1):866–8.
[52] Morley A, et al. *Pharm J* 1987;238(Jan 17):72–3.
[53] Chenoy R, et al. *Br Med J* 1994;308(Feb19):501–3.
[54] Belch JJF, et al. *Ann Rheum Dis* 1988;47:96.
[55] Brzeski M, et al. *Br J Rheumatol* 1991;30:370.
[56] Joe L, et al. *DICP* 1993;27(Dec):1475–7.
[57] Gillbanks L, et al. *N Z Pharm* 1996;16(May):34–7.
[58] Horrobin DF. *Med Hypoth* 1979;5:365.
[59] Field EF. *Lancet* 1978;1:780

[60] Millar JHD, et al. *Br Med J* 1973;1:765.
[61] Field EF, Joyce G. *Eur Neurol* 1983;22:78.
[62] Schalin-Karrila M. *Br J Dermatol* 1987;117:11.
[63] Wright S, Burton JL. *Lancet* 1982;2:1120.
[64] Lovell C, et al. *Lancet* 1981;1(Jan 31):278.
[65] Bordoni A, et al. *Drugs Exp Clin Res* 1988;14(4):291–7.
[66] Biagli P, et al. *Drugs Exp Clin Res* 1988;14(4):285–90.
[67] Humphreys F, et al. *Eur J Dermatol* 1994;4(8):598–603.
[68] Morse P, et al. *Br J Dermatol* 1989;121(Jul):75–90.
[69] Kerscher MJ, Horting HC. *Clin Investig* 1992;70:167.
[70] Biagli P, et al. *Drugs Exp Clin Res* 1994;20(2):77–84.
[71] Schafer L, Kragballe K. *Lipids* 1991;26:557.
[72] Berth-Jones J. *Lancet* 1993;341(Jun 19):1557–60.
[73] Thomas J. *Aust J Pharm* 1994;75(Aug):739–40.
[74] Jamal GA. *Lancet* 1986;1:1098.
[75] Arisaka M, et al. *Prostaglandins Leukot Essent Fatty Acids* 1991;43:197.
[76] Simpson L. *N Z Pharm* 1985;5(Jan):14.
[77] O'Brien P, et al. *Br J Clin Pharmacol* 1985;19(Mar):335–42.
[78] Novak E. *Can Med Assoc J* 1988;139(Jul 1):14.
[79] van der Merwe CF, et al. *Prostaglandins Leukot Essent Fatty Acids* 1990;40:199.
[80] Ballentine C, et al. *FDA Consumer* 1987;21(Nov):34–5.
[81] Sinclair B. *N Z Pharm* 1988;8(Jan):28–9,31.
[82] Barber A. *Pharm J* 1988;240(Jun 4):723–5.
[83] Anonymous. *S Afr Pharm J* 1989;56(Feb):55–75.
[84] Barber A. *Ir Pharm Union Rev* 1989;14(Apr):121–2, 124.
[85] Kleijnen J. *Pharm Weekbl* 1989;124(Jun 9):418–23.
[86] Po A. *Pharm J* 1991;246(Jun 1):676–8.
[87] Pittit J. *Ir Pharm Union Rev* 1991;16(Oct):248,250–1, 253–6,258–9.
[88] Anonymous. *Ir Pharm Union Rev* 1992;17(Sep):199,201.
[89] Docherty M. *Aust J Pharm* 1994;75(Jan):48–53.
[90] Kleijnen J. *Br Med J* 1994;309(Oct 1):824–5.
[91] Carter JP. *Food Technol* 1988;(6):72.

Eyebright

SCIENTIFIC NAME(S): *Euphrasia officinale* L. Other species include *E. rostkoviana* Hayne and *E. stricta* J.P. Wolff ex J.F. Lehm. Family: Scrophulariaceae

COMMON NAME(S): Eyebright

BOTANY: This small annual plant grows to about one foot. It has oval leaves but can have a variable appearance. Its flowers are arranged in a spike; the white petals often have a red tinge, but may be purple-veined or have a yellow spot on the lower petal. It blooms from July to September. The flowers have the appearance of bloodshot eyes. It is believed to have originated from European wild plants.

HISTORY: Eyebright was used as early as Theophrastus and Dioscorides, who prescribed infusions for topical application in the treatment of eye infections. This was in large part due to the similarity of the "bloodshot" petals to irritated eyes. The plant has been used in homeopathy to treat conjunctivitis and other ocular inflammations. The plant continues to find use in black herbal medicine.[1]

Further historic data on the use of Euphrasia includes a 14th century cure for "all evils of the eye." An eyebright ale was described in Queen Elizabeth's era. It was a component of British Herbal Tobacco, which was smoked for chronic bronchial conditions and colds. Other early uses include treatments for allergies, cancers, coughs, conjunctivitis, earaches, epilepsy, headaches, hoarseness, inflammation, jaundice, ophthalmia, rhinitis, skin ailments and sore throats.

CHEMISTRY: Eyebright contains the glycoside aucuboside. In addition, the plant contains a tannin, aucubin, caffeic and ferulic acids, sterols, choline, some basic compounds and a volatile oil.[2]

Other components include vitamin C, β-carotene, glycosides, nonacosame, ceryl alcohol, beta-sitosterol, oleic-, and linoleic-, palmitic- and stearic- acids, fumaric acid, isoquercitrin, quercetin and rutin.[3] Additionally, the iridoid glycosides catalpol, euphroside and ixoroside, the lignan dehydrodiconiferlyl alcohol 4–β-D-glucoside, the phenylpropane glycoside eukovoside, the flavonoid apigenin, gallotannins, traces of tertiary alkaloids, steam-volatile substances and a range of free and combined phenol-carboxylic acids, principally caffeic, p-hydroxy-phenylpyruvic and vanillic acids.

Tannins, aucuboside (aucubin),[4] seven known iridoid glycosides and the new compound, eurostoside[5] as well as seven flavonoids[6] have all been isolated from *E. rostkoviana*.

PHARMACOLOGY: None of the chemical components of eyebright have been associated with a significant therapeutic effect. There are no controlled studies in man to evaluate its effectiveness in the treatment of ocular irritations.

Eyebright is commonly used in European folk medicine for blepharitis and conjunctivitis, as well as for a poultice for styes and the general management of eye fatigue. They also use it internally for coughs and hoarseness, as well as a homeopathic remedy for conjunctivitis.[7] The phenol-carboxylic acids are thought to play a role in the antibacterial effects of eyebright.

TOXICOLOGY: While there are no known risks associated with eyebright, its purported activities have not been clinically substantiated and the folkloric use is unacceptable on hygenic grounds.

German studies suggest that 10 to 60 drops of eyebright tincture could induce confusion, cephalalgia, violent pressure in the eyes with tearing, itching, redness and swelling of the margins of the lids, photophobia, dim vision, weakness, sneezing, coryza, nausea, toothache, constipation, hoarseness, cough, expectoration, dyspnea, yawning, insomnia, polyuria and diaphoresis.[3] Hence, ophthalmic use of this material is strongly discouraged.

SUMMARY: Eyebright is an herbal remedy that continues to find use among herbal enthusiasts. Although many adverse effects have been reported with its use, there appears to be little or no evidence in today's scientific literature for its effectiveness.

PATIENT INFORMATION – Eyebright

Uses: Eyebright preparations have been used to treat a variety of complaints, especially inflammatory eye disease.

Side Effects: The range of adverse effects is considered to outweigh the dubious benefits.

[1] Boyd EL, et al. Home Remedies and the Black Elderly. Ann Arbor: University of Michigan, 1984.

[2] Harkiss KJ, Timmins P. Studies in the Scrophulariaceae. 8. Phytochemical investigation of Euphrasis officinalis. *Planta Med* 1973;23(4):342.

[3] Duke JA. Handbook of Medicinal Herbs. Boca Raton, FL: CRC Press, 1985.

[4] Sodzawiczny K, et al. Content of Tannins and Aucuboside in *Herba euphrasiae* from Southern Poland. *Herba Polonica* 1984;30(3–4):165.

[5] Salama O, Sticher O. Iridoid Glucosides from *Euphrasia rostkoviana*. Part 4. Glycosides from *Euphrasia* species. *Planta Med* 1983;47:90.

[6] Matlawska I, et al. Flavonoid Compound in *Herba euphrasiae*. *Herba Polonica* 1988;34(3):97.

[7] Bisset NG, ed. Herbal Drugs and Phytopharmaceuticals. Stuttgart: Medpharm Scientific Publishers, 1994.

False Unicorn

SCIENTIFIC NAME(S): *Chamaelirium luteum* (L.) Gray, Family: Liliaceae (Lilies)

COMMON NAME(S): False unicorn, helonias root, devil's b t, blazing star, drooping starwort, rattlesnake, fairy-wand

BOTANY: *Chamaelirium luteum* is a native lily of the eastern US. It is considered a threatened species because of a loss of habitat and effects of collection from the wild for herbal use. Cultivation is considered possible, but has not yet become commercially important. The root is collected in autumn. *C. luteum* is a dioecious species (ie, the male and female flowers are borne on separate plants). The plant has been confused with the lilies *Helonias bullata* and *Aletris farinosa* (true unicorn root), because of several shared common names.[1,2,3]

HISTORY: False unicorn root was used by the Eclectic medical movement of the late 19th and early 20th centuries. Its chief use was for female complaints or as a uterine tonic in the treatment of amenorrhea or morning sickness. It has also been used for appetite stimulation and as a diuretic, vermifuge, emetic, and insecticide.[2,3,4,5,6]

CHEMISTRY: The root contains ≈ 10% of a saponin, chamaelirin ($C_{36}H_{62}O_{18}$), but neither its structure nor composition have been fully elucidated. Diosgenin was isolated from a hydrolyzate of the root extract, indicating that some components of the saponin may be based on this genin.[7] The fatty acids oleic, linoleic, and stearic acid were isolated from the root.[8]

PHARMACOLOGY: The fluid extract of false unicorn root was examined for its effects on isolated guinea pig uterus; however, no stimulant or relaxant effect was detected.[9,10,11] Similar experiments in the intact dog were also negative.[12] Nevertheless, a water extract did not block gonadotropin release in the rat.[13] A recent observation suggests, that false unicorn root may act through increasing human chorionic gonadotropin.[14] The notion that the occurrence of diosgenin might be responsible for hormonal effects is incorrect because the parent saponin is unlikely to be hydrolyzed to a free sterol in vivo. An understanding of false unicorn root's effects must await additional modern chemical and pharmacological studies.

TOXICOLOGY: False unicorn root is emetic at high doses. Cattle have died from consumption of the plant.[4] The safety of the plant for use in pregnancy has not been established.

SUMMARY: False unicorn has been used as a uterine stimulant; however, there is no chemical or pharmacological literature that substantiates this use. Its safety cannot be guaranteed in pregnancy; however, its century-long history of use contradicts serious acute toxicity. A monograph of false unicorn can be found in the *British Herbal Pharmacopoeia*, vol. 1.[15]

PATIENT INFORMATION – False Unicorn

Uses: Historically, false unicorn has been used as a uterine toric for treatment of amenorrhea and morning sickness, as an appetite stimulant, diuretic, vermifuge, emetic, and insecticide.

Side effects: False unicorn can be emetic at high doses. Safety has not been established during pregnancy.

---

[1] Clause E. *Pharmacognosy*, 3rd ed. Philadelphia, PA: Lea & Febiger, 1956.
[2] Foster S. False unicorn. *Herbs for Health* 1999 Jan/Feb;22.
[3] Grieve M. *A Modern Herbal* London, England: Jonathan Cape, 1931.
[4] Meyer C. *The Herbalist*, 3rd ed. 1976.
[5] Harding Ar. *Ginseng and other Medicinal Plants* Columbus, OH: A.R. Harding Publishing Co., 1908.
[6] Brinker FA. Comparative review of Eclectic femal regulators. *J Naturopathic Med* 1997;7(1):11.
[7] Marker RE, et al. Sterols. CXLVI. Sapogenins. LX. Some new sources of diosgenin. *J Am Chem Soc* 1942;64:1283.
[8] Cataline EL, et al. The phytochemistry of *Helonias* I. Preliminary examination of the drug. *J Amer Pharm Assoc* 1942;31:519.
[9] Pilcher JD. The action of various female remedies on the excised uterus of the guinea pig. *J Am Med Assoc* 1916;67:490.
[10] Pilcher JD, et al. The action of so-called female remedies on the excised uterus of the guinea pig. *Arch Intern Med* 1916;18:557.
[11] Pilcher JD. The action of certain drugs on the excised uterus of the guinea pig. *J Pharmacol* 1916;8:110.
[12] Pilcher JD, et al. The action of "female remedies" on intact uteri of animals. *Surg Gynecol Obstet* 1918;27:97.
[13] Graham RCB, et al. Comparison of in vitro activity of various species of *Lithospermum* and other plants to inactivate gonadatropin. *Endocrinology* 1955;56:239.
[14] Brandt D. A clinician's view. *HerbalGram* 1996;36:75.
[15] *British Herbal Pharmacopoeia*, vol 1. Great Britain: British Herbal Medicine Association, 1996.

Fennel

SCIENTIFIC NAME(S): *Foeniculum vulgare* Mill. syn. *F. officinale* All. and *Anethum foeniculum* Family: Apiaceae (Umbelliferae) A number of subspecies have been identified and their names add to the potential confusion surrounding the terminology of these plants.

COMMON NAME(S): Common, sweet or bitter fennel, carosella, Florence fennel, finocchio, garden fennel, large fennel, wild fennel[1,2]

BOTANY: Fennel is an herb native to southern Europe and Asia Minor. It is also cultivated in the United States, Great Britain and temperate areas of Eurasia. All parts of the plant are aromatic. When cultivated, fennel stalks grow to a height of about three feet. Plants have finely divided leaves composed of many linear or awl-shaped segments. Grayish, compound umbels bear small, yellowish flowers. The fruits or seeds are oblong ovals about 6 mm long and greenish or yellowish brown in color; they have five prominent dorsal ridges. The seeds have a taste resembling that of anise. Besides *F. vulgare*, *F. dulce* ("carosella") is grown for its stalks, while *F. vulgare* var azoricum Thell. ("finocchio") is grown for its bulbous stalk bases.

HISTORY: According to Greek legend, man received knowledge from Mount Olympus as a fiery coal enclosed in a stalk of fennel. The herb was known to the ancient Chinese, Indian, Egyptian and Greek civilizations, and Pliny recommended it for improving the eyesight. The name "foeniculum" is from the Latin word for "fragrant hay." Fennel was in great demand during the Middle Ages. The rich added the seed to fish and vegetable dishes, while the poor reserved it as an appetite suppressant to be eaten on feast days. The plant was introduced to North America by Spanish priests and the English brought it to their early settlements in Virginia.[3] All parts of the plant have been used for flavorings, and the stalks have been eaten as a vegetable. The seeds serve as a traditional carminative. Fennel has been used to flavor candies, liqueurs, medicines and food, and it is especially favored for pastries, sweet pickles and fish. The oil can be used to protect stored fruits and vegetables against infection by pathogenic fungi.[4] Beekeepers have grown it as a honey plant.[3] Health claims have included its use as a purported antidote to poisonous herbs, mushrooms and snakebites[5] and for the treatment of gastroenteritis, indigestion, to stimulate lactation and as an expectorant and an emmenagogue.[1] Tea made from crushed fennel seeds has been used as an eyewash.[3] Powdered fennel is said to drive fleas away from kennels and stables.[4]

CHEMISTRY: The oils of sweet and bitter fennel contain up to 90% trans-anethole, up to 20% fenchone and small amounts of limonene, camphor, alpha-pinene and about a half dozen additional minor volatile compounds.[6] The seeds contain between 3% and 6% of an essential oil and about 20% of a fixed oil composed of petroselinic acid, oleic acid and tocopherols.

Sweet fennel contains derivatives of caffeic acid and hydroxybenzoic acid.[7] The fruits (seeds) and leaves have been shown to contain a number of flavonoid compounds. These include quercetin 3-glucuronide, isoquercetin, kaempferol 3-glucuronide and kaempferol 3-arabinoside. Low concentrations of isorhammetin glycosides occur in the leaves.[8]

PHARMACOLOGY: An acetone extract of the seeds of *F. vulgare* has been shown to have estrogenic effects on the genital organs of male and female rats.[9] As an herbal medicine, fennel is reputed to increase milk secretion, promote menstruation, facilitate birth, ease the male climacteric and increase the libido. These supposed properties led to research on fennel for the development of synthetic estrogens during the 1930s. The principal estrogenic component of fennel was originally thought to be anethole, but it is now believed to be a polymer of anethole, such as dianethole or photoanethole.[10] The volatile oil of fennel increases the phasic contraction of ileal and tracheal smooth muscle in the guinea pig. The effect was generally greater with ileal muscle.[11] Administration of the volatile oil to rats has exacerbated experimentally-induced liver damage.[12]

TOXICOLOGY: Ingestion of the volatile oil may induce nausea, vomiting, seizures and pulmonary edema.[13] Its therapeutic use in Morocco has occasionally induced epileptiform madness and hallucinations.[4] The principal hazards with fennel itself are photodermatitis and contact dermatitis. Some individuals exhibit cross-reactivity to several species of Apiaceae, characteristic of the so-called celery-carrot-mugwort-condiment syndrome.[14] Rare allergic reactions have been reported following the ingestion of fennel.

Fennel oil was found to be genotoxic in the *Bacillus subtilis* DNA-repair test.[15] Estragole, present in the volatile oil, has been shown to cause tumors in animals.

A survey of fennel samples in Italy found viable aerobic bacteria, including coliforms, fecal streptococci and *Salmonella* species suggesting the plant may serve as a vector of infectious gastrointestinal diseases.[16]

A serious hazard associated with fennel is that poison hemlock can easily be mistaken for the herb. Hemlock contains highly narcotic coniine, and a small amount of hemlock juice can cause vomiting, paralysis and death.[5]

SUMMARY: Fennel is a popular herb that has been known since ancient times. It is widely used as a flavoring and scent and has served as an herbal remedy. Fennel oil contains compounds with estrogenic activity. The principal hazards associated with the plant are allergic reactions, photodermatitis and contact dermatitis in sensitive individuals, and some samples may be contaminated with pathogenic bacteria. However, poison hemlock can be mistakenly identified as fennel.

PATIENT INFORMATION – Fennel

Uses: Fennel has been used as a flavoring, scent, insect repellent, herbal remedy for poisoning and GI conditions, and as a stimulant to promote lactation and menstruation.

Side Effects: Fennel may cause photodermatitis, contact dermatitis and cross reactions. The oil may induce hallucinations, seizures, etc. Poison hemlock may be mistaken for fennel.

---

[1] Locock RA. *CPJ/RPC* 93/94;12/1:503.
[2] Meyer JE. The Herbalist. Hammond, IN: Hammond Book Co., 1934.
[3] Dobelis IN, ed. Magic and Medicine of Plants. Pleasantville, NY: Reader's Digest Assoc., 1986.
[4] Duke JA. Handbook of Medicinal Herbs. Boca Raton, FL: CRC Press, 1985.
[5] Loewenfeld C, Back P. The Complete Book of Herbs and Spices. London: David E. Charles, 1974.
[6] Lawrence PM. *Perfum Flavor* 1979;4:49.
[7] Schmidtlein H, Hermann K. *Z Lebensm Unters Forsch* 1975;159:255.
[8] Kunzemann J, Hermann K. *Z Lebensm Unters Forsch* 1977;164:194.
[9] Malini T, et al. *Indian J Physiol Pharmacol* 1985;29:21.
[10] Albert-Puleo M. *J Ethnopharmacol* 1980;2:337.
[11] Reiter M, Brandt W. *Arzneimforsch* 1985;35(1A):408.
[12] Gershbein LL. *Food Cosmet Toxicol* 1977;15:173.
[13] Marcus C, Lichtenstein EP. *J Agric Food Chem* 1979;27:1217.
[14] Wuthrich B, Hofer T. *Dtsch Med Wochenschr* 1984;109:981.
[15] Sekizawa J, Shibamoto T. *Mutat Res* 1982;101:127.
[16] Ercolani GL. *Appl Environ Microbiol* 1976;31:847.

Fenugreek

SCIENTIFIC NAME(S): *Trigonella foenum-graecum* L. Family: Leguminosae

COMMON NAME(S): Fenugreek

BOTANY: Fenugreek spice is commonly sold as the dried ripe seed. The plant is an annual that is native to Asia and southeastern Europe.

HISTORY: The European herb fenugreek has been used for centuries as a cooking spice and has been used in folk medicine for almost as long. The herb has been used in folk medicine in the treatment of boils, diabetes, cellulitis and tuberculosis. Extracts of the seeds are used to flavor maple syrup substitutes. The seeds are rich in protein and the plant is grown as an animal forage. Following commercial extraction of diosgenin (which is used as a natural precursor in commercial steroid synthesis), the nitrogen and potassium-rich seed residue is used as an agricultural fertilizer.

CHEMISTRY: The leaves of the plant contain at least seven saponins called graecunins. These compounds are glycosides of diosgenin.[1] Seeds contain from 0.1% to 0.9% diosgenin and are extracted on a commercial basis.[2,3] Plant tissue cultures from seeds grown under optimal conditions have been found to produce up to 2% diosgenin with smaller amounts of gitongenin and trigogenin. The seeds also contain the saponin fenugrin B.[4]

Several coumarin compounds have been identified in fenugreek seeds.[5] The seeds contain a number of alkaloids (trigonelline, gentianine, carpaine). A large portion of the trigonelline is degraded to nicotinic acid and related pyridines during roasting of the seed. These degradation products are in part responsible for the flavor of the seed. The seeds also yield up to 8% of a fixed, foul-smelling oil.

Several C-glycoside flavones have been identified in the seeds of fenugreek. These include vitexin, vitexin glycoside and an arabinoside of orientin (iso-orientin).[6] Three new minor steroidal sapogenins have also been found in fenugreek seeds: Smilagenin, sarsasapogenin and yuccagenin.[7] The mucilages of the seeds of several plants, including fenugreek, have been determined and their hydrolysates analyzed.[8]

Fenugreek is the source of a galactomannan-like mucilage. Because the seeds contain up to 50% of mucilaginous fiber, they have been used in the preparation of topical poultices and emollients and internally because of their ability to swell and relieve constipation and diarrhea.

PHARMACOLOGY: Fenugreek seeds reduce serum cholesterol levels in lab animals. In one study, fractions of fenugreek seeds were added to the diets of diabetic hypercholesterolemic and normal dogs for 8 days. The defatted fraction, which is rich in fibers (about 54%) and contains about 5% steroidal saponins, significantly lowered plasma cholesterol, blood glucose and plasma glucagon levels from pretreatment values in both diabetic hypercholesterolemic and normal dogs.[9] The hypocholesterolemic effect has also been reproduced in rats. When fenugreek seeds replaced 50% of their diet for 2 weeks, normal rats showed a 42% decreased and hypercholesterolemic rats showed a 58% decrease from baseline in cholesterol levels.[10]

The hypoglycemic effect of the seeds was evaluated further in dogs. Fractions of the seeds were administered orally to normal and diabetic dogs for 8 days. The lipid extract had no pharmacologic effects. The defatted fraction lowered blood glucose levels, plasma glucagon, and somatostatin levels and reduced carbohydrate-induced hyperglycemia. When this fraction was added to the insulin treatment of diabetic dogs, a decrease in hyperglycemia and insulin dose was noted. It is not clear if these changes are due to the common effect of dietary fiber on blood glucose or if the changes are due to a pharmacologically active compound.[11]

Water and alcoholic extracts have been shown to stimulate the isolated guinea pig uterus, indicating that these extracts may have oxytocic activity.

A French patent (2,073,285 Oct 1972) has been granted to a product purported to have antitumor activity, especially against "fibromas." The product contains extracts of tansy, juniper berries, fenugreek seeds, cinnamon, sedum, St. John's wort flowers, bitter orange rind and hydrated ferric oxide. No clinical studies have been reported using this or any other fenugreek extract in the treatment of cancers.

Fenugreek extracts have been shown to exhibit some anti-inflammatory and diuretic activity in animal models.[12] Fenugreek leaf extracts have been shown to repel numerous common insects.[13]

A recent study demonstrated that the steroid saponins of fenugreek enhance food consumption and motivation to eat, and reduce plasma cholesterol levels in rats.[14] Studies continue on the ability of fenugreek to lower blood glucose both in normal as well as in diabetic rats, dogs and humans.[15,19] Similarly, the hypocholesterolemic properties of fenugreek continue to be studies.[20,21] Another property of the plant is under investigation, namely its ability to decrease the quantity of calcium oxalate deposited in the kidneys.[22]

TOXICOLOGY: When ingested in usual culinary quantities, fenugreek is essentially devoid of adverse reactions. An interesting syndrome was noted in a nine-day-old boy who was admitted to the hospital for the treatment of gastroenteritis. Nurses noted that the boy's urine and entire body smelled distinctly of maple syrup. Laboratory tests ruled out the presence of "maple syrup urine" disease (an inborn error of metabolism that results in the abnormal accumulation of leucine, isoleucine and valine and their ketoacid metabolites in the blood and urine).

The mother told the physicians that she had been giving the child a tea prepared by boiling fenugreek seeds in water, a common Ethiopian folk remedy for diarrhea and vomiting. The smell of the tea was found to be indistinguishable from that of the child's urine.[23]

The acute toxicity from a large dose of fenugreek has not been characterized, but may result in potentially severe hypoglycemia. Fenugreek may also cause a new type of occupational asthma.[24] Finally, myositis and peritonitis have occurred in chickens given fenugreek crude saponins intramuscularly or intraperitoneally.[25]

SUMMARY: Fenugreek seeds are used as a culinary spice and their extracts as flavorings. Folk uses include the treatment of boils, diabetes, cellulitis, tuberculosis and gastrointestinal problems. Investigations in animals have found the seeds to reduce serum cholesterol and glucose levels. It is not known if these effects are due to the high fiber content or to the saponins or alkaloids found in the seed. Studies continue to elucidate the mechanism of fenugreek's abilities to lower cholesterol and glucose levels. Recent studies also show the ability of the plant to decrease the quantity of calcium oxalate deposited in the kidneys.

PATIENT INFORMATION – Fenugreek

Uses: Fenugreek has been used as a flavoring, animal forage, insect repellent and folk medicine for boils, diabetes and tuberculosis. In lab animals, it has been shown to lower blood cholesterol and glucose, and to exert anti-inflammatory and diuretic effects.

Side Effects: Unusual quantities may result in hypoglycemia.

---

[1] Varchney JP, Jani DC. *Natl Acad Sci Lett* 1979;2:331.
[2] Sauvaire Y, Baccou JC. *Lloydia* 1978;41:247.
[3] Elujoba AA, Hardman R. *Fitotherapia* 1985;56:368.
[4] Gangrade H, Kaushal R. *Indian Drugs* 1979;16:149.
[5] Parmer V, et al. *Z Naturforsh* 1982;37B:521.
[6] Adamska M, Lutomski J. *Planta Med* 1971;20:224.
[7] Gupta RK, et al. *J Nat Prod* 1986;49:1153.
[8] Karawya MS, et al. *Planta Med* 1980;38:73.
[9] Valette G, et al. *Atherosclerosis* 1984;50(1):105.
[10] Singhal PC, et al. *Curr Sci* 1982;51:136.
[11] Ribes G, et al. *Ann Nutr Metab* 1984;28(1):37.
[12] Totte J, Vlietinck AJ. *Farm Tijdschr Belg* 1983;60:203.
[13] Jilani G, Su HCF. *J Econ Entomol* 1983;76:154.

[14] Petit PR, et al. *Steroids* 1995;60(10):674.
[15] Khosla P, et al. *Indian J Physiol Pharmacol* 1995;39(2):173.
[16] Sharma RD, et al. *Eur J Clin Nutr* 1990;44(4):301.
[17] Madar Z, et al. *Eur J Clin Nutr* 1988;42(1):51.
[18] Ajabnoor MA, Tilmisany AK. *J Ethnopharmacol* 1988;22(1):45.
[19] Ribes G, et al. *Proc Soc Exp Biol Med* 1986;182(2):159.
[20] Stark A, Madar Z. *Br J Nutr* 1993;69(1):277.
[21] Sauvaire Y, et al. *Lipids* 1991;26(3):191.
[22] Ahsan SK, et al. *J Ethnopharmacol* 1989;26(3):249.
[23] Bartley GB, et al. *N Engl J Med* 1981;305(8):467.
[24] Dugue P, et al. *Presse Med* 1993;22(19):922.
[25] Nakhla HB, et al. *Vet Hum Toxicol* 1991;33(6):561.

Feverfew

SCIENTIFIC NAME(S): *Tanacetum parthenium* Schulz-Bip. synonymous with *Chrysanthemum parthenium* L. Bernh., *Leucanthemum parthenium* (L.) Gren and Godron, and *Pyrethrum parthenium* (L.) Sm.[1] Alternately described as a member of the genus *Matricaria*. Family: Asteraceae Compositae.

COMMON NAME(S): Feverfew, featherfew, altamisa, bachelor's button, featherfoil, febrifuge plant, midsummer daisy, nosebleed, Santa Maria, wild chamomile, wild quinine[2-5]

BOTANY: A short bushy perennial that grows from 15 to 60 cm tall along fields and roadsides. Its yellow-green leaves and yellow flowers resemble those of chamomile *(Matricaria chamomilla),* for which it is sometimes confused. The flowers bloom from July to October.

HISTORY: The herb feverfew has had a long history of use in traditional and folk medicine, especially among Greek and early European herbalists. However, during the last few hundred years feverfew had fallen into general disuse, until recently.[6] It has now become popular as a prophylactic treatment for migraine headaches and its extracts have been claimed to relieve menstrual pain, asthma, dermatitis and arthritis. Traditionally, the herb has been used as an antipyretic, from which its common name is derived. The leaves are ingested fresh or dried, with a typical daily dose of 2 to 3 leaves. These are bitter and are often sweetened before ingestion. It has also been planted around houses to purify the air due to its strong, lasting odor, and a tincture of its blossoms doubles as an insect repellant and balm for their bites.[3] It was once used as an antidote for overindulgence in opium.[2]

CHEMISTRY: The chemistry of feverfew is now well-defined. The plant is rich in sesquiterpene lactones, the principal one being parthenolide.[7] Parthenolide comprises up to 85% of the total sesquiterpene content.[1] Other active sesquiterpene lactones are canin, seco-tanapartholide A, artecanin, and 3-beta-hydroxyparthenolide.[8] Other members of this class have been isolated and have been shown to possess spasmolytic activity perhaps through an inhibition of the influx of extracellular calcium into vascular smooth muscle cells. The plant contains several flavonoid glycosides, the main ones being luteolin and apigenin.[9]

PHARMACOLOGY: Feverfew action does not appear to be limited to a single major mechanism; rather, plant extracts affect a wide variety of physiologic pathways.

In vitro: Feverfew appears to be an inhibitor of prostaglandin synthesis. Extracts of the above-ground portions of the plant suppress prostaglandin production by up to 88%; leaf extracts inhibit prostaglandin production to a lesser extent (58%). Neither the whole plant nor leaf extracts inhibit cyclooxygenation of arachidonic acid, the first step in prostaglandin synthesis.[10]

Aqueous extracts prevent the release of arachidonic acid and inhibit in vitro aggregation of platelets stimulated by ADP or thrombin.[11] Whether these extracts block the synthesis of thromboxane, a prostaglandin involved in platelet aggregation, is controversial.[12,13] Data suggest that feverfew's inhibition of prostaglandin synthesis differs in mechanism from that of the salicylates. Extracts may inhibit platelet behavior via effects on platelet sulfhydryl groups.[14,15]

Feverfew extracts are potent inhibitors of serotonin release from platelets and polymorphonuclear leucocyte granules, providing a possible connection between the claimed benefit of feverfew in migraines and arthritis. Feverfew may produce and antimigraine effect in a manner similar to methysergide maleate (*Sansert*), a known serotonin antagonist.[16,17] Extracts of the plant also inhibit the release of enzymes from white cells found in inflamed joints, a similar anti-inflammatory effect may occur in the skin, providing a rationale for the traditional use of feverfew in psoriasis.

In addition, feverfew extracts inhibit phagocytosis, inhibit the deposition of platelets on collagen surfaces, exhibit antithrombotic potential, have in vitro antibacterial activity, inhibit mast cell release of histamine[18] and exhibit cytotoxic activity.[9] Monoterpenes in the plant may exert insecticidal activity, and alpha-pinene derivatives may possess sedative and mild tranquilizing effects.

Clinical Uses: Much interest has been focused on the activity of feverfew in the treatment and prevention of migraine headaches.[19] The first significant, modern, public account of its use as a preventative for migraine appeared in 1978. This story, reported in the British health magazine, *Prevention*, concerned a Mrs. Jenkins who had suffered from severe migraine since the age of 16. At the age of 68, she began using three leaves of feverfew daily, and after 10 months her headaches ceased altogether. This case prompted studies by Dr. E. Stewart Johnson.[6]

A study in eight feverfew-treated patients and nine placebo-controlled patients found that fewer headaches were reported by patients taking feverfew, for up to six months of treatment. Patients in both groups had self-medicated with feverfew for several years before enrolling in the study. The incidence of headaches remained constant in those patients taking feverfew but increased almost three-fold in those switched to placebo during the trial (p < 0.02).[20] The abrupt discontinuation of feverfew in patients switched to placebo caused incapacitating headaches in some patients. Nausea and vomiting were reduced in patients taking feverfew. The statistical analysis has been questioned but the results provide a unique insight into the activity of feverfew.[21] These results were confirmed in a more recent placebo-controlled study in 72 patients suffering from migraine.[22] On the basis of their research, Johnson, et al, predict that feverfew will be useful not only for the classical migraine and cluster headache, but for premenstrual, menstrual and other headaches, as well.[23]

However, studies at the London Migraine Clinic[24] found that the experimental observations may not be clinically relevant to migraine patients taking feverfew. Ten patients who had taken extracts of the plant for up to 8 years to control migraine headaches were evaluated for physiologic changes that may have been related to the plant. The platelets of all treated patients aggregated characteristically to ADP and thrombin and similarly to those of control patients. However, aggregation in response to serotonin was greatly attenuated in the feverfew users.

Feverfew has been investigated in the treatment of rheumatoid arthritis. In one major study, 41 female patients received feverfew (70 to 86 mg) or placebo once daily for 6 weeks under double-blind conditions. No significant differences were observed in more than 15 parameters between the test groups suggesting no apparent benefit from oral feverfew therapy.[25]

Canada's Health Protection Branch has granted a Drug Identification Number (DIN) for a British feverfew (*Tanacetum parthenium*) product. This allows the product's manufacturer, Herbal Laboratories, Ltd., to make the claim, as a nonprescription drug, for effectiveness in the prevention of migraine headache. Canada's Health Protection Branch recommends a daily dosage of 125 mg of a dried feverfew leaf preparation, from authenticated *Tanacetum parthenium* containing at least 0.2% parthenolide for the prevention of migraine.[26]

TOXICOLOGY: Much has been learned about the safety of feverfew over the last decade. In the study conducted by Johnson, et al, patients received 50 mg/day, roughly equivalent to two leaves. Adverse effects noted during 6 months of continued feverfew treatment were mild and did not result in discontinuation. Four of the eight patients taking the plant had no adverse effects. Heart rate increased dramatically (by up to 26 beats/min) in two treated patients. There were no differences between treatment groups in laboratory test results.

Patients who had been switched to placebo after taking feverfew for several years experienced a cluster of nervous system reactions (rebound of migraine symptoms, anxiety, poor sleep patterns) along with muscle and joint stiffness; Johnson refers to this as the "postfeverfew syndrome."

In a larger series of feverfew users, 18% reported adverse effects, the most troublesome being mouth ulceration (11%). Feverfew can induce more widespread inflammation of the oral mucosa and tongue, often with lip swelling and loss of taste.[20] Dermatitis has been associated with this plant.[27,18]

No studies of chronic toxicity have yet been performed on the plant and the safety of long-term use has not been established scientifically. The plant should not be used by pregnant women, as the leaves have been shown to possess potential emmenagogue activity and is not recommended for lactating mothers or children under the age of 2.[26] Although an interaction with anticoagulants is undocumented, this may be clinically important in sensitive patients.

One study has evaluated the potential genotoxic effects of chronic feverfew ingestion. Analysis of the frequency of chromosomal aberrations and sister chromatid exchanges in circulating lymphocytes from patients who ingested feverfew for 11 months found no unexpected aberrations suggesting that the plant does not induce chromosomal abnormalities.[29]

SUMMARY: Feverfew has been used for the treatment of disorders often controlled by aspirin, such as fever, rheumatic inflammations and headache. The chemistry and pharmacology of feverfew have been reasonable well defined. The ability of the plant to aid in the control of migraine has been under close study. To date, the studies comparing the plant to placebo have generally found a significant clinical benefit from the administration of feverfew. Preliminary safety data from clinical trials suggest that the plant is relatively safe, although the incidence of mouth ulcers has been disturbingly high in some trials. The plant does not appear to be mutagenic and should not be used by pregnant women.

PATIENT INFORMATION – Feverfew

Uses: Traditionally an antipyretic, feverfew has been used in recent times to avert migraines and relieve menstrual pain, asthma, dermatitis and arthritis.

Side Effects: Patients withdrawn from feverfew experienced a syndrome of ill effects. Most adverse effects of treatment with feverfew are mild, although some patients have experienced increased heart rate. Feverfew should not be used by pregnant or lactating women or children under age 2. Feverfew may possibly interact with anticoagulants.

---

[1] Awang DVC. *Can Pharm J* 1989;122:266.

[2] Duke JA. *Handbook of Medicinal Herbs.* Boca Raton, FL: CRC Press, 1985.

[3] Dobelis IN, ed. *Magic and Medicine of Plants.* Pleasantville, NY: Reader's Digest Assoc., 1986.

[4] Meyer JE. *The Herbalist.* Hammond, IN: Hammond Book Co., 1934.

[5] Castleman M. *The healing Herbs.* Emmaus, PA: Rodale Press, 1991.

[6] Hobbs C. *National Headache Foundation Newsletter* Winter 1990:11.

[7] Bohlmann F, Zdero C. *Phytochemistry* 1982;21:2543.

[8] Groenewegen WA, et al. *J Pharm Pharmacol* 1986;38:709.

[9] Hobbs C. *HerbalGram* 1989;20:26.

[10] Collier HOJ, et al. *Lancet* 1980;2:922. Letter.

[11] Loecshe EW, et al. *Folia Haematol* 1988;115:181.

[12] Makheja AN, Bailey JM. *Lancet* 1981;2:1054. Letter.

[13] Heptinstall S, et al. *Lancet* 1985;1:1071.

[14] Heptinstall S, et al. *J Pharm Pharmacol* 1987;39:459.

[15] Voyno-Yesenetskaya TA, et al. *J Pharm Pharmacol* 1988;40:501.

[16] Tyler VE. *The New Honest Herbal.* Philadelphia, PA: GF Stickley Co., 1987.

[17] Olin BR, Hebel SK, eds. *Drug Facts and Comparisons.* St. Louis: Facts and Comparisons, Oct 1991:257.

[18] Hayes NA, Foreman JC. *J Pharm Pharmacol* 1987;39:466.

[19] Feverfew-a new drug or an old wives' remedy. *Lancet* 1985;1:1084. Editorial.

[20] Johnson ES, et al. *Br Med J* 1985;291:569.

[21] Waller PC, Ramsay LE. *Br Med J* 1985;291:1128. Letter.

[22] Murphy JJ, et al. *Lancet* 1988;2:189.

[23] Hobbs C. *National Headache Foundation Newsletter* Winter 1990:10.

[24] Biggs, et al. *Lancet* 1982;2:776. Letter.

[25] Pattrick M, et al. *Ann Rheum Dis* 1989;48:547.

[26] Awang DVC. *HerbalGram* 1993;29:34.

[27] Vickers HR. *Br Med J* 1985;291:827. Letter.

[28] Schmidt RJ, Kingston T. *Contact Derm* 1985;13:120.

[29] Anderson D, et al. *Human Toxicol* 1988;7:145.

Flax

SCIENTIFIC NAME(S): *Linum usitatissimum* L. Family: Linaceae. Numerous additional members of the genus *Linum* are used throughout the world for their fiber and oil content.

COMMON NAME(S): Flax, flaxseed, linseed, lint bells,[1] linum

BOTANY: The flax plant grows as a slender annual and reaches 1 to 3 feet in height. It branches at the top and has small, pale-green alternate leaves that grow on the stems and branches. Flax was introduced to the North American continent from Europe, and it now grows widely in Canada and the northwestern United States. Each branch is tipped with one or two delicate blue flowers that bloom from February through September.[2]

HISTORY: Flax has been used for more than 10 thousand years as a source of fiber for weaving or clothing.[2] It was one of the earliest plants that man recognized could be used for purposes other than as food. Flax is prepared from the fibers in the stem of the plant.[3] Linseed oil, derived from the flaxseed, has been used as a topical demulcent and emollient and as a laxative, particularly for animals. Linseed oil is used in paints and varnishes and as a waterproofing agent. Flaxseed cakes have been used as cattle feed.

Traditional medicinal uses of the plant have been varied and, at times bizarre; one text notes that the seeds have been used to remove foreign material from the eye. A moistened seed would be placed under the closed eyelid for a few moments, allowing the material to adhere to the seed, thereby facilitating removal.[4] Other uses include the treatment of coughs and colds, constipation and urinary tract infections.[2] The related *L. catharticum* yields a purgative decoction.[4]

CHEMISTRY: Linseed oil is a drying oil obtained by the expression of linseed. It is mainly composed of unsaturated fatty acids including linolenic, linoleic and oleic acids.[5] Flaxseed and linseed oil are among the best natural sources of alpha-linolenic acid. Flaxseed is a source of a soluble fiber mucilage, which is also obtained from other members of the *Linum* genus. It is composed of D-xylose, L-galactose, L-rhamnose and D-galacturonic acid.[6] Linusitamarin, a phenylpropanoid glucoside, has also been isolated from flaxseed.[7] Flax leaves and seed chaff contain the cyanogenic glycosides linamarin, linustatin and neolinustatin, from which the enzyme linamarase is capable of releasing cyanide.[4,10]

PHARMACOLOGY: Significant interest has centered on the ability of diets rich in flax to improve the blood lipid profile. Preliminary work indicated that egg yolk was enriched with alpha-linolenic acid by feeding hens diets containing flax. Furthermore, the cholesterol content of the liver tissue of the chicks born to the flax-fed hens was lower ($p > 0.05$) than in chicks hatched from control hens.[8]

More recent evidence indicates that flax-supplemented diets reduce the atherogenic risk factors in humans. When hyperlipemic subjects ate three slices of bread containing flaxseed plus 15 g of ground flaxseed daily for 3 months, serum total and low-density lipoprotein cholesterol levels were reduced significantly; high-density lipoprotein cholesterol levels, however, did not change. In addition, thrombin-stimulated platelet aggregation decreased with the flax supplement. These changes suggest beneficial improvement in plasma lipid and related cardiovascular risk factors.[9]

When healthy female volunteers supplemented their diet with 50 g of ground flaxseed/day for 4 weeks, the diet raised alpha-linolenic acid levels in both plasma and erythrocytes; serum total cholesterol decreased by 9% and low density lipoprotein cholesterol dropped by 18%. Similar results were obtained when either flaxseed oil or flour were used, suggesting high bioavailability of the alpha-linolenic acid from ground flaxseed. No cyanogenic glucosides were detected in baked flax muffins.[10]

Flax contains lignans (phytochemicals shown to have weakly estrogenic and antiestrogenic properties). When healthy women ingested flaxseed powder for three menstrual cycles, the ovulatory flax cycles were consistently associated with a longer luteal phase. There were no differences between control and flax-cycles in estradiol or estrone levels, although the luteal phase progesterone/estradiol ratios were significantly higher during the flax cycles. These findings suggest a specific role for flax lignans in the relationship between diet and sex steroid action, and possibly between diet and the risk of breast and other hormone-dependent cancers.[11]

Preliminary evidence derived from a mouse model of lupus indicates that diets supplemented with 15% flaxseed for 14 weeks delayed the onset of proteinuria and significantly reduced overall mortality compared with controls.[12]

TOXICOLOGY: The cyanogenic properties of some of the constituents of flax suggest that ingestion of large amounts of the plant may be harmful; this, however, is primarily a veterinary problem encountered in grazing animals.

Approximately half of the workers exposed to flax at their jobs demonstrated immunologically positive antigen tests in one survey.[13] No other significant toxicity has been associated with dietary levels of flax.

SUMMARY: Flax and its seed are economically important products that find use in medicine, in the paint and varnish industry and in the manufacture of fibers for apparel and other weaving. Preliminary evidence suggests that diets supplemented with the ground seed can improve the lipid profile of hypercholesterolemic patients, reducing certain atherogenic risk factors.

PATIENT INFORMATION – Flax

Uses: Linseed oil, derived from flaxseed, has been used as a topical demulcent and emollient, as a laxative, and as treatment for coughs, colds and urinary tract infections. Flaxseed cakes have been used as cattle feed. Research suggests dietary flaxseed may improve blood lipid profile.

Side Effects: Ingestion of large amounts may be harmful. Many workers exposed to flax show immunologically positive antigens.

---

[1] Meyer JE. *The Herbalist*. Hammond, IN: Hammond Book Co., 1934.

[2] Dobelis IN. *Magic and Medicine of Plants*. Pleasantville, NY: Reader's Digest Association, 1986.

[3] Lewis WH, Elvin-Lewis MPF. *Medical Botany: Plants affecting man's health*. New York: John Wiley & Sons, 1977.

[4] Evans WC. *Trease and Evans' Pharmacognosy*. 13th ed. London: Balliere Tindall, 1989.

[5] Morton JF. *Major Medicinal Plants*. Springfield, IL: Charles C. Thomas, 1977.

[6] Robinson T. *The Organic Constituents of Higher Plants*, 6th Ed. North Amherst, MA: Cordus Press, 1991.

[7] Luyengi L, et al. *J Nat Prod* 1993;56:2012.

[8] Cherian G, Sim JS. *Lipids* 1992;27:706.

[9] Bierenbaum ML, et al. *J Am Coll Nutr* 1993;12:501.

[10] Cunnane SC, et al. *Br J Nutr* 1993;69:443.

[11] Phipps WR, et al. *J Clin Endocrinol Metab* 1993;77:1215.

[12] Hall AV, et al. *Am J Kidney Dis* 1993;22:326.

[13] Zuskin E, et al. *Environ Res* 1992;59:350.

Fo-ti

SCIENTIFIC NAME(S): *Polygonum multiflorum Thunb.* (Polygonaceae)

COMMON NAME(S): He shou wu (Chinese), flowery knotweed, climbing knotweed, Chinese cornbind. This plant should not be confused with the commercial product Fo-ti Tieng, which does not contain fo-ti.

BOTANY: Fo-ti is native to central and southern China and is distributed in Japan and Taiwan. It is a perennial climbing herb, which can grow to 30 feet in height. The plant has red stems, heart-shaped leaves and white or pink flowers. The roots of 3- to 4-year-old plants are dried in autumn. The stems and leaves are used also.[1,2]

HISTORY: Fo-ti is a popular Chinese tonic herb, dating back to 713 A.D.[1] It is considered one of the country's great four herbal tonics (along with angelica, lycium and panax).[3] Regarded as a rejuvenating plant, fo-ti has been thought to prevent aging and to promote longevity. According to folklore, the older and larger roots have the most power.[1] One source quotes "...300-year-old (root) product makes one immortal."[3]

CHEMISTRY: Fo-ti contains chrysophanic acid, chrysophanic acid anthrone and chrysophanol. Anthraquinones emodin and rhein are also present. Lecithin has also been found in the plant.[1,3] A stilbene glucoside from fo-ti has been identified.[4] A spectrophotometric assay of stilbene glucoside in another report may be used for quality control in the plant's processing.[5] Qualitative analysis and content determination of phospholipids in fo-ti drug vs four processed products have been performed.[6] An alcoholic extract from fo-ti roots yielded three bioactive compounds: E-2,3,5,4'-tetrahydroxystilbene 2-O-beta-D-glucopyranoside and cis- and trans-E-3-butylidene-4,5,6,7-tetrahydro-6,7-dihydroxy-1(3H)-isobenzofuranone. Two of these compounds were found to be calcium-ATPase inhibitors.[7]

PHARMACOLOGY: In China, millions take fo-ti regularly for its **rejuvenating** and **toning** properties. It is used to **increase liver and kidney function** and to **cleanse the blood.** The plant is also prescribed for symptoms of **premature aging** such as gray hair.[1] A Chinese-13-herb mixture ("shou xing bu zhi") that includes fo-ti has been studied for its **antisenility** effects in mice. Results showed this mixture was effective in slowing the aging process.[8] It is also indicated for **insomnia, weak bones, constipation** and **atherosclerosis.**[2] Lifespan and lipid studies of fo-ti in quails have been performed.[9] Fo-ti also has been shown to **reduce blood cholesterol levels** in

animals.[1] The root portion of the plant has exhibited an inhibitory effect on triglyceride accumulation and has reduced enlargement of mice livers.[10] In a clinical trial in humans, fo-ti had similar **cholesterol-lowering** effects.[1]

Emodin exhibited **vasodilation** and **immunosuppressive** effects in rats, suggesting its usefulness against **transplantation rejection** and *autoimmune disease.* Extract of he shou wu significantly reduced tumor incidence in rats in another report.[12] The Chinese use the root of the plant for **cancer** as well.[3]

Stilbenes isolated from polygonium species have been evaluated on rat peritoneal polymorphonuclear leukocyte lipoxygenase and cyclooxygenase activity.[13] A mixture including fo-ti has been studied for its effects on glucocorticoid receptor in senile rat thymocyte.[14] The plant has also been shown to **inhibit lipid peroxidation** in isolated rat heart mitochondria.[15] Fo-ti also exhibits antimicrobial properties against tuberculosis bacillus and malaria.[1]

Other uses of the plant include: To **increase fertility**,[1] to **increase blood sugar levels**,[1] to treat **anemia** and to relieve **muscle aches.**[3]

TOXICOLOGY: There is little information in the area of toxicology from fo-ti. However, all plants that contain anthraquinone cathartic compounds should be used cautiously to prevent developing dependence on their laxative effects. One case report describes herb-induced hepatitis in a 31-year-old pregnant Chinese woman from medicine prepared from the plant.[16] The use of these compounds in pregnant women should be discouraged.

SUMMARY: Fo-ti is a widely used herb in ancient and current Chinese medicine. It is known for its rejuvenating and tonic properties, to increase liver and kidney function, to cleanse the blood and to slow down signs of premature aging. The plant also exhibits cholesterol-lowering effects and immunosuppressive actions and has antimicrobial properties. Little is known about the plant's toxicity as more studies are needed.

PATIENT INFORMATION – Fo-ti

Uses: Fo-ti has been used in China for its rejuvenating and toning properties, to increase liver and kidney function and to cleanse the blood. It is also used for insomnia, weak bones, constipation and atherosclerosis. It can increase fertility, increase blood sugar levels and relieve muscle aches and exhibits antimicrobial properties against tuberculosis bacillus and malaria.

Side Effects: Little information exists on fo-ti's side effects. Discourage use in pregnant women.

[1] Chevallier A. *Encyclopedia of Medicinal Plants*. New York, NY: DK Publishing, 1996;121.

[2] Reid D. *Chinese Herbal Medicine*. Boston, MA: Shambhala Publishing, Inc., 1994;150.

[3] Duke J. CRC *Handbook of Medicinal Herbs*. Boca Raton, FL: CRC Press, Inc., 1989;163-64.

[4] Hata K, et al. *Yakugaku Zasshi* 1975;95(2):211-13.

[5] Liu C, et al. *Chung Kuo Chung Yao Tsa Chih* 1991;16(8):469-72.

[6] Ma C, et al. *Chung Kuo Chung Yao Tsa Chih* 1991;16(11):662-64.

[7] Grech J, et al. *J Nat Prod* 1994;57(12):1682-87.

[8] Chen J. *Chung Hsi I Chieh Ho Tsa Chih* 1989;9(4):226-27.

[9] Wang W, et al. *Chung Hsi I Chieh Ho Tsa Chih* 1988;8(4):223-24.

[10] Liu C, et al. *Chung Kuo Chung Yao Tsa Chih* 1992;17(10):595-96.

[11] Huang H, et al. *Eur J Pharmacol* 1991;198(2-3):211-13.

[12] Horikawa K, et al. *Mutagenesis* 1994;9(6):523-26.

[13] Kimura Y, et al. *Biochim Biophys Acta* 1985;834(2):275-78.

[14] Zhao W, et al. *Chung Kuo Chung Hsi I Chieh Ho Tsa Chih* 1995;15(2):92-94.

[15] Hong, et al. *Am J Chin Med* 1994;22(1):63-70.

[16] But P, et al. *Vet Hum Toxicol* 1996;38(4):280-82.

Fruit Acids

SCIENTIFIC NAME(S): Alpha hydroxy acids, malic acid, lactic acid, gluconolactone

COMMON NAME(S): Fruit acids

SOURCE: As the name indicates, these acidic organic compounds are derived primarily from fruit sources. Juices and fruit pulps may be rich in malic and lactic acids, although other sources may be used for commercial production of these acids (ie, starch, glucose or other sugars).

HISTORY: Organic acids such as lactic acid have long been used in dermatologic preparations as humectants to improve the moisturization of the top skin layers. Organic acids have also been used to de-hair and to tan animal hides.[1]

Most organic acids can be caustic in sufficiently high concentrations. As agents that modify the keratinization process (see Pharmacology), alpha hydroxy acids may be useful for the treatment of acne and other skin disorders.[2] Since they help debride dead cells from the skin, they have been added to a variety of skin cleansers.

A number of cosmetic companies are marketing products that contain alpha hydroxy acids for their anti-aging effects on the skin. While the fruit acids have the ability to promote the sloughing of outer skin layers, there is no evidence that the use of these products, particularly over a long period of time, can "rejuvenate" the skin or alter the basic aging-related changes of the skin. It is possible, however, that removal of top skin layers may enhance the appearance of the skin.

CHEMISTRY: The "fruit acids" are a group of organic acids that share a common chemical structure consisting of a hydroxyl group positioned at the alpha-carbon position. Consequently, these compounds are often referred to as "alpha hydroxy acids." Common fruit acids include lactic and malic acids. Because of the structural configuration of these acids, they are optically active and only certain forms of the isomers are obtained from natural sources. For example, only (-)malic acid is obtained from fruit juices.[3]

PHARMACOLOGY: Lactic acid (in concentrations of approximately 1% to 2% in creams or lotions) has been reported to be an effective naturally occurring skin humectant, having beneficial effects on dry skin and also in severe hyperkeratotic conditions.

Hyperkeratinization appears to play a role in the development of acne and is often the result of decreases in the rate of skin cell sloughing, which itself is due to an increase in the cohesion of cells known as corneocytes.[4] Alpha hydroxy acids may decrease the cohesiveness of corneocytes by weakening intracellular bonding,[5] thereby freeing skin cells and permitting more efficient cell removal and skin cleansing.[6]

One fruit acid component, gluconolactone, has been found to be as effective as benzoyl peroxide in the treatment of acne.[4] In a double-blind trial of 150 patients, a 14% solution of gluconolactone was compared with benzoyl peroxide 5% lotion and to a placebo vehicle.

Both active treatments significantly reduced the number of inflamed lesions (compared to baseline) during the 12–week study. While there was no significant difference between active treatments during the first 4 weeks, the benzoyl peroxide was significantly better in reducing the number of inflamed lesions by weeks 8 and 12 than was the alpha hydroxy acid. Both groups were similarly effective in reducing the total number of inflamed and noninflamed lesions, but dryness was reported by significantly more patients treated with benzoyl peroxide.

Overall, 50% of the benzoyl peroxide-treated patients reported adverse events, compared to 24% of those treated with gluconolactone and 10% of the placebo-treated patients. Dryness, scaling and burning were the most commonly reported events.

TOXICOLOGY: Depending on the concentrations used, alpha hydroxy acids can cause severe skin irritation, burning and sloughing. Hypersensitive individuals and those with irritated skin should use alpha hydroxy acids with caution.

SUMMARY: The fruit acids are growing in popularity for their topical use as skin cleansers and for the management of disorders such as acne. While natural in their composition, they must be used cautiously because of their potential to irritate skin. Preparations containing lactic acid are available both over-the-counter and by prescription. Many of the consumer-oriented products, however, do not define the composition of the fruit acids used, thereby eliminating the method by which consumers could recognize the presence of potentially irritating substances in the product.

PATIENT INFORMATION – Fruit Acids

Uses: Fruit acids are used for cleansing, moisturizing the top layers of skin and for treating acne.

Side Effects: Dryness, scaling, burning and similar effects may occur in sensitive individuals or with prolonged use.

---

[1] Windholz M, ed. *The Merck Index*, ed. 10. Rahway, NJ: Merck & Co., 1983.
[2] Van Scott EJ, Yu RJ. *Arch Dermatol* 1974;110:586.
[3] Morrison RT, Boyd RN. Organic Chemistry, ed. 3. Boston: Allyn and Bacon, Inc., 1973.

[4] Hunt MJ, Barnetson RS. *Australas J Dermatol* 1992;33:131.
[5] Van Scott EJ, Yu RJ. *J Am Acad Dermatol* 1984;11:867.
[6] Van Scott EJ, Yu RJ. *Cutis* 1989;43:222.

Fumitory

SCIENTIFIC NAME(S): *Fumaria officinalis* L. Family: Fumariaceae

COMMON NAME(S): Fumitory, common fumitory, earth smoke

BOTANY: Fumitory is an annual plant of somewhat variable characteristics, often resembling a bush, but also observed as a low trailing shrub. It has gray pointed leaves that, at a distance, give the plant a wispy appearance of smoke (hence its common name).[1] The pink-purple flower blooms in spring. The plant is widely dispersed and can be found in gardens, on slopes and in wastelands. The flowering plant has traditionally been used in herbal medicine.

HISTORY: Fumitory has been known since antiquity and was described in herbals from the Middle Ages. In traditional medicine, the plant has been used to treat eczema and other dermatologic conditions. It also found use as a laxative and diuretic. Interest in the plant has undergone a resurgence in the past decade based on reports that extracts may be useful in the management of disorders of the cardiovascular system and hepatobiliary tract. The bulk of recent work with the plant has originated in France.

CHEMISTRY: While the composition of related species (ie, *F. parviflora*) has been better investigated, the composition of *F. officinalis* remains poorly defined. A number of flavone heterosides have been identified,[2] but the pharmacologically active components have not been well characterized. An alkaloidal fraction is likely responsible for the cardiovascular activity of the plant.[3]

PHARMACOLOGY: Animal and human investigations have identified several pharmacologic actions of fumitory extracts. Intravenous injection of 1 to 2 mg/kg in dogs reduced ischemia caused by experimental ligation of the circumflex artery. A dose of 5.2 mg/kg prevented ischemic-induced arrhythmias for up to 87 minutes.[3]

In addition, fumitory extracts have been shown to ameliorate bile duct blockage in animals and to assist in the management of similar disorders in man. Fumaria extract typically has been administered by nebulizer and has been investigated in gallbladder calculi in mice and rats.[4,5,6] When investigated in 85 patients with cholecystopathies, a fumaria-containing preparation improved patent status in 70% of the cases overall and in more than 80% of the cases of biliary dyskinesia. Optimum results were obtained following 10 days of therapy and the difference was statistically greater than observed with placebo.[7]

TOXICOLOGY: Fumitory has not been associated with significant toxicity. In one clinical study,[7] no adverse events were reported. Alkaloids found in other members of the Fumariaceae (protopine and others) have been known to cause trembling, convulsions and death when consumed in large quantities.[8]

SUMMARY: Fumitory has a long history of use in traditional medicine and has been investigated for its therapeutic potential in the management of cardiovascular and hepatobiliary disorders. Preliminary animal and human data suggest that the plant has pharmacologic activity, which requires further elucidation. Fumitory has not been associated with significant toxicity.

PATIENT INFORMATION – Fumitory

Uses: Fumitory has been traditionally used as a laxative, diuretic and treatment for dermatologic conditions such as eczema. Evidence suggests it benefits those with cardiovascular and hepatobiliary disorders.

Side Effects: Fumitory is not associated with significant toxicity, but large quantities of other members of the family have caused fatal outcomes.

---

[1] Schauenberg P, Paris F. Guide to Medicinal Plants. New Canaan, CT: Keats Publishing, 1977.
[2] Torck M, et al. *Ann Pharm Fr* 1971;29(12):591.
[3] Gorbunov NP, et al. *Kardiologiia* 1980;20(5):84.
[4] Lagrange E, Aurousseau M. *Ann Pharm Fr* 1973;31(5):357.
[5] Dubarry JJ. *J Med Bord* 1967;144(6):918.
[6] Boucard M, Laubenheimer B. *Therapie* 1966;21(4):903.
[7] Zacharewicz M, et al. *Wien Med Wochenschr* 1979;129(8):221.
[8] Hardin JW, Arena JM. Human Poisoning from Native and Cultivated Plants, ed. 2. Durham, NC: Duke University Press, 1974.

Gamma Oryzanol

SCIENTIFIC NAME(S): *"Oz,"gamma-orizanol, caclate, gammajust 50, gamma-oz, gammariza, gammatsul, guntrin, hi-z, maspiron, oliver, oryvita, oryzaal, thiaminogen*

COMMON NAME(S): Rice bran oil

SOURCE: Gamma oryzanol, a sterol-like structure, is a mixture of ferulic acid esters of sterols and triterpene alcohols, extracted from rice bran oil and other grain oils such as corn and barley.[1] Ferulic acid compounds are also present in many foods, including oats, berries, citrus fruits, tomatoes, olives, and vegetables. Gamma oryzanol serves as an important antioxidant within plant cells.[2]

HISTORY: Early reports are available from the mid-1950s discussing isolation, extraction, and purification methods of gamma oryzanol.[1] However, the Japanese have been using it as a medicine since 1962. It was first used to treat anxiety. In the 1970s it was found to be an effective treatment for menopause. Gamma oryzanol therapy was approved to treat elevated cholesterol and triglyceride levels in the late 1980s.[2]

CHEMISTRY: This mixture of esters of sterols (such as campestrol, stigmasterol, and beta-sitosterol) and triterpene alcohols (such as cycloartanol, cycloartenol, 24-methylenecycloartanol, and cyclobranol) known as gamma oryzanol. Extraction from rice bran, corn, and barley oils has been performed.[1] The Japanese process approximately 7500 tons of gamma oryzanol from rice bran each year.[2] Separation of three major components of gamma oryzanol has yielded "oryzanol A" ($C_{40}H_{58}O_4$), "oryzanol C" ($C_{41}H_{60}O_4$), and "oryzanol B," which has been found to be a mixture of oryzanols A and C.[1] Gamma oryzanol has been laboratory-synthesized.[3] Mass fragmentographic determination of ferulic acid in plasma has been performed.[4] A review is available concerning constituents of rice bran oils as functional foods.[5]

PHARMACOLOGY: The pharmacokinetics of gamma oryzanol have been reported in animals.[6,7]

Gamma oryzanol possesses many therapeutic effects including menopausal, hypolipidemic, gastrointestinal, central nervous system (CNS), endocrine, and "body-building."

Menopausal: Gamma oryzanol has been proven effective to treat symptoms of menopause such as hot flashes.[2] In 40 patients experiencing aging syndromes, gamma oryzanol administration lessened menopausal complaints.[8] A report in oophorectomy patients, given 300 mg of gamma oryzanol daily, found a 50% reduction in menopausal symptoms in about 70% of patients. A later study reported 85% improvement in symptoms with the same 300 mg dosage.[2] The proposed mechanisms of gamma oryzanol are the reduction in secretion of leutinizing hormone by the pituitary gland and promotion of endorphin release by the hypothalamus.[2]

Hypolipidemic: Several studies indicate gamma oryzanol and its related constituents (eg, tocotrienols) in rice bran oil exert marked hypocholesterolemic effects.[9,10,11,12] Positive effects of gamma oryzanol on lipid metabolism in animals have also been extensively reported,[13,14,15] including IV administration of gamma oryzanol increasing excretion of lipids in rat blood,[16] reducing of liver lipids and increasing of HDL cholesterol in rats,[17] and an increase fecal excretion of cholesterol, which lowers the level by 20% in rats.[18] Oryzanol has cholesterol-lowering actions, reducing aortic fatty streak formation in hamsters.[19] However, in another report gamma oryzanol had little or no preventative effects on atherosclerosis in rabbits.[20] Another study concludes that rats fed oryzanol along with a 1% cholesterol diet, inhibited platelet aggregation.[21]

Human studies are also promising. Reduced total cholesterol and triglyceride levels, and increased HDL levels were noted in hyperlipidemic patients given gamma oryzanol.[1,8] Total cholesterol and LDL levels were decreased in 20 schizophrenic dyslipidemic patients with no side effects observed.[22] Another clinical trial involving 67 hyperlipidemic patients given 300 mg of gamma oryzanol for 4 weeks, found cholesterol levels to decrease by approximately 10%, mean triglyceride levels to decrease from 222 mg/dl average to 190 mg/dl average, and HDL levels to slightly elevate.[2] The mechanism of action of gamma oryzanol involves the increase of cholesterol conversion to bile acids, the increase in bile acid excretion and inhibition of cholesterol absorption.[16,18]

Gastrointestinal: In Japan, at least 23 clinical studies have been conducted regarding gamma oryzanol and its effectiveness in treating gastrointestinal disorders.[2] Animal studies include its anti-ulcer effect in rats,[23–25] inhibition of gastric secretion in rats,[26] improvement in gastric lesion and suppression of intestinal propulsion in mice,[28] and its effects on stomach and ileum movement in dogs.[29]

An endocrinological study is available evaluating gastrointestinal symptoms in gastritis patients.[30] The mechanisms by which gamma oryzanol seems to exert its effects appear to be the normalizaton of nervous system control of digestive secretions.[2]

CNS/Endocrine: Gamma oryzanol's effects on the CNS and endocrine systems have been sporadically reported. The results primarily concern mechanisms more than specific beneficial therapeutic actions. More human clinical trials are needed. The overall importance of these effects has not been fully determined.

Gamma oryzanol component, "cycloartenol ferulic acid ester," has suppressant effects on the CNS, different from existing tranquilizers. However, it may serve to be a cerebral activator because of its efficacy in models of cerebral dysfunction.[31] Gamma oryzanol has also been found to increase brain norepinephrine content in rats by inhibiting degradation or release of this neurotransmitter.[32] Gamma oryzanol's endocrine effects include a rat pituitary study,[33] suppression of growth hormone synthesis and prolactin release,[34] potent inhibition of LH release and weak inhibition of prolactin in rats,[35-37] and in humans, its inhibition of serum TSH levels in patients with primary hypothyroidism, possibly by a direct action at the hypothalmus.[38] From these studies, one can conclude that gamma oryzanol's actions are mainly on the hypothalmus and pituitary gland. It produces certain effects on these control hormones, but does not appear to alter the level of hormones they control.[2]

Bodybuilding: Gamma oryzanol supplementation in bodybuilding has been addressed.[39] Some studies suggest that gamma oryzanol is poorly absorbed, the major-

ity being excreted in the feces. Endocrinological studies in animals, as previously mentioned, indicate that gamma oryzanol suppresses leutinizing hormone release, reduces growth hormone and increases of neurotransmitters in the brain. Gamma oryzanol may even reduce testosterone production.[40]

Few well controlled human trials exist. However, in one well controlled study, weight lifters taking ferulic acid esters (vs placebo) for 8 weeks, experienced increases both in body weight and strength (as measured by repetitious weight lifting). Another double-blinded study found increases in beta endorphin levels after ferulic acid supplementation, indicative of gamma oryzanol's actions on the hypothalmus.[2] In a later study, however, 9 weeks of 500 mg/day of gamma oryzanol supplementation did not influence performance during resistance exercise training.[41]

Other: At least two reports are available on gamma oryzanol's role as an antioxidant.[3]

TOXICOLOGY: Gamma oryzanol has been shown to be very safe. No side effects have been reported in either animal or human studies.[2] In one report, gamma oryzanol was not damaging to DNA nor mutagenic nor clastogenic.[44] In addition, it was not carcinogenic in mice[45] or rats.[46]

SUMMARY: Gamma oryzanol is a mixture of ferulic acid esterols of sterols and triterpene alcohols. It is a natural product extracted from rice bran oil and other grains. Therapeutic benefits, although unproven, include treatment of menopausal symptoms, hyperlipidemias, and gastrointestinal problems. Gamma oryzanol has been demonstrated to be safe in both animal and human studies.

PATIENT INFORMATION – Gamma Oryzanol

Uses: Gamma oryzanol has been used to treat menopausal symptoms, hyperlipidemias, and GI problems. It is being studied for effects on the CNS and endocrine systems and also as a supplementation in bodybuilding.

Side Effects: No known side effects.

---

[1] Budavari S, et al. *The Merck Index*, 11th Ed. Rahway: Merck and Co., 1989.
[2] Murray M. *Encyclopedia of Nutritional Supplements*, Rocklin, CA: Prima Publishing, Inc, 1996;332–35.
[3] Sato A, et al. *Radioisotopes* 1981;30(3):156–58.
[4] Fujiwara S, et al. *Chem Pharm Bull* 1982;30(3):973–79.
[5] deDeckere E, et al. *Nutr Rev* 1996;54(11 Pt. 2):S120–26.
[6] Fujiwara S, et al. *Yakugaku Zasshi* 1980;100(10):1011–18.
[7] Fujiwara S, et al. *Chem Pharm Bull* 1983;31(2):645–52.

[8] Ishihara M, et al. *Nippon Sanka Fujinka Gakkai Zasshi* 1982;34(2):243–51.
[9] Kiribuchi M, et al. *J Nutr Sci Vitaminol* 1983;29(1):35–43.
[10] Rukmini C, et al. *J Am Coll Nutr* 1991;10(6):593–601.
[11] Sugano M, et al. *Biomed Environ Sci* 1996;9(2–3):242–46.
[12] Sugano M, et al. *J Nutr* 1997;127(3):5215–45.
[13] Shinomiya M, et al. *Tchoku J Exp Med* 1983;141(2):191–97.
[14] Nakayama S, et al. *Jpn J Pharmacol* 1987;44(2):135–43.
[15] Seetharamaiah G, et al. *Indian J Med Res* 1988;88:278–81.

[16] Sakamoto K, et al. *Jpn J Pharmacol* 1987; 45(4):559–65.
[17] Seetharamaiah G, et al. *Atherosclerosis* 1989;78(2–3):219–23.
[18] Seetharamaiah G, et al. *Indian J Med Res* 1990;92:471–75.
[19] Rong N, et al. *Lipids* 1997;32(3):303–09.
[20] Hiramatsu K, et al. *Tokai J Exp Clin Med* 1990;15(4):299–305.
[21] Seetharamaiah G, et al. *J Nutr Sci Vitaminol* 1990;36(3):291–97.
[22] Sasaki J, et al. *Clin Ther* 1990;12(3):263–68.
[23] Itaya K, et al. *Nippon Yakurigaku Zasshi* 1976;72(4):475–81.
[24] Itaya K, et al. *Nippon Yakurigaku Zasshi* 1976;72(8):1001–11.
[25] Itaya K, et al. *Nippon Yakurigaku Zasshi* 1977;73(4):457–63.
[26] Mizuta K, et al. *Nippon Yakurigaku Zasshi* 1978;74(2):285–95.
[27] Mizuta K, et al. *Nippon Yakurigaku Zasshi* 1978;74(4):517–24.
[28] Ichimaru Y, et al. *Nippon Yakurigaku Zasshi* 1984;84(6):537–42.
[29] Mizonishi T, et al. *Nippon Heikatsukin Gakkai Zasshi* 1980;16(1):47–55.
[30] Arai T. *Horumon To Rinsho* 1982;30(3):271–79.
[31] Hiraga Y, et al. *Arzneimittelforschung* 1993;43(7):715–21.

[32] Kaneta H, et al *Nippon Yakurigaku Zasshi* 1979;75(4):399–403.
[33] Ishihama A, et al. *Yokohama Med Bull* 1966;17(5):183–89.
[34] Ieiri T, et al. *Nippon Naibunpi Gakkai Zasshi* 1982;58(10):1350–56.
[35] Yamauchi J, et al. *Nippon Naibunpi Gakkai Zasshi* 1980;56(8):1130–39.
[36] Takayanagi H, et al. *Horumon To Rinsho* 1981;29(1):91–93.
[37] Yamauchi J, et al. *Horm Metab Res* 1981;13(3):185.
[38] Shimomura Y, et al. *Endocrinol Jpn* 1980;27(1):83–86.
[39] Grunewald K, et al. *Sports Med* 1993;15(2):90–103.
[40] Wheeler K, et al. *Int J Sport Nutr* 1991;1(2):170–77.
[41] Fry A, et al. *Int J Sport Nutr* 1997;7(4):318–29.
[42] Hirose M, et al. *Carcinogenesis* 1991;12(10):1917–21.
[43] Kim S, et al. *Biosci Biotechnol Biochem* 1995;59(5):822–26.
[44] Tsushimoto G, et al. *J Toxicol Sci* 1991;16(4):191–202.
[45] Tamagawa M, et al. *Food Chem Toxicol* 1992;30(1):49–56.
[46] Tamagawa M, et al. *Food Chem Toxicol* 1992;30(1):41–48.

Garlic

SCIENTIFIC NAME(S): *Allium sativum* L. Family: Liliacea

COMMON NAME(S): Garlic, allium, stinking rose, rustic treacle, nectar of the gods, camphor of the poor, poor man's treacle

BOTANY: A perennial bulb with a tall, erect flowering stem that grows to 2 to 3 feet. The plant produces pink to purple flowers that bloom from July to September. The bulb is odiferous.

HISTORY: The name *Allium* comes from the Celtic word "all" meaning burning or smarting. Garlic was valued as an exchange medium in ancient Egypt and its virtues were described in inscriptions on the Cheops pyramid. The folk uses of garlic have ranged from the treatment of leprosy in humans to managing clotting disorders in horses. Physicians prescribed the herb during the Middle Ages to cure deafness, and the American Indians used garlic as a remedy for earaches, flatulence and scurvy.

CHEMISTRY: Fresh garlic is a source of numerous vitamins, minerals and trace elements, although most are found in only minute quantities. Garlic contains the highest sulfur content of any member of the *Allium* genus. Two trace elements, germanium and selenium, are found in detectable quantities and have been postulated to play a role in the herb's antitumor effect.

Garlic contains about 0.5% of a volatile oil which is composed of sulfur-containing compounds (diallyldisulphide, diallyltrisulphide, methylallyltrisulphide).[2] The bulbs contain an odorless, colorless, sulfur-containing amino acid called alliin (S-allyl-L-cysteine sulfoxide), which has no pharmacologic activity.[3] When the bulb is ground, the enzyme allinase is released, which results in the conversion of alliin to 2-propenesulfenic acid, which dimerizes to form allicin. Allicin gives the pungent characteristic odor to crushed garlic and is believed to be responsible for some of the pharmacologic activity of the plant.

PHARMACOLOGY: Researchers at Shandong Academy of Medical Science reported the effects of allicin as an antioxidant. They discovered that allicin increased the levels of two important antioxidant enzymes in the blood: Catylase and glutathione peroxidase. This discovery confirmed the antioxidant and free-radical scavenging potential of allicin. Researchers in Japan studied the sulfur compounds in aged garlic extract (a popular deodorized form of garlic) and found five sulfur compounds that

inhibited lipid peroxidation in the liver, preventing a reaction that is considered to be one of the main features of aging in liver cells. According to the findings of the research, the sulfur compounds "appear to be approximately 1000 times more potent in antioxidant activity than the crude, aged garlic extract."[4]

Garlic has received attention in the lay press and the scientific literature for its ability to slow the process of atherosclerosis and to control hypertension. In animal studies, garlic extracts effectively counteracted the hyperlipidemic effects of high sucrose diets. When rats were fed high sugar diets for a 2-month period, serum and tissue cholesterol and triglyceride levels increased approximately 50%. A matched group of rats fed 100 mg/kg/day of garlic oil showed decreases or only slight increases in mean serum and tissue cholesterol, triglycerides and total lipid levels.[5] Oral administration of the essential oil and defatted residue of garlic was found to reduce serum and liver cholesterol levels in rats fed the material for 7 weeks.[6]

Similar results have been observed in humans. In a short-term study, 10 healthy subjects received a fatty meal containing 100 g of butter either alone or concomitantly with the juice of 50 g of garlic. After 3 hours, the garlic-treated group showed mean serum cholesterol levels 7% lower than baseline compared to the untreated group which was 7% above baseline (the changes were significant, $p < 0.001$, for both groups). Furthermore, the garlic-treated group had a 15% increase in fibrinolytic activity compared to controls (49% decrease) ($p < 0.001$ for both groups).[7]

These effects have been duplicated in larger trials. In one study, 20 healthy subjects were fed garlic (0.25 mg/kg/day of oil in two divided doses) for 6 months. The oil significantly lowered mean serum cholesterol and triglyceride levels while raising high-density lipoprotein (HDL) levels. Sixty-two patients with coronary artery diseases and elevated cholesterol levels were also randomly assigned to two subgroups: one group was fed garlic for 10 months and the second group served as the untreated controls. Garlic decreased the serum cholesterol, triglyceride and low-density lipoprotein levels significantly ($p < 0.05$) while increasing the HDL fraction ($p < 0.001$).[8]

The organic disulphides found in the oil can reduce the activity of the thiol group found in many enzymes and can oxidize NADPH. As such, these compounds can inactivate thiol enzymes such as coenzyme A and HMG coenzyme A reductase, and can oxidize NADPH, all of which are factors normally required for lipid synthesis.

It is well documented that garlic oil inhibits platelet function, probably by interfering with thromboxane synthesis.[9] Ariga et al[2] isolated a component of garlic oil that inhibits platelet aggregation and identified it as methylallyltrisulphide (MATS). MATS is present in natural oil in a concentration of 4% to 10%. The purified compound inhibits ADP-induced platelet aggregation at a concentration of less than 10 umol/L in plasma.

Further studies indicated that the most potent antithrombotic compound in garlic is 4,5,9, trithiadodeca-1,6,11-triene 9-oxide, also known as ajoene. This compound is formed by an acid-catalyzed reaction of two allicin molecules followed by rearrangement; the compound can be synthesized commercially. Unlike other antithrombotics now under investigation, ajoene appears to inhibit platelet aggregation regardless of the mechanism of induction.[10]

Scientists at Venezuela's Laboratory of Thrombosis Experimentation were able to demonstrate the effect of ajoene in preventing clot formation caused by vascular damage. The experiment was set up to mimic the conditions of blood flow in small- and medium-sized arteries by varying the velocity of the blood; the compound proved to be effective in both conditions. The authors went on to suggest that the compound may be useful in situations where emergency treatment is needed to prevent clot formation produced by vascular damage.[4]

The inhibition of platelet aggregation is also observed in persons who ingest fresh garlic. In one study, the platelets from health subjects who had eaten garlic cloves (100 to 150 mg/kg) showed complete inhibition to aggregation induced by 5-hydroxytryptamine. The effect was no longer detectable 2.5 hours after ingestion.[11]

Although an earlier study concluded that dried garlic, administered in the form of sugar-coated tablets, had no effect on blood lipids, apolipoproteins, and blood coagulation parameters (in a double-blind trial in 85 patients with primary hyperlipoproteinemia).[12] More recent studies have found that garlic tablets produce a significantly greater reduction in TC and LDL-C than with placebo.

A study conducted by Tulane University stated that total cholesterol levels in those taking garlic tablets dropped by 6% and LDL cholesterol was reduced by 11%. Researchers at the University of Kansas discovered that garlic tablets reduced the susceptibility of LDL oxidation by 34% compared with the placebo group.[13,14]

Garlic administration has been reported to increases fibrinolytic activity. Some investigators believe that garlic's ability to reduce cholesterol, triglycerides and LDL, increase HDL, reduce platelet adhesiveness and increase fibrinolytic activity can combine to significantly decrease the risk of atherosclerotic disease.[13] Some demographic data suggest that the lower-than-normal incidence of atherosclerotic disease in parts of Spain and Italy may in part be due to the routine consumption of garlic in those regions.

A recent study made by researchers at the Clinical Research Center in New Orleans concluded that a garlic preparation of 1.3% allicin appeared to lower diastolic blood pressure in a large dose. Although no statistical significance was achieved in systolic blood pressure, researchers believed a definite trend was observed.[15]

Oral administration of the oil (0.1 ml/10 g) in mice reduced the gastric transit time of a charcoal meal by 75% and prevented castor oil-induced diarrhea for up to 3 hours.[16] The investigators concluded that garlic oil should be investigated for its effectiveness in the managment of hypermotile intestinal disorders.

Garlic has been shown to reduce blood-sugar levels in both animals and humans.[3] Researchers noted an increase in serum insulin and improvement in liver glycogen storage after garlic administration.[17]

The antiseptic and antibacterial properties of garlic have been known for centuries. As recently as World War II, garlic extracts were used to disinfect wounds. During the 1800s, physicians routinely prescribed garlic inhalaton for the treatment of tuberculosis. Garlic extracts inhibit the growth of numerous strains of *Mycobacterium*, but at concentrations that may be difficult to achieve in human tissues.[17]

Preparations containing garlic extracts are used widely in Russia and Japan. Both gram positive and gram negative organisms are inhibited in vitro by garlic extracts. The potency of garlic is such that 1 mg is equivalent to 15 Oxford units of penicillin, making garlic about 1% as active as penicillin.[17]

Garlic extracts have shown antifungal activity when tested in vitro.[17] and their use has been suggested in the treatment of oral and vaginal candidiasis. In an attempt to quantitate the in vivo activity of garlic extracts, Caporaso et al[18] administered 25 ml of fresh garlic extract orally to volunteers. Serum and urine samples were tested for antifungal activity against 15 species of fungal pathogens. While serum exhibited anticandidal and anticryptococcal activity within 30 minutes after ingestion, no biological activity was found in urine. The findings suggest that while garlic extracts may exhibit some antifungal activity in vivo, they are probably of limited use in the treatment of systemic infections.

The antineoplastic activity of garlic has been studied in mice injected with cancer cells that had been pretreated with a garlic extract. No deaths occurred in this treatment group for up to 6 months, while mice injected with untreated cancer cells died within 16 days.[17] It is believed that the reaction of allicin with sulfhydryl groups (the concentration of which increases rapidly in dividing cells) may contribute to this inhibitory effect.

Garlic contains the trace elements germanium and selenium, which have been thought to play a role in improving host immunity and "normalizing" the oxygen utilization of neoplastic cells. Researchers at South Dakota State University studied the effects of garlic oil in preventing skin tumors. The study found that two oil soluble compounds from garlic, diallyl sulfide and diallyl disulfide, when applied topically succeeded in protecting mice against carcinogen-induced skin tumors and increased survival rate.[4]

TOXICOLOGY: Although garlic is used extensively for culinary purposes with essentially no ill effects, the safety of the long-term use of concentrated extracts is unclear. In one rat study, reductions in the protein levels of the liver and kidney were noted after 2 months of treatment with the extract.[5] The clinical significance of these changes is unknown.

A single 25 ml dose of fresh garlic extract has caused burning of the mouth, esophagus and stomach, nausea, sweating and lightheadedness and the safety of repeated doses of this amount has not been defined. Repeated exposure to garlic dust can induce asthmatic reactions.[17] It is understandable why the inhalation of garlic powder was abandoned as a treatment for tuberculosis.

There are no studies that evaluate the effect of garlic and its extracts in persons who require stringent blood glucose control or in patients being treated with anticoagulants (coumarins, salicylates, "antiplatelet" drugs), but the potential for serious interactions should be kept in mind.

Garlic preparations are available commercially as oil-filled capsules, as capsules containing "deodorized" oil, and as tablets (often with parsley to decrease odor). The antibacterial and antilipemic activities of garlic appear to reside in the odiferous constituents, and the therapeutic value of "deodorized" garlic has been disputed.

SUMMARY: Garlic is a common herb used in cooking throughout the world. Garlic and its extracts have a long history of folk use and recent research has indicated that the herb has significant pharmacologic activity when administered even in small doses. These include effects on blood sugar, cholesterol and lipid levels, and a distinct antithrombotic effect.

PATIENT INFORMATION – Garlic

Uses: Evidence suggests garlic beneficially affects levels of blood sugar, cholesterol and lipids. Among its traditional uses, it has been employed for its antiseptic and antibacterial properties.

Side Effects: Garlic may affect those requiring stringent blood glucose control or being treated with anticoagulants.

---

[1] Dobelis IN. *Magic and Medicine of Plants.* Pleasantville, NY: The Reader's Digest Association, 1986.
[2] Ariga T, et al. *Lancet* 1980;i:150.
[3] Castleman M. *The Healing Herbs.* Emmaus, PA: Rodale Press, 1991.
[4] McCaleb R. *Herbal Gram* 1993;29:18.
[5] Adamu L, et al. *Experientia* 1982;38:899.
[6] Kamanna VS, Chandrasekhara N. *Ind J Med Res* 1984;79:580.
[7] Bordia A, Bansal HC. *Lancet* 1973;ii:1491.
[8] Bordia A. *Am J Clin Nutr* 1981;34:2100.
[9] Makheja AN, et al. *Lancet* 1979;i:781.
[10] *Chem Eng News* 1985;63(1):34.
[11] Boullin DJ. *Lancet* 1981;i:776.
[12] Luley C, et al. *Arznm Forsch* 1986;36:766.
[13] Jain AK, et al. *Am J Med* 1993;94:632.
[14] Glorious Garlic. *NARD Journal* 1993;9:13.
[15] McMahon FG, Vargas R, et al. *Pharmacotherapy* 1993;13(4):406.
[16] Joshi DJ, et al. *Phytotherapy Res* 1987;1:141.
[17] Pareddy SR, Rosenberg JM. *Hospital Pharmacist Report* 1993;8:27.
[18] Caporaso, et al. *Antimicrob Agents Chemother* 1983;23:700.
[19] Osol A, Farrar GE Jr, ed. The Dispensatory of the United States of America, 25th ed. Philadelphia: JB Lippincott, 1955:1538.

Gelsemium

SCIENTIFIC NAME(S): *Gelsemium sempervirens* (L.) Ait. Synonymous with *G. nitidum* Michx. and *Bignonia sempervirens* L. Family: Loganiaceaea or Spigeliaceae. Not to be confused with true jasmine (*Jasminum grandiflorum* L.)

COMMON NAME(S): Gelsemium, yellow or Carolina jasmine, wild, yellow or Carolina jessamine, woodbine, evening trumpet flower

BOTANY: Gelsemium is a climbing, woody evergreen vine characterized by very fragrant, bright yellow flowers. Although native to the southwest United States, it also grows in Mexico and parts of Central America where it is widely cultivated as an ornamental.[1]

HISTORY: Gelsemium has been used as an ingredient in some analgesic and homeopathic products, but its use has been limited due to its toxicity. At the turn of the century, it was a popular ingredient in asthma and respiratory remedies.[2] Related species have been used in traditional Chinese medicine to treat neuralgia and various painful conditions. It is the state flower of South Carolina.

CHEMISTRY: The active components of gelsemium are the alkaloids, which are present in a concentration of about 0.5%. These consist primarily of gelsemine, with lesser amounts of related compounds (gelsemicine, gelsedine, etc).[1] Other compounds found in the plant include scopoletin (also called gelsemic acid), a small amount of volatile oil, fatty acid and tannins.[1]

PHARMACOLOGY: Gelsemium and its principle alkaloid gelsemine have been reported to exert central stimulant and analgesic effects, being able to potentiate the effects of aspirin and phenacetin.[1] The plant has been investigated for its anticancer properties.

TOXICOLOGY: All parts of the plant contain toxic alkaloids that can cause paralysis and death, and should never be ingested. Gelsemium alkaloids are highly toxic. Ingestion of as little as 4 ml of a fluid extract has been reported to be fatal. Toxic symptoms include giddiness, weakness, ptosis, dilated pupils and respiratory depression. Gelsemicine is more toxic than gelsemine.[3]

Toxicity has been reported in animals that have grazed on gelsemium, and bees that pollinate the plant have been poisoned.[2] Honey derived from the plant nectar has been reported to be toxic.[2]

SUMMARY: Gelsemium is a beautiful yet highly toxic plant. Although it has been used in traditional medicine, its narrow safety margin limits its use. Today, the plant is widely cultivated for its ornamental flowers.

PATIENT INFORMATION – Gelsemium

Uses: Gelsemium has been traditionally used to treat pain and respiratory ailments.

Side Effects: All parts of the gelsemium are toxic and can cause death when ingested.

---

[1] Leung AY. *Encyclopedia of Common Natural Ingredients Used in Food, Drugs, and Cosmetics*. New York, NY: J. Wiley and Sons, 1980.
[2] Dobelis IN. *Magic and Medicine of Plants*. Pleasantville, NY: Readers Digest Books, 1986.
[3] Evans WC. *Trease and Evans' Pharmacognosy*, ed. 13. London, England: Balliere Tindall, 1989.

Gentian

SCIENTIFIC NAME(S): *Gentiana lutea* L. Stemless gentian is derived from *G. acaulis* L. Family: Gentianaceae

COMMON NAME(S): Gentian, stemless gentian, yellow gentian, bitter root, pale gentian, gall weed

BOTANY: Native to Europe and western Asia, *G. lutea* is a perennial herb with erect stems and oval leaves, which grows to 1.8 meters in height. The plant produces a cluster of fragrant orange-yellow flowers. *G. acaulis* is a small herb with a basal rosette of lance-shaped leaves and generally grows to only 10 cm in height. It is native to the European Alps at 3000 to 5000 feet above sea level. The roots and rhizomes are nearly cylindrical, sometimes branched, varying in thickness from 5 to 40 mm. The root and rhizome portions are longitudinally wrinkled. The color of the rhizomes, ranging from dark brown to light tan, appears to be related to its bitter principal content, the darker roots having more of a persistent bitter taste.[1] The roots and rhizome of *G. lutea* are used medicinally, whereas the entire plant of *G. acaulis* is used.

HISTORY: The gentians have been used for centuries as bitters to stimulate the appetite, improve digestion and to treat a variety of gastrointestinal complaints (eg, heartburn, vomiting, stomach ache, diarrhea).[2,3] Both gentian and stemless gentian are approved for food use. Stemless gentian usually is consumed as a tea or alcoholic extract such as *Angostura Bitters*. The extracts are used in a variety of foods, cosmetics and some antismoking products. The plant has been used externally to treat wounds and internally to treat sore throat, arthritic inflammations and jaundice.

CHEMISTRY: The most characteristic aspect of gentian is its bitter taste. This is imparted by a number of bitter compounds, primarily amarogentin, gentiopicrin (about 1.5% in fresh roots),[4] gentiopicroside and swertiamarin. Amarogentin is one of the most strongly bitter compounds known. The speed of drying of the roots affects its use as a medicinal bitter. Slow drying permits enzymatic hydrolysis of gentiopicrin into gentiogenin and glucose, thus reducing the bitter nature of the product.[5] Gentian extract is used in concentrations of about 0.02% in nonalcoholic beverages. In addition, the plant contains numerous alkaloids (gentianine and gentialutine), xanthones, triterpenes, common sugars and a small amount of a volatile oil.[6] Stemless gentian also contains the xanthone glycoside gentiacauloside. It should be noted that the dye, gentian violet, is not derived from this plant.

PHARMACOLOGY: Bitter substances ingested before eating are reputed to improve the appetite and aid digestion by stimulating the flow of gastric juices and bile. However, since gentian is most often consumed as an alcoholic beverage, it is difficult to distinguish the effects of gentian from those of alcohol, which are quite similar when alcohol is consumed in moderate amounts.[7]

Gentianine has been shown to exert a measurable anti-inflammatory effect in animals.

TOXICOLOGY: Although the extract usually is taken in very small doses that do not appear to cause adverse effects, at least one author has suggested that gentian may not be well tolerated by persons with hypertension or by women who are pregnant.[6] The extract may cause gastric irritation, resulting in nausea and vomiting.

The highly toxic white hellebore (*Veratrum album* L.) often grows in close proximity to gentian. At least five cases of acute veratrum alkaloid poisoning have been reported in persons who prepared homemade gentian wine that had been accidentally contaminated by veratrum.[8]

SUMMARY: Gentian is a widely recognized plant that has been used as a bitter tonic for centuries. It is believed that a small amount of the extract (usually mixed with alcohol) can stimulate appetite and improve digestion. Aside from this, none of the other professed effects is well documented in humans.

PATIENT INFORMATION – Gentian

Uses: Gentian is used in bitters to stimulate appetite, improve digestion and treat GI complaints. It has also been used to treat wounds, sore throat, arthritic inflammations and jaundice.

Side Effects: The extract may cause gastric irritation and may not be tolerated by pregnant women or hypertensive patients.

---

[1] Meyer JE. *The Herbalist*. Hammond, IN: Hammond Book Co., 1934.
[2] Leung AY. *Encyclopedia of Common Natural Ingredients Used in Food, Drugs, and Cosmetics*. New York, NY: John Wiley and Sons, 1980.
[3] DerMarderosian A, Liberti L. *Natural Product Medicine*. Philadelphia, PA: G.F. Stickley Co., 1988.
[4] Spoerke DG. *Herbal Medications*. Santa Barbara, CA: Woodbridge Press, 1980.

[5] Tyler VE, et al. *Pharmacognosy*, ed. 9. Philadelphia, PA: Lea & Febiger, 1988.
[6] Tyler VE. *The Honest Herbal*. Philadelphia, PA: G.F. Stickley Co., 1982.
[7] Tyler VE. *The New Honest Herbal*. Philadelphia, PA: G.F. Stickley Co., 1987.
[8] Garnier R, et al. *Ann Med Interne* 1985;136:125.

Ginger

SCIENTIFIC NAME(S): *Zingiber officinale* Roscoe; occasionally *Z. capitatum* Smith.[1] Family: Zingiberaceae

COMMON NAME(S): Ginger, ginger root, black ginger, zingiberis rhizoma

BOTANY: A native of tropical Asia, this perennial is cultivated in tropical climates such as Australia, Brazil, China, India, Jamaica, West Africa, and parts of the US.[1] The term "root" is actually a misnomer because it is the rhizome that is used medicinally and as a culinary spice. Cultivation with natural manuring is thought to increase the spiciness of the rhizome and is therefore preferred to wild crafting.[1] The rhizome is harvested between 6 and 20 months; taste and pungency increase with maturity.[1] The plant carries a green-purple flower in terminal spikes; the flowers are similar to orchids.[1,2]

HISTORY: Medicinal use of ginger dates back to ancient China and India; references to its use are found in Chinese pharmacopoeias, the Sesruta scriptures of Ayurvedic medicine as well as Sanskrit writings.[1] Once its culinary properties were discovered in the 13th century, use of this herb became widespread throughout Europe. In the Middle Ages, it held a firm place in apothecaries for travel sickness, nausea, hangovers, and flatulence.[1]

Ginger and its constituents are stated to have antiemetic, cardiotonic, antithrombotic, antibacterial, antioxidant, antitussive, antihepatotoxic, anti-inflammatory, antimutagenic, stimulant, diaphoretic, diuretic, spasmolytic, immunostimulant, carminative, and cholagogue actions as well as to promote gastric secretions, increase intestinal peristalsis, lower cholesterol levels, raise blood glucose, and stimulate peripheral circulation.[1,3,4] Traditionally, ginger is used as an acrid bitter to strengthen and stimulate digestion.[1] Modern uses include prophylaxis for nausea and vomiting (associated with motion sickness, hyperemesis gravidarum and surgical anesthesia), dyspepsia, lack of appetite, anorexia, colic, bronchitis, and rheumatic complaints.[1,3-5] The food industry uses ginger oil as a spice and ginger extract in the manufacturing of ginger ale.[1,5] In China, ginger root and stem are used as pesticides against aphids and fungal spores.[6]

Ginger is in the official pharmacopoeias of Austria, China, Egypt, Great Britain, India, Japan, the Netherlands, and Switzerland.[1,4,5] It is approved as a nonprescription drug in Germany and as a dietary supplement in the US.[4] Only scraped or unscraped, unbleached ginger is accepted as a medicinal-grade drug, often combined with at least

1.5% volatile oil.[1] Langner et al consider Jamaican and Cochin ginger to be the best varieties, and report the Japanese plant to be of inferior quality and do not recommend it for medicinal use.[1] Standards of quality for ginger can be found in *The United States Pharmacopeia National Formulary*.

Powder, alcoholic solutions, and freshly pressed juice and oil are found in pharmaceutical preparations. Ginger as a spice, seasoning, flavoring, oil, extract, and oleoresin is considered "Generally Recognized As Safe" (GRAS) by the FDA.[7,8] Deliberate or accidental adulterants include exhausted (overprocessed) ginger, Japanese ginger, *Z. cassummunar*, *Z. zerumbet*, and other foreign substances.[1]

CHEMISTRY: It had long been believed that the "pungent principles" of ginger were also responsible for its pharmacologic activity, and this has been found to be accurate. The characteristic aroma of ginger is due mainly to the presence of a zingiberol volatile oil.[1,9]

The major constituents in ginger rhizomes are carbohydrates (50 to 70%), which are present as starch. The concentration of lipids is 3 to 8% and includes free fatty acids (eg, palmitic, oleic, linoleic, linolenic, capric, lauric, myristic), triglycerides, and lecithins. Oleoresin provides 4 to 7.5% of pungent substances as gingerol homologues, shogaol homologues, zingerone, and volatile oils.[1] Volatile oils are present in 1 to 3% concentrations and consist mainly of the sesquiterpenes beta-besabolene and zingiberene; other sesquiterpenes include zingiberol and zingiberenol; numerous monoterpenes are also found. Amino acids, raw fiber, ash, protein, phytosterols, vitamins (ie, nicotinic acid and vitamin A), and minerals are among the other constituents.[1,6]

Analyses of the oleoresins have resulted in the identification of a class of structurally related cardiotonic compounds called gingerols, which upon dehydration, form shogaols and degrade further to zingerone.[1,6] [6]-gingerol and [6]-shogaol are the main components however, the pharmacologically active compounds [6]- and [10]-dehydrogingerdione, and [6]- and [10]-gingerdione have also been identified.[1,10,11]

PHARMACOLOGY: The gingerols and the related compound shogaol have been found to possess cardiotonic activity. Crude methanol extracts of ginger were known to have a strong positive inotropic effect on animal hearts. The gingerols have been found to exert a dose-dependent positive inotropic action at doses as low as 10^{-4} g/ml when applied to isolated atrial tissue.[12] Cardiac workload is further decreased by dilation of blood vessels via stimulation of prostacyclin biosynthesis.[1]

Administration of [6]-gingerol and [6]-shogaol (1.75 to 3.5 mg/kg IV and 70 to 140 mg/kg orally) inhibited spontaneous motor activity, produced antipyretic and analgesic effects, and prolonged hexobarbital-induced sleeping time in laboratory animals. [6]-shogaol was generally more potent than [6]-gingerol and showed an intense antitussive effect when compared with dihydrocodeine phosphate. Interestingly, [6]-shogaol inhibited intestinal motility when given IV, but facilitated GI motility after oral administration. Both compounds were cardiodepressant at low doses and cardiotonic at higher doses.[10]

[6]-gingerol, the dehydrogingerdiones, and the gingerdiones are potent inhibitors of prostaglandin biosynthesis through the inhibition of prostaglandin synthetase (cyclooxygenase).[11] Inhibition of thromboxane synthesis results in inhibition of platelet aggregation, but evidence indicates this is dose dependent or may only occur with fresh ginger.[1,13] The only 2 in vivo reports of impaired platelet function involved consumption of large quantities of raw ginger; 1 subject consumed large quantities of marmalade containing 15% ginger, and 1 study administered 5 g raw fresh ginger daily for 1 week.[13] One study was unable to detect measurable changes in bleeding time, platelet count, or platelet aggregation following a single 2 g dose of dried ginger in 8 healthy males.[13]

Ginger has been reported to have weak fungicidal, strong antibacterial, and anthelmintic properties. Active constituents have been shown to inhibit reproduction of *Escherichia coli*, *Proteus* species, staphylococci, streptococci, and *Salmonella* but to stimulate lactobacilli growth.[1] In vitro anthelmintic activity has been documented for the volatile oil of *Z. purpureum* Roxb against *Ascaridia galli* Schrank.[5] Activity has also been reported against parasites, such as *Schistosoma* and *Anisakis*.[1]

The cytotoxic compound zerumbone and its epoxide have been isolated from the rhizomes of *Z. zerumbet*. This plant, also a member of the family Zingiberaceae, has been used traditionally in China as an antineoplastic. The isolates inhibited the growth of a hepatoma tissue culture.[14] In addition, juice prepared from ginger root has been found to inactivate the mutagenicity of tryptophan pyrolysis products in vitro.[15]

Human clinical trials have examined ginger's antiemetic effects related to kinetosis (motion sickness), perioperative anesthesia, and hyperemesis gravidarum. However, little is still known regarding its human pharmacology in these settings. Animal studies have described enhanced GI transport as well as anti-5-hydroxytryptamine ($5HT_3$) and possible CNS antiemetic effects.[17]

One clinical trial (n = 12) employed gastroduodenal manometry to evaluate prokinetic effects of ginger in fasting and postprandial healthy subjects. A significant increase in antral motility and in corpus motor response with a trend toward increased motor response in all regions was found.[18] However, no effect of ginger on gastric motility using an acetaminophen absorption technique was found in 16 healthy volunteers.[19]

Kinetosis: One double-blind study (n = 36) compared the effect of 940 mg powdered ginger root, 100 mg dimenhydrinate, and placebo (chickweed herb) in the prevention of motion sickness. Preparations were administered 20-25 minutes prior to placing blindfolded subjects in a rotating chair. Those receiving ginger root remained in the chair longer (average of 5.5 minutes, compared with 3.5 and 1.5 minutes for the dimenhydrinate and placebo groups, respectively), and 50% remained in the chair for the full 6 minutes of the test; none of the subjects in the other groups completed the test. In general, it took longer for the ginger group to begin feeling sick, but once the vomiting center was activated, sensations of nausea and vomiting progressed at the same rate in all groups.[20]

A double-blind, placebo-controlled study in seasick marine cadets (n = 79) reported significant reductions in symptoms (vomiting and cold sweats) and noticeably suppressed dizziness following administration of 1 g ginger rhizome. Nystagmus was reported as unchanged.[1] A study involving 1741 participants on an ocean sailing tour described the administration of 250 mg ginger prior to departure to be as effective as cinnarizine, scopolamine, dimenhydrinate, meclizine, and cyclizine.[1] Ginger (500 mg every 4 hours) and dimenhydrinate (100 mg every 4 hours) were compared in another double-blind study with similar protective effects, however those receiving ginger reported no side effects.[1]

Other trials have shown no significant differences among ginger, antiemetics, and placebo with regard to gastric as well as nongastric symptoms. Two separate investigations showed no effect of ginger on the CNS impairment caused by kinetosis as subjects retained the ability to perform certain head and eye movements. A scopolamine/*d*-amphetamine combination proved most effective but resulted in definite side effects.[1]

Another placebo-controlled study evaluated participants' ability to tolerate head movements in a rotating chair while blindfolded.[21] Ginger was compared against scopolamine (0.6 mg orally) in several small groups of test subjects. It was concluded that ginger administered as 500 to 1000 mg powdered root or 1000 mg fresh root provided no protection against motion sickness under various test conditions, while the scopolamine group was able to tolerate a significant increase in number of head movements. In this same study, gastric emptying and gastric electrical activity (via electrogastrogram [EGG]) were evaluated in 2 more small groups of subjects. Ginger partially inhibited and stabilized tachygastria but did not affect EGG amplitude. The authors concluded that symptoms of motion sickness can be dissociated from gastric electrical activity and that the partial tachygastric effects of ginger offer little to relieve the onset or severity of these symptoms.[21]

It has been proposed that, unlike antihistamines which act on the CNS, the aromatic, carminative, and possibly absorbent properties of ginger ameliorate the effects of motion sickness in the GI tract directly.[16,20] It may increase gastric motility and block GI reactions and subsequent nausea feedback.[20]

Postoperative nausea and vomiting (PONV): The antiemetic effects of ginger have been compared with metoclopramide and droperidol in prevention of PONV.[22,23] One prospective, randomized, double-blind trial (n = 120) evaluated 1 g powdered ginger root and 10 mg metoclopramide administered 1 hour prior to anesthesia in women undergoing gynecological laparoscopy; anesthesia was induced with propofol, fentanyl, and atracurium. Findings supported those of previous studies; ginger and metoclopramide were equally effective and were more effective than placebo in reducing the incidence of PONV (21%, 27%, and 41%, respectively). The need for postoperative antiemetics was significantly reduced in those receiving ginger over the placebo group (15% vs 38%, p = 0.006).[22]

In a placebo-controlled comparison against droperidol, no statistically significant difference was found with ginger root or ginger root plus droperidol in the incidence of PONV in 120 women undergoing outpatient gynecological laparoscopy; anesthesia was induced with thiopental fentanyl, and succinylcholine. Patients were given droperidol (1.25 mg IV), oral ginger root (1 g given 1 hour prior to induction of anesthesia and 1 g given 30 minutes prior to discharge), ginger plus droperidol or placebo. While incidences of postoperative nausea (20%, 22%, 33%, and 32%) and vomiting (13%, 25%, 25%, and 35%) did not reach statistical significance, the figures do appear to have potential clinical importance.[23]

A dosage study (randomized, double-blind, placebo-controlled) concluded that 0.5 g and 1 g powdered ginger root were ineffective in reducing the incidence of PONV in 108 patients. However, study methods in this particular trial could be questioned. To allow the identifying aroma of the ginger capsules to dissipate, capsules were removed from their original container and stored in pairs for 2 days in plastic bags until the odor disappeared. It has already been noted that the pungent principles (including the sesquiterpenes lending ginger its characteristic aroma) are responsible for ginger's pharmacological activity.[24]

Hyperemesis gravidarum: Pregnant women suffering from hyperemesis gravidarum received ginger (250 mg 4 times daily) or placebo for 4 days. About 70% of women subjectively preferred ginger treatment, with greater symptomatic relief being observed compared with placebo.[25]

Selective serotonin reuptake inhibitor discontinuation syndrome: One case report describes the successful use of ginger in one female patient with subsequent beneficial use in over 20 additional patients for the amelioration of symptoms (eg, disequilibrium, nausea) associated with abrupt discontinuation or intermittent noncompliance of selective serotonin reuptake inhibitors. Administration of 1100 mg ginger root 3 times daily at the onset of discontinuation-induced symptoms resulted in partial to complete relief of symptoms within 24 to 48 hours; ginger therapy was continued for approximately 2 weeks, the time required for symptoms to usually abate.[26]

TOXICOLOGY: There are no reports of severe toxicity in humans from the ingestion of ginger root. In culinary quantities, the root is generally devoid of activity. Large overdoses carry the potential for causing CNS depression. Inhibition of platelet aggregation has been reported after consumption of large (clinically impractical) amounts of ginger but returned to normal within one week of discontinuation.[13] Cardiotonic and cardiodepressant activity have been demonstrated in animals. Reports that ginger extracts may be mutagenic or antimutagenic in experimental test models require confirmation.[1,25]

There is no convincing evidence regarding the safety of ingesting large amounts of ginger by pregnant women. The German Commission E contraindicates ginger for the use of morning sickness, however, data are lacking to support toxic effects in pregnant women.[1,3,4] The FDA considers ginger as a food supplement as generally recognized as safe (GRAS).[7,8]

SUMMARY: Ginger root is an ancient spice that has had a role in herbal medicine for thousands of years. Evidence appears to support its usefulness in symptoms of motion sickness, postoperative nausea and vomiting, and GI disturbances. These effects seem to be associated with direct actions of ginger on the GI tract and less, if at all, on the CNS. Studies have been conducted in pregnant women with benefit shown over placebo for symptoms of morning sickness. Ginger has extremely low toxicity and is devoid of side effects at normal doses.

PATIENT INFORMATION – Ginger

Uses: Ginger and its constituents have antiemetic, cardiotonic, antithrombotic, antibacterial, antioxidant, antitussive, antihepatotoxic, anti-inflammatory, antimutagenic, stimulant, diaphoretic, diuretic, spasmolytic, immunostimulant, carminative, and cholagogue actions. Ginger is used to promote gastric secretions, increase intestinal peristalsis, lower cholesterol levels, raise blood glucose, and stimulate peripheral circulation. Traditionally used to stimulate digestion, its modern uses include prophylaxis for nausea and vomiting (associated with motion sickness, hypermesis gravidarum, and anesthesia), dyspepsia, lack of appetite, anorexia, colic, bronchitis, and rheumatic complaints. Ginger can be used as a flavoring or spice as well as a fungicide and pesticide.

Side Effects: Excessive amounts may cause CNS depression and may interfere with cardiac function or anticoagulant activity.

---

[1] Langner E, et al. Ginger: history and use. *Adv Ther* 1998;15(1):25-44.

[2] Schauenberg P, et al. *Guide to Medicinal Plants.* New Canaan, CT: Keats Publishing, Inc., 1977.

[3] Blumenthal M, et al. 1997. *German Commission E Monographs: Therapeutic Monographs on Medicinal Plants for Human Use.* Austin, TX: American Botanical Council.

[4] Blumenthal M. 1997. *Popular Herbs in the US Market: Therapeutic Monographs.* Austin, TX: American Botanical Council.

[5] Newall C, et al. 1996. *Herbal Medicines: A Guide for Healthcare Professionals.* London: Pharmaceutical Press.

[6] Yang R, et al. *Economic Botany* 1988;42(3):376.

[7] Food and Drug Administration, Department of Health and Human Services. Code of Federal Regulations, 21CFR182.10. Accessed via http://www.access.gpo.gov/nara/cfr/cfr-table-search.html. March 2000.

[8] *Herb safety and drug interactions.* 1998. Boulder, CO: Herb Research Foundation.

[9] Tyler V. *The New Honest Herbal.* Philadelphia, PA: GF Stickley Co., 1987.

[10] Suekawa M, et al. Pharmacological studies on ginger. *J Pharmacobiodyn* 1984;7(11):836–48.

[11] Kiuchi F, et al. Inhibitors of prostaglandin biosynthesis from ginger. *Chem Pharm Bull* 1982;30(2):754–57.

[12] Shoji N, et al. Cardiotoninc principles of ginger (*Zingiber officinale* Roscoe). *J Pharm Sci* 1982;71(1):1174–75.

[13] Lumb A. Effect of dried ginger on human platelet function. *Thromb Haemost* 1994;71(1):110-11.

[14] Matthes H, et al. *Phytochemistry* 1980;19:2643.

[15] Morita K, et al. *Agric Biol Chem* 1978;42(6):1235.

[16] Babbar O. Protective patterns of different interferons: possible efficacy of chick embryo and plant interferons against microbial infections and malignancies of animals. *Indian J Exp Biol* 1982;20:572-76.

[17] Lumb A. Mechanism of antiemetic effect of ginger. *Anaesthesia* 1993;48(12):1118.

[18] Micklefield G, et al. Effects of ginger on gastroduodenal motility. *Int J Clin Pharmacol Ther* 1999;37(7):341-46.

[19] Phillips S, et al. Zingiber officinale does not affect gastric emptying rate: a randomized, placebo-controlled, crossover trial. *Anaesthesia* 1993;48(5):393-95.

[20] Mowrey D, et al. Motion sickness, ginger, and psychophysics. *Lancet* 1982;1(8273):655-57.

[21] Stewart J, et al. Effects of ginger on motion sickness susceptibility and gastric function. *Pharmacology* 1991;42(2):111-20.

[22] Phillips S, et al. Zingiber officinale (ginger)-an antiemetic for day case surgery. *Anaesthesia* 1993;48(8):715-7.

[23] Visalyaputra S, et al. The efficacy of ginger root in the prevention of postoperative nausea and vomiting after outpatient gynaecological laparoscopy. *Anaesthesia* 1998;53:506-10.

[24] Arfeen Z, et al. A double-blind randomized controlled trial of ginger for the prevention of postoperative nausea and vomiting. *Anaesth Intensive Care* 1995;23:449-52.

[25] Fischer-Rasmussen W, et al. Ginger treatment of hyperemesis gravidarum. *Eur J Obstet Gynecol Reprod Biol* 1991;38(1):19-24.

[26] Schechter J. Treatment of disequilibrium and nausea in the SRI discontinuation syndrome. *J Clin Psychiatry* 1998;59(8):431-32.

Ginkgo

SCIENTIFIC NAME(S): *Ginkgo biloba* L. Family: Ginkgoaceae

COMMON NAME(S): Ginkgo, maidenhair tree, kew tree, ginkyo, yinhsing (Silver Apricot-Japanese)

BOTANY: The ginkgo is the world's oldest living tree species, and it can be traced back more than 200 million years to the fossils of the Permian period. It is the sole survivor of the family Ginkgoaceae. Individual trees may live as long as 1000 years. They grow to a height of about 125 feet and have fan-shaped leaves. The species is dioecious; male trees more than 20 years old blossom in the spring. Adult female trees produce a plum-like gray-tan fruit that falls in late autumn. Its fleshy pulp has a foul, offensive odor and causes contact dermatitis. The edible inner seed resembles an almond and is sold in oriental markets.[1]

HISTORY: The ginkgo species was almost destroyed during the ice age. The species survived in China, where it was cultivated as a sacred tree, and is still found decorating Buddhist temples throughout Asia. Preparations have been used for medicinal purposes for more than a thousand years. Traditional Chinese physicians used ginkgo leaves to treat asthma and chillblains, which is the swelling of the hands and feet from exposure to damp cold. The ancient Chinese and Japanese ate roasted ginkgo seeds, and considered them a digestive aid and preventive for drunkenness.[2] In the Western world, ginkgo has been used since the 1960s when technology made it possible to isolate its essential compounds. The flavonoids act as free radical scavengers, and the terpenes (ginkgolides) inhibit platelet activating factor.[3] Currently, oral and intravenous forms are available in Europe, where it is one of the most widely prescribed medications. Neither form has been approved for medical use in the United States, although ginkgo is sold as a nutritional supplement.

CHEMISTRY: There is a seasonal variation in the content of active compounds in leaves, with the highest amounts present in autumn.[4] Leaf constituents include amino acid 6–hydroxykynurenic acid, flavonoids (dimeric bioflavones) such as bilobetin, ginkgetin, isoginkgetin, sciadopitysin, and flavonols quercetin, kaempferol and their glycosides.[4,5] About 40 different flavonoids have been indentified so far. Some of these flavonoids are catechins, dehydrocatechins (proanthocyanidins), and flavones (eg, ginkgetin, amentoflavune, bilobetin, sciadopitysin).[6] Also present in ginkgo leaves are terpenoids (diterpenes), such as bilobalide, and gingolides A, B, C, J and M.[5,6] Other leaf components include steroids (sitosterol, stigmasterol), polyprenols, organic acids (shikimic, vanillic, ascorbic, p-coumaric), benzoic acid derivatives, carbohydrates, straight chain hydrocarbons, alcohol, ketones and 2 hexenol.[6]

The seed portion of ginkgo contains carbohydate (38%), protein (4%) and fat (< 2%). Alkaloids such as ginkgotoxin, amino acids, cyanogenetic glycosides and phenols (long-chain, including anacaric acid, bilobol and cardanol) are also present.[5] Ginkgolic acid and related alkylphenols from lipid fraction of the fruit pods has been reviewed.[7] The foul-smelling odor of the fleshy portion of the seeds is caused by high concentrations of butanoic and hexanoic acids. 4–O-methylpyridoxine has also been isolated from the seeds.[6,9]

Biological standardization of ginkgo extracts has been reported.[8]

PHARMACOLOGY: Pharmacokinetic parameter testing of ginkgo has been performed in animals[6,9] and also in humans evaluating three ginkgo forms (capsules, drops and tablets).[10] Behavior of ginkgo after IV and oral administration in humans has been documented.[11]

Numerous studies on the pharmacological actions of ginkgo have been reported, including treatments for **cerebral insufficiency**, **dementia**, **circulatory disorders** and **asthma**. The plant is also known for its antioxidant and neuroprotective effects.

Cerebral insufficiency: Cerebral insufficiency may cause anxiety and stress, memory, concentration and mood impairment, and hearing disorders, all of which may benefit from ginkgo therapy.In man, intravenous injection of ginkgo biloba extract (GBE) increased cerebral blood flow in about 70% of the patients evaluated. This increase was age-related: Patients between the ages of 30 and 50 years had a 20% increase from baseline, compared with 70% in those 50 to 70 years old. Further, the time to reach peak blood flow was shorter in the elderly.[12] Ginkgo leaf improves cerebral metabolism and protects against hypoxic damage in animals with cerebral ischemia.[5] Cerebral insufficiency in 112 patients (average age 70.5 years) treated with ginkgo leaf extract (120 mg) for 1 year, resulted in reduced symptoms such as headache, dizziness, short-term memory, vigilance and disturbance.[5] Electroencephalographic effects of different preparations of GBE have been performed.[13] A review of 40 clinical trials was performed, most evaluating 120 mg GBE per day for 4 to 6 weeks, reporting positive results in treating cerebral insufficiency. Only eight studies did not have major methodological flaws; the results from these studies were, nevertheless, difficult to interpret. They suggested that long-term treatment (greater than 6 weeks) is required and that any effect is similar to that observed following treatment with ergoloids.[14] A meta-analysis of 11 placebo controlled, randomized, double-blinded studies, concluded GBE (150 mg/day) to be superior to placebo in patients with cerebrovascular insufficiency.[15]

Ginkgo's role as a psychotropic drug is under review.[16]

Anti-anxiety/stress: MAO inhibition in rats produced by extracts of ginkgo (dried and fresh leaves) has been performed, suggesting a mechanism by which the plant exerts its anti-stress actions.[17] Glucocorticoid synthesis, regulated by ACTH (adrenocorticotropic hormone), which accelerates cholesterol transport, can lead to neurotoxicity. Ginkgolides A and B, through a series of events, decrease cholesterol transport, resulting in decreased corticosteroid synthesis. The anti-stress and neuroprotective effects of GBE may also be caused by this mechanism of action.[18]

GBE in combination with *Zingiber officinale*, was compared to diazepam to study anxiolytic effects in animals. Results showed these effects to be comparable to those of diazepam, but in high doses, the combination may have anxiolytic properties.[19] Social behavior in animals has been evaluated using GBE, diazepam and ethyl beta-carboline-3-carboxylate.[20]

Memory improvement: Oral administration of GBE (alone and in combination with panax ginseng) improved retention of learned behavior using conditioned-reflex methods (punishment or positive reinforcement) in young and old rats.[21] GBE can help improve behavioral adaptation despite adverse environmental events, as shown in rats taught reward vs punishment (stress) testing to obtain drinking water. This supports clinical use of the plant to treat cognitive impairment in the elderly population.[22]

In elderly men with slight age-related memory loss, ginkgo supplementation reduced the time required to process visual information.[23] Effects of GBE on event-related potentials in 48 patients with age-associated memory impairment has been performed.[24] Significant improvement in memory (as measured by a series of psychological testing), in 8 patients (average age, 32 years) was found one hour after administration of 600 mg GBE vs placebo, again confirming the plant's usefulness in this area.[5]

Tinnitus hearing disorder therapy: Because of the diverse etiology of tinnitus, and lack of objective method to measure its symptoms, results using GBE for treatment of this disease are contradictory. GBE may have positive effects in some individuals.[25] In animals with salicylate-induced tinnitus, GBE resulted in a statistically significant decrease of behavioral manifestations of tinnitus.[26]

In patients with hearing disorders secondary to vascular insufficiency of the ear, about 40% of those treated orally with a leaf extract for 2 to 6 months showed improvement in auditory measurements. The extract also was extremely effective in relieving vertigo associated with vestibular dysfunction.[27]

Dementias: Clinical application of ginkgo biloba in dementia syndromes has been reported, and therapeutic effectiveness of the plant in this area has been demonstrated.[28,29] One report recommends early GBE therapy in dementias, especially because there are not side effects associated with other dementia drugs.[30]

Effects of 240 mg/day GBE in approximately 200 patients with dementia of Alzheimer type and multi-infarct dementia, have been investigated in a randomized, double-blinded, placebo controlled, multi-center study. Parameters such as psychopathological assessment, attention, memory and behavior were monitored, resulting in clinical efficacy of the extract in dementias of both types.[31] In another set of patients with moderate dementias (of Alzheimer, vascular or mixed type), short-term IV infusion therapy with GBE also had positive results, improving psychopathology and cognitive performance.[32] In a 52-week, randomized, double-blinded, placebo controlled, multi-center study, mild to severe Alzheimer or multi-infarct dementia patients received 120 mg/day GBE vs placebo. Results of this report again confirm improved cognitive performance and social functioning in a number of cases.[33]

Circulatory disorders/asthma: Ginkgolides competitively inhibit the binding of platelet-activating factor (PAF) to its membrane receptor.[5,6] Effects of this mechanism are useful in the treatment of allergic reaction and inflammation (asthma and bronchospasm) and also in circulatory diseases.

Ginkgolides have been proven effective in both early and late phases of airway hyperactivity in one double-blinded, randomized, crossover study in asthma patients.[5]

A meta-analysis evaluating GBE in peripheral arterial disease, concludes a highly significant therapeutic effect of the plant in this area.[34] Numerous studies are available concerning GBE and circulatory disorders including its ability to protect against cardiac ischemia reperfusion injury,[35] to adjust fibrinolytic activity[36] and, in combination with aspirin, to treat thrombosis.[37] It also appears useful in management of peripheral vascular disorders such as Raynaud's disease, acrocyanosis and post-phlebitis syndrome.[27] In man, IV injection of 50 to 200 mg of ginkgo extract caused a dose-dependent increase in microcirculation and blood viscoelasticity in patients with pathologic blood flow disorders.[38]

A 6-month, double-blind trial suggested some efficacy in treating obliterative arterial disease of the lower limbs. Patients who received extract showed a clinically and statistically significant improvement in pain-free walking distance, maximum walking distance and plethysmographic recordings of peripheral blood flow.[39] GBE improves walking performance in 60 patients with intermittent claudication, with good tolerance to the drug.[40] However, another report concludes GBE (120 mg/day) to have no effect on walking distance or leg pain in intermittent claudication patients (but finds other cognitive functions to be improved).[41] A review of 10 controlled trials evaluating treatment of the plant for this condition, found poor methodological quality, but did note all the studies to show clinical effectiveness of GBE in treating intermittent claudication.[42]

Antioxidant/neuroprotective effects: GBE is known to improve diseases associated with free radical generation. The ginkgolides may contribute to neuroprotective effects. The flavonoid fraction contains free radical scavengers, both of which are important in areas such as hypoxia, seizure activity and peripheral nerve damage.[43]

GBE exerts a restorative effect in aged rats caused by its protective action on neuronal membrane.[44] It was also shown to protect rat cerebellar neurons suffering from oxidative stress induced by hydrogen peroxide.[45] GBE may be a potent inhibitor of nitric oxide production under tissue-damaging inflammatory conditions in murine macrophage cell lines.[46] GBE was found to be more effective than water-soluble antioxidants and as effective as lipid-soluble antioxidants, in an in vitro model using human erythrocyte suspensions.[47]

Other numerous reports exist concerning this topic, including GBE's effect against lipid peroxidation and cell necrosis in rat hepatocytes,[48] its effect as an oxygen radical scavenger and antioxidant,[49] and its powerful effects on copper-mediated LDL oxidative modification.[50] In Chernobyl accident recovery workers, GBE's antioxidant effects were also studied. Clastogenic factors (risk factors for development of late effects of irradiation) were successfully reduced by the plant.[51]

A number of other potentially beneficial pharmacologic effects have been observed for ginkgo, including its ability to prevent the deterioration of lipid profiles when subjects were challenged with high-cholesterol meals over an extended holiday season,[52] improvement in the symptoms of PMS, particularly breast-related symptoms.[53] GBE's use in eye problems[6] and its scavenging abilities to reduce functional and morphological retina impairments.[54] In addition, GBE has in vitro and in vivo activity against *Pneumocystis carinii*[55] and has been studied in animals with diabetes[56,57] and in human diabetic patients. When GBE extract was given, peripheral blood flow increased by 40% to 45%, compared with an increase of 35% after administration of nicotinic acid.[58] Other reports suggest GBE to be effective in arresting fibrosis development (in 86 chronic hepatitis patients),[59] promoting hair regrowth in mice[60] and relaxing both animal and human penile tissue, suggesting a possible use as a drug for impotence.[61] Long-chain phenols from ginkgo biloba seeds are active against sarcoma 180 ascites in mice.[5] Seed extracts of the plant possess antibacterial and antifungal activity.[6]

TOXICOLOGY: Ingestion of the extract has not been associated with severe side effects. Adverse events from clinical trials of up to 160 mg/day for 4 to 6 weeks did not differ from placebo group. German literature lists ginkgo's possible side effects as headache, dizziness, heart palpitations and GI and dermatologic reactions. Injectable forms of ginkgo may cause circulatory disturbances, skin allergy or phlebitis. Willmar Schwabe Co. has withdrawn its parenteral ginkgo product *Tebonin* from the market because of the possible severity of side effects from this form.[6]

A toxic syndrome, ("Gin-nan" food poisoning) has been recognized in the Orient in children who have ingested ginkgo seeds. Approximately 50 seeds produce tonic/clonic seizures and loss of consciousness.[62] Seventy reports (between 1930 and 1960) found 27% lethality, with infants being most vulnerable. Ginkgotoxin (4-O-methylpyridoxine), found only in the seeds, was considered responsible for this toxicity.[5,6]

Contact with the fleshy fruit pulp has been known since ancient times to be a skin irritant. Constituents alkylbenzoic acid, alkylphenol and their derivatives cause reactions of this type. Allergic dermatitis such as erythema, edema, blisters and itching have all been reported.[6] A cross-allergenicity exists between ginkgo fruit pulp and poison ivy. Ginkgolic acid and bilobin are structurally similar to the allergens of poison ivy, mango rind and cashew nut shell oil. Contact with the fruit pulp causes erythema and edema, with the rapid formation of vesicles accompanied by severe itching. The symptoms last 7 to 10 days. Ingestion of as little as two pieces of pulp has been reported to cause perioral erythema, rectal burning and tenesmus (painful spasms of the anal sphincter).[1]

Allergans ginkgols and ginkgolic acids can also cause contact reactions of mucous membranes, resulting in cheilitis and GI irritation. Oral ingestion of ginkgo preparations, however, do not have this ability.[5,6] Ginkgo pollen can also be strongly allergenic.[63]

In one report, spontaneous bilateral subdural hematomas have, in addition, been associated with ingestion of the plant.[64]

In animal experimentation, no mutagenic or teratogenic effects were found. Oral administration of up to 1600 mg/kg/day of GBE to rats did not produce teratogenic effects. Other animal toxicity data is available including lethal dosing and other studies performed in mice, rats, guinea pigs, rabbits and dogs.[6]

No human data is yet available concerning pregnancy and lactation, so ginkgo should be avoided by this population.[5,6]

SUMMARY: The ginkgo is the oldest known living tree species. An extract of the leaves has been shown to have pharmacologic activity in the areas of cerebral insufficiency, dementias, circulatory disorders and bronchoconstriction. The plant also is known for its antioxidant and neuroprotective effects. Ingestion of ginkgo extract has not been associated with severe side effects, but contact with the fleshy fruit pulp causes allergic dermatitis, similar to poison ivy. In animals, ginkgo does not produce teratogenicity, but limited human data is available on this subject, suggesting avoidance of use during pregnancy and lactation.

PATIENT INFORMATION – Ginkgo

Uses: Ginkgo has been used in treating Raynaud's disease, cerebral insufficiency, anxiety/stress, tinnitus, dementias, circulatory disorders/asthma. It has positive effects on memory and diseases associated with free radical generation.

Side Effects: Severe side effects are rare; possible effects include headache, dizziness, heart palpitations and GI and dermatologic reactions. Ginkgo pollen can be strongly allergenic. Contact with the fleshy fruit pulp causes allergic dermatitis, similar to poison ivy.

---

[1] Becker LE, Skipworth GB. JAMA 1975;231:1162.
[2] Castleman M. The Herb Quarterly 1990 Spring:26.
[3] Z'Brun A. Schweiz Rundsch Med Prax 1995;84(1):1–6.
[4] Briancon-Scheid F, et al. J Med Plant Res 1983;49:204.
[5] Newall C, et al. Herbal Medicines. London, England: Pharmaceutical Press 1996;138–40.
[6] DeSmet P, et al. Ginkgo Biloba. Berlin: Springer-Verlag 1997;51–66.
[7] Jaggy H, et al. Pharmazie 1997;52(10):735–38.
[8] Steinke B, et al. Planta Med 1993;59(2):155–60.
[9] Pietta P, et al. J Chromatogr B Biomed Appl 1995;673(1):75–80.
[10] Wojcicki J, et al. Mater Med Pol 1995;27(4):141–46.
[11] Fourtillan J, et al. Therapie 1995;50(2):137–44.
[12] Pistolese GR. Minerva Med 1973;79:4166.
[13] Kunkel H. Neuropsychobiology 1993;27(1):40–45.
[14] Kleijnen J, et al. Br J Clin Pharmacol 1992;34(4):352–58.
[15] Hopfenmuller W. Arzneimittelforschung 1994;44(9):1005–13.
[16] Cott J. Psychopharmacol Bull 1995;31(4):745–51.
[17] White H, et al. Life Sci 1996;58(16):1315–21.
[18] Amri H, et al. Endocrinology 1996;137(12):5707–18.
[19] Hasenohrl R, et al. Pharmacol Biochem Behav 1996;53(2):271–75.
[20] Chermat R, et al. Pharmacol Biochem Behav 1997;56(2):333–39.
[21] Petkov V, et al. Planta Med 1993;59(2):106–14.
[22] Rapin J, et al. Gen Pharmacol 1994;25(5):1009–16.
[23] Allain H, et al. Clin Ther 1993;15:549-58.
[24] Semlitsch H, et al. Pharmacopsychiatry 1995;28(4):134–42.
[25] Holgers K, et al. Audiology 1994;33(2):85–92.
[26] Jastreboff P, et al. Audiol Neurootol 1997;2(4):197–212.
[27] Nazzaro P, Dicarlo A. Minerva Med 1973;79:4198.
[28] Herrschaft H. Pharm Unserer Zeit 1992;21(6):266–75.
[29] Itil T, et al. Psychopharmacol Bull 1995;31(1):147–58.
[30] Reisecker F. Wien Med Wochenschr 1996;146(21–22):546–48.
[31] Kanowski S, et al. Pharmacopsychiatry 1996;29(2):47–56.
[32] Haase J, et al. Z Gerontol Geriatr 1996;29(4):302–9.
[33] LeBars P, et al. JAMA 1997;278(16):1327–32.
[34] Schneider B. Arzneimittelforschung 1992;42(4):428–36.
[35] Haramaki N, et al. Free Radic Biol Med 1994;16(6):789–94.
[36] Shen J, et al. Biochem Mol Biol Int 1995;35(1):125–34.
[37] Belougne E, et al. Thromb Res 1996;82(5):453–58.
[38] Koltringer P, et al. Fortschr Med 1993;111:170.
[39] Bauer U. Arzneim Forsch 1984;34:716.
[40] Blume J, et al. VASA 1996;25(3):265–74.
[41] Drabaek H, et al. Ugeskr Laeger 1996;158(27):3928–31.
[42] Ernst E. Fortschr Med 1996;114(8):85–87.
[43] Smith P, et al. J Ethnopharmacol 1996;50(3):131–39.
[44] Huguet F, et al. J Pharm Pharmacol 1994;46(4):316–18.
[45] Oyama Y, et al. Brain Res 1996;712(2):349–52.
[46] Kobuchi H, et al. Biochem Pharmacol 1997;53(6):897–903.
[47] Kose K, et al. J Int Med Res 1995;23(1):9–18.
[48] Joyeux M, et al. Planta Med 1995;61(2):126–29.
[49] Maitra I, et al. Biochem Pharmacol 1995;49(11):1649–55.
[50] Yan L, et al. Biochem Biophys Res Commun 1995;212(2):360–66.
[51] Emerit I, et al. Radiat Res 1995;144(2):198–205.
[52] Kenzelmann R, Kade F. Arzneim Forsch 1993;43:978.
[53] Tamborini A, Taurelle R. Ref Fr Gynecol Obstet 1993;88:447-57.
[54] Droy-Lefaix M, et al. Int J Tissue React 1995;17(3):93–100.
[55] Atzori C, et al. Antimicrob Agents Chemother 1993;37:1492.
[56] Agar A, et al. Int J Neurosci 1994;76(3–4):259–66.
[57] Punkt K, et al. ACTA Histochem 1997;99(3):291–99.

[58] Bartolo M. *Minerva Med* 1973;79:4192.
[59] Li W, et al. *Chung Kuo Chung Hsi I Chieh Ho Tsa Chih* 1995;15(10):593–95.
[60] Kobayashi N, et al. *Yakugaku Zasshi* 1993;113(10):718–24.
[61] Paick J, et al. *J Urol* 1996;156(5):1876–80.

[62] Yagi M, et al. *Yakugaku Zasshi* 1993;113:596.
[63] Long R, et al. *Hua Hsi I Ko Ta Hsueh Hsueh Pao* 1992;23:429.
[64] Rowin J, et al. *Neurology* 1996;46(6):1775–76.

Ginseng

BOTANY: Ginseng commonly refers to *Panax quinquefolium* L. or *Panax ginseng* C. A. Meyer, two members of the family Araliaceae. The ginsengs were classified as members of the genus *Aralia* in older texts. A number of species of ginseng grow around the world and are used in local traditional medicine. The roots or rhizomes of these plants are used medicinally.

Scientific Name	Common Name	Distribution
P. quinquefolium L.	American ginseng	USA
P. ginseng C. A. Meyer	Korean ginseng	N.E. China, Korea, East Siberia
P. pseudoginseng Wall. var. notoginseng	Sanchi ginseng	S.W. China
P. pseudoginseng var. major	Zhuzishen	China
P. pseudoginseng (Will.) subsp. japonicus	Chikusetsu ginseng	Japan
P. pseudoginseng subsp. himalaicus	Himalayan ginseng	Japan
P. trifolius L.	Dwarf ginseng	USA

In the USA, ginseng is found in rich, cool woods; a significant crop is also grown commercially. The short plant grows from 3 to 7 compound leaves that drop in the fall. It bears a cluster of red or yellowish fruits from June to July. The roots mature slowly and are usually harvested only after the first 3 years of growth. The shape of the root can vary between species and has been used to distinguish types of ginseng.

Approximately 45,000 kg of dried cultivated *P. quinquefolium* root and an equal amount of wild root are shipped abroad from the US annually, primarily to markets in the orient. About 5% of the root crop is retained for domestic use.[1]

HISTORY: Ginseng is perhaps the most widely recognized plant used in traditional medicine and now plays a major role in the herbal health care market. For more than two thousand years, various forms have been used in medicine. The name Panax, derives from the Greek word "all healing" and its properties have been no less touted. Ginseng root's man-shaped figure (shen-seng means "man-root") led proponents of the "Doctrine of Signatures" to believe that the root could strengthen any part of the body. Through the ages the root has been used in the treatment of asthenia, atherosclerosis, blood and bleeding disorders, colitis and to relieve the symptoms of aging, cancer and senility.

Evidence that the root possesses a general strengthening effect, raises mental and physical capacity, exerts a protectant effect against experimental diabetes, neurosis, radiation sickness and some cancers has been reported. Today, its popularity is due to the "adaptogenic effect" (stress-protective) of the saponin content.

CHEMISTRY: The first study of the plant was reported in 1854 when a saponin called panaquilon was isolated from *P. quinquefolium*.[2] The analysis of ginseng has focused on a group of compounds known as ginsenosides or panaxosides. These steroid-like compounds are saponin (a steroidal compound that froths in solution) glycosides (often linked to sugars).[3,4] About 12 major panaxosides have been isolated.[5] However, several dozen minor glycosides have been identified. The composition varies based on the species, age of the root, location, season and curing method.[6] Panaxosides are found in only minute quantities and are difficult to purify on a large scale. Therefore, the whole root is used in herbal preparations.

Many other minor components have been isolated and may contribute to the pharmacologic effects. These include a volatile oil, beta-elemine, sterols, flavonoids, peptides, vitamins and minerals, enzymes and choline.[7]

COMMERCIAL PRODUCTS: A wide range of ginseng products are available over-the-counter. These range from fresh and dried roots to extracts, solutions, capsules, tablets, cosmetics, sodas and teas. The taste of ginseng is disagreeable to many. Physical and chemical analyses have shown that while some commercial products closely resemble the whole root in composition, many contain little or no detectable ginsenoside concentrations.[8,9] Some preparations have been adulterated with phenylbutazone, aminopyrine or mandrake root.[10,11] Other preparations labelled "native American ginseng" were found not to contain any species of *Panax*. The root of Siberian ginseng (*Acanthopanax senticosus* Harms. or *Eleutherococcus senticosus* Maxim) is sometimes used in herbal medicine for the same purposes as traditional ginseng. This plant contains related compounds and is described in more detail in its own monograph (see Eleutherococcus q.v.).

PHARMACOLOGY: From the earliest times it has been claimed that ginseng exerts a strengthening effect while also raising physical and mental capacity for work. These properties have been defined as an "adaptogenic effect" or a non-specific increase in resistance to the noxious effects of physical, chemical or biological stress.[12] Animal studies have shown that ginseng extracts can prolong swimming time, prevent stress-induced ulcers, stimulate the proliferation of hepatic ribosomes, increase natural killer cell activity and may enhance the production of interferons.[13] The steroidal panaxosides may alter the activity of hormones produced by the pituitary,[14] adrenal[15] or gonadal tissue.[16] However, a study in mice found no adaptogenic effects.[17]

Over the past 30 years, in vitro and animal screenings have identified a diverse array of pharmacologic effects. Ginseng exerts its effects when taken orally. These effects vary with dose, duration of treatment, and animal species and include CNS depression or stimulation, variable effects on systemic blood pressure, a papaverine-like action on smooth muscle, analgesic and anti-inflammatory activity.[18] Because most studies have used whole root preparations, there has likely been considerable variation among these preparations (uncertain species identification, age of the roots, curing process used, etc). Also, most of its properties appear to manifest only after prolonged use.[19]

Despite the shortcomings of many animal studies, a significant body of experience describes some of the pharmacologic effects of the panaxosides. For example, ginsenoside Rb-1 has CNS activity (depressant, anticonvulsant, analgesic, antipsychotic), protects against the development of stress ulcers and accelerates glycolysis and nuclear RNA synthesis. In one study, ginsenoside Rd promoted the incorporation of leucine into serum protein. Prolonged doses of mixed ginsenosides have decreased cholesterol and triglyceride levels in rats. Ginseng appears to potentiate the normal function of the adrenal gland, for some "anti-stress" activity.

A number of generally small and poorly designed trials in man have been reported from eastern Europe and Asia.

These trials indicate that ginseng has a variety of beneficial effects; ie, it appears to reduce plasma glucose levels and increase the level of high density cholesterol. Five glycans with strong hypoglycemic activity have been isolated from the root.[20,21] Ginsenoside Rg-1 given to post-operative gynecologic patients caused a greater increase in hemoglobin and hematocrit levels among treated women than in placebo-treated controls. Serum protein and body weight also increased to a greater degree in the treated patients. The adaptogenic effect has not been well documented in humans, although there is a strong body of evidence from traditional medicine.

TOXICOLOGY: Through its extensive history of use in popular herbal products, ginseng has established a remarkable record of safety. It is estimated that more than 6 million people ingest ginseng regularly in the USA alone. Nevertheless, there have been a few reports of severe reactions. One controversial report described a "ginseng abuse syndrome" among 133 patients who took relatively large doses of the root (more than 3 g/day) for up to 2 years.[22] Patients reported a feeling of stimulation, well being and increased motor and cognitive efficiency, but also often noted diarrhea, skin eruptions, nervousness, sleeplessness and hypertension. This was an open study and the intake of concomitant drugs (eg, caffeine) confounded interpretation of the data.

Several other reports have implicated ginseng as having an estrogen-like effect in women.[23] One case of diffuse mammary nodularity has been reported,[24] as has been a case of vaginal bleeding in a 72-year-old woman.[25]

The most commonly reported side effects of ginseng are nervousness and excitation, which usually diminish after the first few days of use or with dosage reduction. Inability to concentrate has also been reported following long term use.[26]

The hypoglycemic effect of the whole root and individual panaxosides has been reported by many investigators. Although no cases of serious reactions in diabetic patients have been reported, those who must control their blood glucose levels should take ginseng with caution.

SUMMARY: Ginseng is one of the oldest and most widely recognized herbal products. At least six species and varieties of *Panax* have been used in traditional medicine. Today, ginseng is a popular ingredient in herbal teas and cosmetics. It is available in a variety of dosage forms and is promoted for its "anti-stress" effects. Numerous animal studies have confirmed this "adaptogenic effect" and preliminary clinical evidence also indicates this effect is demonstrable in man. However, establishing the proper dose and duration of use remains poorly defined. Ginseng is not usually associated with serious adverse reactions, although a potential "ginseng abuse syndrome" has been reported.

Those wishing to obtain additional information about ginseng may contact:

Ginseng Research Institute of America
Attn: Robert Duwe, President
500 Third Street, Suite 208-2
Wausau, WI 54401
(715) 845-7300

PATIENT INFORMATION – Ginseng

Uses: Ginseng is widely used in various ingestible forms and in cosmetics. Research evidence lends some support to its virtue as an antistress treatment. It seems to lower cholesterol and blood sugar, resist infection and have an estrogen-like effect on women. Among its other reputed benefits, it is credited with increasing strength, endurance and mental acuity. Ginseng may depress or stimulate the CNS.

Side Effects: Nervous excitation induced by ginseng use reportedly diminishes with acclimation or dose adjustment. Difficulty concentrating has been reported following long use. Diabetics should use ginseng with caution because of the hypoglycemic effects.

---

[1] Lewis WH. *JAMA* 1980;243:31.
[2] Garriques S. *Ann Chem Pharm* 1854;90:231.
[3] Brekhman II, Dardymov IV. *Lloydia* 1969;32:46.
[4] Sandberg F. *Planta Medica* 1973;24:392.
[5] Kim SK, et al. *Planta Medica* 1981;42:181.
[6] Lui JHC, Staba EJ. *J Nat Prod* 1980;43:340.
[7] Gstirner F, Vogt HJ. *Arch Pharmazie* 1967;300:371.
[8] Liberti LE, DerMarderosian AH. *J Pharm Sci* 1978;67:1487.
[9] Lui JHC, Staba EJ. *J Nat Prod* 1980;43:340.
[10] Reis CA, Sahud MA. *JAMA* 1975;231:352.
[11] *Medical Letter* 1979;21:29.
[12] Brekhman II, Dardymov IV. *Lloydia* 1969;32:46.
[13] Singh VK, et al. *Planta Medica* 1984;50:462.
[14] Fulder SJ. *Am J Chinese Med* 1981;9:112.

[15] Hiai S, et al. *Endocrinol Jap* 1979;26:737.
[16] Fahim MS, et al. *Arch Androl* 1982;8:261.
[17] Lewis WH, et al. *J Ethnopharm* 1983;8:209.
[18] Chong SKF, et al. *Lancet* 1982;2:663.
[19] DerMarderosian AH, Liberti LE. *Natural Product Medicine*, Philadelphia: G.F. Stickley Co, 1988.
[20] Konno C, et al. *Planta Medica* 1984;50:434.
[21] Masashi T, et al. *Planta Medica* 1984;50:436.
[22] Siegal RK. *JAMA* 1979;241:1614.
[23] Punnonen R, Lukola A. *Br Med J* 1980;281:1110.
[24] Palmer BV, et al. *Br Med J* 19781:1284.
[25] Greenspan EM. *JAMA* 1983;249:2018.
[26] Hammond TG, Whitworth JA. *Med J Aust* 1981;1:492.

Glucomannan

SCIENTIFIC NAME(S): *Amorphophallus konjac* Koch. Family: Araceae

COMMON NAME(S): Konjac, Konjac mannan, glucomannan

SOURCE: Konjac mannan is a polysaccharide derived from the tubers of konjac. It is purified from konjac flour by repeated treatment with cupric hydroxide and subsequent washings with ethanol[1] or by dialysis against water (US patents 3, 973,008 [Aug 3, 1976] and 3, 856, 945 [Dec 24, 1974]).

CHEMISTRY: Glucomannan is composed of glucose and mannose combined by beta-1,4 glucosidic linkages in a molecular ratio of 1:1.6 and is often referred to as glucomannan. The polysaccharide is easily "denatured" through enzymatic cleavage or treatment with weak alkaline solutions, becoming irreversibly water insoluble. In Japan, this coagulated product is called "konnyaku" and is commonly used as a foodstuff.

PHARMACOLOGY: Polysaccharides such as guar gum (composed of galactose and mannose; galactomannan), tragacanth, cellulose, methylcellulose, pectin, and wheat bran have found use as foodstuffs and, more recently, as dietary and therapeutic agents. Their ability to swell by the absorption of water has made them useful as laxatives. Konjac mannan has been reported to alleviate moderate constipation in 1 to 2 days and reduces fecal flora by a factor of 1000 in 10 days. Research on microflora in mice and rats suggests that a diet that includes konjac mannan alters the microbial metabolism in the intestine.[2] The study noted that in animals bearing human microflora, the differences in microbial composition were only slight despite the metabolic differences observed.

By increasing the viscosity of the intestinal contents, slowing gastric emptying time, and acting as a barrier to diffusion, agents such as guar gum have been shown to delay the absorption of glucose from the intestines.[3] Several small studies have shown that diabetics fed a diet consisting largely of raw vegetables, uncooked seeds, fruits and goat's milk, were able to reduce or discontinue their insulin requirements.[4] Similarly, konjac mannan has been reported to reduce the need for hypoglycemic agents. When 13 diabetic patients received 3.6 or 7.2 g of konjac mannan daily for 90 days, their mean fasting glucose levels fell by 29% and insulin or hypoglycemic agent doses were reduced in most patients.[5] Five healthy men enrolled in the same study underwent a glucose tolerance test with or without a single dose of 2.6 g konjac mannan. The polysaccharide reduced mean blood glucose levels by 7.3% at 30 minutes with a concomitant decrease in serum insulin concentration. Another study of 72 type II diabetic patients showed a significant reduction in fasting blood glucose and postprandial blood glucose after consuming konjac food 30 and 65 days.[6]

Konjac mannan is gaining popularity as a weight-reducing agent and is often included in "grapefruit diet" tablets. One U.S. patent claims that its use resulted in weight loss without appetite changes; however, no weights were reported. Some research has indicated that patients treated with oral glucomannan have decreased body weight compared with control groups. In one study involving an 8–week cardiac rehabilitation program, patients were given 1.5 grams of glucomannan twice daily.[7] Body weight among treated patients decreased by 1.5 kg at the end of 4 weeks and by 2.2 kg at the end of 8 weeks. These losses were significant when compared with the placebo group. In contrast, other research conducted with overweight children has found no significant difference in weight loss between children treated with 1 g glucomannan twice daily and those given a placebo.[8]

Hydrophilic gums have found some use as diet aids based on the theory that the feeling of fullness provided by their swelling leads to a decrease in appetite. Such agents are generally considered to be only marginally effective.

Konjac mannan has been shown to reduce plasma cholesterol levels in rats.[9] Interestingly, only water-soluble konjac mannan retains this effect. The hypocholesteremic effect is completely eliminated when the mannan is coagulated to a water-insoluble form. Rats fed high cholesterol diets containing 3% crude konjac mannan for 7 days exhibited plasma cholesterol levels 16% lower than control rats fed only the high cholesterol diet. Rats fed highly purified konjac mannan had plasma cholesterol levels 23% lower than the controls. Rats treated with konjac mannan that had been coagulated with cellulase had mean cholesterol levels greater than the controls. The implication is that the foodstuff konnyaku (coagulated water-insoluble product) most likely has no cholesterol-reducing activity.

In a study of 10 overweight patients, the daily administration of 100 ml of 1% solution of konjac mannan for 11 weeks resulted in decreases in serum cholesterol levels of 0% to 39% (mean, 18%) (US patent 3,973,008). In a separate double-blind crossover trial involving 63 men, total cholesterol was reduced by 10% among subjects given a daily dose of 3.9 g of konjac glucomannan for a 4–week period.[10] Interestingly, no significant change in high-density lipoprotein (HDL) cholesterol was observed as a result of the treatment. The diabetic patients treated in another study[5] showed a reduction in mean serum cholesterol levels of 11% after 20 days of konjac mannan treatment. Several other studies confirm the effects of konjac mannan on lipid metabolism.[11,12,13]

The activity of this polysaccharide cannot be explained by a simple interaction with bile acids since konjac mannan shows no in vitro or in vivo bile-binding activity. Rather, it appears to inhibit the active transport of cholesterol in the jejunum and the absorption of bile acids in the ileum.[14] A study on bile output in rats fed a diet of 5% konjac mannan showed an increase in the volume of bile juice secreted and the release of bile acids, protease and amylase compared to animals fed a control diet without fiber.[15] This effect was only observed for prolonged feeding of the experimental diet with konjac mannan and could not be produced with a single dose.

A Chinese study has investigated the ability of konjac powder to inhibit lung cancers in mice.[16] Mice fed a diet of 8% Konjaku powder, mixed in with a common diet, showed a reduction in cancer rate from 70.87% in the positive control group to 19.38% in the group fed with konjac powder. Lung tumors were induced with MNNG. The study reported no adverse reactions to the konjaku powder.[16]

TOXICOLOGY: Four cases of severe esophageal obstruction due to glucomannan diet tablets have been reported.[17,18] Seven additional cases were noted during 1984/85 by the Australian Adverse Drug Reactions Advisory Committee.[19] Glucomannan-containing tablets have been banned in Australia since May 1985 because these also carry the potential for inducing lower gastrointestinal obstruction. Encapsulated and powder forms remain available.

Glucomannan use is associated with a reduction in the need for hypoglycemic agents, and the product may result in a loss of glycemic control in diabetic patients. It should be used with great care by diabetic patients.

SUMMARY: Konjac mannan (glucomannan) has been shown to possess many of the pharmacologic characteristics of other polysaccharides. In large doses it has laxative activity and may alter the metabolism of microflora in the intestine. It should be used with care by diabetics, in whom its use may result in altered insulin or hypoglycemic requirements. Konjac mannan may be effective in reducing serum cholesterol levels in man and animals. There is conflicting evidence regarding its use as a weight-reduction aid though it does appear to alter lipid metabolism.

PATIENT INFORMATION – Glucomannan

Uses: Glucomannan reportedly alleviates constipation, reduces intestinal flora, lowers blood sugar and cholesterol and may possibly promote weight loss and inhibit cancer.

Side Effects: Severe esophageal and GI obstruction have been reported due to glucomannan tablets. The hypoglycemic effects are potentially dangerous to diabetics.

---

[1] Kiriyama S, et al. *J Nutr* 1972;102(12):1689.
[2] Fujiwara S, et al. *Food Chem Toxicol* 1991;29(9):601.
[3] Jenkins DJ, et al. *Br Med J* 1978;1(6124):1392.
[4] Anonymous. *Med Letter* 1979;21(12):51.
[5] Doi K, et al. *Lancet* 1979;1(May 5):987.
[6] Huang CY, et al. *Biomed Environ Sci* 1990;3(2):123.
[7] Reffo GC, et al. *Curr Ther Res* 1990;47(May):753.
[8] Vido L, et al. *Padiatr Padol* 1993;28(5):133.
[9] Kiriyama S, et al. *J Nutr* 1969;97(3):382.
[10] Arvill A, Bodin L. *Am J Clin Nutr* 1995;61(3):585.

[11] Zhang MY, et al. *Biomed Environ Sci* 1990;3(1):99.
[12] Hou YH, et al. *Biomed Environ Sci* 1990;3(3):306.
[13] Shimizu H, et al. *J Pharmacobiodyn* 1991;14(7):371.
[14] Kiriyama S, et al. *J Nutr* 1974;104(1):69.
[15] Ikegami S, et al. *J Nutr Sci Vitaminol* 1984;30(6):515.
[16] Luo DY. *Chung-Hua Chung Liu Tsa Chih [Chin J Oncol]* 1992;14(1):48.
[17] Fung M. *Med J Austr* 1984;140(6):350.
[18] Gaudry P. *Med J Austr* 1985;142(3):204.
[19] Henry DA, et al. *Br Med J* 1986;292(6520):591.

Glucosamine

SCIENTIFIC NAME(S): 2–Amino-2–deoxyglucose

COMMON NAME(S): Chitosamine

BIOLOGY: Glucosamine is found in mucopolysaccharides, mucoproteins and chitin. Chitin is found in yeasts, fungi, arthropods and various marine invertebrates as a major component of the exoskeleton. It also occurs in other lower animals and members of the plant kingdom.[1]

CHEMISTRY: Chemically, chitin is a biopolymer which is cellulose-like, but differs in that it is made up of predominantly unbranched chains of beta (1–4)-2–acetamido-2–deoxy-D-glucose or N-acetyl-D-glucosamine residues. Basically, it can be perceived as a cellulose derivative where the C-2 hydroxyl groups of the polymer have been replaced by acetamido moieties. Glucosamine is isolated from chitin and is chemically 2–amino-2–deoxyglucose.[2] It can also be prepared synthetically. Glucosamine sulfate is the preferred form. N-acetyl-D-glucosamine (NAG) is also sold but has no advantages over glucosamine.[3]

PHARMACOLOGY: Chitin has been described as a vulnerary or wound-healing polymer,[2] while glucosamine has been referred to as a **pharmaceutical aid** and **antiarthritic**.[1] In osteoarthritis (the most common form of arthritis) there is a progressive degeneration of cartilage glycosaminoglycans (GAG). The idea of using glucosamine orally is to provide a "building block" for its regeneration. Glucosamine is the rate-limiting step in GAG biosynthesis. It is biochemically formed from the glycolytic intermediate fructose-6–phosphate by way of amination of glutamine as the donor, ultimately yielding glucosamine-6–phosphate. This is subsequently converted and/or acetylated to galactosamine before being incorporated into growing GAG. Hopefully, this will stimulate the production of cartilage components and bring about joint repair.[3] Several double-blind studies indicate that glucosamine sulfate may be better than some non-steroidal anti-inflammatory drugs (NSAIDs) and placebos in relieving both pain and inflammation due to osteoarthritis.[3–5] The efficacy and safety of intramuscular glucosamine sulfate in osteoarthritis of the knee was studied in a randomized, placebo controlled double-blind study and revealed that the treatment was well tolerated and effective.[4] Other double-blind clinical studies of intra-articular glucosamine were conducted and resulted in reduced pain, increased angle of joint flexion and restored articular function compared with placebo.[5] The

relative efficacy of ibuprofen and glucosamine sulfate was compared in the management of osteoarthritis of the knee.[6] At 8 weeks, glucosamine was more effective in reducing pain (1.5 g daily dose orally). Oral glucosamine sulfate therapy vs placebo in osteoarthritis were studied and researchers found (80 patients, 1.5 g daily dose orally) decreased symptoms and improved autonomous motility with glucosamine.[7] These investigators also employed electron microscopy studies on cartilage and found that patients who had placebo showed a typical picture of established osteoarthrosis while those on glucosamine showed a picture similar to healthy cartilage. They concluded that glucosamine tends to rebuild damaged cartilage, thus restoring articular function in most chronic arthrosic patients.

At least 15 other studies showed that glucosamine can be safe and effective in the treatment of various forms of osteoarthritis. At least one researcher has decried the fact that physicians in the US have totally ignored this rational and safe therapeutic strategy. Standard drug therapy is only of palliative benefit and may worsen loss of cartilage. Glucosamine is an intermediate in mucopolysaccharide synthesis, and its availability in cartilage tissue culture can be rate-limiting for proteoglycan production. Reviews of related literature also demonstrate glucosamine's effectiveness in decreasing pain and improving mobility in osteoarthritis without side effects. Further, by mechanisms still unknown, the natural methyl donor 5–adenosylmethionine also promotes production of cartilage proteoglycans and is likewise therapeutically beneficial in osteoarthritis in well-tolerated oral doses. One researcher promotes the use of glucosamine and other safe nutritional measures supporting proteoglycan synthesis because these may offer a practical method of preventing or postponing the onset of osteoarthritis in athletes and older people.[8]

Other studies on glucosamine show its pharmacokinetics in dog and man (radiolabeled glucosamine was quickly and completely absorbed either orally or by IV);[9] attempt to synthesize derivatives of glucosamine which have immunomodulating activity;[10] demonstrate the ability of glucosamine to inhibit the development of viral cytopathic effects and the production of infective viral particles,[11] and show the inhibitory effects of D-glucosamine on a carcinoma and protein, RNA and DNA synthesis.[12]

TOXICOLOGY: No direct toxic effects of glucosamine could be found in the scientific literature, however, one report shows potential bronchopulmonary complications of antirheumatic drugs including glucosamine.[13]

SUMMARY: Glucosamine appears to be a safe and effective approach to the management of various categories of osteoarthritis. Further studies are warranted on various dosage regimens (IV, oral, etc) and potential long-term effects.

PATIENT INFORMATION – Glucosamine

Uses: Glucosamine is being investigated extensively as an antiarthritic in osteoarthritis.

Side Effects: Well-tolerated. No side effects have been directly associated with glucosamine.

---

[1] Budavari S, ed. *The Merck Index* ; 11th edition, Merck & Co., Inc., N.J. 1989;4353.
[2] Budavari S, ed. *The Merck Index* ; 11th edition, Merck & Co., Inc., N.J. 1989;2049.
[3] Anonymous. *Am J Natl Med* 1994;1(1):10–14.
[4] Reichelt A, et al. *Arzneimittel-Forschung* 1994;44(1):75–80.
[5] Vajaradul Y. *Clin Ther* 1981;3(5):336–43.
[6] Vaz A. *Current Med Res Op* 1982;8(3):145–9.

[7] Drovanti A, et al. *Clin Ther* 1980;3(4):260–72.
[8] McCarty M. *Med Hyp* 1994;42(5):323–37.
[9] Setnikar I, et al. *Arzneimittel-Forschung* (Apr):1986;36:729–35.
[10] Valcavi U, et al. *Arzneimittel-Forschung* 1989;39(10):190–5.
[11] Delgadillo R, et al. *J Pharm Pharmacol* (Jul):1988;40:488–93.
[12] Bekesi J, et al. *Can Res* (Dec.)1970;30:2905–912.
[13] Larget-Piet B, et al. *Ther* 1986;41(4):269–77.

Goldenseal

SCIENTIFIC NAME(S): *Hydrastis canadensis* L. Family: Ranunculaceae

COMMON NAME(S): Goldenseal, yellowroot, orangeroot, eyebalm, eyeroot, goldenroot, ground raspberry, Indian turmeric, yellow puccoon, jaundice root, sceau d'or

BOTANY: Goldenseal is a perennial herb found in the rich woods of the Ohio River valley and other locations in the northeastern US. The single, green-white flower, which has no petals, appears in the spring on a hairy stem above a basal leaf and 2 palmate, wrinkled leaves. The flower develops into a red seeded berry. The plant grows from horizontal, bright yellow rhizomes, which have a twisted, knotty appearance.

HISTORY: Goldenseal root was used medicinally by American Indians of the Cherokee, Catawba, Iroquois, and Kickapoo tribes as an insect repellent, a diuretic, a stimulant, and a wash for sore or inflamed eyes.[1] It was used to treat arrow wounds and ulcers,[2] as well as to produce a yellow dye. Early settlers learned of these uses from the Indians and the root found its way into most 19th century pharmacopeias. The Eclectic medical movement was particularly enthusiastic in its adoption of goldenseal for gonorrhea and urinary tract infections. The widespread harvesting of *Hydrastis* in the 19th century, coupled with loss of habitat, resulted in depletion of wild populations. In 1997, *Hydrastis* was listed under Appendix II of the Convention on International Trade in Endangered Species of Wild Fauna and Flora (CITES), which controls exports of the root to other countries. The final listing included roots or live plants but excluded finished products. As an alternative to wild harvesting, goldenseal was cultivated in the Skagit Valley of Washington state and is being promoted as a cash crop in New York, North Carolina,[3] and Canada. Because of its high price, goldenseal, like other expensive herbs, has often been adulterated. Common adulterants include species of Coptis and *Xanthorrhiza,*[4] both of which also contain large amounts of the yellow alkaloid berberine. The popular notion that goldenseal can be used to affect the outcome of urinalysis for illicit drugs evolved from the novel *Stringtown on the Pike* by pharmacist John Uri Lloyd, in which goldenseal bitters are mistaken for strychnine in a simple alkaloid test by an expert witness in a murder trial.[5] Goldenseal can be variously ingested prior to testing or added to the urine sample after collection. It is one of several adulterants commonly detected in urinalysis samples.[6]

CHEMISTRY: The isoquinoline alkaloids hydrastine (4%), berberine (up to 6%), and canadine are present in goldenseal root and are viewed as the principle bioactive components.[7] Other minor alkaloids such as canadaline.[8] and canadinic acid[9] have been isolated. Quinic acid esters were elucidated.[10] Quantitation of the alkaloids has been accomplished in a variety of ways including spectrophotometry,[11] thin-layer chromatography,[12] ion-pair dye colorimetry,[13] high-performance liquid chromatography (HPLC),[14] capillary electrophoresis,[15] and CE-mass spectrometry.[16]

PHARMACOLOGY: While berberine is widely distributed in plants, hydrastine is characteristic of goldenseal root and is considered to be the most important bioactive alkaloid. There is extensive pharmacologic literature on hydrastine and berberine. The alkaloids are poorly absorbed when taken orally, so studies of parenterally administered goldenseal alkaloids must be interpreted with care. Goldenseal alkaloids have modest antimicrobial activity, which may be relevant when applied topically. Berberine, canadine, and canadaline had disinfectant activity against 6 strains of bacteria, while hydrastine was inactive.[17] Berberine sulfate was bactericidal against *Vibrio cholerae* but bacteriostatic to *Staphylococcus aureus*.[18] Berberine sulfate has been shown to block adherence of *Streptococcus pyogenes* to epithelial cells, which may be a reasonable mode of action for topical antimicrobial use.[19] Berberine has been identified as the active component of *Hydrastis* in an antitubercular assay.[10] while hydrastine and other isolated compounds had no activity. Berberine has been reported to inhibit uptake of glucose by cancer cells,[20] and to inhibit tumor promotion by phorbol esters in a mouse skin carcinogenesis model.[21] Berberine showed weak activity in an antioxidant model.[22] Palmery investigated the inhibitory activity of *Hydrastis* alkaloids on isolated rabbit aorta stimulated by epinephrine, finding a weak synergistic effect for berberine, canadine, and canadaline, but no activity in hydrastine.[23] In isolated guinea pig ileum preparations, the same group found that berberine, canadine, and canadaline evoked contractions, while hydrastine again was inactive.[24] A third study found a relaxant effect of berberine on rabbit prostate strips stimulated by norepinephrine or phenylephrine,[25] however, an adrenergic mechanism was considered unlikely. While hydrastine is closely related to the convulsant isoquinoline alkaloid bicuculline, hydrastine had no activity in a GABA-receptor binding assay at high concentrations.[26]

Very high doses of goldenseal may rarely induce nausea, anxiety, depression, seizures, or paralysis. Hydrastine was once used as a uterine hemostatic[7] but was found inferior to ergot in the treatment of postpartum hemorrhage. Goldenseal is generally contraindicated for use in pregnancy. Because of hypertensive actions of the alkaloids, it is also contraindicated in cardiovascular patients.

SUMMARY: A *Hydrastis* monograph is under preparation by the American Herbal Pharmacopeia. *Hydrastis* was official in the US Phamacopeia from 1860 to 1926, and in the National Formulary from 1936 to 1955.

Goldenseal's popularity is out of proportion to its scientifically documented worth. It may be of use in topical infections and is still used as an eyewash. While contraindicated in pregnancy and hypertension, adverse effects to usual doses are rare.

PATIENT INFORMATION – Goldenseal

Uses: Goldenseal may be of use in topical infections and is used as an eyewash. Goldenseal has been included in cold and flu preparations for its anticatarrhal effects but little evidence supports this use and its effects are debatable.

Side Effects: Goldenseal is contraindicated in pregnancy and hypertension; adverse effects to usual doses are rare.

---

[1] Hobbs C. Goldenseal in early American medical botany. *Pharmacy in History* 1990;32:79.

[2] Bolyard J. *Medicinal Plants and Home Remedies of Appalachia.* Springfield, IL: Charles C. Thomas,1981.

[3] Davis J. *Advances in goldenseal cultivation.* North Carolina Cooperative Extension Service, Horticultural Information Leaflet No. 131, 1996.

[4] Blaque G, et al. Les falsifications actuelles de l' "*Hydrastis canadensis.*" *Bull Sci Phar* 1926;33:375.

[5] Foster S. Goldenseal. *Hydrastis canadensis. Botanical Series,* No. 309, 2nd ed. Austin, TX: American Botanical Council, 1996.

[6] Mikkelsen S, et al. Adulterants causing false negatives in illicit drug testing. *Clin Chem* 1988;34:2333-36.

[7] Genest K. Natural products in Canadian pharmaceuticals. IV. *Hydrastis canadensis. Can J Pharm Sci* 1969;4:41-45.

[8] Gleye J, et al. La canadine: nouvel alcloide d'*Hydrastis canadensis. Phytochemistry* 1974;13:675-76.

[9] Galeffi C, et al. Canadinic acid: An alkaloid from *Hydrastis canadensis. Planta Med* 1997;63:194.

[10] Gentry E, et al. Antitubercular natural products: berberine from the roots of commercial *Hydrastis canadensis* powder. Isolation of inactive 8-oxotetrahydrothalifendine, canadine, beta-hydrastine, and two new quinic acid esters, hycandinic acid esters-1 and -2. *J Nat Prod* 1998;61:1187-93.

[11] Caille G, et al. Dosage spectrophotofluormetrique des alcaloides berberine, tetrahydroberberine, hydrastine et application a l'extrait sec et a la teinture d'*Hydrastis canadensis* L. *Can J Pharm Sci* 1970;5:55.

[12] Datta D, et al. Thin layer chromatography and UV spectrophotometry of alcoholic extracts of *Hydrastis canadensis. Planta Med* 1971;19:258-63.

[13] El-Masry S, et al. Colorimetric and spectrophotometric determinations of *Hydrastis* alkaloids in pharmaceutical preparations. *J Pharm Sci* 1980;69:597-98.

[14] Leone M, et al. HPLC determination of the major alkaloids extracted from *Hydrastis canadensis* L. *Phytother Res* 1996;10:S45-46.

[15] Unger M, et al. Improved detection of alkaloids in crude extracts applying capillary electrophoresis with field amplified sample injection. *J Chromatogr A* 1997;791:323-331.

[16] Sturm S, et al. Analysis of isoquinoline alkaloids in medicinal plants by capillary electrophoresis-mass spectrometry. *Electrophoresis* 1998;19:3026-32.

[17] Scazzocchio F, et al. Antimicrobial activity of *Hydrastis canadensis* extract and its major isolated alkaloids. *Fitoterapia* 1998;64:58.

[18] Amin A, et al. Berberine sulfate: antimicrobial activity, bioassay, and mode of action. *Can J Microbiol* 1969;15:1067-76.

[19] Sun D, et al. Berberine sulfate blocks adherence of *Streptococcus pyogenes* to epithelial cells, fibronectin, and hexadecane. *Antimicrobial Agents Chemother* 1988;32:1370-74.

[20] Creasey W. Biochemical effects of berberine. *Biochem Pharmacol* 1979;28:1081-84.

[21] Nishino H, et al. Berberine sulfate inhibits tumor-promoting activity of teleocidin in two-stage carcinogenesis on mouse skin. *Oncology* 1986;43:131-34.

[22] Misík V, et al. Lipoxygenase inhibition and antioxidant properties of protoberberine and aporphine alkaloids isolated from *Mahonia aquifolium. Planta Med* 1995;61:372-73.

[23] Palmery M, et al. Further studies of the adrenolytic activity of the major alkaloids from *Hydrastis canadensis* L. on isolated rabbit aorta. *Phytother Res* 1996;10:S47-49.

[24] Cometa M, et al. Acute effect of alkaloids from *Hydrastis canadensis* L. on guinea pig ileum: structure-activity relationships. *Phytother Res* 1996;10:S56-58.

[25] Baldazzi C, et al. Effects of the major alkaloid of *Hydrastis canadensis* L., berberine, on rabbit prostate strips. *Phytother Res* 1998;12:589-91.

[26] Kardos J, et al. Inhibition of [3H] GABA binding to rat brain synaptic membranes by bicuculline related alkaloids. *Biochem Pharmacol* 1984;33:3537-45.

Gossypol

SCIENTIFIC NAME(S): Gossypol is commonly derived from members of the family Malvaceae. Cotton (*Gossypium* spp.) represents the most common source.

HISTORY: Gossypol was first identified as an antifertility agent as a result of epidemiologic studies conducted in China during the 1950s. Investigators had been puzzled by the extremely low birth rates in a particular geographic region. The men had very low sperm counts and many women had amenorrhea. Eventually the phenomenon was related to the exclusive use of crude cottonseed oil for cooking. Further investigation revealed that the anti-fertility component was gossypol, a potentially toxic phenolic pigment found in the seed, stem and root of the cotton plant.[1]

CHEMISTRY: Gossypol is a natural product that can be made synthetically[2] or produced inexpensively on a very large scale by the extraction of cottonseed. Estimates have placed US gossypol production at more than 50,000 tons per year, all as a by-product of cottonseed oil production.[3] Cotton represents perhaps the most well-known source of this compound. The seeds of species of *Gossypium* vary widely in their gossypol content with levels ranging from 0.13% to 6.6%.[2]

PHARMACOLOGY: Gossypol has been shown to be an active antifertility agent in male hamsters and rats.[4] Large-scale clinical trials in men by Chinese investigators have found gossypol to be orally active and relatively safe and effective. Gossypol is a nonsteroidal compound that acts by inhibiting sperm production and motility in a variety of male animal species and humans. It does not affect sex hormone levels or libido, and its mechanism is somewhat distinct from that of steroidal oral contraceptives used by women.

Gossypol exerts its contraceptive action by inhibiting an enzyme that plays a crucial role in energy metabolism in sperm and spermatogenic cells. The target enzyme, lactate dehydrogenase X, is found only in sperm and male gonadal cells. It is involved in glycolysis and plays a role in inducing mitochondria to produce energy. A variety of lactate dehydrogenases are found throughout the body and gossypol exerts a degree of inhibition on many of these. However, the drug exhibits its greatest inhibitory effect on lactate dehydrogenase X.

Sperm recovered from the epididymis of rats and hamsters treated with gossypol for as little as 6 weeks were immotile with detached heads or tails.[5] Gossypol does not demonstrate estrogenic or androgenic activity but does potentiate the androgenicity of methyltestosterone.[6]

Male contraception: The clinical testing of gossypol began in the early 1970s in China, and to date the drug has been studied extensively in thousands of men. The usual daily dose is 20 mg until the sperm count is reduced below 4 million/ml; this usually requires 2 to 3 months of treatment. Maintenance doses of 75 to 100 mg are subsequently taken twice a month. A proposed contraceptive dose is 3 g/man/year.

Wu.[7] published a comprehensive review of the clinical trials of gossypol. Clinical trials have found the drug's antifertility effect to be more than 99%. Sperm counts usually return to normal within 3 months after termination of therapy, and men treated with gossypol have fathered normal children. However, long-term follow-up studies indicate that inhibition of spermatogenesis may continue following discontinuation in up to 20% of men after 2 years. Spermatogenesis does not return to normal in some men. Concerns regarding the lack of predictable reversible effects have delayed the further clinical development of gossypol in western countries.

Female contraception: Although gossypol is generally considered to be a male antifertility agent, it is effective when given to female animals. The intramuscular injection of gossypol to female rats inhibited implantation and the maintenance of normal pregnancy, most likely by affecting luteinizing hormone levels.[8] Gossypol is also an inhibitor of platelet activating factor and leukotrienes.[9]

Gossypol has also shown effects that suggest some inhibition of ovarian function and cytotoxicity in endometrial cells.[10]

Gossypol has been evaluated as a topical spermicide. Solutions of gossypol or gossypol acetate do not decrease sperm motility. However, a solution of gossypol-PVP coprecipitate completely immobilized all spermatozoa within 3 minutes at a concentration of 5 mg/ml and within 20 seconds at 40 mg/ml. The spermicidal activity of gossypol was found to be equal to or greater than that of the commercially available creams *Delfin* and *Preceptin* and *Encare Oval* vaginal suppositories.[11] A gelatin coprecipitate of gossypol is an effective spermicide in monkeys.[12] A gossypol-containing gel decreased the number and rapidly immobilized sperm when tested in healthy women.[13] The topical use of gossypol has been recommended because it has low systemic toxicity, it acts in micromolar concentrations and is effective in the presence of cervical mucus.[14]

Other clinical uses: Gossypol has been investigated for the treatment of uterine myoma, endometriosis and dysfunctional uterine bleeding. Gossypol and its derivatives are active against the HIV virus[15] and the herpes simplex virus type 2.[16] A trial is now under way to evaluate the therapeutic efficacy of gossypol for the treatment of metastatic carcinoma of the endometrium or ovary, and as an antiviral and interferon inducer in patients with AIDS.[7]

TOXICOLOGY: Commercial cotton seed oil is processed in order to remove its gossypol content.

A low incidence of side effects was originally reported in men treated with gossypol. Some men develop a transient weakness during the first days of administration and this appears to be related to hypokalemia induced by gossypol. This may be caused by renal loss of potassium during therapy and can be managed effectively with oral potassium supplementation. Some men notice changes in appetite. Gossypol also inhibits malate dehydrogenase in animals and glutathione-S-transferase in both animals and man. This latter enzyme is involved in the detoxification of potentially toxic and carcinogenic compounds. At high doses (100 to 700 times the contraceptive dose)

gossypol may cause diarrhea, hair discoloration, malnutrition, circulatory problems and heart failure. The compound has not been found to be mutagenic when tested in the Ames salmonella microsome test,[17] but questions still remain about is genotoxic characteristics.[18]

The results of more recent well-controlled studies found that the incidence of adverse events was significantly high as to warrant abandoning the development of gossypol as a male contraceptive.[19]

Gossypol is found in two isomeric forms. Only (-) gossypol shows antispermatogenic effects in animals; the (+) form appears to be associated with hypokalemia. Therefore, administration of a purified (-) form may provide efficacy while reducing certain side effects.

Gossypol toxicity is a potential veterinary problem and as little as 200 ppm of free gossypol could kill a calf.[18] Non-ruminant animals are more sensitive to the toxic effects of gossypol than ruminants.[21]

SUMMARY: Gossypol is a toxic component contained in cottonseed. This compound has been shown to be an orally effective male contraceptive. Although it has been used widely in China, its development has not been pursued in the West primarily because its inhibitory effects on spermatogenesis are not predictably reversible. A reduction in dosage may be associated with a lower incidence of permanent sterility. The drug is effective when used as a topical spermicidal cream or gel.

PATIENT INFORMATION – Gossypol

Uses: Gossypol acts as a male and female contraceptive. It may be a treatment for certain gynecological problems and viral infections.

Side Effects: It is potentially toxic. Contraceptive effects may not be reversible.

---

[1] Maugh TH. *Science* 1981;212:314.
[2] Adams R, et al. *Chem Rev* 1960;60:555.
[3] Rawls R. *Chem Eng News* 1981;59:36.
[4] Waller DP, et al. *Contraception* 1981;23:653.
[5] Chang MC. *Contraception* 1980;21:461.
[6] Hahn DW, et al. *Contraception* 1981;24:97.
[7] Wu. *Drugs* 1989;38:333.
[8] Lin YC, et al. *Life Sciences* 1985;37:39.
[9] Touvay C, et al. *J Pharm Pharmacol* 1987;39:454.
[10] Peng-di Z, et al. *Am J Obstet Gyn* 1984;149:780.
[11] Waller DP, et al. *Contraception* 1980;22:183.
[12] Cameron SM, et al. *Fertil Steril* 1982;37:273.
[13] Ratsula K, et al. *Contraception* 1983;27:571.
[14] Poso, et al. *Lancet* 1980;i:885.
[15] Prusoff W, et al. *Pharmacol Ther* 1993;60:315–29.
[16] Wichmann K, et al. *Am J Obstet Gyn* 1982;142;593.
[17] dePeyster A, et al. *N Engl J Med* 1979;301:275.
[18] dePeyster A, et al. *Mutat Res* 1993;297:293.
[19] Comhaire FH. *Human Reprod* 1994;586.
[20] Morgan SE. *Vet Clin North Am Food Anim Pract* 1989;5:251.
[21] Rondel RD, et al. *J Anim Sci* 1992;70:1628.

Gotu Kola

SCIENTIFIC NAME(S): *Centella asiatica* (L.) Urb. Also: *Hydrocotyle asiatica* Family: Umbelliferae (Apiaceae).

COMMON NAME(S): Gotu kola, hydrocotyle, Indian pennywort, talepetrako

BOTANY: *Centella asiatica* is a slender, creeping plant that grows commonly in swampy areas of India, Sri Lanka, Madagascar, South Africa and the tropics.

HISTORY: Gotu kola has been widely used to treat a variety of illnesses, particularly in traditional Eastern medicine. Sri Lankans noticed that elephants, renowned for their longevity, munched on the leaves of the plant. Thus the leaves became known as a promoter of long life, with a suggested "dosage" of a few leaves each day. Among the ailments purported to be cured or controlled by gotu kola are mental problems, high blood pressure, abscesses, rheumatism, fever, ulcers, leprosy, skin eruptions, nervous disorders and jaundice. Gotu kola has been touted as an aphrodisiac. Gotu kola should not be confused with the dried seed of *Cola nitide* (Vent.) (also known as kolanuts, kola or cola), the plant used in cola beverages. *Cola nitida* contains caffeine and is a stimulant, while gotu kola has no caffeine and has sedative properties.[1]

CHEMISTRY: Extracts of gotu kola contain the active principle madecassol, as well as asiatic acid and the glycoside asiaticoside.[2] Also present is isothankuniside. This compound has been used to derive another substance called BK compound (methyl 5–hydroxy-3,6–dioxo-23 (or 24)-nor-urs-12–ene-28–oate).[3] Below-ground parts of *C. asiatica* have been found to contain small amounts of at least 14 different polyacetylenes. The molecular structures of five of these have been determined: (1) 2,9–pentadecadiene-4,6–diyn-1–ol, acetate; (2) pentadeca-1,9–diene-4,6–diyne-3,8–diol, 8–monoacetate; (3) pentadeca-1,9–diene-4,6–diyne-3,8 diol, diacetate; (4) pentadeca-1,8–diene-4,6–diyne-3,10–diol, 10–monoacetate and (5) pentadeca (1,8)-diene-4,6–diyne-3,10–diol. Nine other polyacetylenes have been partially characterized.[4]

A recent phytochemical of *C. asiatica* revealed the presence of amino acids, flavonols, fatty acids, alkaloids, sterols, saccharides and inorganic salts. The bio-stimulant activity is attributed to asiaticoside, asiatic acid and madecassic acid.[5] A study of powdered gotu kola by microscopic and chemical identification methods has also recently been done.[6]

PHARMACOLOGY:

Wound healing: *C. asiatica* extracts have been found to promote wound healing.[7] Cell culture experiments have shown that the total triterpenoid fraction of the extracts, at a concentration of 25 mcg/ml does not affect cell proliferation, total cell protein synthesis or the biosynthesis of proteoglycans in human skin fibroblasts. However, the fraction does significantly increase the collagen content of cell layer fibronectin, which may explain the action in wound healing.[8] The glycoside madecassoside has anti-inflammatory properties, while asiaticoside appears to stimulate wound healing. Experiments with rats showed that wounds heal by a process involving a dilation phase followed by a contraction phase. These phases were prolonged in rats undergoing repeated experimental wounding. Titrated extract of *C. asiatica* (TECA, 100 mg/kg), however, accelerated healing time.[7] A study employing rats and mice found that topically applied TECA rapidly penetrated to subcutaneous tissues and abdominal muscle in high concentrations, and had a greater effect on wound healing than oral administration. Asiatic acid was absorbed later than madecassic acid. The topical preparations of TECA were also able to penetrate to the plasma and deeper tissues.[9]

Other Topical Uses: TECA has been used as a scarring agent to stimulate wound healing in patients with chronic lesions such as cutaneous ulcers, surgical wounds, fistulas and gynecologic lesions. A clinical study evaluated TECA for treating bladder lesions in 102 patients with biharzial infections. Injections of TECA 2%, usually administered intramuscularly, for 1 to 3 months, produced cure or improvement in 75% of the cases, as determined from symptoms, urinary findings and cystoscopic findings. Healing occurred with little scar formation, thus avoiding much of the loss of bladder capacity that can result from biharzial infections.[10]

C. asiatica has also shown promise in treatment of psoriasis. When creams containing oil and water extracts of the leaves were administered each morning to seven psoriatic patients, five showed complete clearance of lesions within 3 to 7 weeks. One patient showed clearance of most lesions, and one showed improvement without clearance. One patient experienced a mild recurrence 4 months after treatment. Although this study was not controlled, a placebo effect was considered unlikely. Experience indicated that the creams were nontoxic and cosmetically acceptable, making them suitable for long-term use.[1]

Antifertility Effects: Crude extract of *C. asiatica* isothankuniside and BK compound were all found capable of significantly reducing the fertility of female Swiss albino mice when administered orally. The effective dosages were 20 to 80 mg of whole plant/kg body weight for the crude extract, 40 to 120 mg/kg for isothankuniside, and 5 mg/kg for BK compound. BK compound thus had the strongest effect.[3] Because this was only a preliminary screening study, the mechanism for this effect was not investigated.

Antihypertensive Effects: The efficacy of Centellase from *C. asiatica* in the treatment of venous hypertension has been evaluated, using a combined microcirculatory model.[11] The researchers conducted a single blind, placebo controlled randomized study of the effects of the total triterpenoid fraction (Centellase) in 89 patients with venous hypertension microangiopathy. The effects of Centellase were found significantly different from placebo in hypotensive activity on all the microcirculatory parameters investigated. No side effects were noted.

Varicose Veins: The effects of gotu kola extract on mucopolysaccharide metabolism were noted in subjects with varicose veins.[12] The total triterpenic fraction of the plant (60 mg/day for 3 months) elevated the basal levels of uronic acids and of lysosomal enzymes, indicating an increased mucopolysaccharide turnover in varicose vein patients. These results confirm the regulatory properties of *C. asiatica* extract on the metabolism in the connective tissue of the vascular wall.

Anticancer Effect: Perhaps the most interesting recent study on gotu kola is the finding that Centella is effective in destroying cultured cancer tumor cells.[13] The extract, a 5:1 concentrate extracted with methanol, was effective at a level of 100 mcg/ml. In addition, practically no toxic effects were detected in normal human lymphocytes.

Micellaneous Effects: A French preliminary study showed TECA to produce histologic improvement in 5 of 12 patients with chronic hepatic disorders.[14]

A double-blind, placebo controlled study of 94 patients with venous insufficiency of the lower limbs indicated that TECA produced clinical improvement in this condition. The patients received 12 or 60 mg/day for 8 weeks.

Improvement occurred in the subjective measures of the sensation of heaviness and pain in the legs, edema and overall patient assessment of efficacy, and in the objective measure of vein distensibility. The researchers concluded that TECA stimulated collagen synthesis in the vein wall, thus increasing vein tonicity and reducing the capacity of the vein to distend. In contrast, patients receiving placebo exhibited an increase in vein distensibility. Although there were no statistically significant differences between the two TECA dosage groups, data trends suggested that the effect of TECA was dose-related.[15]

The pharmacokinetics of the total triterpenic fraction of gotu kola have been studied, after single and multiple administrations to healthy volunteers.[16] Using a new HPLC procedure for detection of asiatic acid, the researchers found that after chronic treatment of two doses, the peak plasma concentration, AUC (area under the curve) and half-life were significantly higher than those observed after the corresponding single dose administration.

TOXICOLOGY: Preparations of *C. asiatica* have a reputation for having a relative lack of toxicity. However, contact dermatitis has been reported in some patients using preparations of fresh or dried parts of the plant.[2] This is not surprising in light of the topical irritant qualities of certain components of the plant. In the cited study of biharzial patients, some who received subcutaneous injections rather than intramuscular injections experienced pain at the injection site, and there was blackish discoloration of the subcutaneous tissues. These side effects may have been diminished with intramuscular injections.[10]

Relatively large doses of extract have been found to be sedative in small animals; this property is attributed to the presence of two saponin glycosides, brahmoside and brahminoside.

SUMMARY: Gotu kola is a plant widely used in traditional Eastern medicine and other forms of herbal therapy. Its most important pharmacologic effect appears to be the promotion of wound healing, particularly in chronic lesions. There is evidence to support the folk medicine use of gotu kola to promote wound healing and as an antifertility agent. Plant extracts appear to be of a low order of toxicity, although hypersensitivity reactions may occur in some people. Recent studies show that gotu kola has selective toxicity against tumor cells in vitro.

PATIENT INFORMATION – Gotu Kola

Uses: Traditionally used as treatment for a variety of ills and as aphrodisiac, gotu kola has demonstrated some efficacy treating wounds and varicose veins and destroying cancer cells in lab research. Evidence suggests is has antifertility, hypotensive and sedative effects.

Side Effects: Gotu kola causes contact dermatitis in some individuals.

[1] Natarajan S, Paily PP. *Ind J Dermatol* 1973;18(4):82.
[2] Eun HC, Lee AY. *Contact Dermatitis* 1985;13(5):310.
[3] Dutta T, Basu UP. *Ind J Exp Biol* 1968;6(3):181.
[4] Schulte KE, et al. *Arch Pharm* 1973;306:197.
[5] Castellani C, et al. *Boll Chim Farm* 1981;120:570.
[6] Sappakun N, Ungwitayatom J. *Mahidol Univ J Pharm Sci* 1982;9:53.
[7] Poizot A, Dumez D. *C R Acad Sci* 1978;286(10):789.
[8] Tenni R, et al. *Ital J Biochem* 1988;37(2):69.

[9] Viala A, et al. *Therapie* 1977;32(5):573.
[10] Fam A. *Intern Surg* 1973;58:451.
[11] Becaro G, et al. *Current Therapeutic Res* 1989;46:1015.
[12] Arpaia MR, et al. *Int J Clin Pharma Res* 1990;10(4):229.
[13] Babu TD, et al. *J Ethnopharmacol* 1995;48:53.
[14] Darnis F, et al. *Sem Hop* 1979;55(37–38):1749.
[15] Pointel JP, et al. *Angiology* 1987;38(1 Pt 1):46.
[16] Grimaldi R, et al. *J Ethnopharmacol* 1990;28(2):235.

Grapefruit

SCIENTIFIC NAME(S): *Citrus Paradisi* Macfad., Rutaceae

COMMON NAME(S): Grapefruit

BOTANY: The grapefruit is a large, dimpled, round citrus fruit, measuring 3 to 6 inches in diameter. It descends from a cross between a pomelo (pummelo) or shaddock (*C. Grandis*), a large Malaysian citrus, and a sweet orange. Some believe the grapefruit could also have arisen as a mutation of another type of citrus tree. The fruit grows in clusters similar to grapes, and this may be the reason why the "grapefruit" was so named. The two main varieties of grapefruit include the Duncan (many seeds and good flavor) and the Marsh (seedless with less flavor). The pink varieties followed; the Foster (1907; seeded) and the Thompson (1913; seedless). The Ruby red-pulped grapefruit was developed in the late twenties in McAllen, Texas. Grapefruits can be considered a "New World" product, a species only a few hundred years old.[1-3] The juice of the fruit, including concentrate, accounts for approximately 42% of all US processed grapefruit products.[2]

HISTORY: In 1310 B.C., Greek historian Theophrastus wrote of how Citron was thought to be an antidote to poison and how it could also "sweeten the breath." Later, Pliny, a Roman naturalist, used the word "citrus" for the first time and labeled the fruit as a medicine.[4] The grapefruit, then called "small shaddock," was first mentioned by Griffith Hughes in 1750, as the "forbidden fruit" of Barbados.[1,2] The name "grapefruit" was said to have been first used in Jamaica in 1814. In 1823, the grapefruit was introduced in Florida by a French count, Odette Phillippe, but did not begin to gain popularity until the end of the nineteenth century.[1] Worldwide production of grapefruit today averages 4.3 million metric tons.[2]

In the 1930's, Hollywood's "Grapefruit Diet" came into vogue, including calorie intake to approximately 800 per day, and including grapefruit consumption at each meal. Weight was lost from this diet, but any diet based primarily on one food is too restrictive to be healthy because too many other important nutrients may be missing.[5]

Analysis of grapefruit seed extract has been performed.[6]

CHEMISTRY: The chemistry of citrus fruits has been reviewed. Components of citrus fruits include sugars, polysaccharides, organic acids, nitrogenous constituents, lipids, carotenoids (that contribute to color), vitamins, minerals, flavonoids and volatile components (that contribute to aroma).[7,8]

Grapefruit is high in water and fiber.[5] The whole fruit is also a good source of potassium, vitamin C, inositol, bioflavonoids and pectin.[2] However, the juice alone is not high in pectin.[4] In addition, grapefruit has no fat and is low in calories and sodium. The pink variety contains beta-carotene.[5] Folic acid is also present in grapefruit. The peel contains citral, an aldehyde that antagonizes the effects of vitamin A.[2]

Other constituents in grapefruit have been found to affect liver enzymes. $6^1,7^1$-dihydroxybergamottin, a cytochrome P450 inhibitor, has been identified.[9] Naringin, naringenin, limonin and obacunone also exhibit inhibitory effects in human liver microsomes (see Pharmacology).[10]

PHARMACOLOGY: In the US, the grapefruit is popular as a breakfast fruit, usually eaten in halves. Approximately one-half of the world grapefruit crop is made into juice.[2]

Nutrition studies have been performed that discovered grapefruit to be of value as a dietary supplement.[11] Grapefruit has also been used as a nutritional supplement for patients experiencing potassium loss.[12]

Grapefruit pectin has been found to reduce cholesterol and to promote regression of atherosclerosis.[4,13] Because the pectin resides in the cell walls of the fruit and not in the juice, the juice itself does not decrease blood cholesterol.[4] Other blood effects of grapefruit include induction of red cell aggregation by constituent naringin (per in vitro observation) and reduction of hematocrits in 36 human subjects who ingested one grapefruit per day.[14]

The Swedes have studied grapefruit for its anti-cancer effects. In a 1986 analysis, subjects who consumed citrus fruit daily had lower incidences of pancreatic cancer.[2]

A pharmacokinetic study suggests citrus flavanones to undergo glucuronidation before urinary excretion.[15]

A report discussing treatment of psoriasis with cyclosporine and grapefruit juice is available.[16]

Grapefruit juice has been found to increase the bioavailability of certain drugs by inhibition of the cytochrome P450 3A4 (CYP3A4) isozyme found in the liver and gut wall.[17-21] However, the effects of grapefruit juice are primarily on the isozyme found in the gut wall. As a result of this inhibition, more of the drug is absorbed and the plasma concentration increases. The elevated drug concentration may lead to an increase in the drug's activity and side effects. In some instances, the increase in drug concentration may be beneficial (see Toxicology).

TOXICOLOGY: Grapefruit juice has been reported to interact with certain nonsedating antihistamines, benzodiazepines, the dihydropyridine class of calcium channel blockers, cyclosporine, estrogens and quinidine. The mechanism of the interaction probably involves inhibition of gut wall enzymes, specifically the CYP3A4 isozyme.

Antihistamines: In humans, grapefruit ingestion may increase the bioavailability of terfenadine (no longer available in US)[33-36] and probably astemizole. Altered cardiac repolarization (in poor metabolizers of terfenadine)[34] and increases in the QT interval[33] have been reported when terfenadine was taken with grapefruit juice compared with water. More than one metabolic pathway appears to be inhibited.[36] There is considerable patient variability in the pharmacokinetic effect of the interaction.[36] The clinical importance of this interaction has not been determined.

Benzodiazepines: In healthy human subjects, taking midazolam or triazolam with grapefruit juice has been reported to increase plasma concentrations and the area under the plasma concentration-time curve (AUC) of these benzodiazepines.[46,51] However, the clinical effects of taking midazolam or triazolam with grapefruit juice are likely to be minor.[46,47,51]

Calcium channel blockers: In humans, the bioavailability of the dihydropyridine calcium channel blockers, including amlodipine, felodipine, nifedipine, nimodipine and nisoldipine, may be increased by concurrent ingestion of grapefruit juice.[23-30,49,50] While the increases in peak plasma concentrations for amlodipine were slight (15%),[29] peak plasma concentrations of felodipine increased more than 300%.[23,24,27,32] nifedipine increased by nearly 35% and the hypotensive effects were enhanced,[51] nimodipine levels increased by 24%,[29] and nisoldipine plasma levels increased by 400%.[20] The bioavailability of diltiazem, a different class of calcium channel blocker (eg, a benzothiazepine) was not affected by grapefruit juice ingestion.[31]

Cyclosporine: Human studies have demonstrated that grapefruit juice alters the pharmacokinetics of cyclosporine.[22,37-40] Taking cyclosporine with grapefruit juice may result in an increase in plasma concentrations[39,40] and AUC of cyclosporine.[22,40] In addition, concentrations of a cyclosporine metabolite may be increased.[40] An increase in neurologic side effects, including tremors, was reported when cyclosporine was taken with grapefruit juice.[40] Some patients are instructed by their physicians to take cyclosporine with grapefruit juice in order to administer a lower dose of cyclosporine and reduce cost to the patient.[22] Thus, grapefruit juice may provide an inexpensive, nontoxic alternative to drugs given to reduce the cyclosporine dose.[22] In this situation, patients should avoid fluctuations in their grapefruit juice ingestion.

Estrogens: In 13 healthy female volunteers, grapefruit juice increased plasma concentration of ethinyl estradiol by 37% and the AUC by 28% compared with ingestion of the estrogen with herbal tea.[43]

Quinidine: When studied in 12 healthy male volunteers, administration of quinidine with grapefruit juice, compared with water, delayed the absorption of quinidine and inhibited the metabolism of quinidine to its major metabolite (3-hydroxyquinidine).[44] The effects of quinidine on the QT_c interval were delayed and reduced by ingestion with grapefruit juice.

Miscellaneous: Other reports are available regarding the effect of grapefruit juice on caffeine metabolism,[41] inhibition of 11-beta-hydroxysteroid dehydrogenase,[42] and shifting the metabolic ratios of clomipramine.[45] Grapefruit juice has been associated with hypotension in one patient.[48]

SUMMARY: The grapefruit is a popular breakfast fruit in the US. Approximately one-half of the world's grapefruit crop is made into juice. Grapefruit juice has been found to increase bioavailability of certain drugs by inhibition of the CYP3A4 gut wall enzyme system. Drugs affected by this system include some calcium channel blockers, terfenadine, cyclosporine and others. These drug-food interactions are important and warrant the counseling of patients by pharmacists and other healthcare workers.

PATIENT INFORMATION – Grapefruit

Uses: Grapefruit juice is used as a nutritional supplement for potassium loss. Grapefruit pectin can help reduce cholesterol and promote regression of atherosclerosis. Other effects include induction of red cell aggregation by constituent naringin, reduction of hemocrits and possible anti-cancer effects.

Side Effects: Grapefruit juice can create adverse effects by altering drugs metabolized by the CYP3A4 enzyme system (eg, some nonsedating antihistamines, benzodiazepines, selected calcium channel blockers, estrogens, quinidine, and cyclosporine). A case report exists about grapefruit juice-induced hypotension.

[1] Davidson A, et al. *Grapefruit, Pomelo, Ugli. Fruit-A Connoiseur's Guide and Cookbook.* New York, NY: Simon and Schuster Inc. 1991:66.
[2] Ensminger A, et al. *Grapefruit Foods and Nutrition Encyclopedia* 2nd ed. CRC Press Inc., Boca Raton, FL 1994; 1097-99.
[3] Simpson B, et al. *Fruits and Nuts of Warm Regions. Economic Botany-Plants in our World.* New York, NY: McGraw-Hill Inc. 1995:124.
[4] Carper J. *Grapefruit. The Food Pharmacy.* New York, NY: Bantam Books. 1988:213-15.
[5] http://countryliving.com/gh/health/07nutrb3.htm
[6] Sakamoto S, et al. *Eisei Shikenjo Hokoku* 1996;114:38-42.
[7] Ranganna S, et al. *Crit Rev Food Sci Nutr* 1983;18(4):313-86.
[8] Ranganna S, et al. *Crit Rev Food Sci Nutr* 1983;19(1):1-98.
[9] Edwards D, et al. *Drug Metab Dispos* 1996;24(12):1287-90.
[10] Fukuda K, et al. *Biol Pharm Bull* 1997;20(5):560-64.
[11] Staroscik J, et al. *J Am Diet Assoc* 1980;77(5):567-69.
[12] Boner G, et al. *Harefuah* 1980;98(6):251-52.
[13] Cerda J. *Trans Am Clin Climatol Assoc* 1987;99:203-13.
[14] Robbins R, et al. *Int J Vitam Nutr Res* 1988;58(4):414-17.
[15] Ameer B, et al. *Clin Pharmacol Ther* 1996;60(1):34-40.
[16] Taniguchi S, et al. *Arch Dermatol* 1996;132(10):1249.
[17] Bailey D, et al. *Clin Pharmacokinet* 1994;26(2):91-98.
[18] Anon. *Med Lett Drugs Ther* 1995;37(955):73-74.
[19] Fuhr U, et al. *Clin Pharmacol Ther* 1995;58(4):365-73.
[20] Spence J. *Clin Pharmacol Ther* 1997;61(4):395-400.
[21] Ameer B, et al. *Clin Pharmacokinet* 1997;33(2):103-21.
[22] Yee G, et al. *Lancet* 1995;345(8955):955-56.
[23] Bailey D, et al. *Lancet* 1991;337(8736):268-69.
[24] Edgar B, et al. *Eur J Clin Pharmacol* 1992;42(3):313-17.
[25] Miniscalco A, et al. *J Pharmacol Exp Ther* 1992;261(3):1195-99.
[26] Bailey D, et al. *Clin Pharmacol Ther* 1993;54(6):589-94.
[27] Bailey D, et al. *Br J Clin Pharmacol* 1995;40(2):135-40.
[28] Rashid T, et al. *Br J Clin Pharmacol* 1995;40(1):51-58.
[29] Josefsson M, et al. *Eur J Clin Pharmacol* 1996;51(2):189-93.
[30] Lundahl J, et al. *Eur J Clin Pharmacol* 1997;52(2):139-45.
[31] Sigusch H, et al. *Pharmazie* 1994;49(9):675-79.
[32] Bailey D, et al. *Clin Pharmacol Ther* 1996;60(1):25-33.
[33] Benton R, et al. *Clin Pharmacol Ther* 1996;59(4):383-88.
[34] Honig P, et al. *J Clin Pharmacol* 1996;36(4):345-51.
[35] Clifford C, et al. *Eur J Clin Pharmacol* 1997;52(4):311-15.
[36] Rau S, et al. *Clin Pharmacol Ther* 1997;61(4):401-09.
[37] Bennett W. *Pediatr Nephrol* 1995;9(1):10.
[38] Majeed A, et al. *Pediatr Nephrol* 1996;10(3):395-96.
[39] Hollander A, et al. *Clin Pharmacol Ther* 1995;57(3):318-24.
[40] Ioannides-Demos L, et al. *J Rheumatol* 1997;24(1):49-54.
[41] Fuhr U, et al. *Int J Clin Pharmacol Ther* 1995;33(6):311-14.
[42] Lee Y, et al. *Clin Pharmacol Ther* 1996;59(1):62-71.
[43] Weber A, et al. *Contraception* 1996;53(1):41-47.
[44] Min D, et al. *J Clin Pharmacol* 1996;36(5):469-76.
[45] Oesterheld J. *J Clin Psychopharmacol* 1997;17(1):62-63.
[46] Hukkinen S, et al. *Clin Pharmacol Ther* 1995;58(2):127-31.
[47] Vanakowski J, et al. *Eur J Clin Pharmacol* 1996;50(6):501-08.
[48] Nilsson I. *Lakartidningen* 1997;94(3):112-13.
[49] Fuhr U, et al. *Int J Clin Pharmacol Ther* 1998;36(3):126-32.
[50] Pisarik P. *Arch Fam Med* 1996;5(7):413-16.
[51] Kupferschmidt MHT, et al. *Clin Pharmacol Ther* 1995;58(1):20-28.

Grape Seed

SCIENTIFIC NAME(S): *Vitis vinifera* L. and *V. coignetiae* Family: Vitaceae

COMMON NAME(S): Grape seed, muskat

SOURCE: Red grape seeds are generally obtained as a by-product of wine production. When ground, these seeds become the source of grape seed oil.

CHEMISTRY: Grape seed oil contains nutritionally useful essential fatty acids and tocopherols (vitamin E).[1] The methanol extract of the oriental species (*Vitis coignetiae*) contains epsilon-viniferin, oligostilbenes, ampelopsins A, C, F and the mixture of vitisin A and cis-vitisin A.[2] Dietary grape seed tannins are reported,[3] as well as procyanidines (polyphenol oligomers).[4] New 5'-nucleotidase inhibitors designated as NPF-88BU-IA and NPF-88BU-IB (all polyphenolic compounds), respectively, have been isolated from the seeds and skin of the wine grape.[5]

PHARMACOLOGY: The wine grape seeds can be used as "health oils" because of their high content of essential fatty acids and tocopherols.[1] A methanol extract of the Oriental medicinal plant *Vitis coignetiae* indicated protective effects for liver cells in the in vitro assay method using primary cultured rat hepatocytes. Activity-guided fractionation of this extract produced epsilon-viniferin as an active principle. It also showed protection against carbon tetrachloride-induced hepatic injury in mice, shown by serum enzyme assay and pathological examination. Ampelopsin C and the mixture of vitisin A and cis-vitisin A were found to be strong hepatotoxins.[2]

Vallet et al[3] have studied the effects of dietary grape seed tannins on nutritional balance and on some enzymic activities along the crypt-villus axis of rat small intestine. This study did not reveal a significant tannin toxicity, except for a reduced dry matter and nitrogen digestibility. However, the tannins directly interfere with mucosal proteins, stimulating the cell renewal.[3]

Maffei et al[4] have studied the scavenging by procyanidines from *Vitis vinifera* seeds of reactive oxygen species involved in the onset and the maintenance of microvascular injury. They report that procyanidines have a remarkable dose-dependent antilipoperoxidant activity. They also inhibit xanthine oxidase activity (the enzyme which triggers the oxy radical cascade). In addition, procyanidines non-competitively inhibit the proteolytic enzymes collagenase and elastase and the glycosidases hyaluronidase and beta-glucuronidase. These are involved in the turnover of the main structural components of the extravascular matrix collagen, elastin and hyaluronic acid.[4]

Studies by Toukairin et al[5] have shown that polyphenolic substances from the seeds and skin of the wine grapes ("Koshu") can: Strongly inhibit 5'nucleotidase activities from snake venom and rat liver membrane; have significant therapeutic activity in Ehrlich ascites carcinoma; have inhibitory action against the growth of *Streptococcus mutans*, a cariogenic bacteria; and inhibit glucan formation from sucrose. These last two actions may indicate that these principles can aid in the prevention of dental caries.[5] Interestingly, grape seed oil has been shown to be a safe and efficient hand cleansing agent.[6]

TOXICOLOGY: No human toxicity has been reported in recent literature for the grape seed, the oil or its isolated constituents, except for hepatotoxicity in mice (discussed in Pharmacology).[2]

SUMMARY: Grape seed oil appears to be safe and potentially useful as a dietary source of essential fatty acids and tocopherols. Interestingly, some compounds from *Vitis coignetiae* show hepatoprotective activity while others show hepatotoxic effects. Seed tannins directly interfere with mucosal proteins, thereby stimulating cell renewal. Procyanidines from the seeds may have the ability to maintain the microvascular system and the main structural components of the skins. Polyphenolic derivatives in the seeds and skin have interesting anti-enzyme properties and significant therapeutic potential against Ehrlich ascites carcinoma. In addition, these substances may be useful in preventing dental caries.

PATIENT INFORMATION – Grape Seed

Uses: Grape seed oil has shown promise in lab research as a cleansing agents, anti-enzyme, nutritional supplement and inhibitor of tooth decay.

Side Effects: Research has indicated hepatoxicity in mice.

[1] El-Mallah MH, Murui T. *Seifen-Oele-Fette-Wachse* 1993;119:45.
[2] Oshima Y, et al. *Experientia* 1995;51(1):63.
[3] Vallet J, et al. *Ann Nutr Metab* 1994;38(2):75.
[4] Maffei Facino R, et al. *Arzneimittel-Forschung* 1994;44(5):592.
[5] Toukairin T, et al. *Chem Pharm Bull* 1991;39(6):1480.
[6] Krogsrud NE, Larsen Al. *Contact Dermatitis* 1992;26(3):208.

Green Tea

SCIENTIFIC NAME(S): *Camellia sinensis* L. Kuntze. Family: Theaceae

COMMON NAME(S): Tea, green tea

BOTANY: *C. sinensis* is a large shrub with evergreen leaves native to eastern Asia, where it is cultivated extensively. The plant has leathery, dark green leaves, and fragrant, white flowers with 6 to 9 petals. Cultivated tea plants are trimmed to about 1.5 m to facilitate the harvest.[1,2]

HISTORY: The dried, cured leaves of *C. sinensis* have been used to prepare beverages for more than 4000 years.[3] The method of curing determines the nature of the tea to be used for infusion, and green tea is 1 type of cured tea. Green tea is prepared from the steamed and dried leaves; by comparison, black tea leaves are withered, rolled, fermented, and then dried.[4] Oolong tea is semifermented and considered to be intermediate in composition between green and black teas.[2,5] Green tea is less popular in America and Europe than the black tea varieties.[6] Tea has been used medicinally for centuries, and the Chinese regarded the drink as a cure for cancer, although the tannin component is believed to be carcinogenic. Tea has been known to act as a diuretic and has been used to relieve headaches.

Research stems from people believing tea may have positive healing benefits because of its continued use as a fluid supply for those suffering from illness and disease. Focused investigations on therapeutic effects began in Japan and China, and continued in Europe and the US. The polyphenol presence in tea may play a role in lowering heart disease and cancer risk.[3]

CHEMISTRY: The chemistry of tea is complex because of the numerous components that are formed during the curing and drying process. Tea leaves contain varying amounts of polyphenols (flavonols, depsides such as chlorogenic acid, coumarylquinic acid, and theogallin), and catechins (the flavonol group of polyphenols).[5] Separation of catechins in green tea using HPLC[7,8] and other mass spectrometric methods (eg, EIMS, FABMS, LC/ESIMS) has been performed.[9] Structure (-)-epigallocatechin gallate has been detected as well, and was found to be an acetyl-CoA carboxylase inhibitor.[10]

The method of preparing green tea precludes the oxidation of the green leaf polyphenols. The composition of green tea is very similar to that of the fresh leaf, except for a few enzymatically catalyzed changes that occur extremely rapidly following plucking.[5]

Other tea constituents include tannins (evaluation of content has been reported),[11] caffeine (1% to 4% = 10 to 50 mg/180 ml), theophylline, theobromine, other methylxanthines (in small amounts), protein (15% to 20%), fiber, sugars (5%), B-vitamins, ascorbic acid (present in fresh leaf but destroyed in making black tea), amino acid theanine, malic and oxalic acids, and fats.[2,4,5,6] Lignans and isoflavonoid concentrations have been analyzed in tea.[12] Essential oil constituents of green tea dihydroactinidiolide and p-vinylphenol have been isolated.[13] Other volatile oil components include hexenal, hexenol, aldehydes, phenylethyl alcohols, phenols, and geraniol.[4] The folacin content of tea has also been reported.[14]

PHARMACOLOGY: Areas of current pharmacologic interest concerning green tea include pharmacokinetic studies, **lipid effects**, **dental caries inhibition**, **antimicrobial actions**, **antimutagenic** and **antioxidative actions**, a wide variety of **anticancer** studies, and other miscellaneous effects.

Pharmacokinetics: The pharmacokinetics of green tea have been reported. Blood and urine levels have been investigated in humans.[15] Drinking green tea daily may maintain significant plasma catechin levels, which may exert antioxidant activity against lipoproteins in blood circulation.[16] HPLC determination of catechins and polyphenol components have been performed.[16-19]

Lipid effects: Green tea appears to have promising effects in lowering lipid levels in vitro and in animal studies. However, research in humans does not support these claims. In vitro testing found that green tea markedly delays lipid peroxidation, with the polyphenol components having the strongest actions.[20] Green tea was also found to possess significant serum and liver cholesterol-lowering effects in (diet-induced) hypercholesterclemic rats. HDL-total cholesterol ratio was increased while HDL and triglyceride levels were not affected.[21] Another report investigating effects of green and black tea vs other dietary antioxidants in hypercholesterolemic rabbits concluded that green tea consumption reduced aortic lesion formation by 31%. Black tea, vitamin E, and beta carotene had no effect.[22] Human consumption of green tea has been associated with a decrease in total cholesterol levels but not in triglycerides or HDL cholesterol levels,[10] in this survey, 9 or more cups of tea had to be consumed per day for a significant effect to be noted.[23] A report investigating green tea intake and its effect on cholesterol levels in 1000 Japanese patients did not support the tea's beneficial actions on serum lipid levels.[24]

Dental caries: Green tea exhibits antimicrobial actions against oral bacteria.[25] After 5 minutes of contact with a 0.1% green tea polyphenol solution, *Streptococcus mutans* was completely inhibited. Plaque and gingival index were decreased after a 0.2% solution was used to rinse and brush teeth.[26] In vitro and in vivo data suggest green tea's fluoride content (although in low concentrations), may increase the cariostatic action along with the other tea components.[27] A report in animal models also suggests fluoride content in conjunction with other tea constituents, such as tannins, to decrease the rate of caries formation.[28] After rinsing with green tea extract, the catechin components present in human saliva have been determined by HPLC, and were present in the saliva for up to 1 hour.[29] Green tea consumption may also be effective in reducing the cariogenic potential of starch-containing foods by inhibiting salivary amylase, which hydrolyzes food starch to fermentable carbohydrates.[30]

Antimicrobial: Green tea's antimicrobial effects have been well documented. Green tea inhibited the growth of diarrhea-causing bacteria *Staphlococcus aureus*, *S. epidermidis*, *Vibrio cholerae* O1, *V. cholerae* non O1, *V. parahaemolyticus*, *V. mimicus*, *Campylobacter jejuni*, and *Plesiomonas shigelloides*.[31] In vitro antibiosis of green tea was demonstrated against 5 pathogenic fungi. When dilutions of 1:100 of culture filtrate green tea isolate were sprayed on infected plants, insect populations were also successfully controlled.[32] Green tea extract also inhibits a wide range of pathogenic bacteria including MRSA (methicillin-resistant *S. aureus*). This activity may be caused by the catechin and theaflavin (and its gallates) components.[33] In mice inoculated with green tea extract, inhibition of *E. coli* bacterial growth was demonstrated.[34] In addition, when tested in human infected root canals, green tea extract had antibacterial actions against 24 bacterial strains.[35]

Antimutagenic: Antimutagenic activity against a variety of organisms has been evaluated from different tea components.[36,37] Flavonol constituents in both green and black teas contributed to antimutagenic potential against dietary carcinogens.[38] The catechin components have been shown to contribute to antimutagenicity as well.[39] The antimutagenic potential of green tea extracts may be caused by 2 different proposed mechanisms, 1 of which may involve a direct interaction between reactive genotoxic species of various promutagens and nucleophilic tea components present in the aqueous extracts.[40] The tea tannins have been shown to modify chromosomal changes in mutagen-treated cells and mice.[41]

Antioxidative: Tea antioxidants have been well recognized.[42-44] Antioxidative activity was studied in 25 tea types, the actions due, in part, to the catechins present.[45] Tea consumed with milk may affect in vivo antioxidation thought to be caused by the complexation of tea polyphenols by milk proteins.[46] An evaluation of longevity of 3300 Japanese women practitioners of chanoyu (a Japanese tea ceremony) suggests that their intake of green tea contributes to their longevity[41] by providing a degree of protection against fatal diseases.[47]

Anticancer: Studies and reviews in the general area of anticancer effects from green tea and its various components are vast.[42,48-52] Some reports find that tea possesses anticarcinogenic effects, protecting animals and humans against cancer risk.[42,48-52] One epidemiologic review explains favorable effects from tea only if high intake occurs in high-risk populations.[53] Another study (prospective cohort) finds data unsupportive in the hypothesis that black tea consumption protects against 4 major human cancers.[54] In another report, no consistent patterns of evidence were found concerning black tea consumption influencing cancer rates.[55] One other epidemiological study suggests modest anticancer benefits with several investigations leading to the possibility of decreased risks of digestive tract cancer from tea consumption.[56]

The polyphenol components of green tea (including flavanones, flavonols, isoflavones, and catechins) may possess chemopreventative properties.[57-64] The polyphenol content of green tea has been shown to inhibit the in vitro and in vivo formation of N-nitrosation by-products, which have been established as cancer-inducing compounds.[65] Various catechins exhibit inhibitory actions on human tumor cell lines, including breast, colon, lung, and melanoma.[66] A report on the nonpolyphenolic fraction of green tea finds pheophytins to be potent antigenotoxic substances as well.[67]

Additive effects of tea and other components have been documented. Tea and curcumin (constituent from the spice turmeric, an inhibitor of cyclooxygenase and lipoxygenase) used in combination on certain cell types were noted to have a synergistic effect in chemoprevention.[68,69] Green tea in combination with anticancer drug doxorubicin enhanced inhibitory effects on tumor growth by 2.5-fold when tested in mice.[70]

There are many proposed mechanisms as to how green tea expresses its anticancer effects. Some of these include antioxidative reactions, enzyme activities, inhibition of pathways such as lipid peroxidation, irradiation, and TPA-induced epidermal ornithine decarboxylase, inhibition of protein kinase and cellular proliferation, anti-inflammatory activity, and enhancement of gap junction intercellular communication.[42,58,59,62,64]

Anticancer, GI reports: Several reports conclude the possibility of lowered risk of digestive tract cancers in consumers of green tea.[56] Animal studies support these claims. Green tea extract inhibited GI tumors in rats (induced by N-methyl-N'-nitro-n-nitrosoguanidine) by 88%. Green tea catechols combine with the N-nitro-compounds to reduce their carcinogenic activity.[71] Green tea and its catechins have also prevented GI carcinoma in mice[72] and displayed a preventative and blocking effect on esophageal cancer in rats as well.[73] The theaflavin fraction of tea was also tested in rat esophageal cancer models, significantly reducing tumor formation.[74]

Most human studies confirm green tea's positive effects in cancer prevention. Consumption of green tea may offer protective effects against digestive tract cancers.[75] A case control study in over 1000 patients with esophageal cancer suggests a protective effect against this type of carcinogenesis from tea consumption.[76] Findings of another report evaluating 931 colon cancer cases, 884 rectum cancer cases, and 451 pancreas cancer cases concluded that green tea consumption may lower the risk of these cancers as well.[77] Affected human stomach cells treated with green tea catechin extract led to growth inhibition and induction of apoptosis, suggesting possible stomach cancer protection.[78] Catechins have also contributed to inhibition of small intestine carcinogenesis.[79] In tube-fed patients given 1 cup of green tea (100 mg catechins) 3 times daily for 3 weeks, positive effects were seen against colon carcinoma.[80] One conflicting study found a direct correlation between drinking 5 or more cups of green tea a day and the preference for salty foods as a risk factor for pancreatic cancer among Japanese men.[81] A tutorial is available on chemoprevention of aerodigestive cancers.[82]

Anticancer, skin: Green tea offers chemopreventative effects against skin cancers of varying stages and is useful against inflammatory responses in cancers caused by known skin tumor promoters such as chemicals or radiation.[83] Green tea and its polyphenol fractions display a protective effect against mouse skin papilloma.[84] UV radiation-induced skin cancer in animal and human models.[85] and have inhibited photocarcinogenesis in mice in topical applications.[86]

Anticancer, various: Green tea's chemopreventative activities against hepatic and pulmonary carcinogenesis have been addressed.[87,88] The tea's anticancer effects against lung tumorigenesis,[89] smoke-induced mutations in humans,[90] pancreatic carcinogenesis,[91] and leukemia[92] have all been reported. Green tea can inhibit the carcinogenic effects of female hormones as well.[93] A recent Canadian report is available concerning the unconventional use of green tea to treat breast cancer.[94]

Miscellaneous effects: Two well-known components of green tea from a pharmacologic basis are caffeine and tannin. Caffeine is an effective central nervous system stimulant that can induce nervousness, insomnia, tachycardia, elevated blood sugar and cholesterol levels, high levels of stomach acid, and heartburn.[6] These components are also useful for headaches, enhancement of renal excretion of water, weight loss, and as a cardiotonic. Green tea is also used as an astringent, for wounds and skin disorders, and soothing insect bites, itching, and sunburn. Tea is also a sweat-inducer, a nerve tonic, and has been used for functional asthenia, eye problems (as a poultice for baggy or tired eyes), and as an analgesic.[1,2,4] Green tea has been employed in hepatitis treatment and for protection of the liver, as with induced injury by carbon tetrachloride in rats.[1,95] The plant has also reduced methylguanidine levels, thus slowing the progression of renal failure in rats as well.[96] Green tea's role in stroke prevention,[97] as a thromboxane inhibitor,[98] as a radioprotective in mice to prolong lifespan,[99] and as a hypotensive (from hot water extracts)[100] has been described.

TOXICOLOGY: There is evidence that in animals caffeine can be teratogenic, and the FDA has advised that women who are or may become pregnant should avoid caffeine-containing products.[6] However, studies in humans drinking moderate amounts of caffeine have shown inconsistent results, with more recent studies not demonstrating adverse effects on the fetus.[101,102] Caffeine-containing beverages may also alter female hormone levels, including estradiol.[103]

There is evidence that condensed catechin tannin of tea is linked to a high rate of esophageal cancer in regions of heavy tea consumption. This effect may be overcome by adding milk, which binds the tannin, possibly preventing its detrimental effects.[4] Catechins have also been linked to tea-induced asthma[104] and with rat hepatic microsomal cytochrome P450 enzyme interactions.[105] One study reports that catechins may have antiallergic effects, inhibiting type I allergic reactions.[106] Certain green tea workers experienced shortness of breath, stiffness, pain in neck and arms, and other occupation-related problems.[107]

The daily consumption of an average of 250 ml of tea by infants has been shown to impair iron metabolism, resulting in a high incidence of microcytic anemia.[108] However, in another report, no inhibitory effects on iron absorption were found in elderly patients.[109]

SUMMARY: Green tea is a widely popular beverage, particularly in Asia. Because of its unique preparation process, green tea retains many of the chemical characteristics of the fresh leaf. Pharmacologically, a wealth of information is available concerning green tea's effects on lipid levels, dental caries prevention, antimicrobial, antimutagenic, and antioxidative actions. It appears that green tea components may exert a chemoprotective effect that may contribute to a reduced incidence of cancers and other life-threatening diseases. Because of the caffeine present in the tea, it should be avoided by pregnant women. The tea may be an asthma-inducing agent.

PATIENT INFORMATION – Green Tea

Uses: Traditionally consumed as a beverage, green tea retains many chemicals of the fresh leaf. It is thought to reduce cancer and other fatal diseases, lower lipid levels, help prevent dental caries, and possess antimicrobial, antimutagenic, antioxidative, and other effects.

Side Effects: The FDA advises those who are or may become pregnant to avoid caffeine. Heavy consumption may be associated with esophageal cancer. Tea may impair iron metabolism.

---

[1] Chevallier A. *Encyclopedia of Medicinal Plants.* New York, NY: DK Publishing, 1996;179.

[2] Bruneton J. *Pharmacognosy, Phytochemistry, Medicinal Plants.* Paris, France: Lavoisier, 1995; 885-87.

[3] Weisburger J. Tea and health: a historical perspective. *Cancer Lett* 1997; 114(1-2):315-17.

[4] Duke JA. *Handbook of Medicinal Herbs.* Boca Raton, FL: CRC Press, 1985.

[5] Graham H. Green tea composition, consumption, and polyphenol chemistry. *Prev Med* 1992; 21(3):334–50.

[6] Tyler V. *The New Honest Herbal.* Philadelphia, PA: G.F. Stickley Co., 1987.

[7] Khokhar S, et al. A RP-HPLC method for the determination of tea catechins. *Cancer Lett* 1997; 114(1-2):171-72.

[8] Dalluge J, et al. Selection of column and gradient elution system for the separation of catechins in green tea using high-performance liquid chromatography. *J Chromatogr A* 1998; 793(2):265-74.

[9] Miketova P, et al. Mass spectrometry of selected components of biological interest in green tea extracts. *J Nat Prod* 1998; 61(4):461-67.

[10] Watanabe J, et al. Isolation and identification of acetyl-CoA carboxylase inhibitors from green tea. *Biosci Biotechnol Biochem* 1998;62(3):532-34.

[11] Savolainen H. Tannin content of tea and coffee. *J Appl Toxicol* 1992; 12(3):191-92.

[12] Mazur W, et al. Lignan and isoflavonoid concentrations in tea and coffee. *Br J Nutr* 1998; 79(1):37-45.

[13] Fukushima S, et al. Studies on the essential oil of green tea. *Yakugaku Zasshi* 1969; 89(12):1729-31.

[14] Chen T, et al. Folacin content of tea. *J Am Diet Assoc* 1983; 82(6):627-32.

[15] Yang CS, et al. Blood and urine levels of tea catechins after ingestion of different amounts of green tea by human volunteers. *Cancer Epidemiol Biomarkers Prev* 1998;7(4):351-54.

[16] Nakagawa K, et al. Dose-dependent incorporation of tea catechins, (-)-epigallocatechin-3-gallate and (-)-epigallocatechin, into human plasma. *Biosci Biotechnol Biochem* 1997;61(12):1981-85.

[17] Unno T, et al. Analysis of (-)-epigallocatechin gallate in human serum obtained after ingesting green tea. *Biosci Biotechnol Biochem* 1996;60(12):2066-68.

[18] Dalluge J, et al. Capillary liquid chromatography/electrospray mass spectrometry for the separation and detection of catechins in green tea and human plasma. *Rapid Commun Mass Spectrom* 1997;11(16):1753-56.

[19] Maiani G, et al. Application of a new high-performance liquid chromatographic method for measuring selected polyphenols in human plasma. *J Chromatogr B Biomed Sci Appl* 1997;692(2):311-17.

[20] Yokozawa T, et al. Influence of green tea and its 3 major components upon low-density lipoprotein oxidation. *Exp Toxicol Pathol* 1997;49(5):329-35.

[21] Yang T, et al. Hypocholesterolemic effects of Chinese tea. *Pharmacol Res* 1997;35(6):505-12.

[22] Tijburg L, et al. Effects of green tea, black tea, and dietary lipophilic antioxidants on LDL oxidizability and atherosclerosis in hypercholesterolaemic rabbits. *Atherosclerosis* 1997;135(1):37-47.

[23] Kono S, et al. Green tea consumption and serum lipid profiles. *Prev Med* 1992;21(4):526.

[24] Tsubono Y, et al. Green tea intake in relation to serum lipid levels in Middle-aged Japanese men and women. *Ann Epidemiol* 1997;7(4):280-84.

[25] Saeki Y, et al. Antimicrobial action of green tea extract, flavono flavor, and copper chlorophyll against oral bacteria. *Bull Tokyo Dent Coll* 1993;34(1):33-37.

[26] You S. Study on feasibility of Chinese green tea polyphenols (CTP) for preventing dental caries. *Chung Hua Kou Hsueh Tsa Chih* 1993;28(4):197-99.

[27] Yu H, et al. Anticariogenic effects of green tea. *Fukuoka Igaku Zasshi* 1992;83(4):174-80.

[28] Rosen S, et al. Anticariogenic effects of tea in rats. *J Dent Res* 1984;63(5):658.

[29] Tsuchiya H, et al. Simultaneous determination of catechins in human saliva by high-performance liquid chromatography. *J Chromatogr B Biomed Sci Appl* 1997:703(1-2):253-58.

[30] Zhang J, et al. Inhibition of salivary amylase by black and green teas and their effects on the intraoral hydrolysis of starch. *Caries Res* 1998;32(3):233-38.

[31] Toda M, et al. Antibacterial and bactericidal activities of Japanese green tea. *Nippon Saikingaku Zasshi* 1989;44(4):669-72.

[32] Bezbaruah B, et al. Fungicidal and insect controlling properties of Proteus strain RRLJ 16, isolated from tea, *Camellia sinensis* (L) O Kuntze, plantations. *Indian J Exp Biol* 1996;34(7):706-09.

[33] Yam T, et al. Microbiological activity of whole and fractionated crude extracts of tea and of tea components. *FEMS Microbiol Lett* 1997;152(1):169-74.

[34] Isogai E, et al. Protective effect of Japanese green tea extract on gnotobiotic mice infected with an *Escherichia coli* O157:H7 strain. *Microbiol Immunol* 1998;42(2):125-28.

[35] Horiba N, et al. A pilot study of Japanese green tea as a medicament: antibacterial and bactericidal effects. *J Endod* 1991;17(3):122-24.

[36] Nagao M, et al. Mutagens in coffee and other beverages. *Mutat Res* 1979;68(2):101-06.

[37] Yen G, et al. Relationship between antimutagenic activity and major components of various teas. *Mutagenesis* 1996;11(1):37-41.

[38] Bu-Abbas A, et al. A comparison of the antimutagenic potential of green, black, and decaffeinated teas: contribution of flavanols to the antimutagenic effect. *Mutagenesis* 1996;11(6):597-603.

[39] Constable A, et al. Antimutagenicity and catechin content of soluble instant teas. *Mutagenesis* 1996;11(2):189-94.

40 Bu-Abbas A, et al. Marked antimutagenic potential of aqueous green tea extracts: mechanism of action. *Mutagenesis* 1994;9(4):325-31.

41 Imanishi H, et al. Tea tannin components modify the induction of sister-chromatid exchanges and chromosome aberrations in mutagen-treated cultured mammalian cells and mice. *Mutat Res* 1991;259(1):79.

42 Katiyar S, et al. Tea antioxidants in cancer chemoprevention. *J Cell Biochem Suppl* 1997;(27):59-67.

43 Cheng T. Antioxidants in Chinese green tea. *J Am Coll Cardiol* 1998;31(5):1214.

44 Yamanaka N, et al. Green tea catechins such as (-)-epicatechin and (-)-epigallocatechin accelerate Cu2+-induced low density lipoprotein oxidation in propagation phase. *FEBS Lett* 1997;401(2-3):230-34.

45 Kumamoto M, et al. Evaluation of the antioxidative activity of tea by an oxygen electrode method. *Biosci Biotechnol Biochem* 1998;62(1):175-77.

46 Serafini M, et al. In vivo antioxidant effect of green and black tea in man. *Eur J Clin Nutr* 1996;50(1):28-32.

47 Sadakata S, et al. Mortality among female practitioners of Chanoyu. *Tohoku J Exp Med* 1992;166(4):475.

48 Mukhtar H, et al. Tea components: antimutagenic and anticarcinogenic effects. *Prev Med* 1992;21(3):351-60.

49 Yang C, et al. Tea and cancer. *J Natl Cancer Inst* 1993;85(13):1038-49.

50 Mukhtar H, et al. Cancer chemoprevention by green tea components. *Adv Exp Med Biol* 1994;354:123-24.

51 Mitscher L, et al. Chemoprotection: a review of the potential therapeutic antioxidant properties of green tea and certain of its constituents. *Med Res Rev* 1997;17(4):327-65.

52 Dreosti I, et al. Inhibition of carcinogenesis by tea. *Crit Rev Food Sci Nutr* 1997;37(8):761-70.

53 Kohlmeier L, et al. Tea and cancer prevention. *Nutr Cancer* 1997;27(1):1-13.

54 Goldbohm R, et al. Consumption of black tea and cancer risk. *J Natl Cancer Inst* 1996;88(2):93-100.

55 Blot W, et al. Cancer rates among drinkers of black tea. *Crit Rev Food Sci Nutr* 1997;37(8):739-60.

56 Blot W, et al. Tea and cancer. *Eur J Cancer Prev* 1996;5(6):425-38.

57 Cheng S, et al. Progress in studies on the antimutagenicity and anticarcinogenicity of green tea epicatechins. *Chin Med Sci J* 1991;6(4):233-38.

58 Komori A, et al. Anticarcinogenic activity of green tea polyphenols. *Jpn J Clin Oncol* 1993;23(3):186-90.

59 Stoner G, et al. Polyphenols as cancer chemopreventive agents. *J Cell Biochem Suppl* 1995;22:169-80.

60 Han C. Screening of anticarcinogenic ingredients in tea polyphenols. *Cancer Lett* 1997;114(1-2):153-58.

61 Yang C, et al. Polyphenols as inhibitors of carcinogenesis. *Environ Health Perspect* 1997;105 (Suppl. 4):971-76.

62 Chan M, et al. Inhibition of inducible nitric oxide synthase gene expression and enzyme activity by epigallocatechin gallate, a natural product from green tea. *Biochem Pharmacol* 1997;54(12):1281-86.

63 Ahmad N, et al. Green tea constituent epigallocatechin-3-gallate and induction of apoptosis and cell cycle arrest in human carcinoma cells. *J Natl Cancer Inst* 1997;89(24):1881-86.

64 Tanaka K, et al. Inhibition of N-nitrosation of secondary amines in vitro by tea extracts and catechins. *Mutat Res* 1998;412(1):91-98.

65 Wang H, et al. Inhibitory effect of Chinese tea on N-nitrosation in vitro and in vivo. *IARC Sci Publ* 1991;105:546.

66 Valcic S, et al. Inhibitory effect of 6 green tea catechins and caffeine on the growth of 4 selected human tumor cell lines. *Anticancer Drugs* 1996;7(4):461-68.

67 Okai Y, et al. Potent suppressing activity of the non-polyphenolic fraction of green tea against genotoxin-induced umu C gene expression in *Salmonella typhimurium* —association with pheophytins a and b. *Cancer Lett* 1997;120(1):117-23.

68 Khafif A, et al. Quantitation of chemopreventive synergism between (-)-epigallocatechin-3-gallate and curcumin in normal, premalignant, and malignant human oral epithelial cells. *Carcinogenesis* 1998;19(3):419-24.

69 Conney A, et al. Some perspectives on dietary inhibition of carcinogenesis: studies with curcumin and tea. *Proc Soc Exp Biol Med* 1997;216(2):234-45.

70 Sadzuka Y, et al. Modulation of cancer chemotherapy by green tea. *Clin Cancer Res* 1998;4(1):153-56.

71 Yan Y. The experiment of tumor-inhibiting effect of green tea extract in animal and human body. *Chung Hua Yu Fang I Hsueh Tsa Chih* 1993;27(3):129-31.

72 Yamane T, et al. Inhibitory effects and toxicity of green tea polyphenols for gastrointestinal carcinogenesis. *Cancer* 1996;77(Suppl. 8):1662-67.

73 Wang C, et al. A preliminary study of the preventive and blocking effect of green tea grown in mengding mountain area on the esophageal cancer in rats. *Hua Hsi I Ko Ta Hsueh Hsueh Pao* 1996;27(2):206-08.

74 Morse M, et al. Effects of theaflavins on N-nitrosomethylbenzylamine-induced esophageal tumorigenesis. *Nutr Cancer* 1997;29(1):7-12.

75 Inoue M, et al. Tea and coffee consumption and the risk of digestive tract cancers. *Cancer Causes Control* 1998;9(2):209-16.

76 Gao Y, et al. Reduced risk of esophageal cancer associated with green tea consumption. *J Natl Cancer Inst* 1994;86(11):855-58.

77 Ji B, et al. Green tea consumption and the risk of pancreatic and colorectal cancers. *Int J Cancer* 1997;70(3):255-58.

78 Hibasami H, et al. Induction of apoptosis in human stomach cancer cells by green tea catechins. *Oncol Rep* 1998;5(2):527-29.

79 Ito N, et al. Strategy of research for cancer-chemoprevention. *Teratogenesis Carcinog Mutagen* 1992;12(2):79.

80 Hara Y. Influence of tea catechins on the digestive tract. *J Cell Biochem Suppl* 1997;27:52-58.

81 Mizuno S, et al. A multi-institute case-control study on the risk factors of developing pancreatic cancer. *Jpn J Clin Oncol* 1992;22(4):286.

82 Berwick M, et al. Chemoprevention of aerodigestive cancer. *Cancer Metastasis Rev* 1997;16(3-4):329-47.

83 Mukhtar H, et al. Green tea and skin—anticarcinogenic effects. *J Invest Dermatol* 1994;102(1):3-7.

84 Katiyar S, et al. Protection against induction of mouse skin papillomas with low and high risk of conversion to malignancy by green tea and polyphenols. *Carcinogenesis* 1997;18(3):497-502.

85 Ley R, et al. Chemoprevention of ultraviolet radiation-induced skin cancer. *Environ Health Perspect* 1997;105(Suppl 4):981-84.

86 Gensler H, et al. Prevention of photocarcinogenesis by topical administration of pure epigallocatechin gallate isolated from green tea. *Nutr Cancer* 1996;26(3):325-35.

87 Klaunig J, et al. Chemopreventive effects of green tea components on hepatic carcinogenesis. *Prev Med* 1992;21(4):510-19.

88 Cao J, et al. Chemopreventive effects of green and black tea on pulmonary and hepatic carcinogenesis. *Fundam Appl Toxicol* 1996;29(2):244-50.

89 Katiyar S, et al. Protection against N-nitrosodiethylamine and benzopyrene-induced forestomach and lung tumorigenesis in A/J mice by green tea. *Carcinogenesis* 1993;14(5):849-55.

90 Lee I, et al. Chemopreventive effect of green tea against cigarette smoke-induced mutations in humans. *J Cell Biochem Suppl* 1997;27:68-75.

91 Majima T, et al. Inhibitory effects of beta-carotene, palm carotene, and green tea polyphenols on pancreatic carcinogenesis initiated by N-nitrosobis(2-oxopropyl)amine in Syrian golden hamsters. *Pancreas* 1998;16(1):13-18.

92 Asano Y, et al. Effect of (-)-epigallocatechin gallate on leukemic blast cells from patients with acute myeloblastic leukemia. *Life Sci* 1997;60(2):135-42.

93 Gao F, et al. Studies on mechanisms and blockade of carcinogenic action of female sex hormones. *SCI CHINA B* 1994;37(4):418-29.

94 Kaegie E. Unconventional therapies for cancer: 2. Green tea. *CMAJ* 1998;158(8):1033-35.

95 Sugiyama K, et al. Green tea suppresses D-galactosamine-induced liver injury in rats. *Biosci Biotechnol Biochem* 1998;62(3):609-11.

96 Yokozawa T, et al. Proof that green tea tannin suppresses the increase in the blood methylguanidine level associated with renal failure. *Exp Toxicol Pathol* 1997;49(1-2):117-22.

97 Sato Y, et al. Possible contribution of green tea drinking habits to the prevention of stroke. *Tohoku J Exp Med* 1989;157(4):337-43.

98 Ali M, et al. A potent thromboxane formation inhibitor in green tea leaves. *Prostaglandins Leukot Essent Fatty Acids* 1990;40(4):281-83.

99 Yutoku S, et al. Radioprotective effects of (-)-epigallocatechin 3-O-gallate in mice. *Life Sci* 1992;50(2):147-52.

100 Taniguchi T, et al. A hypotensive constituent in hot water extracts of green tea. *Yakugaku Zasshi* 1988;108(1):77-81.

101 Briggs G, et al. Drugs in Pregnancy and Lactation, ed. 3. Baltimore, MD: Williams and Wilkins, 1990.

102 Mills J, et al. Moderate caffeine use and the risk of spontaneous abortion and intrauterine growth retardation. *JAMA* 1993;269(5):593.

103 Nagata C, et al. Association of coffee, green tea, and caffeine intakes with serum concentrations of estradiol and sex hormone-binding globulin in premenopausal Japanese women. *Nutr Cancer* 1998;30(1):21-24.

104 Shirai T, et al. Epigallocatechin gallate-induced histamine release in patients with green tea-induced asthma. *Ann Allergy Asthma Immunol* 1997;79(1):65-69.

105 Wang Z, et al. Interaction of epicatechins derived from green tea with rat hepatic cytochrome P-450. *Drug Metab Dispos* 1988;16(1):98-103.

106 Shiozaki T, et al. Effect of tea extracts, catechin, and caffeine against type-I allergic reaction. *Yakugaku Zasshi* 1997;117(7):448-54.

107 Mirbod S, et al. Some aspects of occupational safety and health in green tea workers. *Ind Health* 1995;33(3):101-17.

108 Merhav H, et al. Tea drinking and microcytic anemia in infants. *Am J Clin Nutr* 1985;41:1210.

109 Kubota K, et al. Effect of green tea on iron absorption in elderly patients with iron deficiency anemia. *Nippon Ronen Igakkai Zasshi* 1990;27(5):555-58.

Guar Gum

SCIENTIFIC NAME(S): *Cyamopsis tetragonolobus* (L.) Taub. synonymous with *C. psoralioides* DC. Family: Fabaceae or Leguminosae.

COMMON NAME(S): Guar, guar flour, jaguar gum

BOTANY: The guar plant is a small nitrogen-fixing annual that bears pods, each containing a number of seeds. Native to tropical Asia, the plant grows throughout India and Pakistan and has been grown in the southern United States since the beginning of the twentieth century.[1]

HISTORY: Guar gum is a dietary fiber obtained from the endosperm of the Indian cluster bean. The endosperm can account for more than 40% of the seed weight and is separated and ground to form commercial guar gum.

Guar gum has been used for centuries as a thickening agent for foods and pharmaceuticals. It continues to find extensive use for these applications and also is used by the paper, textile and oil drilling industries.

CHEMISTRY: Guar is a polysaccharide galactomannan that forms a viscous gel when placed in contact with water. It forms solutions that range from slightly acidic to neutral pH. Even at low concentrations (1% to 2%) guar gum forms gels in water. The viscosity of these gels is generally unaffected by the pH of the solution.

Food grade guar gum contains approximately 80% guaran (a galactomannan composed of D-mannose and D-galactose units) with a molecular weight of about 220,000. Guar gum is not a uniform product, however, and its viscosity may vary in proportion to the degree of galactomannan cross-linking.

PHARMACOLOGY:

Hyperlipidemia: Guar gum has been shown to decrease serum total cholesterol levels by about 10% to 15% and low density lipoprotein-cholesterol (LDL-cholesterol) by up to 25% without any significant effect on triglycerides or high density lipoprotein-cholesterol (HDL-cholesterol) levels.[2] In their comprehensive review of the lipid lowering effects of guargum, Todd et al described a general hypothesis for the mechanism of this action: guar reduces cholesterol absorption and increases bile excretion leading to increased hepatic turnover of cholesterol. It has been suggested that the effects of guar on LDL-cholesterol metabolism are similar to those of the bile-sequestering agents.[3] Alterations in appetite and dietary intake also may contribute to the lipid lowering effects of guar. Studies of the hypocholesterolemic effects of guar have generally enrolled a small number of patients treated for short periods of time (up to 3 months). Placebo-controlled trials using uncoated granules have demonstrated decreases of up to 15% in total cholesterol[4] while at least one study found no significant change from baseline after 4 months of treatment.[5] Other formulations (powders, crispbread, flavored formulas) have demonstrated decreases of 10% to 15% in total cholesterol and LDL-cholesterol following as little as 2 weeks of treatment.[6] Doses generally have ranged from 12 to 15 g/day. Mixtures of water-soluble dietary fibers (psyllium, pectin, guar, locust bean gum) have been shown to decrease plasma total cholesterol by 10% after 4 weeks with a 14% reduction in LDL-cholesterol; no changes were observed in HDL-cholesterol, VLD-cholesterol, or triglycerides.[7] The addition of guar gum to lovastatin (*Mevacor*) therapy resulted in a larger decrease in total cholesterol levels (44%) compared to lovastatin alone (34%) after 18 weeks of treatment.[8]

Diabetes mellitus: The ability of guar to affect gastrointestinal transit may contribute to its hypoglycemic activity. Guar reduces post-prandial glucose and insulin levels in both healthy and diabetic subjects and may be a useful adjunct in the treatment of non-insulin-dependent diabetes.[9-13] These effects seem to be most pronounced when large amounts of guar gum are added to the diet, however, and when the fiber is administered with the glucose or food.[14] Furthermore, when dietary fats and proteins are not adequately controlled in the diabetic diet, the addition of guar has been shown to have little effect on postprandial glucose or C-peptide responses.[15]

Weight Loss/GI Uses: Preparations containing guar gum have been used extensively to promote normal gastrointestinal motility and to maintain fecal bulk.[16] Guar preparations may significantly delay gastric emptying time or gastrointestinal transit, but these effects seem most related to the nature of the meal and diet. Because bulk-forming fibers may impart a "feeling of fullness," they have been used to help curb appetite. Although the effectiveness of fiber products as appetite suppressants is controversial, they remain important ingredients in over-the-counter weight loss preparations. Even in the absence of weight loss, guar supplementation for 2 weeks reduced blood pressure by 9% in moderately overweight men.[17] Enzymatically modified guar gum added to enteral formulas has been shown to increase gastrointestinal transit time and to increase fecal nitrogen excretion.[18]

TOXICOLOGY: In the colon, guar gum is fermented to short-chain fatty acids. Both guar and its resultant by-products do not appear to be absorbed by the gut. The most common adverse effects, therefore, are gastrointestinal, including gastrointestinal pain, nausea, diarrhea, and flatulence. Approximately half of those taking guar experience flatulence; this usually occurs early in treatment and resolves with continued use. Starting with doses of about 3 g three times a day, not to exceed 15 g per day, can minimize gastrointestinal effects.[19]

Guar gum may affect the absorption of concomitantly administered drugs. Bezafibrate, acetaminophen (eg, *Tylenol*), digoxin (eg, *Lanoxin*), glipizide (eg, *Glucotrol*) or glyburide (eg, *DiaBeta*, *Micronase*)[20] are generally unaffected by concomitant administration.[2] The ingestion of more than 30 g of guar per day by diabetic patients did not adversely affect mineral balances after 6 months.[21]

Guar gum in a weight-loss product has been implicated in esophageal obstruction in a patient who exceeded the recommended dosage.[22] In a recent review, 18 cases of esophageal obstruction, seven cases of small bowel obstruction, and possibly one death were associated with the use of *Cal-Ban 3000*, a guar gum-containing diet pill.[23] The water-retaining capacity of the gum permits it to swell to 10- to 20-fold and may lead to luminal obstruction, particularly when an anatomic predisposition exists. Guar always should be taken with large amounts of liquid. Occupational asthma has been observed among those working with guar gum.[24]

Because of its potential to affect glycemic control, guar gum should be used cautiously by diabetic patients.

Guar gum is not teratogenic nor does it significantly affect reproduction in rats.[25]

SUMMARY: Guar gum forms a mucilaginous mass when hydrated. This material has been shown to reduce total serum cholesterol and LDL-cholesterol levels by approximately 10% to 15% when taken for 3 months. In addition, guar has been found to reduce post-prandial insulin and glucose levels and appears to be a useful adjunct in the management of non-insulin-dependent diabetes mellitus. Guar is used as a common food additive and is not associated with adverse effects in the low quantities generally used in foods. Severe gastrointestinal obstructions have been reported with the use of some guar-containing dietary supplements.

PATIENT INFORMATION – Guar Gum

Uses: Guar gum is a food additive shown to reduce serum cholesterol with prolonged use. It appears useful for managing blood glucose. It has been used to promote weight loss.

Side Effects: Guar gum may cause GI obstruction. It should be used cautiously with diabetics. Flatulence and other forms of GI distress are common during initial use.

---

[1] Leung AY, *Encyclopedia of Common Natural Ingredients Used in Food, Drugs and Cosmetics.* New York, NY: John Wiley and Sons, 1980.
[2] Todd PA, et al. *Drugs* 1990;39:917.
[3] Turner PR, et al. *Atherosclerosis* 1990;81:145.
[4] Aro A, et al. *Am J Clin Nutr* 1984;39:911.
[5] Tuomilehto J, et al. *Acta Med Scand* 1980;208:45.
[6] Jenkins DJA, et al. *Am J Clin Nutr* 1979;32:16.
[7] Jensen CD, et al. *J Am Coll Nutr* 1993;12:147.
[8] Uusitupa MI, et al. *Arterioscler Throm* 1992;12:806.
[9] Smith U and Holm G. *Atherosclerosis* 1982;45:1.
[10] Aro A, et al. *Diabetologia* 1981;21:29.
[11] Lakhdar A, et al. *Br Med J* 1988;296:1471.
[12] Kirsten R, et al. *Int J Clin Pharmacol Ther Toxicol* 1992;30:582.
[13] Landin K, et al. *Am J Clin Nutr* 1992;56:1061.
[14] Nuttall FQ. *Diabetes* 1993;42:503.
[15] Sels JP, et al. *Horm Metab Res Suppl* 1992;26:52.
[16] Rajala SA, et al. *Comp Gerontol* 1988;2:83.
[17] Krotkiewski M. *Acta Med Scand* 1987;222:43.
[18] Lampe JW, et al. *J Parenter Enteral Nut* 1992;16:538.
[19] Tuomilehto J, et al. *Atherosclerosis* 1989;76:71.
[20] Uusitupa M, et al. *Int J Clin Pharmacol Ther Toxicol* 1990;28:153.
[21] Behall KM, et al. *Diabetes Care* 1989;12:357.
[22] *Australian Adverse Drug Reactions Bulletin* August, 1989.
[23] Lewis JH. *Am J Gastroenterol* 1992;87:1424.
[24] Lagier F, et al. *J Allergy Clin Immunol* 1990;85:785.
[25] Collins TF, et al. *Food Chem Toxicol* 1987;25:807.

Guarana

SCIENTIFIC NAME(S): Paullinia cupana Kunth var. *sorbilis* (Mart.) Ducke or *P. sorbilis* (L.) Mart. Family: Sapindaceae

COMMON NAME(S): Guarana, guarana paste or gum, Brazilian cocoa, Zoom

BOTANY: Guarana is the dried paste made from the crushed seeds of *P. cupana* or *P. sorbilis*, a fast-growing woody perennial shrub native to Brazil and other regions of the Amazon.[1] It bears orange-yellow fruits that contain up to 3 seeds each. The seeds are collected and dry-roasted over fire. The kernels are ground to a paste with cassava and molded into cylindrical sticks, which are then sun-dried. Today, the most common forms of guarana include syrups, extracts, and distillates used as flavorings and a source of caffeine by the soft drink industry. Guarana also is used as an ingredient in herbal weight loss preparations usually in combination with ma huang.

HISTORY: Guarana has played an important role in the Amazonian Indians' society. It is often taken during periods of fasting to improve tolerance of dietary restrictions. In certain regions, the extract is believed to be an aphrodisiac and to protect from malaria and dysentery.[2,3] In the 19th century, guarana became popular as a stimulating drink in France,[1] and in 1880 was introduced as an official drug in the US Pharmacopeia, where it remained listed until 1910.[4] Natural diet aids, which rely on daily doses of guarana, have been advertised in the lay press. Guarana is occasionally combined with glucomannan in natural weight loss tablets. The advertisements indicate that the ingredients in guarana have the same chemical makeup as caffeine and cocaine but can be used for weight reduction without any of the side effects of these drugs. This is not entirely correct.

The stems, leaves, and roots of guarana are used as a fish-killing drug in Central and South America.

PHARMACOLOGY: Guarana is used by Brazilian Indians in a stimulating beverage used like tea or coffee; it is sometimes mixed with alcohol to prepare a more intoxicating beverage. In 1840, caffeine was identified as guarana's principal constituent, with a level ranging from 3% to greater than 5% by dry weight.[2]

By comparison, coffee beans contain ≈ 1% to 2% caffeine and dried tea leaves vary from 1% to 4% caffeine content.[5] The related alkaloids theophylline and theobromine have also been identified in the plant. Guarana is

also high in tannins (primarily catechutannic acid and catechol), present in a concentration of 5% to 6% dry weight; these impart an astringent taste to the product. Guarana contains no cocaine.

The appetite suppressant effect is related to the caffeine content. The "zap of energy" that guarana tablets are reported to give is also due to caffeine. This stimulating effect is so widely recognized that guarana is sometimes called "Zoom."

Trace amounts of a saponin known as timbonine, related to compounds reported in timbo fish poisons used by Amazonian Indians, have been reported.[2]

Guarana extracts have been shown to inhibit aggregation of rabbit and human platelets following either parenteral or oral administration, possibly due to inhibition of platelet thromboxane synthesis.[6]

Some researchers claim that part of the revitalizing effects of guarana may be because of its antioxidant action.[7]

Numerous investigational studies have shown the ability of the sympathetic stimulant ephedrine, when coupled with caffeine, to have a synergistic effect on increasing metabolic rates with subsequent increased energy expenditure (thermogenesis), and to have lipolytic effects.[8] These effects have resulted in a statistically significant weight loss in animal and human trials when combined with diet.

In one animal study, behavioral effects in rats and mice subsequent to acute and chronic guarana administration were observed.[7] In this study, groups of animals treated with guarana in doses of 2000 mg/kg showed no difference when compared with control groups for the parameters of motor activity, tremor, or salivation. Another study showed an increase in physical capacity when mice were subjected to a stressful situation, such as forced swimming, after 3 to 6 months of guarana treatment.[9]

There are few human clinical trials concerning the safety and efficacy of guarana. In a small study, 3 groups of normal volunteers ranging from 20 to 35 years of age were given either placebo, 25 mg caffeine, or 1000 mg of guarana containing 2.1% caffeine daily. After 4 days, no reproducible improvement in cognition was noted in any group using neuropsychological testing, assessment of sleep quality, and a State-Trait Anxiety Inventory.[10] In another study, the effects of long-term administration of guarana on the cognition of healthy, elderly volunteers were studied. Guarana did not cause statistically significant memory improvement.[11]

TOXICOLOGY: There are no published reports describing severe toxicity from guarana, but people sensitive to caffeine should use guarana with caution. This includes patients taking herbal weight loss preparations. Guarana use has led to excessive nervousness and insomnia. Use

of guarana is contraindicated in pregnancy and lactation.[12] Given its high tannin content, excessive use may lead to an increased risk of cancer of the oropharynx.

SUMMARY: Guarana contains high concentrations of caffeine and related alkaloids and its pharmacologic effects are similar to those of coffee or tea. Commercially available weight-reduction products containing caffeine offer standardized quantities of caffeine at often lower prices than those containing guarana. Use guarana with caution in people with cardiovascular disease. The use of guarana as a natural energizer and weight loss aid cannot be recommended and should be discouraged unless used as a flavoring agent in beverages and in patients without contraindications to caffeine ingestion.

PATIENT INFORMATION – Guarana

Uses: Guarana has been used as a natural energizer, cognitive stimulant, flavoring for beverages, and as a component in natural weight loss products; however, it cannot be recommended as a natural energizer or weight loss aid.

Side Effects: Excessive nervousness, insomnia, and other health risks in patients sensitive to caffeine.

---

[1] Angelucci E, et al. Chemical evaluation of guarana seed (Paullinia cupana var. *sorbilis* Ducke). *Bol Inst Tecnol Aliment* 1978;56:183-92.

[2] Henman A. Guarana (Paullinia cupana var. *sorbilis*): ecological and social perspectives on an economic plant of the central Amazon basin. *J Ethnopharmacol* 1982;6(3):311-38.

[3] Lewis W, et al. *Medical Botany: Plants Affecting Man's Health.* New York: Wiley, 1977.

[4] Steinmetz E. Guarana. *Quart J Crude Drug Res* 1965:749-51.

[5] Der Marderosian A, et al. *Natural Product Medicine: A Scientific Guide to Foods, Drugs, Cosmetics.* Philadelphia, PA: G.F. Stickley Co., 1988.

[6] Bydlowski S, et al. An aqueous extract of guarana (Paullinia cupana) decreases platelet thromboxane synthesis. *Braz J Med Biol Res* 1991;24(4):421-24.

[7] Mattei R, et al. Guarana (Paullinia cupana): toxic behavioral effects in laboratory animals and antioxidants activity in vitro. *J Ethnopharmacol* 1998;60(2):111-16.

[8] Breum L, et al. Comparison of an ephedrine/caffeine combination and dexfenfluramine in the treatment of obesity. A double-blind multi-centre trial in general practice. *Int J Obes Relat Metab Disord* 1994;18(2):99-103.

[9] Espinola E, et al. Pharmacological activity of Guarana (Paullinia cupana Mart.) in laboratory animals. *J Ethnopharmacol* 1997;55(3):223-29.

[10] Galduroz J, et al. Acute effects of the Paulinia cupana, "Guarana" on the cognition of normal volunteers. *Rev Paul Med* 1994;112(3):607-11.

[11] Galduroz J, et al. The effects of long-term administration of guarana on the cognition of normal, elderly volunteers. *Rev Paul Med* 1996;114(1):1073-78.

[12] Brinker F. *Herb Contraindications and Drug Interactions.* 2nd ed. Sandy, OR: Eclectic Medical Publications, 1998.

Guayule

SCIENTIFIC NAME(S): *Parthenium argentatum* A. Gray Family: Asteraceae

COMMON NAME(S): Guayule (pronounced "why-oo-lay")

BOTANY: Guayule is a common shrub native to the Chihuahuan desert of northern Mexico and the adjacent Big Bend region of Texas. The plant can be readily grown in the arid regions of the southwestern US.

HISTORY: Guayule had a history as a domestic source of rubber. In the early 1900s, guayule accounted for almost 50% of all the natural rubber consumed in the US and 10% of consumption worldwide.[1] A variety of factors, including the Great Depression and the Mexican Revolution, combined to destroy the industry. The US mounted an intensive research program under the Emergency Rubber Project to identify a domestic source of natural rubber as supplies from Southeast Asia dwindled because of World War II. The work led to the re-evaluation of guayule. The project was ended after the war, following the development of synthetic rubber and the return of cheap *Hevea* rubber. In 1977, interest in guayule was renewed when the National Research Council noted that the increasing demand for imported natural rubber could result in domestic shortages. The escalating price and variable supply of foreign petroleum, along with the great advantage that guayule can be harvested mechanically, made guayule rubber production attractive from both economic and national security standpoints.[2]

CHEMISTRY: The physical and chemical properties of guayule rubber, which is composed of polymeric cisisoprenoid units, are essentially identical to those of *Hevea* rubber. Guayule rubber is found in parenchymatous cells of the stem and root tissue as a latex.[3] Studies of over 75 native guayule plants have identified at least three prominent plant forms, termed Groups I, II and III, which differ in their leaf shape, trichome morphology and rubber content.[4] Rubber levels range from about 17% in Group I to 6% in Group III. Guayule grows in close association with a related desert plant, *P. incanum* (mariola). Morphologic and biochemical data indicate the presence of mariola genes in Group II and III guayule, resulting in morphologic changes and decreased rubber content. Group II plants are the most common, and the development of higher rubber-bearing plants should be guided by genetic assessments of guayule stock. Cross-breeding methods have been used to develop improved-yield varieties, and the application of bioinducers can stimulate the production of latex, with a resultant 2– to 6–fold increase in the amount of rubber.[5]

The processing of guayule plants leaves behind several by-products that may add to the economic value of guayule rubber production. The process yields large amounts of woody fiber (bagasse), which may serve as a fuel or in the manufacture of paper. To obtain a high-quality rubber, it is necessary to deresinate the crude product. The resin fraction may equal the rubber content. This resin has too high a boiling point to be used as gasoline, but it might be converted to an automotive diesel fuel.[6] Acetone extracts of woody guayule tissue have as their major components sesquiterpene esters composing 10% to 15% of the total, triterpenoids accounting for 27% and fatty acid triglycerides accounting for 7% to 19%. The sesquiterpenes are in part artifacts of heat processing. The major triterpene compounds are C-30 argentatins. Organic acid content varies, but the major aromatic acid is cinnamic acid and the major fatty acid is linoleic acid.

Aqueous extraction yields polysaccharides accounting for 63% of the extract. These are not a good source of fermentable sugars.[7] Guayule had been seen as a potential economic boon to poor native American Indians. Similar to proposals for jojoba, guayule represents an easily grown, economically sound, renewable resource that may be cultivated in economically depressed areas of the southwest.

In recent studies, researchers have found that guayule plants accumulate large amounts of rubber inside the stem tissue parenchyma cells. The rubber particles develop packed within discrete organelles. These are made up mainly of a lipophilic, cis-polyisoprene core, small amounts of lipids and various proteins (most abundant is the M53,000 rubber particle proteins [RPP]). Based on cDNA cloning and spectroscopic analyses, RPP has been placed in the CYP74 family of P450s and further established it as the first P450 localized in rubber particles as well as the first eukaryotic P450 to be identified outside endoplasmic reticulums, mitochondrion or plastids. One researcher has described the sesquiterpenes, guayulins C and D in guayule.

TOXICOLOGY: Guayule contains a potent contact allergen, long known to pose a hazard to guayule farmers and processing-plant employees.[10] More recent investigations of acetone extracts resulted in the isolation of guayulin-A, a potent elicitor of contact dermatitis. This sesquiterpene cinnamic acid ester induces strong erythema in animals within 24 hours of application in concentrations as low as 0.003% (0.5 nM), which persists for almost 2 weeks. The compound is present in stems and leaves at levels of 0.05% to 0.3%. Guayule processing plants are now designed to minimize worker contact with resins. The allergenicity of guayulin-A may cause unexpected difficulties in the cross-breeding of *Parthenium* species to develop high-yield strains. Guayule readily undergoes hybridization with mariola and *P. tomentosum* var. stramonium, close desert relatives. These species contain sesquiterpene lactones that are cytotoxic and produce skin reactions in persons sensitized to other species of Asteraceae. Preliminary investigations of crosses of *P. tomentosum* with guayule indicate the presence of guayulin-A and stramonin-B (a cytotoxic pseudoguaianolide) in the first generation of experimental hybrids.[11]

SUMMARY: Guayule is slowly becoming an economically important rubber substitute, although its commercial development has not been as rapid as once hoped. Its more widespread cultivation may result in an increased incidence of allergic dermatitis among guayule farmers.

Guayule rubber plant is made up of a cis-polyisoprene core. The sesquiterpenes guayulin C and D have been described.

PATIENT INFORMATION – Guayule

Uses: Guayale is used in the production of rubber. Its use as a fuel is being investigated.

Side effects: Contact with Guayule can cause strong erythema. The potency of its allergen (guayulin A) has been equated to that of poison ivy.

---

[1] Maugh TH. *Science* 1977;196:1189.
[2] McIntyre D. *Rubber World* 1979;(Sep):50.
[3] Loyd FE. *Plant Physiol* 1932;7:31.
[4] Mehta IJ, et al. *Am J Botany* 1979;66:796.
[5] Yokoyama H, et al. *Science* 1977;197:1076–7.
[6] Lipinsky ES. *Science* 1978;199:644–5.
[7] Schloman WW, et al. *J Agr Food Chem* 1983;31:873.
[8] Pan Z. *J Biol Chem* 1995;270(15):8487–94.
[9] Martinez M, et al. *J Nat Prod* 1986;49(6):1102–3.
[10] Smith LM, Hughes RP. *Arch Derm & Syph* 1938;38:778.
[11] Rodriguez E, et al. *Science* 1981;211:1444–5.

Guggul

SCIENTIFIC NAME(S): *Commiphora mukul* Family: Burseracaea.

COMMON NAME(S): Guggul, guggal, gum guggal, gum guggulu

BOTANY: The guggul plant is widely distributed throughout India and adjacent regions. It is in the same genus as *C. myrrha*, the myrrh of the Bible.

HISTORY: The plant has been used in traditional Ayurvedic medicine (Asiatic Indian plant medicine) for centuries in the treatment of a variety of disorders,[1] most notable arthritis and as a weight-reducing agent in obesity.[2] More recently, extracts of the plant have been investigated for their ability to reduce serum lipid levels. A commercial product (*Guggulow*) has been introduced in the US touting the cholesterol-lowering properties of the plant. This has raised interest in the activity of the plant.

CHEMISTRY: Essentially, all of the published research on the plant and its extracts has originated in India. Several pharmacologically active components have been identified in the plant, including guggulsterone[3] and gugulipid (found in the ethyl acetate extract of the plant).[4]

PHARMACOLOGY: A number of studies have investigated the lipid-lowering activity of guggulsterone and guggul extract. In rats, ingestion of guggulsterone resulted in hypolipidemic activity, which was mediated primarily through an increase of up to 87% in hepatic binding sites for LDL-cholesterol.[3] These findings have been confirmed in other animal studies in which the ethyl acetate extract of guggul, given together with extracts of *Allium sativum* and *Allium cepa*, prevented significant rises in serum cholesterol and serum triglyceride levels induced by an atherogenic diet.[5] These treatments also conferred protection against diet-induced atherosclerosis. By comparison, a mixture of guggul and garlic powder was more effective in reducing lipid levels in dogs and monkeys than treatment with guggul alone.[6]

Similar findings have been observed in man. When treated with 500 mg of gugulipid for 12 weeks, a significant lowering of serum cholesterol (24% average) and serum triglycerides (23% average) was observed in 80% of patients.[7] A crossover follow-up to this preliminary investigation compared gugulipid to the antihyperlipidemic drug clofibrate (eg, *Atromid-S*) in 233 patients. With gugulipid, the average fall in serum cholesterol and triglycerides was 11% and 17%, respectively. These effects were evident within 3 to 4 weeks of starting therapy. Hypercholesterolemic patients responded better to the gugulipid therapy than did hypertriglyceridemic patients. HDL-cholesterol increased in 60% of responders to gugulipid therapy, but clofibrate had no effect on this parameter.[7]

Furthermore, guggulsterone has been shown to exhibit thyroid-stimulating activity.[8] It has also been shown to exert a protective effect on cardiac enzymes and the cytochrome P450 system against drug-induced myocardial necrosis.[9] Extracts of the plant also have an anti-inflammatory action and inhibit carrageenan-induced rat paw edema.[10]

TOXICOLOGY: While the human safety profile of the extract has not been well described, no significant adverse events were reported in clinical studies; the reported events were primarily gastrointestinal in nature.

SUMMARY: Guggul and its extracts have been used for centuries in traditional Indian medicine. A growing body of evidence suggests that components of the plant can exert a lipid-lowering effect possible equivalent to that of the drug clofibrate.

PATIENT INFORMATION – Guggul

Uses: Traditionally used to treat arthritis, obesity and other disorders, guggul has been shown to lower cholesterol and triglycerides and to stimulate thyroid activity.

Side Effects: Adverse GI effects have been reported.

---

[1] Antarkar DS, et al. *J Postgrad Med* 1984;30:111.
[2] Satyavati GV. *Indian J Med Res* 1988;87:327.
[3] Singh V, et al. *Pharmacol Res* 1990;22:37.
[4] Gopal K, et al. *Assoc Physicians India* 1986;34:249.
[5] Lata S, et al. *J Postgrad Med* 1991;37:132.
[6] Dixit VP, et al. *Biochem Exp Biol* 1980;16:421.
[7] Niyanand S, et al. *J Assoc Physicians India* 1989;3:323.
[8] Tripathi YB, et al. *Planta Med* 1984;1:78,
[9] Kaul S, et al. *Indian J Med Res* 1989;90:62.
[10] Duwiejua M, et al. *Planta Med* 1993;59:12.

Gymnema

SCIENTIFIC NAME(S): *Gymnema sylvestre* R.Br. It has been referred to in some texts as *Asclepias geminata* Roxb., *Gymnema melicida* Edg., and *Periploca sylvestris* Willd.[1] Family: Asclepiadaceae

COMMON NAME(S): Meshashringi, gurmar, merasingi

BOTANY: *Gymnema sylvestre* is commonly found in Africa and India. Its distribution has become worldwide however, and it is recognized in the traditional medicinal literature of many countries including Australia, Japan and Vietnam. The leaves are most commonly used, but the stem also appears to have some pharmacologic action.

HISTORY: Gymnema has played an important role in Ayurvedic medicine for centuries. Its use has been confined primarily to the management of diabetes and similar hypo/hyperglycemic conditions. As early as 1930 the pharmacologic effect of the plant was being investigated.[2] The plant has been used alone and as a component of the Ayurvedic medicinal compound "Tribang shila," a mixture of tin, lead, zinc, *G. sylvestre* leaves, neem (*Melia azadirachta*) leaves, *Enicostemma littorale*, and jambul (*Eugenia jambolana*) seeds. The plant also is used in traditional African medicine.

More recently, the plant has been identified by the natural products industry in North America and Europe and a number of commercial over-the-counter herbal products are now available that contain varying amounts of gymnema. These products generally are associated with an ability to control blood glucose levels or to contribute to overall metabolic control.

CHEMISTRY: Few studies have closely investigated the details of the composition of *G. sylvestre*. It appears that the compound gymnemic acid (gymnemin) maybe responsible for most of the plant's pharmacologic activity. Gymnemic acid also has been identified in a number of related members of the Asclepiadaceae and represents a mixture of at least nine closely related acidic glycosides, the major component being gymnemic acid A1.[3]

PHARMACOLOGY: A number of studies have evaluated the effects of *G. sylvestre* on blood sugar in animals.[4] In one typical study, rats were administered an alcoholic extract of *G. sylvestre* (100 mg/kg daily for one month) through a stomach tube. The rats were made diabetic by the administration of anterior pituitary extract.

By the second week, the mean blood sugar level was significantly lower among the animals receiving the gymnema extract (74 mg/dL) than among those who did not (106 mg/dL). This difference was maintained for the duration of the study. The blood glucose level among these treated animals was no different from a control group that did not receive pituitary or gymnema extract. These data indicated that extracts of the plant could exert a clinically measurable hypoglycemic effect in diabetic animals.[5]

In another study, *G. sylvestre* extract (100 mg/kg daily) was compared to tolbutamide (eg, *Orinase*) (5 mg/kg daily) given to rats for a month. Both treatments caused a statistically significant reduction in blood glucose levels compared to controls in normal rats after one month. Both drugs also effectively reduced blood sugar levels in diabetic rats after one month (controls: 88 mg/dL; *G. sylvestre*: 74 mg/dL; tolbutamide: 73 mg/dL).[6] These results suggested that gymnema extracts exerted a hypoglycemic effect following oral administration and that the pharmacologic effect approximated that of tolbutamide. It should be noted that the doses used would be equivalent to a 7 g dose of extract for a typical man. A more dramatic effect was noted when the extract was administered parenterally to rats.[7]

Although the exact mechanism of the plant's hypoglycemic activity has not been established, it appears to act in a manner similar to that of the sulfonylurea drugs, stimulating the release of endogenous insulin stores or perhaps by sensitizing cells to the effects of insulin.

A solution of gymnemic acid inhibits the ability to taste bitter or sweet flavors (such as quinine or sugar), but maintains the ability to taste sour, astringent or pungent substances. It is not clear whether gymnemic acid also is responsible for the hypoglycemic effect of the drug, although most evidence points in this direction.

TOXICOLOGY: Little is known about the safety of this plant. The animal studies that reported the hypoglycemic efficacy of the plant did not provide details of animal safety. The plant has not been associated with published reports of human toxicity. Because of its documented hypoglycemic effect, it is possible that as few as a dozen tablets of some otc preparations could cause a demonstrable hypoglycemic reaction in humans.

SUMMARY: *Gymnema sylvestre* is a plant that has found use in the traditional medicine of a number of societies for the management of blood sugar disorders. Pharmacologic evaluations of the plant have found it to possess hypoglycemic activity approximating that of tolbutamide. Little is known about the long-term safety of the plant, but it generally has not been associated with human toxicity. It represents one of a number of plants that should be investigated in more detail for its potential as a hypoglycemic agent.

PATIENT INFORMATION – Gymnema

Uses: The plant has been used in traditional medicine, most notably to control blood glucose.

Side Effects: Gymnema is not known to be toxic, but caution should be exercised as to its hypoglycemic effect. Gymnemic acid inhibits the ability to taste bitterness or sweetness.

---

[1] Penso G. *Inventory of Medicinal Plants Used In the Different Countries*, World Health Organization, 1982.
[2] Mhaskar KS, Caius JF. *Indian Med Res Memoirs* 1930; #16.
[3] Windholz M, ed. *The Merck Index*, ed. 10 Rahway, NJ: Merck & Co., 1983.
[4] Rahman AU, Zaman K. *J Ethropharm* 1989;26:73.
[5] Gupta SS, et al. *Indian J Med Res* 1962; Sep. 50:1.
[6] Gupta SS, Seth CB. *Indian J Med Res* 1962; Sep. 50:708.
[7] Gupta SS, Variyar MC. *Indian J Med Res* 1964; Feb. 52:200.

Hawthorn

SCIENTIFIC NAME(S): *Crataegus oxyacantha* L., *C. laevigata* (Poir.) DC, and *C. monogyna* Jacquin. Family: Rosaceae

COMMON NAME(S): Hawthorn, English hawthorn, haw, maybush, whitethorn[1]

BOTANY: Hawthorn is a spiny bush or small tree that grows up to 7.5 m in height. Its deciduous leaves are divided into three to five lobes. The white, strong-smelling flowers grow in large bunches and bloom from April to June. The spherical bright red fruit contains one nut (*C. monogyna*) or two to three nuts (*C. oxyacantha*).[1] Morphological and microscopical observation of certain Chinese hawthorn species has been performed.[2]

HISTORY: The use of hawthorn dates back to Dioscorides, but the plant gained widespread popularity in European and American herbal medicine only toward the end of the 19th century. The flowers, leaves, and fruits have been used in the treatment of either high or low blood pressure, tachycardia, or arrhythmias.[3] The plant is purported to have antispasmodic and sedative effects. Hawthorn has been used in the treatment of atherosclerosis and angina pectoris. Preparations containing hawthorn remain popular in Europe[4,5] and have gained some acceptance in the US.[6]

CHEMISTRY: The leaves, flowers, bark, and fruits contain the flavonoid pigments hyperoside and vitexin-rhamnoside, leucoanthocyanidins, and the lactone crataeguslactone (a mixture of ursolic, oleanic, and crataegolic acids).[4,7] Flavonoid constituents from hawthorn have been frequently reported.[8,9,10,11] Glycoflavonoid structural characteristics have been evaluated.[12] Procyanidine and 2,3-cis-procyanidin have been isolated from hawthorn.[13,14] Chlorogenic acid from *C. pyracantha Pers.* has been found.[15] Analysis of active hawthorn components has been reviewed.[16]

PHARMACOLOGY: Hawthorn's beneficial roles in cardiovascular disease have been extensively reviewed.[17,18,19,20] Pharmacokinetic, pharmacodynamic, and metabolic studies on hawthorn have been performed.[21,22,23]

Because of its strong cardiac activity, hawthorn has been suggested to be of use in CHF[24,25] and cardiac performance.[26] The plant is known to contain cardiotonic amines.[27] The flavonoids cause an increase in coronary flow and heart rate and a positive inotropic effect. In isolated animal hearts, the inhibition of the enzyme 3',5'-cyclic adenosine menophosphate phosphodiesterase may be a mechanism by which hawthorn exerts its cardiac actions.[28] When tested in rat cardiac myocytes, hawthorn produced strong contraction of heart tissue, along with increases in energy turnover in certain processes.[29] Another study evaluated hawthorn in combination with digoxin to treat heart disease.[30] At least one report exists on the plant's potential antiarrhythmic effects.[31]

Hawthorn flavonoid components also possess vasodilatory action.[28,32] Extracts of hawthorn dilate blood vessels, in particular coronary blood vessels, resulting in reduced peripheral resistance and increased coronary circulation. In vitro increases in coronary circulation ranging from 20% to 140% have been observed following the administration of a dose equal to ≈ 1 mg of the dry extract.[17]

Hawthorn also exhibited vasorelaxant effects in isolated rat mesenteric arteries.[33] A double-blind study of the related species *C. pinnatifida* and its effect on 46 angina cases has been performed.[34]

Hawthorn is also known to be beneficial in myocardial ischemia.[35,36] The flavonoid, monoacetyl-vitexinrhamnoside, possesses marked anti-ischemic properties in several in vitro models, suggesting improvement in myocardial perfusion.[37] Hawthorn's effects on oxygen-deprived rat heart cells have been reported.[38] The plant's influence on myocardial ischemia in dogs has also been evaluated.[39,40] Other studies concerning circulation aspects have been addressed, including peripheral arterial circulation disorder[41] and varicose symptom complex.[42]

Hawthorn has been studied in the prevention and treatment of atherosclerosis. A hawthorn preparation in combination was administered to animals, resulting in lower cholesterol, triglycerides, blood viscosity, and fibrinogen levels vs controls.[43] Another report finds tincture of hawthorn to increase bile acid excretion and decrease cholesterol synthesis in rats. The mechanism involves an up-regulation of hepatic LDL-receptors, resulting in a greater influx of cholesterol into the liver. Hawthorn was also found to enhance cholesterol degradation.[44] A drink containing hawthorn has lipid-lowering effects when studied in rats and humans.[45]

Hawthorn has been studied for its effects on hypertension.[46,47] The plant has active components which cause vasorelaxation in rat mesenteric arteries.[33]

Other effects of hawthorn include oxygen species scavenging activity,[48] anticomplementary activity,[49] and the ability to effectively treat elective mutism, a rare syndrome in which children with normal verbal capabilities refuse to speak for prolonged time periods.[50]

TOXICOLOGY: The acute parenteral LD_{50} of *Crataegus* preparations has been reported to be in the range of 18 to 34 mg/kg, with that of individual constituents ranging from 50 to 2600 mg/kg.[17] Acute oral toxicity has been reported to be in the range of 18.5 to 33.8 mg/kg.[51] In humans, low doses of hawthorn are usually devoid of adverse effects.[17] No serious adverse drug reactions have been reported from hawthorn, and it appears to be safe and effective for CHF.[24] However, higher doses have the potential to induce hypotension and sedation. The health professional and user must be aware of the potential of hawthorn to affect heart rate and blood pressure. Hawthorn may pharmacodynamically interfere with digoxin or digoxin monitoring.[52] This proposed interaction has not been documented clinically. Since digoxin has a narrow therapeutic index, it would be prudent for patients taking digoxin to avoid hawthorn.

Hawthorn extract may increase the intracellular concentrations of cyclic AMP by influencing the activity of the enzyme phosphodiesterase, and it also may influence other mechanisms that activate adenylcyclase.[17] At least one report is available on hypersensitivity reaction to hawthorn,[53] and toxiderma as a result of the fruits of the plant.[54] Hawthorn toxicity in general has been evaluated.[51]

SUMMARY: Hawthorn is often found in popular herbal remedies, in particular those marketed in Europe. It is not as popular in the US, where the literature contains relatively few *otc* products or herbal product information, although some health food stores carry the product. Hawthorn seems to have beneficial effects in cardiovascular disease such as ischemia, angina, and atherosclerosis. The plant also possesses lipid-lowering and antihypertensive actions. No major toxicities have been reported. More studies are needed to fully evaluate its potential in these conditions.

PATIENT INFORMATION – Hawthorn

Uses: Hawthorn has been used to regulate blood pressure and heart rhythm, to treat atherosclerosis and angina pectoris, and as an antispasmodic and sedative.

Drug Interactions: Hawthorn may pharmacodynamically interfere with digoxin or digoxin monitoring.

Side Effects: Hawthorn is reportedly toxic in high doses, which may induce hypotension and sedation.

---

[1] Dobelis IN. Magic and Medicine of Plants. Pleasantville, NY: Reader's Digest Association, 1986.

[2] Gao G, et al. Comparison of morphological and microscopical diagnostic characters of hawthorn fruits (*Crataegus* species). *Yao Hsueh Hsueh Pao* 1995;30(10):781-88.

[3] Stepka W, et al. A survey of the genus *Crataegus* for hypotensive activity. *Lloydia* 1973;36:431.

[4] Duke J. Handbook of Medicinal Herbs. Boca Raton, FL: CRC Press, 1985.

[5] Tyler V. The Honest Herbal: A Sensible Guide to the Use of Herbs and Related Remedies. Binghamton, NY: The Haworth Press, 1993.

[6] Rodale J. The Hawthorn Berry for the Heart. Emmaus, PA: Rodale Books, 1971.

[7] Thompson E, et al. Preliminary study of potential antiarrhythmic effects of *Crataegus monogyna*. *J Pharm Sci* 1974;63(12):1936-37.

[8] Fisel J. New flavonoids from *Crataegus* 1. Isolation of an acetylated vitexin-4′-rhamnoside from *Crataegus monogyna* L. *Arzneimittelforschung* 1965;15(12):1417-21.

[9] Fisel J. New flavonoids from *Crataegus*. 2. The isolation of a mixture from rutin and quercetin-3-rhamnogalactoside from *Crataegus monogyna* L. *Arzneimittelforschung* 1966;16(1):80-82.

[10] Lewak S. Flavonoids of hawthorn. *Postepy Biochem* 1969;15(3):425-34.

[11] Kery A, et al. Comparative study of flavonoids from *Crataegus oxyacantha* L. and *Crataegus monogyna* Jacq. *Acta Pharm Hung* 1977;47(1):11-23.

[12] Nikolov N, et al. Some structural characteristics of hawthorn glycoflavonoids. *Farm Zh* 1973;28(1):78-81.

[13] Rewerski W, et al. Pharmacological properties of oligomeric procyanidine isolated from hawthorn (*Crataegus oxyacantha*). *Arzneimittelforschung* 1971;21(6):886-88.

[14] Vanhaelen M, et al. TLC-densitometric determination of 2,3-cis-procyanidin monomer and oligomers from hawthorn (*Crataegus laevigata* and *C. monogyna*). *J Pharm Biomed Anal* 1989;7(12):1871-75.

[15] Paris R, et al. On the polyphenols of *Crataegus pyracantha* Pers.: presence of chlorogenic acid. rutoside and an eriodictyol glycoside. *Ann Pharm Fr* 1965;23(11):627-30.

[16] Oswiecimska M, et al. Therapeutic value of hawthorn extracts in the light of analysis of its active components. *Pol Tyg Lek* 1982;37(28):833-35.

[17] Hamon NW. Hawthorns. *Canad Pharm J* 1988(Nov):708, 724.

[18] Petkov V. Plants and hypotensive, antiatheromatous, and coronarodilatating action. *Am J Chin Med* 1979;7(3):197-236.

[19] Kendler B. Recent nutritional approaches to the prevention and therapy of cardiovascular disease. *Prog Cardiovasc Nurs* 1997;12(3):3-23.

[20] Miller A. Botanical influences on cardiovascular disease. *Altern Med Rev* 1998;3(6):422-31.

21 Ammon H, et al. Crataegus, toxicology, and pharmacology. Part III: Pharmacodynamics and pharmacokinetics. *Planta Med* 1981;43(4)313-22.

22 Ammon H, et al. Crataegus, toxicology, and pharmacology. Part II: Pharmacodynamics. *Planta Med* 1981;43(3):209-39.

23 Hammerl H, et al. Clinico-experimental metabolic studies using a *Crataegus* extract. *Arzneimittelforschung* 1967;21(7):261-64.

24 Weittmayr T, et al. Therapeutic effectiveness of *Crataegus*. *Fortschr Med* 1996;114(1-2):27-29.

25 Gildor A. *Crataegus oxyacantha* and heart failure. *Circulation* 1998;98(19):2098.

26 O'Conolly M, et al. Treatment of decreasing cardiac performance. Therapy using standardized crataegus extract in advanced age. *Fortschr Med* 1986;104(42):805-8.

27 Wagner H, et al. Cardioactive drugs IV. Cardiotonic amines from *Crataegus oxyacantha*. *Planta Med* 1982;45(2):98-101.

28 Schussler M, et al. Myocardial effects of flavonoids from *Crataegus* species. *Arzneimittelforschung* 1995;45(8):842-45.

29 Popping S, et al. Effect of a hawthorn extract on contraction and energy turnover of isolated rat cardiomyocytes. *Arzneimittelforschung* 1995;45(11):1157-61.

30 Wolkerstorfer H. Treatment of heart disease with a digoxin-crataegus combination. *Munch Med Wochenschr* 1966;108(8) 438-41.

31 Thompson E, et al. Preliminary study of potential antiarrhythmic effects of *Crataegus monogyna*. *J Pharm Sci* 1974;63(12):1936-37.

32 Blesken R. Crataegus in cardiology. *Fortschr Med* 1992;110(15):290-92.

33 Chen Z, et al. Endothelium-dependent relaxation induced by hawthorn extract in rat mesenteric artery. *Life Sci* 1998;63(22):1983-91.

34 Weng W, et al. Therapeutic effect of *Crataegus pinnatifida* on 46 cases of angina pectoris—a double blind study. *J Tradit Chin Med* 1984;4(4):293-94.

35 Piotti L, et al. The therapeutic effect of hawthorn extract in myocardial hypoxia. *Med Klin* 1965;60(53):2142-45.

36 Massoni G. On the use of hawthorn extract (*Crataegus*) in the treatment of certain ischemic myocardial diseases in old age. *G Gerontol* 1968;16(9):979-84.

37 Schussler M, et al. Functional and antiischaemic effects of Monoacetyl-vitexinrhamnoside in different in vitro models. *Gen Pharmacol* 1995;26(7):1565-70.

38 Li L, et al. Studies on hawthorn and its active principle. II. Effects on cultured rat heart cells deprived of oxygen and glucose. *J Trad Chin Med* 1984;4(4):289-92.

39 Li L, et al. Studies on hawthorn and its active principle. I. Effect on myocardial ischemia and hemodynamics in dogs. *J Trad Chin Med* 1984;4(4):283-88.

40 Lievre M, et al. Cardiovascular effects of hyperoside extracted from hawthorn in anesthetized dogs. *Ann Pharm Fr* 1985;43(5):471-77.

41 Di Renzi L, et al. On the use of injectable crataegus extracts in therapy of disorders of peripheral arterial circulation in subjects with obliterating arteriopathy of the lower extremities. *Boll Soc Ital Cardiol* 1969;14(4):577-85.

42 Gehrels P. Therapy of varicose symptom complex with Rexiluven. *Ther Ggw* 1970;109(8):1163-66.

43 He G. Effect of the prevention and treatment of atherosclerosis of a mixture of Hawthorn and Motherwort. *Chung Hsi i Chieh Ho Tsa Chih* 1990;10(6):361, 326.

44 Rajendran S, et al. Effect of tincture of *Crataegus* on the LDL-receptor activity of hepatic plasma membrane of rats fed an atherogenic diet. *Atherosclerosis* 1996;123(1-2):235-41.

45 Chen J, et al. Hawthorn (shan zha) drink and its lowering effect on blood lipid levels in humans and rats. *World Rev Nutr Diet* 1995;77:147-54.

46 Rigo J, et al. The effect of magnesium-enriched hawthorn syrup (Viroma) on experimental hypertension. *Orv Hetil* 1968;109(37):2059-60.

47 Iwamoto M, et al. Klinische wirkung con Crataegutt bein herzerhrankungen ischamischer une/oder hypertensiver genese. *Planta Med* 1981;42:1.

48 Bahorun T, et al. Oxygen species scavenging activity of phenolic extracts from hawthorn fresh plant organs and pharmaceutical preparations. *Arzneimittelforschung* 1996;46(11):1086-89.

49 Shahat T, et al. Anti-complementary activity of *Crataegus sinaica*. *Planta Medica* 1996;62(1):10-13.

50 Krohn D, et al. A study of the effectiveness of a specific treatment for elective mutism. *J Amer Acad Child Adolesc Psychiatry* 1992;31(4):711-18.

51 Ammon H, et al. Crataegus toxicology and pharmacology. *Planta Med* 1981;43:105.

52 Miller L. Herbal medicinals: selected clinical considerations focusing on known or potential drug-herb interactions. *Arch Intern Med* 1998;158(20):2200-11.

53 Steinman H, et al. Immediate-type hypersensitivity to *Crataegus monogyna*. *Contact Dermatitis* 1984;11(5):321.

54 Rogov V. Toxiderma due to the fruits of the hawthorn. *Vestn Dermatol Venerol* 1984;7:46-47.

Hibiscus

SCIENTIFIC NAME(S): *Hibiscus sabdariffa* L. Family: Malvaceae

COMMON NAME(S): Hibiscus, karkade, red tea, red sorrel, Jamaica sorrel, rosella

BOTANY: Hibiscus is native to tropical Africa but today grows throughout many tropical climates. This strong annual herb grows to 5 feet or more and produces elegant red flowers. The flowers (calyx and bract portions) are collected when slightly immature. The major producing countries are Jamaica and Mexico.[1]

HISTORY: The hibiscus has had a long history of use in Africa and neighboring tropical countries. Its fragrant flowers have been used in sachets and perfumes. Fiber from *H. sabdariffa* has been used to fashion rope as a jute substitute and the fleshy red calyx is used in the preparation of teas, drinks, jams and jellies, and the leaves have been used like spinach.[2] The plant is used widely in Egypt for the treatment of cardiac and nerve diseases[3] and has been described as a diuretic. It has been used in the treatment of cancers.[1] The mucilagenous leaves are used as a topical emollient in Africa.[4] In western countries, hibiscus flowers are often found as components of herbal tea mixtures.

CHEMISTRY: A variety of compounds have been isolated from the hibiscus plant. As expected from their vivid color, hibiscus flowers contain various anthocyanins (about 1.5%) and other pigments. Oxalic, malic, citric and tartaric acids have been identified. These, along with 15% to 28% of hibiscic acid (the lactone of a hydroxycitric acid) most likely contribute to the tartness of the herb and its teas. The flowers contain beta-sitosterol, traces of an alkaloid[5] and sitosterol-beta-D-glucoside.[6]

PHARMACOLOGY: The plant has been used as a mild laxative, an effect that may be in part due to the acids described above. However, the pharmacologic evaluation of the extract suggests that hibiscus is not an effective laxative. A 5% solution caused a slight increase in intestinal motility in vitro, while higher concentrations reduced it. Complete inhibition of intestinal motility was observed in vitro with more concentrated water extracts.[5]

When injected intravenously in dogs, a 10% aqueous extract of the flowers caused a rapid but short-lived dose-dependent decrease in mean blood pressure. The extract reduced uterine motility in vitro and had essentially no effect on respiratory rate.[5]

There is no evidence that doses of hibiscus from teas have a sedative effect.

Aqueous extracts of hibiscus appear to exert a slight antibacterial effect. Extracts have been found to inhibit the movement of human and canine taenias and a 4% solution killed the worms in about one-half hour in vitro.[5] A 15% aqueous extract prevented the growth of *Mycobacterium tuberculosis* in vitro, and 10 ml doses of a 20% extract prevented growth of the bacillus in infected rabbits.[7] However, these data require confirmation and the antibacterial effect of the plant should not be considered to be clinically relevant.

TOXICOLOGY: Hibiscus flowers are generally considered to be relatively non-toxic. However, a 30% aqueous extract of the flowers had an LD-50 of 0.4 to 0.6 ml in mice following intraperitoneal injection.[5] Animals injected with this toxic dose were dull and apathetic and died within 24 hours.

SUMMARY: Hibiscus is a popular plant whose flowers are found in numerous herbal tea preparations. The flowers contribute color and a pleasant taste to beverages. In normal concentrations, the teas would not be expected to exert any pharmacologic action.

PATIENT INFORMATION – Hibiscus

Uses: The leaves and calyxes have been used as food and the flowers steeped for tea. Hibiscus has been used in folk medicine as a diuretic, mild laxative and treatment for cardiac and nerve diseases and cancer. Mucilaginous leaves have been used as topical emollient.

Side Effects: The flowers are considered relatively non-toxic, although an injected extract killed mice within 24 hours.

[1] Leung AY. Encyclopedia of Common Natural Ingredients Used in Food, Drugs and Cosmetics. NY: J Wiley and Sons, 1980.

[2] Mabberley DJ. The PlantBook. Cambridge University Press, 1987.

[3] Osman AM et al, *Phytochemistry* 14:829, 1975.

[4] Duke JA. Handbook of Medicinal Herbs. Boca Raton, FL: CRC Press, 1985.

[5] Sharaf A, *Planta Medica* 10:48, 1962.

[6] Osman AM; Ahmad ZA et al, *Planta Med* 53:579, 1987.

[7] Sharaf A and Gineidi A, *Planta Med* 11:109, 1963.

Holly

SCIENTIFIC NAME(S): *Ilex*, *I. aquifolium*, *I. opaca* and *I. vomitoria*. Family: Aquifoliaceae

COMMON NAME(S): A number of members of the genus *Ilex* are referred to as "holly." Holly, English holly, Oregon holly and American holly are the species most often associated with the ornamental Christmas holly. Yaupon, Appalachian tea, cassena, deer berry, Indian holly, Indian black drink are also commonly discussed with the hollies.

BOTANY: The *Ilex* species are evergreen trees or shrubs with stiff leathery leaves. The flowers are often white and produce fruits that range in color from black to bright red to yellow. The plants are found throughout most of the eastern and southern United States.

The genus *Ilex* consists of over 400 species worldwide. It requires a wet and equable climate and shows a worldwide distribution, except in arctic or arid regions. The major areas of distribution are Central and South America, with Brazil alone having 60 species, and Asia which has at least 112 different species. The North American species are largely ornamental and derived from Central and South America.[1]

HISTORY: The plants in the holly family have been used as ornamentals and in herbal medicine for centuries. Early history records the European pagans offering holly branches as gifts during the Saturnalia. Early Christians decorated their homes with holly during Christmas, a practice still continued today.[1] The early settlers in the southeastern United States made yaupon tea from *I. vomitoria*, reserving a stronger decoction for use as an emetic. *I. opaca* fruit tea had been used as a cardiac stimulant by the American Indians; the Chinese had used it to treat coronary disease.

One of the most economically important species, *I. paraguayensis* or Maté tea (see separate monograph) has long been cultivated and used in Brazil and Paraguay as a tea-like beverage containing caffeine. The mixed leaves of *I. cassine*, *I. vomitoria* and *I. dahoon* were also used for another hot drink called yaupon or black drink. Drinkers used it ceremonially to "cleanse" themselves, probably due to its sweat- and vomiting-inducing effects. Another beverage made from the leaves of *I. cassine* and *I. vomitoria* was used as a stimulant tea in the Southern US during the Civil War.[1]

CHEMISTRY: A fair amount has been written about the chemistry of the holly. Most contain tannins. Analyses done on the leaves of *I. aquifolium* described the pres-ence of tannic acid, a bitter glycoside (ilicin), ilexanthin (rutin), and ilicic acid.[2] Some members of the genus, such as *I. paraguayensis* St. Hill (yerba mate) contain xanthine alkaloids such as caffeine in levels as high as 2%. Other species contain saponins and triterpenes.[3]

One review on the chemistry of *Ilex* documented hundreds of compounds isolated from *Ilex* from the late 1800s up to 1987. Selected examples of the various classes of chemical constituents include phenols and phenolic acids (p-hydroxybenzoic acid, arbutin), anthocyanins (pelargondin 3–bioside, cyanidin 3–glucoside), flavonols and flavons (rutin, kaempferol), terpenoids (alpha-amyrin, ursolic acid), sterols (sitosterol, ergosterol), purine alkaloids (caffeine, theobromine), amino acids (aspartic acid, glutamic acid), miscellaneous nitrogen compounds (trigonelline, choline), fatty acids (oleic, linolenic), alkanes and alcohols (nonacosane, mellisyl alcohol), carbohydrates (sugar alcohols, sucrose), vitamins and carotenoids (ascorbic acid, thiamine).

PHARMACOLOGY: Many *Ilex* species seem to be devoid of significant pharmacologic activity; however, some are capable of **inducing vomiting** through a local irritant action. Saponins are found in some species of *Ilex* but their absorption through intact mucosa is minimal. Saponins generally cause severe **diarrhea** and **GI upset.**

One extensive review provides a cosmopolitan view of the folkloric uses of *Ilex*. These include the use of *I. pubescens* in the traditional medicine of China for treating coronary heart disease, *I. cornuta* for dizziness and hypertension, *I. aquifolium* leaves for intermittent fevers and rheumatism as well as for its antipyretic, astringent, diuretic and expectorant properties, and the use of *I. opaca* leaves as a diuretic, tonic, purgative and cardiac stimulant. Earlier reports from the early 1930s indicate that the dried powder emulsion made from the leaves and berries of *I. aquifolium* and *I. opaca* possessed the pharmacological activity of digitalis. Several studies have confirmed the depurative, stimulant and diuretic actions of *I. paraguayensis* and related these effects to its high purine content. More recent studies have shown that *I.*

asprella constituents (asprellic acids A and C) have shown cytotoxicity against RPMI-7951 and KB cells, whereas asprellic acid B was inactive.

TOXICOLOGY: Although they are not usually considered to be poisonous, ingestion of the holly berry may cause gastrointestinal disturbances such as vomiting and diarrhea, and may result in stupor if eaten in quantity.[5] Their ingestion should be considered dangerous to small children with the probable fatal dose having been estimated to be 20 to 30 berries.[6]

A case of 2-year-old identical twins who ingested a "handful" of holly berries (*I. opaca*) has been reported.[7] Both children vomited for more than 6 hours and one became drowsy; 20 hours after ingestion, both had an episode of green watery diarrhea. Both were asymptomatic 30 hours after ingestion of the berries. This report indicated that the gastrointestinal effects associated with this plant could be so severe that its presence could cause dehydration and electrolyte imbalance. The drowsiness experienced by one of the children may have been induced by ipecac.

General schemes are available for treating holly poisoning. They involve induction of vomiting if large quantities of berries are ingested, followed by activated charcoal and a saline cathartic. Excess stimulation caused by theobromine may be countered with barbiturates or benzodiazepines. The central nervous system should be monitored.

The leaves of most species are generally considered to be nontoxic, although the spines of some leaves may tear or puncture skin and mucous membranes.

SUMMARY: Holly leaves and berries are used as common ornamentals, particularly at Christmas time. The ingestion of small amounts of holly berries may not induce toxicity; however, because of the potential for severe vomiting and diarrhea, all cases of holly berry ingestion should be referred to a physician. The leaves of some species of holly have been used to make herbal teas, but there is no evidence to indicate that they are effective in the treatment of any disorder.

While several chemical studies and some folkloric studies reveal potential for the development of medications from holly, none have reached the clinical stage to the extent that any *Ilex* can be recommended for the treatment of any disorder. One species (*I. asprella*) has antitumor properties, but it also needs further examination. *I. paraguayensis* is used in Paraguay and Brazil and is covered under a separate monograph, Maté tea.

PATIENT INFORMATION – Holly

Uses: Primarily used as a holiday decoration. Historically used in teas as an emetic and a CNS stimulant.

Side effects: Although no fatalities have been reported, 20 to 30 berries is the estimated lethal dose in small children. Ingestion can cause vomiting, diarrhea, stupor, dehydration and electrolyte imbalance.

---

[1] Alikaridis F. *J. Ethnopharmacol* 1987;20:121–44.
[2] Fournier P. *Plantes medicinales et veneneuses de France. P. [French]* Le Chevalier, Paris, 1948.
[3] West LG, et al. *Phytochemistry*, ed. 16. 1977:1846.
[4] Kashiwada Y, et al. Antitumor agents. Part 145. *J. Nat Prod* 1993 Dec;56:2077–82.

[5] Arena JA. *JAMA* 1979;242:2341.
[6] Ellis MD. *Hosp Phys* 1972 Dec 2;42–3.
[7] Rodriguez TD, et al. *Vet Hum Toxicol.* 1984;26:157.
[8] Turner N, et al. Common Poisonous Plants and Mushrooms of North America. Portland: Timber Press. 1991:155–56.

Honey

SCIENTIFIC NAME(S): Honey, clarified a strained honey, mel

COMMON NAME(S): Honey, purified honey, miel blanc (French), honig (German)

BOTANY: Honey is a bee-concentrated and processed product of the nectar of flowers of numerous plants. This saccharine secretion is deposited in honeycombs by bees (*Apis mellifera* L., Fam. *Apidae*). Most desired and flavorful honeys come from the nectar of the white clover blossom, raspberry blossom, basswood flower and many others.[1] Purified honey is prepared by melting honey at a moderate temperature, skimming off any impurities and diluting with water to a weight per milliliter of 1.35 - 1.36 g at 20°C.

HISTORY: The common and once official honey of the National Formulary used for flavoring medicinals was first known historically as a flavored sweeting agent. Its use dates back to ancient times, with Egyptian medical texts (circa between 2600 and 2200 BC) mentioning honey in at least 900 remedies.[2] Almost all early cultures universally hailed honey for its sweetening and nutritive qualities, as well as its topical healing properties for sores, wounds and skin ulcers. During wartime it was used on wounds as an antiseptic by the ancient Egyptians, Asyrians, Greeks, Romans, Chinese and even by the Germans as late as World War I.

The 1811 edition of The Edinburgh New Dispensatory states, "From the earliest ages, honey has been employed as a medicine . . . it forms an excellent gargle and facilitates the expectoration of viscid phlegm; and is sometimes employed as an emollient application to abscesses, and as a detergent to ulcers."[2] It has consistently appeared in modern use for the same purposes by the laity and medical profession alike. Today, bees are commonly kept in Europe, the Americas, Africa and Asia; at least 300,000 tons are produced annually. Honey is used directly as a sweetener or fermented into a sweet-tasting mead or *methgeiyn* beer.[3]

CHEMISTRY: Bees and other insects extract a thin, aqueous fluid (nectar) from the nectaries of various flowers. The composition of the nectar varies, but certain flowers offer distinct flavors to the different honeys. The color of honey also varies. Some honeys can be poisonous if the nectar is obtained from poisonous plants (eg, mountain laurel, jimson weed, etc). When taken in by the bee, the nectar is modified by the secretions from glands in the head and thorax so that levulose, dextrose and sucrose are formed. Honey is a thick, syrup-like liquid ranging in color from light yellow to golden borwn. It is translucent when fresh, but darkens to opacity when old and even can become granular through the crystallization of dextrose. Generally, honey has a characteristic odor and a sweet, faintly acrid taste. Honey is levorotatory and naturally mildly acidic. While honey varies a little in composition, its principle constituents are a mixture of dextrose and levulose in almost equal amounts ranging from 65 to 80 percent of one or the other. Sucrose ranges from 0.5 up to 8 percent; dextrin from 1 up to 10 percent.[1]

In recent literature there have been numerous reports on an antimicrobial honey distillate fraction and related antifungal compounds.[4,5,6,7] These studies have shown that the activity is not simply due to the high sugar content. Thus far, the active anti-microbial principles have not been fully identified.

PHARMACOLOGY: Today, as in earlier times, honey has been used as an ingredient in various cough preparations. Other reported uses include: inducing sleep, curing diarrhea and treating asthma.[2] A review of the literature from 1984 to 1995 found at least 20 scientific articles verifying honey's wound and topical ulcer healing powers. A representative sample of these include articles by: Postmes et al[8] on honey for wounds, ulcers and skin graft preservation; Ndayisaba et al[9] on an analysis of 40 cases where honey was used on wounds and which showed a positive (88% healing) effect; Bourne[10] on honey and its healing properties for leg ulcers; Greenwood[11] on the successful use of honey for superficial wounds and ulcers; and Kolmos[12] on honey as a wound-healing agent with antibacterial activity. A number of related activities and unique medical applications include: the successful use of honey for treating the gastric ulcer causative agent *Helicobacter pylori*;[13,14] its effectiveness in treating burns;[15,16,17] its usefulness in managing abdominal wound disruption in 15 patients after Caesarean section;[18] its use in treating senile cataracts[19] and postherpetic opacities of the cornea;[20] and moderate antitumor and pronounced antimetastic effects in rat and mice tumors.[21]

Interestingly, potent antibacterial peptides (apidaecins and abaecin) have been isolated and characterized in the honeybee (*apis mellifera*) itself,[22,23] and a new potent antibacterial protein named royalisin has been found in the royal jelly of the honeybee.[24]

TOXICOLOGY: Generally, honey is considered very safe as a sweet food product, a gargle and cough soothing agent, and a topical product for minor sores and wounds. However, the medical reports still show that honey can be a problem when fed to infants because some batches contain spores of *Clostridium botulinum* which can multiply in the intestines and result in botulism poisoning.[25,26] Infant botulism is seen most commonly in 2- to 3–month old infants after ingestion of botulinal spores which colonize in the gastrointestinal tract and toxin production in vivo. Infant botulism is not produced by ingestion of preformed toxin, as is the case in foodborne botulism. Clinical symptoms include constipation followed by neuromuscular paralysis (starting with the cranial nerves, then proceeding to the peripheral and respiratory musculature). Cases are frequently related to ingestion of contaminated honey, house dust and soil. Intense management under hospital emergency conditions and trivalent antitoxin are available, although use of the latter in infant botulism has not been adequately investigated.[27]

SUMMARY: Honey is widely used as a nutritive agent for its flavor and caloric value. Its topical use for various wounds and skin ulcers is very old and has been recently verified as to its efficacy. Ongoing standardization and double-blind clinical trials should continue to prove its usefulness as an antibacterial and healing agent. Care should be taken in its use in infant formulations, since botulism may result from *Clostridium botulinum* spores present in contaminated samples. Pollen in honey may also cause allergic reactions in some individuals. Recent studies on antibacterial peptides (apidaecins and abaecin) from the honeybee itself, may help explain its pharmacological activity.

PATIENT INFORMATION – Honey

Uses: Honey has been used as remedy for hundreds of ills, including as a gargle and as topical treatment for sores and wounds. Modern research lends support for this use, both in statistical findings and in isolation of antimicrobial and antifungal elements. There has been successful use of honey treating *Helicobacter pylori*, burns, wound disruption in C-section patients, senile cataracts and corneal opacities, and tumors in rats and mice.

Side Effects: Contaminated honey containing botulism spores can poison infants. Some may have allergic reactions to pollen in honey. Honey from poisonous plants can be poisonous.

---

[1] Osol A, et al. The Dispensatory of the United States of America, ed. 25. Philadelphia: Lippincott, 1960.

[2] Carper J. The Food Pharmacy. New York: Bantam Books, 1988.

[3] Klein R. The Green World: An Introduction to Plants and People, ed. 2. New York: Harper & Row, 1987.

[4] Obaseiki-Ebor E, et al. In vitro evaluation of the anticandidiasis activity of honey distillate (HY-1) compared with that of some antimycotic agents. J Pharm Pharmacol 1984;36(4):283.

[5] Radwan SS, et al. Experimental evidence for the occurrence in honey of specific substances active against microorganisms. Zentralbl Mikrobiol 1984;139(4):249.

[6] Elbagoury EF, Rasmy S. Antibacterial action of natural honey on anaerobic bacteroides. Egyptian Dental J 1993;39(1):381.

[7] Efem SE, et al. The antimicrobial spectrum of honey and its clinical significance. Infection 1992;20(4):227.

[8] Postmes T, et al. Honey for wounds, ulcers, and skin graft preservation [letter]. Lancet 1993;341(8847):756.

[9] Ndayisaba G, et al. [Clinical and bacteriological outcome of wounds treated with honey. An analysis of a series of 40 cases.] [French] Rev Chir Orthop 1993;79(2):111.

[10] Bourne IH. Honey and healing of leg ulcers [letter; comment]. J R Soc Med 1991;84(11):693.

[11] Greenwood D. Honey for superficial wounds and ulcers. Lancet 1993;341(8837):90.

[12] Kolmos HJ. [Honey: A potential wound-healing agent with antibacterial activity.] [Danish] Ugeskr Laeger 1993;155(42):3397.

[13] al Somal N, et al. Susceptibility of Helicobacter pylori to the antibacterial activity of manuka honey. J R Soc Med 1994;87(1):9.

[14] Ali AT, et al. Inhibitory effect of natural honey on Helicobacter pylori. Trop Gastroenterol 1991;12(3):139.

[15] Subrahmanyam M. Honey-impregnated gauze versus amniotic membrane in the treatment of burns. Burns 1994;20(4):331.

[16] Subrahmanyam M. Honey-impregnated gauze versus polyurethane film (OpSite) in the treatment of burns — a prospective randomised study. Br J Plast Surg 1993;46(4):322.

[17] Subrahmanyam M. Topical application of honey in treatment of burns. Br J Surg 1991;78(4):497.

[18] Phuapradit W, Saropala N. Topical application of honey in treatment of abdominal wound disruption. Aust Nz J Obstet Gynecol 1992;32(4):381.

[19] Golychev VN. [Use of honey in conservative treatment of senile cataracts]. [Russian] Vestn Oftalmol 1990;106(6):59.

[20] Mozherenkov VP. Honey treatment of postherpetic opacities of the cornea. Oftalmol Zh 1984;3:188.

[21] Gribel NV, Pashinskii VG. [The antitumor properties of honey]. [Russian] Vopr Onkol 1990;36(6):704.

[22] Casteels P, et al. Apidaecins: antibacterial peptides from honeybees. EMBO J 1989;8(8):2387.

[23] Casteels P, et al. Isolation and characterization of abaecin, a major antibacterial response peptide in the honeybe (Apis mellifera). Eur J Biochem 1990 187(2):381.

[24] Fugiwara S, et al. A potent antibacterial protein in royal jelly. Purification and determination of the primary structure of royalisin. J Biol Chem 1990;265(19):11333.

[25] Anonymous. A case of infant botulism. Communicable Disease Report. CDR Weekly 1994;4(12):53.

[26] Fenicia L, et al. A case of infant botulism associated with honey feeding in Italy. Eur J Epidemiol 1993;9(6):671.

[27] Berkow R. The Merck Manual, ed. 15. Rahway, NJ: Merck Co, 1987.

Hops

SCIENTIFIC NAME(S): *Humulus lupulus* L. Family: Moraceae or Cannabaceae

COMMON NAME(S): Hops, European hops, common hops, lupulin

BOTANY: Hops are climbing perennial plants with male and female flowers on separate plants. Hops can attain heights of 25 ft.[1] The plant is cultivated throughout the world. Commercially, the female cone-like flowering parts are collected and dried. Lupulin is composed of the separated glandular hairs, and contains more resins and volatile oil than hops, although it may also contain more adulterants.

HISTORY: The major use of hops is in the production of beer, where oxidation of the bitter principle humulene yields the characteristic flavor.[2] Extracts are used as flavors in the food and beverage industry. Traditionally, hops had been used as a diuretic and in the treatment of intestinal cramping, tuberculosis, cancer and cystitis.[1] Brewery sludge baths had been used medicinally for their rejuvenating effects and for the treatment of menstrual problems.[3]

As sedation was sometimes observed in hop pickers, the flowers were used as sedatives and were sometimes placed in pillows to relieve nervous conditions.[4] Some extracts are used as emollients in skin preparations.

CHEMISTRY: A complex mixture of compounds has been identified in hops and hops volatile oil, with more than 100 compounds having been characterized. The oil comprises approximately 1% of the plant. Resinous bitter principles are found in the plant and are composed of bitter acids including humulone and related compounds, lupulone and related compounds, and other resins.[1]

The volatile oil comprises primarily humulene (alpha-caryophyllene), myrcene, beta-caryophyllene and farnesene, which account for more than 90% of the oil fraction.[5] The gas chromatographic analysis of the essential oil often permits the identification of hops varieties, an often difficult task to accomplish using standard botanical characteristics.[6]

PHARMACOLOGY: A number of pharmacologic activities have been ascribed to hops extracts. The bitter acids (lupulone, humulone, etc) are reported to have antimicrobial activity,[1] with the more hydrophobic compounds being the most active.

In addition the extracts are said to inhibit smooth muscle spasticity. A volatile alcohol, 2-methyl-3-butene-2-ol may account in part for the sedative and hypnotic effects of the plant.[4]

A number of reports have suggested that hops contain compounds that impart estrogenic activity. An early study by Zenisek and Bednar[3] found a high level of estrogenic activity in the beta-bitter acid fraction of the plant. One poorly designed study (which subsequently became something of a legend) reported that women who participated in hops collection often began menstruating 2 days after starting to reap the hops. However, neither estrogenic nor any other hormonal activity has been observed in a variety of hops extracts tested in several animal models under carefully controlled conditions.[7]

Hops are closely related botanically to marijuana, and the smoking of hops as a mild sedative has been described.[4]

TOXICOLOGY: Extracts can be allergenic with contact dermatitis having been reported after exposure to hops pollen.[1] However, bronchial hyperresponsiveness among hops packagers occurred with an incidence similar to that observed in the normal population.[8]

SUMMARY: Hops are used widely in the commercial preparation of beer, where the degradation of certain components yields the characteristic flavor. Hops extracts have been used for a variety of medicinal purposes throughout the ages, although most of these uses have not persisted. Although hops had been used in the management of numerous ''female disorders,'' there is no evidence that hops possess estrogenic or other hormonal activity.

PATIENT INFORMATION – Hops

Uses: Hops have been used as a flavoring, diuretic, sedative and treatment for intestinal cramping, tuberculosis, cancer, cystitis, menstrual problems and nervous conditions.

Side Effects: Contact dermatitis has been reported after exposure to hops pollen.

[1] Leung AY. Encyclopedia of Common Natural Ingredients Used in Food, Drugs, and Cosmetics. New York, NY: J. Wiley and Sons, 1980.

[2] Lam KC, Deinzer ML. Tentative Identification of Humulene Diepoxides by Capillary Gas Chromatography/Chemical Ionization Mass Spectrometry. *J Agric Food Chem* 1987;35:57.

[3] Zenisek A, et al. Contribution to the Identification of the Estrogen Activity of Hops. *Am Perfumer Arom* 1960;75:61.

[4] Tyler VE. The New Honest Herbal. Philadelphia, PA: G.F. Stickley Co., 1987.

[5] Lam KC, et al. A Rapid Solvent Extraction Method for Hop Essential Oils. *J Agric Food Chem* 1986;34:63.

[6] Buttery RG, Ling LC. Identification of Hop Varieties by Gas Chromatographic Analysis of Their Essential Oils. *J Agric Food Chem* 1967;15(3):531.

[7] Fenselau C, Talalay P. Is Oestrogenic Activity Present in Hops? *Food Cosmet Toxicol* 1973;11:597.

[8] Meznar B, Kajba S. Bronchial responsiveness in hops processing workers. *Plucne Bolesti* 1990;42(1-2):27.

Horehound

SCIENTIFIC NAME(S): *Marrubium vulgare* (Tourn.) L. Family: Labiatae

COMMON NAME(S): Horehound, hoarhound, white horehound

BOTANY: Horehound is native to Europe and Asia and has been naturalized to other areas, including the United States.[1] It is a perennial aromatic herb of the mint family. The plant grows to a height of about three feet and has oval leaves covered with white, woolly hairs. Horehound bears small, white flowers in dense whorls which bloom from June to August.

HISTORY: The leaves and flower tops of the horehound have long been used in home remedies as a bitter tonic for the common cold. They are now used primarily as flavorings in liqueurs, candies and cough drops. In addition, extracts of the plant had been used for the treatment of intestinal parasites and as a diaphoretic and diuretic. A different genus, the black horehound (*Ballota nigra*), is a fetid-odored perennial native to the Mediterranean area that is sometimes used as an adulterant of white horehound.

CHEMISTRY: The bitter principle of horehound is the volatile oil marrubiin, a diterpene lactone. Some researchers believe, however, that marrubiin is an artifact, generated from premarrubiin during isolation. In addition to marrubiin, horehound contains a sterol in an esterified form that is related to compounds found in other plants of the Labiatae family, and a sesquiterpene that has two nonconjugated double bonds and can be isolated from the nonsaponifiable fraction of extracts.[2]

At least six flavonoids have been isolated from the herb: Apigerin, luteolin, apigerin 7–glycoside, luteolin 7–glycoside, quercetin 3–glycoside and quercetin 3–rhamnoglycoside. Two crystalline precipitates from horehound have been found to contain four additional unidentified flavonoids.[3] Horehound contains normal alkanes and four types of branched alkanes: 2– methylalkanes, 3–methylalkanes, 2-(omega-1)-dimethylalkanes and 3-(omega-9)-dimethylalkanes. These molecules are in the C27–C33 series, with odd-numbered chains predominant. Two- and 3- methylalkanes are present in approximately equal proportions in short-chain compounds.[4]

In a related species, *Marrubium alysson*, five known glycosides: verbascoside, leucoseptoside A, martyno-side, forsythoside B, leucosceptoside B and a new phenylpropanoid glycoside, alyssonoside, were isolated.[5]

Further constituents of horehound are essential oil made up of 0.06% mono and sesquiterpenes, 2.6% to 2.9% tannic acid, resinous substances (eg, ursolic acid), sterols (eg, beta-sitosterol), mucilaginous materials, bitter glycosides and pure marrubina (1,2,5-trimethylnaftalene).[6]

PHARMACOLOGY: Horehound has been used traditionally as an expectorant and continues to find a place in cough lozenges and cold preparations. The volatile oil has been reported to have expectorant and vasodilatory effects. Similarly, marrubiin stimulates secretion by the bronchial mucosa.[7]

A study in rats tested the hypothesis that marrubiin stimulates bile secretion. There was no evidence of this, but marrubiin acid, prduced by saponification of marrubiin, and the sodium salt of marrubiin acid did stimulate bile secretion. This effect was temporary.[8] Aqueous extracts of horehound are said to be serotonin-antagonists in vitro.[9]

In a recent study using rabbits, *Marribium vulgare* was found to have hypoglycemic effects.[10] This may be important for possible use as an antidiabetic agent.

TOXICOLOGY: Marrubiin has an LD_{50} of 370 mg/kg when administered orally to rats.[8] While marrubiin has been reported to have antiarrhythmic properties, it may also induce cardiac irregularities in larger doses.

SUMMARY: Horehound is an aromatic herb that has been widely used in folk remedies. It is most often classified as an expectorant. The active principle of the plant is marrubiin, metabolites of which may also influence bile secretion. Recently, a hypoglycemic effect has been reported. Although widely known, horehound has not been the subject of a large body of literature in the West.

PATIENT INFORMATION – Horehound

Uses: Horehound has been used as a flavoring, expectorant, vasodilator, diaphoretic, diuretic and treatment for intestinal parasites. It reportedly has hypoglycemic effects and influences bile secretion.

Side Effects: Large doses may induce cardiac irregularities.

[1] Windholz M, ed. Merck Index, ed 10. Rahway, NJ: Merck and Co., 1983.
[2] Nicholas H. Isolation of Marrubiin, a Sterol, and a Sesquiterpene from *Marrubium vulgare*. *J Pharm Sci* 1964;53:895.
[3] Kowalewska Z, et al. *Herba Polonica* 1978;24:183.
[4] Brieskem CI, et al. *Phytochem* 1968;7:485.
[5] Calis I, et al. Phenylpropanoid Glycosides from *Marrubium alysson*. *Phytochem* 1992:31(10):3624.
[6] Bartarelli M. [Il *Marrubium vulgare* e le sue applicazioni farmaceutiche. Parte I.] [Italian] *Boll Chim Farm* 1966:105(11):787.

[7] Tyler VE. The New Honest Herbal. Philadelphia: GF Stickley, 1987.
[8] Krejci I, et al. *Planta Med* 1959;7:1.
[9] Cahen R. Pharmacological Spectrum of *Planta Med* 1959;7:1.
[10] Cahen R. Pharmacological Spectrum of *Marrubium vulgare*. *CR Soc Biol* 1970;164(7):1467.
[11] Roman R, et al. Hypoglycemic Effect of Plants Used in Mexico as Antidiabetics. *Arch Med Res* 1992;23(1):59.

Horse Chestnut

SCIENTIFIC NAME(S): *Aesculus* Family: Hippocastanaceae. The most common members of the genus in the US and Europe are *A. hippocastanum* L. (horse chestnut), *A. californica* Nutt. (California buckeye) and *A. glabra* Willd. (Ohio buckeye).

COMMON NAME(S): Chestnut, horse chestnut, California buckeye, Ohio buckeye, buckeye.

BOTANY: Members of the genus *Aesculus* grow as trees and shrubs, often attaining heights of 75 feet. The fruit is designated a capsule with a thick, leathery husk that contains from 1 to 6 dark seeds (the nuts). As the husk dries, the nuts are released. The pink and white flowers of the plant grow in clusters. The tree is native to the Balkan woods and western Asia, but is now cultivated worldwide.[1]

HISTORY: Because of their widespread prevalence, chestnuts have been used in traditional medicine and for a variety of other commercial applications for centuries. Extracts of the bark have been used as a yellow dye, and the wood has been used for furniture and packing cases. In the western US, the crushed unripe seeds of the California buckeye were scattered into streams to stupefy fish, and leaves were steeped as a tea to remedy congestion. The horse chestnut has been used as a traditional remedy for arthritis and rheumatism.[2] Extracts are available commercially for oral, topical, and parenteral administration for the management of varicose veins and hemorrhoids.[2]

Even though the seeds are toxic, several traditional methods were employed to rid them of their toxicity. Seeds were buried in swampy, cold ground during the winter to free them of toxic bitter components, then eaten in the spring after boiling.[3] Indians roasted the poisonous nuts, peeled, and mashed them, then leached the meal in lime water for several days, creating a meal used to make breads.[4]

CHEMISTRY: The seeds of *Aesculus* contain a variety of complex constituents. The seed oil contains 65% to 70% oleic acid.[5] The seeds contain protein, ash, and 74% carbohydrate.[4] In addition, 5 triterpene oligoglycosides from horse chestnut seeds have been isolated.[6] The main anti-inflammatory constituent aescin (escin) is present in the plant.[1] This mixture of triterpene glycosides has been radioimmunoassayed,[7] and investigated by HPLC where it was obtained from both cotyledon and stem parts.[8] Triterpenoid saponins are also present in the plant.[1] Sapogenols hippocaesculin and barringtogenol-C 21–an-

gelate have been obtained from fruit parts.[9] Flavonol glycosides quercitrin and its aglycone are also found. Coumarin glycosides found in horse chestnut include fraxin, scopolin, and their aglycones.[10] From the seeds, a lectin and its amino acid composition have been determined.[11] Other constituents include allantoin, sterols, leucocyanidin, leucodelphinidin, tannins, adenine, adenosine, carotin, choline, citric, and uric acids.[4,10] Members of the genus produce the toxic glycoside esculin (aesculin in some texts). This poorly characterized toxin is found in the twigs, sprouts, leaves, and nuts.[5]

PHARMACOLOGY: Commerical extracts of horse chestnut have been evaluated in the treatment of a number of disease states, primarily by European investigators. An extract of the plant (containing 50 mg of triterpene glycosides) decreases venous capillary permeability and appears to have a "tonic" effect on the circulatory system.[12] Constituent aescin inhibits the increase of (induced) vascular permeability in mice and rats.[13] A commercial horse chestnut extract, which contains 70% aescin, has been found to possess a number of pharmacologic properties in vitro and in vivo, including the ability to contract the canine saphenous isolated vein and to potentiate the contractile response to norepinephrine.[14] The bark yields aesculin, which improves **vascular resistance** and aids in toning vein walls. This is desirable for such ailments as hemorrhoids, varicose or problematic veins, leg ulcers, or frostbite.[1] Triterpene and steroid saponins from horse chestnut are effective in treating or preventing venous insufficiency in another report. Enzyme studies demonstrate that elastase (enzymes involved in turnover or perivascular substances) inhibition may be a mechanism involved.[15] Aesculin reduces capillary wall permeability by decreasing fluid retention, by increasing the permeability of capillaries, and allowing reabsorption of excess fluid back into the circulatory system.[1] Aescin displayed moderated diuretic activity in rats, markedly increasing renal loss of sodium, chloride, and potassium.[16] **Anti-inflammatory effects** of horse chestnut preparations also have been reported.[1,17] One reference reported a dosage of 20 mg/day (max) IV administration of preparation aescin to be effective in preventing or treating post-op edema.[18] Aescin extract reduces cutaneous capillary hyperpermeability induced by histamine or serotonin, and it decreases the formation of chemically induced rat paw edema.[14] In patients with chronic venous insufficiency, these extracts have been found to be effective in reducing patient complaints, along with objective measures of edema.[19] In a placebo controlled study, horse-chestnut seed extract improved edema signs and symptoms in patients suffering from venous edema of chronic deep vein incompetence.[20]

The bark of the horse chestnut has been found to possess anti-inflammatory activity, primarily due to the presence of the steroids stigmasterol, alpha-spinasterol, and beta-sitosterol.[21]

Other varied pharmacological effects of horse chestnut preparations include: Treatment of whooping cough from a decoction of the leaves,[1] hypoglycemic activity in rats,[22] fever reduction,[1,4] ability to absorb the skin-damaging UV-B radiation in suntan products,[10] trophic effect on rat muscle by constituent proanthocyanioin-A2,[23] and antimicrobial actions from recently isolated antifungal proteins.[24]

The pharmacology, pharmacokinetics, and toxicology of horse chestnut saponin (escin) has been reviewed.[25,26]

TOXICOLOGY: *Aesculus* (horse chestnut) is classified by the FDA as an unsafe herb;[4] all members of this genus should be considered potentially toxic.[27] A number of components have been attributed toxic properties, including glycosides and saponins. Potential toxins identified in the genus include nicotine, quercitin, quercitrin, rutin, saponin, and shikimic acid.[4]

The most significant toxic principle is esculin. Poisoning is characterized by muscle twitching, weakness, lack of coordination, dilated pupils, vomiting, diarrhea, depression, paralysis, and stupor.[28] The nut is the most toxic part of the plant.[29] Children have been poisoned by drinking tea made from the leaves and twigs, and by eating the seeds; deaths have been reported following such inges-

tion. Amounts as little as 1% of a child's weight may be poisonous. Gastric lavage and symptomatic treatment have also been suggested.[28]

The LD_{50} of a single dose of the water-soluble portion of alcoholic extracts of horse chestnut seeds was calculated to be 10.6 mg/g body weight in chicks and 10.7 mg/g in hamsters. Extracts of the seeds of the Ohio buckeye were nontoxic to chicks and hamsters fed 80 mg/g in this study.[30]

Honey made mainly from the California buckeye has been reported to be toxic. A potential association between nasal cancer and long-term exposure to wood dusts, including dust from chestnut trees, has been reported.[31] Aflatoxins have been identified in some commercial skin cleansing products containing horse chestnut. Since aflatoxins are potent carcinogens that can be absorbed through the skin, it is imperative that strict quality control be applied to topical products containing potentially contaminated horse chestnut material.[32]

Horse chestnut pollen is allergenic and often associated with the development of allergic sensitization, particularly in urban children.[33]

A case report describes drug-induced hepatic injury to a 37-year-old male, induced by venoplant (horse chestnut extract preparation) given for treatment of bone fracture inflammation.[34]

An analysis of serious plant poisonings in Switzerland from 1966 to 1994 reveals horse chestnut to be responsible for 3 allergies and 2 anaphylactic shock episodes.[35]

SUMMARY: Chestnuts of the genus *Aesculus* should be considered toxic and cannot be recommended for internal use. However, they have a long history in traditional medicine, and recent research suggests that components of the horse chestnut may improve venous compliance and reduce edema in patients with chronic venous insufficiency.

PATIENT INFORMATION – Horse Chestnut

Uses: Sweet chestnuts, used as food, are of a separate genus than the horse chestnuts or buckeyes of traditional medicine, which are potentially useful against edema, inflammation, and venous insufficiency.

Side Effects: All parts of plants in the *Aesculus* family are potentially toxic, especially the seeds. Horse chestnut has been classified by the FDA as an unsafe herb. Buckeye sawdust and horse chestnut components in skin cleansers are potentially carcinogenic. Even buckeye honey may be toxic.

---

[1] Chevallier A. Encyclopedia of Medicinal Plants. New York, NY: DK Publishing, 1996;159.

[2] Tyler V, et al. Pharmacognosy. Philadelphia, PA: Lea & Febiger, 1988.

[3] Sweet M. Common Edible & Useful Plants of the West. Healdsburg, CA: Naturegraph Publishers, 1976.

[4] Duke J. Handbook of Medicinal Herbs. Boca Raton, FL: CRC Press, 1985.

[5] Evans W. Trease and Evans' Pharmacognosy, ed. 13. London, England: Bailliere Tindall, 1989.

[6] Yoshikawa M, et al. Chem Pharm Bull 1994;42(6):1357-59.

[7] Lehtola T, et al. J Immunoassay 1990;11(1):17-30.

[8] Profumo P, et al. J Pharm Pharmacol 1994;46(11):924-25.

[9] Konoshima T, et al. J Nat Prod 1986;49(4):650-56.

[10] Bisset N. Herbal Drugs and Phytopharmaceuticals. Stuttgart, Germany: CRC Press, 1994;268-72.

[11] Antoniuk V. UKR Biokhim Zh 1992;64(5):47-52.

[12] Bisler H, et al. Dtsch Med Wochenschr 1986;111(35):1321.

[13] Matsuda H, et al. Biol Pharm Bull 1997;20(10):1092-95.

[14] Guillaume M, et al. Arzneimittleforschung 1994;44:25.

[15] Facino R, et al. Arch Pharm 1995;328(10):720-24.

[16] Martin M, et al. Ann Pharm Fr 1990;48(6):306-11.

[17] Tsutsumi S, et al. Shikwa Gakuho 1967;67(11):1324-28.

[18] Reynolds J, ed. Martindale: The Extra Pharmacopoeia, ed. 31. Royal Pharmaceutical Society, London, England, 1996:1670.

[19] Hitzenberger G. Wien Med Wochenschr 1989;139(17):385.

[20] Diehm C, et al. Vasa 1992;21:188.

[21] Senatore F, et al. Boll Soc Ital Biol Sper 1989;65(2):137.

[22] Yoshikawa M, et al. Chem Pharm Bull 1996;44(8):1454-64.

[23] Ambrogini P, et al. Boll Soc Ital Biol Sper 1995;71(7-8):227-34.

[24] Osborn R, et al. Febs Lett 1995;368(2):257-62.

[25] Panigati, D. Boll Chim Farm 1992;131(7):284-93.

[26] Panigati, D. Boll Chim Farm 1992;131(8):320-21.

[27] Nagy M. JAMA (letter) 1973;226(2):213.

[28] Hardin J, et al. Human Poisoning From Native and Cultivated Plants, ed. 2. Durham, NC: Duke University Press, 1974.

[29] Anon. Vet Hum Toxicol 1983;25:80.

[30] Williams M, et al. Am J Vet Res 1984;45(3):539.

[31] Battista G, et al. Scand J Work Environ Health 1983;9(1):25.

[32] el-Dessouki S. Food Chem Toxicol 1992;30:993.

[33] Popp W, et al. Allergy 1992;47:380.

[34] Takegoshi K, et al Gastroenterol Jpn 1986;21(1):62-65.

[35] Jaspersen-Schib R, et al. Schweiz Med Wochenschr 1996;126(25):1085-98.

Horseradish

SCIENTIFIC NAME(S): *Armoracia rusticana* Gaertn., Mey. and Scherb. sometimes referred to as *A. lapathiofolia* Gilib. More than 20 plants have been called "horseradish" throughout the ages. Family: Cruciferae

COMMON NAME(S): Horseradish, pepperrot

BOTANY: Horseradish is a large-leafed hardy perennial. It is cultivated commercially for its thick, fleshy white roots which possess an intense pungent taste. Horseradish is believed to be native to Europe.[1] The plant reaches a height of 3 feet, bearing white flowers in the late spring. Some hybrids may be sterile and therefore the plant is generally propagated through root cuttings.

HISTORY: Horseradish has been cultivated for approximately 2000 years. Early settlers brought the horseradish plant to America, and the plant was commonplace in gardens by the early 1800s. Through plant selection, hardy varieties were obtained that could be grown easily in the Midwest. The root has a long history of use in traditional medicine. Early uses included reducing pain from sciatica, expelling afterbirth, relieving colic, increasing urination and killing intestinal worms in children.[1] Young tender leaves have been used as a potherb and as a salad green. Horseradish is one of the "five bitter herbs" (horseradish, coriander, horehound, lettuce and nettle) of Passover.

CHEMISTRY: The pungency of horseradish is due to the release of allylisothiocyanate and butylthiocyanate, which occur in combination with the glucosinolates sinigrin and 2-phenylethylglycosinolate. The pungency is released only upon crushing. The isothiocyanates are released from glucosinolates by the action of thioglucosidases, which are commonly referred to as myrosinase.[2] More than one-half dozen volatile glucosinolates have been identified using GC-MS analysis.[3]

To preserve the quality of horseradish, the root is commonly dehydrated, freeze-dried and powdered.[4]

Peroxidase enzyme is extracted from the root and is used as an oxidizer in commercial chemical tests such as blood glucose determinations.[5] The enzyme has also been used as a molecular probe in rheumatoid arthritis studies.[6]

PHARMACOLOGY: Horseradish is widely known for its pungent, burning flavor. The isothiocyanates may irritate mucous membranes upon contact or inhalation. Ingestion of large amounts can cause bloody vomiting and diarrhea.[7] Despite the potential for severe irritation, horseradish is generally recognized as safe for human consumption as a natural seasoning and flavoring.

An extract of horseradish has been shown to inhibit the enzyme cholinesterase.[8]

SUMMARY: Horseradish is a commonly used spice, the use of which dates back more than 2000 years. Although not used to any extent in herbal medicine today, the plant has a long history of traditional use. The pungency of the root develops upon enzymatic hydrolysis of thiocyanate-containing compounds. These irritants may cause severe inflammation to mucous membranes.

PATIENT INFORMATION – Horseradish

Uses: Horseradish has been used as a vegetable, condiment, diuretic, vermifuge and treatment for colic and sciatic pain.

Side Effects: Horseradish may irritate mucosa. Large amounts may cause bloody vomiting and diarrhea.

---

[1] Courter JW and Rhodes AM. Historical Notes on Horseradish. *Economic Botany* 1968:156.
[2] Korb KA and Chism GW. A rapid method for determining allylisothiocyanate in horseradish-containing products. *J Food Sci* 1989;54:778.
[3] Grob K and Matile P. Capillary GC of glucosinolate-derived horseradish constituents. *Phytochemistry* 1980;19:1789.
[4] Sahasrabudhe MR and Mullin WJ. Dehydration of Horseradish Roots. *J Food Sci* 1980;45:1440.
[5] Jamnicky B, et al. Application of horse-raddish peroxidase to glucose determination in body fluids. *Acta Pharm Jugo* 1988;38:53.
[6] Shiozawa S, et al. Presence of HLA-DR antigen on synovial type A and B cells: an immunoelectron microscopic study in rheumatoid arthritis, osteoarthritis and normal traumatic joints. *immunology* 1983;50:587.
[7] Simon JE. Herbs: an indexed bibliography, 1971-1980. Hamden, CT: Shoestring Press, 1984.
[8] Leiner IE. Toxic Constituents of Plant Foodstuffs. New York, NY: Academic Press, 1980.

Horsetail

SCIENTIFIC NAME(S): *Equisetum arvense* L. Family: Equisetaceae

COMMON NAME(S): Horsetail, souring rush, bottle brush, scouring rush, shave grass

BOTANY: Horsetail is a pteridophyte more closely related to ferns than to flowering plants. This rush-like perennial grows to about 1 foot and has hollow jointed stems and scale-like leaves.

HISTORY: Horsetail had been used as a metal polisher owing to the abrasive nature of its high silica content. Traditionally, the plant has been used as a diuretic, as an antitubercular drug, and in the treatment of kidney and bladder disturbances. Externally, it has been used in cosmetics[1] and as an astringent to stop bleeding[2] and stimulate wound healing.[3]

CHEMISTRY: The stems of horsetail contain 5% to 8% of silica and silicic acids. The plant contains about 5% of a saponin called equisetonin in addition to the flavone glycosides isoquercitrin, equisetrin and galuteolin.[4] The sterol fraction of *E. arvense* contains beta-sitosterol, campestrol, isofucosterol and trace amounts of cholesterol.[5] Nicotine is present in minute amounts (less than 1 ppm)[4] but may account for a portion of the pharmacologic activity of the plant. The cytokinin isopentenyladenosine has been identified in fertile fronds.[6]

PHARMACOLOGY: The plant exerts a slight diuretic activity, which is most probably due to the combined effects of equisetonin and the flavone glycosides. There are no data to support the use of horsetail in the treatment of urological disorders, tuberculosis or to enhance wound healing.[4]

TOXICOLOGY: Horsetail has been listed as an herb of undefined safety by the FDA.[7] Ingestion of large amounts of the fern may be toxic. Children have been reported to have been poisoned by using the stems as blow guns or whistles. In animals, the ingestion of horsetail produces muscle weakness, ataxia, weight loss, abnormal pulse rate, cold extremities and fever;[8] these symptoms are similar to those seen in nicotine intoxication. Hay composed of 20% or more *E. arvense* produced these symptoms in 2 to 5 weeks.[3] Cattle appear to recognize the odor of horsetail and have been documented to have refused hay contaminated with about 12% horsetail.[9]

Seborrheic dermatitis has been reported to have been induced by horsetail.[10]

SUMMARY: Horsetail continues to find some use in OTC herbal preparations. It contains small amounts of nicotine and other physiologically active compounds and is a marginally effective diuretic.

PATIENT INFORMATION – Horsetail

Uses: Horsetail has been used as a diuretic and treatment of kidney and bladder disturbances, as an astringent to stop bleeding and stimulate healing, as an antitubercular drug and as a cosmetic component.

Side Effects: Horsetail is of undefined safety and may be toxic, especially to children.

---

[1] L. Boruch T, et al. Extracts of plants and their cosmetic application, Part V. Extracts from Equisetum arvense. *Chem Abstracts* 1984;100.

[2] Schauenberg P, Paris F. Guide to Medicinal Plants. New Canaan, CT: Keats Publishing, 1977.

[3] Duke JA. Handbook of Medicinal Herbs. Boca Raton, FL: CRC Press, 1985.

[4] Tyler VE. The New Honest Herbal. Philadelphia, PA: G.F. Stickley Co., 1987.

[5] D'Agostino M, et al. Sterols From Equisetum arvense. *Boll Soc Ital Biol Sper* 1984;60(12):1241.

[6] Yamane H, et al. Identification of cytokinins in two species of pteridophyte sporophytes. *Plant Cell Physiol* 1983;24(6):1027.

[7] Der Marderosian AH, Liberti LE. Natural Product Medicine. Philadelphia, PA: G.F. Stickley Co., 1988.

[8] Spoerke DG. Herbal Medications. Santa Barbara, CA: Woodbridge Press, 1980.

[9] Kamphues J. Refusal of breeding bulls to eat hay contaminated with horsetail (Equisetum palustre). *Tierarztl Prax* 1990;18(4):349.

[10] Sudan BJL. Seborrhoeic dermatitis induced by nicotine of horsetails (Equisetum arvense L.). *Contact Dermatitis* 1985;13(3):201.

Hyssop

SCIENTIFIC NAME(S): *Hyssopus officinalis* L. Family: Labiatae

COMMON NAME(S): Hyssop. It should be noted that there are a number of other common plants found in North America that go by a variation of the name "hyssop." These include giant hyssop (*Agastache* sp.), hedge hyssop (*Gratiola officinalis* L.), and water hyssop (*Bacopa* sp.): none of these plants are members of the genus *Hyssopus*, nor are they all members of the Family: Labiatae.

BOTANY: Hyssop is a perennial plant which is native to the Mediterranean region and has been imported to and naturalized in the United States and Canada. It grows along roadsides and is sometimes found as a garden herb. Its thin pointed leaves extend onto a central herbaceous stem that is sessile in form. The tubular flowers grow from the upper leaf axils and bloom small blue flowers from July to October. The fruit contains four "nutlets," each having one seed. Hyssop is quite similar in appearance to other members of the mint family. It grows to about 2 feet. Its volatile oil imparts a highly aromatic camphor-like smell.[1]

HISTORY: Hyssop has been noted for centuries in herbal medicine. In addition, there are a number of references in the Bible to plants called "hyssop," although there is considerable controversy regarding the actual identity of these plants. There is little evidence that the plant mentioned in Bible was actually "*H. officinalis.*"

The ancient use of this plant was an insecticide, insect repellent and pediculicide.[2] The plant has been used in herbal medicine for the treatment of sore throats, colds, hoarseness and as an expectorant.[3] Some herbalists also believe that hyssop has beneficial effects for asthma, urinary tract inflammation and appetite stimulation.[1] Its effectiveness in relieving gas and colic are also listed under its medicinal uses.[2]

Although an extract of the leaves has been suggested for the treatment of wounds, there does not appear to be strong evidence for its effectiveness as an antibacterial.

Extracts of plant have been used in perfumes and to flavor liqueurs, sauces, puddings and candies.[4]

CHEMISTRY: As a member of the mint family, hyssop contains a number of fragrant, volatile components. Pinocamphone, isopinocamphone, alpha- and beta-pinene, camphene and alpha-terpinene make up about 70% of the volatile oil.[5] The plant contains 0.3% to 2% of this volatile oil. Other constituents include glycosides (hyssopin as well as the flavonoid glycosides, hesperidin and diosmine), 5% to 8% tannin, oleanolic acid, ursolic acid, β-sitosterol, marrubiin and resins. Other substituents reported are pinocampheol, cineole, linalool, terpineol, terpinyl acetate, bornyl acetate, *cis*-pinic acid, *cis*-pinonic acid, myrtenic acid, myrtenol methyl ether, *d*-2-hydroxy-isopinocamphone, methyl myrtenate, cadinene and other unidentified compounds totalling more than 50 in number.[4]

Crude hyssop also contains 0.5% rosmarinic acid and total hydroxycinnamic derivatives at 2.2%.[4] Another recent gas chromatographic study confirms the presence of the above constituents of *H. officinalis* and states percentage values for them, the most prevalent being pinocamphone (69.1%).[6]

PHARMACOLOGY: Still used today by herbalists for its beneficial effects, hyssop's volatile oil represents the most important fraction of this plant. It may have some small beneficial effect in the treatment of sore throats and as an expectorant.

Hyssop oil is used to fragrance perfumes and soaps. It was found to be nonirritating to the skin in both animal and human studies.[4]

Extracts of dried leaves of *H. officinalis* exhibit strong antiviral activity against HIV, probably due to the caffeic acid, tannins and unidentified high molecular weight compounds present.[7] Anti-HIV activity was also recently found in a study where an isolated polysaccharide inhibited HIV-1 replication.[8] Both studies suggest this anti-HIV activity may be useful in healing AIDS patients.

TOXICOLOGY: Hyssop is classified among plants "generally recognized as safe (GRAS)" by the FDA; however, three recent studies demonstrate convulsant actions associated with the plant's use in rats. Commercial preparations of hyssop essential oils produced convulsions in rats at 0.13 g/kg and death at 1.25 g/kg.[9]

The neurotoxicity of hyssop appears to be related to two terpene ketones: Pinocamphone and isopinocamphone.[9] In a similar study, IP injections of hyssop essential oil, ranging from 200 mcl/kg to 4 mcl/kg, produced a generalized crisis in rats that led from convulsions to death. The authors concluded that hyssop essential oils are not as safe as most people believe.[10] The convulsions were later determined, by electrocortical evidence, to be of CNS origin.[11]

SUMMARY: Hyssop represents a useful herbal compound. It is used commercially as a flavoring agent and as an ingredient in cough and cold preparations. It appears to exert its demulcent and expectorant effects through the action of its volatile oil. However, it must be used with caution because of its convulsive effects.

More studies are needed to verify the reported antiviral therapeutic efficacy which may be of use in HIV infected patients.

PATIENT INFORMATION – Hyssop

Uses: Hyssop is used as flavoring, fragrance, insecticide, insect repellent and cough and cold treatment.

Side Effects: The essential oils have produced fatal convulsions in rats.

---

[1] Bunney S, ed. The Illustrated Encyclopedia of Herbs. New York: Dorset Press, 1984.

[2] Polunin M, Robbins C. The Natural Pharmacy: An illustrated guide to natural medicine. New York: Collier Books, 1992.

[3] Bianchini F, Corbetta F. Health Plants of the World: Atlas of medicinal plants. New York: Newsweek Books, 1975.

[4] Leung AY, Foster S. Encyclopedia of Natural Ingredients, ed. 2. New York: John Wiley & Sons, 1996.

[5] Tyler VE. The Honest Herbal. Philadelphia: GF Stickley Co, 1981.

[6] Shath NC, et al. Gas Chromatographic Examination of Oil of *Hyssopus officinalis. Parfuemerie Kosmetik* 1986;67:116.

[7] Kreis W, et al. Inhibition of HIV Replication by *Hyssopus officinalis* Extracts. *Antiviral Res* 1990:14(6):323.

[8] Gollapudi S, et al. Isolation of a Previously Unidentified Polysaccharide (MAR-10) from *Hyssop officinalis* That Exhibits Strong Activity Against Human Immunodeficiency Virus Type 1. *Biochem Biophys Res Comm* 1995;210(1):145.

[9] Millet Y, et al. [Experimental Study of the Toxic Convulsant Properties of Commercial Preparations of Essences of Sage and Hyssop.] [French] *Rev Electroenceph Neurophys Clin* 1979;9(1):12.

[10] Millet Y, et al. Study of the Toxicity of Essential Vegetable Oils: Hyssop oil and sage oil. *Med Leg Toxicol* 1980;23:9.

[11] Millet Y, et al. Toxicity of Some Essential Plant Oils. Clinical and experimental study. *Clin Toxicol* 1981;18(12):1485.

Iboga

SCIENTIFIC NAME(S): *Tabernanthe iboga.* Family: Apocyanaceae.

COMMON NAME(S): Iboga

BOTANY: The iboga plant is native to Gabon, Zaire and the Congo and is the only member of the dogbane family known to be used as an hallucinogen.[1] The plant is cultivated throughout west Africa.[2] The yellow-colored root is used in traditional medicine and is the source of the hallucinogenic principle.

HISTORY: The growing use of iboga has been said to be an important force against the spread of Christianity and Islam in its native growing regions.[1] The root of the plant is used in initiation rites of some African cultures. The plant is believed to be an aphrodisiac and stimulant. Large doses are used to induce a euphoric state in which people are said to be able to communicate with the spirits of their ancestors. In addition, the plant is consumed by those who believe it can reveal objects reputedly buried by individuals subjected to the intoxicant during their former lives. Failure to retrieve these hidden treasures has resulted in "sudden and mysterious deaths" among villagers.[2] The use of iboga is legally prohibited in the United States.[3]

CHEMISTRY: Indole alkaloids comprise approximately 6% of the root[3] and ibogaine is the principle indole alkaloid among the dozen or more identified to date.[4] Other related alkaloids include ibogamone, tabernanthine, and iboluteine.[3] The root contains a tannin.

PHARMACOLOGY: The dried root bark is chopped into a fine powder often mixed with other hallucinogenic plants. Alternately, the root is chewed to obtain the desired effect.

Ibogaine is a cholinesterase inhibitor.[3] As such, the effects of iboga are secondary to increases in synaptic concentrations of acetylcholine.

The pharmacologic effects are dose-dependent and range from mild excitation and euphoria to visual and auditory hallucinations. Related pharmacologic effects of cholinergic hyperactivity include slowing of the heart rate, hypotension, convulsions, paralysis, and respiratory arrest.[1,3] Hallucinations are typically accompanied by anxiety and apprehension and may only occur with doses large enough to cause death.[3]

Tabernanthine demonstrates cardiac conduction effects characteristic of a calcium channel antagonist; it also has other pharmacologic actions that are due to the inhibition of cellular calcium metabolism and are related to the turnover of intracellular calcium that is released by noradrenaline.[5,6]

SUMMARY: Iboga is an hallucinogen that is popular in western and central Africa. While it is considered a powerful drug, the hallucinatory effects are usually only experienced at the highest doses, which are also the doses most likely to induce death. Ibogaine is a cholinesterase inhibitor and related alkaloids also exhibit calcium channel blocking activity.

PATIENT INFORMATION – Iboga

Uses: Iboga is used ritually as a hallucinogen.

Side Effects: Iboga is illegal in the United States. It can cause paralysis and eventually death.

---

[1] Schultes RE. Hallucinogenic Plants. New York: Golden Press, 1976.
[2] Duke JA. Handbook of Medicinal Herbs. Boca Raton, FL: CRC Press, 1985.
[3] Lewis WH, Elvin-Lewis MPF. Medica Botany: Plants affecting man's health. New York: John Wiley & Sons, 1977.
[4] Evans, WC. Trease and Evans' Pharmacognosy. 13th ed. London: Balliere Tindall, 1989

[5] Ha,o-Tello N, Dupont C, Weppierre J, Cohen Y, et al. Effects of tabernanthine on calcium and catecholamine stimulated contractions of isolated vascular and cardiac muscles. *Arch Int Pharmacodyn Ther* 1985:276:35.
[6] Miller RC, Godfraind T. The action of tabernanthine on noradrenaline-stimulated contractions of 45Ca movements in rat isolated vascular smooth muscle. *Eur J Pharmacol* 1983;96:251.

Indian Frankincense Tree

SCIENTIFIC NAME(S): *Boswellia serrata* Roxb. Family: Burseraceae

COMMON NAME(S): Indian frankincense tree, "salai guggal" (term for the gum resin of the tree)

BOTANY: The *Burseraceae* family of trees and shrubs has 18 genera and 540 species that grow mostly in tropical regions of America, North Africa and Arabia. Most species contain resin ducts in the bark, which yield the products myrrh and frankincense.[1] The *Boswellia serrata* tree grows on dry hilly areas throughout most of India. When the bark is cut, the "aromatic balsam" or "gum resin" oozes out and is used for medicinal purposes.[2]

HISTORY: The Indian frankincense tree is related to the tree that brought forth the frankincense given as a gift to baby Jesus by the wise men. Ayurvedic medicine has been practiced in India for thousands of years, using different parts of the tree for asthma, rheumatism, dysentery, skin ailments, ulcers, blood purification, bronchial conditions and wound treatment.[2] Frankincense is also used to perfume clothes, hair and rooms. It is enjoyed at traditional festivities such as weddings or religious celebrations.[1]

CHEMISTRY: The gum resin of *Boswellia serrata* contains the biologically active boswellic acid (3-alpha-hydroxy-urs-12-en-23-oic acid) and its derivatives.[3]

Boswellin (patented product of Sabinsa Corporation)[2] is the standardized ethanol extract of *Boswellia serrata* gum resin. It contains 60% to 65% boswellic acids and can be found in health food stores.[2]

Isolation and identification of a 4-O-methyl-glucuronoarabinogalactan from *Boswellia serrata* have been performed.[4]

Other compounds found in the gum resin include volatile oils, terpinols, arabinose, xylose, galactose, uronic acids, beta-sitosterin and phlobaphenes.[5]

PHARMACOLOGY: Anti-inflammatory activity has been studied in animals.[3] The plant extract displays marked anti-inflammatory action as well as anti-arthritic activity with no significant side effects in rats.[6] A mixture of boswellic acid and its derivatives is used in India to treat arthritis.[3]

Boswellic acids in vitro are specific inhibitors of 5-lipoxygenase, the key enzyme of leukotriene biosynthesis. Leukotrienes are biochemicals in the body that maintain inflammation. Boswellic acids may offer an alternative to corticosteroid and NSAID therapy in treating such inflammatory conditions as arthritis, tendinitis or bursitis.[2,3] One report evaluates boswellic acid inhibition on leukotriene synthesis (via 5-lipoxygenase), finding it to have no effect on 12-lipoxygenase, cyclooxygenase or the peroxidation of arachnidonic acid by iron and ascorbate, suggesting the boswellic acid component to be a specific, non-redox inhibitor of leukotriene synthesis.[7] Similar results were found in rat peritoneal neutrophils.[8,9]

Boswellia serrata in an herbomineral combination was studied in 42 osteoarthritic patients in a randomized, double blind, placebo controlled crossover study. Pain and disability scores were significantly decreased but radiological assessment showed no change.[10]

In an immunological study, boswellic acids have also been shown to possess **anti-complementary activity** via C3-convertase inhibition.[11] C3-convertase is involved in the production of anaphylatoxin.[16]

Salai guggal, the gum resin exudate of *Boswellia serrata*, has been evaluated for effects on: Glycosaminoglycan metabolism in rats,[12] humoral immune response, inhibiting infiltration of polymorphonuclear leukocytes in rats[13] and some analgesic and psychopharmacological effects.[14]

In patients given *Boswellia serrata* gum resin preparation (350 mg 3 times daily) for 6 weeks compared with sulfasalazine (1 g 3 times daily), parameters of ulcerative colitis (eg, stool properties, histolopathology, rectal biopsies, blood work) were improved. Remission was 82% with the resin and 75% with sulfasalazine. Ulcerative colitis, also an inflammatory disease, seems to benefit from Boswellia's ability to inhibit 5-lipoxygenase as well.[15]

TOXICOLOGY: The limited data available on toxicity of the Indian frankincense tree include: No side effects,[2,5] no cytotoxic effect,[13] no effects on cardiovascular, respiratory or CNS function, no ulcerogenic effects[6] or "side effects observed...did not necessitate withdrawal of treatment."[10]

SUMMARY: The Indian frankincense tree is well known for its gum resin, which is used for frankincense and myrrh. This species (of which there are many), *Boswellia serrata*, has been used in ayurvedic medicine for thousands of years, treating such ailments as asthma, dysentery, skin problem, ulcers and wounds. The constituent boswellic acid is known to be a specific inhibitor of 5-lipoxygenase, an enzyme responsible for synthesis of leukotrienes that maintain inflammation. Clinical trials are available studying its anti-inflammatory effects in the treatment of arthritis and colitis. The toxicity profile is low, with most studies reporting no side effects.

PATIENT INFORMATION – Indian Frankincense Tree

Uses: The extract of Indian frankincense tree has anti-inflammatory activity. Boswellic acids may play a role in preventing formation of anaphylatoxins during severe acute allergic reactions.

Side Effects: Although data are limited, no side effects have been reported that necessitated stopping treatment.

---

[1] Ghazanfar S. Handbook of Arabian Medicinal Plants. Boca Raton, FL: CRC Press 1994:62.
[2] Broadhurst C, et al. *Herbs for Health* 1998;Jan/Feb:20.
[3] Bruneton J. Pharmacognosy, Phytochemistry, Medicinal Plants. Paris, France: Lavoisier Pub 1995:607-8.
[4] Sen A, et al. *Carbohydr Res* 1992;223:321-27.
[5] Ammon H. *Eur J Med Res* 1996;1(8):369-70.
[6] Singh G, et al. *Agents Actions* 1986;18(3-4):407-12.
[7] Ammon H, et al. *J Ethnopharmacol* 1993;38(2-3):113-19.
[8] Ammon H, et al. *Planta Med* 1991;57(3):203-7.
[9] Safayhi H, et al. *J Pharmacol Exp Ther* 1992;261(3):1143-46.
[10] Kulkarni R, et al. *J Ethnopharmacol* 1991;33(1-2):91-95.
[11] Kapil A, et al. *Int J Immunopharmacol* 1992;14(7):1139-43.
[12] Reddy G, et al. *Biochem Pharmacol* 1989;38(20):3527-34.
[13] Sharma M, et al. *Agents Actions* 1988;24(1-2):161-64.
[14] Menon M, et al. *Planta Med* 1971;19(4):333-41.
[15] Gupta I, et al. *Eur J Med Res* 1997;2(1):37-43.
[16] Barrett JT. *Textbook of Immunology, 4th Ed.* St Louis, MO: CV Mosby Company 1983:177.

Indigo

SCIENTIFIC NAME(S): *Indigofera* species including *I. tinctoria* (French indigo) and *I. suffruticosa* Mill. (Guatemalan indigo) formerly known as *I. anil* L. Family: Fabaceae (Leguminosae).

COMMON NAME(S): Common or Indian Indigo; not to be confused with false, wild or bastard indigo (*Baptisia tinctoria* L), a native North American plant from which a blue dye is obtained from the leaves.[1,2]

BOTANY: These plants are perennial shrubs that reach a height of 1 m to 2 m. The French and Guatemalan varieties differ in the shape and size of the leaflets and pods.

HISTORY: Indigo refers to several species of *Indigofera* that are known for the natural blue colors obtained from the leaflets and branches of this herb.[1] Before the development of synthetic aniline and indigo dyes, indigo plants were grown commercially in the East Indies and South and Central America. Indigo was a popular dye during the middle ages.[1] It has been used medicinally as an emetic; the Chinese used the plant to purify the liver, reduce inflammation and fever and to alleviate pain.[1] Extracts of *I. tinctoria* have been reported to have nematicide activity and the leaf and plant juice have been used to treat cancers, particularly of the ovaries and stomach.[3] In addition, the plant has been used for the treatment of numerous ailments ranging from hemorrhoids to scorpion bites.

CHEMISTRY: The blue dye is produced during the fermentation of the leaves, which is commonly accomplished with caustic soda or sodium hydrosulfite.[1] A paste exudes from the fermenting plant material and this is processed into cakes that are finely ground. The blue color develops as the powder is exposed to air.

Indigo dye is a derivative of indican, a glucoside[3] component of numerous *Indigofera* species and this is enzymatically converted to blue indigotin.[1] This colorfast dye is combined with stabilizers and other compounds to produce a wide range of colorants. Today, almost all indigo used commercially is produced synthetically.

PHARMACOLOGY: Little is known about the pharmacologic effects of *Indigofera* species. Preliminary evidence suggests that *I. tinctoria* may have a protective effect against carbon tetrachloride-induced hepatotoxicity,[4] which is opposite to the hepatotoxic effect observed with other members of this genus. The related *I. aspalathoides* has been reported to possess anti-inflammatory activity.[5]

TOXICOLOGY: Indigo appears to be a mild ocular irritant.[3] Dermatitis is common among indigo dyers but there is no direct evidence that this is linked to exposure to the plant or dye.[3] *I. spicata* is recognized as a teratogen due to the presence of indospicine. Indospicine also is hepatotoxic.[6,7] In animals, it causes cleft palate and embryo lethality.[8] *I. endacaphylla* (creeping indigo) has been responsible for livestock poisonings and deaths.[1]

SUMMARY: The *Indigofera* species have been used for centuries as a natural source of an exquisite blue dye. While the medicinal uses and claims for the plants are numerous, there is little evidence to verify these effects. Several species of *Indigofera* are toxic.

PATIENT INFORMATION – Indigo

Uses: Chiefly a source of dye, indigo has also been used as a nematicide and treatment for a range of ills including scorpion bites and ovarian and stomach cancer.

Side Effects: Some species are toxic and cause birth defects.

---

[1] Simon JE. Herbs: an indexed bibliography, 1971-1980. Hamden, CT: Shoe String Press. 1984.
[2] Spoerke DG. Herbal Medications. Santa Barbara, CA: Woodbridge Press, 1980.
[3] Duke JA. Handbook of Medicinal Herbs. Boca Raton, FL: CRC Press, 1985.
[4] Anand KK, Chand D, Ray Ghatak BJ, et al. Histological evidence of protection by *Indigofera tinctoria* Linn. against carbon tetrachloride induced hepatotoxicity — an experimental study. *Indian J Exp Biol* 1981;19:298.

[5] Amala Bhaskar E, Ganga N, Arivudainambi R, et al. Anti-inflammatory activity of *Indigofera aspalathoides* Vahl. *Indian J Med Res* 1982;76(Suppl):115.
[6] Liener IE, ed. Toxic Constituents of Plant Foodstuffs. London; Academic Press, 1980.
[7] Hegarty MP, Kelly WR, McEwan D, et al. Hepatotoxicity to dogs of horse meat contaminated with indospicine. *Aust Vet J* 1988;65:337
[8] Evans WC. Trease and Evans' Pharmacognosy. 13th ed. London; Bailliere Tindall, 1989.

Ipecac

SCIENTIFIC NAME(S): *Cephaelis ipecacuanha* A. Rich. Also known as *Psychotria ipecacuanha*. Other *Cephaelis* species include *C. acuminata* (Cartagena ipecac).[1] Family: Rubiaceae

COMMON NAME(S): Ipecac, ipecacuanha, golden root, Rio or Brazilian ipecac, Matto Grosso ipecac, Costa Rica ipecac

BOTANY: The ipecac is a small perennial tropical plant that grows to about 2 feet in height. Horizontal roots extend from its slender underground stem. At maturity, the roots have a dark brown or red covering, a bitter taste and a musty odor. The plant is native to the humid forests of Bolivia and Brazil where large plantations have been established to commercialize the collection of ipecac root. Much of the root crop continues to be harvested from the wild, particularly in South America.[2] India is also an important producer of ipecac.

HISTORY: Brazilian Indians valued ipecac as a remedy for dysentery and this information was brought to Europe by Portuguese missionaries.[3] The dried root and rhizome are the source of the medicinally useful products. Ipecac has been widely used in its syrup form as a potent and effective emetic. Ipecac powder had been used to induce sweating at the onset of influenza and small amounts of the extract have been incorporated into cough syrups as expectorants. Emetine, derived from the root, has been used for more than a century to treat dysentery.[1]

CHEMISTRY: The root and rhizomes of ipecac contain a number of closely related isoquinoline alkaloids in a total concentration of up to 2.5% by weight of the root.[1] These are primarily emetine, cephaeline and psychotrine. Because leaves contain less than 0.5% emetine, they are usually not processed commercially. More than a half-dozen additional alkaloids are distributed thoughout parts of the plant. Emetine may be manufactured commercially by the chemical modification of either cephaeline or psychotrine.

PHARMACOLOGY: The syrup induces vomiting in 15 to 60 minutes, and is most effective when accompanied by fluid intake. Ipecac induces vomiting both by an irritant action on the intestinal mucosa and produces reflex vomiting and diarrhea; it also exerts a central emetic action.[5] Emetine has primarily a central action on the chemoreceptor trigger zone.

Both cephaeline and emetine are active amebicides, although emetine is more active. Emetine injected intra-muscularly is distributed systemically and kills the motile trophozoites of *Entamoeba histolytica* in doses smaller than are effective against cysts.[5] The drug inhibits cell protein synthesis.[5] The drug does not reach high levels in the gut and therefore is not effective against amebic dysentery. It is useful for amebic abscesses and hepatitis.

TOXICOLOGY: Ipecac extracts can be highly toxic when given either acutely or chronically. Powdered ipecac is a respiratory irritant and pharmacists may develop rhinitis or asthma following repeated exposure to the powder during compounding procedures.[1]

Cephaeline is more toxic than emetine, causing more nausea and vomiting.[4] Emetine, which constitutes more than half of the total ipecac content, is a cardiotoxin.[4] If given over a period of time or in total doses exceeding 1 g, the cumulative effect of emetine may lead to myositis at the injection site, gastrointestinal and nervous system symptoms, hematuria and circulatory collapse. Emetine is therefore given in low doses for a short period of time, with a break of several weeks between treatment regimens. Emetine can irritate skin if applied topically. The synthetic compound 2,3–dihydroemetine is often used to treat amebiasis; it may lead to less cardiotoxicity but may be less effective than emetine.[1,5]

Fluid extract of ipecac had largely been abandoned because of the large number of fatal overdoses that were occurring when the product was mistaken for syrup of ipecac. The fluid extract is 14 times more concentrated than the syrup and as little as 10 ml has been fatal.[4] By comparison, syrup of ipecac, which is kept in most households as a first-aid emetic, has demonstrated a remarkable safety profile. As much as 105 ml of the syrup has been retained in a child with only minor changes in the ECG. However, at least one fatality has been reported with the syrup, this in a 26–year-old woman who had drank 3 to 4 bottles of the syrup each night over a 3-month period in order to lose weight.[6] Another case described a woman who ingested 200 ml ipecac syrup per week for 3 months to lose weight who developed myopathy, which resolved to normal 4 months after stopping ipecac use.[7] This myopathy may be accompanied by cardiomyopathy.[8]

to treat dysentery. Ipecac and its constituents should be used cautiously because their misuse can lead to serious acute and chronic toxicities.

SUMMARY: Ipecac is a widely used natural product that is an effective emetic whose components have been used

---

PATIENT INFORMATION – Ipecac

Uses: Ipecac has been used as an emetic and treatment for dysentery. It has amebicidal components.

Side Effects: Ipecac extracts can be highly toxic and should not be confused with syrup of ipecac.

---

[1] Morton JF. Major Medicinal Plants. Springfield, IL: Charles C. Thomas, 1977.
[2] Dobelis IN. Magic and Medicine of Plants. Pleasantville, NY: Reader's Digest Association, 1986.
[3] Evans, WC. Trease and Evans' Pharmacognosy, 13th ed. London: Balliere Tindall, 1989.
[4] Kink, WD. Syrup of ipecac: A drug review. *Clin Toxicol* 1980;17:353.
[5] Bowman WC. Textbook of Pharmacology, 2nd ed. St. Louis, MO: Blackwell Mosby Book Distributors, 1980.

[6] Adler AG, et al. Death resulting from ipecac syrup poisoning. *JAMA* 1980;243:1927.
[7] Thyagarajan D, et al. Emetine myopathy in a patient with an eating disorder. *Med J Aust* 1993;159:757.
[8] Dresser LP, et al. Ipecac myopathy and cardiomyopathy. *J Neurol Neurosurg Psychiatry* 1993;56:560.

Jewelweed

SCIENTIFIC NAME(S): *Impatiens* L. Several members of this genus (ie, *I. balsamina*, *I. capensis*[1] and *I. biflora*[2]) have been referred to as jewelweed. Some texts indicate that jewelweed can refer to any member of the genus. Family: Balsaminaceae.

COMMON NAME(S): Jewelweed, jewel weed, jewel balsam weed, touch-me-not, garden balsam[3]

BOTANY: The *Impatiens* are tender, succulent herbs that are commonly grown as bedding and house plants. Jewelweed is sometimes called the "touch-me-not." This name alludes to the presence of a seed capsule made of a soft fleshy tissue that tends to expell its contents if touched or shaken.

HISTORY: Jewelweed has long been recognized as an herbal remedy for the treatment of topical irritation, most notably for the treatment of poison ivy rash. The juice (sap) of the jewelweed has been used by Native Americans, particularly those living in Appalachia, as a prophylactic against poison ivy rash and as a treatment after the eruptions have occurred.[1] Jewelweed extracts are not generally found in commercial topical products.

CHEMISTRY: While little is known about the chemical composition of many of the *Impatiens* species, it has been reported that the compound 2–methoxynaphthoquinone, derived from *I. balsamina*, demonstrates antifungal activity.[1]

PHARMACOLOGY: Several attempts have been made to verify that jewelweed extracts, when applied topically, have a beneficial effect on poison ivy eruptions. However, the scant data available to date indicate that jewelweed extract is not particularly effective for this indication.

Results of a recent *Prevention* [magazine] Home-Remedy Survey found that only 53% of the respondents who applied jewelweed to poison ivy rash obtained "good" relief from itching. (These findings were derived from approximately 350 respondents who had tried jewelweed, 7% of the total survey group.)[4]

Another small, uncontrolled study compared the effects of an aqueous jewelweed extract and water in reducing poison ivy irritation. In both subjects, the reaction remained significant after 3 days; in one of the subjects, areas treated with *I. biflora* extract demonstrated more severe and widespread reactions than control areas or those areas treated with water. Since water is believed to degrade *Toxicodendron* oleoresin and possibly have a small clinical effect of its own, any benefit could be due to the water rather than to the jewelweed.[2]

TOXICOLOGY: There are no published reports of significant toxicity associated with the topical use of jewelweed extracts. The safety of internal ingestion of jewelweed is not well-defined.

SUMMARY: Jewelweed is a popular herbal remedy for topical irritation, such as that produced by poison ivy. However, results of small, poorly controlled assessments of the herb's activity suggest that it has little or no significant beneficial effect against itching or other topical manifestations of the irritation.

PATIENT INFORMATION – Jewelweed

Uses: Jewelweed has traditionally been used as topical prevention and treatment for poison ivy rash.

Side Effects: None known for topical use.

---

[1] Lewis WH, Elvin-Lewis MPF. *Medical Botany: Plants affecting man's health.* New York: John Wiley & Sons, 1977.
[2] Guin JD, Reynolds R. Jewelweed treatment of poison ivy dermatitis. *Contact Derm.* 1980;6:287.
[3] Mabberley DJ. *The Plant-book.* Cambridge, England: Cambridge University Press, 1987.
[4] Zarrow S, et al. Reader-tested home remedies. *Prevention.* 1991;Dec:33.

Jiaogulan

SCIENTIFIC NAME(S): *Gynostemma pentaphyllum* (Thunb.) Makino. Family: Cucurbitaceae (Squashes)

COMMON NAME(S): Jiaogulan, Penta tea, Amachazuru (Japan), Southern ginseng, Dungkulcha (Korea)

BOTANY: *Gynostemma pentaphyllum* is a climbing, perennial vine native to China, Japan, and parts of southeast Asia. The plant is dioecious, that is, it carries male and female flowers on separate plants. While the plant grows abundantly and is harvested from the wild, it has been brought under cultivation and tissue culture has been achieved.[1-4] Adulteration by *Cayratia japonica* has been noted.[3]

HISTORY: Jiaogulan has been incorporated into traditional Chinese medicine only in the last 20 years. The plant has a history of folk use in the Guizhou province in China. Its properties are said to have been investigated when a Chinese census revealed a large number of elderly people in the province reported using the plant. Investigation as a potential sweetening agent stimulated chemical investigations in Japan. Commercialization and scientific study of the leaves have been promoted by provincial Chinese authorities, and the discovery that several ginseng saponins occur in the leaves has prompted aggressive promotion of the product as a substitute for ginseng. The appearance of jiaogulan in American commerce has been heralded by publication of a popular book.[5]

CHEMISTRY: A large series of dammarane triterpene saponins, gypenosides 1-82, have been isolated from the leaves, principally by Takemoto's group.[7-14] Several of these saponins are identical to those found in ginseng. Specifically, gypenoside 3 is identical to ginsenoside Rb1, gypenoside 4 is identical to ginsenoside Rb3, gypenoside 8 is identical to ginsenoside Rd, and gypenoside 12 is identical to ginsenoside F2. Many of the other gypenosides are closely related structurally to the ginsenosides and include the 6'-malonyl derivatives characteristic of ginseng.[15] The content of saponins is comparable to that of ginseng roots. However, wide variation in the amount and nature of gypenosides has made production of a product standardized with specific gypenosides somewhat problematic. Most current products are standardized on total saponin content. The reasons for this variation have been investigated but have not been fully elucidated.

Other constituents reported from *Gynostemma pentaphyllum* include sterols with the ergostane, cholestane, and stigmastane skeletons,[16-20] with several examples containing an acetylenic functionality, which is considered unusual in plants.[21] The flavonoid glycosides rutin, ombuoside,[22] and yixingensin[23,24] have also been identified.

The related species *G. compressum* Chen and Liang have yielded dammarane saponins related to the gypenosides.[25]

PHARMACOLOGY: Though the plant contains ginseng and ginseng-like saponins, it has not been reported to contain the other types of biologically active compounds, acetylenes, and polysaccharides found in ginseng. Thus, while ginseng pharmacology presents a reasonable starting point for investigation, jiaogulan cannot be considered as pharmacologically identical to ginseng.

Hyperlipidemia: Oral administration of a gynostemma decoction in combination with *Nelumbo nucifera* and *Crataegus cuneata* was found to lower triglycerides and cholesterol in rats and quail. However, a dose response was not demonstrated.[26] Administration of an aqueous extract of the whole plant to rats in chow over 12 weeks resulted in a reduction in serum levels of total cholesterol and beta-lipoproteins.[27] A second study in mice and rats given 200 mg/kg PO of the crude saponin demonstrated lower total cholesterol (TC) and VLDL but increased HDL/LDL.[28] A clinical study of hyperlipoproteinemic subjects also found a decrease in TC with increased HDL/TC at a dose of 10 mg given 3 times daily for 30 days.[29] A study of 105 patients confirmed these effects.[30]

Lipid peroxidation: An antioxidant effect of gypenosides was reported in phagocyte, endothelial cell, and liver microsome systems.[31] Further study by the same group[32] explored these effects in vascular endothelial cells injured by hydrogen peroxide. Rat microsome studies also have found similar effects for crude gypenosides.[33]

Adaptogenic: Despite the wide reputation of ginseng as an adaptogen, few studies have been published on the topic. Chen[34] found an increased tolerance to fatigue in forced swimming and hanging models in mice, and enhanced tolerance to anoxia, along with potentiation of pentobarbital hypnosis.

Cardio- and cerebrovascular effects: The hot water extract of *Gynostemma pentaphyllum* was found to activate platelet aggregation. However, the active principle was not elucidated.[35] Gypenosides inhibited platelet aggregation in another study.[36] In rabbits, crude gypenosides decreased heart rate, increased stroke volume, dilated blood vessels, and reduced blood pressure while slightly increasing cardiac output.[37] Purified gypenosides 5 and 10 were found to lower systolic and diastolic blood pressure, decrease coronary, brain, and peripheral blood vessel resistance, raise coronary flow, and lower heart rate in dogs.[38] Crude gypenosides protected against cerebral ischemic damage in a rabbit model.[39]

Cancer and immunologic effects: An extract of *Gynostemma* inhibited the growth of a rectal adenocarcinoma cell line,[40] while total gypenosides inhibited growth of A549, Calu 1, and 592/9 carcinoma cells more potently (1 to 10 mg/L) than Hela and Colo 205 cells.[41] Both callus and field grown *Gynostemma* increased the lifespan of mice bearing Ehrlich's ascites carcinoma, an effect attributed to immune enhancement.[42] Crude gypenosides also had activity versus S-180 cells both in vitro and in vivo.[43] Gypenosides protected against cyclophosphamide-induced bone marrow and spermatozoal mutagenesis when given orally at 40 to 160 mg/kg to mice.[44] Similar treatments enhanced immune function in another

report.[45] Cancer patients given jiaogulan granules after chemotherapy showed improved immune function by several endpoints.[46]

Other: Experimental senility in mice induced by D-galactose was attenuated by intraperitoneal (IP) injection of *Gynostemma* aqueous extract.[47]

TOXICOLOGY: The LD50 in mice for the aqueous extract has been reported as 2.8 g/kg IP. However, LD50 for the oral route could not be determined.[34] Another study found an oral LD50 of 49 g/kg for the crude extract with no organ toxicity at 4 g/kg daily for 90 days.[48] A third study of two different extracts found an LD50 of 1 to 2 g/kg IP in mice.[49] A rat LD50 of 1.9 g/kg IP has also been reported.[34] Side effects reported in clinical studies included severe nausea and increased bowel movements.[50]

SUMMARY: *Gynostemma pentaphyllum* and its extracts are relatively nontoxic, with extensive chemical characterization and numerous pharmacologic studies supporting use in hyperlipidemia and as an immune stimulant. Several of its bioactive saponins are identical and most are closely related to the ginsenosides found in ginseng.

PATIENT INFORMATION – Jiaogulan

Uses: Studies on *Gynostemma* have found that the plant is effective in regulating blood pressure, strengthening the immune system, lowering cholesterol, and in increasing stamina and endurance properties. *Gynostemma* has also been found to have hyperlipidemic, lipid peroxidation adaptogenic, anticancer, cardio- and cerebrovascular effects.

Side effects: The side effects of *Gynostemma* include severe nausea and increased bowel movements.

---

[1] Zhang ZH, et al. Propagation of *Gynostemma pentaphyllum* by tissue culture. *China J Chinese Materia Medica* 1989; 14(6):335–36.

[2] Liu X, et al. Tissue culture and plantlet regeneration of *Gynostemma pentaphyllum*. *Journal of Chinese Medicinal Materials* 1989; 12(6):8–10.

[3] Wu M, et al. Pharmacognosy of *Gynostemma pentaphyllum* and *Cayratia japonica*. *Zhongyaocai* 1987; (4):22–25.

[4] Ding S, et al. Pharmacognostical study of *Gynostemma* (Cucurbitaceae) in China. *Chinese Pharmaceutical Journal* 1994; 29(2):79–83.

[5] Blumert M, et al. *Jiaogulan* (*Gynostemma pentaphyllum*) China's immortality herb. Badger, CA: Torchlight Publishing, 1999.

[6] Nagai M, et al. Two glycosides of a novel dammarane alcohol from *Gynostemma pentaphyllum*. *Chem Pharm Bull* 1981; 29(3):779–83.

[7] Takemoto T, et al. Studies on the constituents of *Gynostemma pentaphyllum* Makino. I. Structures of gypenosides. I-XIV. *Yakugaku Zasshi* 1983; 103:173

[8] Takemoto T, et al. Studies on the constituents of *Gynostemma pentaphyllum* Makino. II. Structures of gypenosides. XV-XXI. *Yakugaku Zasshi* 1983; 103(10):1015–23.

[9] Takemoto T, et al. Studies on the constituents of Cucurbitaceae plants. XI. On the saponin constituents of *Gynostemma pentaphyllum* Makino. *Yakugaku Zasshi* 1984; 104(10):1043–49.

[10] Takemoto T, et al. Studies on the constituents of Cucurbitaceae plants. XII. On the saponin constituents of *Gynostemma pentaphyllum* Makino. *Yakugaku Zasshi* 1984; 104(11):1155–62.

[11] Takemoto T, et al. Studies on the constituents of Cucurbitaceae plants. XIV. On the saponin constituents of *Gynostemma pentaphyllum* Makino. *Yakugaku Zasshi* 1986; 106(8):664–70.

[12] Yoshikawa K, et al. Studies on the constituents of Cucurbitaceae plants. XV. On the saponin constituents of *Gynostemma pentaphyllum* Makino. *Yakugaku Zasshi* 1986; 106(9):758–63.

[13] Yoshikawa K, et al. Studies on the constituents of Cucurbitaceae plants. XVI. On the saponin constituents of *Gynostemma pentaphyllum* Makino. *Yakugaku Zasshi* 1987; 107(4):262–67.

[14] Yoshikawa K, et al. Studies on the constituents of Cucurbitaceae plants. XVII. On the saponin constituents of *Gynostemma pentaphyllum* Makino. *Yakugaku Zasshi* 1987; 107(5):361.

[15] Kuwahara M, et al. Dammarane saponins of *Gynostemma pentaphyllum* Makino and the isolation of malonylginsenosides-Rb1, Rd, and malonylgypenoside V. *Chem Pharm Bull* 1989; 37(1):135–39.

[16] Akihisa T, et al. 14α-methyl-5α-ergosta-9(11),24(28)-dien-3β-ol, a sterol from *Gynostemma pentaphyllum*. *Phytochemistry* 1987; 26(8):2412–13.

[17] Akihisa T, et al. 24,24-Dimethyl-5α-cholestan-3β-ol, a sterol from *Gynostemma pentaphyllum*. *Phytochemistry* 1988; 27(9):2931–33.

[18] Akihisa T, et al. 24,24-Dimethyl-5α-cholest-8–en–3β-ol, a new sterol from *Gynostemma pentaphyllum*. *Yukagaku* 1988; 37(8):659–62.

[19] Akihisa T, et al. (24R)-and (24S)-14α-methyl-5α-ergost-9(11)-en 3β-ols from *Gynostemma pentaphyllum*. *Phytochemistry* 1989;28(4):1271–73.

[20] Akihisa T, et al. 4α, 14α-dimethyl-5α-ergosta-7,9(11),24(28)trien-3β-ol from *Phaseolus vulgaris* and *Gynostemma pentaphyllum*. *Phytochemistry* 1990; 29(5):1647–51.

[21] Akihisa T, et al. Isolation of acetylenic sterols from a higher plant. Further evidence that marine sterols are not unique. *J Org Chem* 1989; 54:606–10.

[22] Hu L, et al. Dammarane-type glycosides from *Gynostemma pentaphyllum*. *Phytochemistry* 1997; 44(4):667.

[23] Fang Z, et al. Isolation and identification of flavonoids glycosides and organic acids from *Gynostemma pentaphyllum*. *China J of Chinese Materia Medica* 1989; 14(11):676–78.

[24] Si J, et al. Isolation and identification of flavonoids from *Gynostemma yixingense*. *Zhiwu Xuebao* 1994; 36(3):239.

[25] Ding S, et al. Gycomoside I: a new dammarane saponin from *Gynostemma compressum*. *Planta Med* 1993; 373.

[26] La Cour B, et al. Traditional Chinese medicine in treatment of hyperlipidaemia. *J Ethnopharmacol* 1995; 46:125–29.

[27] Geng W, et al. Effects of *Gynostemma pentaphyllum* extract on T-lymphocyte and lipid metabolism in rats. *Guangxi Med J* 1988; 10(1):8–9.

[28] Dai H, et al. Effects of the total saponin of *Gynostemma pentaphyllum* on lipoproteins. *Chinese Tradit Herbal Drugs* 1989; 20(4):172–73.

[29] Hu X, et al. Antilipemic effect *Gynostemma pentaphyllum* in patients. *Fujian Medical Journal* 1988; 10(5):4–6.

[30] Zhou H, et al. Treatment of hyperlipidemia with *Gynostemma pentaphyllum* <Jiaogulan>. *Hunan Med J* 1991; 8(5):259–60.

[31] Li L, et al. Protective effect of gypenosides against oxidative stress in phagocytes, vascular endothelial cells, and liver microsomes. *Cancer Biother* 1993; 8(3):263–272.

[32] Li L, et al. Protection of vascular endothelial cells from hydrogen peroxide-induced oxidant injury by gypenosides saponins of *Gynostemma pentaphyllum*. *Phytother Res* 1993; 7(4):299–304.

[33] Li L, et al. Protective effects of gypenosides on rat hepatic lipid peroxidation and membrane fluidity damage: in vitro studies. *Chinese Pharm Bull* 1991; 7(5):341–44.

[34] Chen J, et al. Antistress action of *Gynostemma pentaphyllum*. *Chinese Tradit Patent Med* 1989; 11(1):31–32.

[35] Takagi J, et al. A new platelet aggregation factor from *Gynostemma pentaphyllum* Makino. *Chem Pharm Bull* 1985; 33(12):5568–71.

[36] Wu J, et al. Effects of gypenosides on platelet aggregation, release, and cAMP level in rabbits. *Chinese J Pharmacol Toxicol* 1990; 4(1):54–57.

[37] Li Y, et al. Effects of total gypenosides on heart function and blood pressure of rabbits. *Acta Academiae Medicinae Shandong* 1990; 28(3):34–36.

[38] Chen L, et al. Comparison between the effects of gypenosides and ginsenosides on cardiac function and hemodynamics in dogs. *Chinese J Pharmacol Toxicol* 1990; 4(1):17–20.

[39] Wang Z, et al. Protective effect of gypenoside on acute incomplete cerebral ischemia in rabbits. *Chinese J Pharmacol Toxicol* 1992; 6(3):204–06.

[40] Jin M, et al. Effects of extract of *Gynostemma pentaphyllum* on human rectal adenocarcinoma cell. *Modern Applied Pharmacy* 1992; 9(2):49–52.

[41] Liu H, et al. Suppression effects of gypenosides on cultured human carcinoma cells. *Journal of Xi'an Medical University* 1994; 15(4):346–48.

[42] Wang Z, et al. Inhibitory effect of *Gynostemma pentaphyllum* on Ehrlich's ascites carcinoma. *Tumor* 1990; 10(6):246–49.

[43] Wang Y, et al. Antineoplastic action of gypenosides. *Chinese J Integrated Tradit Western Med* 1988; 8(5):286.

[44] Wang Y, et al. Effects of gypenosides on mutagenesis induced by cyclophosphamide in mice. *Chinese Pharmacol Bull* 1994; 10(6):457–59.

[45] Tong K, et al. Immunological effects of *Gynostemma pentaphyllum* in mice. *Jiangsu Journal of Traditional Chinese Medicine* 1989; (4):184–86.

[46] Wang J, et al. Immunological effects of jiaogulan granule in 19 cancer patients. *Zhejiang Journal of Traditional Chinese Medicine* 1989; 24(10):449.

[47] Xu F, et al. Anti-aging actions of *Gynostemma pentaphyllum* and its compound formula. *Chinese Tradit Patent Med* 1989; 11(5):29–30.

[48] Li R, et al. Chemical and pharmacological studies on *Gynostemma pentaphyllum*. *Journal of New Chinese Medicine* 1988; 20(4):51–53.

[49] Liu X, et al. Pharmacological studies on the total saponin of *Gynostemma pentaphyllum* from Guangxi. *Chinese Tradit Patent Med* 1989; 11(8):27–29.

[50] Chen Z, et al. Progress in the research on the pharmacology of *Gynostemma pentaphyllum*. *Journal of Chinese Medicinal Materials* 1989; 12(6):42–44.

Jojoba

SCIENTIFIC NAME(S): *Simmondsia chinensis* (Link) Schneider and *S. californica* Nutall. Family: Buxaceae

COMMON NAME(S): Jojoba

BOTANY: *Simmondsia chinensis* is a desert shrub indigenous to Arizona, California and Northern Mexico. It grows in a number of deserts worldwide including Israel's Negev Desert. A woody evergreen shrub with thick, leathery, bluish-green leaves and dark brown nutlike fruit. Male and female flowers are borne on separate plants, the number of each being about equal. The plant can withstand extreme daily fluctuations of temperature. It thrives in well-drained, coarse desert soils and coarse mixtures of gravels and clays.[1] The mature plant produces about 5 to 10 pounds of seeds, which range between the coffee bean and peanut in size. It is an important forage plant for desert bighorn sheep and mule deer. While birds and rodents eat the seeds, it is toxic to humans and most animals.[2]

HISTORY: Indians and Mexicans have for a long time used jojoba oil as a hair conditioner and restorer, and in medicine, cooking and rituals. In the United States, jojoba is considered a viable cash crop for the southwestern Indians, and the Bureau of Indian Affairs has funded most of the studies in this area.[2,3]

With the banning of the sale of sperm whale oil in 1973, the cosmetic industry turned to jojoba oil for use in shampoos, moisturizers, sunscreens and conditioners. It has further potential as an industrial lubricant, since it does not break down under high temperature or pressure.[4] A major disadvantage to its use is its relatively high cost.

CHEMISTRY: Jojoba seeds produce 50% by weight a colorless, odorless oil. The oil is almost completely (97%) composed of straight chain monoesters of C-20 and C-22 acids and alcohols with two double bonds. The acids have been identified as mixture of cis-11–eicosenoic (C-20) and cis-13–docosenoic (C-22, erucic) acids. The alcohols have been identified as mixtures of cis-11–eicosenol, cis-13–docosenol and cis-15–tetracosenol (C-24)[5] These alcohols are potentially valuable in the production of detergents, wetting agents and dibasic acids.[3] Also included are small quantities of sterols (less than 0.5% of a total mixture of Campesterol, Stigmasterol and Sitosterol). Jojoba oil is essentially triglyceride-free.[1,5]

PHARMACOLOGY: Jojoba is most commonly recognized as an ingredient in cosmetics and other topical preparations. JMC Technologies, a jojoba marketing and research cooperative, reports that studies with jojoba oil conducted at Ben Gurion University Medical Center (Israel) indicate that the wax may be of value in the management of acne and psoriasis.[6] Other topical irritations such as sunburn and chapped skin appear to respond to topical jojoba therapy. While this data is largely unpublished and requires confirmation, there is a substantial body of anecdotal evidence that suggests the wax is beneficial in alleviating minor skin irritations.

There has also been considerable interest and success in marketing jojoba preparations promoted to stimulate hair growth and rejuvenation. Jojoba oil penetrates skin and skin oils easily—unclogging hair follicles and preventing sebum buildup which could lead to hair loss.[7]

In a rabbit study, ingestion of jojoba oil as a 2% supplement to an atherogenic diet produced a 40% reduction of blood cholesterol, although the mechanism by which this occurred was not determined.[8]

Recent study has shown antioxidant activity of jojoba. This activity is related to the content of α-tocopherol found in the leaves.[9]

Jojoba oil is presently used in cosmetic and personal care products. Recommended oil ingredient levels include: skin care preparations, 5–10%; shampoos and conditioners, 1–2%; bar soaps, 0.5-3.0%.[7]

TOXICOLOGY: The LD-50 of crude jojoba wax is greater than 160 g/kg in mice.[10] In ocular tests, it was only slightly irritating (comparable to olive oil) and its application resulted in less irritation than liquid paraffin. Hypoallergenic sensitivity to the wax has been reported,[10] and cases of contact dermatitis have been reported in persons using jojoba oil as shampoo or hair conditioner.[4]

Topical administration of the refined wax to guinea pigs for 20 weeks resulted in no systemic effects; a reversible swelling accompanied by reduced skin flexibility and an increased sensitivity to shaving was observed. There were, however, no histological changes in skin tissues. These effects were most likely due to an occlusive-like action created by the wax. This mechanism is inconsistent with data provided by JMC Technologies which indicate that jojoba's effects result from percutaneous absorption and subsequent incorporation into dermal tissue.

Subcutaneous injection of 1 mL/kg for 7 weeks in test animals resulted in no systemic effects, although some systemic accumulation was observed.[11]

Jojoba oil is 14% erucic acid, a causative factor in myocardial fibrosis.[8] Although no direct relationship has been established between this compound and jojoba toxicity, jojoba should not be ingested in any form. *Lactobacillus acidophilus* and *Lactobacillus bulgaricus* grow well on jojoba seed meal, metabolizing toxic simmondsin and other toxicants remaining in the meal after removal of the oil. The treated meal is nontoxic to mice, poultry, sheep and cattle.[12,13]

SUMMARY: A combination of social, economic and political factors have generated increased interest in the use of jojoba oil in cosmetics and industrial lubricants. If its hypocholesterolemic potential is to be realized, long-term studies must be undertaken.

PATIENT INFORMATION – Jojoba

Uses: Jojoba oil has traditionally been used in cosmetics, medicine and cooking. It appears to alleviate skin irritations and help guard against hair loss.

Side Effects: Jojoba should not be ingested. Seeds are toxic. One component contributes to myocardial fibrosis. Sensitive individuals may develop contact dermatitis.

---

[1] Wisniak J. Jojoba oil and derivatives. *Prog Chem Fats Other Lipids* 1977;15(3):167.
[2] Office of Arid Lands Studies, University of Arizona. Jojoba: What is it? (leaflet). 1979;June.
[3] Majgh TH. Guayule and Jojoba: Agriculture in Semiarid Regions. *Science* 1977;196:1189.
[4] Scott MJ, Scott MJ Jr. Jojoba oil. *J Am Acad Der* 1982;6(4 Pt 1):545.
[5] McKeown EC. Jojoba: A Botanical with Proven Functionality. *Cosmet Toiletries* 1983;98(6):81.
[6] Mosovich B. Treatment of acne and psoriasis, Proceedings of the 6th International Jojoba Conference, Ben Gurion University, Israel. 1984;October 21–26.
[7] Arndt GJ. Jojoba. *Cosmet Toiletries* 1987;102(6):68.
[8] Clarke JA, Yermanos DM. Effects of ingestion of jojoba oil on blood cholesterol levels and lipoprotein patterns in New Zealand white rabbits. *Biochem Biophys Res Com* 1981;102(4):1409.

[9] Mallet JF, et al. Antioxidant activity of plant leaves in relation to their α-tocopherol content. *Food Chem* 1994;49(1):61.
[10] Taguchi M, Kunimoto T. Toxicity studies on jojoba oil for cosmetic uses. *Cosmet Toiletries* 1977;92(9):53.
[11] Yaron A, et al. Physiological toleration of jojoba wax in laboratory animals. *J Soc Cos Chem* 1982;33(5-6):141.
[12] Verbiscar AJ, et al. Detoxification of jojoba meal by Lactobacilli. *J Agri Food Chem* 1981;29(2):296.
[13] Perez-Gil F, et al. [Chemical composition and content of antiphysiological factors of jojoba (Simmondsia chinensis) residual meal]. [Spanish]. *Archivos Latinoamericanos de Nutricion* 1989;39(4):591.

Juniper

SCIENTIFIC NAME(S): *Juniperus communis* Family: Cupressacea

COMMON NAME(S): Juniper

BOTANY: The genus *Juniperus* includes 60 to 70 species of aromatic evergreens native to Northern Europe, Asia and North America. The plants bear blue or reddish fruit variously described as berries or berry-like cones. Junipers are widely used as ornamental trees. The cone is a small green berry during its first year of growth and turns blue-black during the second year. The small flowers bloom from May to June.

HISTORY: Juniper berries (the mature female cone) have long been used as a flavoring in foods and alcoholic beverages such as gin. Production by apothecaries and other historical uses for gin have been reported.[1] Gin's original preparation used juniper for kidney ailments. The berries also serve as seasonings, for pickling meats and as flavoring for liqueurs and bitters. Other uses include perfumery and cosmetics. Oil of juniper, also known as oil of sabinal, is used for preserving catgut ligatures.[2] Juniper tar is also used for its gin-like flavor and in perfumery. In herbal medicine, juniper has been used as a carminative and as a steam inhalant in the management of bronchitis. It has also been used to control arthritis.

CHEMISTRY: Juniper berries contain about 2% volatile oil, juniperin, resin (about 10%), proteins, and formic, acetic, and malic acids. In addition, fatty acid, sterol and terpene content has been analyzed by gas chromatography, identified from extracts of ripe and unripe juniper berries.[3] The dried ripe fruit contains oil of juniper, pinene, cadinenes, camphene and a number of diterpene acids.

The volatile oil is composed of more than 50% monoterpenes (pinene, myrcene, sabinene) with many minor constituents. Variability in juniper oil is seen, particularly between first year fruits vs third year fruits.[4] Steam distillation of the berries yields mono- and sesquiterpenes from the oil.[5] In other studies, isolation, chemical characterization and composition of the essential oil of juniper are described, revealing 23 compounds.[6,7]

Isolates of dimeric proanthocyanidins (tannin-producing), from bark extracts of *Juniperus communis* have also been reported,[8] as well as determination of polyprenols in the juniper pine needles.[9]

PHARMACOLOGY: Juniper berry oil has been used as a **diuretic**. This activity is most likely due to the action of terpinen-4-ol, which is known to increase renal glomerular filtration rate.[10] This activity appears to be a local irritant effect. Juniper berries are often found in herbal diuretic products. The effects of juniper berry oil with regard to urinary tract disease has also been reported.[11]

Juniper has been used in phytotherapy and cosmetics in the eastern Mediterranean area.[12] Reported therapeutic uses of juniper include juniper baths for treatment of **neurasthenic neurosis**[13] and management of scalp **psoriasis** in its tar form in combination with other tars.[14]

In traditional Swedish medicine, *Juniperus communis* has been used to treat wounds and inflammatory diseases. A recent study evaluates its **inhibitory activity on prostaglandin biosynthesis** and **platelet activating factor** (PAF)-induced exocytosis in vitro.[15]

Dried berries of juniper and juniper decoction have been evaluated into recent animal studies. Results support hypoglycemic activity in streptozotocin-diabetic mice.[16,17] Further proof is necessary to determine if this effect can be beneficial for human diabetics.

Berry extracts increase uterine tone and should, therefore, not be ingested by pregnant women. Anti-implantation/anti-fertility activity has been determined in female rats by three similar studies, with one study reporting 60% to 70% efficacy.[18,19,20]

In a recent study, the antioxidative effects of juniper are discussed.[21]

Of interest in veterinary medicine, treatment of psoroptic mange in sheep with extract of *Juniperus communis* has been reported.[22]

TOXICOLOGY: Adverse effects in humans are generally of an allergic nature. These include occupational allergy affecting the skin and respiratory tract[23] through a sensitivity to airborne juniper pollen.[24] Two reports note that

Chinese, Japanese and Filipinos tend to be more sensitive to juniper pollens than Caucasians.[25,26] Juniper and other related pollens affect 13% to 36% of patients with pollen allergies.[27]

Epidermal contact with juniper tar (eg, preparation for psoriasis treatment) can cause potentially carcinogenic DNA damage in human tissue.[28]

Single large doses of juniper berries may cause catharsis, and repeated large doses may be associated with convulsions and renal damage.[2]

Kidney irritation from juniper oil is examined in one report, that relates this effect to 1–terpinen-4–ol content.[29]

Because the berries are known to exert their diuretic effect by irritating the renal tissue, products containing juniper should be used with caution by all and should never be used by those with reduced renal function. Safer and more effective diuretic and carminative drugs exist. The oil can induce gastric irritation and may induce diarrhea. Therefore, its use is limited to low concentrations (less than 0.01%) as a beverage flavor.

Juniper tar has an oral lethal dose of 8014 mg/kg in the rat.[2]

SUMMARY: Junipers are evergreen trees found widely in the northern hemisphere. The dried ripe fruit is commonly used as a flavoring in foods and alcoholic beverages, particularly gin, and in cosmetics and perfumes. Juniper berries and their extracts have been used with some success as diuretics. Juniper may have some promise in diabetic treatment, but further study is necessary. Juniper has an extensive toxicology profile, and therefore must be used with caution.

PATIENT INFORMATION – Juniper

Uses: Juniper berries have long been used as a flavoring for beverages and as a seasoning for cooking. It is also used as a diuretic and in the management of bronchitis and arthritis.

Side Effects: Skin and respiratory allergic reactions, potentially carcinogenic DNA damage and, in large doses, convulsions and renal damage. Use is limited to low concentrations. Juniper should not be ingested by pregnant women.

---

[1] Clutton DW. *Flavour Ind* 1972;3(Sep):454–6.
[2] Windholz M, et al. *The Merck Index*, 10th edition, Merck and Co., Rahway, 1983.
[3] Guerra-Hernandez EJ, et al. *Cience Ind Farm* 1988;7(Jan):8–13.
[4] Horster H. *Planta Medica* 1974;25(Feb):73–79.
[5] Lamparsky D, et al. *Parfuemerie Und Kosmetik* 1985;66(Sep):553–6,558–60.
[6] Da Proenca Cunha A. *Revista Portuguesa de Farmacia* 1989;39:(Jul-Sep):18–20.
[7] Proenca Da Cunha A. *Journal of Essential Oil Research* 1989;1(Jan-Feb):15–17.
[8] Engelshowe R. *Planta Medica* 1983;49(Nov):170–5.
[9] Sasak W, et al. *FEBS Letters* 1976;64(1):55-8.
[10] Janku J, et al. *Experientia* 1957;13:255.
[11] Schilcher H. *Medizinische Monatsschrift Fur Pharmazeuten* 1995;18(7):198-9.
[12] Tammaro F, Xepapadakis G. *J Ethnopharmacol* 1986;16:167.
[13] Jonkov S, Naidenov G. *Folia Med* (Plovdiv) 1974;16:291.
[14] Cunliffe WJ, et al. *British Journal of Clinical Practice* 1974;28(Sep):314-316.
[15] Tunon H, et al. *Journal of Ethnopharmacology* 1995;48(2):61-76.
[16] Swanston-Flatt SK, et al. *Diabetologia* 1990;33(8):462-4.
[17] Sanchez de Medina F, et al. *Planta Medica* 1994;60(3):197-200.
[18] Agrawal OP, et al. *Planta Medica* 1980;SUPPL:98-101.
[19] Prakash AO, et al. *ACTA Europaea Fertilitatis*. 1985;16(6):441–8.
[20] Prakash AO. *International Journal of Crude Drug Research* 1986;24(Mar):16-24.
[21] Takacsova M, et al. *Nahrung* 1985;39(3):241-3.
[22] Srivastava SC, et al. *Indian Veterinary Journal* 1969;46(9):826-8.
[23] Rothe A, et al. *Berufsdermatosen* (Germany, West) 1973;21:11.
[24] Anderson JH. *Ann Allergy* 1985;54:390.
[25] Kaufman HS, et al. *Ann Allergy* 1984;53:135.
[26] Kaufman HS, et al. *Ann Allergy* 1988;60(1):53-6.
[27] Bousquet J, et al. *Clin Allergy* 1984;14:249.
[28] Schoket B, et al. *Journal of Investigative Dermatology* 1990;94(2):241-6.
[29] Schilcher H, et al. *PZ Wissenschaft* 1993;138(3-4):85–91.

Kaolin

SCIENTIFIC NAME(S): Kaolin, hydrated aluminum silicate

COMMON NAME(S): Heavy or light kaolin, China clay, bolus alba, porcelain clay, white bole, argilla[1]

SOURCE: Kaolin is a hydrated aluminum silicate. It is a naturally occurring clay that is prepared for pharmaceutical purposes by washing with water to remove sand and other impurities.

HISTORY: Kaolin has been used commercially and medicinally for hundreds of years. It is currently found in the manufacture of pottery, bricks, cement, plastering material, color lakes (insoluble dyes) and insulators. It is also used in pharmaceutical preparations as a filtering agent to clarify liquids. When applied topically, it serves as an emollient and drying agent. When ingested, it acts as an adsorbent to bind gastrointestinal toxins and to control diarrhea.

Kaolin has been added to dusting powders and is used as a tablet excipient. Kaolin is also utilized in a variety of automated laboratory chemistry tests, including the determination of activated coagulation time (ACT)[2] and in the serodiagnosis of tuberculosis, using the kaolin agglutination test (KAT).[3]

CHEMISTRY: Kaolin has the approximate chemical formula of $H_2 Al_2 Si_2 O_8 (H_2O)$. It is a white or yellow-white powder that has a slightly oily feel to the touch. It is insoluble in water.[1] Light kaolin is the preferred material for use in pharmaceutical preparations. The finely divided particles of kaolin yield a very large surface area that adsorbs a wide variety of compounds.

PHARMACOLOGY: When given orally, kaolin (especially light kaolin) adsorbs substances from the gastrointestinal tract and increases the bulk of feces.[4] Therefore, antidiarrheal preparations containing kaolin have been used in the treatment of enteritis, cholera and dysentery. Kaolin preparations, however, have no intrinsic antibacterial activity and should not be used as the sole treatment in infectious diarrheas. A dose of 15 to 60 g is typically administered to adults to assist in the control of diarrhea.

TOXICOLOGY: Because kaolin actively adsorbs a wide variety of substances to its surface, it should not be administered with drugs that may adhere (ie, digoxin, lincomycin, phenothiazines, etc).[4] This is a particular concern when formulating new dosage forms, in that it must be assured that the kaolin diluent does not reduce the bioavailability of the active drug substance.[4]

Kaolin is highly insoluble and is not absorbed systemically. Therefore, it is not generally associated with severe toxicity.

Inhalation of nonfibrous silicate compounds such as kaolin may predispose miners to pulmonary diseases.[5]

SUMMARY: Kaolin is a widely used natural mineral that finds its most common pharmaceutical application as an adsorbent in antidiarrheal preparations. Kaolin is believed to exert it effects by adsorbing toxins that may have initiated the diarrheal episode by providing bulk to the stool. Kaolin may adsorb certain drugs, thereby reducing their bioavailability.

PATIENT INFORMATION – Kaolin

Uses: Kaolin is used internally to control diarrhea and topically as an emollient and drying agent.

Side Effects: Kaolin may adsorb certain drugs and reduce their bioavailability.

---

[1] Windholz M, ed. *The Merck Index, 10th ed.* Rahway, NJ: Merck & Co., 1983.
[2] Huyzen RJ, et al. Alternative perioperative anticoagulation monitored during cardiopulmonary bypass in aprotinin-treated patients. *J Cardiothorac Vasc Anesth* 1994;8:153.
[3] Sarnaik RM, et al. Serodiagnosis of tuberculosis: assessment of kaolin agglutination test. *Tuber Lung Dis* 1993;74 405.
[4] Bowman WC. *Textbook of Pharmacology, 2nd ed.* London: Blackwell Scientfic Publications, 1980.
[5] Short SR, Petsonk EL. Respiratory health risks among nonmetal miners. *Occup Med* 1993;8:57.

Karaya Gum

SCIENTIFIC NAME(S): *Sterculia urens* Roxb. Family: Sterculiaceae. The gum may also be obtained from *S. villosa*, *S. tragacantha* or other species of *Sterculia.*[1]

COMMON NAME(S): Karaya, sterculia, Indian tragacanth, Bassora tragacanth, kadaya, mucara, kadira, katila, kullo [2,3,4,5]

BOTANY: The Sterculia is a soft wooded tree that grows to approximately 30 ft. It is native to India and Pakistan and grows there almost exclusively, where it is cultivated for karaya production. All parts of the tree exude a soft gum when injured. Karaya gum is produced by charring or scarring the tree trunk and removing a piece of bark or by drilling holes into the trunk. The gum seeps from the scars and is collected, washed and dried. The tree bears a star-like fruit and flowers bloom from February to March.[3]

HISTORY: The use of karaya gum became widespread during the early 20th century, when it was used as an adulterant for tragacanth gum. However, experience indicated that karaya possessed certain physiochemical properties that made it more useful than tragacanth; furthermore, karaya gum was less expensive. Today the gum is used in a variety of products to provide bulk, including cosmetics, hair sprays and lotions.[6] The bark is astringent and has been used traditionally.[3]

CHEMISTRY: The quality of karaya gum depends on how well impurities have been removed. Food-grade gum is usually a white to pinkish gray powder with a slight vinegar smell.[2] Pharmaceutical grades of karaya may be almost clear or translucent.[3]

Karaya gum is the least soluble of the commercial plant exudates but it absorbs water rapidly and swells to form viscous colloidal solutions even at low concentrations (1%).[2] When used in higher concentrations in water (up to 4%), karaya forms gels or pastes. Unlike other gums, karaya swells in 60% alcohol, but remains insoluble in other organic solvents. Karaya may absorb up to 100 times its weight in water.[2]

The polysaccharide component of karaya has a high molecular weight and is composed of residues containing galacturonic acid, beta-D-galactose, glucuronic acid, L-rhamnose and other residues.[1,2,3]

Because the gum is partially acetylated, upon degrading it may release acetic acid.[2]

PHARMACOLOGY: Karaya gum is not digested, nor is it absorbed systemically. Medicinally, it is used primarily as a bulk laxative[7] and as an adhesive for dental fixtures and ostomy equipment.[4] The gum has been used as a base for salicylic acid patches.[8] Karaya gum is essentially inert and is not associated with any pharmacologic activity per se. Some preliminary studies suggest that gums may normalize blood sugar and plasma lipid levels,[9] but this has not been well investigated with karaya gum.

The demulcent properties of the gum make it useful as an ingredient in lozenges to relieve sore throat.[3] A protective coating of karaya gum applied to dentures has been shown to reduce bacterial adhesion by 98%.[10]

TOXICOLOGY: Karaya gum is generally recognized as safe for internal consumption. Widespread experience with the product throughout the US and Europe has not been associated with any significant adverse experiences.[11]

SUMMARY: Karaya gum finds widespread use in the food and pharmaceutical industries. Its ability to absorb large amounts of water make it useful in the production of gels and as a bulk laxative. The gum has not been associated with any significant toxicity and is essentially inert when ingested.

PATIENT INFORMATION – Karaya Gum

Uses: Karaya gum is used in cosmetics and food, and in pharmaceuticals as a laxative and adhesive.

Side Effects: Karaya gum is generally recognized as safe.

---

[1] Tyler VE, et al. *Pharmacognosy.* Philadelphia, PA: Lea & Febiger, 1981.

[2] Leung AY. *Encyclopedia of Common Natural Ingredients Used In Food, Drugs, and Cosmetics.* New York, NY: J. Wiley and Sons, 1980.

[3] Morton JF. *Major Medicinal Plants.* Springfield, IL: CC Thomas, 1977.

[4] Evans WC. *Trease and Evans' Pharmacognosy, 13th ed.* London, England: Bailliere Tindall, 1989.

[5] Osol A, Farrar GE Jr, eds. *The Dispensatory of the United States of America, 25th ed.* Philadelphia, PA: J.B. Lippincott Co., 1955.

[6] Der Marderosian AH, Liberti LE. *Natural Product Medicine.* Philadelphia, PA: G.F. Stickley Co., 1988.

[7] Meier P, et al. Bulk-forming agents as laxatives in geriatric patients. *Schweiz Med Wochenschr* 1990;120(9):314.

[8] Bart BJ, et al. Salicylic acid in karaya gum patch as a treatment for verruca vulgaris. *J Am Acad Dermatol* 1989;20(1):74.

[9] Behall KM. Effect of soluble fibers on plasma lipids, glucose tolerance and mineral balance. *Adv Exp Med Biol* 1990;270:7.

[10] Wilson M, Harvey W. Prevention of bacterial adhesion to denture acrylic. *J Dent* 1989;17(4):166.

[11] Anderson DM. Evidence for the safety of gum karaya (*Sterculia* spp.) as a food additive. *Food Addit Contam* 1989;6(2):189.

Kava

SCIENTIFIC NAME(S): *Piper methysticum* Forst. f. Family: Piperaceae

COMMON NAME(S): Kava, kawa, kava-kava, awa, yangona

BOTANY: Kava is the dried rhizome and roots of *Piper methysticum*, a large shrub widely cultivated in many Pacific islands ranging from Hawaii and Tahiti to New Guinea.[1] It has large, heart-shaped leaves and is propagated exclusively by root cuttings. It is thought to be derived from the wild species *P. wichmannii* C. DC.[2] Many kava cultivars are recognized, and the comparative chemistry and ethnopharmacology have been studied in detail by Lebot,[3] who grouped 121 named cultivars from 51 islands into 6 chemotypes.

HISTORY: The kava beverage is prepared from the roots of the plant, which were traditionally chewed or pulverized and steeped in water. The cloudy mixture is filtered and served at room temperature. Kava has been an important part of the Pacific island ceremonial cultures for many centuries, with elaborate rituals attending its consumption.[4] Traces of kava extract on artifacts from Fiji have been identified by mass spectrometry.[5] Its main use has been as a relaxation inducer in kava ceremony participants, facilitating discussion and interaction.

CHEMISTRY: Lewin's monograph on kava[6] stimulated research on kava and isolation of the kava lactones, the primary bioactive constituents of kava root. There are 6 major kava lactones: Kawain, dihydrokawain, methysticin, dihydromethysticin, yangonin, and demethoxyyangonin,[7] which occur in varying proportions in different cultivars. Borsche's group was the first to elucidate the structures of the kava lactones in the 1930s,[8] although many of the pure compounds were first isolated in the 19th century. They were later synthesized in racemic and optically pure form.[9-11] While the kava lactones are characteristic of *P. methysticum*, individual kava lactones have more recently been found in other plant families (*Lauraceae*, *Gesneriaceae*, and *Zingiberaceae*[12]). A process for the commercial production of kava extract has been patented by the Schwabe company,[13] and the use of supercritical fluid extraction for removing kava lactones from the root has been demonstrated.[14] Many methods have been developed for the analysis of kava lactones. These include thin layer chromatography,[15] gas chromatography,[16] HPLC,[17-19] GC-MS,[12,20-22] chiral HPLC,[23] HPLC-MS,[24] and micellar electrokinetic chromatography.[25] The metabolism of the kava lactones has been studied in rats[26] and humans[27] while the uptake into mouse brain of kava lactones has also been studied.[28] The latter study found elevated brain levels of kawain when the whole resin was administered, compared with kawain alone. This supported the observation that the total kava resin has greater pharmacologic effect than the sum of the individual kava lactones, presumably because of saturation of common metabolic pathways utilized by these compounds.

Other constituents of kava include 2 chalcones, flavokawains A and B,[29] which Shulgin later postulated to be the cause of a dermopathy seen in heavy kava users.[30] The Schwabe patent[13] claims production of an extract with very low chalcone content. Several minor alkaloids have also been isolated from kava roots[31] and leaf.[32]

PHARMACOLOGY: Chewing kava causes numbness in the mouth due to a local anesthetic action of the kava lactones. In addition, it produces a mild euphoria characterized by feelings of contentment and fluent and lively speech. Higher doses may lead to muscle weakness, especially in the legs, although some observers relate this to sitting for long periods during the kava ceremony rather than to kava itself. Very high doses may induce a deep sleep. Kava lactones, especially kawain, have been shown to have modest anticonvulsant activity in electroshock and metrazol models.[33]

The molecular mechanism of action of kava lactones and kava is not entirely clear. Kava lactones at concentrations from 0.1 to 100 mcM were found to enhance the binding of bicuculline to the GABA receptor by only 20% to 30%.[34] Another study found weak displacement of diazepam from rat brain membranes by kava lactones but no effect on binding of GABA or of baclofen.[35] The observation that strychnine-induced convulsions are effectively antagonized by several kava lactones supports a possible effect on the glycine receptor.[36] Kava extract and methysticin also protect rats against ischemic brain damage, although several kava lactones were not active in this model.[37] This could point to antagonism of the excitatory amino acids glutamate and aspartate. Inhibition of uptake of noradrenaline but not serotonin by kava lactones at high doses was observed.[38] No effect on dopamine or serotonin levels occurred in a chronic experiment with kava lactones in rats.[39]

A somewhat more persuasive mechanism involves kava lactone inhibition of various neuronal sodium channels. Patch clamp experiments with voltage-gated sodium channels of rat hippocampal neurons found that kava lactones could rapidly and reversibly lower peak amplitudes of sodium currents.[40] A noncompetitive inhibition of the binding of batrachotoxinin benzoate to voltage-gated sodium channels by kava lactones was demonstrated in saturation-binding experiments.[41] Less potently, kava lactones blocked veratridine-activated sodium channels but had no effect on glutamate release from brain slices.[42] In rat brain synaptosomes, kava lactones appeared to interact with voltage-dependent sodium and calcium channels.[43] High concentrations of synthetic kavain relaxed evoked contractile activity in a guinea pig ileum preparation, showing that smooth muscle also is affected by kava lactones.[44]

Neurophysiological studies of sleep-wakefulness in cats showed a decrease in muscle tone, marked changes in EEG, and decreased duration of wakefulness and increased sleep. Involvement of the amygdala and other limbic structures of the brain was deduced.[45] These effects were distinct from those of tricyclic antidepressants and benzodiazepines.

Kavain had an antithrombotic effect on platelets, dose-dependently blocking platelet aggregation, ATP release, and synthesis of prostaglandins at high micromolar concentrations.[46] Despite a reputation as an antimicrobial agent in urinary tract infections, kava extracts showed minimal antifungal, and no antimicrobial or antiviral activity.[47]

Concerns about impaired performance under the influence of kava have motivated several studies in humans. Prescott, et al,[48] found insignificant changes in cognitive function under kava, with only the extent of body sway showing an increase. Subjects' rating of intoxication under kava was low to moderate, while respiration, heart rate, and blood pressure were unaffected. Kava lowered arousal rating without affecting the stress rating, although the decrease was not statistically significant.[48] Another small study compared kava with oxazepam in their effects on behavior and event-related potentials in a word recognition task. While oxazepam produced pronounced effects on performance, no effects were seen with kava.[49] A

study of reaction time by the same authors concluded that kava may increase attention slightly, in contrast to oxazepam, which impaired attention.[50] In EEG studies, kavain showed mild sedation at high doses (600 mg) but not at lower doses (200 mg).[51] Kava had no effect on alertness and long-term memory in a further study.[52] Minor changes in vision and balance were detected with kava in a single subject.[53]

Clinical studies on kava have produced evidence of substantial efficacy in mild-to-moderate anxiety. Several studies have been reviewed in comparison with other CNS-active herbal products by Schulz.[54] Kavain was compared with oxazepam in a double-blind study and was equally effective and safe.[55] Over 4 weeks, kava extract progressively reduced anxiety compared with placebo with no reported side effects.[56] Menopause-related anxiety was successfully treated with kava extract in an 8-week study, with rapid onset of efficacy.[57] A longer, 25-week, double-blind, placebo-controlled study of 101 patients with anxiety disorders found that Hamilton Anxiety Scale scores decreased faster than with placebo.[58] A similar 4-week study using HAMA and CGI scores found kava extract effective.[59] All of the preceding studies were conducted in Germany. The first US study of kava in anxiety was recently reported at a conference but has not yet been published. It found similar therapeutic effects of kava extract under double-blind, placebo-controlled conditions.[60]

TOXICOLOGY: Kava's actions are additive with those of alcohol and benzodiazepines, although this well-known interaction is poorly documented in the clinical toxicology literature.[61,62] Heavy consumption of kava produces a scaly skin rash similar to pellagra. However, supplementation with niacin did not reverse the condition.[63] Cessation of kava use causes reduction or disappearance of the dermopathy. Shulgin suggested that the flavokawain pigments were responsible for this toxicity;[30] despite the lack of any scientific proof, these pigments are commonly removed in the production of commercial extracts.[13] Poor nutritional status and other general adverse effects were seen in an Australian aboriginal community where (non-traditional) kava consumption was very heavy.[64] Disturbances in visual accomodation have also been described.[53]

Kava is contraindicated in pregnancy and lactation and should not be used in patients with depression. Do not use while operating heavy machinery. There is a possible interaction between kava and other sedatives and levodopa. Limit kava use to 3 months to avoid habituation.

SUMMARY: Kava has long been a popular social and ceremonial drink in many South Pacific islands. Kava lactones are the chemical principles responsible for its mild sedative effects, which are additive with those of alcohol or benzodiazepines. Heavy use can cause a characteristic skin condition and visual disturbances. Reviews of its chemistry and pharmacology are extensive.[1,6,30,65-70]

Kava root is approved for conditions of nervous anxiety, stress, and restlessness by the German Commission E, and is also monographed in the *British Herbal Pharmacopeia* (vol. 2) and by WHO (vol. 2).

PATIENT INFORMATION – Kava

Indications: Kava is used in the treatment of mild-to-moderate anxiety and for sedation.

Side Effects: Kava is contraindicated in pregnancy and lactation and should not be used in patients with depression. Heavy consumptoms of kava can produce a scaly skin rash similar to pellagra; however, supplementation with niacin did not reverse the condition. Disturbances in visual accomodation have been described.

---

1 Singh Y. Kava: An overview. *J Ethnopharmacol* 1992;37:13.

2 Lebot V, et al. Evidence for conspecificity of *Piper methysticum* Forst. f. and *Piper wichmannii* C. DC. *Biochem Syst Ecol* 1996;24:775.

3 Lebot V, et al. Genetic control of kavalactone chemotypes in *Piper methysticum* cultivars. *Phytochem* 1996;43:397.

4 Holmes L. The function of kava in modern Samoan culture. In: Efron DH, *Ethnopharmacologic Search for Psychoactive Drugs*. Washington, DC: Public Health Service Pub. No. 1645,1967;107.

5 Hocart C, et al. Chemical archaeology of kava, a potent brew. *Rapid Comm Mass Spectrom* 1993;7:219.

6 Lewin L. *Über Piper methysticum (kawa-kawa)*. Berlin: Medical Society,1886.

7 Smith R. Kava lactones in *Piper methysticum* from Fiji. *Phytochem* 1983;22:1055.

8 Borsche W, et al. Constituents of kava root X. Kawain and dihydrokawain. *Chem Ber* 1930;63B:2414.

9 Klohs M, et al. *Piper methysticum* Forst. II. The synthesis of dl-methysticin and dl-dihydromethysticin. *J Org Chem* 1959;24:1829.

10 Israili Z, et al. Synthesis of kavain, dihydrokavain, and analogs. *J Org Chem* 1976;41:4070.

11 Spino C, et al. Enantioselective synthesis of (+)- and (-)-dihydrokawain. *Tetrahedron Lett* 1996;37:6503.

12 Kuster R, et al. GC-MS determination of kava-pyrones in *Alpinia zerumbet* leaves. *HRC Journal of High Resolution Chromatography* 1999;22:129.

13 Schwabe K-P. *Kava-kava extract, process for the production thereof and use thereof*. 1994;United States Patent No.5296224.

14 Lopez-Avila V, et al. Supercritical fluid extraction of kava lactones from *Piper methysticum* (Kava) herb. *HRC Journal of High Resolution Chromatography* 1997;20:555.

15 Gracza L, et al. Eifache methode zur trennung und quantitativen bestimmung von kawa-laktonen durch hochleistungs-flüssigkeits-chromatographie. *J Chromatogr* 1980;193:486.

16 Duve R. Gas-liquid chromatographic determination of major constituents of *Piper methysticum*. *Analyst* 1981;106:160.

17 Smith R, et al. High-performance liquid chromatography of kava lactones from *Piper methysticum*. *J Chromatogr* 1984;283:303.

18 Häberlein H, et al. *Piper methysticum*: Enantiomeric separation of kavapyrones by high performance liquid chromatography. *Planta Med* 1997;63:63.

19 Shao Y, et al. Reversed-phase high-performance liquid chromatographic method for quantitative analysis of the six major kavalactones in *Piper methysticum*. *J Chromatogr* 1998;A,825:1.

20 Duffield A, et al. Analysis of kava resin by gas chromatography and electron impact and methane negative ion chemical ionization mass spectrometry. *Biomed Environ Mass Spectrom* 1986;13:621.

21 Cheng D, et al. Identification by methane chemical ionization gas chromatography/mass spectrometry of the products obtained by steam distillation and aqueous acid extraction of commercial *Piper methysticum*. *Biomed Environ Mass Spectrom* 1988;17:371.

22 Duffield A, et al. Analysis of the constituents of *Piper methysticum* by gas chromatography methane chemical ionization mass spectrometry. *Biomed Environ Mass Spectrom* 1986;13:305.

23 Boonen G, et al. Contribution to the quantitative and enantioselective determination of kavapyrones by high-performance liquid chromatography on ChiraSpher NT material. *J Chromatogr* 1997;B702:240.

24 He K, et al. Electrospray high performance liquid chromatography-mass spectrometry in phytochemical analysis of kava (*Piper methysticum*) extract. *Planta Med* 1997;63:70.

25 Lechtenberg M, et al. Qualitative and quantitative micellar electrokinetic chromatography of kavalactones from dry extracts of *Piper methysticum* Forst. and commercial drugs. *J Chromatogr* 1999;A,848:457.

26 Rasmussen A, et al. Metabolism of some kava pyrones in the rat. *Xenobiotica* 1979;9:1.

27 Duffield A, et al. Identification of some human urinary metabolites of the intoxicating beverage kava. *J Chromatogr* 1989;475:273.

28 Keledjian J, et al. Uptake into mouse brain of four compounds present in the psychoactive beverage kava. *J Pharm Sci* 1988;77:1003.

29 Hänsel R, et al. Isolation and characterization of two new pigments from *Piper methysticum* rhizomes. *Arch Pharm* 1961;294:739.

30 Shulgin A. Narcotic pepper. Chemistry and pharmacology of *Piper methysticum* and related species. *Bull Narc* 1973;25:59.

31 Smith R. Pipermethysticine, a novel pyridone alkaloid from *Piper methysticum*. *Tetrahedron* 1979;35:437.

32 Jaggy H, et al. Cepharadione A from *Piper methysticum*. *Planta Med* 1992;58:111.

33 Furgiuele A, et al. Central activity of aqueous extracts of *Piper methysticum* (kava). *J Pharm Sci* 1965;54:247.

34 Boonen G, et al. Influence of genuine kavapyrone enantiomers on the GABA-A binding site. *Planta Med* 1998;64:504.

35 Davies L, et al. Effects of kava on benzodiazepine and GABA receptor binding. *Eur J Pharmacol* 1990;183:558.

36 Kretzschmar R, et al. Strychnine antagonistic potency of pyrone compounds of the kavaroot (*Piper methysticum* Forst.). *Experientia* 1970;26:283.

37 Backhauss C, et al. Extract of kava (*Piper methysticum*) and its methysticin constituents protect brain tissue against ischemic damage in rodents. *Eur J Pharmacol* 1992;215:265.

38 Seitz U, et al. [³ H]-Monoamine uptake inhibition properties of kava pyrones. *Planta Med* 1997;63:548.

39 Boonen G, et al. In vivo effects of the kavapyrones (+)-dihydromethysticin and (±)-kavain on dopamine, 3,4-dihydroxyphenylacetic acid, serotonin and 5-hydroxyindoleacetic acid levels in striatal and cortical brain regions. *Planta Med* 1998;64:507.

40 Magura EI, et al. Kava extract ingredients, (+)-methysticin and (±)-kavain inhibit voltage-operated Na+-channels in rat CA1 hippocampal neurons. *Neuroscience* 1997;81:345.

41 Friese J, et al. Kavain, dihydrokavain and dihydromethysticin non-competitively inhibit the specific binding of [³ H]-batrachotoxin-A 20-α-benzoate to receptor site 2 of voltage-gated Na+ channels. *Planta Med* 1998;64:458.

42 Gleitz J, et al. Kavain inhibits non-stereospecifically veratridine-activated Na+ channels. *Planta Med* 1996;62:580.

43 Gleitz J, et al. Anticonvulsive action of (±)-kavain estimated from its properties on stimulated synaptosomes and Na+ channel receptor sites. *Eur J Pharmacol* 1996;315:89.

44 Seitz U, et al. Relaxation of evoked contractile activity of isolated guinea-pig ileum by (±)-kavain. *Planta Med* 1997;63:303.

45 Holm E, et al. Studies on the profile of neurophysiological effects of D,L-kavain. Cerebral sites of action and sleep-wakefulness-rhythm in animals. *Arzneim-Forsch* 1991;41:673.

46 Gleitz J, et al. Antithrombotic action of the kava pyrone (+)-kavain prepared from *Piper methysticum* on human platelets. *Planta Med* 1997;63:27.

47 Locher CP, et al. Antimicrobial activity and anti-complement activity of extracts obtained from selected Hawaiian medicinal plants. *J Ethnopharmacol* 1995;49:23.

48 Prescott J, et al. Acute effects of kava on measures of cognitive performance, physiological function and mood. *Drug and Alcohol Review* 1993;12:49.

49 Münte T, et al. Effects of oxazepam and an extract of kava roots (*Piper methysticum*) on event-related potentials in a word recognition task. *Neuropsychobiology* 1993;27:46.

50 Heinze H, et al. Pharmacopsychological effects of oxazepam and kava extract in a visual search paradigm assessed with event-related potentials. *Pharmacopsychiatry* 1994;27:224.

51 Saletu B, et al. EEG-brain mapping, psychometric and psychophysiological studies on central effects of kavain - A kava plant derivative. *Human Psychopharmacology* 1989;4:169.

52 Russell P, et al. The effects of kava on alerting and speed of access of information from long-term memory. *Bulletin of the Psychonomic Society* 1987;25:236.

53 Garner L, et al. Some visual effects caused by the beverage kava. *J Ethnopharmacol* 1985;13:307.

54 Schulz V, et al. Clinical trials with phyto-psychopharmacological agents. *Phytomedicine* 1997;4:379.

55 Lindenberg D, et al. D,L-kavain in comparison with oxazepam in anxiety states, a double blind clinical trial. *Fortschr Med* 1990;108:31.

56 Kinzler E, et al. Clinical efficacy of kava extracts in patients with anxiety syndrome, a double-blind, placebo controlled study over 4 weeks. *Arzneim-Forsch* 1991;41:584.

57 Warnecke V. Neurovegetative dystonia in the female climacteric. Studies in the clinical efficacy and tolerance of kava extract WS 1490. *Fortschr Med* 1991;109:119.

58 Volz H, et al. Kava-kava extract WS 1490 versus placebo in anxiety disorders - A randomized placebo-controlled 25-week outpatient trial. *Pharmacopsychiatry* 1997;30:1.

59 Lehmann E, et al. Efficacy of a special kava extract (*Piper methysticum*) in patients with states of anxiety, tension, and excitedness of non-mental origin - A double-blind, placebo controlled study of four weeks treatment. *Phytomedicine* 1996;3:113.

60 Singh N, et al. A double-blind, placebo controlled study of the effects of kava (*Kavatrol*) on daily stress and anxiety in adults. *Alternative Therapies* 1998;4:97.

61 Almeida J, et al. Coma from the health food store: Interaction between kava and alprazolam. *Ann Intern Med* 1996;125:940.

62 Miller L. Herbal medicinals: selected clinical considerations focusing on known or potential drug-herb interactions. *Arch Intern Med* 1998;158:2200.

63 Ruze P. Kava-induced dermopathy: a niacin deficiency? *Lancet* 1990;335:1442.

64 Mathews J, et al. Effects of the heavy usage of kava on physical health: Summary of a pilot survey in an aboriginal community. *Med J Aust* 1988;148:548.

65 Buckley J, et al. Pharmacology of kava. In: Efron DH, *Ethnopharmacologic Search for Psychoactive Drugs*. Washington, DC: Public Health Service Pub. No. 1645,1967,141.

66 Keller F, et al. A review of the chemistry and pharmacology of the constituents of *Piper methysticum*. *Lloydia* 1963;26:1.

67 Meyer H. Pharmacology of kava. In: Efron DH, Holmstedt B, Kline NS, *Ethnopharmacologic Search for Psychoactive Drugs*. Washington, DC: GPO,1967,133.

68 Mors W, et al. Naturally occurring aromatic derivatives of monocyclic α-pyrones. In: *Prog. Chem. Org. Natural Products*, Zeichmeister L, ed., Berlin: Springer-Verlag,1962,131.

69 Lebot V, et al. *Kava: The Pacific Drug*. New Haven, CT: Yale University Press,1992.

70 Hänsel R. Kava-kava (*Piper methysticum* G. Forster) in contemporary medicinal research. *Eur J Herbal Med* 1996;17.

KH-3

SCIENTIFIC NAME(S): Procaine HCl

COMMON NAME(S): KH-3, Gerovital-H3, GH-3, Gero-vita

HISTORY: The last 25 years have seen the publication of sometimes incredible claims for a product that is often better known to patients than to their health professionals. These products have been administered parenterally and orally for the treatment of cerebral atherosclerosis, progressive dementia, arthritis, hair loss, hypertension, sexual dysfunction and to impart an overall rejuvenating effect.

KH-3 was developed in Germany in the 1960s and has been popularized by Rumanian and other Eastern block researchers.[1,2] Procaine-containing products are available over-the-counter and by mail order in the United States and parts of Europe.

CHEMISTRY and SOURCE: Preparations based primarily on the purported pharmacologic effects of procaine HCl are often marketed as mixtures of procaine, buffers (benzoic acid, potassium metabisulfite, etc), analgesics and nutritional supplements.[2] Most products contain approximately 2% procaine HCl. One German preparation contains procaine, hematoporphyrin to aid absorption, magnesium carbonate, sodium hydrogen phosphate, potassium HCl and other compounds.

PHARMACOLOGY: Procaine has been used for decades as a local anesthetic and antiarrhythmic. The compound has a number of pharmacologic characteristics, including the ability to decrease membrane excitability and alter membrane ionic transmission. Procaine is hydrolyzed rapidly to inactive compounds by plasma enzymes.[2]

Some authors suggest that procaine may act as an inhibitor of monoamine oxidase,[3] thereby relieving depression, although this finding is controversial.

To date, numerous studies have been conducted to evaluate the efficacy of procaine HCl or commercially available mixtures of this compound for the treatment of elderly patients with a variety of organic diseases. The results have been conflicting, but generally indicate that these compounds are ineffective in the treatment of any disease.[4]

Procaine is only poorly absorbed following oral administration, with a considerable amount of the drug being metabolized quickly after absorption. Hematoporphyrin is added to some oral preparations and is said to inhibit intestinal hydrolysis of procaine. There is no evidence that pharmacologic levels of procaine are attained in the brain or other target organs following oral administration of KH-3 or similar products.

As early as 1977, a comprehensive review of the use of procaine in over 100,000 patients found no evidence for its efficacy.[5] Of eight studies published prior to 1980, six found no effect. In one study of hospitalized geriatric patients, digit span and memory improved slightly compared with placebo after 1 year of treatment, and the other study found slight mood improvement in elderly depressed patients.[2] Although a slight antidepressant activity was considered possible by Ostfeld and colleagues,[5] they suggest that this may have accounted for the occasional reports of improvement in complaints related to the musculoskeletal, cardiovascular and gastrointestinal symptoms.

Reports of the effect of procaine on blood cholesterol levels are inconsistent, with some studies showing a reduction in cholesterol and many others showing little beneficial effect.[6]

TOXICOLOGY: Procaine HCl is generally contraindicated in patients who have shown a hypersensitivity to it or related compounds. The drug should not be administered to patients taking concurrent anticholinesterase medications (eg, neostigmine) or who have a known pseudocholinesterase deficiency. It should not be taken during pregnancy.

Procaine may interact with sulfonamides, inhibiting the bacteriostatic action of the antibiotic.[2]

Published reports have described heartburn, migraine and systemic lupus erythematosus following treatment with KH-3, although no adverse events have been reported in other studies.[2]

SUMMARY: Procaine HCl has been available for several decades in preparations designed for the amelioration of chronic diseases associated with aging. Although a number of published reports have described its use, these have generally been poorly designed and their results have been inconclusive. There is no valid evidence for a pharmacologic effect of these compounds in the elderly.

PATIENT INFORMATION – KH-3

Uses: Without much supporting data, KH-3 has been credited with inhibiting diseases of aging.

Side Effects: KH-3 is contraindicated in those sensitive to related compounds or in cholinesterase therapy.

---

[1] Kent S. A look at Gerovital-the "youth" drug. *Geriatrics* 1976;31:95.
[2] Brodaty H. Rejuvenation with KH3. *New Ethicals* 1990;Feb:11.
[3] MacFarlane MD. Procaine HCl (Gerovital H3): A weak, reversible, fully competitive inhibitor of monoamine oxidase. *Fed Proc* 1975;34(1):108.
[4] Orgogozo JM, Spiegel R. Critical review of clinical trials in senile dementia I. *Postgrad Med J* 1987;63:237.

[5] Ostfeld A, et al. The Systemic Use of Procaine in the Treatment of the Elderly: A Review. *J Am Geriatr Soc* 1977;25(1):1.
[6] Jarvik LF, Milne JF. Gerovital-H3 - A Review of the Literature. *Psychopharmacol Bull* 1975;11(4):51.

Khat

SCIENTIFIC NAME(S): *Catha edulis* Forsk. Family: Celastraceae

COMMON NAME(S): Khat, qut, kat, chaat, Kus es Salahin, Tchaad, Tschut, Tohat, Tohai, Gat

BOTANY: A tall plant (9 to 12 feet) with a natural distribution limited to East Africa and the Arabian Peninsula (Kenya, the Yemens and Ethiopia). It grows best at high elevations, and its tender twigs and leaves are harvested almost year-round. Freshly harvested khat is wrapped in leaves and exported by air to neighboring African countries.

HISTORY: One of the most common forms of drug abuse in many East African nations involves chewing parts of the khat plant. Khat use has increased steadily over the last 50 years and has become a problem of significant social and medical importance. Because of its social acceptability and euphoriant effects, khat chewing often plays a dominant role in celebrations, meetings, marriages and other gatherings. Khat use is even prevalent in the Somali military. It is frequently issued to soldiers in their daily rations with the intention of inhibiting their need for food and sleep, as well as increasing their aggression.[1] The amount of khat chewed is variable but is usually about 2 ounces. The tender leaves and stems, which lose their potency one day after harvest, are chewed and the juice is swallowed.[1] It has a sweetish taste and astringent action.[2] Large amounts of liquids are consumed while chewing because of the dryness induced by the plant.

Khat leaves have been used in traditional medicine for the treatment of depression, fatigue, obesity and gastric ulcers.

CHEMISTRY: Studies of the chemical constituents of this plant date to the late 1800s, when European investigators isolated the alkaloid fraction "katin." It had a stimulating effect on the frog heart and caused dilation of the frog pupil. Katin was later renamed cathine and was identified as (+)-norpseudoephedrine (also designated S(-)-alpha-aminopropiophenone).[3] This amphetamine-like compound has been isolated from the genus *Ephedra*, the biologic effects of which are, in many respects, similar to those of khat. The cathine content of dried khat leaves ranges from 0.1% to 0.2%.[4] Cathine has about one-tenth the stimulant activity of d-amphetamine. It decreased food intake and increased locomotor activity in rat studies. The compound has been confused with d,1-norephedrine in the literature, although the two compounds differ significantly in pharmacologic properties.[5]

Cathinone (alpha-aminopropiophenone) has been isolated in variable quantities from fresh leaves. This compound is a more powerful stimulant than cathine and generally is considered to be the most important component; however, it is unstable in the presence of oxygen.

The "red" type of khat, considered superior by users, contains more cathinone than the "white" type and fresh leaves contain more than the dried plant. More than 30 other minor compounds (cathinine, cathidine, eduline, ephedrine, etc.) have been isolated from khat leaves. Khat contains khatamines (phenylpropyl and phenylpentenylamines) in amounts that vary according to the origin, type and quality of the product.[6] Khat leaves and twigs contain large amounts of tannins (up to 14% of dry weight).[7] One hundred grams of fresh leaves contain 130 to 160 mg. After oral administration, 22% to 52% of synthetic cathinone is excreted in 24-hour urine samples, the principal metabolites being aminoalcohols. S-(-)-cathinone is metabolized primarily to R/S-(-)-norephedrine, and R-(+)-cathinone is metabolized primarily to R/R-(-)-norpseudoephedrine.[8]

PHARMACOLOGY: Questioning of khat users indicates that the subjective effects of khat are euphoria, intellectual efficiency and alertness in most subjects, with others reporting only dysphoria and mild sedation. The expression of these effects appears to be affected by environmental factors.[9]

In studies of skeletal muscle, (-)-cathinone and d-norpseudoephedrine antagonized the actions of physostigmine but not those of d-tubocurarine, suggesting that the two compounds have a direct action on the neuromuscular junction independent of cholinergic and adrenergic transmission.[10] In the toad heart, a khat extract produced a dose-dependent chronotropic effect and increased the amplitude of the ventricular action potential in acute treatment. Chronic treatment had the opposite effects. These results are related to the catecholamine-releasing effects of the extract.[11]

The psychotropic effects of khat are caused by the amphetamine-like compounds, of which cathine is found in highest concentration. The stimulating effects of khat lie somewhere between caffeine and amphetamine. Although amphetamine and cathinone act on different regions of the brain, they both share common pharmacologic effects, including an interaction with the dopaminergic pathways.[12]

Central stimulation by khat is manifested by euphoria, increased alertness, garrulousness, hyperactivity, excitement, aggressiveness, anxiety, elevated blood pressure and manic behavior, effects that have been verified in a double-blind trial of a single dose of khat.[13] Insomnia, malaise and a lack of concentration almost always follow. True psychotic reactions occur with much less frequency than with amphetamines. This is most likely because of the self-limiting dose of khat, which does not permit blood levels of the active compounds to rise high enough for toxic psychosis to occur. Physical dependence to khat does not occur, and mental depression, sedation and social separation that may follow withdrawal are a rebound phenomenon rather than an abstinence syndrome. The psychic dependence that occurs is less than that with amphetamines but makes daily use of khat the norm.

Cardiovascular effects occur within 15 to 30 minutes after ingestion, suggesting absorption of active principles through the oral mucosa. Effects include tachycardia, palpitations and increased blood pressure.

Chronic use of khat has been implicated as a contributing factor to hypertension in young adults; spontaneous improvement follows cessation of use. Other physiological effects include increased respiratory rate, hyperthermia, sweating, pupil dilation and decreased intraocular pressure. Gastrointestinal side effects are often encountered with khat use. Stomatitis, esophagitis and gastritis noted in chronic users are most likely due to the presence of the strongly astringent tannins. One report has noted an exceptionally high rate of periodontal disease in Yemeni males who chewed khat.[14] A more recent report, however, states that khat use is associated with some temporomandibular joint dysfunction and keratosis of the buccal mucosa.[15]

Constipation is perhaps the most common GI symptom and is caused by the tannins and the sympathomimetic effects of the alkaloids. The relationship between khat use and constipation is so strong that when a ban was imposed on khat in Aden in 1957, the sales of laxatives decreased by 90%, but returned to the original levels soon after the ban was lifted.[4]

Khat has little effect on blood sugar levels. Although hypoglycemia has been noted in rabbits after subcutaneous injections of khat leaf extracts, no changes in blood sugar were found in 15 healthy males after khat ingestion.[16] Interviews of 7500 khat users in Somalia[17] did not reveal any beneficial effect of khat in diabetics. The overall effect of khat on diabetic patients is deleterious. Its appetite-suppressant effect leads to the omission of meals; the uncooperative khat user is less likely to follow dietary advice, and the consumption of sweetened beverages while using khat aggravates hyperglycemia.[18] Anorexia is a socially important effect of khat abuse. The WHO implicates khat in a vicious cycle of khat use, destitution, hunger, anorexia, malnutrition and digestive troubles.

Norpseudoephedrine has been found in breast milk from mothers who use khat and in the urine of at least one infant of such a mother. Until research into health hazards is completed, use of khat by lactating mothers should be discouraged.

Experimental therapeutic use: In experiments with albino rats, a flavonoid fraction isolated from khat, at a dosage of 200 mg/kg, significantly reduced paw edema induced by carrageenan and cotton-pellet granuloma. The substance had an anti-inflammatory activity comparable to that of oxyphenbutazone.[19]

TOXICOLOGY: Severe adverse effects have been associated with khat use; migraine, cerebral hemorrhage, myocardial infarction and pulmonary edema have been described, particularly in older and predisposed individuals. Hepatic cirrhosis of unknown etiology has been noted in khat users; poor diets and the potentially hepatotoxic effects of khat tannins may be contributing factors. Anaphrodesia is reported frequently by men during khat use. Although libido initially may be increased, a loss of sexual drive, spermatorrhea and subsequent impotence soon follow. In females, however, the situation is very different. Seventy-two percent of female users in one survey reported increased sexual desire, followed by an improvement in sexual performance in 78% of the respondents.[16]

In vitro studies have demonstrated that a chloroform extract of khat leaves is cytotoxic in cultures of KB, 1BR.3, and XP2B1 mammalian cells. This cytotoxicity appears to be due to inhibition of de novo RNA synthesis affecting all the cell strains tested; KB cells possessed some resistance to the toxicity.[20] Oral cancers in certain regions of Saudia Arabia have been found to occur mostly among patients who had been chronic khat chewers.[21]

Data from *Allium cepa* root tips suggest that (-)-cathinone is responsible for teratogenic and mutagenic effects of khat, since it caused clumping and condensation of chromosomes, sticky metaphases and anaphasic bridges.[22] Animal studies indicate that cathinone can depress testosterone levels, degenerate testicular tissue and decrease sperm count and motility.[23]

Several studies of full-term human newborns has shown that khat use by the mother is associated with significantly lower birth weight,[24] but no differences in the rates of stillborns or congenital malformations were observed.[25] A study of guinea pigs suggests that (+)-norpseudoephedrine in khat may reduce placental blood flow, impairing fetal growth.

A report of two cases has described bilateral optic atrophy in two khat users who consumed amounts larger than usual. This may have been an idiosyncratic reaction to khat.[26]

SOCIAL NOTES: In his excellent review of the use of khat in Somalia, Elmi[16] warns that "the pleasant stimulation obtained when chewing khat induces many to abuse the drug. This may have damaging effects from a social and economic point of view. Some people may arrive at spending a great part of their earnings on khat, thus failing to ensure for themselves and their families important and vital needs. Excess of khat chewing may lead to family disintegration. The chewer shows (very often) irritability and spends much of the time away from home. These facts and the failure of sexual intercourse after chewing may endanger family life. For some countries where khat imports account for the loss of a sizable portion of the national income, there may be a serious economic balance of payments problem."

SUMMARY: Khat is a plant product produced and consumed in East Africa and the Arabian Peninsula. Chewed for its euphoric effects, khat does not induce physical dependence. It does, however, induce psychological dependence and can cause serious physical and psychological side effects. Khat is now being exported worldwide and can represent a serious economic problem, with considerable social costs, for users.

PATIENT INFORMATION – Khat

Uses: Khat leaves are chewed for stimulant and euphoriant effects, and used to treat obesity and gastric ulcers. Some users experience dysphoria and sedation.

Side Effects: Khat may cause oral cancer, cerebral hemorrhage, myocardial infarction, hypertension, testicular degeneration, low birth weight and a variety of other severe effects, including psychological addiction and the attendant ills.

---

[1] Randall T. Khat Abuse Fuels Somali Conflict, Drains Economy. *JAMA* 1992;269:12.

[2] Osol A, Farrar GE Jr. The Dispensatory of the United States of America, 25th ed. Philadelphia, PA: JB Lippincott Co., 1955.

[3] Kalix P. Cathinone, a natural amphetamine. *Pharmacol Toxicol* 1992;70:77.

[4] Halbach H. Medical aspects of the chewing of khat leaves. *Bull World Health Organ* 1972;47:21.

[5] Eisenberg MS, et al. A comparison of the effects of phenylpropanolamine, d-amphetamine and d-norpseudoephedrine on open-field locomotion and food intake in the rat. *Appetite* 1987;9:31.

[6] Geisshusler S, Brenneisen R. The content of psychoactive phenylpropyl and phenylpentenyl khatamines in *Catha edulis* Forsk. of different origin. *J Ethnopharmacol* 1987;19:269.

[7] Paris MR, Moyes H. *Bull Narcotics* 1958;10:29.

[8] Brenneisen R et al. Metabolism of cathinone to (e-)-norephedrine and (-)-norpseudoephedrine. *J Pharm Pharmacol* 1986;38:298.

[9] Nencini P, et al. Subjective effects of khat chewing in humans. *Drug Alcohol Depend* 1986;18:97.

[10] Guantai AN, et al. Effects of the active constituents of *Catha edulis* on the neuromuscular junction. *Neuropharmacology* 1987;26:401.

[11] Nabil Z, et al. Effects of an extract of khat (*Catha edulis*) on the toad heart. *J Ethnopharmacol* 1986;18:245.

[12] Pehek EA, et al. Effects of cathinone and amphetamine on the neurochemistry of dopamine in vivo. *Neuropharmacology* 1990;29:1171.

[13] Brenneisen R, et al. Amphetamine-like effects in humans of the khat alkaloid cathinone. *Br J Clin Pharmacol* 1990;30:825.

[14] Rosenzweig KA, Smith P. *Periodont Res* 1966;1:250.

[15] Hill CM and Gibson A. The oral and dental effects of q'at chewing. *Oral Surg Oral Med Oral Pathol* 1987;63:433.

[16] Elmi AS. *J Ethnopharmacol.* 1983;8:163.

[17] Ibid. 1983;8:331.

[18] Luqman W. The Use of Khat (*Catha edulis*) in Yemen Social and Medical Observations. *Ann Intern Med* 1976;85:246.

[19] Al-Meshal IA, et al. *Agents Actions* 1986;17:379.

[20] Al-Ahhdal, et al. Cytotoxicity of Khat (*Catha edulis*) extract on cultured mammalian cells: effects on macromolecule biosynthesis. *Mutat Res* 1988;204:317.

[21] Soufi HE, et al. Khat and oral cancer. *J Laryngol Otol* 1991;105:643.

[22] Al-Meshal IA. Mitodepressive effect of (-)-cathinone, from *Catha edulis* (Khat), on the meristematic region of Allium cepa root tips. *Toxicon* 1987;25:451.

[23] Islam MW, et al. An evaluation of the male reproductive toxicity of cathinone. *Toxicology* 1990;60:223.

[24] Abdul Ghani N, et al. The influence of khat-chewing on birth weight in full-term infants. *Soc Sci Med* 1987;24:625.

[25] Eriksson M, et al. Khat chewing during pregnancy-effect upon the off-spring and some characteristics of the chewers. *East Afr Med J* 1991;68:106.

[26] Roper JP. The presumed neurotoxic effects of *Catha edulis* -an exotic plant now available in the United Kingdom. *Br J Ophthalmol* 1986;70:779.

Kinetin

SCIENTIFIC NAME(S): N6-furfuryladenine, N-(2-furanylmethyl)-1H-purin-6-amine, 6-furfurylaminopurine

COMMON NAME(S): Kinetin

BOTANY: Kinetin, a cytokinin and plant hormone, is a cell division factor found in plant parts and yeast.[1] Kinetin has also been detected in freshly extracted DNA from human cells.[2]

HISTORY: Plant hormones, or cytokinins, were named for their ability to stimulate cell division (cytokinesis).[3] The first known cytokinin was a component of coconut milk. This was used as a standard additive to plant tissue cultures in the lab because of its ability to make plants divide. Cytokinins were eventually isolated from coconut milk, immature organs of corn, and various other sources.[4] Studies dating back to the mid-1950s describe the structure and synthesis of kinetin specifically.[1]

Kinetin has been advertised as an antiaging product for wrinkled skin treatment. *Kinerase* is a cream/lotion containing a 0.1% kinetin concentration.[5]

CHEMISTRY: Cytokinins are N6-substituted adenine derivatives.[6] The furfuryl moiety of kinetin is reported to originate from furfural, a primary oxidation product of the deoxyribose in DNA.[7] N6-furfuryladenine has electrochemical properties. Electrochemical assignments have been confirmed from kinetin using mass-spectrometric analysis.[2]

Studies have reported the following: Isolation of kinetin from autoclaved water slurries of DNA, structure determination, and physiologic activity at high dilutions in the presence of auxin.[1]

PHARMACOLOGY: Cytokinins function as essential growth hormones, which can influence cell growth and differentiation in plant and non-plant tissues.[6,7] Kinetin can be formed in vivo, neutralizing harmful properties of hydroxyl radical reaction products. This is a defense mechanism in response to oxidative stress of cells.[3] Degradation of sugar residues in DNA is a major route of this cellular damage.[7] Kinetin-activated, major nucleolar organizer regions in basal, equatorial, and near-apical tissue of onion (leaf base) suggest it to be a regulator.[9] Single-celled yeast, *Saccharomyces cerevisiae*, used as a model, demonstrated spore formation at micromolar concentrations of kinetin.[6] Another report finds kinetin to delay aging and prolong lifespan of the fruitfly *Zaprionus paravittiger*.[10] Addition of kinetin in a culture medium of human cells can delay and offset aging characteristics such as growth rate and cell size.[11] The amount of DNA in the nucleii of the fibroblast cells increased in the presence of kinetin from human skin.[12]

The skin care product *Kinerase* claims to be a "nature-identical" plant growth factor, which "delays and improves unwanted changes in appearance and texture of photo-damaged skin." It allegedly reduces wrinkles and improves skin texture, telangiectasia, and mottled hyperpigmentation. Results are typically seen in 4 to 6 weeks. Product literature compares *Kinerase* with the prescription cream *Renova* (0.05% tretinoin), finding *Kinerase* to be superior to *Renova* parameters by patient self-assessment at a 24-week period. There was an incidence of side effects using *Kinerase* vs *Renova* (eg, erythema, peeling, burning, and stinging).[5]

TOXICOLOGY: Computer literature searches found no information on toxicology of kinetin. The makers of *Kinerase* claim its use is associated with virtually no skin irritation, no thinning of the skin, no restrictions in pregnant or nursing women, no restrictions on duration of use, etc. The product is reportedly hypoallergenic and non-comedogenic and has no known interactions with drugs or other products.[5]

SUMMARY: Kinetin is a cytokinin, a plant hormone, with the ability to influence cell growth and differentiation in plant and non-plant tissues. It has gained some popularity with the introduction of the product *Kinerase*, which supposedly improves wrinkles, skin texture, and color. Very low incidence of adverse effects have been reported in studies with use of the product. Further research in human clinical trials are warranted.

PATIENT INFORMATION – Kinetin

Uses: Kinetin functions as an essential growth hormone, which can influence cell growth and differentiation. It can delay and offset aging characteristics such as cell growth rate and size. It is claimed to reduce wrinkles and improve skin texture, telangiectasia, and mottled hyperpigmentation.

Side effects: There is a very low incidence of side effects.

[1] Budavari S, et al, eds. *The Merck Index 11th ed*. Rahway, NJ: Merck & Co., Inc. 1989;5195.

[2] Barciszewski J, et al. Evidence for the presence of kinetin in DNA and cell extracts. *FEBS Letters*. 1996;393(2-3):197-200.

[3] Starr C, et al. *Biology — The Unity and Diversity of Life, 4th ed*. Belmont, CA: Wadsworth Publishing Co. 1987;286.

[4] Arms K, et al. *Biology, 2nd ed*. New York, NY: Saunders Publishing, Co. 1982:786.

[5] http://www.dermcosmetic.com/kinerase.html.

[6] Laten H. Cytokinins affect spore formation but not cell division in the yeast *Saccharomyces cerevisiae*. *Biochimica et Biophysica Acta* 1995;1266(1):45-49.

[7] Barciszewski J, et al. Furfural, a precursor of the cytokinin hormone kinetin, and base propenals are formed by hydroxyl radical damage of DNA. *Biochem Biophys Res Commun* 1997;238(2):317-19.

[8] Barciszewski J, et al. A mechanism for the in vivo formation of N6-furfuryladenine, kinetin, as a secondary oxidative damage product of DNA. *FEBS Lett* 1997;414(2):457-60.

[9] Karagiannis C, et al. Effect of abscisic acid, gibberellic acid, indoleacetic acid, and kinetin on selective ribosomal cistron regulation in quiescent and senescent onion leaf base tissue. *Mech Ageing Dev* 1994;76(2-3):145-55.

[10] Sharma S, et al. Plant growth hormone kinetin delays ageing, prolongs the lifespan, and slows down development of the fruitfly *Zaprionus paravittiger*. *Biochem Biophys Res Commun* 1995;216(3):1067-71.

[11] Rattan S, et al. Kinetin delays the onset of ageing characteristics in human fibroblasts. *Biochem Biophys Res Commun* 1994;201(2):665-72.

[12] Kowalska E. Influence of kinetin (6-furfurylo-amino-purine) on human fibroblasts in the cell culture. *Folia Morphol (Warsz)* 1992;51(2):109-18.

Kiwi Fruit

SCIENTIFIC NAME(S): *Actinidia chinensis* Planchon. Family: Actinidiaceae

COMMON NAME(S): Kiwi fruit, Chinese gooseberry, China gooseberry

BOTANY: The kiwi is native to eastern Asia, but today is widely cultivated for its fruit. Major producers of the kiwi fruit include New Zealand and Italy, although a significant harvest is obtained from other temperate countries including France and Israel. The bisexual plant grows as a trained vine and is often cultivated as an ornamental.[1]

HISTORY: The kiwi fruit has been used in China as the basis for a flavorful wine. It has a long tradition of use as a fruit beverage.

CHEMISTRY: An enzyme inhibitor and a proteolytic enzyme have been isolated from the kiwi fruit. A glycoprotein inhibitor specific for pectin methylesterase has been isolated from the fruit.[2] This enzyme inhibitor is ineffective against other polysaccharide-degrading enzymes such as polygalacturonase and amylase.

The proteolytic enzyme, actinidin, is derived from the kiwi fruit.[3] The nucleotide sequence of this enzyme has been established.[3,4,5] The proteolytic activity of actinidin is similar to, but not identical to, that of papain. Kiwi fruit juice has been used in some cultures as a traditional meat tenderizer.

Kiwi fruits have high concentrations of vitamin C, and the serotonin concentration of the fruit is approximately twice that of tomatoes and one-third that of bananas.[6] Ingestion of kiwi fruits, therefore, can increase urinary 5-hydroxyindoleacetic acid excretion and may interfere with laboratory analyses for this serotonin by-product.

PHARMACOLOGY: Kiwi fruit has no inherent pharmacologic activity. However, the action of the proteolytic enzymes can result in activity that may lead to toxic events (see Toxicology).

One study reported the effects of a kiwi fruit-based drink supplement given to athletes training in hot environments.[7] In athletes riding a Monark ergometer, the mean work time to exhaustion was longer (149 min) compared to placebo (120 min), and the work load was larger (947 KJ vs 833 KJ) ($p < 0.001$). The kiwi-based drink supplement resulted in an expansion of blood volume; hematocrit increased significantly after exercise in athletes taking placebo, but did not change significantly in those consuming the supplement. Furthermore, based on the urinary excretion of vitamin C, it appeared that the vitamin C status of supplemented athletes improved compared to placebo. The drink was found to be "fragrant, tasty, refreshing and thirst quenching," and it did not appear to have any side effects.

TOXICOLOGY: The enzymatic components appear to be largely responsible for the toxicities associated with kiwi fruit. These events are typically manifested as food allergies.[8] This hypersensitivity manifests as oral/buccal reactions that occur a few minutes after ingesting the fruit.[9] More severe reactions, including dysphagia, vomiting and urticaria, have occurred immediately following ingestion of the fruit.[10]

Contact urticaria has also been reported.[11]

SUMMARY: The kiwi fruit is a widely cultivated, popular fruit throughout the world. It serves as the base for flavorful juices. It contains a proteolytic enzyme that has been used as a traditional meat tenderizer, but which may also be responsible for an increasing number of allergic events to the fruit.

PATIENT INFORMATION – Kiwi Fruit

Uses: Kiwi fruit is used as food, meat tenderizer and basis of a "sports drink."

Side Effects: Some experience severe allergic reactions immediately after consumption.

[1] Mabberley DJ. *The Plant-Book*. New York, NY: Cambridge University Press, 1987.

[2] Balestrieri C, et al. A glycoprotein inhibitor of pectin methylesterase in kiwi fruit (*Actinidia chinesis*). *Eur J Biochem* 1990;193:183.

[3] Varughese KI, et al. Crystal structure of an actinidin-E-64 complex. *Biochemistry* 1992;31:5172.

[4] Naylor S, et al. Paid determination of sequence variations in actinidin isolated from *Actinidia chinesis* (var. Hayward) using fast atom bombardment mapping mass spectrometry and gas phase microsequencing. *Biomed Envir Mass Spectrom* 1989;18:424.

[5] Podivinsky E, et al. Nucleotide sequence of actinidin, a kiwi fruit protease. *Nucleic Acid Res* 1989;17:8363.

[6] Feldman JM, Lee EM. Serotonin content of foods: effect on urinary excretion of 5-hydroxyindoleacetic acid. *Am J Clin Nutr* 1985;42:639.

[7] Chen JD, et al. The effects of actinidia sinensis planch (kiwi) drink supplementation on athletes training in hot environments. *J Sports Med Phys Fitness* 1990;30:181.

[8] Joral A, Garmendia J. Dietary allergy to kiwi (letter). *Med Clin* 1992;98:197.

[9] Dore P, et al. Allergy to kiwi: an unrecognized allergy. *Allerg Immunol* 1990;22:20.

[10] Garcia BE, et al. A rare case of food allergy: monosensitivity to kiwi (*Actinidia chinesis*). *Allergol Immunopathol* 1989;17:217.

[11] Veraldi S, Schianchi-Veraldi R. Contact urticaria from kiwi fruit. *Contact Dermatitis* 1990;22:244.

Kombucha

SCIENTIFIC NAME(S): Yeast/bacteria fungal symbiot

COMMON NAME(S): Kombucha tea, kombucha mushroom, Manchurian tea, Combucha tea, Spumonto, Tschambucco, Teekwass, Kwassan, Kargasok tea. "Fungus" Japonicus, Manchurian "fungus, " Dr. Sklenar's kombucha mushroom infusion, Champagne of life, T'Chai from the sea

BOTANY: Kombucha is not a fungus or a mushroom, but rather a gray, pancake-shaped patty that grows up to six inches in diameter. The patty is placed in a mixture of black tea and sugar to ferment. Technically, the fermentation becomes a mixture of yeast and bacteria (ie, *Bacterium xylinum*, *Bacterium gluconicum*, *Acetobacter ketogenum* and *Pichia fermentans*).

HISTORY: Kombucha tea has grown rapidly in popularity over the past year and has been touted as a miracle cure for a wide variety of illnesses, ranging from memory loss to premenstrual syndrome.[1]

The name kombucha is derived from the Japanese in that it is brewed in a seaweed (kombu) tea (cha).[2] In Western countries, the product is typically propagated in black tea. Users float growing spores on the surface of brewed, sweetened black tea. The mycelium double in mass approximately every week. The mass is then divided and the new portion is propagated on a new tea media. In this manner, kombucha mycelium can be propagated at a rapid rate for commercial distribution. Units of the fungus can sell for $50 each.[2]

As the growth matures, it ferments the beverage slightly. This fermented tea is drunk for its purported medicinal properties. Drinking fermented teas has long been popular in Eastern countries, and the use of this particular mycelial growth may date back several centuries.

Despite extravagant claims for its pharmacologic activity, some experts believe that the tea fulfills the FDA criteria identifying a *fraudulent* product, including: reference to non-US medical studies, an appeal to a person's vanity, ancient origins and alleged cures for a wide variety of ailments.[1] Some of these claims include curing cancer, rheumatism, aging and intestinal disorders.

CHEMISTRY: The fermentation process induced by kombucha is said to produce substantial amounts of glucuronic acid, which is normally synthesized by the body.[1]

Fermentation products may also include alcohol (0.5%), hyaluronic acid, chondroitin-sulfate acid, mukoitin sulfate, heparin, lactic acid[3] and usnic acid.[1]

PHARMACOLOGY: There is no good evidence to support the pharmacologic claims for kombucha. Because kombucha tea is a product of bacterial fermentation, it may contain compounds that affect the bacterial flora of the gut.

One report on Dr. Sklenar's kombucha mushroom infusion (1960s) as a cancer therapy indicated that there was no solid medical data available on its usefulness in cancer treatment.[4]

Screening of "Kargasok tea" (kombucha tea) for anorexia and obesity has also been reported, but not validated.[5]

TOXICOLOGY: Cases of nausea and allergic responses have been reported. No kombucha-related deaths have occurred, although Iowa health officials have reported the first suspected death linked to the tea.[6] Regulatory agencies are investigating the possibility that kombucha may be a source of bacterial pathogens.[2] In one case, an 83-year-old person with multiple health problems drank 0.5 cup of a kombucha mixture for a 3–week period. Upon examination, laboratory results indicated AST/MLT greater than 2000 IU/L, lactate dehydrogenase peaking at 4000 IU/L and a prothrombin time over 25 seconds. The APAP (acetaminophen) level was "trace."[3]

SUMMARY: Kombucha is a popular natural product that is used to ferment tea. However, it is not approved by the FDA for medical purposes. Kombucha tea is covered widely in the popular press. The fermented liquid is purported to have a wide variety of medicinal properties, but there is no good evidence supporting any clinically relevant pharmacologic activity. No significant adverse events have been associated with drinking the fungal tea, although one suspected death linked to it has been reported.

PATIENT INFORMATION – Kombucha

Uses: There is no good evidence to support the pharmacologic claims for kombucha.

Side Effects: The fermented tea associated with kombucha has been suspected as fatal in one user.

[1] Foster RD. Kombucha: Mushroom with a Mission. *Natural Health* 1995;March/April:52.

[2] Marin R, Biddle NA. Trends: Taking the Fungal-Tea Plunge. *Newsweek* 1995;Jan 9:64.

[3] Kombucha Tea, *Poisindex*, Product Reference: 4985284.

[4] Hauser SP. [Dr. Sklenar's Kombucha mushroom infusion - a biological cancer therapy. Documentation No. 18 (German)]. *Schweizerische Rundschau fur Medizin Praxis* 1990;79(9):243.

[5] Kwanashie HO, et al. Screening of 'kargasok tea' I: Anorexia and obesity. *Biochem Soc Trans* 1989;17(6):1132.

[6] Hearn W. Mushroom tea: Toxicity concerns about new 'cure-all.' *American Medical News* 1995;38(17):16.

Kudzu

SCIENTIFIC NAME(S): *Pueraria lobata* (Willd) Ohwi. Also known as *P. thunbergiana*. Family: Leguminosae. Other species include the following: *P. mirifica* (Thailand herb known as kwaao khruea, used for hormonal content),[1] *P. tuberosa* DC (also studied for hormonal effects),[2,3] and *P. thomsonii* Benth.[4]

COMMON NAME(S): Japanese arrowroot, kudzu vine[5], ge gen (Chinese)

BOTANY: Kudzu is a fast-growing vine native to the tropics of China and Japan. It has been used as fodder and as a ground cover crop. Because it produces long stems that can attain 20 m in length and extensive roots, it has been used to control soil erosion. The plant was introduced into the US where it has become established and proliferates particularly in the moist southern regions. It is in the southern regions that it grows vigorously and is now considered a pest. The leaves of the plant contain 3 broad oval leaflets with purple flowers and curling tendril spikes.[6]

HISTORY: Although kudzu has been widely recognized as a ground cover and fodder crop in the Western world, the plant has a long history of medicinal use in Asian cultures. As far back as the 6th century BC, Chinese herbalists have used the plant for muscular pain and for the treatment of measles.[6] Kudzu is cited in botanical herbals from Japan, China, and Fiji.[7] The Chinese have also used extracts of the plant to treat alcoholism.[6,8]

CHEMISTRY: Numerous reports are available identifying chemical constituents of various plant parts of kudzu.[9-11] Flavonoid, isoflavonoid, and isoflavone content have been identified in kudzu roots and flowers.[12-18] A report discusses kudzu as an excellent food source for both genistein and daidzein, 2 anticancer isoflavones.[19] Oleanene-type triterpene glycosides, termed "kudzu saponins," have been isolated from the plant as well.[20,21]

Analysis of isoflavonoid aglycones and their glycosides has been performed.[22] Robinin in kudzu leaf has also been reported.[23] Other constituents reported include daidzin, formononetin, biochanin A, puerarin, and plant sterols.[6,8,24-26] In addition, morphological and anatomical identification of kudzu have been performed.[27]

PHARMACOLOGY: Pharmacokinetic studies on urinary and biliary metabolites of kudzu have been performed in rats.[28,29]

Kudzu has gained attention because the isoflavones contained in the root have been found to be **reversible inhibitors of the enzyme alcohol dehydrogenase.** Derivatives of these compounds are also potent inhibitors of aldehyde dehydrogenase. Both of these enzymes are required for the normal metabolic degradation of alcohol and its byproducts.[25]

In one controlled study, an extract of kudzu reduced alcohol consumption in Syrian Golden hamsters, which are bred for their desire for alcohol. After establishing baseline intakes of water and a 15% ethanol solution, animals were injected with crude kudzu extract, daidzein or daidzin for 6 days. In each group, the volume of ingested alcohol solution decreased by ≥ 50% during the treatment phase. Alcohol consumption returned to pretreatment levels after the study was stopped. This in vivo activity is likely because of the inhibition of enzymes that metabolize alcohol.[30] Isoflavones daidzin and daidzein were later determined to account for this suppression of ethanol intake.[31] In animal experimentation, these same compounds have also decreased blood alcohol levels, and shortened alcohol-induced sleep.[32,33] Certain saponins from kudzu have also demonstrated in vitro liver protective effects when tested in rat hepatocytes.[34,35]

Traditional Chinese medicine still employs kudzu for treatment of **muscular aches** and pain, such as neck pain and stiffness and upper back problems.[6] It is also a traditional remedy for gastritis, dysentery, and the flu.[26] *P. lobata* and *P. omeiensis* have significantly inhibited induced fever in rats.[36]

Kudzu's beneficial effects on **heart disease** and related disorders have been documented. Plant extracts increased cerebral blood flow in arteriosclerosis patients,[6] decreased oxygen consumption by myocardium, exerted spasmolytic activity,[26] and have caused relaxation in induced contractions in cat vascular smooth muscle.[37] Kudzu has been used in the treatment of hypertension,[38] arrhythmia,[39] ischemia,[36] angina pectoris, and migraines.[26] At least one report is available discussing one kudzu glycoside and its antioxidant activity.[40]

Related species *P. mirifica* and *P. tuberosa* have been studied for their contraceptive effects.[6] One of these reports investigates *P. mirifica* for birth control in pigeons.[41]

TOXICOLOGY: Kudzu has been used as a medicinal herb for centuries without any reported toxic side effects.[25] However, the safety profile of the plant and its extracts has yet to be defined through systematic pharmacologic screens. The Chinese Materia Medica, through pharmacological and clinical experimentation, has been published to establish safety information for just under 4700 known specimens used in traditional medicine of which kudzu is discussed.[38] Acute toxicity of 4 species of *Pueraria* has been comparatively studied.[36]

SUMMARY: Kudzu is a fast-growing plant native to Asia that has been naturalized to the southern US. It has been used as a ground cover and for fodder and in Asian medicine for the management of alcoholism. Several compounds in kudzu root can inhibit enzymes involved in alcohol metabolism, thereby inducing a reduction in alcohol consumption in animal models. Kudzu is also used for muscular aches, heart disease, and related disorders. Its toxicity profile is low. More clinical studies in humans are needed to verify its wide use in numerous medical conditions.

PATIENT INFORMATION – Kudzu

Uses: Kudzu has been used as a ground cover, fodder, and medicinal herb especially for treating alcoholism. It is also used for muscular aches, heart disease, and related disorders.

Side Effects: No known toxic effects; safety undefined.

---

1 http://www.ostc-was.org.
2 Mathur R, et al. Effect of *Pueraria tuberosa* DC on the oestrous cycle of adult rats. *Acta Eur Fertil* 1984;15(5):393-94.
3 Prakash A, et al. Contraceptive potency of *Pueraria tuberosa* DC and its hormonal status. *Acta Eur Fertil* 1985;16(1):59-65.
4 Yu S, et al. Comparison of constituents in *Pueraria thomsonii* Benth before and after processing. *Chung Kuo Chung Yao Tsa Chih* 1992;17(9):534-36, 575.
5 Mabberley D. *The Plant-Book*. Cambridge: Cambridge University Press, 1987.
6 Chevallier A. *Encyclopedia of Medicinal Plants*. New York: DK Publishing, 1996;256.
7 Penso G. *Inventory of Medicinal Plants Used in the Different Countries*. World Health Organization, 1982.
8 Anonymous. Kudzu extract shows potential for moderating alcohol abuse. *Am J Hosp Pharm* 1994;51:750.
9 Kurihara T, et al. Studies on the constituents of flowers. I. On the components of flower of *Pueraria thunbergiana* Benth. *Yakugaku Zasshi* 1973;93(9):1201-205.
10 Kurihara T, et al. Studies on the constituents of flowers. VI. On the components of the flower of *Pueraria thubergiana* Benth. *Yakugaku Zasshi* 1976;96(12):1486-488.
11 Chen M. Studies on the chemical constituents of *Pueraria lobata*. *Chung Yao-tung Pao* 1985;10(6):34-36.
12 Saiiad S, et al. Flavonoids of the flowers of *Pueraria lobata*. *Farm Zh* 1978;(6):83-84.
13 Saiiad S, et al. Flavonoids of the rhizomes of *Pueraria*. *Farm Zh* 1979;(2):76-77.
14 Xu L, et al. Differential pulse polarographic determination of flavonoids in *Pueraria lobata*. *Yao Hsueh Hsueh Pao* 1987;22(3):208-11.
15 Ohshima Y, et al. Isolation and high performance liquid chromatography (HPLC) of isoflavonoids from the *Pueraria* root. *Planta Med* 1988;54(3):250-54.
16 Kubo M, et al. Isolation of a new isoflavone from Chinese *Pueraria* flowers. *Chem Pharm Bull* 1975;23(10):2449-451.
17 Kurihara T, et al. Studies on the constituents of flowers. V. On the components of flower of *Pueraria thunbergiana* benth. (2). Isolation of a new isoflavone glycoside. *Yakugaku Zasshi* 1975;95(11):1283-285.
18 Zhao S, et al. Quantitative TLC-densitometry of isoflavones in *Pueraria lobata* (Willd) Ohwi. *Yao Hsueh Hsueh Pao* 1985;20(3):203-208.
19 Kaufman P, et al. A comparative survey of leguminous plants as sources of the isoflavones, genistein and daidzein: implications for human nutrition and health. *J Altern Complement Med* 1997;3(1):7-12.
20 Arao T, et al. Oleanene-type triterpene glycosides from *Puerariae* radix. II. Isolation of saponins and the application of tandem mass spectrometry to their structure determination. *Chem Pharm Bull* 1995;43(7):1176-179.
21 Arao T, et al. Oleanene-type triterpene glycosides from *Puerariae* radix. IV. Six new saponins from *Pueraria lobata*. *Chem Pharm Bull* 1997;45(2):362-66.
22 Rong H, et al. Narrow-bore HPLC analysis of isoflavonoid aglycones and their O- and C-glycosides from *Pueraria lobata*. *Biomed Chromatogr* 1998;12(3):170-71.
23 Saiiad S, et al. Isolation, identification, and quantitative determination of robinin in the leaves of *Pueraria lobata*. *Farm Zh* 1979;(4):52-55.
24 Keung W, et al. Daidzin: a potent, selective inhibitor of human mitochondrial aldehyde dehydrogenase. *Proc Natl Acad Sci USA* 1993;90:1247.
25 Keung W. Biochemical studies of a new class of alcohol dehydrogenase inhibitors from *Radix puerariae*. *Alcohol Clin Exp Res* 1993;17:1254.
26 Bruneton J. *Pharmacognosy, Phytochemistry, Medicinal Plants*. Paris: Lavoisier Publishing, 1995;298.
27 Kartmazova D, et al. Morphological and anatomical diagnosis of the subterranean vegetative organs of *Pueraria lobata*. I. *Farm Zh* 1980;(3):61-63.
28 Yasuda T, et al. Urinary and biliary metabolites of daidzin and daidzein in rats. *Biol Pharm Bull* 1994;17(10):1369-374.
29 Yasuda T, et al. Urinary and biliary metabolites of puerarin in rats. *Biol Pharm Bull* 1995;18(2):300-303.
30 Keung W, et al. Daidzin and daidzein suppress free-choice ethanol intake by Syrian Golden hamsters. *Proc Natl Acad Sci USA* 1993;90:10008-12.
31 Keung W, et al. Kudzu root: an ancient Chinese source of modern antidipsotropic agents. *Phytochemistry* 1998;47(4):499-506.
32 Xie C, et al. Daidzin, an antioxidant isoflavonoid, decreases blood alcohol levels and shortens sleep time induced by ethanol intoxication. *Alcohol Clin Exp Res* 1994;18(6):1443-447.
33 Lin R, et al. Effects of isoflavones on alcohol pharmacokinetics and alcohol-drinking behavior in rats. *Am J Clin Nutr* 1998;68(6 Suppl):1512S-515S.
34 Arao T, et al. Preventive effects of saponins from *Puerariae radix* (the root of *Pueraria lobata* Ohwi) on in vitro immunological injury of rat primary hepatocyte cultures. *Biol Pharm Bull* 1997;20(9):988-91.
35 Arao T, et al. Preventive effects of saponins from the *Pueraria lobata* root on in vitro immunological liver injury of rat primary hepatocyte cultures. *Planta Med* 1998;64(5):413-16.
36 Zhou Y, et al. Comparative study on pharmacological effects of various species of *Pueraria*. *Chung Kuo Chung Yao Tsa Chih* 1995;20(10):619-21, 640.
37 Wang L, et al. Effects of puerarin on cat vascular smooth muscle in vitro. *Chung Kuo Yao Li Hsueh Pao* 1994;15(2):180-82.
38 Qicheng F. Some current study and research approaches relating to the use of plants in the traditional Chinese medicine. *J Ethnopharmacol* 1980;2(1):57-63.
39 Lai X, et al. Recent advances in the experimental study and clinical application of *Pueraria lobata* (Willd) Ohwi. *Chung Kuo Chung Yao Tsa Chih* 1989;14(5):277, 308-11.
40 Sato T, et al. Mechanism of antioxidant action of *pueraria* glycoside (PG)-1 (an isoflavonoid) and magiferin (a xanthonoid). *Chem Pharm Bull* 1992;40(3):721-24.
41 Smitasiri Y, et al. The means of application of *Pueraria mirifica* for pigeon (*Columba* sp.) birth control. *J Sci Technol* 1995;(2):89-96.

Labrador Tea

SCIENTIFIC NAME(S): Several Ledum species have been used medicinally including *L. groenlandicum, L. latifolium, Jacq.*, and *L. palustre*, L. Family: *Ericaceae*.

COMMON NAME(S): Labrador tea, James tea, Marsh tea, Wild rosemary and Continental tea

BOTANY: *L. groenlandicum* is a short (1-6 ft. high), aromatic, evergreen shrub common to North America, primarily found in Greenland and Canada, where it thrives in wet, peaty soils. It has bright-green, 1-3" alternate leaves with a leathery dorsal surface, and a rust colored, hair-like underside. The leaves curl inward and have a bluntly pointed tip. The small (12 mm), white, bell-shaped, scented flowers grow from slender stalks in terminal clusters. The fruit is a many seeded capsule.[1-3]

HISTORY: Labrador Tea (*L. latifolium, Jacq.*) is named after the swamps of Greenland and Labrador, where it grows in profusion. During the American Revolution, it was one of the several herbs used as a pleasant-tasting substitute for commercial tea. Germans once added the leaves to their beer to make it more intoxicating. Although Labrador tea is found as far south as Wisconsin and Pennsylvania, it is listed as rare and could become an endangered species. Medical literature gives full credit to Labrador tea use in folk medicine, though it has been rarely studied clinically. It has been used for coughs, chest ailments, headache, kidney, rheumatisim, diarrhea, sore throat and malignancies.[1-3,4]

CHEMISTRY: Reported constituents of *L. latifolium* include tannic acid, arbutin, resin, and mineral salts.[2] Leaves contain 0.3–2.5% volatile oil, including ledum camphor (ledol), palustrol, (a stearopten), with valeric and volatile acids, ericolin, and ericinol.[4]

PHARMACOLOGY: The leaves of the *L. groenlandicum* have been used as an **astringent.** They were once used to treat dysentery and diarrhea.[2] It is also said to be very useful in coughs and colds, as well as bronchial and pulmonary infections. A tea can be prepared by adding 1 teaspoonful of dried leaves to one cup of boiling water.

A stronger decoction has been recommended externally for itching and redness from skin ailments. Homeopaths have used Labrador tea for various ailments such as insect bites and stings, acne, prickly heat, varicella and wounds. Homeopathic use also includes asthma, hand and foot pain, gout, rheumatism, ear inflammation, tinnitus and tuberculosis.[3] Other references discuss use of the leaves by Koreans to treat female disorders.[4] It is rarely used today as it once was used historically.[2]

TOXICOLOGY: Labrador tea has narcotic properties. Evidence suggests that excessive use of the tea may cause delirium or poisoning.[2] Labrador tea contains andromedotoxin, more recently designated as grayanotoxin. This toxic diterpene causes symptoms of intoxication, such as slow pulse, lowering of blood pressure, lack of coordination, convulsions, paralysis and death.[5] It is apparently safe in a weak tea solution, but should not be made too strong.[6]

SUMMARY: Labrador tea is an aromatic evergreen, native to Greenland and Canada. It has been used in folk medicine for upper respiratory ailments, and by homeopaths for skin infections and asthma. It contains grayanotoxin which causes symptoms of intoxication and can lead to paralysis and death in high concentrations. Further clinical investigation is welcome in order to assess more of the potentially useful properties of Labrador tea.

PATIENT INFORMATION – Labrador Tea

Uses: Labrador tea has been used historically and folklorically for a variety of ailments ranging from skin complaints to malignancies. It can be made safely into a weak tea, but care must be taken not to make concentrations too high. A tea for coughs, colds, bronchial infections and pulmonary infections can be made by adding one teaspoonful of dried leaves to one cup of boiling water.

Side Effects: Labrador tea has narcotic properties. If taken in concentrations that are too high, it can cause symptoms of intoxication that can lead to paralysis and death. If Labrador tea is to be used, be sure to take only in small doses with weak concentrations.

[1] Whiteford R. 1996; savebiosvoicenet.com.

[2] Stuart M, ed. *The encyclopedia of herbs and herbalism*. Crescent Books, NY. 1987;213.

[3] Hutchens AR. *Indian herbalogy of North America*. Shambhala Publications, Boston, MA. 1991;172–3.

[4] Duke JA. *Handbook of Medicinal Herbs*. Boca Raton, FL: CRC Press, Inc., 1985;275.

[5] Lewis WH, et al. *Medical botany, plants affecting man's health*. John Wiley and Sons, Inc. NY. 1977;35.

[6] Turner NJ, et al. *Common poisonous plants and mushrooms of North America*. Timber Press, Portland, OR. 1991;267.

Laminaria

SCIENTIFIC NAME(S): *Laminaria digitata* Lamour or *L. japonica*. Family: Laminariaceae

COMMON NAME(S): Kelp, brown algae, laminaria, horsetail, sea girdles[1]

BOTANY: The marine kelps derived from *Laminaria* species are found primarily in the cold waters of the North Atlantic and North Pacific oceans.

HISTORY: Laminaria for cervical dilation is used in the form of "tents." A tent is any material, usually hygroscopic (readily absorbs water), which is placed in a canal or chamber to maintain the opening or cause dilation. Laminaria tents are made from the dried stems of *Laminaria* seaweeds. When dried and rounded into a stick-like shape, the tent is approximately 6 cm (2 1/2 inches) long with a diameter of 0.3 to 0.5 cm. A strong thread is attached to one end and a collar prevents its migration into the uterus. The stem is hygroscopic and can swell to 3 to 5 times its original diameter within 12 to 24 hours. Other natural products have been used in the past as tents, including sponges, dried corn stalks, slippery elm bark and tupelo wood.[2] The use of laminaria became popular in the 1800s; hollow laminaria tents were developed to improve uterine drainage and laminaria coated with wax was designed to release antiseptics as it melted.

Tents fell into disuse because of complications due to infections. This was especially evident in tents derived from land plants because of the inability to sterilize *Clostridium* spores (the causative agents of tetanus, botulism and gas gangrene). Although laminaria from the ocean contain relatively nonpathogenic bacterial contaminants, polluted waters and poor packaging extended the problems of infection to its use. However, with the advent of ethylene oxide and gamma irradiation sterilization techniques, interest in laminaria tents returned.

CHEMISTRY: Laminarin (laminaran) is a polysaccharide found in *Laminaria* spp. A soluble and insoluble form are found in the plants.[3] Kelp (of which *Laminaria* are one species) are rich in algin, a high molecular weight polysaccharide that forms viscous colloidal solutions or gels in water. This property has led to the use of kelp derivatives as bulk laxatives.[4]

PHARMACOLOGY:

Cervical ripening: When inserted into the cervix, laminaria tents absorb surrounding moisture and gradually swell to a diameter of approximately 1/2 inch. While most of the swelling occurs in the first 4 to 6 hours, swelling may continue for up to 24 hours. Since this is a gradual process, the patient rarely notices pain. At the same time, the cervix is induced to ripening (becoming soft and flexible). The effect is often limited to local cervical ripening; however, stimulation of the cervix can induce labor. The mechanism of action may be similar to that of a foreign body which, when inserted into the cervical canal, disturbs the normal chorioamniotic balance and initiates a cascade of prostaglandin synthesis. This in turn has myometrial contracting and cervical ripening effects.[5] Others suggest that the activity of laminaria may be due to its high levels of the prostaglandin precursor arachidonic acid.[6] Cervical dilation may also be the result of partial placental detachment induced by laminaria.[7]

Laminaria tents have been used to dilate narrow cervixes prior to D&C and diagnostic procedures,[8] to provide relief from cervical stenosis, to ripen the near-term or term cervix, especially in primagravidas, to facilitate labor,[9] to induce labor at term with the adjunctive use of prostaglandins[10] and to induce first-trimester abortions.[11] Laminaria tents have been inserted before the placement and removal of intrauterine devices and to facilitate the placement of therapeutic radium within the uterus.[2]

The effectiveness of laminaria in dilating the cervix and inducing labor has been evaluated in a number of clinical trials. In one study, the effectiveness of laminaria on the preinduction ripening of the cervix was compared to untreated control patients. Although laminaria was effective in reducing the duration of induction, there was no difference in the incidence of cesarean births. Endometritis occurred in 15 of 25 mothers treated with laminaria and 3 of 28 in the control group ($p < 0.05$). Furthermore, 5 of the 25 neonates from the laminaria group had bacterial sepsis compared to none of the controls ($p < 0.05$). Three of the five septic neonates died.[5] In another study 28 of 32 women were induced successfully with laminaria compared to 4 of 32 untreated controls ($p < 0.001$). The mean induction-to-delivery time was significantly shorter (12 1/3 hours vs 2 1/2 days) in the laminaria group.[9]

Miscellaneous Pharmacologic Properties: Seaweeds of the species *Laminaria* have other pharmacologic properties. Laminarin, a complex polysaccharide, has antilipemic activity when partially sulfated and exerts anticoagulant activity similar to that of heparin when sulfated more extensively. The basal parts of the blades of *L. japonica* and *L. angustata* have been used as a hypotensive agent (ne-kombu) in Japanese folk medicine. Chemical analysis of the blades suggests that histamine and the amino acid laminine may be responsible for this hypotensive effect.[12] Alginate-containing algae and kelp have been shown to reduce the absorption of radioactive strontium in both animals and man and are used in the management of radioactive intoxications.[13]

TOXICOLOGY: A review of the findings from the early studies with laminaria suggests that it may be associated with a risk of neonatal and maternal infection. One manufacturer recommends swabbing the cervical canal with a suitable lubricant and antibacterial agent prior to inserting the tent, then packing the canal with antibacterial gel. The followup of 17 women who had laminaria tents inserted for the induction of abortion and then decided to continue the pregnancy found no evidence of infection at term.[14]

The spontaneous uterine contractions that may accompany the use of laminaria have been implicated in the induction of fetal hypoxia and subsequent intrauterine death.[10] Fetal activity should be monitored closely. Other potential problems with the use of laminaria include difficulty removing the tent, breaking the tent during removal[15] or rupturing the cervical wall and subsequent infection. Blood loss does not appear to increase following the use of laminaria tents in first-trimester abortions.[16]

Although laminaria tents possess many qualities of an ideal cervical dilator (easy to insert/remove, slow expansion, painless dilation), persistent problems of infection and cervical injury have spurred the search for alternate types of dilators. Synthetic laminaria tents prepared from hydrophilic polymers provide increased levels of structure stability.[17] Synthetic tents have efficacy similar to that of prostaglandin E2 tablets.[18]

SUMMARY: Laminaria tents are effective in stimulating the dilation of the cervical canal and in ripening the cervix at term. Their effectiveness in facilitating labor is variable. Clinical studies suggest that laminaria tents may increase the incidence of maternal and neonatal infections. Other pharmacologic properties of laminaria derivatives include the ability to limit the absorption of radioactive strontium and to impart anticoagulant properties.

PATIENT INFORMATION – Laminaria

Uses: Laminaria has been used as a hygroscopic cervical dilator and inducer of labor.

Side Effects: Laminaria may cause or contribute to maternal and neonatal infection.

---

[1] Morton JF. *Major Medicinal Plants*. Springfield, IL: CC Thomas, 1977.
[2] Newton BW. Laminaria tent: relic of the past or modern medical device? *Am J Obstet Gynecol* 1972;113:442.
[3] *The Merck Index*, 10th ed. Rahway, NJ: Merck and Co., Inc., 1983.
[4] Tyler VE. *The New Honest Herbal*. Philadelphia, PA: G.F. Stickley Co., 1987.
[5] Kazzi GM, et al. Efficacy and safety of *Laminaria digitata* for preinduction ripening of the cervix. *Obstet Gynecol* 1982;60(4):440.
[6] Crawford MA, et al. *Comp Biochem Physiol* 1976;54B:395.
[7] Jonasson A, et al. Placental and decidual u-PA, t-PA, PAI-1 and PAI-2 concentrations, as affected by cervical dilatation with laminaria tents or Hegar dilators. *Thromb Res* 1989;53(2):91.
[8] Manabe Y. Laminaria tent for gradual and safe cervical dilatation. *Obstet Gynecol* 1971;110(5):743.
[9] Tohan N, et al. Ripening of the term cervix with laminaria. *Obstet Gynecol* 1979;54(5):588.
[10] Agress RL, Benedetti TJ. Intrauterine fetal death during cervical ripening with laminaria. *Am J Obstet Gynecol* 1981;141(5):587.
[11] Propping D, et al. Uterine rupture following midtrimester abortion by laminaria, prostaglandin F and oxytocin: report of two cases. *Am J Obstet Gynecol* 1977;123(6):689.

[12] Funayama S, Hikino H. Hypotensive principle of laminaria and allied seaweeds. *Planta Med* 1981;41:29.
[13] Gong YF, et al. Suppression of radioactive strontium absorption by sodium alginate in animals and human subjects. *Biomed Environ Sci* 1991;4(3):273.
[14] Schneider D, et al. Outcome of continued pregnancies after first- and second-trimester cervical dilation by laminaria tents. *Obstet Gynecol* 1991;78(6):1121.
[15] Borgotta L, Barad D. Prolonged retention of laminaria fragments: an unusual complication of laminaria usage. *Obstet Gynecol* 1991;78(5 pt. 2):988.
[16] Jonasson A, et al. The effect of cervical dilatation by laminaria tent in first trimester legal abortions on blood loss related to fibrinolytic activity in the decidua and placenta. *Int J Gynaecol Obstet* 1989;29(1):73.
[17] Chvapil M, et al. Instruments and methods-new synthetic laminaria. *Obstet Gynecol* 1982;60(6):729.
[18] Bagratee JS, Moodley J. Synthetic laminaria tent for cervical ripening. *S Afr Med J* 1990;78(12):738.

Larch

SCIENTIFIC NAME(S): Larch (*Larix*) species include: *L. dahurica* L., *L. decidua* Mill (*L. europaea*), *L. eurolepis* Gord., *L. gmelinii*, *L. kaempferi* , *L. laricina* Koch., *L. leptolepis* (Sieb. et Zucc.) Gord., *L. occidentalis* Nutt., and *L. sibirica ledeb.* Family: Pinaceae.

COMMON NAME(S): Larch, Larix, Mongolian Larchwood (*L. dahurica*)

BOTANY: Larch trees are deciduous conifers. One example, *L. decidua*, grows to 50 m and has needle-like leaves and small, light brown cones.[1]

HISTORY: Larch trees were said to have been introduced into Great Britain in 1639 and cultivated there since the early 19th century. The tree is grown mainly for its timber, but the inner bark and resin are also used.[1] Arabinogalactan constituents from certain *Larix* species have gained popularity because of their ability to enhance the immune system.[2]

CHEMISTRY: Arabinogalactans are present in species *L. dahurica* and *L. occidentalis*.[3-5] Arabinogalactans are long, densely branched, highly molecular polysaccharides found throughout the plant kingdom and in some microbial systems. They are abundant in the genus *Larix* and are most often covalently linked to pectin and protein.[2,3] The powdered extract from the pine bark of the western larch tree, for example, is 98% arabinogalactan. This substance has a pine odor, a sweet taste, and is easily soluble in water.[2] All arabinogalactans isolated thus far from *Larix*, are the 3,6-beta-D-galactan type.[3] The extract is harvested from already fallen trees, otherwise a waste product from the lumber industry. A benefit of this natural polymer is that it possesses great uniformity. Batch variation is not a problem among larch trees that it is with other natural products.[2] Arabinogalactans from *L. occidentalis* have been isolated, characterized, and purified as discussed in one report.[5] Properties of arabinogalactans from *L. dahurica* have been documented as well, finding a homogeneous product with very narrow molecular weight distribution.[3]

Other constituents from *Larix* have been identified. *Larix* flavonoids from various species have been analyzed, including flavanones (naringenin, hesperitin, hesperidin), flavones (apigenin, vitexin), and flavonols (kaempferols, quercetins, isorhamnetins, myricetins, and syringetins).[6] *L. decidua* contains lignans, resins, and volatile oil (mainly alpha- and betapinene and limonene).[1] 18-nor-abietatrienes and diterpenes, including abietane-type diterpenes (eg, 7alpha,15-dihydroxyabieta-8,11,13-trien-18-al), have been isolated from species *L. kaempferi*.[7,8] Phenolics (flavonoids) from *L. leptolepis* have been reported.[9] Resin constituent diterpene from *L. europaea* has been documented.[10]

PHARMACOLOGY: Arabinogalactan displays moisture retention, flavor encapsulation, film-forming capabilities, and desirable viscosities for a pleasant feeling in the mouth as both a natural and functional food ingredient.[2] Also, its role as a dietary fiber and its solubility properties make arabinogalactan an important polysaccharide. Its properties may be influenced by different side chain moieties on the molecule.[3]

Arabinogalactan's role as an immune-boosting phytochemical has gained popularity. It has been reported to stimulate macrophages and other immune system components better than echinacea, although echinacea contains some arabinogalactans. Arabinogalactans have also been reported to increase the release of interferons, tumor necrosis factors, and interleukins, all of which are known to enhance immune function. Liver metastases in animals have been inhibited by arabinogalactans.[2] Human peripheral blood mononuclear cells and other cell lines have shown enhancement of natural killer cytotoxicity against certain tumor cells when pretreated with arabinogalactans extracted from *L. occidentalis* .[11]

Arabinogalactan has properties that make it an ideal carrier to deliver agents to hepatocytes via the asialoglycoprotein receptors. Of radiolabeled arabinogalactans, 52.5% (4 mg/kg) were identified in the livers of rats receiving IV injection.[4] Arabinogalactan is highly bound to this receptor in both in vitro and in vivo experimentation. In one study, it was reported that those arabinogalactans with a lower molecular weight may be more desirable for hepatic drug delivery than others.[5] In another study, arabinogalactan conjugated with the antiviral vidarabine was effective in suppressing serum viral DNA titers in woodchucks infected with the hepatitis virus.[12]

Arabinogalactan has also been reported to exhibit anti-inflammatory actions, and it may enhance vascular permeability.[2]

L. laricina inhibited xanthine oxidase, thereby reducing uric acid formation, in a study of plant remedies used for gout. This was the greatest inhibition seen among the 26 species from 18 families that were evaluated.[13]

Larchwood (*L. decidua*) also possesses astringent and diuretic actions. Its antiseptic actions may be useful in treating cystitis, respiratory infections, and wounds.[1]

TOXICOLOGY: There is no apparent allergy or toxicity to larch-derived arabinogalactans.[2] Arabinogalactan produced no adverse reactions in single IV doses administered to mice at 5000 mg/kg or at repeated doses in rats for 90 days at 500 mg/kg/day.[4] One source advises caution with the use of *L. decidua* in patients suffering from kidney disease.[1]

SUMMARY: Larch is a genus of conifers that has many species. It has gained popularity because of its high yield of the polysaccharide arabinogalactan from certain species, which has been reported to enhance the immune system. Arabinogalacten attains high concentrations in the liver, making it ideal to deliver agents there. Species *L. laricina* may be helpful in treating gout. *L. decidua* possesses antiseptic actions. No toxicity has been reported from larch arabinogalactans. Use *L. decidua* with caution in patients with kidney disease.

PATIENT INFORMATION – Larch

Uses: Arabinogalactan, present in some larch species, has been reported to stimulate the immune system, to exhibit anti-inflammatory actions, and may enhance vascular permeability. Larchwood possesses astringent and diuretic actions. Its antiseptic actions may be useful in treating cystitis, respiratory problems, and wounds.

Side Effects: No adverse effects have been reported with use. Use with caution in patients with kidney disease.

---

[1] Chevallier A. Larch. *Encyclopedia of Medicinal Plants*. New York: DK Publishing, 1996;224.

[2] Benedikt H. Arabinogalactans: New Immune Boosting Fiber. *Natural Pharmacy* 1999;3:12.

[3] Odonmazig P, et al. Structural and molecular peoperties of the arabinogalactan isolated from Mongolian larchwood (*Larix dahurica* L.). *Carbohydr Res* 1994;252:317-24.

[4] Groman E, et al. Arabinogalactan for hepatic drug delivery. *Bioconjug Chem* 1994;5(6):547-56.

[5] Prescott J, et al. Larch arabinogalactan for hepatic drug delivery: isolation and characterization of a 9 kDa arabinogalactan fragment. *Carbohydr Res* 1995;278(1):113-28.

[6] Niemann G, et al. Phenolics from Larix needles. XIII. Analysis of main Larix flavonoids by high-pressure liquid chromatography. *Planta Med* 1977;31(3):297-301.

[7] Ohtsu H, et al. 18-nor-Abietatrienes from the cones of Larix kaempferi. *J Nat Prod* 1998;61(3):406-408.

[8] Ohtsu H, et al. Abietane diterpenoids from the cones of larix kaempferi. *J Nat Prod* 1998;61(10):1307-9.

[9] Niemann G. Phenolics from Larix needles. 8. Flavonoids of L. leptolepis. *Planta Med* 1974;26(2):101-3.

[10] Bruns K. Diterpene. VI. Neutral constituent of the resin from Larix europaea D.C. *Tetrahedron* 1969;25(8):1771-75.

[11] Hauer J, et al. Mechanism of stimulation of human natural killer cytotoxicity by arabinogalactan from Larix occidentalis. *Cancer Immunol Immunother* 1993;36(4):237-44.

[12] Enriquez P, et al. Conjugation of adenine arabinoside 5'-monophosphate to arabinogalactan: synthesis, characterization, and antiviral activity. *Bioconjug Chem* 1995;6(2):195–202.

[13] Owen P, et al. Xanthine oxidase inhibitory activity of northeastern North American plant remedies used for gout. *J Ethnopharmacol* 1999;64(2):149-60.

Lathyrus

SCIENTIFIC NAME(S): Various species of *Lathyrus*, most commonly *L. sativus* (chickling vetch or chick-pea), *L. odoratus* (sweet pea), *L. cicera* (flat-podded vetch), *L. hirsutus* (caley pea), *L. sylvestris* (everlasting pea), *L. clymenum* (spanish vetchling), *L. incanus* (wild pea) and *L. pusillus* (singletary pea). Family: Leguminosae[1,2]

COMMON NAME(S): Chickling vetch, chick-pea, sweet pea, flat-podded vetch, caley pea, everlasting pea, spanish vetchling, wild pea, singletary pea and others, depending on species

BOTANY: *Lathyrus* is a widespread genus with species that grow throughout the world.

HISTORY: The *Lathyrus* species are generally cultivated for food, fodder and as ornamentals. For example, flowers of the sweet pea, *L. odoratus* (not to be confused with the common garden pea, *Pisum* spp.), are cultivated for their color and fragrance. The seeds of the *Lathyrus* species are commonly eaten by large populations in India, parts of Africa, France, Italy, Spain and other countries.[1] *L. sativus* is used to prepare unleavened Indian bread and is sometimes eaten raw as pasteballs or cooked.[1] However, ingestion of certain species, particularly *L. sativus*, *L. cicera* and *L. clymenum*, can result in a toxic syndrome known as neurolathyrism. This disease has been recognized for more than a century in Europe, Africa and Asia; most commonly in Asia. Because of the potential for public health problems, the sale of *L. sativus* has been banned in many states in India; despite these efforts, distribution persists.[1] Lathyrism remains a common problem among grazing animals in some countries.

CHEMISTRY: A variety of compounds with potential neurotoxic effects have been identified and are discussed below. Other compounds isolated from seeds of the *Lathyrus* species include phytates, divicine and a mixture of alkaloids. The lack of vitamins A, B and C from these seeds may enhance the neurotoxic potential.[1]

PHARMACOLOGY: Lathyrism appears to be the result of toxicity caused by several compounds, including beta-N-oxalyl-L-alpha,beta-diaminopropionic acid (ODAP) and beta-aminopropionitrile (BAPN).

ODAP is a neurotoxin that is associated with the animal and human neurotoxic manifestations of the disease neurolathyrism. BAPN induces skeletal abnormalities in animals; this compound and related compounds appear to be responsible for osteolathyrism (damage to the skeleton), which has not been observed in man. BAPN induces osteolathyrism and angiolathyrism (damage to the blood vessels) without inducing neurotoxic effects.[3] *L. odoratus* is more commonly associated with osteolathyrism than other species[1] and a separate term, odoratism, has been proposed for this syndrome.

TOXICOLOGY: Osteolathyrism, evidenced by skeletal deformities and aortic rupture, has been induced in rats given a 50% diet of sweet peas or diets containing 0.1-0.2% BAPN.[1] The toxicity appears to be related to structural defects in collagen induced by the *Lathyrus* toxins.

Neurolathyrism occurs in many animal species, but some (eg, the squirrel monkey) appear to be particularly resistant to the toxic effects of *Lathyrus*.[4] Human neurolathyrism remains a significant public health problem in India, particularly among the poor for whom *L. sativus* forms the main part of the diet. The disease generally occurs when a diet consisting of one-third to one-half *L. sativus* seeds in consumed for 3 to 6 months. Muscular rigidity and spasticity, weakness, paralysis of leg muscles, weak pulse, shallow breathing, convulsions or death may occur.[1,5,6] Prolonged neurotoxicity lasting more than 40 years, characterized by poor central motor coordination and reduced nerve conduction in the lower limbs, has been observed in persons suffering from the effects of neurolathyrism.[7]

There does not appear to be a common mechanism for the mode of action of the neurolathyrogens. Some propose that these compounds may affect glutamine concentrations or activity in the central nervous system.[1]

Pyramidal tract involvement has been observed in primates fed beta-N-oxalylamino-L-alanine (BOAA), a potent neuroexcitatory amino acid found in chickling peas and an inhibitor of glutamate.[8] Others have proposed that the neurotoxin may function as a zinc carrier and that cerebral zinc deficiency may play a role in the disease.[9]

Several procedures have been used in an attempt to deactivate the toxin prior to ingestion. Typically, these involve soaking seeds in water, followed by steaming or sun drying. Roasting the seeds at high temperatures for 20 minutes also seems to help destroy the neurotoxic factors. These procedures, however, only destroy 80–85% of the toxin.[1]

Preliminary findings suggest that treatment with the centrally acting muscle relaxant tolperisone can significantly reduce the spasticity in neurolathyrism.[10]

SUMMARY: Seeds of many *Lathyrus* species play an important role as foodstuffs and animal fodder throughout much of the developing world. Unfortunately, numerous species of these plants contain toxic compounds that can induce severe neurotoxicity in both animals and man when ingested at high levels for prolonged periods. This toxic syndrome is rare in Western countries, but remains common in Asia and may be observed in Asian immigrants to Western countries. No effective therapy is available for this toxicity.

PATIENT INFORMATION – Lathyrus

Uses: Some *Lathryus* species are eaten.

Side Effects: Some species are neurotoxic.

---

[1] Liener IE, ed. *Toxic Constituents of Plant Foodstuffs*, 2nd ed. New York: Academic Press, 1980.

[2] Lewis WH, Elvin-Lewis MPF. *Medical Botany: Plants affecting man's health.* New York: John Wiley & Sons, 1977.

[3] Spencer PS, Schaumburg HH. Lathyrism: a neurotoxic disease. *Neurobehav Toxicol Teratol* 1983;5(6):625.

[4] Mehta T, et al. The *Lathyrus sativus* Neurotoxin: Resistance of the Squirrel Monkey to Prolonged Oral High Doses. *Toxicol Appl Pharmacol* 1983;69:480.

[5] Hardin JW, Arena JM. Human Poisoning from Native and Cultivated Plants, 2nd ed. Durham, NC: Duke University Press, 1974.

[6] Misra UK, Pandey CM. H reflex studies in neurolatyrism. *Electroencephalogr Clin Neurophysiol* 1994;93(4):281.

[7] Hugon J, et al. Studies of the etiology and pathogenesis of motor neuron disease. III. Magnetic cortical stimulation in patients with lathyrism. *Acta Neurol Scand* 1993;88(6):412.

[8] Spencer PS, et al. Lathyrism: evidence for role of the neuroexcitatory aminoacid BOAA. *Lancet* 1986;2(8515):1066.

[9] Lambein F, et al. From soil to brain: zinc deficiency increases the neurotoxicity of Lathyrus sativus and may affect the susceptibility for the motorneurone disease neurolathyrism. *Toxicon* 1994;32(4):461.

[10] Haque A, et al. New findings and symptomatic treatment for neurolathyrism, a motor neuron disease occuring in north west Bangladesh. *Paraplegia* 1994;32(3):193.

Lavender

SCIENTIFIC NAME(S): Several Lavandula species have been used medicinally, including *L. angustifolia* Mill. (syn. *L. officinalis* Chaix. and *L. spica* L.), *L. stoechas*, *L. dentata*, *L. latifolia* and *L. pubescens* Decne. Family: Lamiaceae

COMMON NAME(S): Aspic, lavandin (usually refers to particular hybrids), lavender, spike lavender, true lavender

BOTANY: Lavender plants are aromatic evergreen sub-shrubs that grow to about 3 feet high. The plants are native to the Mediterranean region. Fresh flowering tops are collected, and the essential oil is distilled or extracts are obtained by solvent extraction.[1] The plant has small blue or purple flowers. The narrow leaves are fuzzy and gray when young and turn green as they mature.[2] Lavender is cultivated extensively for use as a perfume, potpourri and as an ornamental.

HISTORY: Lavender has long found a role in folk medicine. The plant has been used as an antispasmodic, carminative, diuretic and general tonic. Extracts have been used to treat conditions ranging from acne to migraines.[1] Although the plant has been known to increase bile flow output and flow into the intestine, its greatest value is not in the treatment of biliary conditions.[2] Lavender has been used quite extensively as an antidiabetic agent in parts of Spain and is included in some commercial herbal antidiabetic preparations.[3] Fresh leaves and flowers are applied to the forehead to relieve headaches and to joints to treat rheumatic pain. The vapors of steamed flowers are used as a cold remedy.[4] Chileans drink the tea to induce or increase menstrual flow.[5]

Lavender is usually administered in the form of an infusion, decoction or oil and is either taken internally or applied topically for relief of neuralgia. Today, lavender oil and extracts are used as pharmaceutical fragrances and in cosmetics. Spike lavender oil is often used in soaps because it is inexpensive but of lower quality than true lavender oil. Lavandin oil, lavender absolute (an extract) and spike lavender oil are used in concentrations of up to 1.2% in perfumes.[1] Small amounts (0.002% to 0.004%) of the oil are used to flavor food.

Lavender's versatility is seen in its various applications as a fragrance in perfumes, bath and shower products, hair care products, toiletry soaps, detergents, typical formulations, synthetic derivatives and production figures.[6]

CHEMISTRY: Lavender flowers contain between 1% to 3% essential oil.[7] Lavandin hybrids contain a higher volatile oil content, but its composition is extremely variable. The oil is a complex mixture of more than 150 compounds, the most abundant of which are linaloyl acetate (30% to 55%), linalool (20% to 35%), cineole, camphor, beta-ocimene, limonene, caproic acid, caryophyllene oxide and tannins (5% to 10%).[1,7] However, the relative amounts of these compounds can vary widely between species.[8,9] Perillyl alcohol, a distillate of *L. angustifolia* has been shown to exert anticancer effects.[10] Several articles on lavender are available, discussing analysis methods,[11-13] enantiomeric purity and distinctiveness,[14-16] variety deviation,[17-20] essential oil quality,[21,22] GC retention indices,[23] and lavender content in perfumes.[24]

PHARMACOLOGY: One report investigated the effects of lavender oil aromatherapy for insomnia and concluded that it is comparable to hypnotics or tranquilizers.[25] Lavender aromatherapy has also been utilized to increase mental capacity and diminish fatigue,[26] and to improve mood and perceived levels of anxiety.[27] Oils of different lavender species yield different results.[28] The German Commission E Monograph lists among lavender's uses, to be helpful for **restlessness** and **difficulties in sleeping**.[7] Lavender EEG studies, which have shown various alpha wave responses to different odors, can be used for psychophysiological response evaluation.[30] Spike lavender oil has a spasmolytic effect on animal smooth muscle. These effects are consistent with the pharmacologic activities of many other common volatile oils. In mice, lavender oil exhibits **CNS depressant** activity, characterized by anticonvulsant activity and a potentiation of chloral hydrate-induced sleep. Another report on aromatherapy finds "exposure time-dependent" decreases in motility in mice after inhalation of lavender fragrance. This helps to confirm folk remedies such as herbal pillow use to facilitate rest or minimize stress in people.[29]

The infusion and suspension of *L. stoechas* cause hypoglycemia in normoglycemic rats, reaching maximum activity 30 minutes after administration.[3] Further studies with *L. dentata* and *L. latifolia* have found the active hypoglycemic components to be partially water soluble.

Furthermore, the extracts were not active in rats with alloxan-induced diabetes, indicating the need for intact pancreatic cells for a pharmacologic effect to occur. The active components have not been chemically classified.[31]

There is little direct evidence to support the use of lavender oil as a choleretic or for the treatment of GI disorders. A Bulgarian report discusses choleretic and cholagogic action of Bulgarian lavender oil.[32] Many volatile oils also may share these common actions. One of lavender's uses listed in the German Commission E Monograph includes helping in functional disorders of the upper abdomen with irritable stomach and intestinal disorders of nervous origin. Its effects are both calming and antiflatulent.[7]

Extracts of lavender are used in Europe as insect repellents. This effect appears to be related to compounds in the volatile oil.[33]

A study of percutaneous absorption of lavender oil in massage found that within 5 minutes after application, main constituents of the oil were detected in the blood. After this rapid absorption, most of the lavender oil was excreted within 90 minutes.[34]

Another report evaluated the role of lavender oil as a bath additive to relieve perineal discomfort after childbirth. When compared with placebo and synthetic oil, analysis of daily discomfort scores show less discomfort between days 3 to 5 with true lavender oil use.[35]

Herbal research finds perillyl alcohol, a compound distilled from lavender (also found in cherries, mint and celery seeds) to possess anticancer activities.[10] This monoterpene is being tested in clinical trials to study its role in cancer chemoprevention and therapy.[36-37]

A variety of mechanisms are proposed to explain perillyl alcohol's chemopreventative and chemotherapeutic effects. One such mechanism is that it promotes "apoptosis," a self-destructing ability the cell has when its DNA is severely damaged. In cancer, these cells lack this self-destructing ability, resulting in abnormal cell growth.[10] In one report, liver tumor formation was not promoted by perillyl alcohol, but its growth was inhibited by this apoptosis mechanism by enhancing tumor cell loss.[38] In another report, the rate of apoptosis was more than 6–fold higher with perillyl alcohol treated pancreatic adenocarcinoma cells than in untreated cells.[39]

Another proposed mechanism of monoterpenes is inhibition of post-translational isoprenylation of cell growth-regulatory proteins (such as Ras).[40] Perillyl alcohol has inhibited in vivo prenylation of specific proteins in one report,[41] and has altered RAS protein synthesis and degradation in another. Interfering with these pathways can regulate malignant cell proliferation.[42] Monoterpene-treated rat mammary tumors have been remodeled and redifferentiated to more benign phenotypes.[40] Perillyl alcohol treatment resulted in 70% to 99% inhibition of "aberrant hyperproliferation," a late occurring event preceding mammory tumorigenesis in vivo.[43]

Other cancers where perillyl alcohol has been effective include: murine melanoma growth suppression in vitro and in vivo;[44] pancreatic carcinoma in hamsters;[45-46] colon carcinogenesis in rats;[47] mammary cancer in rats;[40,48] liver tumors in rats;[38] and lung cancer in rats.[10]

With such promising results from animal studies, human clinical trials are under way to treat patients with breast, ovarian and prostate cancers. Results are not yet available.[10]

Besides anticancer effects, perillyl alcohol has been used orally in rabbits to reduce vein graft intimal hyperplasia.[49] It was also found to suppress hepatic HMG-CoA reductase activity, a rate limiting step in cholesterol synthesis, lowering serum cholesterol.[50]

TOXICOLOGY: Lavender oil exhibited a low order of toxicity when administered subcutaneously to animals. Although lavender absolute has been reported to be a skin sensitizer, no human phototoxicity has been reported. Lavender and lavandin oil have been reported to be nonirritating and nonsensitizing to human skin.[1]

However, three reports discuss allergic contact dermatitis from lavender oil and fragrance.[51-53] These examples are few, probably because the oil is used in small quantities in foods and cosmetics and has not been associated with major toxicity during normal use. The German Commission E Monograph lists no known side effects or contraindications.[7]

One report in mice observes an interaction between a 1/60 dilution of lavender oil, and pentobarbital, where sleeping time is increased.[54]

SUMMARY: Lavender is an aromatic plant that has been used in herbal medicine for centuries. It has been known to exhibit CNS depressant activity and is used for insomnia or to relieve anxiety and stress. It may also be helpful in GI disorders to reduce sugar and cholesterol levels and aid in grafting surgery. Lately, lavender compound perillyl alcohol is being studied for its promising effects in cancer prevention. Lavender has a low toxicity profile.

PATIENT INFORMATION – Lavender

Uses: Therapeutic: Antispasmotic, carminative, antidiabetic agent, restlessness and insect repellant. Nutritional: Food flavoring agent.

Drug Interactions: May increase or potentiate the CNS depressant effects of sedative-hypnotics.

Side Effects: Allergic contact dermatitis.

---

[1] Leung AY. *Encyclopedia of Common Natural Ingredients Used in Food, Drugs and Cosmetics.* J Wiley and Sons. 1980.
[2] Weiss RF. Herbal Medicine, Hippokrates Verlag, 1988.
[3] Gamez MJ, et al. *Pharmazie* 1987;42:706.
[4] Abulafaith HA. *Econ Bot* 1987;41:354.
[5] San Martin JA. *Econ Bot* 1983;37:216.
[6] Lamparsky, D. Lavender. *Perf & Flav* 1986;11(Aug-Sep):7-8, 10, 12-13, 15-20.
[7] Bisset NL. *Lavandulae Floes.* Herbal Drugs and Phytopharmaceuticals, CRC Press, Stuttgart, Germany, 1994;292-94.
[8] Mesonero MM, et al. *Boll Chim Pharm* 1974;113:131.
[9] Szabolcs N, et al. *Acta Pharm Hung* 1985;55:49.
[10] Jones C. *Herbs for Health* 1998;(Jan/Feb):17.
[11] Boelens, MH. *Perf & Flav* 1986;11(Oct-Nov):43-54, 56,58-60, 62-63.
[12] Kustrak D, et al. *Pharma Acta Helv* 1975;50(11)373-78.
[13] Ikechukwu E, et al. *J Chromatogr B Biomed Appl* 1997;688(2):354-58.
[14] Kreis P, et al. *PZ Wissenchaft* 1993;138(5-6):149-55.
[15] Ognyanov I, et al. *Rev Ital Ess Profumi Piante Officinali Aromi Saponi Cosmetici Aerosol* 1973;9(Sep):560-64.
[16] Mizrahi I, et al. *Soap, Perfumery & Cosmetics* 1970;43(Jun):379-88.
[17] Djarmati S, et al. *Arch Farmaciju* 1987;37(5):229-33.
[18] Prager MJ, et al. *Perf & Flav* 1981;6(Apr-May):53-58.
[19] Agnel R, et al. *Perf & Flav* 1984;9(Oct-Nov):53-56.
[20] Ahmed A, et al. *Revi Itali Ess Profumi Piante Oficinali Aromi Saponi Cosmetici Aerosol* 1980;62(Sep-Oct):293-96.
[21] Rouzet M. *Lab Pharma Probl Tech* 1984;32(Jun):462-66.
[22] Denny EFK. *Soap, Perfumery & Cosmetics* 1969;42(Oct):737-38.
[23] Nviredy S, et al. *Acta Pharm Hung* 1985;55(Mar) 49-58.
[24] Cabo J, et al. *ARS Pharmaceutica* 1982;23(4):501-06.
[25] Hardy M, et al. *Lancet* 1995;346(Sept 9):701.
[26] Leshchinskaia I, et al. *Kosm Med* 1983;17(2):80-83.
[27] Dunn C, et al. *J Ad Nurs* 1995;21(1):34-40.
[28] Buckle J. *Nurs Times* 1993;89(20):32-35.
[29] Buchbauer G, et al. *Z Naturforsch* 1991;46(11-12):1067-72.
[30] Lee CF, et al. *Ann Physiol Anthropol* 1994;13(5):281-91.
[31] Gamez MJ, et al. *Pharmazie* 1988,43:441.
[32] Gruncharov V. *Vutr Boles* 1973;12(3):90-96.
[33] Secey DM, Smith AE. *Econ Bot* 1983;37:28.
[34] Jager W et al. *J Soc Cosm Chem* 1992;43(Jan-Feb):49-54.
[35] Dale A, et al. *J Adv Nurs* 1994;19(1):89-96.
[36] Kellof G et al. *J Cell Biochem Suppl* 1996;26:1-28.
[37] Gould M. *Environ Health Perspect* 1997;105(Suppl)4:977-79.
[38] Mills J, et al. *Cancer Res* 1995;55(5):979-83.
[39] Staybrook K, et al. *Carcinogenesis* 1997;18(8):1655-58.
[40] Crowell F et al. *Adv Exp Med Biol* 1996;401:131-36
[41] Ren Z, et al. *Biochem Pharmacol* 1997;54(1):113-20.
[42] Hohl R, et al. *Adv Exp Med Biol* 1996;401:137-46.
[43] Katdare M. *Cancer Lett* 1997;111(1-2):141-47.
[44] He L, et al. *J Nutr* 1997;127(5):668-74.
[45] Stark M, et al. *Cancer Lett* 1995;96(1):15-21.
[46] Burke Y, et al. *Lipids* 1997;32(2):151-56.
[47] Reddy B, et al. *Cancer Res* 1997;57(3):420-25.
[48] Gould, M. *J Cell Biochem Suppl* 1995;22:139-44.
[49] Fulton G, et al. *J Surg Res* 1997;69(1):128-34.
[50] Elson C, et al. *J Nutr* 1994;124(5):607-14.
[51] Brandao FM. *Contact Derm* 1986;15(4):249-50.
[52] Rademaker M. *Contact Derm* 1994;31(1):58-59.
[53] Schaller M, et al. *Clin & Exp Derm* 1995;20(2):143-45.
[54] Guillemain J. *Ann Pharm Fr* 1989;47(6):337-43.

Lecithin

SCIENTIFIC NAME(S): 1,2-diacyl-sn-glycero-3-phosphatidylcholine

COMMON NAME(S): Lecithin, lecithol, vitellin, kelecin, granulestin

SOURCE: Lecithin is found in many animal and vegetable sources including beef liver, steak, eggs, peanuts, cauliflower, and oranges.[1] Commercial sources for lecithin can come from soybeans, egg yolk, or brain tissue.[3,4] Some commercial lecithin and lecithin supplements contain between 10% and 35% phosphatidylcholine.[1]

HISTORY: Lecithin originated from the Greek "Lekithos." Lecithin is used today to treat liver ailments, hypercholesterolemia and neurologic diseases.[1,2] It is also used in the food processing industry.[3,5] Lecithin is a common compound found in cells of all living organisms, its presence being required for proper biological function.[6]

CHEMISTRY: Lecithin is a phospholipid mixture of acetone insoluble phosphatides consisting mainly of phosphatidylcholine, phosphatidyl ethanolamine, phosphatidyl serine, phosphatidyl inositol combined with various other substances including fatty acids and carbohydrates.[2] Lecithin is the common name for a series of related compounds called phosphatidylcholines.[5] Lecithin is defined chemically as a mixture of the diglycerides of stearic, palmitic, and oleic acids, linked to the choline ester of phosphoric acid (eg, soybean lecithin contains 4% stearic, 11.7% palmitic, 9.8% oleic acids, along with others). Lecithins also contain phosphorous and nitrogenous (eg, choline) compounds.[5]

Physical properties of lecithin can vary depending upon acid value. It is a waxy mass at acid value 20 and a thick pourable fluid at acid value 30. The color is white when freshly made but turns yellow to brown in air. It is an edible and digestible surfactant and emulsifier.[3]

PHARMACOLOGY:

Use: Lecithin is used as an emulsifying and stabilizing agent in the food (eg, margarine, chocolate production), pharmaceutical, and cosmetic (eg, creams, lipsticks, conditioners) industries.[2,3,5]

Pharmacological use of lecithin primarily includes treatments for hypercholesterolemia, neurologic disorders, and liver ailments.

Hypercholesterolemia: Lecithin seems to possess beneficial properties in reducing cholesterol levels and controlling or preventing atherosclerosis. However, studies done in the late 1970's to early 1980's provide insufficient clinical or epidemiologic evidence to entirely support its positive effects against atherosclerosis. Although other studies from this time appear promising and have found results such as "18% cholesterol reduction," or "lowered cholesterol levels along with changes in lipid metabolism," no study is reliable with respect to atherosclerosis progression.[5]

Four months of soybean lecithin administration was found to reduce total serum lipids, cholesterol, and triglycerides in 21 hyperlipidemic patients.[6] The mechanism appears to be enhancement of cholesterol metabolism in the digestive system.

Neurology: Variable results occur using lecithin supplementation for treatment of neurologic disorders.

Lecithin is a good source of choline for treatment in dementias.[2] Phosphatidylcholine is thought to be a precursor for acetylcholine (Ach) synthesis.[5] Choline increases the accumulation of Ach within the brain. Ach is important for many brain functions including memory, so increasing concentration of this neurotransmitter can result in improved memory.[1] Positive effect on long-term memory has been demonstrated after administration of 35 g lecithin for 4 to 6 weeks.[5] However, another report shows no improvement from lecithin in memory disorders when taken in 30 mg/day dosages.[7]

Lecithin supplementation has also been studied in Alzheimer's disease, starting with memory difficulties. Three of 7 Alzheimer's patients receiving 25 g lecithin showed improvement in learning ability (coinciding with peak choline levels).[8] Combination tacrine and lecithin therapy conducted in a 32-patient double-blinded trial yielded poor results.[9] In a multicenter study, this combination did not improve mental status in 67 Alzheimer's patients.[10]

Ach deficiencies are also associated with other neurological disorders including tardive dyskinesia, Huntington's chorea, Friedreich's ataxia, myasthenia gravis, and other brain atrophies. In 2 patients with tardive dyskinesia, lecithin administration reduced abnormal movements. Ten cases of Friedreich's ataxia were also improved by lecithin supplementation.[11] One study failed to show any beneficial response in 12 patients with Friedreich's ataxia taking 25 g lecithin daily.[12]

Liver: In Germany, a product called *Essentiale*, (phosphatidylcholine) is marketed for liver disorders including acute and chronic hepatitis, cirrhosis, diabetic fatty liver, and toxic liver damage. Documentation supporting these claims have been authorized by the BGA (the German equivalent of the FDA). One report describes supplementation with phosphatidylcholine and how it protects against alcoholic cirrhosis in baboons.[1]

Other: Lecithin has also modified the immune system, activating specific and nonspecific defense systems in 20 patients receiving 1 teaspoonful 3 times daily for 30 days.[13] Another report discusses gallstone dissolution in 2 of 7 patients treated with lecithin and oral cholic acid. One patient experienced stone size reduction.[14]

TOXICOLOGY: Adverse effects generally have not been associated with lecithin as a nutritional supplement.[5] Some studies had no observable side effects, as well.[4,6,11] Six of 12 patients complained of anorexia and nausea when taking 25 g lecithin daily; one of these patients also noted excessive salivation.[12] Gastrointestinal side effects and hepatitis were experienced from the study in Alzheimer's patients taking both tacrine and lecithin.[10] One report in rats observes biochemical alterations and impaired sensorimotor development in offspring of rats fed a diet including 5% crude lecithin, suggesting its consumption is inadvisable during pregnancy.[5]

SUMMARY: Lecithin is a phospholipid mixture naturally occurring in nervous tissue and certain plants. It is used for its emulsifying properties in the food, pharmaceutical, and cosmetic industries. Pharmacological use of lecithin includes treatment for hypercholesterolemia, neurologic disorders, and liver ailments, all with variable to poor results. Toxicity profile appears to be low, with some exceptions. Its use in crude form is not recommended during pregnancy.

PATIENT INFORMATION – Lecithin

Uses: Lecithin is used for its emulsifying properties in the food, pharmaceutical, and cosmetic industries. Pharmacological use of lecithin includes treatment for hypercholesterolemia, neurologic disorders, and liver ailments. It has also been used to modify the immune system by activating specific and nonspecific defense systems.

Side Effects: Adverse effects are usually not associated with lecithin. However, there have been reports of anorexia, nausea, increased salivation, other GI effects, and hepatitis. Use during pregnancy is not recommended.

---

[1] Murray M. *Encyclopedia of Nutritional Supplements*. Rocklin, CA: Prima Publishing, 1996.

[2] Reynolds J, ed. *Martindale, The Extra Pharmacopoeia*, ed. 31. London, Eng.: Royal Pharm. Society, 1996.

[3] Budavari S, ed. The Merck Index, ed. 11. Rahway, NJ: Merck and Co., 1989.

[4] Venturella US. Natural Products. Gennaro AR, ed. *Remington: The Science and Practice of Pharmacy*, ed. 19. Easton, PA: Mack Publishing Co., 1995.

[5] DerMarderosian A, et al. *Natural Product Medicine*, Philadelphia, PA: George F. Stickley Co., 1988;121-22,140,313-15.

[6] Saba P, et al. *Current Therapeutic Research, Clinical & Experimental*, 1978 Aug;24:299-306.

[7] Caine E. *NEJM* 1980 Sep 4;303:585-86.

[8] Etienne P, et al. *Lancet* 1978 Dec 2;2:1206.

[9] Maltby N, et al. *BMJ* 1994 Apr 2;308:879-83.

[10] Chatellier G, et al. *BMJ* 1990 Feb 24;300:495-99.

[11] Barbeau A, et al. *NEJM* 1978 Jul 27;299:200-1.

[12] Pentland B, et al. *BMJ* 1981 Apr 11;282:1197-98.

[13] Pawlik A, et al. *Herba Polonica* 1996;42(1):42-46.

[14] Toouli J, et al. *Lancet* 1975 Dec 6;2:1124-26.

Leeches

SCIENTIFIC NAME(S): *Hirudo medicinalis* L. Phylum: Annelida

COMMON NAME(S): Fresh water leech, medicinal leech

HISTORY: The medicinal uses of leeches date back to more than two centuries before Christ. The 19th century heralded the widespread use of leeches for "bloodletting," a practice that grew so quickly that by the 1830s a leech shortage arose in France requiring the importation of more than 40 million Mexican leeches.[1] The last 45 years have seen a resurgence in the use of leeches, particularly as adjuncts in post-surgical wound healing procedures.

THERAPEUTIC USES: Medicinal leeches are used to stimulate the flow of blood at post-operative surgical sites, a procedure that has been claimed to increase the success of tissue transplants, reduction mammoplasty and the surgical reattachment of amputated extremities.[2]

The application of leeches to the area immediately surrounding the surgical wound temporarily reestablishes venous blood flow, thereby allowing the nutritive perfusion of the wound site by fresh blood. Blood stasis is a major contributor to unsuccessful reconstructive surgery. It is believed that if sufficient blood flow is maintained at the site until permanent adequate natural perfusion is established, the affected tissue has a significantly improved survival rate.

After attaching to the site, leeches secrete compounds that reduce blood viscosity; they also draw from 20 to 50 ml of blood from each bite. The leeches provide the drainage needed to permit decongestion and to preserve tissue viability until normal venous flow is established (about 5 to 7 days after the surgery).[3]

Application method: Leeches obtained from commercial breeders are easily maintained in a chlorine-free salt solution at 10°C to 20° C. Under such conditions, leeches can survive for up to 18 months.

Patients undergoing leech therapy should be administered a broad-spectrum antibiotic such as an aminoglycoside or third-generation cephalosporin to prevent infection by *Aeromonas hydrophilia*, which is found in the leech gut.[4,5] This is of particular importance considering that wild species are being investigated and that these leeches have been reported to contain a variety of potentially pathogenic bacteria.[6] In one study, blood from collected African leeches tested positive for HIV and hepatitis B, and leeches bought in German pharmacies contained up to 11 species of bacteria; viruses and protozoans have been shown to survive for months in the gut of the leech and as such, the leech should be considered a vector for infectious diseases.[7]

In practice, the area is washed well and covered by gauze or transparent dressing with a precut 1 cm hole to reveal adhesion site. The leech is then placed near the site. The biting end of the leech is generally the smaller of the two ends and moves in a "searching" fashion.[4] If attachment does not occur readily, the leech can be induced by pricking the skin with a pin to draw a drop of blood or the area can be dabbed with a sugar solution. The bite has been described as virtually painless or similar to a mosquito bite. A detailed description of the application technique has been outlined by Abrutyn.[8]

One leech is applied from 2 to 4 times a day for up to a week.[9] Feeding is complete in about 20 minutes, at which time the leech drops off. The feeding may suffice the leech for months. Removal of the leech may be hastened by applying solutions of salt, vinegar, a match or a local anesthetic, but the leech should not be forcibly removed. Bleeding from the attachment site usually continues for several hours.[10] Reuse of leeches is discouraged to minimize cross-infection.

PHARMACOLOGY: Medicinal leeches have an anterior and posterior sucker; within the anterior sucker is a y-shaped mouth with marginal teeth for biting. Following attachment, the leech secretes hirudin, a selective thrombin inhibitor, which enhances bleeding and prevents coagulation.

Hirudin was first described more than a century ago. It has recently been identified as a 65-amino acid peptide with antithrombokinase activity. Therapeutic studies of hirudin have been limited by its low natural yield, but the compound has recently been produced in quantities by recombinant gene techniques.[11,12] Recombinant hirudin binds very efficiently with thrombin, thus low doses are needed to inhibit venous thrombosis in animals. Extracts from leeches have been marketed as a cream for topical application, but their efficacy is unproven.

Recombinant hirudin has been used successfully in the treatment of Kasabach-Merritt Syndrome which leads to loss of circulating platelets and fibrinogen. Paradoxically, low-dose subcutaneous hirudin normalized fibrinogen and platelet activity.[11]

In addition to hirudin, leeches secrete a vasodilator, a hyaluronidase, a collagenase and two fibrinases (one disrupts clots, the other atherosclerotic plaque). The compound calin has also been isolated from leeches. By binding to collagen to interfere with the platelet-collagen interaction, this inhibitor of von Willebrand factor causes an antithrombotic effect in vitro and in hamster models.[13,14] There is conflicting evidence as to whether an anesthetic is secreted.

A number of studies have confirmed that the use of medicinal leeches improves venous drainage of wound sites in patients who have undergone reattachment surgery after amputation.[15,16] The ability of leeches to improve blood flow across congested surgical flaps has been documented using Doppler laser perfusion monitoring in pigs. Within one hour of applying leeches, blood flow through the surgical area increased 142% at surface probes and 491% at implanted probes. The average change for untreated control flaps was 6%.[1]

One study, however, found no changes in ipsilateral activated partial thromboplastin or prothrombin times when leeches were applied to an intact hand.[17] These findings suggest that significant systemic or local anticoagulation is not likely to occur and the risk of interference with other therapies may be small.

Salivary extracts of the giant leech (*Haementeria*) interfere with the metastatic growth of lung tumors.[2]

TOXICOLOGY: Leeches may draw up to 50 ml of blood per feeding. Repeated leeching may decrease hemoglobin levels dramatically. Drops of 1 to 2 gm% during a 5-day course are common. Decreases of up to 7 gm% have been observed following a 6-day course and required tranfusion therapy.[9] Following removal of leeches, the wound site will continue to bleed for up to 4 hours.

Several reports have documented severe wound and systemic infections caused by *Aeromonas hydrophila* (a Gram negative rod) harbored by leeches, and *Providentia* has been isolated in transport water.[18]

Local allergic reactions and anaphylaxis have been reported.[10] A unique case of nasal bleeding was reported in Spain, where a man was found to have a leech in his nostril. It is believed that the leech was transmitted through water from a rural drinking fountain.[19]

SUMMARY: Leeches have been used medicinally for centuries and interest in their use continues today. They are used most widely in post-surgical wound management. Although their use is not painful, it has been associated with severe anemia and systemic infections. The clinical development of hirudin and other leech-derived anticoagulant compounds may eventually supplant the use of leeches. Experience with the leech continues to grow and to become well documented.

PATIENT INFORMATION – Leeches

Uses: Leeches have been used for bloodletting, wound healing and stimulating blood flow at post-surgical sites.

Side Effects: Allergic reactions, anaphylaxis and infection, possibly even with hepatitis and HIV, may develop.

[1] Hayden RE, et al. Objective monitoring of altered perfusion in congested flaps. *Arch Otolaryngol Head Neck Surg* 1988;114:1395.
[2] Lent C. New medical and scientific uses of the leech. *Nature* 1986;323:494.
[3] Abrutyn E. Hospital-associated infection from leeches. *Ann Int Med* 1988;109:356.
[4] Kourt B, et al. When the prescription says leeches. *Am J Hosp Pharm* 1994;51:2113.
[5] Bickel KD, et al. Intestinal flora of the medicinal leech Hirudinaria manillensis. *J Reconstr Microsurg* 1994;10:83.
[6] Wilken GB, Appleton CC. Bacteriological investigation of the occurrence and antibiotic sensitivities of the gut-flora of the potential southern African medicinal leech, Asiaticobdella buntonensis (Hirudinidae). *J Hosp Infect* 1993;23:223.
[7] Nehili M, et al. Experiments on the possible role of leeches as vectors of animal and human pathogens: a light and electron microscopy study. *Parasitol Res* 1994;80:277.
[8] Abrutyn. *Am J Hosp Pharm* 1988;109:356.
[9] Rao P, et al. Leechmania in microsurgery. *Practitioner* 1985;229:901.
[10] Adams SL. The emergency management of a medicinal leech bite. *Annals Emerg Med* 1989;18:316.
[11] Wallis RB Hirudins and the role of thrombin: lessons from leeches. *Trends in Pharmacol Sci* 1988;9:245.
[12] Hard R, et al. A Review of the Pharmacology, Clinical Applications, and Toxicology of Hirudin and Hirulog. *Transgenica: The Journal of Clinical Biotechnology* 1994;1:1.
[13] Deckmyn H, et al. Calin from Hirudo medicinalis, an inhibitor of platelet adhesion to collagen, prevents platelet-rich thrombosis in hamsters. *Blood* 1995;85:712
[14] Harsfavi J, et al. Calin from Hirudo medicinalis, an inhibitor of von Willebrand factor binding to collagen under static and flow conditions. *Blood* 1995 85:705.
[15] Soucacos PN, et al. The use of medicinal leeches, Hirudo medicinalis, to restore venous circulation in trauma and reconstructive microsurgery. *Int Angiol* 1994;13:251.
[16] Soucacos PN, et al. Successful treatment of venous congestion in free skin flaps using medical leeches. *Microsurgery* 1994;15:496.
[17] Blackshear JL Ebener MK. Leeching, hirudin, and coagulation tests [letter]. *Ann Intern Med* 1994;121:151.
[18] Dickson P, et al. An unusual source of hospital wound infection. *Brit Med J* 1984;289:1727.
[19] Bergua A, et al. Unavoidable epistaxis in the nasal infection of leeches. *Acta Otorrinolaringol Esp* 1993;44:391.

Lemon

SCIENTIFIC NAME(S): *Citrus limon* (L.), family *Rutaceae*

COMMON NAME(S): Lemon

BOTANY: The lemon tree is an evergreen, growing to over 6 m in height. Its toothed leaves are light green. The citrus fruit (lemon) is small, green to yellow in color, and oval in shape. Unlike other citrus varieties, the lemon tree bears fruit continuously. The plant is cultivated in Mediterranean and subtropical climates worldwide.[1-2]

HISTORY: The lemon originated in southeast Asia, probably in India or southern China. Its history is sometimes unclear because of the confusion with the similarly appearing "citron," a closely related species. The lemon was thought to have been depicted in Roman artwork as early as the first century A.D.[2] Other sources state that the fruit was first grown in Europe in the second century A.D.[1]

In the 1600s, physicians became aware that daily intake of lemon juice would prevent outbreaks of scurvy among sailors on long sea voyages. Scurvy is a vitamin deficiency disease characterized by muscle wasting, inability of wound healing, bruising, and gum deterioration.[3] English ships were required by law to carry enough lemon or lime juice for each sailor to get 1 ounce daily, earning them the nickname "limeys."[3]

The California lemon industry began after the Gold Rush of 1849. From 1940 to 1965, production increased. Today, California and Arizona are the major lemon producers, making the US a major source ahead of Mexico and Italy.

More than 50% of the US lemon crop is processed into juice and other drink products. The peel, pulp, and seeds are also used to make oils, pectin, or other products. Lemon juice has long been used as a diuretic, diaphoretic, astringent, tonic, lotion, and gargle.[2]

CHEMISTRY: Citrus fruits in general contain sugars, polysaccharides, organic acids, lipids, carotenoids (responsible for color), vitamins, minerals, flavonoids, limonoids (causing bitterness), and volatile components.[4-5]

The lemon is a good source of potassium (145 mg/100 g of fruit), bioflavonoids, and vitamin C (40 to 50 mg/100 g, twice as much as oranges).[1-2] The isolation of vitamin C from lemon juice has been performed.[6] Calcium (61 mg) is also present, along with vitamins A, B_1, B_2, and B_3. The fruit is also low in calories, containing 27 Kcal/100 g.[1,2,7]

Other constituents of lemon include volatile oil (2.5% of the peel), limonene ($\leq$ 70%), alpha-terpinene, alpha-pinene, citral, coumarins, mucilage, pectins, and bioflavonoids (mostly from pith and peel).[1] Flavonoids eriocitrin and hesperidan have been evaluated.[8] When purchasing supplements for bioflavonoid benefits, it is also important to note content. Low-cost powdered lemon (and other citrus fruit) peels contain only 1% to 2% flavonoids, where standardized products contain 10% to 90% flavonoids. The percentage may not be stated on the label.[9] Adulteration of lemon juice has been reported.[10]

PHARMACOLOGY: Pharmacologically, the lemon is also important for its nutritional value. Vitamin C is necessary to sustain the body's resistance to infection and heal wounds. The potassium content in the fruit is useful to offset the potassium loss caused by blood-pressure lowering drugs in some patients.[11] In addition, lemon juice may increase iron absorption as described in a report of 234 women.[12]

Lemons also play a role as antioxidants. German studies in the late 1980s related this effect to the peel.[3] Bioflavonoids eriocitrin and hesperidan reduced oxidative stress in diabetic rats.[8] The pectin fiber and lemon oil also possess antioxidant properties.[11]

Lemons have anticancer properties illustrated in animal and human studies.[7,11] Citrus fruit intake is inversely related to cancer rates, especially stomach cancers. Vitamin C blocks formation of carcinogenic nitrosamines, after consumption of nitrites or nitrates (ie, in smoked food).[11]

The pectin component in lemons, because of the hydrophilic properties, acts to thicken gastric contents, regulating transit. This is useful to treat both vomiting and diarrhea.[13] Pectin also lowers blood cholesterol and aids in prevention of cardiovascular disease.[3,11,13] Bioflavonoids strengthen the inner lining of the blood vessels, including veins and capillaries. This is important for treatment of varicose veins, easy bruising, arteriosclerosis, or bleeding gums.[1]

Lemon's role as an antimicrobial agent has been reported. The volatile oil is said to be both antiseptic and antibacterial.[1] It has inhibited growth of *Aspergillus* mold in 1 report.[14] The juice has been evaluated as a natural biocide to disinfect drinking water.[15] Lemon juice also has sterilized rabies-virus-contaminated areas, to inactivate the virus in patients bitten by affected dogs.[16] The lemon has also been useful for infections, fevers, colds, flu, sore throat, gingivitis, and canker sores. It is also a liver and pancreas tonic.[1]

Skin ailments have also benefitted from lemons. It has been externally used for acne, fungus (ringworm and athlete's foot), sunburn, and warts.[1] One study reports lemon juice in the treatment of keloid, a scarring condition.[17] Application of lemon juice, once thought to have faded tattoos in conjunction with sunlight exposure, was disproven in another report.[18]

Once digested, lemon (despite its acidity) has an alkaline effect in the body, rendering it useful in such conditions as rheumatism, arthritis, and gout, where acidity is a negative contributing factor.[1]

Other actions of lemon preparations include sedative effects in fish,[3] increasing citrate levels inexpensively as therapy in patients with hypocitraturic calcium nephrolithiasis,[19] and behavior modification.[20-24]

TOXICOLOGY: The erosive effects of lemon juice on tooth enamel have also been evaluated.[25-28] One study finds loss of gloss, alteration in enamel color, and irregular dental tissue loss upon morphological analysis.[28]

SUMMARY: The lemon is an important and versatile fruit, dating back to the first or second century A.D. It contains many important vitamins including vitamin C, a necessary factor in preventing infection and healing wounds. Lemon's effects as an antioxidant and antitumor agent have been reported. The pectin component is also beneficial, aiding in cardiovascular health. Lemons also play important roles as antimicrobials, for skin ailments, and in GI health. Toxicology includes erosive effects on tooth enamel.

PATIENT INFORMATION – Lemon

Uses: Lemon has been used in food preparations and the agricultural industry to gel and stabilize foods. Important for its nutritional value, the lemon possesses vitamin C, which is necessary to sustain the body's resistance to infection and heal wounds. The lemon also contains antioxidant, anticancer, hydrophilic, and antimicrobial properties.

Side Effects: Toxicology reports include erosive effects on tooth enamel.

---

[1] Chevallier, A. *Encyclopedia of Medicinal Plants.* New York, NY: DK Publishing 1996;81.

[2] Ensminger A, et al. *Foods & Nutrition Encyclopedia,* 2nd edition. Boca Raton, FL: CRC Press Inc., 1994;1299-1302.

[3] Carper, J. *The Food Pharmacy.* New York, NY: Bantam Publishing, 1988;222-23.

[4] Ranganna S, et al. Citrus fruits–varieties, chemistry, technology, and quality evaluation. *Crit Rev Food Sci Nutr* 1983;18(4):313-86.

[5] Ranganna S, et al. Citrus fruits. Part II. Chemistry, technology, and quality evaluation. *Crit Rev Food Sci Nutr* 1983;19(1):1-98.

[6] King, C. The isolation of vitamin C from lemon juice. *Fed Proc* 1979;38(13):2681-83.

[7] Murray, M. *The Healing Power of Food.* Rocklin, CA: Prima Publishing Co., 1993;143,366.

[8] Miyake Y, et al. Protective effects of lemon flavonoids on oxidative stress in diabetic rats. *Lipids* 1998;33(7):689-95.

[9] Liva, E. Quality of nutritional supplements, Part II: The good news, the bad news. *Natural Pharmacy* 1999;3(1):18.

[10] Lifshitz A, et al. Detection of adulteration of fruit juice. I. Characterization of Israel lemon juice. *J Assoc Off Anal Chem* 1971;54(6):1262-65.

[11] Polunin, M. *Healing Foods.* New York, NY: DK Publishing, 1997;64-65.

[12] Ballot D, et al. The effects of fruit juices and fruits on the absorption of iron from a rice meal. *Br J Nutr* 1987;57(3):331-43.

[13] Bruneton, J. *Pharmacognosy, Phytochemistry, Medicinal Plants.* Paris, France: Lavoisier Publishing, 1995;107-9.

[14] Alderman G, et al. Inhibition of growth and aflatoxin production of *Aspergillus parasiticus* by citrus oils. *Z Lebensm Unters Forsch* 1976;160(4):353-58.

[15] D'Aquino M, et al. Lemon juice as a natural biocide for disinfecting drinking water. *Bull Pan Am Health Organ* 1994;28(4):324-30.

[16] Larghi O, et al. Inactivation of rabies virus by chemical agents. *Rev Asoc Argent Microbiol* 1975;7(3):86-90.

[17] Rueter, G. Treatment with lemon juice in the prevention of recurrences of keloid. *Zentralbl Chir* 1973;98(16):604-6.

[18] Chapel J, et al. Lemon juice, sunlight, and tattoos. *Int J Dermatol* 1983;22(7):434-35.

[19] Setzer M, et al. Dietary manipulation with lemonade to treat hypocitraturic calcium nephrolithiasis. *J Urol* 1996;156(3):907-9.

[20] Eysenck S, et al. Salivary response to lemon juice as a measure of introversion. *Percept Mot Skills* 1967;24(3):1047-53.

[21] Casey J, et al. Salivary response to lemon juice as a measure of introversion in children. *Percept Mot Skills* 1971;33(3):1059-65.

[22] Sajwaj T, et al. Lemon-juice therapy: the control of life-threatening rumination in a 6-month-old infant. *J Appl Behav Anal* 1974;7(4):557-63.

[23] Cook J, et al. Use of contingent lemon juice to eliminate public masturbation by a severely retarded boy. *Behav Res Ther* 1978;16(2):131-33.

[24] Hogg, J. Reduction of self-induced vomiting in a multiply handicapped girl by "lemon juice therapy" and concomitant changes in social behaviour. *Br J Clin Psychol* 1982;21(Pt 3):227-28.

[25] Allan D. Enamel erosion with lemon juice. *Br Dent J* 1967;122(7):300-2.

[26] Takaoka S, et al. Initial changes in human enamel surface caused by the topical application of fresh lemon juice. *Koku Eisei Gakkai Zasshi* 1971;21(1):6-11.

[27] Pias, M. The effects of lemon juice (citric acid) on the surfaces of teeth. *Chronicle* 1972;35(8):217-18.

[28] Grando L, et al. In vitro study of enamel erosion caused by soft drinks and lemon juice in deciduous teeth analysed by steromicroscopy and scanning electron microscopy. *Caries Res* 1996;30(5):373-78.

Lemon Balm

SCIENTIFIC NAME(S): *Melissa officinalis* L. Family Lamiaceae (Mints)

COMMON NAME(S): Lemon balm, balm, melissa, sweet balm

BOTANY: Lemon balm is a low perennial herb with ovate- or heart-shaped leaves that have a lemon odor when bruised. The small yellow or white flowers are attractive to bees and other insects. It is indigenous to the Mediterranean region and western Asia, and widely naturalized in Europe, Asia, and North America. The leaves are harvested before flowering and used medicinally.

HISTORY: Lemon balm has been used in herbal medicine since the times of Pliny, Dioscorides, Paracelsus, and Gerard. The name "melissa" corresponds to the Greek word for bee, while "balm" is a contraction of balsam. The plant has found both culinary and medicinal uses, with the principal historical medicinal uses being carminative, diaphoretic, and antipyretic.

CHEMISTRY: Lemon balm leaves contain 0.2% to 0.3% of a lemon-scented essential oil similar to lemon grass. Major mono- and sesquiterpenes include geranial, neral, b-caryophyllene, b-caryophyllene oxide, linalool, citronellal, nerol, and geraniol.[1-2] R(+)-methyl citronellate is characteristic of melissa oil and distinguishes it from lemon grass oil.[3] Flavonoids,[4] oleanane, and ursane triterpenes[5] also have been isolated from the plant. Major nonvolatile constituents are caffeic acid and its di- and trimeric derivatives, including rosmarinic acid and melitric acids A and B.[6]

PHARMACOLOGY: Lemon balm's traditional medicinal use was as a **sedative** and **antispasmodic**. This activity was formerly attributed to the volatile oil. However, the lyophilized hydroalcoholic extract, which does not contain the volatile oil components, has sedative activity in several mouse models when given intraperitoneally.[7] This extract also was active in an acetic acid writhing analgesia assay but not in the hot plate test. The volatile oil of the plant had much weaker activity or was inactive in the same assays.

Lemon balm has antiviral activity against a variety of viruses, including herpes simplex virus (HSV) and HIV-1. The activity has been attributed to caffeic acid and its di- and trimeric derivatives as well as to tannins.[8-9] A clinical trial of a cream formulation of melissa extract demonstrated evidence of activity against HSV cold sores.[10]

Another use of melissa has been in Graves' disease, in which the thyroid is abnormally activated by thyroid-stimulating immunoglobulin (TSI). Freeze-dried extracts of melissa bound thyrotropin and prevented it and the Graves' TSI from activating its receptor,[11-14] although with less potency than the extracts of *Lithospermum officinales*, *Lycopus virginicus*, and *Lycopus europaeus*. In all cases, the activity was traced to caffeic acid oligomers such as rosmarinic acid and lithospermic acid. Autooxidation of the caffeic acid derivatives to ortho-quinones was postulated to be important for the biological activity.

Rosmarinic acid has also been found to inhibit the C3 and C5 convertase steps in the complement cascade.[15-17] This action may play a role in the anti-inflammatory action of melissa extract, because the action was observed both in vitro and in vivo in rats with oral administration of the compound.

TOXICOLOGY: The antithyroid activity of melissa extract mentioned above is weak enough that it does not present a serious safety concern in patients without Graves' disease. The topical use for herpes cold sores has not produced any reports of dermal toxicity. Melissa extract was not found to be genotoxic in a screen of several medicinal plants.[18]

SUMMARY: Lemon balm may be of use as a topical agent for cold sores, and it appears to have potential use as a mild sedative. No side effects have been reported.

Lemon balm is approved in the German Commission E monographs for nervous sleeping disorders and functional GI complaints. It is also monographed in ESCOP F-2, WHO vol. 2, and BHP vol. 2.[19] An AHP monograph is in progress.

PATIENT INFORMATION – Lemon Balm

Uses: Lemon balm has been used for Graves' disease as a sedative, antispasmodic, and a topical agent for cold sores.

Side Effects: No side effects have been reported.

[1] Adzet T, et al. Content and composition of *M. officinalis* oil in relation to leaf position and harvest time. *Planta Med* 1992;58:562.

[2] Tittel G, et al. über die chemische zusammensetzung von melissenölen. *Planta Med* 1982;46:91.

[3] Hener U, et al. Evaluation of authenticity of balm oil (*Melissa officinalis* L. . *Pharmazie* 1995;50(1):60.

[4] Mulkens A, et al. [Flavonoids of the leaves of *Melissa officinalis* L. (Lamiaceae)]. *Pharma Acta Helv* 1987:62(1):19.

[5] Brieskorn CH, et al. Further triterpenes from *Melissa officinalis* L. *Arch Pharm (Weinheim)* 1974;307(8):603.

[6] Agata I, et al. Meltric acids A and B, new trimeric caffeic acid derivatives from *Melissa officinalis*. *Chem Pharm Bull* 1993;41(9):1608.

[7] Soulimani R, et al. Neurotropic action of the hydroalcoholic extract of *Melissa officinalis* in the mouse. *Planta Med* 1991;57(2):105.

[8] Kucera LS, et al. Antiviral substances in plants of the mint family (Labiatae. Tannin of *Melissa officinalis* . *Proc Soc Exp Biol Med* 1967;124(3):865.

[9] Herrmann EC Jr, et al. Antiviral substances in plants of the mint family (Labiatae). II. Nontannin polyphenol of *Melissa officinalis*. *Proc Soc Exp Biol Med* 1967;124(3):869.

[10] Wöbling RH, et al. Local therapy of Herpes simplex with dried extract from *Melissa officinalis*. *Phytomedicine* 1994;125.

[11] Auf'mkolk M, et al. Inhibition by certain plant extracts of the binding and adenylate cyclas stimulatory effect of bovine thyrotropin in human thyroid membranes. *Endocrinology* 1984;115(2):527.

[12] Auf'mkolk M, et al. Extracts and auto-oxidized constituents of certain plants inhibit the receptor-binding and biological activity of Graves' immunoglobulins. *Endocrinology* 1985;116(5):1687.

[13] Auf'mkolk M, et al. The active principles of plant extracts with antithyrotropic activity: Oxidation products of derivatives of 3,4-dihydroxycinnamic acid. *Endocrinology* 1985;116(5):1677.

[14] Sourgens H, et al. Antihormonal effects of plant extracts. TSH- and prolactin-suppressing properties of Lithospermum officinale and other plants. *Planta Med* 1982;45:78.

[15] Rampart M, et al. Complement-dependent stimulation of prostacyclin biosynthesis: Inhibition by rosmarinic acid. *Biochem Pharmacol* 1986;35(8):1397.

[16] Engelberger W, et al. Rosmarinic acid: A new inhibitor of complement C3-convertase with antiinflammatory activity. *Int J Immunopharmacol* 1988;10(6):729.

[17] Peake PW, et al. The inhibitory effect of rosmarinic acid on complement involves the C5 convertase. *Int J Immunopharmacol* 1991;13(7):853.

[18] Ramos Ruiz A, et al. Screening of medicinal plants for induction of somatic segregation activity in *Aspergillus nidulans*. *J Ethnopharmacol* 1996;52(3):123.

[19] Barrett, M. CRN: Reference on Evaluating Botanicals. Washington, D.C.: Council for Responsible Nutrition, 1998.

Lemon Verbena

SCIENTIFIC NAME(S): *Aloysia triphylla* (L'Her.) Britt. Formerly described as *A. citriodora* (Cav.) Ort., *Verbena citriodora* Cav., *V. triphylla*, *Lippia citriodora* (Ort.) HBK Family: Verbenaceae

COMMON NAME(S): Lemon verbena, louisa

BOTANY: Lemon verbena is an aromatic plant native to Argentina and Chile.[1] It is a deciduous plant that is commonly cultivated in the tropics and Europe. It is grown commercially in France and North Africa. The plant grows to 3 meters and is characterized by the presence of fragrant, lemon-scented narrow leaves. It bears small white flowers in terminal panicles.[1]

HISTORY: Lemon verbena has been used as a medicinal plant for centuries, having been touted for use as an antispasmodic, antipyretic, carminative, sedative and stomachic. The leaves and flowering tops are used in teas and as beverage flavors. Its fragrance is used in perfumery. Although the plant is grown as an ornamental, it requires shelter during cold periods.[1]

CHEMISTRY: An essential oil, which is present in small quantities (0.42% to 0.65%), is extracted from the leaves by steam distillation.[2] Known as oil of verbena, it contains a variety of fragrant compounds including citral (35%), methyl heptenone, carvone, l-limonene, dipentene and geraniol.[1,2] Because the pure oil can be expensive, it is sometimes adulterated with distillates from other plants.

PHARMACOLOGY: The essential oil is said to be acaricidal and bactericidal. An alcoholic leaf extract has been reported to have antibiotic activity in vitro against *Escherichia coli*, *Mycobacterium tuberculosis* and *Staphylococcus aureus*, although it had no antimalarial activity. A 2% emulsion of the oil has been reported to kill mites and aphids.[2]

A component of the related plant, *Verbena officinalis*, has been reported by Chinese investigators to have antitussive activity.[3]

TOXICOLOGY: Lemon verbena generally is recognized as safe for human consumption and for use as a flavor in alcoholic beverages. Contact hypersensitivity has been associated with members of the related *Verbena genus*.

SUMMARY: Lemon verbena is a fragrant plant that finds use in the preparation of teas. Extracts of the plant are used in fragrances and to flavor beverages. No significant toxicity has been associated with the plant.

PATIENT INFORMATION – Lemon Verbena

Uses: Lemon verbena is used in teas, flavorings, fragrances, antispasmodics, carminatives, sedatives and stomachics.

Side Effects: Some individuals may experience contact hypersensitivity.

---

[1] Simon JE, et al. *Herbs: an indexed bibliography*, 1971-1980. Hamden, CT: The Shoe String Press, 1984.
[2] Duke JA. *Handbook of Medicinal Herbs*. Boca Raton, FL: CRC Press, 1985.
[3] Gui CH. Antitussive constituents of *Verbena officinalis*. *Chung Yao Tung Pao* 1985;10:35.

Lemongrass

SCIENTIFIC NAME(S): *Cymbopogon citratus* (DC.) Stapf. *Andropogon citratus* DC, *A. schoenathus. C. flexuosus, A. flexuosus.* Family: Poaceae (Gramineae), Grass.

COMMON NAME(S): Lemongrass. *C. citratus,* is known as Guatemala, West Indian, or Madagascar lemongrass; *C. flexuosus* is known as cochin lemongrass, British Indian lemongrass, East Indian lemongrass, or French Indian verbena.

BOTANY: *Cymbopogon* is a tall, aromatic perennial grass that is native to tropical Asia. *C. citratus* is cultivated in the West Indies, Central and South America, and tropical regions. The linear leaves can grow up to 90 cm in height and 5 mm wide. Freshly cut and partially dried leaves are used medicinally and are the source of the essential oil.[1-2]

HISTORY: Lemongrass is one of the most widely used traditional plants in South American folk medicine. It is used as an antispasmodic, analgesic, for the management of nervous and GI disorders, to treat fevers, and as an antiemetic. In India, it is commonly used as an antitussive, antirheumatic, and antiseptic. It is usually taken by ingesting an infusion made by pouring boiling water on fresh or dried leaves. Lemongrass is an important part of Southeast Asian cuisine, especially in Thai food and has been used in flavoring. In Chinese medicine, lemongrass is used in the treatment for headaches, stomachaches, abdominal pain, and rheumatic pain.[3]

CHEMISTRY: Fresh *C. citratus* grass contains about 0.4% of volatile oil.[3] The oil contains 65% to 85% of citral (a mixture of 2 geometric isomers, geraniol and neral). Citral is used as a flavoring to fortify lemon oil and in perfumes and colognes for its lemon scent.[4] Accumulation of citral in certain lemongrass leaf structures has been studied.[5] The yield of essential oil and citral content in the plant has been evaluated.[6] Certain citral isolated from *C. citratus* from Laguna was found to be of good quality with 93.7% purity.[7] GC analysis in 1 report finds geraniol and neral, along with related geraniol, geranic acid, and nerolic acid.[8]

Other compounds found in the oil include myrcene (12% to 25%), diterpenes, methylheptenone, citronellol, linalol, farnesol, other alcohols, aldehydes, linalool, terpineol, and more than a dozen other minor fragrant components.[1,4,9-11] Reports concerning chemical analyses of *C. citratus* specific to country of origin are available, finding some similarities to the above components. Philippine lemongrass has been found to contain alpha and beta pinene, limonene, phellandrene, and others,[12,13] findings of 21 components such as anisaldehyde, cinnamaldehyde, catechol, and hydroquinone from certain fractions of this species from Bangladesh,[14] and various constituents from this species and others (including *C. winterianus, C. jwarancusa*) from China[15] and Morocco.[16]

Other species' chemical components have been reported. *C. flexuosus* grass contains ≈ 0.5% volatile oil, which in some strains contains up to 85% citral. However, many strains have a higher concentration of geraniol (50%) with citral (10% to 20%) and methyl eugenol as minor components. Yet another type of East Indian lemongrass is reported to contain no citral but up to 30% borneol.[1,3] In 1 report analyzing essential oil samples, *C. jwarancusa* contains 70% piperitone; *C. distans,* 40% piperitone; *C. matrini,* geranol, and geranyl acetate; *C. tortius,* Me eugenol; *C. caesius,* 30% carvone.[15]

Nonvolatile components of *C. citratus* consist of luteolins, homo-orientin, chlorogenic acid, caffeic acid, P-coumaric acid, fructose, sucrose, octacosanol, and others.[17] Flavonoids luteolin and 6-C-glucoside have also been isolated.[18] One study reports high concentrations of cobalt.[19]

PHARMACOLOGY: Lemongrass has been widely used in South American traditional medicine. A report of Guatemalan use lists lemongrass as a popular medicinal plant.[20] Brazilian folk medicine uses the plant for nervous conditions or GI disturbances.[21] Traditional Indian medicine employs lemongrass for fever, infection, and sedation.[1] Other uses include as an astringent, fragrance in beauty products, food flavoring, and treatment for skin conditions, muscle pain, infections, fever, colitis, and indigestion.[1-2] However, effectiveness of lemongrass has not been sufficiently evaluated to help substantiate these claims.

The general lack of pharmacologic activity of oral doses of lemongrass have been substantiated in humans. Volunteers who took a single oral dose or 2 weeks of oral intake of the tea showed no changes in any hematologic or urinary tests, or in EEG or ECG tracings. Some subjects showed mild elevations of direct bilirubin and amylase levels, but none were accompanied by any clinical manifestations. The hypnotic effect was further investigated in 50 volunteers who ingested a tea prepared under double-blind conditions 3 nights 3 to 5 days apart. The parameters tested (sleep induction time, sleep quality, dream recall, reawakening) did not show any effect of lemongrass compared with placebo. Furthermore, 18 patients with documented anxiety traits showed no differences in their anxiety scores after taking a single 150 ml dose of lemongrass tea under double-blind conditions.[21]

A peripheral, dose-dependent, analgesic effect was found in studies including rat paw testing, which may explain certain "sedative" folk uses of the plant.[22] Similarly, when rats were fed the 20% decoction, rat paw edema was inhibited by 19% vs control; however, indomethacin inhibited the edema by 59%. The study concluded that the antirheumatic effects of lemongrass after oral administration were too weak to be considered of any clinical usefulness.[23]

Antimicrobial effects: Several reports demonstrating the antimicrobial effects of lemongrass are available discussing its activity against animal and plant pathogens, gram-positive and gram-negative bacteria, and fungus.[24] Constituents geraniol (alpha-citral) and neral (beta-citral) were found to possess these antibacterial effects in 1 report.[25] The citral content in the oil greatly affected the antibacterial actions as shown in another report testing fresh oil against oils up to 12 years old.[26] Some organisms inhibited by lemongrass oil include *Acinetobacter baumanii, Aeromonas veronii, Candida albicans, Enterococcus faecalis, Escherichia coli, Klebsiella pneumoniae, Pseudomonas aeruginosa, Salmonella enterica, Serratia marcescens, Staphlycoccus aureus,* and *Proteus mirabilis.*[27,28] One mechanism of action explained in a report evaluating lemongrass oil and its antibacterial effects on *E. coli* determined that the oil elicits morphological alterations on the host, including filamentation, inhibition of septum formation, production of bulging, abnormal shaping of cells, as well as cell lysis, all of which deter bacterial growth.[29]

Antifungal effects: Antifungal effects of the oil have been studied as well, and include actions against such dermatophytes as *Trichophyton mentagrophytes, T. rubrum, Epidermophyton floccosum,* and *Microsporum gypseum.*[30] In a 13-oil study, lemongrass oil was found to be among the most active against human dermatophyte strains, inhibiting 80% of strains, with inhibition zones greater than 10 mm in diameter.[31] Other studies report lemongrass actions against keratinophilic fungi,[32] ringworm fungi,[33,34] and food storage fungi.[35] Lemongrass oil is discussed as being effective as an herbicide[36] and an insecticide[37,38] because of these naturally occurring antimicrobial effects.

Anticarcinogenic effects: There are also numerous reports demonstrating the anticarcinogenic (or antitumor) properties of lemongrass. Edible plants (including lemongrass), in general, are discussed.[39,40] Active compounds in lemongrass include d-limonene and geraniol.[41] Essential oil from *C. citratus* leaves and constituent citral were both proven to be toxic against P388 mouse leukemia cells.[42,43] Another report finds the plant extract to possess antimutagenic properties against certain *S. typimurium* strains.[44] Lemongrass extract also inhibits DNA adduct formation in rat colon.[45] Another report on aflatoxin-albumin adduct formation influenced by the plant finds no alteration in this area.[46] A Japanese patent application discusses how constituent geraniol markedly inhibits Epstein-Barr virus.[47] Oil of *C. citrans* possessed high antiradical power, as well as some antioxidant activity.[48]

Other effects: Other reported effects of lemongrass include a 1975 report on fever reduction,[49] dose-related hypotensive effects in rats, weak diuretic actions,[50] and myrcene's ability to induce antinociception in mice.[51]

TOXICOLOGY: Lemongrass is "Generally Recognized As Safe" (GRAS) in the US.

Topical application of lemongrass has rarely led to an allergic reaction. Two cases of toxic alveolitis have been reported from inhalation of the oil.[2] No laboratory test abnormalities were noted after ingestion of lemongrass tea. Oral doses equivalent to 208 times the normal human dose did not potentiate the sleep-time of sodium pentobarbital in mice.[22,52] An infusion of lemongrass given orally to rats for 2 months in doses up to 20 times the corresponding human dose did not induce any toxic effects. The tea did not affect male rats in any way. Similarly, female rats showed no abnormality in the estrus cycle, nor did doses interfere with fertility, pregnancy, or the development of the offspring. No external malformations were noted in the pups. The authors concluded that the lack of toxicity and pharmacologic activity made lemongrass a valuable placebo.[53] Achara, an herbal tea made from dried lemongrass leaves, was found to be atoxic.[54] Substance beta-myrcene was found not to be genotoxic in another report.[55] Aqueous extracts of the plant used as an insecticide led to some mitotic abnormalities in *Allium cepa* root tips grown in these extracts, which may have implications in humans.[56] In addition, constituent beta-myrcene was found in reports to interfere with cytochrome P450 liver enzymes, suggesting possible toxicities.[57-59]

Lemongrass should not be used in pregnancy because of uterine and menstrual flow stimulation.[60]

SUMMARY: Lemongrass is widely used in South American folk medicine for analgesia, nervousness, and GI disorders. In India, it is used for inflammation and as an antiseptic. Lemongrass is also used as a food flavoring and fragrance in beauty products. The plant possesses marked antibacterial and antifungal effects, as well as anticarcinogenic actions. Lemongrass is generally considered to be of low toxic potential, but may alter certain liver enzymes.

PATIENT INFORMATION – Lemongrass

Uses: Lemongrass is used as a fragrance and flavoring, and in folk medicine as an antispasmodic, hypotensive, anticonvulsant, analgesic, antiemetic, antitussive, antirheumatic, antiseptic, and treatment for nervous and GI disorders and fevers. Because there is little human evidence to support its effectiveness in an oral dosage, lemongrass may be considered a placebo.

Side Effects: Lemongrass is considered to be of low toxicity. Constituent beta-myrcene was found to interfere with cytochrome P450 liver enzymes, suggesting possible toxicities.

---

[1] Lawless, J. *The Illustrated Encyclopedia of Essential Oils.* Element Books, Inc. Rockport, MA 1995;132.

[2] Blumenthal, M, ed. *The Complete German Commission E Monographs.* American Botanical Council, Austin TX; 1998;341-42.

[3] Leung A. *Encyclopedia of Common Natural Ingredients Used in Food, Drugs, and Cosmetics.* New York, NY: J Wiley and Sons, 1980.

[4] Windholz M, ed. *The Merck Index,* 10th ed. Rahway, NJ: Merck and Co, 1983.

[5] Lewinsohn E, et al. Histochemical localization of citral accumulation in lemongrass leaves (*Cymbopogon citratus* (DC.) Stapf., Poaceae). *Ann Bot* (London) 1998;81(1):35-39.

[6] Ming L, et al. Yield of essential oil of citral content in different parts of lemongrass leaves (*Cymbopogon citratus* (DC.) Stapf.) Poaceae. *Acta Hortic* 1996;426 (International Symposium on Medicinal and Aromatic Plants), 555-59.

[7] Torres R. Citral from *Cymbopogon citratus* (DC) Stapf (lemongrass) oil. *Philipp J Sci* 1993;122(3):269-87.

[8] Sargenti S, et al. Supercritical fluid extraction of *Cymbopogon citratus.* *Chromatographia* 1997;46(5/6):285-90.

[9] Kasumov F, et al. Components of the essential oil of *Cymbopogon citratus* Stapf. *Khim Pnr Soedin* 1983;(1):108-09.

[10] Ansan S, et al. Thin layer gas liquid chromatographic analysis of lemongrass oil. *Indian J Nat Prod* 1986;2(2):3-7.

[11] Viturro C, et al. Composition of the essential oil of *Cymbopogon citratus.* *An Asoc Quim Argent* 1998;86(1-2):45-48.

[12] Torres R, et al. Extraction and characterization of the essential oil of Philippine *Cymbopogon citratus* (DC) Stapf. *Philipp J Sci* 1994;123(1):51-63.

[13] Torres R, et al. Chemical composition of the essential oil of Philippine *Cymbopogon citratus* (DC) Stapf. *Philipp J Sci* 1996;125(2):147-56.

[14] Faruq M, et al. TLC technique in the component characterization and quality determination of Bangladeshi lemongrass oil (*Cymbopogon citratus* Stapf.) *Bangladesh J Sci Ind Res* 1994;29(2):27-38.

[15] Liu C, et al. Chemical studies of the essential oils of *Cymbopogon* genus. *Huaxue Xuebao* 1981;(Zengikan):241-47.

[16] Idrissi A, et al. Composition of the essential oil of lemongrass (*Cymbopogon citratus* DC. Stapf) grown in Morocco. *Plant Med Phytothe* r 1993;26(4):274-77.

[17] De Matouschek. Phytochemical studies on non-volatile constituents of *Cymbopogon citratus* (DC.) Stapf grown in Morocco. *Pharm Acta Helv* 1991;66(9-10):242-45.

[18] Guanasingh C, et al. Flavonoids of *Cymbopogon citratus.* *Indian J Pharm Sci* 1981;43(3):115.

[19] Ahmed I. Multielemental analysis of lemongrass by inductively coupled plasma spectrometry. *J Chem Soc Pak* 1989;11(3):251-55.

[20] Giron L, et al. Ethnobotanical survey of the medicinal flora used by the Caribs of Guatemala. *J Ethnopharmacol* 1991;34(2-3):173-87.

[21] Leite J, et al. Pharmacology of lemongrass (*Cymbopogon citratus* Stapf.) III. Assessment of eventual toxic, hypnotic and anxiolytic effects on humans. *J Ethnopharmacol* 1986;17(1):75-83.

[22] Lorenzetti B, et al. Myrcene mimics the peripheral analgesic activity of lemongrass tea. *J Ethnopharmacol* 1991;34(1):43-48.

[23] Carbajal D, et al. Pharmacological study of *Cymbopogon citratus* leaves. *J Ethnopharmacol* 1989;25:103-07.

[24] Baratta M, et al. Antimicrobial and antioxidant properties of some commercial essential oils. *Flavour Fragrance J* 1998;13(4):235-44.

[25] Onawunmi G, et al. Antibacterial constituents in the essential oil of *Cymbopogon citratus* (DC.) Stapf. *J Ethnopharmacol* 1984;12(3):279-86.

[26] Syed M, et al. Essential oils of the family *Gramineae* with antibacterial activity. Part 2. The antibacterial activity of a local variety of *Cymbopogon citratus* oil and its dependence on the duration of storage. *Pak J Sci Ind Res* 1995;38(3/4):146-48.

[27] Hammer K, et al. Antimicrobial activity of essential oils and other plant extracts. *J Appl Microbiol* 1999;86(6):985-90.

[28] Chalcat J, et al. Correlation between chemical composition and antimicrobial activity. VI. Activity of some African essential oils. *J Essent Oil Res* 1997;9(1):67-75.

[29] Ogunlana E, et al. Effects of lemongrass oil on the morphological characteristics and peptidoglycan synthesis of *Escherichia coli* cells. *Microbios* 1987;50(202):43-59.

[30] Wannissorn B, et al. Antifungal activity of lemon grass and lemon grass oil cream. *Phytother Res* 1996;10(7):551-54.

[31] Lima E, et al. In vitro antifungal activity of essential oils obtained from official plants against dermatophytes. *Mycoses* 1993;36(9-10):333-36.

[32] Qureshi S, et al. In vitro evaluation of inhibitory nature of extracts of 18–plant species of Chhindwara against 3-keratinophilic fungi. *Hindustan Antibiot Bull* 1997;39(1-4):56-60.

[33] Yadav P, et al. Screening some essential oils against ringworm fungi. *Indian J Pharm Sci* 1994;56(6):227-30.

[34] Kishore N, et al. Fungitoxicity of essential oils against dermatophytes. *Mycoses* 1993;36(5-6):211-15.

[35] Mishra A, et al. Evaluation of some essential oils for their toxicity against fungi causing deterioration of stored food commodities. *Appl Environ Microbiol* 1994;60(4):1101-5.

[36] Dudai N, et al. Essential oils as allochemicals and their potential use as bioherbicides. *J Chem Ecol* 1999;25(5):1079-89.

[37] Ahmad F, et al. Repellancy of essential oils against the domiciliary cockroach, *Periplanta americana. Insect Sci Its Appl* 1995;16(3/4):391-93.

[38] Gilbert B, et al. Activities of the Pharmaceutical Technology Institute of the Oswaldo Cruz Foundation with medicinal, insecticidal and insect repellant plants. *An Acad Bras Cienc* 1999;71(2):265-71.

[39] Murakami A, et al. Possible anti-tumor promoting properties of Thai edible plants and some of their active constituents. *Fragrance J* 1994;22(7):71-79.

[40] Murakami A, et al. Cancer chemopreventive potentials of edible Thai plants and some of their active constituents. *Mem Sch Biol-Oriented Sci Technol Kinki Univ.* 1997;1-23.

[41] Zheng G, et al. Potential anticarcinogenic natural products isolated from lemongrass oil and galanga root oil. *J Agric Food Chem* 1993; 41(2):153-56.

42 Dubey N, et al. Cytotoxicity of the essential oils of *Cymbopogon citratus* and *Ocium gratissimum*. *Indian J Pharm Sci* 1997;59(5):263-64.

43 Dubey N, et al. Citral: a cytotoxic principle isolated from the essential oil of *Cymbopogon citratus* against P388 leukemia cells. *Curr Sci* 1997;73(1):22-24.

44 Vinitketkumnuen U, et al. Antimutagenicity of lemon grass (*Cymbopogon citratus* Stapf) to various known mutagens in salmonella mutation assay. *Mutat Res* 1994;341(1):71-75.

45 Suaeyun R, et al. Inhibitory effects of lemongrass (*Cymbopogon citratus* Stapf) on formation of azoxymethane-induced DNA adducts and abberant crypt foci in the rat colon. *Carcinogenesis* 1997;18(5):949-55.

46 Vinitketkumnuen U, et al. Aflatoxin-albumin adduct formation after single and multiple doses of aflatoxin B(1) in rats treated with Thai medicinal plants. *Mutat Res* 1999;428(1-2):345-51.

47 Nagamine K et al. Tumor promotion-inhibiting compositions and foods. *Jpn Kokai Tokkyo Koho*. 1994 (4pp). App number: JP 93-71649 19930330.

48 Menut C, et al. Aromatic plants of Tropical West Africa. XI. Chemical composition, antioxidant and antiradical properties of the essential oils of three *Cymbopogon* species from Burkina Faso. *J Essent Oil Res* 2000;12(2):207-12.

49 Olaniyi A, et al. Phytochemical investigation of some Nigerian plants used against fevers. II. *Cymbopogon citratus*. *Planta Med* 1975;28(2):186-89.

50 Carbajal D, et al. Pharmacological study of *Cymbopogon citratus* leaves. *J Ethnopharmacol* 1989;25(1):103-07.

51 Rao V, et al. Effect of myrcene on nociception in mice. *J Pharm Pharmacol* 1990;42(12):877-78.

52 Carlini E, et al. Pharmacology of lemongrass (*Cymbopogon citratus* Stapf.). I. Effects of teas prepared from the leaves on laboratory animals. *J Ethnopharmacol* 1986;17:37-64.

53 Souza Formigoni M, et al. Pharmacology of lemongrass (*Cymbopogon citratus* Stapf). II. Effects of daily two month administration in male and female rats and in offspring exposed "in utero." *J Ethnopharmacol* 1986;17:65-74.

54 Orisakwe O, et al. Plasma levels of aluminum after lemon-grass (*Cymbopogon citratus*) ingestion in healthy volunteers. *Asia Pac J Pharmacol* 1998;13(2 and 3):79-82.

55 Zamith H, et al. Absence of genotoxic activity of beta-myrcene in the in vivo cytogenetic bone marow assay. *Braz J Med Biol Res* 1993;26(1):93-98.

56 Williams G, et al. Mitotic effects of the aqueous leaf extract of *Cymbopogon citratus* in *Allium cepa* root tips. *Cytobios* 1996;87(350):161-68.

57 Kauderer B, et al. Evaluation of the mutagenicity of beta-myrcene in mammalian cells in vitro. *Environ Mol Mutagen* 1991;18(1):28-34.

58 De-Oliveira A, et al. In vitro inhibition of CYP2B1 monooxygenase by beta-myrcene and other monoterpenoid compounds. *Toxicol Lett* 1997;92(1):39-46.

59 De-Oliveira A, et al. Induction of liver monooxygenase by beta-myrcene. *Toxicology* 1997;124(2):135-40.

60 McGuffin M, et al. *American Herbal Products Association's Botanical Safety Handbook*. Boca Raton, FL: CRC Press; 1997.

Lentinan

SCIENTIFIC NAME(S): *Lentinula edodes* (Berk.) Pegler, synonymous with Tricholomopsis edodes Sing.

COMMON NAME(S): Shiitake, snake butter, pasania fungus, forest mushroom, hua gu

BOTANY: Lentinan is a polysaccharide derived from the vegetative parts of the edible Japanese Shiitake mushroom. It is the cell wall constituent extracted from the fruiting bodies or mycelium of *L. edodes* (Berk.). The mushroom is synonymous with *Cortinellus edodes* (Berk.) *S. Ito* and *Imai, Armillaria edodes* (Berk.) *Sacc.* and *Cortinellus shiitake* (Takeda) Henn.[1] The light, amber fungi are found on fallen broadleaf trees, such as chestnut, beech or mulberry. They have decurrent, even or ragged gills, a stem, and are covered with delicate, white flocking.[2] Shiitake mushrooms are commonly sold in food markets in the Orient and are now widely available in the United States, Canada and Europe.

HISTORY: Lentinan is a complex polysaccharide that has been found to possess immunostimulating antitumor properties. Lentinan was isolated from edible Shiitake mushrooms that have been used in traditional oriental cooking and herbal medicine. Shiitake has been renowned in Japan and China as both a food and medicine for thousands of years. It is now commonplace throughout the world. Extracts of these mushrooms are now being incorporated into over-the-counter dietary supplements designed to improve the status of the immune system.

CHEMISTRY: Lentinan is found in very low concentrations in fresh Shiitake mushrooms. In one study, 200 kg of fresh mushrooms yielded 31 g of lentinan (0.02%). Lentinan is a water-soluble beta-1,3 glucan polysaccharide characterized by beta-1,6 branched glucan linkages. At least five additional polysaccharides have been isolated from *L. edodes*.[1] Lentinan is a high molecular weight polysaccharide in a triple helix structure, containing only glucose molecules with mostly (1–3)-β-D-Glucan linkages in the regularly branched main chain with two β (1,6)-D-glucopyranoside branchings for every five β-(1,3)-glucopyranoside linear linkages.[2]

PHARMACOLOGY: The **antitumor** activity of lentinan has been recognized for almost 30 years. Because a number of naturally occurring polysaccharides had previously been found to have antitumor activity, lentinan was considered for detailed evaluation. In addition to antitumor activity, lentinan also possesses **immune-regulatory** effects, **anti-viral** activity, **antimicrobial** properties and **cholesterol-lowering** effects. The pharmacology available on lentinan is vast. The following is a brief outline of key aspects.

Antitumor Activity: When administered by intraperitoneal (IP) injection to mice implanted with Sarcoma 180, lentinan showed striking antitumor activity. Ten daily doses as low as 1 mg/kg/dose resulted in tumor growth inhibition of 95% to 100% depending on the strain of mouse tested. Although one other polysaccharide fraction from *L. edodes* inhibited tumor growth, most other fractions were devoid of activity.[1]

In rats with a model of colon cancer, lentinan was found highly effective in extending their lifespan. When treated with five IP injections 2 days apart, (2 mg/kg), 11 of 20 rats were found to be tumor-free at autopsy on day 42 of the study. Furthermore, lentinan significantly increased the lifespan of carcinomatous rats. In the control group, 50% of the rats lived 42 days compared with 70 days in the treated group. Four of 10 treated rats were still alive on day 210 of the study while all of the controls had died by day 70.[3]

Therapeutic effects of lentinan in the GI tract have been noted. A case study reports reduced primary tumor size, in a 63–year-old patient treated with lentinan combination therapy. Metastasis disappeared, and only mild thrombocytopenia occured as a side effect.[4] Lentinan used as an agent for post-operative adjuvant therapy was investigated in GI patients with stages II-IV cancer. Stage IV patients had higher lymphocyte counts than control patients, suggesting lentinan's immuno-potentiating efficacy in advanced GI cancer.[5] Another study reports lifespan prolongation in stomach cancer patients, using lentinan combination therapy.[6] Other successful chemotherapies using lentinan include: CDDP and 5-FU,[7] mitomycin and 5-FU,[3] cisplatin with radiation[8] and interleukin 2.[9] Another study involving gastric cancer describes how lentinan causes marked development of reticular fibers related to anti-tumor effect and enhanced interstitial response.[10] Intracavitary injection of lentinan is a useful treatment for malignant effusions in gastric carcinoma patients.[11] Resistance to lentinan chemoimmunotherapy is also reported.[12]

Lentinan's effects in other cancers have also been reported. In prostatic cancer, lentinan 2 mg weekly in combination with Tegafur was evaluated. A five year average survival rate of treated patients was 43% compared with 29% in the control group.[13] Another report referred to the safety and efficacy of lentinan post-treatment with surgical therapy in 33 breast cancer patients.[14] Lentinan has also been evaluated in cervical cancer patients.[15–17]

Another study has reported effective results for lentinan in metastasis inhibition.[19] In combination therapy with IL-2, lentinan exhibited a synergistic effect against induced fibrosarcoma in mice.[19] The same combination again in mice had similar results against lung metastases.[20]

Survival rates using lentinan therapies have increased. One study reports 129 days vs. 49 days in malignant ascites and pleural effusion patients given lentinan 4 mg/week for 4 weeks.[21] A four-year follow-up survey of stomach cancer patients reports survival at 1, 2 and 3 years, with few reported side effects.[6]

Immune System Effects: Although not directly cytotoxic, beta-1,3 glucan has been shown to enhance natural protective immunity. When administered IP to mice with implanted tumors, lentinan effectively increased the activity of cytotoxic peritoneal exudate cells.[22] Kurokawa, et al draws a similar conclusion when reporting direct action of lentinan on tumor cells in mice by scanning electron microscopy. Lentinan contributes to antitumor immunity enhancement, but not to direct killing activity against tumor cells.[23] Evidence suggests that lentinan preferentially acts on T-cells and may enhance T-helper cell function. Furthermore, lentinan augments natural killer cell activity and activates macrophages.[24] Lentinan also triggers production of interleukin 1 by a direct action on macrophages or indirectly by augmenting colony stimulating factor.[25] Many other studies are available where lentinan is found to improve immune function by stimulating T-cell/killer cell/monocyte production,[5,9,11,26-31] increasing natural cell-mediated cytotoxicity,[32] stimulating production of acute-phase transport proteins,[33] affecting lymphocyte and enzyme concentrations[34] and activating complement.[35]

Anti-viral Activity: Lentinan has antiviral activity and has been found to protect against encephalitis caused by the intranasally infected vesicular stomatitis virus in mice.[36] Lentinan enhances AZT's effects when used in combination against HIV for in vitro studies.[37] Additional discussion of lentinan's mechanism against HIV is reported in an article by the same authors.[38]

Antimicrobial Properties: Tsujinaka, et al report that rabbits with induced septic insult without lentinan treatment had low platelet counts, elevated bilirubin and creatinine. In lentinan-treated septic animals, platelet counts did not decrease, and elevation of plasma bilirubin and creatinine levels were less prominent. Findings suggest a modified septic process by administration of lentinan.[39] Host resistance against microbial infection by lentinan is reviewed in another report by Kaneko, et al.[40]

Cholesterol-Lowering Effects: The compound lentinacin has been shown to reduce cholesterol levels in rats by 25% after 7 days of oral administration in a dose as low as 0.005% of feed intake.[41] Other compounds isolated from Shiitake have also been shown to lower blood cholesterol and lipids as well.[42]

TOXICOLOGY: The Shiitake mushroom is edible and has not been associated with toxicity. In animals, lentinan shows little toxicity. In mice, the LD-50 is greater than 1,500 mg/kg (IP). In a phase I study conducted in 50 patients with advanced cancer, minor side effects were observed in 3 patients; in a study of 185 patients, 17 experienced minor adverse reactions.[3] Animal studies have been remarkable for lack of significant toxicity.[1] Few toxic effects are mentioned in two reports of lentinan use.[43,44]

SUMMARY: Lentinan is a polysaccharide derived from the edible Shiitake mushroom. It is found to have anti-tumor, immune-regulatory, anti-viral, antimicrobial and cholesterol-lowering effects. Studies show little toxicity associated with lentinan's use.

PATIENT INFORMATION – Lentinan

Uses: Lentinan is proving to be a valuable component in cancer and infection treatments. It has also demonstrated cholesterol-lowering and immune-regulatory properties.

Side Effects: Lentinan is derived from the Shiitake mushroom, which is edible and is not generally associated with side effects. Lentinan side effects are rarely reported.

[1] Chihara G, et al. *Cancer Res* 1970;30:2776.
[2] Hobbs C. *Medicinal Mushrooms*, Botanica Press, Santa Cruz, CA. 1995;125.
[3] Jeannin JF, et al. *Int J Immunopharm* 1988;10:855.
[4] Maekawa S, et al. *Gan to Kagaku Ryoho* 1990;17(1):137–40.
[5] Tanabe H, et al. *Nippon Gan Chiryo Gakki Shi* 1990;25(80):1657–67.
[6] Tagachi T. *Cancer Detection & Prevention* 1987;1(Supp):333–49.
[7] Mio H, et al. *Gan To Kagaku Ryoho* 1994;21(4):531–4.
[8] Egawa S, et al. *Nippon Hinyokika Gakki Zasshi* 1989;8(2):249–55.
[9] Suzuki M, et al. *Int J Immunopharm* 1990;12(6):613–23.
[10] Ogawa K, et al. *Gan To Kagaku Ryoho* 1994;21(13):2101–4.
[11] Hazama S, et al. *Gan To Kagaku Ryoho* 1995;22(11):1595–97.
[12] Hamuro J, et al. *British Journal of Cancer* 1996;73(4):465–71.
[13] Tani K, et al. *Hinyokika Kiyo-Acta Urologica Japonica* 1994;40(2):199–23.
[14] Kosaka A, et al. *Gan To Kagaku Ryoho* 1987;14(2):516–22.
[15] Shimizu H, et al. *Nippon Sanka Fujinka Gakkai Zasshi* 1988;40(12):1899–900.
[16] Shimizu Y, et al. *Nippon Sanka Fujinka Gakkai Zasshi* 1988;40(10):1557–8.
[17] Shimizu Y, et al. *Nippon Sanka Fujinka Gakkai Zasshi* 1990;42(1):37–44.
[18] Lapis K, et al. *Archiv Fur Geschwulstforschung* 1990;60(2):97–102.
[19] Hamuro J, et al. *Japanese Journal of Cancer Research* 1994;85(12):1288–97.
[20] Yamasaki K, et al. *Cancer Immunology, Immunotherapy* 1989;29(2):87–92.
[21] Oka M, et al. *Biotherapy* 1992;5(2):107–12.
[22] Hamuro J et al, *Immunology* 1980;39:551.
[23] Kurokawa T, et al. *Nippon Gan Chiryo Gakki Shi* 1990;25(12):2822–7.
[24] Reed FC, et al. *Int J Immunopharm* 1982;4:264.
[25] Hamuro J, Chihara G. *Int J Immunopharm* 1982;4:267.
[26] Hanaue H, et al. *Nippon Gan Chiryo Gakki Shi* 1989;24(8):1566–71.
[27] Hanaue H, et al. *Clinical Therapeutics* 1989;11(5):614–22.
[28] Tani M, et al. *Anticancer Research* 1993;13(5C):1773–6.
[29] Tani M, et al. *Eur J Clin Pharmacol* 1992;42(6):623–7.
[30] Arinaga S, et al. *Int J Immunopharm* 1992;14(4):535–9.
[31] Arinaga S, et al. *Int J Immunopharm* 1992;14(1):43–7.
[32] Peter G, et al. *Immunopharm & Immunotox* 1988;10(2):157–63.
[33] Suga T, et al. *Int J Immunopharm* 1986;8(7):691–9.
[34] Feher J, et al. *Immunopharm & Immunotox* 1989;11(1):55–62.
[35] Takeshita K, et al. *Nippon Geka Gakkai Zasshi* 1991;92(1):5–11.
[36] Chang KSS, *Int J Immunopharm* 1982;4:267.
[37] Tochikura T, et al. *Japanese Journal of Cancer Research* 1987;78(6):583–9.
[38] Yoshida O, et al. *Biochemical Pharmacology* 1988;37(15):2887–91.
[39] Tsujinaka T, et al. *European Surgical Research* 1990;22(6):340–6.
[40] Kaneko Y, et al. *Advances in Experimental Medicine & Biology* 1992;319:201–15.
[41] Chibata I et al, *Experientia* 1969;25:1237.
[42] Hobbs C. *Medicinal Mushrooms*, Botanica Press, Santa Cruz, CA. 1995;p. 133–4.
[43] Chihara G, et al. *Cancer Detection & Prevention* 1987;1:423–43.
[44] Chihara G. *Developments in Biological Standardization* 1992;77:191–7.

Lettuce Opium

SCIENTIFIC NAME(S): Lettuce opium is a product obtained from the milky white sap of *Lactuca virosa* L. (wild lettuce) and *L. sativa* var *capitata* L. (garden lettuce), but related species are sometimes used. Family: Compositae

COMMON NAME(S): Wild lettuce, German lactucarium, garden lettuce, lettuce opium, strong-scented lettuce, green endive, acrid lettuce, greater prickly lettuce.

BOTANY: Widely cultivated, lettuce flowers from July to September. This biennial herb grows to 6 feet. The large leaves can attain lengths of 18 inches. The stalks are rich in a milky-white sap that flows freely when the stems are broken.

HISTORY: Lettuce opium has been used in folk medicine for indications ranging from aiding circulation to treating swollen genitals. In Europe it is used as a substitute for opium in cough mixtures.[1] In homeopathy, a tincture has been used for laryngitis, bronchitis, asthma, cough and infections of the urinary tract.[2] The juice of the stem covering yields a medicinal extract known as *thridace*, the use and effectiveness of which is widely disputed.[3]

Chinese medicine has made wide use of lettuce preparations. The dried juice has been recommended as a topical wound antiseptic and the seeds have been used as a galactogogue (to increase the flow of milk in nursing mothers). It has been claimed the flowers and seeds are effective in reducing fevers.[4] More recently, lettuce opium products have been marketed as legal highs, or narcotic substitutes intended to be smoked alone or in combination with marijuana to enhance potency and flavor.[5] Its analgesic and sedative attributes seem more based on fiction than fact.

CHEMISTRY: Some confusion exists regarding the nomenclature of the products derived from *L. virosa* and related plants. Flowering lettuce plants contain large amounts of a milky-white sap which has a bitter taste and strong opiate-like odor. The juice is collected, and when exposed to air develops a brown color. This brown mass is called *lactucarium*, a mixture of compounds to which the touted narcotic properties of the product have been ascribed. Lactucarium has been reported to contain lactucin (approximately 0.2%), a sesquiterpinoid lactone. Additionally, the mixture contains a volatile oil, caoutchouc, mannitol and lactucerol (taraxasterol) (approximately 50%). Lactucerin, also found in the latex, is the acetyl derivative of taraxasterol, a widely distributed triterpene.[4,6]

Reports that lactucarium contains hyoscyamine have been refuted.[7] A report that *L. virosa* contains N-methyl-beta-phenylethylamine[8] has also been refuted.[5]

PHARMACOLOGY: A variety of legal alternate "hallucinogenic" products containing lettuce opium have been available on the market. Brand names of such products include *Lettucine*, *Black Gold*, *Lettucene*, *Lettuce Hash* and *Lopium*. These products contain a lettuce derivative or lactucarium, which are either smoked in pipes or heated in small bowls, and the vapors generated are inhaled. These extracts are sometimes combined with *Damiana* distillates, African yohimbe bark or catnip distillates. The "hallucinogenic" effect is usually mild and appears to be related to the degree of user expectation. There is no pharmacologic basis for the purported hallucinogenic effects of lettuce opium.

Lettuce leaf cigarettes have been marketed as nicotine-free tobacco substitutes. Support for such alternatives has been variable due to slow acceptance of the unique flavor and the lack of a nicotine-induced kick.

Phytochemical and biological screening of several *Lactuca* species indicates that the genus has no significant antimicrobial activity, slight antitumor activity and can produce gross CNS effects in mice.[9,10] While lactucin and lactucopicrin have been reported to have depressant and sedative activity on the central nervous system, these compounds are chemically unstable and commercial lactucarium contains little, if any, of these.[11] Latex of *L. sativa* has been shown to inhibit the growth of *Candida albicans* in vitro.[12] Extracts of *L. sativa* resulted in hypotension when administered to dogs.[5]

TOXICOLOGY: No reports of significant adverse effects due to smoking lettuce opium have been reported. However, a possible association exists between lettuce ingestion and a localized oral allergic reaction.[13]

SUMMARY: Lettuce opium is an antiquated folk remedy which finds little value in modern medicine. The "hallucinogenic" effect of lettuce opium and other lettuce derivatives has not been substantiated. The effects appear to be more psychological rather than physiological and are proportional to the user's expectations.

PATIENT INFORMATION – Lettuce Opium

Uses: Lettuce opium has been used as topical antiseptic, as folk medicine to ameliorate a variety of conditions, and as a narcotic substitute or enhancer.

Side Effects: Ingestion may be associated with allergic reactions.

---

[1] Lewis WH. *Medical Botany*. New York, NY: J. Wiley and Sons, 1977.

[2] Schauenberg P, Paris F. *Guide to Medicinal Plant* s. New Canaan, CT: Keats Publishing, 1977.

[3] Grieve MA. *Modern Herbal*. New York, NY: Dover Publications, 1971.

[4] Brown JK, Malone MH. Legal highs-constituents, activity, toxicology and herbal folklore. *Pacific Information Service on Street Drugs* 1977;5(21):36

[5] Kinghorn AD, Farnsworth NR. Studies on herbal remedies I: Analysis of herbal smoking preparations alleged to contain lettuce (*Lactuca sativa* L.) and other natural products. *J Pharm Sci* (letter) 1982;71(2):270.

[6] Bachelor FW, Ito S. A revision of the sterochemistry of Lactucin. *Can J Chem* 1973;51:3626.

[7] Willaman JJ, Li HL. *Lloydia* 1970;33:1.

[8] Marquardt P, et al. *Arzneimittelforschung* 1976;26:2001.

[9] Bhakuni DS, et al. Screening of Indian plants for biological activity: Part III. *Indian J Exp Biol* 1971;9:91.

[10] Fong HHS, et al. Biological and phytochemical evaluation of plants. X. Test results from a third two-hundred accessions. *Lloydia* 1972;35(1):35.

[11] Tyler VE. *The New Honest Herbal*. Philadelphia, PA: G.F. Stickley Co., 1987.

[12] Moulin-Traffort J, et al. Antifungal action of latex saps from *Lactuca sativa* L. and *Asclepias curassavica* L. *Mycoses* 1990;33(7-8):383.

[13] Bernton HS. Oral allergy after lettuce ingestion. *JAMA* (letter) 1974;230(4):613.

Levant Berry

SCIENTIFIC NAME(S): *Anamirta cocculus* Wight & Arn. Also described as *A. paniculata, Menispermum cocculus, M. lacunosum, Cocculus suberosus* and *C. lacunosus.* Family: Menispermaceae.

COMMON NAME(S): The levant berry goes by a large number of synonyms including fish killer, fishberry, hockle elderberry, Indian berry, louseberry and poisonberry. The dried fruit is called "cocculus fructus" or "cocculus indicus" in commercial trade.[1]

BOTANY: The levant berry is a climbing woody shrub that is native to India, Burma and other parts of Malaysia. It has wide thick leaves and rootlets that ooze a white milky latex. The fragrant flowers produce U-shaped seeds. The fruit dries to a bitter, nearly black wrinkled shape.[1]

HISTORY: The fruits are gathered from the wild and sun-dried for export. In India, the leaves are inhaled as a snuff to relieve malaria, and the leaf juice is used in combination with other natural products as a vermifuge.[1] Extracts of the plant are applied topically for lice, but the toxic nature of the components (in particular picrotoxin) make this a dangerous use, especially when the skin is abraded or irritated. Although picrotoxin had been considered an official remedy for epilepsy at the turn of the century in the US, it is no longer used for this treatment because of severe toxicity. It had found use as a stimulant for the management of morphine poisoning.[1]

CHEMISTRY: The fruit flesh contains the nontoxic alkaloids menispermine and paramenispermine.[1] The seed, however, contains the bitter, toxic principle picrotoxin (1.5% to 5.0%).[2,3] This compound can be separated into picrotoxinin, an oxygenated sesquiterpene derivative, and picrotin. The tasteless compounds anamirtin and cocculin are also present along with a fixed oil (11% to 24% of the seed).[1] The seed is also rich in fatty acids.

PHARMACOLOGY: Picrotoxin in doses of 0.3 mg to 0.6 mg has been used to manage epilepsy and in slightly higher doses to manage night sweating.[1] Picrotoxin continues to find use in experimental models of central nervous system stimulation, but its use in medicine has largely been abandoned in the US and Europe.

TOXICOLOGY: Picrotoxin stimulates the central nervous system and is a gastrointestinal irritant.[1] High doses can cause salivation, vomiting, purging, rapid shallow respiration, palpitations or heart slowing, stupor, loss of consciousness and death. the lethal dose is approximately 30 mg/kg body weight.

In some societies, ground whole dried fruits have been used to kill birds or dogs and to stupefy fish and game. A seed paste is applied to arrow tips by some jungle tribes.[1]

SUMMARY: The levant berry is not widely used in the US and Europe, but remains a popular folk remedy in Asia and adjacent regions. The berry contains the toxic principle picrotoxin and should not be ingested or applied topically to abraded skin.

PATIENT INFORMATION – Levant Berry

Uses: Levant berry is used to relieve malaria, treat lice, stun or kill fish and game, and manage epilepsy.

Side Effects: Levant berry should not be used on abraded skins or ingested. It is potentially lethal.

---

[1] Morton JF. *Major Medicinal Plants.* Springfield, IL: Charles C. Thomas, 1977.
[2] Evans WC. *Trease and Evans' Pharmacognosy.* 13th ed. London: Balliere Tindall, 1989.
[3] Osol A, Farrar GE Jr, eds. The Dispensatory of the United States of America. 25th ed. Philadelphia: J.B. Lippincott. 1955, 1642.

Licorice

SCIENTIFIC NAME(S): *Glycyrrhiza glabra* L., *G. uralensis*, *G. palidiflora* Family: Leguminosae

COMMON NAME(S): Licorice, Spanish licorice, Russian licorice

BOTANY: *Glycyrrhiza glabra* is a 4- to 5-foot shrub that grows in subtropical climates having rich soil. The name glycyrrhiza is derived from Greek words meaning "sweet roots." It is the roots of the plant that are harvested to produce licorice. Most commercial licorice is extracted from varieties of *G. glabra*. The most common variety, *G. glabra var. typica* (Spanish licorice), is characterized by blue flowers, while the variety *G. glabra var. glandulifera* (Russian licorice) has violet blossoms. Turkey, Greece and Asia Minor supply most commercial licorice.

HISTORY: Therapeutic use of licorice dates back to the Roman empire. Hippocrates and Theophratus extolled its uses, and Pliny the Elder (23 A.D.) recommended it as an expectorant and carminative. Licorice also figures prominently in Chinese herbal medicine as a "drug of first class" — an agent that exerts godly influence on the body and acts to lengthen life. Licorice is used in modern medicinals chiefly as a flavoring agent that masks bitter agents, such as quinine, and in cough and cold preparations for its expectorant activity. Most recently, a sample of historic licorice from 756 A.D. was analyzed and was found to still contain active principles even after 1200 years.[1]

CHEMISTRY: Licorice root contains a variety of chemical agents including ammonia and oleanane triterpenoids. However, it is for the glycoside glycyrrhizin that the root is cultivated. The amount of glycyrrhizin varies from 7% to 10% depending on growing conditions. The root also contains various starches and sugars, among them glucose, mannose and sucrose. Raggi, et al have published an HPLC method to compare the bioavailability of glycyrrhizic acid whether in licorice root or in pure glycyrrhiza extract. These can now be tested in blood, urine and bile.[2]

PHARMACOLOGY: As a result of licorice's extensive folk history for gastric irritation, it has undergone extensive research for use as an **anti-ulcerogenic** agent. These investigations have centered on a semi-synthetic succinic acid ester of 18B glycyrrhetic acid, carbenoxolone. While the specific mechanism of action is unknown, carbenoxolone does not act to enhance mucous secretions, increase the lifespan of gastric epithelial cells, inhibit back diffusion of hydrogen ions induced by bile and possibly inhibit peptic activity.

Controlled trials comparing carbenoxolone with cimetidine indicate it is less effective in treating gastric and duodenal disease. In one study, 78% of patients receiving cimetidine demonstrated ulcer improvement by gastroscopy compared with 52% receiving carbenoxolone. Additionally, those patients receiving carbenoxolone experienced more side effects including edema, hypertension and hypokalemia. These side effects are more pronounced in elderly patients, as well as those with underlying renal, hepatic or cardiovascular disease. A proposed mechanism of action for these side effects involves the action of carbenoxolone on the renin-aldosterone-angiotensin axis. Spironolactone relieves the side effects but also attenuates the therapeutic effects.

Another licorice product tested as an anti-ulcer agent is deglycyrrhizinated licorice (DGL), which consists of licorice that has had virtually all of its glycyrrhizin removed. Several studies have evaluated the efficacy of DGL but all have been inconclusive. While these agents have not shown consistent results, neither do they show the serious side effects exhibited by carbenoxolone.

Another use for glycyrrhizins is in **suppression of scalp sebum secretion.** A 10% glycyrrhizin shampoo prevented sebum secretion for 1 week compared with citric acid shampoo, which delayed oil accumulation by 1 day.

Alcohol extracts of *G. glabra* also have in vitro antibacterial activity and weak in vivo antiviral activity.

Glycyrrhetic acid has shown anti-inflammatory and anti-arthritic activity in animal studies. These actions may be caused by PGE_2 inhibitive qualities demonstrated by several glycyrrhizin analogues.

Prepared Chinese licorice, "Zhigancao," was found to have anti-arrhythmic effects, such as prolonging P-R and Q-T intervals.[3] Japanese researchers Matsumoto, et al, tested to see if increased immune complex levels could be lowered by adding licorice to a person's regimen. This was tested on mice and was found to aid in the clearance of excess immune complexes, which are produced in systemic lupus erythematosus. The study was the first of its kind to work on reducing immune complexes in vivo.[4]

TOXICOLOGY: The toxic manifestations of excess licorice ingestion are well documented. One case documented the ingestion of 30 to 40 g of licorice per day for 9 months as a diet food. The subject became increasingly lethargic, having flaccid weakness and dulled reflexes. She also suffered from hypokalemia and myoglobinuria. Treatment with potassium supplements reversed her symptoms. Excessive licorice intake can result in sodium and fluid retention as well as hypertension and inhibition of the renin-angiotensin system.[5]

After consuming large amounts of licorice, human intoxication caused by aldosterone-like effects was found.[6]

A 70-year-old patient with hypertension and hypokalemia caused by chronic licorice intoxication in excess of around 80 candies (2.5 g each having 0.3 glycyrrhizic acid) per day over the past 4 to 5 years, discontinued use one week before hospital admission. After discontinuing the use of licorice and monitoring a treatment plan including licorice, it was found that the activity of 11–β-hydroxysteroid dehydrogenase was suppressed when the patient had been without licorice, but the 11–β-hydroxysteroid dehydrogenase increased as the levels of urinary glycyrrhetic acid decreased.[7]

Other documented complications include paraparesis, hypertensive encephalopathy and one case of quadriplegia. Products that contain licorice as a flavoring, such as chewing tobacco, have also been implicated in cases of toxicity. Hypersensitivity reactions to glycyrrhiza-containing products have also been noted.

SUMMARY: Licorice is widely used as a candy and flavoring agent. Consumption of 30 to 40 grams per day for extended periods may lead to severe and potentially dangerous electrolyte imbalances. Patients with pre-existing renal, hepatic or cardiovascular diseases should be warned of potential toxicities associated with excessive consumption. Also, the retention of sodium and fluids, as well as human intoxications are relevant in terms of toxicities. A recent animal study indicates that licorice may be useful in treating lupus.

PATIENT INFORMATION – Licorice

Uses: Used historically for gastrointestinal complaints, licorice is used today as a flavoring and in shampoos. It is being investigated as an anti-inflammatory and as a treatment for lupus.

Side Effects: Large amounts of licorice taken daily for a long time can cause a range of side effects from lethargy to quadriplegia (body paralysis). Do not over-consume licorice.

---

[1] Shibata S. *Int J Pharmacog* 1994;32(1):75-89.
[2] Raggi M, et al. *Bollettino Chimico Farmaceutico* 1994;133(12):704-8.
[3] Chen RX, et al. *China Journal of Chinese Materia Medica* 1991;16(10):617-19.
[4] Matsumoto T, et al. *J Ethnopharm* 1996;53:1-4.
[5] Sigurjonsdottir HA, et al. *J Human Hyperten* 1995;9(5):345-48.
[6] Bielenberg J. *Pharmazeutische Zeitung* 1989;134(12):9-12.
[7] Farese RV, et al. *N Engl J Med* 1991;325(10):1223-27.

Life Root

SCIENTIFIC NAME(S): *Senecio aureus* L. Family: Asteraceae (Compositae)

COMMON NAME(S): Life root, golden groundsel, golden senecio, ragwort, false valerian, coughweed, cocashweed, female regulator, grundy-swallow[1-5]

BOTANY: Life root is a perennial herb with a slender, erect stem that bears bright yellow flower heads. It grows to a height of about ≈1.2 meters in swampy thickets and moist ground in the eastern and central U. S. The lower leaves are heart-shaped. The entire dried plant, not only the roots, is used medicinally.[2,3,5]

HISTORY: Do not confuse life root with a variety of other plants that have been ascribed broad healing powers, including the mandrake root and ginseng root. Life root has played an important role in traditional Native American herbal medicine and was used by the Catawba women as a tea to relieve the pain of childbirth as well as to hasten labor.[6] The plant has been used to treat a variety of illnesses, including hemorrhage and colds.[1] Despite concern about its safety, this plant continues to be found in some herbal preparations designed to control irregular menses and other gynecologic disturbances.[7]

CHEMISTRY: The plant contains a number of pyrrolizidine alkaloids including senecionine (≈0.006% in the root), senecifoline, senecine, otosenine, floridanine, florosenine, and other related compounds. An astringent tannin has been reported to be present.[1,2,7] Chemical composition of other various *Senecio* species has been reported.[8,9]

PHARMACOLOGY: Traditional use of the plant includes treatment for amenorrhea, menopause, and leucorrhea.[7] Life root has also been used for its uterine tonic, diuretic, and mild expectorant properties.[7] Although it is widely recognized that this plant can influence the activity of female reproductive organs (hence the name "female regulator"), there is little pharmacologic evidence that this plant has a uterotonic effect or that it can influence hormone levels in women.[2,4,7]

Antimicrobial analyses of related species *S. graveolens* have been performed on the essential oil.[9]

TOXICOLOGY: Pyrrolizidine alkaloids have been associated with the development of hypertensive pulmonary vascular disease. However, of greatest concern appears to be the association of this class of alkaloids with the development of hepatotoxicity and liver cancer.[10] In general, pyrrolizidine alkaloids have been shown to produce toxic necrosis of the liver, particularly in grazing animals that have ingested large amounts of plants containing these compounds. There is strong evidence that such alkaloids are involved in human liver diseases, including primary liver cancer (see monograph on Comfrey).[2,11] The mechanism of pyrrolizidine alkaloids can lead to veno-occlusive disease and liver congestion leading to acute and chronic liver disease. The *Senecio* species are generally most toxic when young, and there is some indication that the combination of alkaloids in *S. aureus* may be at the lower end of the toxicity scale for this genus.[10] However, because of the presence of pyrrolizidine alkaloids, do not recommended this plant for internal use.

Life root is contraindicated during pregnancy and lactation, partially because of its abortifacient and uterine tonic effects. Animal studies confirm transferring of pyrrolizidine alkaloids into the placenta and breast milk.[7]

SUMMARY: Life root has been used in traditional medicine for the management of disorders of the female reproductive tract, but there is little pharmacologic evidence to support these uses. Furthermore, members of the *Senecio* genus contain hepatotoxic alkaloids. Therefore, the ingestion of this plant cannot be recommended for any purpose.

PATIENT INFORMATION – Life Root

Uses: Life root has been used as a traditional medicine to hasten labor and relieve labor pains. It has also been used to treat a wide range of illnesses, from colds to hemorrhage.

Side Effects: Use is not recommended; the plant is toxic and possibly carcinogenic.

---

[1] Duke J. *Handbook of Medicinal Herbs*. Boca Raton, FL: CRC Press, 1985.

[2] Tyler V. *The New Honest Herbal*. Philadelphia, PA: G.F. Stickley Co., 1987.

[3] Dobelis I, ed. *Magic and Medicine of Plants*. Pleasantville, NY: Reader's Digest Association, Inc., 1986.

[4] Meyer J. *The Herbalist*. Hammond, IN: Hammond Book Co., 1934.

[5] http://newcrop.hort.purdue.edu/newcrop/herbhunters/groundsel.html

[6] Lewis W. *Medical Botany*. New York, NY: J. Wiley and Sons, 1977.

[7] Newall, C. et al. *Herbal Medicines*. London: Pharmaceutical Press, 1996;180.

[8] Dooren, B. et al. Composition of essential oils of some *Senecio* species. *Planta Med* 1981;42:385-9.

[9] Perez, C. et al. The essential oil of *Senecio graveolens (Compositae)*: chemical composition and antimicrobial activity tests. *J Ethnopharmacol* 1999; 66(1):91-6.

[10] Spoerke D, Jr. *Herbal Medications*. Santa Barbara, CA: Woodbridge Press Publishing Co., 1980.

[11] Liener I, ed. *Toxic Constituents of Plant Foodstuffs*. New York, NY: Academic Press, 1980.

Linden

SCIENTIFIC NAME(S): Several species of the genus *Tilia* produce flowers that are used in traditional herbal medicine. In large part, flowers derived from *T. cordata* Mill. and *T. platyphyllos* Scop. are selected for the preparation of teas. Family: Tiliaceae

COMMON NAME(S): Linden, European linden, basswood, lime tree, lime flower.

BOTANY: Linden trees can grow to heights approaching 100 feet. They are native throughout Europe but also found in the wild or purposely planted in gardens. Linden tree bark is smooth and gray, and its leaves are heart-shaped. The five petaled, yellow-white flowers are collected after the spring bloom, dried and preserved under low-moisture conditions. These are the parts used for the drug.[1,2]

HISTORY: Since the Middle Ages, the flowers of the linden tree have been used to promote sweating. In addition, the flowers have been used traditionally as a tranquilizer and to treat headaches, indigestion and diarrhea. Infusions of the flowers make a pleasant-tasting tea. Several sources report the lore that linden flowers were once believed to be so effective in treating epilepsy that one could be cured simply by sitting beneath the tree.[3,4] Sugar is obtained from the sap of the tree and the seed oil resembles olive oil.[4] In Greek mythology, "Philyra," a nymph, was transformed into a linden tree after begging the gods not to leave her among mortals.[2]

CHEMISTRY: Quercitin, kaempferol and other related flavonoid compounds are the major components found in linden flowers. These compounds, along with p-coumaric acid, appear to be responsible for the diaphoretic (sweat inducing) effect of the plant. Other constituents include caffeic, chlorogenic and p-coumaric acids and amino acids including alanine, cysteine, cystine and phenylalanine. Also present in the plant are volatile oil components (0.02% to 0.1%) including alkanes and esters, citral, eugenol and limonene. Carbohydrates are also found such as arabinose, galactose, glucose, mannose and xylose. Gum and mucilage polysaccharides (3%) are also seen. Tannins are present as well.[1,2,4,5] The ratio of tannins to mucilage appears to be important in determining the flavor of teas prepared from linden flowers. Those teas with a high (2% or greater) tannin level and low mucilage content produce the more flavorful teas. Flowers from *T. cordata* and *T. platyphyllos* contain relatively more tannin than mucilage.[3]

Traces of benzodiazepine-like compounds have been found in linden.[2]

More than two dozen additional minor compounds have been identified in the wood, flowers and fruits of linden.[1,2,4,5] The fragrant components of the flowers degrade rapidly under conditions of high moisture.

PHARMACOLOGY: The diaphoretic activity of the flowers is caused by quercitin, kaempferol and p-coumaric acid. Where "sweat cures" would be an advantage, linden has been used, mainly for feverish colds and infections.[1] Linden can also reduce nasal congestion and relieve throat irritation and cough.[1,2]

A recent report isolates pharmacologically active benzodiazepine receptor ligands from *Tilia tomentosa*. This may explain the plant's use as an anxiolytic.[6]

Linden is also known to possess sedative effects. These effects were significant upon inhalation of *Tilia* species oil in mice.[7] Other sedative effect therapies include relief of sinus headache and migraines and remedies for insomnia, stress and panic disorders. Linden has been used to treat nervous palpitations and has also lowered high blood pressure brought on by stress and nervous tension.[2,5] Folk medicine has employed linden as an antispasmodic.[2] Animal studies in vitro using rat duodenum has supported this claim.[5] The antispasmodic properties are said to be due to p-coumaric acids and flavonoids present in the plant.[5] Homeopaths use linden for enuresis, incontinence, hemorrhage, prolapsed uterus and epilepsy.[4]

An extract of *Tilia* sp. was found to possess in vitro antibacterial activity against organisms associated with stomatologic infections, and these extracts have been found clinically useful.[8] Lime flower has been reported to have antifungal activity as well.[5]

Linden's emollient quality has been used in lotions for itchy skin.[2] It also has been employed for rheumatism. A recent report discusses *Tilia sylvestris'* anti-inflammatory and wound healing properties.[9]

Other effects of linden include diuretic and astringent,[5] and possibly antidiabetic.[10] *Tilia* has also promoted iron absorption in rats, which may be helpful in iron deficiency anemia.[11]

TOXICOLOGY: There is no evidence to support the belief that old linden flowers may induce narcotic intoxication.[3] Frequent use of linden flower teas has been associated with cardiac damage. This rare event suggests that linden teas should not be ingested by those patients with a history of heart disease.[3-5]

Many sources list few side effects from linden. However, reports do exist on specific toxicology such as: Contact urticaria,[12] allergy from certain *Tilia* species' fruit oils in rats,[13] organochlorine pesticide residues in linden-con-taining beverages[14] and soft wood dust exposure from linden, containing volatile and unsteady substances which are micronucleus-inducing matters in peripheral lymphocytes.[15]

SUMMARY: *Tilia* flowers have been used for the preparation of teas and medicinally to induce sweating. Linden has been used to treat colds, infections, throat irritation and cough. It also possesses sedative effects and can treat palpitations, headaches and insomnia. Its antispasmodic qualities make linden useful in incontinence and hemorrhage as well. The use of linden flowers has not generally been associated with toxicity, although several authors have raised concerns about the potential for cardiotoxicity following long-term ingestion of the tea.

PATIENT INFORMATION – Linden

Uses: Linden has been used to induce sweating for feverish colds and infections and can reduce nasal congestion and relieve throat irritation and cough. It possesses sedative effects and can treat nervous palpitations and high blood pressure. It has also been used in lotions for itchy skin.

Side Effects: Rarely, frequent use of linden flower teas has been associated with cardiac damage.

---

[1] Bisset N. *Herbal Drugs and Phytopharmaceuticals.* Stuttgart, Germany: CRC Press, 1994;496–8.
[2] Chevallier A. *Encyclopedia of Medicinal Plants.* New York: DK Publishing Inc., 1996;275.
[3] Tyler VE. *The New Honest Herbal.* Philadelphia: G.F. Stickley Co., 1987.
[4] Duke JA. *Handbook of Medicinal Herbs.* Boca Raton, FL: CRC Press, 1985.
[5] Newall C, et al. *Herbal Medicine* London, England: Pharmaceutical Press, 1996;181.
[6] Viola H, et al. *J Ethnopharmacol* 1994;44(1):47-53.
[7] Buchbauer G, et al. *Arch Pharm* 1992;325(Apr):247–8.
[8] Sucie G, et al. *Rev Chir [Chir]* 1988;35:191.
[9] Fleischner A. *Cosmetics and Toiletries.* 1985;100(Oct):45–6,48–1,54–55,58.
[10] Ashaeva L, et al. *Farmatsiia* 1985;34(3):57–60.
[11] El-Shobaki F, et al. *Zeitschrift Ernahrungswiss* 1990;29(4):264–9.
[12] Picardo M, et al. *Contact Dermatitis* 1988;19(1):72–3.
[13] Cristescu E, et al. *Farmacia* 1969;17(Sep):531–8.
[14] Fernandez N, et al. *Bull Environ Contam Toxicol* 1993;50(4):479–85.
[15] Jiang Z, et al. *Biomed Environ Sci.* 1994;7(2):150–3.

Lorenzo's Oil

COMMON NAME(S): Erucic acid and oleic acid; Lorenzo's Oil

HISTORY: A widely publicized movie about the use of Lorenzo's oil to treat a devastating neurological syndrome recently catapulted this compound into the public spotlight. The oil has been touted for the treatment of a rare genetic disease known as adrenoleukodystrophy, when it appears in children, and adrenomyeloneuropathy when it takes a more insidious path in adults. This X-linked recessive disorder is characterized by demyelinizaton of cerebral nerves resulting in a variety of neurologic symptoms ranging from peripheral neuropathy to blindness, spastic tetraplegia and death.[1]

The primary metabolic abnormality in this disease is the accumulation of saturated very-long-chain fatty acids, which occurs because of a genetically impaired ability to degrade them by normal oxidation. In the absence of normal cellular oxidation of these fatty acids, saturated very-long-chain fatty acids accumulate and are believed to be responsible for the neurologic symptoms associated with the disorder.

CHEMISTRY: "Lorenzo's oil" is a combination of erucic acid (a 22-carbon monounsaturated fatty acid) and oleic acid (an 18-carbon monounsaturated fatty acid). These generally are combined in an approximate ratio of 1.4 (erucic acid:oleic acid). Derivatives of these fatty acids, including glycerol trioleate and glycerol trierucate, typically have been used for the clinical evaluation of Lorenzo's oil.

PHARMACOLOGY: One theoretical approach, therefore, to the treatment of these diseases is to reduce the level of saturated very-long-chain fatty acids present in the blood and nerves. In vitro, monounsaturated fatty acids have been shown to inhibit the synthesis of saturated very-long-chain fatty acids and to reduce their accumulation in cells obtained from patients affected by adrenoleukodystrophy.[1] Therefore, the saturated very-long-chain fatty acids that are believed to be toxic even at low concentrations appear to be exchanged for nontoxic monounsaturated fatty acids.

Clinical trials with diets enriched with monounsaturated fatty acids, such as oleic acid, have shown a partial reduction in the plasma levels of saturated very-long-chain fatty acids, and peripheral nerve function seems to have improved in some patients with adrenomyeloneuropathy.[2] The addition of erucic acid to oleic acid (the combination used in Lorenzo's oil) was found to have led to complete normalization of plasma levels of very-long-chain fatty acids and promised to represent an even more effective therapy.[3] Preliminary investigations of the effect of the oil mixture in the childhood form of the disease generally found no consistent effect, presumably because the fulminant childhood form did not permit sufficient time for the lipid-modifying effects of therapy to take effect.[1] A case report described a 5-year-old boy who responded to 5 months therapy with the oil mixture[4] as evidenced by an increased ability to swallow and an improvement in cerebral structure; in contrast, another case report from China described the failure of the oil to prevent clinical deterioration, and the child developed progressive visual loss and spastic tetraparesis despite dietary changes, steroid therapy and gammaglobulin treatment.[5]

It was hoped that the mixture would be effective in adults with the more insidious form of the illness. Recently reported, well-designed studies of the oil, however, suggest that treatment with Lorenzo's oil offers little evidence for a halt or remission of the disease. In one study, in which 24 patients were treated for up to 48 months, the plasma levels of very-long-chain fatty acids declined to nearly normal within the first 10 weeks of treatment.[6] Nonetheless, none of the patients improved; in 9 of 14 adult males, there was a functional deterioration. Because of ethical considerations, this was not a placebo controlled study, and it is not clear if treatment may have slowed the progression of the disease, although not resulting in a measurable improvement. In an analogous but larger open trial of 108 patients,[7] treatment with the oil for up to 1 year found no improvement in nerve transmission as determined by assessment of visual evoked potentials; there was no correlation between the plasma levels of very-long-chain fatty acids and the rate of deterioration of visual function.

TOXICOLOGY: Thrombocytopenia has been reported following treatment with Lorenzo's oil.[8] In the study by Aubourg et al,[6] the platelet count declined in 23 of 24 patients, but this was not correlated with plasma levels of erucic acid or other metabolites. None of the patients had abnormal bleeding or hematoma. Some of the patients had asymptomatic neutropenia. Dietary supplements of safflower and fish oils were given to the patients during this study, and while a 30% decrease in plasma docosahexaenoic acid levels occurred in all patients, none reported symptoms of essential fatty acid deficiency.

SUMMARY: Lorenzo's oil represents a combination of oleic and erucic acids, which are long-chained mounsaturated fatty acids. The use of this preparation in adrenomyeloneuropathy, a genetically transmitted disease, has resulted in generally poor effectiveness. While the use of this combination appears logically based on the pharmacology of the genetic defect, clinical studies to date have not shown a valid clinical effect.

PATIENT INFORMATION – Lorenzo's Oil

Uses: Lorenzo's oil has been used to treat certain rare diseases, without verified success.

Side Effects: Thrombocytopenia has been reported following treatment.

---

[1] Rizzo WB. Lorenzo's oil: Hope and disappointment. *N Engl J Med* 1993;329:801.

[2] Moser HW, Moser AB, Smith KD, et al. Adrenoleukodystrophy: phenotypic variability and implications for therapy. *J Inherit Metab Dis* 1992;15:645.

[3] Rizzo WB, Leshner RT, Odone A, et al. Dietary erucic acid therapy for X-linked adrenoleukodystrophy. *Neurology* 1989;39:1415.

[4] Maeda K, Suzuki Y, Yajima S, et al. Improvement in clinical and MRI findings in a boy with adrenoleukodystrophy by dietary erucic acid therapy. *Brain Dev* 1992;14:409.

[5] Wong V. Adrenoleukodystrophy in a Chinese boy. *Brain Dev* 1992;14:276.

[6] Aubourg P, Adamsbaum C, Lavallard-Rousseau M-C, et al. A two-year trial of oleic and erucic acids ("Lorenzo's oil") as treatment for adrenomyeloneuropathy. *N Engl J Med* 1993;329:745.

[7] Kaplan PW, Tusa RJ, Shankroff J, et al. Visual evoked potentials in adrenoleukodystrophy: a trial with glycerol trioleate and Lorenzo's oil. *Ann Neurol* 1993;34:169.

[8] Zinkham WH, Kickler T, Borel J, et al. Lorenzo's oil and thrombocytopenia in patients with adrenoleukodystrophy. *N Engl J Med* 1993;328:1126.

Lovage

SCIENTIFIC NAME(S): *Levisticum officinale* Koch. syn. *Angelica levisticum* Baillon. Also referred to as *Hipposelinum levisticum* Britt. and Rose in older texts. Family: Umbelliferae

COMMON NAME(S): Lovage, maggi plant, smellage

BOTANY: Lovage is an aromatic umbelliferous perennial that is similar in appearance to angelica. It carries yellow-green flowers arranged in dense clusters, which bloom from July to August on top of the thick, hollow stems. The plants grow up to 2 meters high. Its leaves are divided by sharply toothed leaflets. Its characteristic, strongly aromatic odor resembles celery. It tastes "spicy-sweet" and slightly bitter.[1,2] Lovage is native to Europe, but is found throughout the northeastern US and Canada. This plant should not be confused with *Oenanthe cocata* L. known commonly as water lovage and *O. aquatica* (L.) Lam. (water fennel), toxic members of the family Apiaceae.

HISTORY: Lovage has been used in folk medicine for > 500 years, primarily for its GI effects. It has a reputation for use as a carminative and antiflatulent, but it has also been used as a diuretic and for the management of sore throats and topical boils. It has been used as a breath lozenge, a skin wash and a lotion. The name "lovage" is from the Latin word meaning "from liguria" because, at one time, the herb flourished in this region. Translated to English, it evolved into "love parsley." Misled by its descriptive name, lovage has been included in numerous otc "love tonics."[2] Today it is a common ingredient in commercial herbal teas. Extracts of lovage are used as flavorings for liqueurs, spice extracts and bitter spirits and fragrances for cosmetics. Cooked leaves and roots have been eaten.

CHEMISTRY: Lovage contains approximately 2% of a volatile oil responsible for its characteristic flavor and odor. This oil is composed primarily (70%) of phthalide lactones, (eg, 3–butylphthalide [32%], cis- and trans-butyldenephthalide, cis- and trans-ligustilide [24%], senkyunolide and angeolide). In addition, lesser amounts of compounds such as terpenoids, volatile acids and furocoumarins contribute to the flavor of the extract. Other compounds found are camphene, bergapten, psoralen and caffeic, benzoic and other volatile acids.[1] Several of the compounds identified in lovage have also been found in celery (see monograph), another member of Umbelliferae. HPLC analysis has been performed to determine glycoside content in lovage.[3] Other reports discuss isolation and identification of phthalides from the roots of the plant by chromatographic and spectrometric methods.[4,5] Chemial composition of lovage oil has been reported.[6]

PHARMACOLOGY: Although teas of this plant have been used primarily for their GI effects, there is little documentation for these indications. In general, many volatile oils, including lovage, induce GI hyperemia resulting in a carminative effect; other oils have also been shown to reduce gas within the GI tract. Lovage extracts probably exert their GI effects through common mechanisms, increasing saliva and gastric juice production by their aroma and mildly bitter taste. Lovage is also used to dissolve phlegm in the respiratory tract. Two constituents of lovage, butylphthalide and ligustilide, have been shown to have spasmolytic action.[1] The phthalides have been reported to be sedative in mice, and the furocoumarins have been associated with a phototoxic reaction following ingestion or contact. Following parenteral administration, extracts of lovage were shown to exert a diuretic effect in rabbits.[7] This effect is presumed to be caused by a mild irritation of the renal tubules by the volatile oil.[7] Lovage has been indicated for pedal edema in humans.[1]

TOXICOLOGY: Furocoumarins in plants of the Umbelliferae family may cause photosensitivity resulting in dermatitis.

SUMMARY: Lovage is a fragrant plant that has been used in herbal medicine for centuries. Although there is only limited evidence to support many of its traditional claims the plant contains a volatile oil that most likely contributes to its carminative and diuretic effects. Photosensitivity has been reported with the harvesting of the plant, but not with its therapeutic use.

PATIENT INFORMATION – Lovage

Uses: Lovage has been used historically as an antiflatulent and diuretic. Its extracts are used in flavorings and fragrances.

Side Effects: Lovage can cause photosensitivity with resultant dermatitis at harvest, but not as a therapeutic agent.

---

[1] Bisset N. *Herbal Drugs and Phytopharmaceuticals*, CRC Press, Stuttgart, Germany. 1994;295–7.
[2] Dobelis I, ed. *Reader's Digest Magic and Medicine of Plants*, Reader's Digest Association, USA 1986;239.
[3] Cisowski W. *Acta Poloniae Pharmaceutica* 1988;45(5):441–4.

[4] Gijbels M, et al. *Planta Medica* 1980;39(Suppl. 1):41–7.
[5] Gijbels M, et al. *Planta Medica* 1982;44(Apr):207–11.
[6] Lawrence B. *Perfumer & Flavorist* 1990;15(Sep-Oct):57–60.
[7] Tyler VE. *The New Honest Herbal*, G.F. Stickley Co, 1987.
[8] Ashywood-Smith M, et al. *Contact Dermatitis* 1992;26(5):356–7.

Lycopene

SCIENTIFIC NAME(S): Ψ, Ψ-carotene

COMMON NAME(S): Lycopene

BOTANY: Lycopene is a carotenoid, occurring in ripe fruit, especially tomatoes.[1] Other sources include watermelon, grapefruit, and guava.[2]

HISTORY: The tomato (*Lycopersicon esculentum*) continues to be a popular and highly consumed fruit in the US, second in production to potatoes.[3] Epidemiological evidence finds the constituent lycopene to be associated with a reduced risk of certain diseases and cancers.[4]

CHEMISTRY: Lycopene is the most prominent carotenoid in tomatoes, followed by beta-carotene, gamma-carotene, phytoene, and other minor carotenoids.[3] Lycopene is also responsible for the red color of the fruit.[5] The carotenes exert antioxidant activity. Lycopene exhibits "the highest overall single oxygen-quenching carotenoid, double than that of beta-carotene."[2] The isolation and structure of lycopene have been determined.[1]

Lycopene is relatively resistant to heat-induced geometrical isomerization in the processing of tomatoes.[4] Processed tomato products are a better source of lycopene than fresh tomatoes[6] and are more bioavailable as well.[7] In addition, human uptake of lycopene is greater from heat processed tomato juice vs unprocessed.[8] Raw tomatoes contain 3.1 mg lycopene (per 100 g of fruit) compared with tomato paste or sauce, which contains an average of 6.4 mg.[2]

PHARMACOLOGY: Factors affecting uptake and absorption of carotenoids have been reported.[9] Pharmacokinetic parameters of lycopene have been evaluated in mice,[10] rats,[11,12] monkeys,[11] and humans.[13-21]

Cooking releases desirable antioxidants from tomatoes. Absorption of lycopene, which is lipid soluble, is improved in the presence of oil or fat.[22] Lycopene's protective mechanisms include **antioxidant activity, induction of cell-cell communication**, and **growth control**.[18,23]

Lycopene's antioxidant actions are well documented. Its presence as a supplement in liquid form reduces lipid peroxidation in one report. It is also suggested that it may ameliorate the oxidative stress of cigarette smoke.[24] Another study reports that certain concentrations of lycopene (and other antioxidants) may protect against cognitive impairment.[25] In 19 subjects, lycopene supplementation decreased serum lipid peroxidation and low-density lipoprotein (LDL) oxidation, suggesting a decreased risk for coronary heart disease (CHD).[26] Lycopene demonstrated a protective effect against MI in the EURAMIC study, confirming its **beneficial effects on the heart**.[27] Carotenoid mixtures display synergistic activity against oxidative damage, most pronounced with the presence of both lycopene and lutein.[28] This combination was also found to have potent anticarcinogenic activity.[29]

Oxidative stress is recognized as a major contributor to increased cancer risk. Lycopene's ideal absorption from tomato products act as antioxidants and may also play important roles in **cancer prevention**.[30] It achieves high concentrations in testes, adrenal glands, and prostate. The intake of lycopene and decreased cancer risk association have been observed in prostate, pancreas, and stomach cancers.[31-34] Tocopherol exhibited synergistic inhibitory effects against 2 human prostate carcinoma cell proliferation lines.[35] Lycopene may also play a protective role in the early stages of cervical carcinogenesis as seen in a study.[36] Plasma levels of lycopene and other carotenoids were lower in women with cervical intraepithelial neoplasia and cervical cancer, suggesting protection with higher lycopene concentrations.[13]

Reports are available on the international symposium on lycopene and tomato products in disease prevention.[37,38] Reviews describing lycopene and disease prevention can also be referenced.[39-42]

Literature addressing beta-carotene's positive outcomes in skin problems (including cancer, pigment balance, and photodermatoses) is available,[43-46] but lycopene may not share these effects because of its structural configuration. One report finds beta-carotene to be active in wound healing, where lycopene was inactive.[47]

TOXICOLOGY: No literature on lycopene toxicity was found.

SUMMARY: Lycopene is a carotenoid present mainly in tomatoes. It is an antioxidant and is being studied for its role in cancer prevention including prostate, pancreatic, and stomach cancers. Lycopene has synergistic effects in some cases when used in conjunction with other antioxidants. Processed tomato products are a better source of lycopene than the raw fruit.

PATIENT INFORMATION – Lycopene

Uses: Lycopene has antioxidant activity and may be used in cancer prevention.

Side Effects: No literature on toxicity was found.

---

1 Budavari S, et al. eds. *The Merck Index*, 11th ed. Rahway: Merck and Co. 1989.
2 Murray M. *Encyclopedia of Nutritional Supplements.* Rocklin, CA: Prima Publishing. 1996;27-29.
3 Beecher G. Nutrient content of tomatoes and tomato products. *Proc Soc Exp Biol Med* 1998;218(2):98-100.
4 Nguyen M, et al. Lycopene stability during food processing. *Proc Soc Exp Biol Med* 1998;218(2):101-105.
5 Polunin M. *Healing Foods.* New York, NY: DK Publishing, Inc. 1997;60.
6 Anon. New study shows processed tomato products are a better source of lycopene than fresh tomatoes. *Oncology* 1997;11(12):1802.
7 Gartner C, et al. Lycopene is more bioavailable from tomato paste than from fresh tomatoes. *Am J Clin Nutr* 1997;66(1):116-22.
8 Stahl W, et al. Uptake of lycopene and its geometrical isomers is greater from heat-processed than from unprocessed tomato juice in humans. *J Nutr* 1992;122(11):2161-66.
9 Williams A, et al. Factors influencing the uptake and absorption of carotenoids. *Proc Soc Exp Biol Med* 1998;218(2):106-108.
10 Glise D, et al. Comparative distribution of beta-carotene and lycopene after intraperitoneal administration in mice. *In Vivo* 1998;12(5)447-54.
11 Mathews-Roth M, et al. Distribution of [14C]canthaxanthin and [14C]lycopene in rats and monkeys. *J Nutr* 1990;120(10):1205-13.
12 Zhao Z, et al. Lycopene uptake and tissue disposition in male and female rats. *Proc Soc Exp Biol Med* 1998;218(2):109-14.
13 Palan P, et al. Plasma levels of beta-carotene, lycopene, canthaxanthin, retinol, and alpha- and tau-tocopherol in cervical intraepithelial neoplasia and cancer. *Clin Cancer Res* 1996;2(1):181-85.
14 Johnson E, et al. Ingestion by men of a combined dose of beta-carotene and lycopene does not affect the absorption of beta-carotene but improves that of lycopene. *J Nutr* 1997;127(9):1833-37.
15 O'Neill M, et al. Intestinal absorption of beta-carotene, lycopene, and lutein in men and women following a standard meal. *Br J Nutr* 1998;79(2):149-59.
16 Talwar D, et al. A routine method for the simultaneous measurement of retinol, alpha-tocopherol and five carotenoids in human plasma by reverse phase HPLC. *Clin Chim Acta* 1998;270(2):85-100.
17 Johnson E. Human studies on bioavailability and plasma response of lycopene. *Proc Soc Exp Biol Med* 1998;218(2):115-20.
18 Sies H, et al. Lycopene: antioxidant and biological effects and its bioavailability in the human. *Proc Soc Exp Biol Med* 1998;218(2):121-24.
19 Boucher B. Intestinal absorption of beta-carotene, lycopene, and lutein in men and women following a standard meal. *Br J Nutr* 1998;80(1):115.
20 Mayne S, et al. Effect of supplemental beta-carotene on plasma concentrations of carotenoids, retinol, and alpha-tocopherol in humans. *Am J Clin Nutr* 1998;68(3):642-47.
21 Yeum K, et al. Relationship of plasma carotenoids, retinol, and tocopherols in mothers and newborn infants. *J Am Coll Nutr* 1998;17(5):442-47.
22 Weisburger J. Evaluation of the evidence on the role of tomato products in disease prevention. *Proc Soc Exp Biol Med* 1998;218(2):140-43.
23 Stahl W, et al. Lycopene: a biologically important carotenoid for humans? *Arch Biochem Biophys* 1996;336(1):1-9.
24 Steinberg F, et al. Antioxidant vitamin supplementation and lipid peroxidation in smokers. *Am J Clin Nutr* 1998;68(2):319-27.
25 Schmidt R, et al. Plasma antioxidants and cognitive performance in middle-aged and older adults: results of the Austrian Stroke Prevention Study. *J Am Geriatr Soc* 1998;46(11):1407-10.
26 Agarwal S, et al. Tomato lycopene and low density lipoprotein oxidation. *Lipids* 1998;33(10):981-84.
27 Kohlmeier I, et al. Lycopene and myocardial infarction risk in the EURAMIC study. *Am J Epidemiol* 1997;146(8):618-26.
28 Stahl W, et al. Carotenoid mixtures protect multilamellar liposomes against oxidative damage. *FEBS Lett* 1998;427(2):305-308.
29 Nishino H. Cancer prevention by natural carotenoids. *J Cell Biochem Suppl* 1997;27:86-91.
30 Rao A, et al. Bioavailability and in vivo antioxidant properties of lycopene from tomato products and their possible role in the prevention of cancer. *Nutr Cancer* 1998;31(3):199-203.
31 Gerster H. The potential role of lycopene for human health. *J Am Coll Nutr* 1997;16(2):109-26.
32 Giovannucci E, et al. Intake of carotenoids and retinol in relation to risk of prostate cancer. *J Natl Cancer Inst* 1995 Dec 6;87(23):1767-76.
33 Clinton S, et al. Cis-trans lycopene isomers, carotenoids, and retinol in the human prostate. *Cancer Epidemiol Biomarkers Prev* 1996;5(10):823-33.
34 Giovannucci E, et al. Tomatoes, lycopene, and prostate cancer. *Proc Soc Exp Biol Med* 1998;218(2):129-39
35 Pastori M, et al. Lycopene in association with alpha-tocopherol inhibits at physiological concentrations proliferation of prostate carcinoma cells. *Biochem Biophys Res Commun* 1998;250(3):582-85.
36 Kantesky P, et al. Dietary intake and blood levels of lycopene: association with cervical dysplasia among non-Hispanic, black women. *Nutr Cancer* 1998;31(1):31-40.
37 Hoffmann I, et al. International symposium on the role of lycopene and tomato products in disease prevention. *Cancer Epidemiol Biomarkers Prev* 1997;6(8):643-45.
38 Weisburger J. International symposium on lycopene and tomato products in disease prevention. *Proc Soc Exp Biol Med* 1998;218(2):93-94.
39 Clinton S. Lycopene: chemistry, biology, and implications for human health and disease. *Nutr Rev* 1998;56(2 pt 1):35-51.
40 Krinsky N. Overview of lycopene, carotenoids, and disease prevention. *Proc Soc Exp Biol Med* 1998;218(2):95-97.
41 Singh D, et al. Cancer chemoprevention. *Oncology* 1998;12(11):1643-53,1657-58,1659-60.
42 Michaud I. Chemoprevention: future is here. *ASHP Midyear Clinical Meeting* 1998 Dec;33:PI-95.
43 Pollitt N. Beta-carotene and the photodermatoses. *Br J Dermatol* 1975;93(6):721-24.
44 Pietzcker F, et al. Treatment of acral vitiligo with beta-carotin. *Med Welt* 1977;28(35):1407-1408.
45 Pietzcker F, et al. "Pigment balance" through oral beta carotene. A new therapeutic principle in cosmetic dermatology. *Hautarzt* 1979;30(6):308-11.
46 Anon. Beta carotene to prevent skin cancer. *N Engl J Med* 1991;324(13):923-25.
47 Lee K, et al. Mechanism of action of retinyl compounds on wound healing. *J Pharm Sci* 1970 Jun;59:851-54.

Lysine

SCIENTIFIC NAME(S): 2,6-diaminohexanoic acid, alpha-epsilon-diaminocaproic acid

COMMON NAME(S): Lysine

SOURCE: Lysine can be found in foods such as yogurt, fish, cheese, brewer's yeast, wheat germ, pork and other meats.[1] Lysine can also be synthesized in the laboratory.[2]

HISTORY: Lysine is an essential amino acid, "essential" in human nutrition, meaning the body cannot produce it, and therefore it must be taken in either by diet or by supplementation.[1,2] Lysine was first isolated from casein (a milk phosphoprotein) by Drechsel in 1889.[3]

CHEMISTRY: Amino acids are protein "building blocks." Amino acids combine to form over 50,000 different proteins and 20,000 enzymes.[1] Lysine is a hydrolytic cleavage product of protein, cleaved either by digestion or by boiling with hydrochloric acid.[3] Many forms of lysine exist, including L-lysine dihydrochloride, L-lysine monohydrochloride, calcium lysinate, lysortine (L-lysine monoorotate), L-lysine succinate, and the lysine salt of aspirin, "lysine acetylsalicylate."[2,4-7] The chemical structure of all amino acids contain an amino group ($-NH_2$) and a carboxyl group (-COOH).[2]

PHARMACOLOGY: Amino acids are fundamental constituents of all proteins. They promote protein production, reduce catabolism, promote wound healing and act as buffers in extra- and intracellular fluids.[8]

Lysine improves calcium assimilation. It also may be helpful in Bell's palsy.[1] However, most clinical data are available on its use in the treatment of herpes infection.

One report describes a relationship between lysine and herpes simplex virus (HSV). The amino acid arginine's composition is high in the HSV viral coding, thus, replication of the virus requires high consumption of arginine. Lysine appears to be an "antimetabolite," acting as an analog of arginine, competing for absorption and entrance into tissue cells. Lysine inhibits HSV replication by limiting arginine (by competing with it) during viral replication. Lysine prophylaxis was 100% effective in preventing herpetic labialis in patients suffering from frequent lesion occurrence. Treatment for recurrent aphthous ulcers (RAU; acute painful oral ulcers, "canker sores") was also evaluated in this study. Only 1 of 28 patients did not benefit from lysine therapy. Dosing was 500 mg lysine/day for prevention and 1000 mg every 6 hours upon development of prodrome in both treatments.[9]

Another report in the form of an epidemiological survey (subjective response questionnaire) was mailed out, and 1543 were completed and returned. Data showed 92% of patients with cold sores, 87% of those with canker sores and 81% with genital herpes stated lysine supplementation was effective. Twelve percent reported no effect of lysine against herpes attacks. Others reported shortened healing time and less severe symptoms with supplementation.[10] An earlier report in 45 patients taking 312 to 1200 mg lysine/day demonstrated beneficial effects from treatment in the form of accelerating herpes simplex infection recovery and suppressing recurrence. Tissue culture studies indicate that viral replication is suppressed as the lysine-to-arginine ratio increases.[11]

In contrast, at least 2 other studies report some failure of lysine in herpes treatment. Lysine 500 mg twice daily had no effect on 251 treated episodes of recurrent herpes simplex labialis in 119 patients.[12] Lysine HCl 750 mg/day, administered to 31 herpes simplex labialis or genitalis patients showed no reduction in number of episodes; however, the 1 g dose showed a 47% reduction.[13]

A case report exists concerning lysine supplementation for hyperargininemia in an 11-year-old girl. Lysine 250 mg/kg/day along with ornithine, produced a marked reduction of plasma ammonia and urinary orotic acid during a 6-month therapy period.[14]

Lysine acetylsalicylate has been used to treat rheumatoid arthritis and to detoxify heroin.[4,7]

TOXICOLOGY: Amino acid breakdown increases nitrogen concentration, which must be eliminated by the kidneys and liver. For this reason, the supplementation of lysine is contraindicated in those with kidney or liver disease.[1]

In rats, effects of dietary lysine on toxicity of barbiturates and ethanol have been evaluated. An increase in onset of loss of righting reflex was observed.[15]

Because the average American consumes 6 to 10 g of lysine daily, prophylaxis of 500 to 1000 mg and treatment dose of 4000 mg/day are insignificant amounts comparatively speaking. Dosages such as these have proven to be safe and free of side effects.[9]

Large doses of lysine increase toxicity of aminoglycoside antibiotics.[1]

SUMMARY: Lysine is an essential amino acid, important as a building block for protein synthesis. Controversial reports exist as to whether lysine can be helpful or not in treating herpes infections including cold sores. Patients with kidney or liver disease should not take the supplement; otherwise lysine has been shown to be safe in dosages up to 4000 mg/day.

PATIENT INFORMATION – Lysine

Uses: Lysine has been studied for the prophylaxis and treatment of herpes infections and cold sores. It also improves calcium assimilation and may be helpful in the treatment of Bell's palsy. Lysine acetylsalicylate has been used to treat rheumatoid arthritis and to detoxify heroin.

Drug Interactions: Large doses of lysine have been reported to increase toxicity of aminoglycoside antibiotics.

Side Effects: Dosages up to 4000 mg/day have been proven to be safe and free of side effects. Lysine supplementation is contraindicated in patients with kidney or liver disease.

---

[1] http://www.teleport.comibis/lysine.html.

[2] Budavari S, ed. *The Merck Index.* ed. 11. Rahway, NJ: Merck & Co. Inc., 1989.

[3] Agnew L, ed. *Dorland's Illustrated Medical Dictionary.* ed. 24. Philadelphia, PA: W.B. Saunders Co., 1965.

[4] Vescovi P, et al. *Current Therapeutic Research* 1984 May;35:826-31.

[5] Sinzinger H, et al. *NEJM* 1984 Oct 18;311:1052.

[6] Aarons L, et al. *Pharm Res* 1989 Aug;6:660-66.

[7] Hill J, et al. *J Clin Pharm Ther* 1990;15(3):205-11.

[8] Olin, BR, Hebel SK, eds. *Drug Facts and Comparisons.* St. Louis, MO: Facts and Comparisons, 1997.

[9] Wright E. *General Dentistry* 1994;42(1):40-42.

[10] Wash D, et al. *J Antimicrob Chemother* 1983 Nov;12:489-96.

[11] Griffith R, et al. *Dermatologica* 1978;156(5):257-67.

[12] Milman N, et al. *Lancet* 1978 Oct 28;2:942.

[13] Simon C, et al. *Arch Dermatol* 1985 Feb;121:167.

[14] Kang S, et al. *J Pediatr* 1983 Nov;103:763-65.

[15] Dubroff L, et al. *J Pharm Sci* 1979 Dec;68:1554-57.

Maca

SCIENTIFIC NAME(S): *Lepidium meyenii* Walp. Family: Brassicaceae (Mustards)

COMMON NAME(S): Peruvian ginseng, Maino, Ayuk willku, Ayak chichira

BOTANY: Maca is cultivated in a narrow, high-altitude zone of the Andes Mountains in Peru. The plant's frost tolerance allows it to grow at altitudes of 3500 to 4450 meters above sea level in the puna and suni ecosystems, where only alpine grasses and bitter potatoes can survive.[1] It and several related wild species are also found in the Bolivian Andes.[2] The plant grows from a stout, pear-shaped taproot and has a matlike, creeping system of stems. While traditionally cultivated as a vegetable crop, use for its medicinal properties has become more prominent in Peru. Maca is related to the common garden cress, *Lepidium sativum* L.

HISTORY: Maca was domesticated at least 2000 years ago and has been used commonly as a food by Peruvian peasants who live in high altitudes. It was considered to be a "famine food," but recent analyses have shown that the root is high in nutritional value, containing essential amino acids and important fatty acids.[3] The root can be dried and powdered, after which it is stored for several years without serious deterioration. Dried roots are cooked in water to make a sweet, aromatic porridge known as "mazamorra." According to Peruvian folk belief, maca enhances female fertility in both humans and livestock, countering the reduction in fertility seen in high altitudes.[4] However, maca is believed to have an antiaphrodisiac effect on males.[5]

CHEMISTRY: *Lepidium meyenii* has not been subjected to close chemical scrutiny. Johns reported the isolation of p-methoxybenzyl isothiocyanate from the plant,[6] although a positive alkaloid test has not been confirmed.

Other species of *Lepidium* have been analyzed more thoroughly; *L. sativum* has been found to contain many glucosinolates that have bactericidal, antiviral, and fungicidal activity in in vitro assays, as well as inhibiting tumorigenesis.[7,8] An alkaloid, lepidine, has been isolated from the seeds of *L. sativum*.[9] Evomonoside, a cardiac glycoside, has been isolated in substantial yield from the seeds of *L. apetalum*, a Korean species.[10] Several flavones and flavonoid glycosides have also been isolated from the genus *Lepidium*.[11]

PHARMACOLOGY: Unreferenced data published on a commercial Web site (www.macaperu.com) claims activity of maca in rat adaptogen models that use swimming time and oxygen consumption as endpoints.

Aphrodisiac and antistress properties have also been claimed. The pharmacology of other *Lepidium* species is documented as the following: *L. capitatum* had anti-implantation activity in rats.[12,13] The ethanolic extract of the seeds of *L. sativum* was found to increase collagen deposition in a rat model of fracture healing.[14] *L. latifolium* was found to have diuretic action in rats.[15]

TOXICOLOGY: The presence of substantial amounts of a cardiac glycoside in the related species, *L. apetalum*,[10] is cause for concern. Cardioactive substances have also been detected in *L. sativum*.[16] However, the fact that dried maca roots have been consumed for many years would argue against a risk for cardiotoxicity. *L. virginicum* was inactive in a screen for genotoxicity.[17]

SUMMARY: Maca is promoted for a variety of fertility and adaptogenic uses. However, there is very little scientific information to support its medicinal use. Its long history as a food in the Andes suggests low potential for toxicity.

PATIENT INFORMATION – Maca

Uses: Maca has been used as an aphrodisiac, fertility aid, and to relieve stress.

Side Effects: There is little information on maca's long-term effects. Its long-time use as a food product suggests low potential for toxicity.

[1] Quiros C, et al. Physiological studies and determination of chromosome number in maca. *Lepidium meyenii (Brassicaceae) Econ Bot* 1996;50(2):216.

[2] Toledo J, et al. Genetic variability of *Lepidium meyenii* and other Andean lepidium species (*Brassicaceae*) assessed by molecular markers. *Ann Bot* 1998;82(4):523.

[3] Dini A, et al. Chemical composition of *Lepidium meyenii. Food Chem* 1994;49(4):347.

[4] Eckes L. Altitude adaptation. IV. Fertility and reproduction at high altitudes. *Gegenbaurs Morphol Jahrb* 1976;122(5):761–70.

[5] Johns T. With bitter herbs they shall eat it. Chemical ecology and the origins of human diet and medicine. Tucson: University of Arizona Press, 1990;119–21.

[6] Johns T. The añu and the maca. *J Ethnobiology* 1981;1:208.

[7] Daxenbichler M, et al. Oxazolidinethiones and volatile isothiocyanates in enzyme-treated seed meals for 65 species of *Cruciferae. J Agric Food Chem* 1964;12(2):127.

[8] Hecht S. Chemoprevention of cancer by isothiocyanates, modifiers of carcinogen metabolism. *J Nutr* 1999;129:768S-74S. Review.

[9] Bahroun A, et al.Contribution to the study of *Lepidium sativum (Cruciferae).* Structure of a new compound isolated from the seed: lepidine. *J Soc Chim Tunis* 1985;2:15. *Chem Abs* 104:65910g.

[10] Hyun J, et al. Evomonoside: the cytotoxic cardiac glycoside from *Lepidium apetalum. Planta Med* 1995;61(3):294–5.

[11] Fursa M, et al. Chemical study of flavonol-3, 7–diglycoside of *Lepidium perfoliatum* L. *Farm Zh* 1970;25(4):83–4.

[12] Singh M, et al. Postcoital contraceptive efficacy and hormonal profile of *Lepidium capitatum. Planta Med* 1984;50(2):154–7.

[13] Prakash O, et al. Anti-implantation activity of some indigenous plants in rats. *Acta Eur Fertil* 1985;16(6):441–8.

[14] Ahsan S, et al. Studies on some herbal drugs used in fracture healing. *Int J Crude Drug Res* 1989;27(4):235.

[15] Navarro E, et al. Diuretic action of an aqueous extract of *Lepidium latifolium* L. *J Ethnopharmacol* 1994;41(1–2):65–9.

[16] Vohora S, et al. Pharmacological studies on *Lepidium sativum*, linn. *Indian J Physiol Pharmacol* 1977;21(2):118–20.

[17] Ramos Ruiz A, et al. Screening of medicinal plants for induction of somatic segregation activity in *Aspergillius nidulans. J Ethnopharmacol* 1996;52(3):123–7.

Mace

SCIENTIFIC NAME(S): The dried aril of *Myristica fragrans* Houtt. Family: Myristicaceae

COMMON NAME(S): Mace, muscade (French), seed cover of nutmeg

BOTANY: Mace and nutmeg are two slightly different flavored spices both originating from the fruit of the nutmeg tree, *Myristica fragrans*. The fruit is a drupe which splits open when mature, exposing the nutmeg (stony endocarp or seed) surrounded by a red, slightly fleshy network (aril). Once the aril is peeled off and dried, it is referred to as mace.[1] Botanical mace should not be confused with the same word which also can describe a weapon of offense (iron or steel) capable of breaking through armor or a relatively modern riot control synthetic compound used as an irritating and debilitating spray or gas.[1,2]

The nutmeg tree is a densely foliazed evergreen tea commonly grown in Grenada (West Indies), Indonesia, Ceylon and the Moluccas in the East Indian Archipelago.[2] The trees first produce fruit in about 7 years and then yield approximately 10 pounds of dried shelled nutmeg and 1 pounds of dried mace per tree.[2] At low concentrations, both nutmeg and mace possess a sweet, warm and highly spicy flavor with mace being slightly "stronger." Ground nutmeg is tan in color, while mace has an orange hue.

HISTORY: Both nutmeg and mace have been used in Indian and Indonesian cooking and in folk medicine. Historical medicinal uses of mace range from the treatment of diarrhea to mouth sores, insomnia and rheumatism.

CHEMISTRY: Numegs, depending on origin and condition, yield, on steam distillation, 5–15% of essential oil.[2] The essential oils of nutmeg and mace are very similar in chemical composition and aroma, with wide color difference (brilliant orange to pale yellow). Both nutmeg and mace contain about 4% of a highly toxic substance called myristicin (methoxysafrole).[2] Other compounds isolated include safrole, elemicin, methoxyeugenol, ($\pm$) camphene, β-terpineol, α- and β-pinene, myrcene, ($\pm$)-limonene and sabinene.[3] Recently, two resorcinols, malabaricone B and malabaricone C have been isolated from mace by Orabi et al.[4] New lignans have been isolated by Kuo[5] and Zacchino et al.[6]

PHARMACOLOGY: A number of interesting articles have appeared on potential anti-cancer properties (chemo-preventor effects of chemically induced carcinogenesis) of mace, including: transmammary modulation of xenobiotic metabolizing enzymes in the liver of mouse pups by mace;[7] effect of nutmeg essential oils on activation and detoxification of xenobiotic compounds (chemical carcinogens and mutagens);[8] potential anticarcinogenic role of *Myristica* volatile oils;[9] modulatory effects of mace on hepatic detoxification;[10] reduction of induced skin papilloma incidence via diet containing 1% mace;[11] reduction of induced carcinogenesis in uterine cervix in mice by mace;[12] and increased level of acid-soluble sulfhydryl (SH) groups in the liver of young mice (chemoprotective) by mace.[13]

A number of miscellaneous pharmacological studies show strong antifungal and antibacterial properties of two antimicrobial resorcinols (malabaricone B and C from mace;[4] anti-inflammatory properties of myristicin from mace;[14] antimicrobial action of mace against oral bacteria;[15] and a larvicidal principle in mace.[16]

TOXICOLOGY: The majority of the literature of the last decade continues to verify the possibility of acute intoxication possible with overdoses of nutmeg itself[17] and of contact or systemic contact-type dermatitis to nutmeg as a spice.[18] Very few, if any, articles appear in the recent literature specifically dealing with mace intoxication.

SUMMARY: Mace continues to be used safely in small amounts as a spice flavoring for pound cakes, doughnuts, fish sauces and meat stews.[2] Mace has been shown to possess potential anti-cancer or chemoprotective effects in several animal models. These have been stimulated, no doubt, by recent ethnobotanical and ethnopharmacological studies aimed at verifying human historical medical uses which range from the use of both nutmeg and mace for the treatment of diarrhea, mouth sores, insomnia and rheumatism.[19] Some of these uses seem to have been verified in the studies mentioned above. However, recent human clinical supporting data are much needed. Attention should be paid to high doses of mace, since it may well produce similar effects known as nutmeg during acute poisoning (eg, hallucinations, palpitations, feelings of impending doom)[17] and potential allergy.[18]

PATIENT INFORMATION – Mace

Uses: Mace has been used as a flavoring and folk medicine for a range of ills, such as diarrhea, insomnia, and rheumatism. Studies show anticancer, antifungal, antibacterial, anti-inflammatory, and larvicidal properties.

Side Effects: Large doses may produce acute intoxication. It may cause dermatitis in sensitive individuals.

[1] Simpson B, Ogorzaly M. Economic Botany: Plants in Our World. New York: McGraw-Hill Book Company, 1986.

[2] Rosengarten F, Jr. The Book of Spices. Wynnewood, PA: Livingston Publishing Company, 1969.

[3] Tyler V, et al. Pharmacognosy, 9th ed. Philadelphia: Lea & Febiger, 1988.

[4] Orabi KY, et al. Isolation and characterization of two antimicrobial agents from mace (Myristica fragrans). *J Nat Prod* 1991;54(3):856.

[5] Kuo YH. Studies on several naturally occurring lignans. *Kao-Hsiung I Hsueh Ko Hseuh Tsa Chih* [*Kaohsiung J Med Sc*] 1989;5(11):621.

[6] Zacchino SA, Badano H. Enantioselective synthesis and absolute configuration assignment of erythro-(3,4,5–trimethoxy-7–hydroxy-1'allyl-2',6'-dimethoxy)-8.0.4'-neolignan from *mace (Myristica fragrans)*. *J Nat Prod* 1988;51:1261.

[7] Chhabra SK, Rao AR. Transmammary modulation of xenobiotic metabolizing enzymes in liever of mouse pups by mace (Myristica fragrans Houtt.). *J Ethnopharmacol* 1994;42(3):169.

[8] Banerjee S, et al. Influence of certain essential oils on carcinogen-metabolizing enzymes and acid-soluble sulfhydryls in mouse liver. *Nutr Cancer* 1994;21(3):263.

[9] Hashim S, et al. Modulatory effects of essential oils from spices on the formation of DNA adduct by aflatoxin B1 in vitro. *Nutr Cancer* 1994;21(2):169

[10] Singh A, Rao AR. Modulatory effect of Areca nut on the action of mace (Myristica fragrans, Houtt.) on the hepatic detoxification systems in mice. *Food Chem Toxicol* 1993;31(7):517.

[11] Jannu LN, et al. Chemopreventive action of mace (Myristica fragrans, Houtt.) on DMBA-induced papillomagenesis in the skin of mice. *Cancer Lett* 1991;56(1):59.

[12] Hussain SP, Rao AR. Chemopreventive action of mace (Myristica fragrans, Houtt.) on methylcholanthrene-induced carcinogenesis in the uterine cervix in mice. *Cancer Lett* 1991;56(3):231.

[13] Kumari MV, Rao AR. Effects of mace (Myristica fragrans, Houtt.) on cytosolic glutathione S-transferase activity and acid soluble sulfhydryl level in mouse liver. *Cancer Lett* 1989;46(2):87.

[14] Ozaki Y, et al. Antiinflammatory effect of mace, aril of Myristica fragrans Houtt., and its active principles. *Jpn J Pharmacol* 1989;49(2):155.

[15] Saeki Y, et al. Antimicrobial action of natural substances on oral bacteria. *Bull Tokyo Dental College* 1989;30(3):129.

[16] Nakamura N, et al. Studies on crude drugs effective on visceral larva migrans. V. The larvicidal principle in mace (aril of Myristica fragrans). *Chem Pharm Bull* 1988;36(7):2685.

[17] Abernethy MK, Becker LB. Acute nutmeg intoxication. *Am J Emerg Med* 1992;10(5):429.

[18] Dooms-Goossens A, et al. Contact and systemic contact-type dermatitis to spices. *Dermatol Clin* 1990;8(1):89.

[19] Van Gils C, Cox PA. Ethnobotany of nutmeg in the Spice Islands [Review]. *J Ethnopharmacol* 1994;42(2):117.

Maggots

SCIENTIFIC NAME(S): *Phaenicia sericata*; *Lucilia caesar*, *Pharmia regina*

COMMON NAME(S): Maggot, fly larva, grub, botfly maggot, "viable antiseptic," "living antiseptic," "surgical maggot"

BIOLOGY: Maggots are the larvae of various flies. The species *Phaenicia sericata* (green blow fly) has been used successfully in maggot therapy for many decades.[1] The life cycle of those used in medicine begins with the laying of eggs by the adult female on meat or other substrate suitable for the larvae to feed on. The eggs hatch within one day, and the larvae then proceed to feed and grow. After 5 to 7 days, they become sessile, non-feeding pupae. After about 2 weeks of pupation, the adults emerge and the females begin laying eggs about five days later.[2]

Larvae-rearing in the clinical setting can be a simple, low-cost procedure if done correctly.[3] A report on species *Lucilia sericata* (Meigen) evaluates a sterile mixture of pureed liver and agar as growth medium. This method was not only inexpensive but provided longer storage capacity and no progressive decomposition or odor problems.[4]

HISTORY: The effects of maggots on wounds have been known since the 1500s when Ambroise Paré described their beneficial actions. It was observed that maggots cleaned untreated wounds, removing necrotic tissue without apparent harm to living tissues. Many military surgeons noticed that soldiers' wounds that became maggot-infested did better than non-infested wounds.[1] The first scientific paper on the surgical use of maggots appeared in 1931, and there was significant interest in the technique during the 1930s and early 1940s. Maggot debridement therapy (MDT) was routinely performed in over 300 hospitals during this time.[1] The first civilian use, based on observations during World War I, was in treating four children with osteomyelitis who did not respond to other available treatments. Subsequent occurrence of tetanus in other cases led to the development of bacteriologically sterile maggots. Early uses for maggot therapy included abscesses, burns, cellulitis, gangrene and ulcers.[2]

Around the mid-'40s, use of maggots declined rapidly with the development of antibiotic drugs. Maggot therapy was occasionally employed when all other therapies failed. For example, a 1976 report described use of maggots to treat subacute mastoiditis.[5] In addition, maggots were used to treat women undergoing low-voltage X-ray therapy for cervical carcinoma. The organisms were used to prevent radiation-induced sloughing of the tissues over the sacrum, buttocks and lower abdomen.[6] Actual clinical use of maggots preceded the literature; there was a thriving industry for commercial preparations of maggots at least 10 years before the 1931 report.[2]

PHARMACOLOGY: The mechanisms by which maggots promote wound healing have not been proven conclusively. However, a variety of mechanisms have been suggested. The exudate produced in response to the maggots physically washes bacteria out of the wound. The crawling larvae mechanically stimulate viable tissues to rapidly produce granulation tissue. They also enzymatically liquefy necrotic tissue. Bacteria are destroyed within the alimentary tracts of the larvae, which also use necrotic tissue as food. Maggots may produce antibacterial agents released in their secretions. They also increase the alkalinity of the wound, promoting healthy granulation. Substances proposed as beneficial secretions of maggots include allantoin, ammonium ions and calcium carbonate.[5]

The most common use of maggots in surgery has been to prevent bone destruction, deformities and other effects of recalcitrant osteomyelitis in which topical wounds heal poorly. Treatment begins with debridement of the affected area. The wound is then left unsutured for about 2 days, after which, 200 to 1000 maggots are applied to the wound. The maggots are contained by a dressing or cage. They are removed in 3 to 5 days to prevent pupation in the wound, and fresh maggots are applied as needed. Application of maggots is followed by rapid formation of a serosanguineous exudate. Healing occurs within 6 to 7 weeks in children and may take somewhat longer in adults.[2]

A 1986 report described the use of maggots to treat two patients with severe skin infections. One patient had a large, necrotic, foul-smelling decubitus ulcer of the perianal and presacral areas. The second was an insulin-dependent diabetic with ketoacidosis and a right scrotal ulcer. Excellent wound healing was achieved in both patients although the second patient subsequently died of general debility.[5] Maggot therapy has also been performed effectively for venous stasis ulcers,[7] pressure ulcers in spinal cord injury patients[8] and wound debridement.[9,10,11] A plantar foot ulcer in one patient existed for several years yet resolved after about 13 weeks of MDT.[10] Some patients with severe tissue destruction may also be receiving antibiotics along with MDT. A report evaluates this combination. Larvae survival was decreased when very high doses of gentamicin and cefazolin were administered. Antibiotics showing no change in survival rate included ampicillin, ceftizoxime, clindamycin, mezlocillin and vancomycin.[12]

Analysis of maggots found in decomposing bodies can provide information on the time of death, as well as on the presence of specific drugs in the bodies.[13] Maggots can also provide clues about crime location and circumstances. The study of maggots (and other insects) used in this way is termed "forensic entomology."[1]

TOXICOLOGY: Surgical maggots in themselves do not appear harmful to living tissues although it should be noted that maggots of screwworms can cause serious tissue damage. The surgical organisms, however, produce intense pruritus. Most patients adapt to this, but some require mild sedation.[5]

Non-surgical maggots are commonly used as fishing lures. At least one report has described delayed-onset asthma in an angler who used *Calliphora* (blue bottle) larvae for bait. The patient was found to have circulating IgG antibody to a larval extract, and symptoms suggestive of immune complex disease subsequently developed.[14] It has been suggested that dyes used to enhance the effectiveness of maggots as fishing lures can induce bladder cancer.[15] A case-control study of more than 1800 subjects found no evidence of an association between the dyes and bladder cancer; however, the number of sub-jects who used dyed maggots in fishing was small so that an actual association may have escaped detection.[16]

Maggots can transmit parasitic diseases resulting in severe destruction of tissues of the ears, nose and throat. This problem is common in India, where it occurs most frequently from September to November.[17] This larval invasion has also been reported in the eye. One case report details the invasion of the ocular orbit of a man by maggots. This infestation was treated successfully by classical wound-cleaning therapy.[18] Another case reports *cuterebra larva* in the conjunctiva of a boy suffering from decreased vision and subretinal hemorrhages. Successful removal was performed after positive identification of this offending agent by light microscopy.[19] A third case of ophthalmic invasion by larva is reported, this time with successful removal by photocoagulation with an argon green laser resulting in good visual recovery.[20]

SUMMARY: Maggots have long been known to promote the healing of wounds without generally causing harm to living tissues. The use of surgical maggots experienced a certain popularity among surgeons during the 1930s and 1940s, but this waned with the development of antibiotic drugs. Nevertheless, maggots have been used successfully in recent years when other methods of treatment failed. Examples of maggot therapy include its use in bone destruction/infection and poorly healing wound debridement, including bedsores and other ulcers. Their medical use requires close supervision to ensure that secondary infections or other invasive complications do not arise. Other uses of maggots include "forensic entomology." Surgical maggots may not be harmful to living tissues but may cause itching. Unwanted larval invasion has occurred in the eyes, ears, nose and throat.

PATIENT INFORMATION – Maggots

Uses: Maggots have been used to promote wound healing and also to treat abscesses, burns, cellulitis, gangrene and ulcers. The most common use of maggots in surgery has been to prevent bone destruction, deformities and other effects of recalcitrant osteomyelitis.

Side Effects: Surgical maggots do not appear harmful to living tissues but produce intense pruritus. Maggots can transmit parasitic disease, and larval ocular invasion has occurred.

[1] http://www.com.uci.edu/~path/sherman/home_pg.htm
[2] Chernin E. *South Med J* 1986;79:1143.
[3] Sherman R, et al. *Am J Trop Med Hyg* 1996;54(1):38–41.
[4] Sherman R, et al. *Med Vet Entomol* 1995;9(4):393–8.
[5] Teich S, Myers R. *South Med J* 1986;79:1153.
[6] Diddle AW. *South Med J* 1987;80:1333.
[7] Sherman R, et al. *Arch Dermatol* 1996;132(3):254–6.
[8] Sherman R, et al. *J Spinal Cord Med* 1995;18(2):71–4.
[9] Reames M, et al. *Ann Plast Surg* 1988;21(4):388–91.
[10] Stoddard S, et al. *J Am Podiatr Med Assoc* 1995;85(4):218–21.
[11] Thomas S, et al. *J Wound Care* 1996;5(2):60–9.
[12] Sherman R, et al. *J Med Entomol* 1995;32(5):646–9.
[13] Beyer JC, et al. *J Forensic Sci* 1980;25:411.
[14] Stockley RA. *Clin Allergy* 1982;12:151.
[15] Massey JA, et al. *Br Med J* 1984;289:1451.
[16] Cartwright RA, et al. *Carcinogenesis* 1983;4:111.
[17] Sood VP, et al. *J Laryngol Otol* 1976;90:393.
[18] Mathur SP, Makhija JM. *Br J Ophthalmol* 1967;51:406.
[19] Glasgow B, et al. *Am J Ophthalmol* 1995:119(4):512–14.
[20] Phelan M, et al. *Am J Ophthalmol* 1995;119(1):106–7.

Maitake

SCIENTIFIC NAME(S): *Grifola frondosa* (polyporaceae)

COMMON NAME(S): Maitake, "king of mushrooms," " dancing mushroom," "monkey's bench," "shelf fungi"

BOTANY: The maitake mushroom is from northeastern Japan. It grows in clusters at the foot of oak trees and can reach 20 inches in base diameter. One bunch can weigh up to 100 lbs. Maitake has no cap but has a rippling, flowery appearance, resembling "dancing butterflies" (hence, one of its common names "dancing mushroom").[1]

HISTORY: In China and Japan, maitake mushrooms have been consumed for 3000 years. The maitake is the most valued because of its "near-miraculous" properties. Maitake's scientific name, *Grifola frondosa*, is derived from an Italian mushroom name, referring to a mythological beast, half lion and half eagle. Years ago in Japan, the maitake had monetary value and was worth its weight in silver. This mushroom was offered to Shogun, the national leader, by local lords. In the late 1980s, Japanese scientists identified the maitake to be more potent than lentinan, shiitake, suehirotake and kawaratake mushrooms, all used in traditional oriental medicine for immune function enhancement. It was found that maitake also possesses this quality.

CHEMISTRY: The polysaccharide beta-glucan is present in most of the mushrooms in the polyporaceae family (eg, reishi mushroom) and has been shown to possess anti-tumor activity.[1] The "D fraction" of beta-glucan appears to be the most active and potent form of the polysaccharide, which is the protein-bound extract developed in Japan.[2] Both structure-functional relationship[3] and fractionation by anion exchange chromatography of beta-glucan[4] have been reported. Neutral and acidic polysaccharides have been extracted from maitake[5] and their structure determined.[6] Two different glycan conformations have been obtained from the plant.[7] The beta-1,3-glycan, grifolan's conformation, has been elucidated using magnetic resonance spectroscopy.[8] Ascorbic acid analogs and glycoside studies have been reported.[9] In addition, a lectin from maitake has been isolated and characterized.[10]

Structural characterization of maitake extract constituents[11] and carbon-13 nuclear magnetic resonance spectral analysis of the fruit body's constituents[12] also have been evaluated.

PHARMACOLOGY: Immunostimulant activity is characteristic of many of the medicinal mushrooms, including shiitake, enokitake or kawaratake. Maitake's polysaccharide may be slightly different from beta-glucans found in these. Maitake exerts its effects by activation of natural killer cells, cytotoxic T-cells, interleukin-1 and superoxide anions, all of which aid in anti-cancer activity.[13] It has also been determined that the large molecular weight of the polysaccharide molecule and certain branch structure configurations of this molecule are necessary for its anti-tumor effect or immunological enhancement.[14,15,16]

The following list is a representative summary of information available on maitake's anti-cancer effects. Maitake extract has been studied in *Escherichia coli*;[17] it has activated macrophages, enhancing cytokine production in vivo;[18] maitake has potentiated anti-tumor activity in mice.[13] Also in mice, maitake has enhanced nitric oxide synthesis of peritoneal macrophages,[19] enhanced antigen-specific antibody response[20] and has exhibited marked inhibitory activity against induced sarcoma when administered intraperitoneally but not orally.[21] At least one report is available on anti-tumor actions of orally administered maitake extract in mice.[22] Another report finds dose-dependent anti-tumor activity in mice also dependent on injection routes and timing.[23] Biological response modification affected anti-tumor action in another report.[24] Some pharmacokinetic parameters of beta-D-glucan have been evaluated in mice.[25]

Animal studies indicate that maitake has a role in treatment of metastatic cancer. Metastasis was prevented in 91.3% of mice injected with cancer cells, then given D-fraction injections (1 mg/kg), compared with control mice experiencing no inhibition.[26]

There is a small number of clinical trials investigating maitake's effects in cancer therapy. Some were unpublished, while others were not blinded or placebo controlled. Additional controlled studies are needed. Some of the available studies are summarized here. In a 165-patient study, results suggested that quality of life indicators had improved, including cancer symptoms (eg, nausea, hair loss) and pain reduction.[27] Previous cancers not identified that were improved by maitake in clinical cases include liver, lung, breast, brain and prostate.[1]

A few animal reports on maitake's effects on **diabetes**, **hypertension** and **cholesterol** are available. Upon oral adminstration of maitake powdered fruit body to genetically diabetic mice, blood glucose reduction was observed compared with control groups.[28] Maitake may control blood glucose levels by possible reduction of insulin resistance and enhancement of insulin sensitivity.[1]

Hypertensive rats given 5% maitake mushroom powder had a reduction in blood pressure.[29,30] Similar pressure-lowering activity was seen in another study performed in rats, where maitake extract lowered blood pressure from 200 to 115 mmHg in 4 hours.[31] In an unpublished human trial, 11 patients with documented essential hypertension took 500 mg of maitake mushroom caplets twice daily. A mean decrease in diastolic blood pressure of approximately 8 mmHg and a mean decrease in systolic blood pressure of about 14 mmHg were reported.[32]

Maitake had the ability to alter lipid metabolism by inhibiting both the accumulation of liver lipids and elevation of serum lipids in hyperlipidemic rats.[33] Similar results were seen in rats fed a high cholesterol diet.[34] Total cholesterol and VLDL-cholesterol decreased in rats given powdered mushroom preparation in another report.[29]

At least two studies are available concerning maitake's **anti-obesity** activity. After 18 weeks, overweight rats fed unheated maitake powder lost weight compared with controls.[35] In an observatory trial, 30 patients lost between 7 and 26 pounds from administration of 20 to 500 mg tablets of maitake powder per day for 2 months.[36]

TOXICOLOGY: Little or no information regarding maitake toxicity is available. Most studies report no side effects.[1] Because potential toxicity exists from mistaken mushroom identity, use caution when obtaining this particular natural product. (For more information, see the Mushroom Poisoning Decision Chart monograph).

SUMMARY: Mushrooms have been consumed in Asian countries for thousands of years. Maitake has recently been found to possess anti-cancer qualities because of the polysaccharide beta-glucan. The mushroom not only demonstrates immunostimulant properties but has also been tested in diabetes, hypertension, cholesterol and HIV therapies. Little is known about the plant's toxicity. More research is needed to fully explore and understand the potential of this "king of mushrooms."

PATIENT INFORMATION – Maitake

Uses: Maitake has been used for cancer, diabetes, high blood pressure, cholesterol and obesity.

Side Effects: Most studies report no side effects.

---

[1] Lieberman S, et al. Maitake King of Mushrooms. New Canaan, CT: Keats Publishing, Inc. 1997;7-48.
[2] Nanba H. *J Naturopathic Med* 1993;(4)1:10-15.
[3] Iino K, et al. *Chem Pharm Bull* 1985;33(11):4950-56.
[4] Ohno N, et al. *Chem Pharm Bull* 1986; 34(3):3328-32.
[5] Ohno N, et al. *Chem Pharm Bull* 1985;33(3):1181-86.
[6] Nanba H, et al. *Chem Pharm Bull* 1987;35(3):1162-68.
[7] Ohno N, et al. *Chem Pharm Bull* 1986;34(6):2555-60.
[8] Ohno N, et al. *Chem Pharm Bull* 1987;35(6):2585-88.
[9] Okamura M. *J Nutr Sci Vitaminol* 1994;40(2):81-94.
[10] Kawagishi H. *Biochim Biophys Acta* 1990;1034(3):247-52.
[11] Ohno N, et al. *Chem Pharm Bull* 1985;33(8):3395-401.
[12] Ohno N, et al. *Chem Pharm Bull* 1985;33(4):1557-62.
[13] Adachi K, et al. *Chem Pharm Bull* 1987;35(1):262-70.
[14] Adachi K, et al. *Chem Pharm Bull* 1989;37(7):1838-43.
[15] Adachi K, et al. *Chem Pharm Bull* 1990;38(2):477-81.
[16] Ohno N, et al. *Biol Pharm Bull* 1995;18(1):126-33.
[17] Jin Z, et al. *Chung Hua Yu Fang I Hsueh Tsa Chih* 1994;28(3):147-50.
[18] Adachi Y, et al. *Biol Pharm Bull* 1994;17(12):1554-60.
[19] Ohno N, et al. *Biol Pharm Bull* 1996;19(4):608-12.
[20] Suzuki I, et al. *J Pharmacobiodyn* 1985;8(3):217-26.
[21] Suzuki I, et al. *J Pharmacobiodyn* 1984;7(7):492-500.
[22] Hishida I, et al. *Chem Pharm Bull* 1988;36(5):1819-27.
[23] Suzuki I, et al. *J Pharmacobiodyn* 1987;10(2):72-77.
[24] Ohno N, et al. *J Pharmacobiodyn* 1986;9(10):861-64.
[25] Miura N, et al. *Fems Immunol Med Microbiol* 1996;13(1):51-57.
[26] Nanba H, et al. *Annals of the New York Academy of Sciences* 1995;768:243-45.
[27] Nanba H. *Townsend Letter for Doctors and Patients* 1996;84-85.
[28] Kubo K, et al. *Biol Pharm Bull* 1994;17(8):1106-1110.
[29] Kabir Y, et al. *J Nutr Sci Vitaminol* 1987;33(5):341-46.
[30] Kabir Y, et al. *J Nutr Sci Vitaminol* 1989;35(1):91-94.
[31] Adachi K, et al. *Chem Pharm Bull* 1988;36(3):1000-1006.
[32] Gerson S. (Director of the Foundation for Holistic Medical Research in NYC). 1994 (unpublished).
[33] Kubo K, et al. *Altern Ther Health Med* 1996;2(5):62-66.
[34] Kubo K, et al. *Biol Pharm Bull* 1997;20(7):781-85.
[35] Ohtsuru M. *Anshin* 1992 July:188-200.
[36] Yokota M. *Anshin* 1992 July:202-204.

Marijuana

SCIENTIFIC NAME(S): *Cannabis sativa* More than a dozen other species names have been used to describe marijuana. Family: Cannabaceae

COMMON NAME(S): A variety of common names have been attributed to the plant. There are, however, specific terms for the various plant parts and extracts. These include: anascha and kif(resinous material and flowering tops mixed with the leaves); banji, hemp, cannabis, shesha, dimba, dagga, suma, vingory and machona (entire plant); bhang and sawi (dried mature leaves); charas (resinous material); ganga (flowering tops); hashish and esrar (resinous material with flowering tops); and marijuana or marihuana (leaves and flowering tops). Names vary with local customs.[1]

BOTANY: More than 100 species of cannabis grow wild throughout most temperate climates, although several species have adapted to harsher climactic conditions. Cannabis is a leafy annual, some species of which attain heights of more than 10 feet.

The stalk may grow 3 to 4 inches thick, is square and hollow and has ridges running along its length. Each leaf has 5 to 11 leaflets radiating from the top of the stalk. These are soft-textured, 7 to 10 inches long, narrow and lance-shaped with regular dentation like the sawblade. The plant is dioecious showing male or female flowers. The female plants have a heavy foliage, while the male plants are sparse. The resin mixture is found in the glandular hairs of the leaflets and floral bracts and is called hashish. Hashish is made up of numerous tetrahydrocannabinol compounds. Cannabis is cultivated worldwide for fiber, seed oil and hashish. The controversy over legitimate and illegal use of cannabis persists.[2,3]

HISTORY: The use of cannabis dates back more than 4,000 years. It has been used for the treatment of catarrh, leprosy, fever, dandruff, hemorrhoids, obesity, asthma, urinary tract infections, loss of appetite, inflammatory conditions and cough. It has been used as a source of fiber for ropes and clothing. The plant's sedative effects were recognized by the ancient Chinese, but the widespread use of the plant for its psychoactive effects most likely began only in the past century.[2,4]

The history and details of the health hazards of cannabis have been reviewed.[4]

CHEMISTRY: More than 420 different compounds have been isolated from cannabis and reported in the chemical literature.[5] The most commonly described compounds are the cannabinoids [delta–9–tetrahydrocannabinol (THC), cannabidiol, and numerous related compounds]. In addition, marijuana contains alkaloids, steroidal compounds and mixtures of volatile components.[5]

Feruloyltyramine, a new amide compound, and p-coumaroyltyramine have recently been identified in cannabis seeds.[6] From the fruits, three new acyclic bis-phenylpropane lignan amides have additionally been isolated.[7]

The concentration of THC varies in different parts of the plant, being higher in the bracts, flowers and leaves and lower in the stems, seeds and roots. THC concentration varies from 0.1% in Kansas hemp to 4% or more in Jamaican or Vietnamese specimens.[8]

Analysis of dried cannabis samples from 1896 to 1905, reported the presence of cannabinol.[9] Additional reports on illicit cannabis samples from Great Britain, Northern Ireland and Denmark exist, evaluating THC content, cannabinoid content and locational differences between regions.[10,11] Cannabinoids in hemp (cultivated for fiber production) have also been reported.[12] Analysis of cannabis includes methods such as gas chromatography (GC), high-performance liquid chromatography (HPLC), random amplification of polymorphic DNA (RAPD) and thin layer chromatography (TLC). These methods are of use in sample differentiation, forensic analysis and other applications.[13-16] Radioimmunoassay of hair for marijuana presence in body systems has also been performed.[17]

PHARMACOLOGY: The pharmacology of whole marijuana and many of its individual compounds has been investigated in detail over the past decade. THC appears to contribute most significantly to the pharmacologic effects observed. Cannabinol may potentially contribute to the psychoactivity of the plant. This compound is a degradation product of THC and is not found in the fresh plant. Marijuana exerts its activity following inhalation of the smoke or oral ingestion. When inhaled, THC is absorbed rapidly. The systemic bioavailability of THC following smoking is approximately 18% but higher in heavy users and lower in light users.

THC is distributed rapidly throughout the body, in particular to tissues with high lipid contents. Approximately 80%

to 90% of an IV dose of THC is excreted in urine and the remainder excreted in the feces via the bile.[5]

Cannabinoid metabolites remain detectable in urine for more than 10 days after a single use and for more than 20 days after chronic use. A French report on detection, evaluating newborn infants of addicted mothers, suggests not only urine testing of the infant to detect drug exposure, but to also test meconium and hair as well. Testing all three parameters increases sensitivity of analysis for parenteral drug exposure detection.[18]

Marijuana's effects can be categorized as follows:

Cardiovascular effects: Ingestion or inhalation of marijuana often results in tachycardia (especially supraventricular). ECG changes are not observed regularly in healthy young adults.[19] The drug may reduce exercise tolerance in anginal patients. Although marijuana may raise blood pressure, there is no evidence that the drug may cause permanent deleterious effects on the normal cardiovascular system.[20]

Pulmonary effects: Bronchial and pulmonary irritation are well-documented following smoking of marijuana. Although short-term inhalation has been found to increase bronchodilation and to reduce bronchospasm in asthmatics, long-term administration impairs lung function. Chronic use may result in constrictive lung disease such as interstitial fibrosis. In one study comparing the adverse effects of marijuana and tobacco, smoking less than one marijuana cigarette a day diminished vital capacity as much as smoking 16 tobacco cigarettes.[21] A later report also evaluating marijuana and tobacco smoke, finds that the gas-phase cytotoxins that are present may have no cytotoxic potential when inhaled by humans.[22]

Various types of marijuana may contain up to 50% more polyaromatic hydrocarbons in its smoke than tobacco does, high levels of which are associated with susceptibility to bronchial carcinoma. Marijuana appears to be frequently contaminated with aspergillus mold. In one study, 11 of 12 samples tested were contaminated. Spores of aspergillus pass readily through marijuana cigarettes into smoke,[23] and can result in fungal sensitization.[24] This is important in light of the use of marijuana by immunocompromised patients. Paraquat (a herbicide sprayed to control marijuana growth) toxicity was identified several years ago, but does not appear to be a clinically important problem.[25]

Neoplastic effects: Mouse skin painted with marijuana smoke particles produced metaplasia of the sebaceous glands. In another study, tobacco tar applied to the skin of mice was more carcinogenic than marijuana tar. Bronchial biopsies from humans have identified atypical cells, basal cell hyperplasia and squamous cell metaplasia to the greatest degree in subjects who used both marijuana and tobacco.[19]

Psychomotor/CNS effects: Marijuana intoxication impairs reaction time, motor coordination and visual perception. Marijuana can produce panic reactions, "flashbacks" and other emotional disturbances for which children and adolescents appear to be at highest risk. Distortion of time and distance and visual and auditory hallucinations have been reported.[1] Marijuana's high potential for abuse explains its classification as a schedule I drug under the jurisdiction of the Controlled Substances Act.[26] Humans and other species prefer higher doses (over lower doses) with many drugs of abuse. Subjects choose high-potency marijuana (1.95% THC) more than low-potency (0.63% THC), linking the drug's abuse liability to the content.[27] "Drug liking" and higher THC dose choice in marijuana cigarettes over placebo has similarly been reported.[28]

A structural relationship has been identified between cannabidiol and phenytoin, suggesting that cannabidiol meets the steriochemical requirements suggested for anticonvulsant drug action.[29] At least one report suggests that marijuana smoking can assist in the control of epileptic seizures;[30] however, marijuana use has also been shown to exacerbate grand mal convulsions.[31] THC has induced catalepsy (abnormal maintenance of posture associated with mental state) in mice, but cannabis oil and related cannabinoids have not.[32]

Endocrine effects: Long-term use of marijuana in females may cause abnormal menstruation, including anovulatory cycles. Fetal damage has been reported in animals and appears to occur in humans. THC mediates the secretion of pituitary gonadotropins. In ovariectomized rats, injected THC in relatively low doses suppressed the release of leuteinizing hormone by up to 68%.[33] In males, conflicting data have been reported regarding the lowering of testosterone levels. Although reduced sperm counts have been reported in controlled trials, these are probably less important than the development of sperm structural abnormalities and motility changes induced by marijuana.

Ocular effects: Increased conjunctival vascular congestion is a common feature of marijuana use. Marijuana and THC have been investigated for the reduction of intraocular pressure in glaucoma. Although some studies indicate that the drug is effective, it is not clear whether treatment preserves visual function.[32]

Antiemetic effects: Considerable attention has been given to the evaluation of THC as an antiemetic agent. THC administered as oral capsules appears to be at least as effective as prochlorperazine but may have more CNS side effects. THC is effective in patients refractory to other agents and the drug appears to be particularly useful against the effects of high-dose methotrexate, BCNU (carmustine) or radiotherapy. Only nine cases of serious adverse effects caused by THC therapy were reported in 1565 patients who received THC treatment. These have ranged from agitation and panic to seizure and tachycardia. One analog, nabilone (*Cesamet*) has been found to be effective but may be difficult to use clinically because of the potential for accumulation.[8] Several publications in the popular press have shown that there is a continued conflict between marijuana's schedule I status vs the rights of physicians to prescribe it for medical purposes.

Miscellaneous effects: Marijuana has been associated with xerostomia, nausea and vomiting. The cannabinoids are highly allergenic when evaluated in the guinea pig.[35] Some fractions of marijuana may have trypanocidal effects,[36] and immune system effects.[37]

SUMMARY: Marijuana has been used in traditional medicine for more than 4,000 years. Today it is most widely known as a psychoactive drug. Marijuana's many effects include cardiovascular, pulmonary, neoplastic, CNS, endocrine, ocular and antiemetic. Although more than 400 compounds have been identified in the plant, none of these have been found to have sufficient therapeutic efficacy to warrant a major role in modern therapy. Continued controversy on this point may change its status in the future.

PATIENT INFORMATION – Marijuana

Uses: Marijuana appears to be medicinally useful as an antiemetic, but its potential for abuse has so far outweighed proposals for its use as a therapeutic agent.

Side effects: Marijuana can be harmful to the heart, lungs, brain, endocrine system and eyes. It also has a strong potential for abuse and is classified as a schedule I drug.

---

[1] Allen LV. *US Pharmacist* April:64, 1978.
[2] Nahas G. Marijuana Deceptive Weed. New York: Raven Press, 1973.
[3] Duke J. CRC Handbook of Medicinal Herbs. Boca Raton, FL: CRC Press, 1989;96–97.
[4] Fehr K, et al. Cannabis and Health Hazards. Toronto, Canada: Alcoholism and Drug Addiction Research Foundation, 1983.
[5] Mason AP, et al. *J Forensic Sci* 1985;30;615.
[6] Yamamoto I, et al. *Pharmacol Biochem Behav* 1991;40(3):465–69.
[7] Sakakibara I, et al. *Phytochemistry* 1995;38(4):1003–7.
[8] Earhart RH, et al. *Wisc Med J* 1980;79:47.
[9] Harvey D. *J Ethnopharm* 1990;28(1):117–28.
[10] Kaa E. *Zeitschrift fur Rechtsmedizin* 1989;102(6):367–75.
[11] Pitts J, et al. *J Pharm Pharmacol* 1990;42(12):817–20.
[12] Hanus L, et al. *Acta Univ Palacki Olomuc Fac Med* 1989;122:11–23.
[13] Lercher G, et al. *Farmaco* 1992;47(3):367–78.
[14] Debruyne D, et al. *Bull Narc* 1994;46(2):109–21.
[15] Petri G, et al. *Acta Pharm Hung* 1995;65(3):63–67.
[16] Gillan R, et al. *Science and Justice* 1995;35(3):169–77.
[17] Hindin R, et al. *Int J Addict* 1994;29(6):771–89.
[18] Samperiz S, et al. *Archives de Pediatrie* 1996;3(5):440–44.
[19] Council on Scientific Affairs. *JAMA* 1981;246:1823.
[20] Reynolds ES. *Texas Med* 1983;79:42.
[21] Tashkin DP, et al. *Am Rev Resp Dis* 1978;117:261 (Council on Scientific Affairs).
[22] Huber G, et al. *Pharm Biochem Behav* 1991;40(3):629–36.
[23] Kagen SL. *N Engl J Med* 1981;304:483.
[24] Kagen SL, et al. *J All Clin Immunol* 1983;71:389.
[25] Lardrigan PJ, et al. *A J Publ Health* 1983;73:784.
[26] Gennaro A, ed. Laws governing pharmacy. *Remington's Pharmaceutical Sciences* 19th ed. Easton, PA: Mack Publishing Co., 1995;1900.
[27] Chait L, et al. *Pharmacol Biochem Behav* 1994;49(3):643–47.
[28] Kelly T, et al. *J Exp Anal Behav* 1994;61(2):203–11.
[29] Meyer AY. *J Med Chem* 1980;23:221.
[30] Conroe PF, et al. *JAMA* 1975;234:306.
[31] Keeler MH et al. *Dis Nerv Sys* 1967;28:474.
[32] Formukong E, et al. *J Pharm Pharmacol* 1988;40(2):132–34.
[33] Tyrey L. *J Pharmacol Exp Ther* 1980;213:306.
[34] *JAMA* 1979;242:1962.
[35] Watson ES, et al. *J Pharm Sci* 1983;72:954.
[36] Nok A, et al. *Vet Hum Toxicol* 1994;36(6):522–24.
[37] Pross S, et al. *Dev Comp Immunol* 1990;14(1):131–37.

Mastic

SCIENTIFIC NAME(S): *Pistacia lentiscus* L. Fam. Anacardiaceae

COMMON NAME(S): Mastic, mastick (tree), mastix, mastich, lentisk

BOTANY: Mastic is collected from an evergreen, dioecious shrub, which can grow to ≈ 3 m in height. It is native to the Mediterranean region, primarily in the Greek Island of Chios. Its leaves are green, leather-like, and oval. The small flowers grow in clusters and are reddish to green. The fruit is an orange-red drupe that ripens to black.

Mastic is "tapped" from the tree from June to August by making numerous, longitudinal gouges in the bark. An oleoresin exudes and hardens into an oval tear shape, about the size of a pea (3 mm). The transparent, yellow-green resin is collected every 15 days. If chewed, it becomes "plastic," with a balsamic/turpentine-like odor and taste. A related species is *P. vera*, the pistachio nut.[1-6]

Mastic resembles the resin "sanderach" (obtained from *Tetraclinis articulata*), without the chewable "plastic" qualities of mastic.[4,5]

HISTORY: Mastic resin was used in ancient Egypt as incense and to embalm the dead.[3,7] It has also been used as a preservative and a breath sweetener.[7] Mastic oil was mentioned by Dioskourides in ancient Grecian times and by Christopher Columbus in 1493.[8] Mastic resin is still used as a flavoring in some Greek alcoholic beverages (eg, "retsina" wine) and in chewing gum from the island of Chios.

CHEMISTRY: Mastic is an oleoresin containing ≈ 2% volatile oil.[2,4] The resin contains alpha and beta masticoresins, masticin, mastic acid, masticoresene, and tannins.[3] It is a complex mixture of tri-, tetra-, and pentacyclic triterpene acids and alcohols.[9] Reports of certain fractions from the plant include polymer fraction isolation/characterization,[10,11] and acidic triterpenic fractions of mastic gum.[12]

The essential oil component in mastic contains > 70 compounds, some of the primary constituents being alpha-pinene, myrcene, caryophyllene, beta-pinene, linalool, and germacrene D.[13-17] A later report lists certain percentages of essential oils from galls and aerial parts of the plant, such as sequiterpene hydrocarbons (47%), beta-caryophyllene (13%), and cadinene (8%).[18] Essential oil composition in this species *P. lentiscus* differs from region to region. Reports on this topic from the areas of

Chios,[19] Egypt,[20] and Corsica[21] are available. Changes in essential oil chemical composition in mastic also differ with solidification and storage[22] and with the time of year samples are taken.[23] Chemical composition of various parts of the plant are discussed, including leaves, fruits, and aerial parts.[24-27] Lipids in the bark of *P. lentiscus* are also addressed.[28]

PHARMACOLOGY: The pharmacology and use of mastic is diverse. Mastic's role in improving benign gastric ulcers is discussed.[29] A double-blind clinical trial in 38 patients with duodenal ulcers given 1 g mastic daily (vs placebo) proved to exhibit ulcer healing effects.[30] A report in rats proposed antisecretory and cytoprotective effects of mastic.[31] A letter in the *New England Journal of Medicine* discusses these studies, as well as others, concluding that 1 g of mastic daily for 2 weeks can cure peptic ulcer rapidly. Its antibacterial actions against *Helicobacter pylori* may explain, in part, these beneficial effects.[32]

Mastic's antibacterial effects have been shown in other reports as well. It has actions against gram-positive and gram-negative strains;[33] some organisms include *Sarcina lutea*, *Staphylococcus aureus*, and *Escherichia coli*.[34] Mastic also possesses significant antifungal actions. The growth of the fungi *Candida albicans*, *C. parapsilosis*, *Torulopsis glabrata*, and *Trichophyton* sp. have all been inhibited by mastic.[34,35]

Various reports are available discussing miscellaneous uses and effects of mastic, including use as a drug-release vehicle,[36] improvement of adhesive strength in surgical tapes,[37-39] and aromatherapy.[7] Mastic has also been reported to be useful in the area of dentistry as a tooth cement and in reducing plaque.[2,8] It can also be used as a flavoring agent, perfume additive,[5] chewed as a gum, or used to retouch photographic negatives.[2] Mastic is also reported to possess some hypotensive effects,[10,40] as well as antioxidant actions because of tocopherol content.[41-43] Effects on blood lipids by mastic have been reported.[44] An herbal mixture including mastic was effective in treating diabetic rats.[45] Mastic as an insecticide has proven to be effective.[46] Other uses include the following: To improve circulation, for muscle aches, bronchial problems,[3,5] as skin care for cuts, and as an insect repellant.[5]

TOXICOLOGY: Most toxicity regarding mastic or source *P. lentiscus* involves allergic reactions. The plant pollen is a major source for allergic reactions.[47,48,49] The first report of immunological reactions to pollen extracts of *Pistacia* genus occurred in 1987.[47] A monographic review on mastic discussing chemistry, pharmacology, and toxicity is available.[50] Children ingesting mastic may develop diarrhea.[51]

SUMMARY: Mastic has been used as far back as ancient Egyptian times to embalm the dead. It is an oleo-resin with "plastic" characteristics. Although few studies have been conducted, the use of mastic is widely varied and includes treatment of ulcer disease, antibacterial and antifungal effects, and use in dentistry. Allergic reactions are the most frequently reported toxicity of the plant. Mastic chewing gum is available in some Greek grocery stores usually imported from the island of Chios.

PATIENT INFORMATION – Mastic

Uses: Mastic has been used as a flavoring and a breath sweetener. It has also been studied for the treatment of ulcers. Mastic may also have antibacterial, antihypertensive, antioxidant, and cytoprotective effects.

Side Effects: Allergic reactions have occurred.

---

1 Youngken H. Textbook of Pharmacognosy. 6th ed. Philadelphia, PA: The Blakiston Company, 1950:535-36.

2 Budavari S, et al, eds. The Merck Index. 11th ed. Rahway, NJ: Merck & Co., Inc., 1989:92.

3 Chevallier A. The Encyclopedia of Medicinal Plants. New York, NY: DK Publishing, 1996:249.

4 Evans W. Trease and Evans' Pharmacognosy. 14th ed. Philadelphia, PA: WB Saunders Company Ltd, 1996:290-91.

5 Lawless J. The Illustrated Encyclopedia of Essential Oils. Rockport, MA: Element Books, 1995:203.

6 www.britannica.com

7 www.herbnet.com/magazine/mag0003_p04.htm

8 www.forthnet.gr/mastic/masticoil.htm

9 Marner F, et al. Triterpenoids from gum mastic, the resin of *Pistacia lentiscus*. *Phytochemistry* 1991;30(11):3709-12.

10 Sanz M, et al. Isolation and hypotensive activity of a polymeric procyanidin fraction from *Pistacia lentiscus* L. *Pharmazie* 1992;47(6):466-67.

11 van den Berg K, et al. Cis-1,4-poly-β-myrcene; the structure of the polymeric fraction of mastic resin (*Pistacia lentiscus* L) elucidated. *Tetrahedron Lett* 1998;39(17):2645-48.

12 Papageorgiou V, et al. Gas chromatographic-mass spectroscopic analysis of the acidic triterpenic fraction of mastic gum. *J Chromatogr* 1997;769(2):263-73.

13 Calabro G, et al. Constituents of essential oils. IV. Essence of lentiscus (*Pistacia lentiscus*). *Atti - Conv Naz Olii Essenz Sui Deriv Agrum* 1974:1-2, 8-18.

14 Calabro G, et al. Essential oil constituents. IV. Essence of lentisc. *Essenze Deriv Agrum* 1974;44(2):82-92.

15 Papageorgiou V, et al. GLC-MS computer analysis of the essential oil of mastic gum. *Chem Chron* 1981;10(1):119-23.

16 Papageorgiou V, et al. The chemical composition of the essential oil of mastic gum. *J Essent Oil Res* 1991;3(2):107-10.

17 Magiatis P, et al. Chemical composition and antimicrobial activity of the essential oils of *Pistacia lentiscus* var. chia. *Planta Med* 1999;65(8):749-52.

18 Fernandez A, et al. Composition of the essential oils from galls and aerial parts of *Pistacia lentiscus* L. *J Essent Oil Res* 2000;12(1):19-23.

19 Katsiotis S, et al. Qualitative and quantitative GLC analysis of the essential oil of *Pistacia lentiscus* (Mastix) from different districts of the Chios Island. *Epistm Ekdosis* 1984;10(1):17-28.

20 De Pooter H, et al. Essential oils from the leaves of three *Pistacia* species grown in Egypt. *Flavour Fragrance J* 1991;6(3):229-32.

21 Castola V, et al. Analysis of the chemical composition of essential oil of *Pistacia lentiscus* L. from Corsica. *EPPOS* 1996;7(Spec Num):558-63.

22 Papanicolaou D, et al. Changes in chemical composition of the essential oil of Chios "mastic resin" from *Pistacia lentiscus* var. Chia tree during solidification and storage. *Dev Food Sci* 1995;37A:303-10.

23 Medina Carnicer M, et al. The Mediterranean shrubby vegetation. X. Evolution of chemical composition of *Pistacia lentiscus* L. (Lentisco). *Arch Zootec* 1979;28(110):105-09.

24 Boelens M, et al. Chemical composition of the essential oils from the gum and from various parts of *Pistacia lentiscus* L. (mastic gum tree). *Flavour Fragrance J* 1991;6(4):271-75.

25 Fleisher Z, et al. Volatiles of the mastic tree —*Pistacia lentiscus* L. aromatic plants of the Holy Land and the Sinai. Part X. *J Essent Oil Res* 1992;4(6):663-65.

26 Wyllie S, et al. Volatile components of the fruit of *Pistacia lentiscus*. *J Food Sci* 1990;55(5):1325-26.

27 Bonsignore L, et al. GC-MS and GC-FTIR analysis of the volatile fraction of *Pistacia lentiscus* L. aerial parts. *Boll Chim Farm* 1998;137(11):476-79.

28 Diamantoglou S, et al. The lipid content and fatty acid composition of barks and leaves of *Pistacia lentiscus, Pistacia terebinthus* and *Pistacia vera* during a year. *Z Pflanzenphysiol* 1979;93(3):219-28.

29 Huwez F, et al. Mastic in treatment of benign gastric ulcers. *Gastroenterol Jpn* 1986;21(3):273-4.

30 Al Habbal M, et al. A double-blind controlled clinical trial of mastic and placebo in the treatment of duodenal ulcer. *Clin Exp Pharmacol Physiol* 1984;11(5):541-44.

31 Al-Said M, et al. Evaluation of mastic, a crude drug obtained from *Pistacia lentiscus* for gastric and duodenal anti-ulcer activity. *J Ethnopharmacol* 1986;15(3):271-78.

32 Huwez F, et al. Mastic gum kills *Helicobacter pylori*. *N Engl J Med* 1993;339(26):1946.

33 Tassou C, et al. Antimicrobial activity of the essential oil of mastic gum (*Pistacia lentiscus* var. chia) on gram positive and gram negative bacteria in broth and in model food system. *Int Biodeterior Biodegrad* 1995;36(3/4):411-20.

34 Iauk L, et al. In vitro antimicrobial activity of *Pistacia lentiscus* L. extracts: Preliminary report. *J Chemother* 1996;8(3):207-09.

35 Ali-Shtayeh M, et al. Antifungal activity of plant extracts against dermatophytes. *Mycoses* 1999;42(11-12):665-72.

36 Georgarakis M, et al. Microencapsulation of potassium chloride with mastic. *Pharmazie* 1987;42(7):455-6.

37 Mikhail G, et al. Reinforcement of surgical adhesive strips. *J Dermatol Surg Oncol* 1986;12(9):904-5, 908.

38 Mikhail G, et al. The efficacy of adhesives in the application of wound dressings. *J Burn Care Rehabil* 1989;10(3):216-19.

39 Lesesne C. The postoperative use of wound adhesives. Gum mastic versus benzoin USP. *J Dermatol Surg Oncol* 1992;18(11):990.

40 Sanz M, et al. Pharmacological actions of a new procyanidin polymer from *Pistacia lentiscus* L. *Pharmazie* 1993;48(2):152-53.

41 Abdel-Rahman A, et al. Mastich as an antioxidant. *J Am Oil Chem Soc* 1975;52(10):423.

42 Abdel-Rahman, A. Mastich and olibanum as antioxidants. *Grasas Aceites (Seville)* 1976;27(3):175-77.

43 Cerrati C, et al. α-Tocopherol, a major antioxidant in Mediterranean plants. *Sostanze Grasse* 1992;69(6):317-20.

44 Bamboi G, et al. Total blood lipids and lipoproteins in sheep fed *Pistacia lentiscus* drupe. *Boll Soc Ital Biol Sper* 1988;64(1):93-99. [Italian.]

45 Eskander E, et al. Hypoglycemic effect of a herbal formulation in alloxan induced diabetic rats. *Egypt J Pharm Sci* 1995;36(1-6):253-70.

46 Pascual-Villalobos M, et al. Screening for anti-insect activity in Mediterranean plants. *Ind Crops Prod* 1998;8(3):183-94.

47 Keynan N, et al. Positive skin tests to pollen extracts of four species of *Pistacia* in Israel. *Clin Allergy* 1987;17(3):243-49.

48 Cvitanovic S, et al. Hypersensitivity to pollen allergens on the Adriatic coast. *J Investig Allergol Clin Immunol* 1994;4(2):96-100.

49 Keynan N, et al. Allergenicity of the pollen of *Pistacia*. *Allergy* 1997;52(3):323-30.

50 Ford R, et al. Mastic absolute. *Food Chem Toxicol* 1992;30(Suppl):71S-72S.

Maté

SCIENTIFIC NAME(S): *Ilex paraguariensis* (St. Hill.) Family: Aquifoliaceae

COMMON NAME(S): Maté, yerba maté, Paraguay tea, St. Bartholomew's tea, Jesuit's tea

BOTANY: Maté itself is a beverage, rather than a plant. It is prepared from the leathery leaves of *Ilex paraguariensis*, a species of holly. The genus *Ilex* includes over 400 species of trees and shrubs, many of which are used as ornamentals. They have alternate, simple leaves and single or clustered small berries that may be red, black or yellow. *Ilex* species require a relatively wet, moderate climate and are found worldwide except in polar regions. *I. paraguariensis* is found in Central and South America. The leaves (harvested from May to September) are dried, then powdered to produce the tea. Maté has a faintly aromatic smell and the flavor is astringent and smoky.[1]

HISTORY: Yerba maté was used as a beverage by ancient Indians in Brazil and Paraguay; however, *I. paraguariensis* was first cultivated by Jesuit missionaries. Consumption of maté is common in Brazil south of the Amazon and in Paraguay and Argentina. In those areas, the beverage largely replaces coffee and tea. Preparations are also available in the United States, where they are sold in health food stores. Traditionally, yerba maté is served in a small gourd called a maté. It is drunk through a drinking tube, or bombilla, also with a filter attached to the lower end to prevent consumption of the leaf fragments. Leaves are prepared for use by plunging them briefly into hot water, drying them in a brick oven and fragmenting them. The beverage is prepared by putting a little hot water and some sugar in the gourd. The leaves are then placed in a gourd, then the gourd is filled with boiling water. Burnt sugar, lemon juice or milk may be used to flavor the infusion.[2]

CHEMISTRY: Yerba maté contains phenylpropanoids, including caffetannin, that yield caffeic acid when hydrolyzed, chlorogenic acid, neochlorogenic acid and isochlorogenic acid. The fruits of *I. paraguariensis* contain the anthocyanins cyanidin-3–xylosylglucoside and cyanidin-3–glucoside. The leaves contain rutin. Other components of the leaves include alpha-amyrin, trigonelline, choline and ursolic acid. Maté has been shown to contain sterols resembling cholesterol and ergosterol.[3] In one report, xanthines present in the dried leaf portion using HPLC analysis include 0.56% caffeine, 0.03% theobromine and 0.02% theopylline. A typical amount of caffeine in an average "maté-round" is approximately 100 mg.[4] More

than 15 amino acids are present in the leaves. Oil from the seeds contains lauric, palmitic, arachidic, stearic, palmitoleic, oleic and linoleic acids.[3] A small amount of essential oil and a resin fraction are also present in the plant.[1] Carbohydrates include sucrose, raffinose, glucose and levulose.[3] In 1989, a new saponin, "matésaponin" from *Ilex Paraguayensis* (St. Hill) leaves was isolated.[5] Vitamins and carotenoids present in maté include vitamins C, B_1 and B_5, nicotinic acid and carotene.[3] Analysis of elements present in maté show high content of K, Mg and Mn. Other elements present include Na, Ca, Cu, Fe and Zn.[6] Another report compares yerba maté with *mangifera indica* (mango) and discusses evidence of it being an adulterant.[7]

Chemistry-related research is also being performed on related Ilex species including: studies on the chemical constituents of *I. cornuta*,[8] saponin isolation and identification of *I. pseudobuxus*,[9] *I. taubertiana*[10] and *I. pubescens*,[11] isolation and identification of new p=coumaroyl triterpenes from *I. asprella*,[12] isolation and identification of *I. chinensis* sims[13,14] and *I. rotunda* thunb.[15] Further chemical studies include: xanthine alkaloid constituents of *I. dumosal*, *I. diuretica* and *I. glazoviana*,[16] high caffeine concentration and ritualistic use of *I. guayusa*,[17] proof by thin-layer chromatography and other methods of theobromine presence in *I. perado* AIT.,[18] comparison of flavonoids on six "Australsouthamerican" species of Ilex,[19] and natural constituents and uses of Ilex species.[3]

PHARMACOLOGY: Yerba maté has traditionally been used as a **depurative** (to promote cleansing and excretion of waste), a **stimulant** and **diuretic**.[3] Because of its caffeine content, maté is used as a centrally acting stimulant. A German monograph lists its uses for mental and physical fatigue, having "analeptic, diuretic, positively inotropic, positively chronotropic, glycogenolytic and lipolytic" effects.[1] In patients given maté infusion for 7 days, theophylline was found as a metabolic product of caffeine. After a week, theophylline levels in blood averaged 1.1 mcg/mL.[20] It is reported that in colonial times, some South Americans consumed a diet consisting almost exclusively of meat. The absence of vitamin deficiencies has been attributed to the vitamins present in the widely consumed yerba maté.[3]

Other Ilex species being evaluated include *I. asprella* as an antitumor agent[12] and *I. kudingcha* as a hypotensive agent in animals.[21]

TOXICOLOGY: A Uruguayan case-control study of 226 patients with esophageal cancer and 469 controls showed that heavy use of yerba maté was associated with a significant increase in the risk of esophageal cancer. Among heavy users, the relative risk was 6.5 for men and 34.6 for women. The risk for men was increased synergistically by alcohol consumption and tobacco smoking, but this increase was not evident among women. The increase in cancer risk was dose-dependent for men and women. It has been speculated that carcinogenesis may be cause by tannins (maté contains 7%-14% tannin) or the high temperature of the beverage. Another factor may be the presence of phenanthrene derivatives such as 1,2–benzpyrene.[22] Because of the caffeine content, teas made from this plant should be used with caution by persons with high blood pressure, diabetes or ulcer disease.

Pyrrolizidine alkaloids were recovered from a contaminant in a maté tea sample of a woman who drank the tea for years. The consumption of such large amounts over time was associated with her hepatic disease.[23]

Seven cases of anticholinergic poisoning (some later reversed by physostigmine) occurred within 2 hours of ingestion of a tea labeled commercially as "Paraguay tea." It was found that not *Ilex paraguariensis* itself, but a contaminant containing belladonna alkaloids caused the ill effects. This plant was evidently misidentified as *I. paraguariensis* at harvest and was an isolated incident in these reported cases.[24]

For further toxicology information on other related Ilex species, refer to the "holly" monograph.

SUMMARY: Yerba maté is a beverage made from an infusion of the dried leaves of *Ilex paraguariensis*. It contains many types of compounds with nutritional value and has been used as a depurative, stimulant and diuretic. Among many people in Central and South America, it replaces coffee and tea as a common beverage. Maté has been associated with esophageal cancer and liver disease. Its related species, the "holly" *Ilex aquifolium*, *I. opaca* and *I. vomitoria* are poisonous.

PATIENT INFORMATION – Maté

Uses: Yerba maté has been traditionally used as a stimulant, diuretic and depurative. It is a caffeine- and vitamin-containing beverage that also acts as a centrally-acting stimulant.

Side Effects: Heavy use can increase risk of esophageal cancer, especially in women.

---

[1] Bisset, N. Herbal Drugs and Phytopharmaceuticals, CRC Press, Stuttgart, Germany 1994;319–21.
[2] Hart FL & Fisher HJ. Modern Food Analysis. New York: Springer-Verlag, 1971.
[3] Alikaridis F. *Journal of Ethnopharmacology* 1987;20(Jul):121–44.
[4] Vazquez A, et al. *Journal of Ethnopharmacology* 1986;18(Dec);267–72.
[5] Gosmann G, et al. *Journal of Natural Products* 1989:52(Nov-Dec):1367–70.
[6] Tenorio-Sanz M, et al. *Arch Latinoam Nutr* 1991;41(3):441–54.
[7] Amat A. *Acta Farmaceutica Bonaerense* 1991;19(Jan-Apr):9–13.
[8] Qin W, et al. *Chin Tradit Herbal Drugs* 1988;19(Oct):434–9.
[9] Taketa A, et al. *Acta Farmaceutica Bonaerense* 1944;13(Sep-Dec):159–64.
[10] Cardoso Taketa A, et al. *Revisita Brasileira de Farmacia* 1995;76(Jun-Mar):9–11.
[11] Jiang Z, et al. *Chin Tradit Herbal Drugs* 1991;22(Jul):291–4.

[12] Kashiwada Y, et al. *Journal of Natural Products* 1993;56(Dec):2077–82.
[13] Zhao H, et al. *Chunci-Kuo Chung Yao Tsa Chin* 1993;18(4):226–8.
[14] Yang S, et al. *Acta Pharmaceutica Sinica* 1981;16(Jul):530–4.
[15] Wen D, et al. *Chin Tradit Herbal Drugs* 1991;22(Jun):246–8.
[16] Bohinc P, et al. *Acta Pharm Jugosl* 1978;28(2):55–60.
[17] Lewis W, et al. *Journal of Ethnopharmacology* 1991;33(1–2):25–30.
[18] Bohinc P, et al. *Planta Medica* 1975;28(Dec):374–8.
[19] Riccio R. *Acta Farmaceutica BonAerense* 1991;10(Jan-Apr):29–35.
[20] Pausse H, et al. *Acta Farmaceutica BonAerense* 1991;10(May-Aug):73–7.
[21] Chen Y, et al. *Chinese Tradit Herbal Drugs* 1995;26(May):250–2.
[22] Vassalo A, et al. *JNCI* 1985;75:1005.
[23] McGee J, et al. *J Clin Patitol* 1976;29(9):788–94.
[24] Anonymous. *MMWR-Morbidity & Mortality Weekly Report* 1995;44(11):193–5.

Meadowsweet

SCIENTIFIC NAME(S): *Filipendula ulmaria* L. Maxim., *Spiraea ulmaria* L. Family: Rosaceae

COMMON NAME(S): Meadowsweet, queen of the meadow, dropwort, bridewort, lady of the meadow

BOTANY: Meadowsweet is a herbaceous perennial shrub growing up to 2 m tall. The plant is native to Europe but also grows in North America, preferring damp, moist soil. The erect stem is red-marbled and hollow. The toothed leaves are dark green in color. Meadowsweet's aromatic, ornamental wildflowers are creamy, yellow-white, and contain 5 petals. The flowers are 5 mm in length and have an aroma reminiscent of oil of winter-green. The dried herb consists of flower petals and some unopened buds, which are the parts used as the drug.[1-8]

HISTORY: In 1597, Gerard mentioned how the smell of meadowsweet "delighteth the senses." In 1652, Culpeper wrote about the plant's therapeutic effects on the stomach.[5] In 1682, meadowsweet was mentioned in a Dutch herbal. Holland called the plant "*Filipendula*," while in the rest of Europe, it was known as "*Spiraea*." Queen Elizabeth I adorned her apartments with meadowsweet. The flowers were used to flavor alcoholic beverages in England and Scandinavian countries.[8] In the Middle Ages, meadowsweet was known as "meadwort" because it was used to flavor "mead," an alcoholic drink made by fermenting honey and fruit juices.[5]

In 1838, salicylic acid was isolated from the plant. In the 1890s, salicylic acid was first synthesized to make aspirin.[5] "Aspirin" is derived from "spirin," based on meadowsweet's scientific name, "*Spiraea*."[8]

The plant was used in folk medicine for cancer, tumors, rheumatism, and as a diuretic.[4,7] Today, it is used as a digestive remedy, as supportive therapy for colds, for analgesia, and other indications.

CHEMISTRY: Flavonoids in meadowsweet include the flavonol glycosides rutin, hyperin, and spiraeoside.[1] Spiraeoside has been evaluated in the plant's flowers.[9] Glycoside spiraein (salicylaldehyde primveroside) is present, as are phenol glycosides including gaultherin.[2,8] A phenolic glycoside from meadowsweet flowers has been reported.[10] Quercetin and kaempferol derivatives have also been found in the plant, and hyperoside is present as well, primarily in the leaves and stalks.[1] A report is available on 7 flavonoids isolated from meadowsweet flowers, fruits, leaves, and stalks.[11]

Constituents in meadowsweet also include hexahydroxydiphenic acid esters of glucose and tannins, 10% to 20%.[1,5,7,8] One report finds tannin content to be high compared with other rosaceae species.[12]

The essential oil contains primarily salicylaldehyde (75%), as well as phenylethyl alcohol, benzyl alcohol, anisaldehyde, methyl salicylate, salicin, gaultherin, spiraein, spiraeoside, heliotropin, phenyl acetate, and vanillin.[1,3,4]

Salicylates in the plant include salicylic aldehyde, salicylic acid, salicin, methyl salicylate, and others.[1,3,4,7] HPLC and TLC screening for meadowsweet salicylates has been performed.[13]

Meadowsweet flowers contain heparin, which binds to the plant's proteins, forming a complex.[14] Heparin isolated from meadowsweet shows some similarity to heparin of animal origin.[15]

Other constituents in meadowsweet include mucilage, carbohydrates, ascorbic acid, sugars, and minerals.[3,8]

Phytochemical study of meadowsweet is available.[16]

PHARMACOLOGY: Meadowsweet is used for supportive therapy in colds, probably because of its analgesic, anti-inflammatory, and antipyretic actions.[1,2,6,8] The roots have been used to treat respiratory problems such as hoarseness, cough, and wheezing.[4]

The plant is also useful as a digestive remedy for acid indigestion or peptic ulcers. It protects the inner lining of the stomach while providing the anti-inflammatory benefits of salicylates.[5] A reduction in ulcerogenic action has been documented in rats, promoting the healing of (induced) chronic ulcers and preventing ASA-induced lesions in the stomach.[17] However, meadowsweet also has been reported to potentiate ulcerogenic properties in animals.[3]

Because joint problems may be related to increased acid, the ability of meadowsweet to reduce acidity is also beneficial in treating joint problems.[5] It has also been mentioned that meadowsweet improves the condition of connective tissue of joints.[8] In folk medicine, meadowsweet was used for rheumatism of muscles and joints, and for arthritis.[1]

A heparin-plant protein complex was found to have anticoagulant and fibrinolytic properties.[15] Meadowsweet flowers and seeds demonstrated an increased level of anticoagulant activity in vitro and in vivo in another report.[18] In vitro complement inhibition from the plant's flowers has been studied.[19]

Bacteriostatic activity from meadowsweet flower extracts include actions against *Staphylococcus aureus*, *S. epidermidis*, *Escherichia coli*, *Proteus vulgaris*, and *Pseudomonas aeruginosa*.[3] The salicylic acid in the plant is a known disinfectant used to treat ailments such as skin diseases.[4] Meadowsweet is also a urinary antiseptic, the mechanism of action being its close relation to phenol.[8]

The tannins in the plant possess astringent properties. Root preparations have been used in the treatment of diarrhea.[3,4]

Local administration of a meadowsweet decoction resulted in a 39% decrease in the frequency of induced squamous-cell carcinoma of the cervix and vagina in mice; 67% of patients had a positive response.[20]

Meadowsweet has been used as a sedative and to soothe nerves.[4] Reduction of motor activity and potentiation of narcotic action has also been observed in animals given the herb.[3]

Meadowsweet had no effect on glycemic control when studied in mice for treatment of diabetes.[21]

TOXICOLOGY: The German Commission E Monographs lists no known side effects, contraindications (except those with salicylate sensitivity), or drug interactions with use of meadowsweet.[2] The FDA has classified the plant as an "herb of undefined safety."[4]

Use caution because of the toxicity profile of salicylates. Methyl salicylate can be absorbed through the skin, resulting in fatalities, especially in children.[3,4]

Bronchospasm has also been documented from use of the plant; therefore, use caution in asthmatics. Uteroactivity has also been observed from meadowsweet, warranting avoidance during pregnancy and lactation.[3]

SUMMARY: Meadowsweet is an herb that has been used for centuries and has been granted "approved" status by the German Commission E. It contains salicylate derivatives, which make it useful for analgesia. The plant has been used for cold therapy, GI disturbances, and joint problems. It also possesses bacteriostatic actions and antitumor activity. Few toxic events have been reported.

PATIENT INFORMATION – Meadowsweet

Uses: Meadowsweet has been used for colds and respiratory problems, acid indigestion or peptic ulcers, joint problems, skin diseases, and diarrhea.

Side Effects: Few toxic events have been reported. Do not use in patients with salicylate or sulfite sensitivity, and use caution in asthmatics.

---

[1] Bisset N. Herbal Drugs and Phytopharmceuticals. Stuttgart, Germany: CRC Press, 1994;480-82.

[2] Blumenthal M, ed. The Complete German Commission E Monographs. Boston, MA: American Botanical Council, 1998;169.

[3] Newall C, et al. Herbal Medicines. London, England: Pharmaceutical Press, 1996;191-92.

[4] Duke J. CRC Handbook of Medicinal Herbs. Boca Raton, FL: CRC Press Inc., 1989;196-97.

[5] Chevallier A. Encyclopedia of Medicinal Plants. New York, NY: DK Publishing, 1996;96.

[6] Schulz V, et al. Rational Phytotherapy. Berlin Heidelberg, Germany: Springer-Verlag, 1998;143-44.

[7] Bruneton J. Pharmacognosy, Phytochemistry, Medicinal Plants. Paris, France: Lavoisier, 1995;221-22, 316-18.

[8] Zeylstra H. Filipendula ulmaria. Br J Phytother 1998;5(1):8-12.

[9] Poukens-Renwart P, et al. Densitometric evaluation of spiraeoside after derivatization in flowers of Filipendula ulmaria (L.) Maxim. J Pharm Biomed Anal 1992;10(10-12):1085-88.

[10] Thieme H. [Isolation of a new phenolic glycoside from the blossoms of Filipendula ulmaria (L.) Maxim]. Pharmazie 1966;21(2):123.

[11] Lamaison J, et al. Principal flavonoids of aerial parts of Filipendula ulmaria (L.) Maxim. subsp. ulmaria and subsp. denudata. Pharm Acta Helv 1992;67(8):218-22.

[12] Lamaison J, et al. Tannin content and inhibiting activity of elastase in Rosaceae. Ann Pharm Fr 1990;48(6)335-40.

[13] Meier B, et al. Salicylates in plant drugs: screening methods (HPLC, TLC) for their detection. Deutsche Apotheker Zeitung 1987 Nov 12;127:2401-407.

[14] Kudriashov B, et al. The content of a heparin-like anticoagulant in the flowers of the meadowsweet. Farmakol Toksikol 1990;53(4):39-41.

[15] Kudriashov B, et al. Heparin from the meadowsweet (Filipendula ulmaria) and its properties. Izv Akad Nauk SSSR [Biol] 1991;6:939-43.

[16] Henih H, et al. Phytcchemical study of the dropworts, Filipendula ulmaria and F. nexapetala, from the flora of Lvov Province. Farmatsevtychnyi Zhurnal 1980:(1):50-52.

[17] Barnaulov O, et al. Anti-ulcer action of a decoction of the flowers of the dropwort, Filipendula ulmaria (L.) Maxim. Farmakol Toksikol. 1980;43(6):700-5.

[18] Liapina L, et al. A comparative study of the action on the hemostatic system of extracts from the flowers and seeds of the meadowsweet. Izv Akad Nauk Ser Biol 1993;(4):625-28.

[19] Halkes S, et al. Strong complement inhibitor from the flowers of Filipendula ulmaria (L.) Maxim. Pharm Pharmacol Lett 1997;7(2-3):79-82.

[20] Peresun'ko A, et al. Clinico-experimental study of using plant preparations from the flowers of Filipendula ulmaria (L.) Maxim for the treatment of precancerous changes and prevention of uterine cervical cancer. Voprosy Onkologii 1993;39(7-12):291-95.

[21] Swanston-Flatt S, et al. Evaluation of traditional plant treatments for diabetes: studies in streptozotocin diabetic mice. Acta Diabetol Latina 1989;26(1):51-55.

Melatonin

SCIENTIFIC NAME(S): *Melatonin, MEL*

COMMON NAME(S): Melatonin, MEL

HISTORY: Melatonin (MEL) is one of the hormones of the pineal gland that is also produced by extrapineal tissues. Early animal studies (mid-1960s) revealed its ability to affect sexual function, skin color and other mammalian functions. It is the mediator of photoinduced antigonadotrophic activity in photoperiodic mammals and effects thermoregulation and locomotor activity rhythms in birds. It has also been implicated in time-keeping mechanisms in the pineal gland. Beginning studies showed that diurnal variations in estrogen secretion in rats could be regulated by changes in melatonin synthesis and release, both induced reflexly by the daily cycle of light and dark via the efferent limb of the reflex in the sympathetic innervation of the pineal glad. Continual darkness depresses the estrous cycle.[1,2]

Melatonin secretion is inhibited by environmental light and stimulated by darkness, with secretion starting at 9 pm and peaking between 2 and 4 am. Nocturnal secretion of melatonin is highest in children and decreases with age.[3,4] Studies in the past decade have widely expanded the use of melatonin, in an extemporaneous manner, for easing insomnia, combating jet lag, preventing pregnancy (in large doses), protecting cells from free-radical damage, boosting the immune system, preventing cancer and even extending life.[5]

Although melatonin is not approved for marketing as a drug product, it has been classified as an orphan drug since November 1993 (Sponsor: Dr. Robert Sack, Oregon Health Sciences University)[4] for the treatment of circadian rhythm sleep disorders in blind people with no light perception. It is commercially available as a nutritional supplement either as a synthetic product or derived from animal pineal tissue. Use of the non-synthetic product should be discouraged because of an increased theoretical risk of contamination or viral trasmission. Most commercial brands are available as 300 mcg, 1.5 mg or 3 mg tablets under various names and cost approximately $10.00 for a bottle of 100. Patients should seek medical advice before undertaking therapy.

CHEMISTRY: Chemically, melaton in N-acetamide or N-acetyl-5–methoxytryptamine. It can be isolated from the pineal glands of beef cattle or can be synthesized from 5–methoxyindole as a starting material via two different routes. It is a relatively low molecular weight hormone (M.W. 232.27) and is a pale yellow crystalline material.[1]

PHARMACOLOGY: Pharmacological disruption of melatonin production can occur via beta-1 and alpha-1 receptors due to sympathetic innervation in the pineal gland. Tryptophan is converted to serotonin, the immediate precursor of melatonin.[3,4,6] Once in circulation, melatonin is metabolized in the liver with more than 85% excreted as 6–sulphatoxyMEL, a reliable marker for melatonin production. Plasma half-life is short, 20 to 50 minutes,[3,4,7] and plasma levels return to baseline levels within 24 hours after chronic dosing (< 10 mg/day) has stopped.[4,8] Melatonin doses of 5 mg produce estimated peak blood levels 25 times above physiological levels, but do not alter endogenous melatonin production.[4,8]

In the last decade, dozens of articles have appeared in the medical literature on the various purported activities of melatonin. A selected overview of the most recent studies includes melatonin's role as an antioxidant,[9] use in general health and disease,[3] hypothermic properties,[10] control of seasonality,[11] oncostatic actions on estrogen-responsive MCF-7 human breast cancer cells,[12] its effectiveness as an endogenous radical scavenger and electron donor,[13] involvement of melatonin and serotonin in winter depression,[14] effect on primary headache,[15] direct effect on the immune system,[16] activation of human monocytes,[17] role in gastrointestinal physiology,[18] function in thermoregulatory processes,[19] involvement in the cardiopulmonary system,[20] effects on puberty,[21] its place in human and animal reproduction,[22] studies on human sleep,[23] melatonin modulation of sympathetic neurotransmission,[24] possible role in infant colic,[25] possible role as proconvulsive hormone[26] and purported chronobiotic and anti-aging properties.[27,28]

Suffice it to say that it would be impossible to cover all of these properties in detail in this monograph. Not only are there too many supposed effects, but almost all of the studies are preliminary and await future verification. In the meantime, many health-food manufacturers and some pharmacies and clinics have begun to make this inexpensive hormone available for various medical and related purposes. Among the most common medical claims are entraining the blind, overcoming jet lag, helping to hasten the onset of sleep and dampening the release of estrogen. (It may diminish breast cancer rates and be useful at higher doses, 75 mg, for oral contraception.) Other common claims include its potential anti-oxidant properties (protection of liver cell damage, protection from ionizing radiation and protecting lungs from the herbicide paraquat, all in animals) and boosting the performance of the immune system, which has been diminished with age.

The FDA has not yet controlled melatonin and warns users that taking it "without any assurance that is is safe or that it will have any beneficial effect."

Blind Entrainment: The sleep wake cycle in humans without light-dark cues approximates 25 hours, causing the sleep cycle to shift by one hour each day, so that such individuals are eventually awake at night and asleep during the day. Blind persons with little or no perception of light often develop *free running* circadian rhythms > 24 hours, and subsequently develop sleep disturbances characterized by chronic fatigue and involuntary napping during the day.

In case reports and small controlled studies, oral melatonin (dosage range: 0.5 mg to 10 mg) has been used to entrain free running activity rhythms in the blind by advancing and stabilizing the phase of endogenous melatonin secretion.[4,8,29] Although success has varied in these reports, the importance of melatonin administration time has been recognized. For example, the administration of melatonin (5 mg or 10 mg for 2–4 weeks at bedtime) to an 18–year-old blind man with chronic sleep disturbances produced slightly improved sleep onset, but did not reduce daytime fatigue or hypersomnolence.[4,29]

However, the administration of melatonin (5 mg for 3 weeks) at 2 to 3 hours prior to habitual bedtime decreased sleep onset (approximately 1.4 hours), slightly increased sleep duration (34 minutes) and had a marked improvement in sleep quality and daytime alertness. The authors suggest that there is a Phase Response Curve (PRC) for the exogenous administration of melatonin; the maximum phase advancing effects occur when melatonin is administered about 6 hours prior to onset of endogenous melatonin secretion.[4,30] The average cumulative phase advancement (CPA) of melatonin rhythms after 3 weeks of treatment with 5 mg and 0.5 mg daily was 8.41 and 7 hours, respectively.[4,8]

Jet Lag: Melatonin's ability to modulate circadian rhythms has prompted several studies investigating the use of this agent in the prevention of jet lag.[4,31,32,33]

Although the effects have been variable, most patients have reported general improvement in daytime fatigue, disturbed sleep cycles, mood and recovery times. These studies are limited by the small number of participants and a focus on subjective ratings of effects with little or no evidence of actual changes in circadian shift (ie, changes in oral temperature or cortisol levels). As with entrainment studies in the blind, it appears that timing of administration and the development of optimal regimens require further study.

Several melatonin regimens have been examined (5–10 mg daily) for various durations. In one study, 52 aircraft personnel were randomized to placebo, early or late melatonin groups. The early group started melatonin (5 mg daily) 3 days before departure until 5 days after arrival.[4,32] The late group received melatonin upon arrival and for 4 additional days. When compared to placebo, the late melatonin group self-reported significantly less jet lag, fewer overall sleep disturbances and a faster recovery of energy and alertness. However, the early group (receiving melatonin for 8 days) reported jet lag symptoms similar to the placebo group and a worsened overall recovery.

Additional data from uncontrolled studies suggest that benefits were also experienced by international travelers when melatonin was given on the day or night of departure and for 2 to 3 nights after arrival.[4,31,33] (Note to travelers: Because driving skills may be affected, be aware that you may experience drowsiness within 30 minutes after taking melatonin and then lasting for about 1 hour.)

Insomnia: Although the administration of melatonin has been shown to shift melatonin secretion and circadian rhythm patterns, its direct hypnotic effect, if any, has not been clearly established. Decreased circulating melatonin serum levels have been demonstrated in insomniacs of all ages and in the healthy elderly.[3,4]

In small studies of healthy volunteers or chronic insomniacs, very large doses of melatonin (75–100 mg) administered at night (9–10 pm) have produced serum melatonin levels exceeding normal nocturnal ranges and significant hypnotic effects. These include decreases in sleep onset, fewer nighttime awakenings and increases in Stage 2 sleep and sleep efficiency (percentage of time asleep/time in bed).[4,34,35] Midday administration of large doses have also increased serum melatonin levels beyond normal nocturnal ranges, increased subjective fatigue and decreased cognitive function and vigor.[4,36]

The administration of smaller doses (0.3–5 mg) has produced inconsistent hypnotic results, but this may be due to the inclusion of patients with a variety of sleep disorders, different drug formulations and different administration times (midday to 15 minutes before bedtime).[4,37-42] The time to reach peak hypnotic effect was significantly longer when melatonin (5 mg) was administered at 12 noon vs 9 pm (3.66 hrs vs 1 hr).[4,38] Delayed latency with daytime administration may be related to the already low circulating melatonin levels during the day. Low doses (0.3 mg or 1 mg) administered to healthy volunteers at 6 pm, 8 pm or 9 pm decreased onset latency and latency to Stage 2 sleep, but did not suppress REM sleep nor induce hangover effects.

In patients with difficulty getting to sleep, low doses of melatonin should be sufficient in promoting sleep onset. However, in patients with difficulty maintaining sleep, low doses of melatonin may not produce sufficient blood concentrations to maintain slumber. A 2 mg oral melatonin dose produced peak levels approximately ten times higher than physiological levels, but it remained elevated for only 3–4 hours.[4,7] To maintain effective serum concentrations of melatonin throughout the night, a high dose, repeated low doses or a controlled release formulation may be needed. When compared to placebo in a trial of 12 elderly chronic insomniacs, melatonin significantly increased sleep efficiency (75% vs 83%) and decreased wake time after sleep onset (73 vs 49 minutes).[4,41] However, there were no significant differences between the groups for total sleep time (365 vs 360 minutes) or sleep onset (33 vs 19 minutes).

Sleep onset and sleep maintenance were improved in elderly insomniacs after 1 week of immediate (1 mg) and sustained release (2 mg) melatonin preparations. Sleep onset improved further when the sustained release form was continued for 2 months.[4,42]

Although several case reports have described the use of melatonin (2–5 mg) in children (ages: 6 mos-14 yrs), optimal dosages, safety and efficacy require further study in this age group.[4,43]

Cancer Protection: Melatonin has demonstrated some inhibitory effects on tumor growth in animal models and *in vitro* cancerous breast cells lines.[3] Proposed oncoprotective mechanisms of melatonin include stimulatory effects on circulating natural killer cells and potent antioxidant activity. Preliminary studies have examined the use of melatonin in patients with solid tumors unresponsive to standard therapies, melanoma and as adjunctive amplifier therapy with interleukin in various metastatic tumors (ie, endocrine, colorectal).[4,44-48] European studies on *B-Oval* (containing melatonin) are ongoing, but it appears to slow the growth rate of human tumor cells. A nightly supplement (10 mg of melatonin) has been shown to improve 1-year survival rates with patients having metastatic lung cancer.[3]

Well-controlled trials are needed before the role of melatonin as an oncostatic agent can be confirmed.

Oral Contraceptive: Because melatonin plays a role in the endocrine-reproductive system and reduces circulating LH, the use of melatonin as a contraceptive agent has been studied.[4,49] Melatonin, administered in various dosage combinations with a synthetic progestin in 32 women for 4 months produced significant anovulatory effects.

TOXICOLOGY: Most studies note the absence of adverse events associated with melatonin administration. Minor side effects with doses < 8 mg have included heavy head, headache and transient depression.[4,32,33] In psychiatric patients, melatonin has aggravated depressive symptoms.[3,4,6] Effects associated with long-term administration have not been studied.

Toxicological studies have shown that a LD_{50} could not be obtained even at extremely high doses. Researchers gave human volunteers 6 g (6,000 mg) of melatonin each night for a month and found no major problems, except for stomach discomfort or residual sleepiness.[5]

As is true with all new medications, however, prolonged studies are needed to verify its safety.

SUMMARY: There are numerous recent studies concerning expanding the traditional role which melatonin plays as a normal hormone in the body. These include treatment of insomnia, overcoming jet lag, use as an anti-oxidant and protective agent against certain toxins, improving the effectiveness of the immune system and even possibly preventing cancer and extending life.

Most of the recent studies show some promise in certain of these areas; however, large-scale double-blind studies are needed, particularly in the US, because of concern for potentially adverse long-term effects. Major promise is currently seen in short-term treatment of insomnia at low-dose schedules (a few milligrams) nightly.

Note: A comprehensive listing of Medline articles regarding melatonin and its various uses is available on the internet via: http://aeiveos.wa.com/diet/melatonin/

PATIENT INFORMATION – Melatonin

Uses: Melatonin is used to regulate sleep, protect against cancer, and provide a variety of other benefits.

Side Effects: Possible adverse effects include headache and depression.

---

[1] Windholz M, et al. Merch Index, 11th ed. Rahway, NJ: Merck and Co., 1989.

[2] Bowman WC, Rand MJ. Textbook of Pharmacology, 2nd ed. St. Louis: Blackwell Scientific Publications, 1980.

[3] Webb SM, Puig-Domingo M. Role of melatonin in health and disease. [Review] Clin Endocrinol 1995;42(3):221.

[4] Generali JA. Keeping Up: Melatonin. Drug Newsletter 1996;15(1):3.

[5] Cowley G. Melatonin. Newsweek 1995;Aug 7:46.

[6] Arendt J. Melatonin. Clin Endocrinol 1988;29:205.

[7] Aldhous M, et al. Plasma concentrations of melatonin in man following oral absorption of different preparations. Br J Clin Pharmacol 1985;19:517

[8] Sack RL, et al. Melatonin administration to blind people phase advances and entrainment. J Biol Rhythms 1991;6(3):249.

[9] Reiter RJ, et al. A review of the evidence supporting melatonin's role as an antioxidant. [Review] J Pineal Res 1995;18(1):1.

[10] Cagnacci A, et al. Hypothermic effect of melatonin and nocturnal core body temperature decline are reduced in aged women. J Appl Physiol 1995;78(1):314.

[11] Morgan PJ, Mercer JG. Control of seasonality by melatonin. [Review] Proc Nutr Soc 1994;53(3):483.

[12] Cos S, Blask DE. Melatonin modulates growth factor activity in MCF-7 human breast cancer cells. J Pineal Res 1994;17(1):25.

[13] Poeggeler B, et al. Melatonin–a highly potent endogenous radical scavenger and electron donor: new aspects of the oxidation chemistry of this indole accessed in vitro. Ann NY Acad Sci 1994;738:419.

[14] Partonen T. Involvement of melatonin and serotonin in winter depression. Med Hypotheses 1994;43(3):165.

[15] Leone M. Melatonin and primary headache. [Editorial comment] Cephalalgia 1994;14(3):183.

[16] Poon AM, et al. Evidence for a direct action of melatonin on the immune system. [Review] Biol Signals 1994;3(2):107.

[17] Morrey KM, et al. Activation of human monocytes by the pineal hormone melatonin. J Immunol 1994;153(6):2671.

[18] Bubenik GA, Pang SF. The role of serotonin and melatonin in gastrointestinal physiology: ontogeny, regulation of food intake and mutual serotonin-melatonin feedback. J Pineal Res 1994;16(2):91.

[19] Saarela S, Reiter RJ. Function of melatonin in thermoregulatory processes. [Review] Life Sci 1994;54(5):295.

[20] Pang CS, et al. 2–iodomelatonin binding sites in the lung and heart: a link between the photoperiodic signal, melatonin and the cardiopulmonary system. [Review] Biol Signals 1993;2(4):228.

[21] Cavallo A. Melatonin and human puberty: current perspectives. [Review] J Pineal Res 1993;15(3):115.

[22] Pevet P. [Present and future of melatonin in human and animal reproduction functions.] [Review] [French] Contraception, Fertilite, Sexualite 1993;21(10):727.

[23] Dawson D, Encel N. Melatonin and sleep in humans. [Review] J Pineal Res 1993;15(1):1.

[24] Carneiro RC, et al. Age-related changes in melatonin modulation of sympathetic neurotransmission. J Pharmacol Exp Ther 1993;266(3):1536.

[25] Weissbluth L, Weissbluth M. The photo-biochemical basis of infant colic: pineal intracellular calcium concentrations controlled by light, melatonin and serotonin. Med Hypotheses 1993;40(3):158.

[26] Sandyk R, et al. Melatonin as a proconvulsive hormone in humans. Int J Neurosci 1992;63(1–2):125.

[27] Armstrong SM, Redman JR. Melatonin: a chronobiotic with anti-aging properties? [Review] Med Hypotheses 1991;34(4):300.

[28] Reiter RJ. Pineal function during aging: attenuation of the melatonin rhythm and its neurobiological consequences. [Review] Acta Neurobiol Exp 1994;54 Suppl:31.

[29] Tzischinsky O, et al. The importance of timing in melatonin administration in a blind man. J Pineal Res 1992;12:105.

[30] Lewy AJ, et al. Melatonin shifts human circadian rhythms according to a phase response curve. Chronobiol Int 1992;9(5):380.

[31] Lino A, et al. Melatonin and jet lag: treament schedule. Biol Psychiatry 1993;34:587.

[32] Petrie K, et al. A double-blind trial of melatonin as a treatment for jet lag in international cabin crew. Biol Psychiatry 1993;33:526.

[33] Claustrat B, et al. Melatonin and jet lag: confirmatory result using a simplified protocol. Biol Psychiatry 1992;32:705.

[34] Waldhauser F, et al. Sleep laboratory investigations on hypnotic properties of melatonin. Psychopharmacol 1990;100:222.

[35] MacFarlane JG, et al. The effects of exogenous melatonin on the sleep time and daytime alertness of chronic insomniacs: a preliminary study. Biol Psychiatry 1991;30:371.

[36] Dollins AB, et al. Effect of pharmacological daytime doses of melatonin on human mood and performances. Psychopharmacol 1993;112:490.

[37] James SP, et al. Melatonin administration in insomnia. Neuropsychopharmacol 1989;3:19.

[38] Tzischinsky O, Lavie P. Melatonin possesses time-dependent hypnotic effects. Sleep 1994;17(7):638.

[39] Nave R, et al. Melatonin improves evening napping. Eur J Pharmacol 1995;275:213.

[40] Zhdanova IV, et al. Sleep inducing effects of low doses of melatonin ingested in the evening. Clin Pharmacol & Ther 1995;57:552.

[41] Garfinkel D, et al. Improvement of sleep quality in elderly people by controlled release melatonin. Lancet 1995;346:541.

[42] Haimov I, et al. Melatonin replacement therapy in elderly insomniacs. Sleep 1995;18(7):598.

[43] Jan JE, et al. The treatment of sleep disorders with melatonin. Dev Med and Child Neurol 1994;36:97.

[44] Lissoni P, et al. Clinical results with the pineal hormone melatonin in advanced cancer resistant to standard anti-tumor therapies. Oncology 1991 48:448.

[45] Zumoff B. Hormonal profiles in women with breast cancer. Obstet Gynecol Clin North Am 1994;21(4):751.

[46] Lissoni P, et al. Immunoendocrine therapy with low-dose subcutaneous interleukin-2 plus melatonin of locally advanced or metastatic endocrine tumors. Oncology 1995;52:163.

[47] Lissoni P, et al. A biological study on the efficacy of low dose subcutaneous interleukin-2 plus melatoinin in the treatment of cancer related thrombocytopenia. Oncology 1995;52:360.

[48] Barni S, et al. A radomized study of low dose subcutaneous interleukin-2 plus melatonin versus supportive care alone in metastatic colorectal cancer patients progressing under 5–fluorouracil and folates. Oncology 1995;52:243.

[49] Voordouw BCG, et al. Melatonin and melatonin-progestin combinations alter pituitary-ovarian function in women and can inhibit ovulation. J Clin Endocrinol Metab 1992;74:108.

Methylsulfonylmethane (MSM)

SCIENTIFIC NAME(S): *Methylsulfonylmethane, DMSO2*

COMMON NAME(S): MSM

SOURCE: MSM is a natural chemical in green plants such as *Equisetum arvense*, certain algae, fruits, vegetables, and grains. It is also seen in animals (eg, the adrenal cortex of cattle, human and bovine milk, and urine). MSM is naturally occurring in fresh foods; however, it is destroyed with even moderate food processing, such as heat or dehydration.[1]

HISTORY: Literature searches on MSM provide mostly animal studies. MSM has been suggested for use as a food supplement.

CHEMISTRY: MSM is the normal oxidation product of DMSO (dimethyl sulfoxide). Unlike DMSO, MSM is odor-free and is a dietary factor. MSM has been referred to as "crystalline DMSO."[2] MSM provides a source of sulfur for methionine.[1]

PHARMACOLOGY: MSM has been said to alleviate GI upset, musculoskeletal pain, arthritis, allergies, and to boost the immune system. It is also said to possess antimicrobial effects against such organisms as *Giardia lamblia*, *Trichomonas vaginalis*, and certain fungal infections. The suggested mechanism is that MSM may bind to surface receptor sites, preventing interface between parasite and host.

Tumor onset in colon cancer-induced rats was markedly delayed in animals receiving MSM supplementation vs controls, suggesting a chemopreventative effect.[3] Four percent MSM had a similar delaying effect on rat mammary breast cancer.[4]

MSM showed no effect in preventing diabetes when tested in spontaneously diabetic mice compared with DMSO or dimethylsulfide (DMS).[5]

A 10-day course of MSM also has been evaluated in 13 horses with COPD, and no changes occurred in parameters such as lung sounds, respiratory rate, heart rate, temperature, nasal discharge, or arterial blood gas.[6]

TOXICOLOGY: No important toxicities were noted in animal reports.[3,4]

SUMMARY: MSM is a natural chemical, which may be of some use for skin problems, GI upset, and certain cancers. No toxicities have been reported. Human trials are needed to fully assess MSM's therapeutic benefits.

PATIENT INFORMATION – Methylsulfonylmethane (MSM)

Uses: MSM is said to alleviate GI upset, musculoskeletal pain, arthritis, and allergies; to boost the immune system; and to possess antimicrobial effects.

Side effects: No important toxicities were noted in animal reports.

---

[1] Richmond V. Incorporation of methylsulfonylmethane sulfur into guinea pig serum proteins. *Life Sci* 1986;39(3):263-68.
[2] Bertken R. "Crystalline DMSO:" DMSO2. *Arthritis Rheum* 1983;26(5):693-94.
[3] O'Dwyer P, et al. Use of polar solvents in chemoprevention of 1,2-dimethylhydrazine-induced colon cancer. *Cancer* 1988;62(5):944-48.
[4] McCabe D, et al. Polar solvents in the chemoprevention of dimethylbenzanthracene-induced rat mammary cancer. *Archives of Surgery* 1986;121(12):1455-59.
[5] Klandorf H, et al. Dimethyl sulfoxide modulation of diabetes onset in NOD mice. *Diabetes* 1989;38(2):194-97.
[6] Traub-Dargatz J, et al. Evaluation of clinical signs of disease, bronchoalveolar and tracheal wash analysis, and arterial blood gas tensions in 13 horses with chronic obstructive pulmonary disease treated with prednisone, methyl sulfonmethane, and clenbuterol hydrochloride. *Am J Vet Res* 1992;53(10):1908-16.

Milk Thistle

SCIENTIFIC NAME(S): *Silybum marianum* (L.) Gaertn. Family: Compositae referred to in older texts as *Carduus marianus*. Recently changed to *Carduus marianum*.

COMMON NAME(S): Holy thistle, lady's thistle, marian thistle, Mary thistle, Milk thistle, St. Mary thistle, silybum

BOTANY: This plant is indigenous to Kashmir, but is found in North America from Canada to Mexico. *Silybum* grows from 5 to 10 feet and has large prickly leaves. When broken, the leaves and stems exude a milky sap. The reddish-purple flowers are ridged with sharp spines. The drug consists fo the shiny mottled black or grey-toned seeds (fruit). These make up the "thistle" portion, along with its silvery pappus, which readily falls off.[1]

HISTORY: Milk thistle was once grown in Europe as a vegetable. The de-spined leaves were used in salads and for spinach substitution; the stalks and root parts were also consumed, even the flower portion was eaten "artichoke-style." The roasted seeds were used as a coffee substitute. Various preparations of milk thistle, especially the seeds, have been used medicinally for over 2000 years. Its use as a liver protectant can be traced back to Greek references. Pliny the Elder, a first century Roman writer, (A.C. 23–79) noted that the plant's juice was excellent for "carrying off bile."[2] Culpepper (England's premier herbalist) noted milk thistle to be of use in removing obstructions of liver and spleen, and to be good against jaundice. The Eclectics (19th-20th century) used milk thistle for varicose veins, menstrual difficulty and congestion in liver, spleen and kidneys.[3]

In homeopathy, a tincture of the seeds has been used to treat liver disorders, jaundice, gall stones, peritonitis, hemorrhage, bronchitis and varicose veins.[4]

CHEMISTRY: Silymarin, a mixture of three isomeric flavonolignans, was first isolated from milk thistle seeds in 1968. Silymarin (molecular formula: $C_{25}H_{22}O_{10}$, MW 482.45, 4% to 6% in ripe fruits) consists primarily of three flavonolignans: Silybin (silibinin), silychristin (silichristin) and silidianin.[5] A review of isolation and structure of these flavonolignan components is available.[6] Silybin is the most biologically active component with regard to milk thistle's antioxidant and hepatoprotective properties. A standardized milk thistle extract composed of silymarin and silybin was developed in Europe and is known commercially as *Legalon®*.[7] Other flavonolignans include dehydrosilybin, 3–desoxysilichristin, deoxysilydianin (silymonin), siliandrin, silybinome, silyhermin and neosilyher-

min.[5] The compound 5,7–dihydroxychromone has also been isolated from *Silybum marianum*.[8] Other seed components include apigenin; silybonol, a fixed oil (16% to 18%) consisting largely of linoleic and oleic acids, plus myristic, palmitic and stearic acids; betaine hydrochloride; triamine; histamine and others.[5] From the roots of *Silybum marianum* Gaertn., twelve polyacetylenes and one polyene have been detected.[9]

Silymarin is poorly soluble in water, so aqueous preparations such as teas are ineffective, except for use as supportive treatment in gallbladder disorders because of cholagogic and spasmolytic effects.[10] The drug is best administered parenterally because of poor absorption of silymarin from the gastrointestinal tract (23% to 47%). The drug must be concentrated for oral use.[11]

Many analyses of milk thistle using different isolation techniques have been reported. The following serves as a brief listing of available information that may be helpful in this specific area of interest.

Gel absorption and column chromatography methods have been employed to investigate flavones in milk thistle;[12] constituents from aerial parts and fruits also have been analyzed;[13] betaine hydrochloride was isolated form milk thistle seeds and was analyzed by chemical and spectroscopic methods;[14] spectrophotometric assay to determine flavone lignans from milk thistle and its preparations is described;[15] a NIR reflectance spectroscopic method was capable of identifying silybum samples from different geographical locations;[16] silymarin has been analyzed by extraction in small amounts using liquid carbon dioxide (supercritical conditions) in HPLC-packed columns. The separation by this method may be useful for flavonolignan analysis;[17] solubility and bioequivalence of silymarin products has also be performed.[18]

PHARMACOLOGY: Milk thistle's therapeutic efficacy involves a variety of molecular mechanisms, although the mechanism of action is not clearly understood. Its primary activities are of use as a **hepatoprotectant** and **antioxidant**. The properties of silymarin (the extract from milk thistle seeds containing the three flavonolignans) are due mainly to its flavonolignans content.[19] Medicinal value may also be attributed in part to the presence of trace metals in the plant.[20]

Mechanisms:

1. Actions of silymarin are almost entirely on liver and kidneys. It undergoes pronounced enterohepatic circulation, which allows for a continuous loop between intestine and liver. Silymarin moves from plasma to bile and concentrates in liver cells.[3]

2. In vivo tests proving increased protein synthesis in liver cells due to increased activity of ribosomal RNA were reported in 1980 by Sonnenbichler. Silybin contains a steroid structure that stimulates DNA and RNA synthesis, resulting in activation of the regenerative capacity of the liver through cell development.[21]

3. Silymarin's hepatoprotective effects may be explained by its altering of the outer liver cell membrane structure, as to disallow entrance of toxins into the cell.[2,22] This alteration involves silymarin's ability to block the toxin's binding sites, thus, hindering uptake by the cell.[3] The poisonous Amanita mushroom studies are remarkable examples of this mechanism of action and are discussed later.

4. Hepatoprotection by silymarin can also be attributed to its antioxidant properties by scavenging prooxidant free radicals and increasing intracellular concentration of glutathione, a substance required for detoxicating reactions in liver cells.[23] Silybin also inhibits peroxidizing enzymes like lipoxygenase, thus blocking peroxidation of fatty acids and damage to membrane lipids.[24,25]

The numerous clinical studies performed on silymarin involve: Hepatoprotection from toxins and other drugs, cirrhosis and hepatitis therapies, blood and immunomodulation, lipid and biliary effects and various other effects.

Earlier clinical studies (1969–1989) of silymarin use may be accessed through reference 3. More recent and other selected reports are categorically presented below.

Hepatoprotection: Silymarin protects liver cells against many hepatotoxins in humans and animals. Some Amanitas (eg, *A. phalloides*, the death cup fungus) contain two toxins: Phalloidine, which destroys the hepatocyte cell membrane and alpha-amanatine, which reaches the cell nucleus and inhibits polymerase-b activity, thereby blocking protein synthesis. Silymarin is capable of negating

both of these effects by blocking the toxin's binding sites, increasing the regenerative capacity of liver cells and blocking enterohepatic circulation of the toxin.[3] In one study, 60 patients with severe Amanita poisoning were treated with infusions of 20 mg/kg of silybin with good results. Although the death rate following this type of mushroom poisoning can exceed 50%, none of the patients treated in this series died.[26] In a clinical trial of 205 patients with Amanita toxicity, 46 patients died; however, all 16 patients who received silybin survived.[27] Administration of silybin within 48 hours of ingestion at a dose of 20 to 50 mg/kg/day was an effective prophylactic measure against severe liver damage.[28] A multicenter trial performed in European hospitals between 1979 and 1982 was conducted using silybin in supportive treatment of 220 Amanita poisoning cases. A 12.8% mortality rate was reported.[29] The death rate using other modern supportive measures such as activated charcoal can be 40%.[3] Silymarin alone or in combination with penicillin reduced death rates from ingestion of death cup fungus to 10%.[30]

In addition to mushroom toxin protection, silymarin also offers liver protection against tetracycline-induced lesions in rats,[31] d-galactosamine-induced toxicity,[32] thallium-induced liver damage[33] and erythromycin estolate, amitriptyline, nortriptyline and tert-butylhydroperoxide hepatotoxin exposure of neonatal hepatocyte cell cultures.[34] In a later Italian double-blind, placebo controlled report, silymarin was elevated in 60 women on long-term phenothiazine or butyrophenone therapy. Results suggested that silymarin treatment can reduce lipoperoxidative hepatic damage caused by chronic use of these psychotropic drugs.[35]

Studies on silymarin's liver-protective effects continue to show it protects against carbon tetrachloride (CCl_4)-induced liver cirrhosis in animals and prevents increases in lipid peroxidation by this toxin, among other beneficial alterations.[36,37,38] When injected intravenously in rats and dogs, silymarin has been shown to protect liver destruction following injection with frog virus-3 (a lethal hepatotoxic virus). Although Kupffer cells were injured, the compound protected endothelial cells form destruction, primarily by inhibiting the release or synthesis of hepatotoxic enzymes.[39] Biologically equivalent activities of silybinin at doses of 30 mg/kg are discussed in another report.[40] Cisplatin, (an anti-cancer drug) toxic to nephrons, was injected in rats to induce renal damage for evaluation of silybin's protective effects in the kidney. Using tubular morphology, observation, proteinuria presence, etc, it was found that silybin could be beneficial in this area as well.[41] Specific evaluations of silymarin's mechanism of plasma membrane stability have been reported.[35,42] There is no evidence yet reported on liver enzyme P450 2E1 involvement in the hepatoprotective mechanism of silymarin.[43]

Cirrhosis: Silymarin's mechanisms offer many types of therapeutic benefit in cirrhosis with the main benefit being hepatoprotection. Use of milk thistle, however, is inadvisable in decompensated cirrhosis.[44]

In two one-month, double-blind studies performed on an average of 50 patients with alcoholic cirrhosis treated with silymarin, elevated liver enzyme levels (AST, ALT) and serum bilirubin levels were normalized. It also reduced high levels of gamma-glutamyl transferase, increased lectin-induced lymphoblast transformation and produced other changes not seen in the placebo group.[45,46,47] A report on free-radical scavenger activity of silymarin suggested that hepatoprotection could be due to antioxidant activity.[48] Similar results were obtained in another double-blind study evaluating a six-month treatment at 420 mg/day of silymarin (*Legalon*®).[49] A 41–month double-blind study performed in 170 patients with alcoholic cirrhosis indicated silymarin to be effective in treatment as well.[50] Silymarin ameliorated indices of cytolysis in a study also using ursodeoxycholic acid in active cirrhosis patients.[51] One study, providing contrasting evidence, suggested no change in evolution or mortality of alcoholic liver disease as compared with placebo in a controlled trial of 72 patients using 280 mg/day of silymarin.[52]

Hepatitis: In patients with acute viral hepatitis, silymarin shortened treatment time and showed improvement in serum levels of bilirubin, AST and ALT.[53,54] Biochemical values returned to normal sooner in silymarin-treated patients.[55] Histological improvement was seen in patients with chronic hepatitis vs placebo in another controlled trial.[56]

In a 116–patient double-blind study of silymarin vs placebo, silymarin 420 mg/day given to histologically-proven alcoholic hepatitis patients was shown not to be clinically useful in treating this disease.[57] A later report suggests stable remission in a 6– to 12–month Russian study evaluating treatment of chronic persistent hepatitis.[44] In 20 chronic active hepatitis patients given 240 mg of silybin twice daily vs placebo, improved liver function tests related to hepatocellular necrosis was reported.[58] A Bulgarian report evaluated two silymarin preparations, *Carsil*® and *Legalon*®, in treatment of various hepatitis types. The preparations did not differ much from each other.[59]

Blood and Immunomodulation: Silymarin's immunomodulatory activity in liver disease patients may also be involved in its hepatoprotective action.[60] Silybin can in-

crease activity of superoxide dismutase and glutathione peroxidase, which may also explain its protective effects against free radicals.[61] Silymarin had an anti-inflammatory effect on human blood platelets.[62] Silybin may have anti-allergic activity. Its effect on histamine release from human basophils was reversed and may be due to membrane stabilizing activity.[63] Silybin inhibition of human T-lymphocyte activation is also reported.[64] In vitro effects of silybin on human polymorpho-nuclear leukocyte (PMN) have been reported. Inhibition of hydrogen peroxide may be a mechanism by which silybin inhibits luminol-enhanced chemiluminescence (a biochemical technique) generated by stimulated PMNs.[65] Another report on PMN activity showed silybin to be effective in enhancing spontaneous motility of leukocytes.[66] Prolonged application of silymarin preparations improved immunity by increasing T-lymphoctyes and reducing all classes of immunoglobulins.[44]

Lipid and Biliary Effects: Administration of silymarin 420 mg/day for 3 months to 14 type II hyperlipidemic patients resulted in slightly decreased total cholesterol and HDL-cholesterol levels.[67] Biliary cholesterol and phospho-lipid concentrations in rats were also slightly reduced. Silybin-induced reduction of biliary cholesterol both in rats and humans may be due in part to decreased liver cholesterol synthesis.[68] An anti-aggregant effect of silymarin in cholesterol atherosclerosis in rabbits was also reported.[69]

Biliary excretion of silybin was evaluated by HPLC. Bioavailability of silybin is greater after silipide (a lipophilic silybin-phosphatidylcholine complex) administration than after silymarin administration; therefore, increased delivery of silipide to the liver results.[70] Pharmacokinetics of silybin have also been evaluated in patients with cholestasis.[71] Use of silymarin prevents disturbance of bile secretion, thereby increasing bile secretion, cholate excretion and bilirubin excretion.[44]

Various Other Effects: Silybin and silymarin have also been evaluated (including case reports) in diabetes patients for possible value in prophylaxis of diabetic complications,[72] in combination therapy to treat aged skin[13] and in oral treatment for prevention of ulceration in rats, both by reduction of neutrophils in gastric mucosa and inhibition of mechanisms of enzymatic peroxidation, thus, avoiding leukotriene synthesis.[74,75] Traditional uses of milk thistle include stimulation of milk production in nursing mothers and antidepressant therapy.[19] Other uses include steroide secretory modulation[76] and as therapy of acute promyelocytic leukemia.[77]

Indications for milk thistle are for any liver-based problems such as cirrhosis, jaundice, alcohol abuse, etc. At risk for liver toxins are those exposed to such pollutants as pesticides or heavy metals. Certain occupations such as those of painters, farmers, chemical workers and those in polluted urban environments are all associated with high risk.[3,78]

Extracts, tablets or capsules (35 to 70 mg) standardized to 70% silymarin are available as commercial preparations in average daily doses of 200 to 400 mg.[5]

TOXICOLOGY: Human studies performed with silymarin have shown little need for concern with adverse effects.[19] Tolerability of silymarin is good; only brief disturbances of GI function and mild allergic reactions have been observed, but rarely enough to discontinue treatment.[44] Mild laxative effects in isolated cases have been reported.[7] A case of urticaria with a foreign commercial milk thistle preparation has been noted in a Russian report.[79]

Silymarin has proved nontoxic in rats and mice after oral doses of 2500 or 5000 mg/kg were given without producing symptoms. In a 12–month study, rats received silymarin 50, 500 and 2500 mg/kg. Investigations including urine analysis and post-mortem studies showed no evidence of toxicity. A similar report in dogs was also performed. No evidence of ante- or postnatal toxicity in animals was reported, nor did silymarin affect fertility in rats.[25]

SUMMARY: Milk thistle extract and its major components have been found to be effective in treating toxin-poisoning, cirrhosis and hepatitis. Although data regarding usefulness in the treatment or prevention of alcoholic cirrhosis and hepatitis are equivocal. It also plays a role in blood and immunomodulation, lipid and biliary effects among others. Silymarin's mechanisms are due mainly to its flavonolignan content and involve hepatoprotection, increased regenerative capacity of liver cell turnover, the alteration of cell membranes preventing toxin uptake and scavenging free radicals, thus, limiting liver damage. Human studies with silymarin have shown few adverse effects. Milk thistle shows great promise and has been used medicinally for over 2000 years. It is widely used in Europe for Amanita mushroom poisoning treatment.

PATIENT INFORMATION – Milk Thistle

Uses: Treatment and protection against Amanita mushroom poisoning, reduced liver damage due to long-term treatment with phenothiazine or butyrophenone therapy. Data regarding protection against alcoholic cirrhosis and hepatitis are equivocal. It shortened treatment time in patients with acute viral hepatitis, had an anti-inflammatory effect on human platelets, and slightly decreased total and HDL-cholesterol levels.

Side Effects: Few adverse effects have been seen other than brief GI disturbances and mild allergic reactions; possible urticaria in one patient.

---

[1] Bisset N. Herbal Drugs and Phytopharmaceuticals, CRC Press, London 1994;121–3.
[2] Foster S. Milke thistle-*Silybum marianum*, Botanical Series No. 305. American Botanical Council, Austin, TX 1991;3–7.
[3] Hobbs C. Milk Thistle: The Liver Herb, 2nd ed., Botanica Press, Capitola, CA 1992;1–32.
[4] Schauenberg P, Paris F. Guide to Medicinal Plants, Keats Publishing, New Canaan, CT. 1974.
[5] Leung A, et al. Encyclopedia of Common Natural Ingredients Used in Food, Drugs and Cosmetics. John Wiley & Sons, Inc. New York, NY 1996;366–68.
[6] Morelli I. *Boll Chim Farm* 1978;117(May):258–67.
[7] Brown D. *Drug Store News for the Pharmacist* 1994;4(Nov):58, 60.
[8] Szilagi I, et al. *Planta Medica* 1981;43(Oct):121–7.
[9] Schulte K, et al. *Arch Pharm* 1970;303(Jan):7–17.
[10] Grauds C. *Pharmacy Times* 1996;62(Mar):95.
[11] Tyler V. *Herbalgram* 1994;30:24–30.
[12] Halback G, et al. *Planta Medica* 1971;19(Apr):293–8.
[13] Khafagy S, et al. *Scientia Pharmaceutica* 1981;49(Jun 30):157–61.
[14] Varma P, et al. *Planta Medica* 1980;38(Apr):377–8.
[15] Szilajtis-Obieglo R, et al. *Herba Polonica* 1984;30(1):27–34.
[16] Corti P, et al. *Int J Crude Drug Res* 1990;28(Sep):185–95.
[17] Martinez F. *Ann Pharm Fr* 1989;47(3):162–8.
[18] Schulz H, et al. *Arzneimittel-Forschung* 1995;45(1):61–4.
[19] Awang D. *Can Pharm J* 1993;(Oct):403–4.
[20] Parmar V, et al. *Int J Pharmacognosy* 1993;31(4):324–6.
[21] Sonnenbichler J, et al. Proceedings of the International Bioflavonoid Symposium (Munich, Frg) 1981;477.
[22] Floersheim GL. *Medical Toxicology* 1987;2:1.
[23] Valenzuela A, et al. *Biological Research* 1994;27(2):105–12.
[24] Rui Y. Mem Inst Oswaldo Cruz. 1991;86(Suppl)2:79–85.
[25] Legalon® Booklet, Madaus AG, D-5000 Koln, West Germany 91, 1989;3–42.
[26] Vogel G, Proceeding of the International Bioflavonoid Symposium, Munich 1981.
[27] Floersheim GL, et al. *Schweiz med Wochenschr* 1982;112:1164.
[28] Hruby, et al. *Hum Toxicol* 1983;2:183.
[29] Hruby K. *Forum* 1984;6:23–26.
[30] Hruby K. *Intensivmed* 1987;24:269–74.
[31] Skakun N, et al. *Antibiot Meditsin Biotekh* 1986;31(10):781–4.
[32] Tyutyulkova N, et al. *Methods Find Exp Clin Pharmacol* 1981;3:71.
[33] Mourelle M, et al. *J Appl Toxicol* 1988;8(5):351–4.
[34] Davila J, et al *Toxicology* 1989;57(3):267–86.
[35] Palasciano G, et al. *Curr Ther Res* 1994;55(5):537–45.
[36] Mourelle M, et al. *Fundam Clin Pharmacol* 1989;3(3):183–91.
[37] Letteron P, et al. *Biochem Pharmacol* 1990;39(12):2027–34.
[38] Muriel P, et al. *J Appl Toxicol* 1990;10(4):275–9.
[39] Condrault JL, et al. *Planta Medica* 1989;39:247.
[40] Skakun N, et al. *Farmatsiia* 1987;36(6):13–17.
[41] Gaedeke J, et al. *Nephrol Dial Transplant* 1996;11(1):55–62.
[42] Feher J, et al. *Acta Physiol Hung* 1989;73(2–3):285–91.
[43] Miguez M, et al. *Chem Biol Interact* 1994;91(1):51–63.
[44] Rumyantseva Z. *Vrach Delo* 1991;(5):15–19.
[45] Lang I, et al. *Acta Med Hung* 1988;45(3–4):287–95.
[46] Lang I, et al. *Tokai J Exp Clin Med* 1990;15(2–3):123–7.
[47] Lang I, et al. *Ital J Gastroenterol* 1990;22(5):283–7.
[48] Lang I, et al. *Acta Med Hung* 1988;45(3–4):265–76.
[49] Muzes G, et al. *Orv Hetil* 1990;131(16):863–6.
[50] Ferenci P, et al. *J Hepatol* 1989;9(1):105–13.
[51] Lirussi F, et al. *Acta Physiol Hung* 1992;80(1–4):363–7.

[52] Bunout D, et al. *Rev Med Chil* 1992;120(12):1370–5.
[53] Magliulo E, et al. *Med Klin* 1978;73:1060–65.
[54] Cavalieri S. *Gazz Med Ital* 1974;133:628.
[55] Wilhelm H, et al. *Wien Med Wochenschr* 1973;123:302.
[56] Kriesewetter E, et al. *Leber Magen Darm* 1977;7:318–23.
[57] Trinchet J, et al. *Gastroenterol Clin Biol* 1989;13(2):120–4.
[58] Buzzelli G, et al. *Int J Clin Pharmacol Ther Toxicol* 1993;31(9):456–60.
[59] Brailski K, et al. *Vutr Boles* 1986;25(3):43–9
[60] Deak G, et al. *Orv Hetil* 1990;131(24):1291–2, 1295–6.
[61] Altorjay I, et al. *Acta Physiol Hung* 1992;80(1–4):375–80.
[62] Max B. *Trends Pharmacol Sci* 1986;7(Nov):435–7.
[63] Miadonna A, et al. *Br J Clin Pharmacol* 1987;24(6):747–52.
[64] Meroni P, et al. *Int J Tissue React* 1988;10(3):177–81.
[65] Minonzio F, et al. *Int J Tissue React* 1988;10(4):223–31.
[66] Kalmar L, et al. *Agents Actions* 1990;29(3–4):239–46.
[67] Somogyi A, et al. *Acta Med Hung* 1989;46(4):289–95.
[68] Nassuato G, et al. *J Hepatol* 1991;12(3):290–5.
[69] Falchi M, et al. *Drug Exp Clin Res* 1983;9(6):419–22.
[70] Schandalik R, et al. *Arzneimittel-Forschung* 1992;42(7):964–8.
[71] Schandalik R, et al. *Drugs Exp Clin Res* 1994;20(1):37–42.
[72] Zhang J, et al. *Chung-Kuo Chung Hsi I Chieh Ho Tsa Chih* 1993;13(12):725–6, 708.
[73] Esteve M, et al. *Parfuemerie und Kosmetik* 1991;72(Dec:92), 822, 824, 826, 828–9.
[74] Alarcon de la Lastra C, et al. *J Pharm Pharmacol* 1992;44(11):929–31.
[75] Alarcon de la Lastra C, et al. *Planta Medica* 1995;61(2):116–9.
[76] Racz K, et al. *J Endocrinol* 1990;124(2):341–5.
[77] Invernizzi R, et al. *Haematologica* 1993;78(5):340–1.
[78] Morazzoni P, Bombardelli E. *Fitoterapia* 1995;66(1):3–42.
[79] Mironets V, et al. *Vrach Delo* 1990;(7):86–7.

Mistletoe

SCIENTIFIC NAME(S): *Phoradendron serotinum* (Raf.) M.C. Johnston, *P. flavescens* (Pursh) Nuttal, *P. tomentosum* (DC) Englem., *Viscum album* L. Family: Loranthaceae

COMMON NAME(S): Mistletoe, Bird Lime, All Heal, Devil's Fuge, Golden Bough[1,2]

BOTANY: The mistletoes are generally grouped into two broad descriptive classes, the American mistletoe that comprises the *Phoradendron* species and the European mistletoes *V. album* and the related species *V. abietis* and *V. austriacum*. All mistletoes are semi-parasitic woody perennials commonly found growing on oaks and other deciduous trees. These evergreen plants produce small white berries and are used as Christmas ornaments. These plants should not be confused with the New Zealand mistletoe (*Ileostylus micranthus*), which contains cytotoxic compounds that may be derived from the host tree (Podocarpus totara).[3]

HISTORY: Early pagan custom required hanging mistletoe to inspire passion during the pagan holiday of "Hoeul." Today's custom of kissing under the plant is a mellowed version of this event. The European mistletoe has been used for centuries in traditional medicine and gained wide popularity in the early 1900s as an anticancer treatment.[4]

CHEMISTRY: All parts of the plant contain appreciable amounts of beta-phenylethylamine, tyramine and structurally related compounds. The stems and leaves of both *Phoradendron* and *V. album* contain chemically similar toxic proteins designated phoratoxins and viscotoxins respectively.[5] The amino acid sequence of these proteins has been elucidated, and each has been found to contain 46 amino acid residues with several cystine bridges.[4] A toxic lectin called "viscumin" and related compounds occur in minute quantities in mistletoe.[6] The human toxicity of this compound, especially after oral ingestion, is unknown[7,8] but appears to be comparable to that of the toxic lectins abrin and ricin. A tumor-reducing component in mistletoe extract has been isolated and identified as a peptide of approximate molecular weight 5000.[9]

PHARMACOLOGY: Despite the popular wisdom that the two types of mistletoe have opposite pharmacologic effects (ie, American mistletoe: Stimulates smooth muscle, raises blood pressure, increases uterine and intestinal motility; European mistletoe: Reduces blood pressure, antispasmodic, calming agent) investigations have shown that the stems and leaves of these plants contain the chemically related phoratoxins and viscotox-ins and thus exert similar pharmacologic effects. These compounds produce dose-dependent hypertension or hypotension,[10] bradycardia and increased uterine and intestinal motility,[11] and have been found to produce the same effects in animals as the injection of cardiotoxin from cobra venom—depolarization of skeletal muscle, contraction of smooth muscle, vasoconstriction and cardiac arrest.[12,13] The irreversible depolarization observed in experimental isolated muscle preparations appears to be reversible by the presence of calcium.[13]

A proteinaceous component of *V. album* had been shown to possess antineoplastic activity in vitro.[14] The phoratoxins and viscotoxins are cytotoxic and, along with several other lectins, account for the anticancer activity of the plant.[15] The regular subcutaneous injection of the beta-galactoside-specific lectin from mistletoe extract reduced the number of lung and liver tumors in two experimental models in mice.[16] This activity appears to be in part due to stimulation by lymphokines of enzymes that repair damaged DNA.[17] The lectins increase the secretion of tumor necrosis factor, interleukin-1 and interleukin-6 both in vitro and in man.[18] At least one published report has found that a patient with small cell lung carcinoma responded well to therapy and lived for more than 5 years following subsequent radiotherapy.[19]

TOXICOLOGY: All parts of mistletoe, including the berries and leaves, should be regarded as toxic and symptomatic treatment should be instituted rapidly. Symptoms of human toxicity include nausea, bradycardia, gastroenteritis, hypertension, delirium and hallucinations. Diarrhea and vomiting may lead to serious dehydration. Vasoconstriction and cardiac arrest may occur. Rapid gastric emptying has been suggested even if as few as one or two berries have been ingested.[11] However, a comprehensive analysis of more than 300 reported cases of mistletoe ingestion in the United States found that the majority of patients remained asymptomatic and no deaths occurred. These data lead to the conclusion that ingestion of up to three berries or two leaves is unlikely to produce serious toxicity.[20]

A case of hepatitis following the ingestion of an herbal-compound containing mistletoe has been reported,[21] but other investigators have suggested that based on the lack of documented hepatic toxicity of the components of mistletoe, the reported toxic effect was more likely due to an adulterant.[22] Cases of death have been reported following the ingestion of teas brewed from these plants for use as a tonic or abortifacient.[23,24] A case of allergic rhinitis has been reported in a subject involved in the handling of commercial mistletoe tea (*V. album*).[25]

SUMMARY: The mistletoes are generally grouped as American mistletoe and European mistletoe. Despite its well-known potential for toxicity, mistletoe continues to find its way into herbal remedies. The FDA classifies mistletoe as a food additive that cannot be marketed unless proven safe for consumption and has withheld from sale and destroyed commercial capsules containing the plant.[26] Several components of the plant have been found to possess antineoplastic activity and should be investigated further for their clinical potential.

PATIENT INFORMATION – Mistletoe

Uses: Mistletoe has been used in traditional medicine and as cancer treatment. It has been shown to be hyper- and hypotensive, to increase uterine and intestinal motility, and to have antineoplastic effects.

Side Effects: Mistletoe is acutely toxic and may cause cardiac arrest.

---

[1] Dobelis IN, ed. The Magic and Medicine of Plants. Pleasantville, NY: Readers Digest Association, 1986.
[2] Meyer JE. The Herbalist. Hammond, IN: Hammond Book Co., 1934.
[3] Bloor SJ, Molloy BP. Cytotoxic norditerpene Lactones from *Ileostylus micranthus. J Nat Prod* 1991;54:1326.
[4] Lecompte JTJ, et al. *Biochemistry* 1987;26:1187.
[5] Tyler VE, et al. Pharmacognosy, 8th ed, Philadelphia, PA: Lea and Febiger, 1981.
[6] Holstkog R, et al. *Oncology* 1988;45:172.
[7] Stirpe F. *Lancet* 1983;i(8319):295.
[8] Olsnes S, et al. *J Biol Chem* 1982;257:13263.
[9] Kuttan G, et al. Isolation and identification of a tumour reducing component from mistletoe extract (Iscador). *Cancer Lett* 1988;41:307.
[10] Fukunaga T, et al. *J Pharm Soc Japan* 1989;109:600.
[11] Mack RB. *North Carolina Med J* 1984;45:791.
[12] Andersson KE, Johannson M. *Eur J Pharmacol* 1973;23:223.
[13] Sauviat MP. *Toxicon* 1990;28:83.
[14] Vester F, Nienhaus J. *Experientia* 1965;21:197.
[15] Jung ML, et al. *Cancer Lett* 1990;51:103.
[16] Beuth J. Influence of treatment with the immunomodulatory effective dose of the beta-galactoside-specific lectin from mistletoe on tumor colinization in BALB/c-mice for two experimental model systems. *In vivo* 1991;5:29.
[17] Kovacs E, et al. Improvement of DNA repair in lymphocytes of breast cancer patients treated with Viscum album extract (Iscador). *Eur J Cancer* 1991;27:1672.
[18] Hajto T, et al. *Cancer Research* 1990;50:3322.
[19] Bradley GW, Clover A. *Thorax* 1989;44:1047.
[20] Hall AH, et al. *Ann Emerg Med* 1986;15:1320.
[21] Harvey J, Colin-Jones DG. *Br Med J* 1981;282:186.
[22] Farnsworth N, Loeb WD. *Br Med J* 1981;283:1058.
[23] Cann HM, Verhulst. *Nat Clearinghouse for Poison Control Centers Bulletin* Dec. 1, 1959.
[24] Moore HW. *South Carolina Med Assn* 1963;59:269.
[25] Seidemann W. *Allergologie* 1984;7:461.
[26] *FDA Consumer* 1981;Dec-Jan:36.

Monascus

SCIENTIFIC NAME(S): *Monascus purpureus* Went

COMMON NAME(S): Monascus, ZhiTai, XueZhiKang (China)

HISTORY: Red yeast dates back to 800 AD, where it was described in the ancient Chinese pharmacopeia (published during the Ming Dynasty, 1368–1644). It is a mild, non-poisonous yeast useful for gastric problems such as indigestion, as well as circulation. *Monascus purpureus* yeast is made by a fermentation process using cooked, non-glutinous rice.

CHEMISTRY: The commercial product contains 0.4% naturally occurring HMG-CoA reductase inhibitors, of which lovastatin and biologically active hydroxy-acids are most abundant.[1]

Monascidin A, another constituent of monascus, has been characterized as citrinin by qualitative methods, mass spectra and NMR.[2]

PHARMACOLOGY: The particular inhibitor found in the yeast, competitively inhibits 3-hydroxy-3-methyl-glutaryl-coenzyme A (HMG-CoA) reductase, which is the enzyme that catalyzes HMG-CoA to mevalonate and then to cholesterol. The result of this is **decreased LDL- and VLDL-cholesterol** and **plasma triglycerides**. HDL-cholesterol ("good cholesterol") is increased, which is beneficial to release free cholesterol from extrahepatic tissues.[3,4]

In the late 1970s, it was discovered that monascus metabolites **inhibited HMG-CoA reductase**, the rate-limiting step in cholesterol biosynthesis.[5] ZhiTai (0.25% HMG-CoA reductase inhibitors) and XueZhiKang (the ethanolic extract containing 1.1% HMG-CoA reductase inhibitors) have both been extensively studied in China. Monascus contains both of these.[1] XueZhiKang, in three separate animal studies, was effective in reducing serum cholesterol levels, similar to lovastatin (an HMG-CoA reductase inhibitor available commercially as the prescription drug, *Mevacor* by Merck). XueZhiKang was also found to suppress aortic atherosclerotic plaque formation and lipid accumulation in the animal livers. The dose of 0.4 and 0.8 g/kg in one report reduced serum cholesterol levels by 44% and 59%, respectively.[6]

Seventeen Chinese studies (some unpublished) are available evaluating monascus. One major randomized multicenter trial involved 446 hyperlipidemic patients with cholesterol levels greater than 230 mg/dl. At the end of an 8 week treatment, total serum cholesterol was reduced 23% (average), triglycerides were reduced by 36.5%, LDL-cholesterol was reduced by 28.5% and HDL-cholesterol levels were increased by 19.6%.[7] *Cholestin* product literature recommends its use as a dietary supplement, combined with diet and exercise in healthy men and women, under a physician's care, who are concerned with maintaining desirable cholesterol levels. Although results of the studies appear promising, they have not been evaluated by the Food and Drug Administration and therefore are not intended to "diagnose, treat, cure or prevent any disease."[1]

TOXICOLOGY: Citrinin, produced by *Monascus purpureus* and *Monascus ruber*, is nephrotoxic.[2]

Toxicity studies on monascus show no adverse reactions at doses much greater than typical dosing in both long- and short-term studies. In rats fed monascus 50 times the human dose, results showed no abnormalities in areas such as behavior, blood and urine testing. In human trials, some reported slight digestive tract discomfort.[1,8] The product is not recommended for patients with liver disease. One to two percent of HMG-CoA reductase users in general experience hepatotoxicity and myopathy.[1,8]

SUMMARY: *Monascus purpureus* Went is a yeast developed by a fermentation process. It has recently been evaluated for its cholesterol-lowering effects and has been found to inhibit HMG-CoA reductase, a step in the synthesis of cholesterol. Chinese studies are available, but monascus has not been adequately investigated in the US. The FDA has not evaluated any claims for the product but is investigating whether it should be considered a drug or a dietary supplement. Results from about 20 studies offer promising therapy for hyperlipidemic patients. More research is needed to further evaluate the yeast's effects. Toxicity studies are also needed.

PATIENT INFORMATION – Monascus

Uses: Monascus, marketed as *Cholestin*, has been recommended as a dietary supplement combined with diet and exercise in healthy men and women, under physician care, concerned with maintaining desirable cholesterol levels.

Side effects: Some patients have reported slight digestive tract discomfort. Not recommended for use in patients with liver disease.

---

[1] Gurr J, et al. Scientific product review (of cholestin), Pharmanex. Simi Valley, CA. (800–999–6229) 1997:1–6.

[2] Blanc P, et al. *Int J Food Microbiol* 1995;27(2–3):201–13.

[3] Olin BR, Hebel SK, eds. Drug Facts and Comparisons. St. Louis, MO: Facts and Comparisons, 1997.

[4] Katcher, Young and Koda-Kimble, eds. Applied Therapeutics, 3rd ed. Spokane, WA: Applied Therapeutics Inc. 1987;651–52.

[5] Endo A. *J Antibiot* 1979;32:852–54.

[6] Zhu Y, et al. *Chin J Pharmacol* 1995;30(11):4–8.

[7] Wang et al. *Chin J Exp Ther Prepar Chin Med* 1995;1(1):1–5.

[8] Various informational literature available from Pharmanex. Simi Valley, CA (800–999–6229).

Morinda

SCIENTIFIC NAME(S): *Morinda citrifolia*

COMMON NAME(S): Morinda, noni, hog apple, Indian mulberry, mengkoedoe, mora de la India, pain killer, ruibarbo caribe, wild pine

BOTANY: The morinda plant, native to Asia, Australia and Polynesia (eg, Tahiti), is a 3 to 8 m high tree or shrub. Its evergreen leaves are oblong and 10 to 45 cm in length. The plant's white flowers are tubular, with conelike heads. The fruit is yellow-white in color, oval in shape, about the size of a potato and has a "bumpy" surface. The ripened fruit has a characteristic cheese-like, offensive odor. Each fruit contains 4 seeds, 3 mm in length.[1]

HISTORY: It is believed that Polynesian healers have used morinda fruits for thousands of years to help treat a variety of health problems such as diabetes, high blood pressure, arthritis and aging. Ancient healing manuscripts cite the fruit as a primary ingredient in natural healing formulations. Today, fruit preparations are sold as juice, in dried "fruit-leather" form and as a dry extract in capsules. US patents can also be found, including such patents as processing morinda fruit into powder,[2] and for xeronine, an alkaloid isolated for medical, food and industrial use.[3]

CHEMISTRY: *Morinda citrifolia* fruits contain essential oils with hexoic and octoic acids, paraffin and esters of ethyl and methyl alcohols.[1] Ripe fruit contains n-caproic acid, presumably responsible for its distinctive odor, known to attract insects such as drosophilia sechellia.[4] Fresh plants contain anthraquinones, morindone and alizarin.[1] A new anthraquinone glycoside from morinda heartwood has recently been described.[5] Hawaiian researcher Ralph Heinicke discovered a small plant alkaloid he termed "xeronine."[3] Damnacanthal, morindone and alizarin are present in cell suspension cultures.[1]

PHARMACOLOGY: *Morinda citrifolia* has been used medicinally for heart remedies, arthritis (by wrapping the leaves around affected joints), headache (local application of leaves on forehead), GI and liver ailments.[1]

It has been theorized that xeronine works at a molecular level to repair damaged cells, regulating their function. It is claimed that all body cells and systems, including digestive, respiratory, bone and skin can benefit.[2]

An overview of traditional applications of the plant in Samoan culture is available.[6]

Morinda has been evaluated for its anticancer activity on Lewis lung carcinoma in mice. It increased lifespan repeatedly in different batches of mice, all yielding similar results. The proposed mechanism is enhancement of the immune system, with macrophage and lymphocyte involvement.[7]

Damnacanthal from *M. citrifolia* root induced normal morphology and cytoskeletal structure in Kirsten-ras Normal Rat Kidney transformed cells (precursors to certain cancer types). This extract was found to be most effective in inhibiting reticular activating system (RAS) function among the 500 extracts tested.[8]

Alcoholic extracts of *M. citrifolia* leaves displayed good anthelmintic activity in vitro against human *ascaris lumbricoides*.[9] Lyophilized aqueous root extracts of the plant showed central analgesic activity, among other effects, suggesting sedative properties of the plant as well.[10]

The fruit of the plant is used as a food, layered in sugar. Leaves are also consumed raw or cooked. The roots yield a red dye, the bark, a yellow dye.[1]

TOXICOLOGY: No information is available about the toxicity of *M. citrifolia* or its constituents. The fruit has long been reported as edible.

SUMMARY: *Morinda citrifolia* has been used as a general healing agent for thousands of years in Polynesia. Current literature claims it is beneficial for immune system function, anticancer activity and for its anthelmintic effects. Little is known about toxicity of the plant. *M. citrifolia* is commercially available as juice or in dried form and is widely promoted in health food markets.

PATIENT INFORMATION – Morinda

Uses: Morinda has been used for heart remedies, arthritis headache, digestive and liver ailments.

Side Effects: No information is available on the side effects of morinda.

[1] Morton J. Atlas of Medicinal Plants of Middle America. Springfield, IL: Charles C. Thomas Publ. 1981;868–69.

[2] US patent # 5,288,491, date of patent Feb. 22, 1994.

[3] US patent # 4,409,144, date of patent Oct. 11,1983.

[4] Higa I, et al. *Genetica* 1993;88(2–3):129–36.

[5] Srivastava M, et al. *International Journal of Pharmacognosy* 1993;31(3):182–84.

[6] Dittmar A. *Journal of Herbs, Spices, and Medicinal Plants* 1993;1(3):77–92.

[7] Hirazumi A, et al. *Proc West Pharmacol Soc* 1994;37:145–46.

[8] Hiramatsu T, et al. *Cancer Lett* 1993;73(2–3):161–66.

[9] Raj R. *Indian J Physiol Pharmacol* 1975;19(1):47–49.

[10] Younos C, et al. *Planta Med* 1990;56(5):430–34.

Muira Puama

SCIENTIFIC NAME(S): *Ptychopetalum olacoides* Benth. Olacaceae (Olax family). Less commonly *P. uncinatum* Anselm. and *Liriosma ovata* Miers

COMMON NAME(S): Muira puama, marapuama, potency wood, raiz del macho, potenzholz

BOTANY: *P. olacoides* is a small tree native to the Brazilian Amazon where the stems and roots are used as a tonic for neuromuscular problems. A root decoction is used externally in massages and baths for paralysis and beriberi. Oral use of tea made from the roots for sexual impotence, rheumatism, and GI problems has been noted.[1]

HISTORY: Muira puama is currently promoted as a male aphrodisiac or as a treatment for impotence. This use can be traced back to the 1930s in Europe but has increased with the success of sildenafil (*Viagra*) and the concurrent promotion of "herbal *Viagra*" preparations. It is also a constituent of a popular Brazilian herbal tonic "catuama" consisting of guarana, ginger, *Trichilia catigua*, and *P. olacoides*. Muira puama was official in the Brazilian Pharmacopeia of 1956.

CHEMISTRY: *P. olacoides* root bark produces a volatile oil containing α-pinene, α-humulene, β-pinene, β-caryophyllene, camphene, and camphor as major constituents.[2] Alkaloids have been detected but not fully characterized. TLC of an alkaloid fraction demonstrated the absence of yohimbine. Coumarin was detected.[3] Fatty acid esters of sterols, free fatty acids (C_{21}-C_{25}), and free sterols such as lupeol have been isolated and identified.[3,4,5] Similar compounds were isolated from *L. ovata*.[6]

PHARMACOLOGY: An extract of *P. olacoides* reduced locomotor activity in an open field test in mice when orally given 1 hour before testing; however, the same extract reduced immobility time in a forced swimming test. An α_2-adrenergic mechanism was postulated because clonidine gave similar results and yohimbine antagonized the effects of both clonidine and the extract.[7] A hot water extract of *P. olacoides* did not induce colony stimulating factor or mitogenesis in an ex vivo immunomodulation study of 21 Brazilian plants.[8]

Japanese patents have been issued that claim muira puama preparations are useful against stress-induced gastric ulceration[9] and stress-induced blood calcium elevation.[10]

Pharmacologic investigation of catuama and its constituents found that *P. olacoides* had modest analgesic effects in chemical and thermal mouse models of pain. The combined preparation had an effect on the opioid system, demonstrating morphine cross-tolerance and blockade by naloxone.[11] *P. olacoides* had no vasorelaxant effects in a related study in which the other constituents of catuama were active.[12]

Clinical studies to support the use of muira puama are sparse. Several promotional Web sites cite the work of a French clinician, Jacques Waynberg,[13] to support their claims; however, peer-reviewed publications are currently lacking. Muira puama has been contrasted favorably with yohimbine.[14] A German language review was published many years ago.[15]

TOXICOLOGY: Muira puama does not appear to contain yohimbine, nor to have the serious side effect potential of yohimbine.

SUMMARY: Muira puama is a popular yet poorly studied herbal product promoted for erectile dysfunction.

PATIENT INFORMATION – Muira Puama

Uses: *P. olacoides* is used as a tonic for neuromuscular problems. A root decoction is used externally in massages and baths for paralysis and beriberi. Oral use of tea made from the roots for sexual impotence, rheumatism, and GI problems has been noted. Muira puama is currently promoted as a male aphrodisiac or as a treatment for impotence.

Side Effects: Muira puama does not appear to have the serious side effect potential of yohimbine.

[1] Schultes R, et al. The Healing Forest: Medicinal and Toxic Plants of the Northwest Amazon. Portland, OR: Dioscorides Press,1990, p. 343.

[2] Bucek E, et al. Volatile constituents of *Ptychopetalum olacoides* root oil. *Planta Med* 1987;53:231.

[3] Toyota A, et al. Studies of Brazilian crude drugs. 1. Muira-puama. *Shoyakugaku Zasshi* 1979;33:57.

[4] Ito Y, et al. Constituents from Muira-puama (the roots of *Ptychopetalum olacoides*). *Nat Med* 1995;49:487.

[5] Auterhoff H, et al. Contents of muira puama. *Arch Pharm Ber Dtsch Pharm Ges* 1968;301:481. German.

[6] Iwasa J, et al. Studies on the constituents of muira puama. *Yakugaku Zasshi* 1969;89:1172.

[7] Paiva L, et al. Effects of *Ptychopetalum olacoides* extract on mouse behavior in forced swimming and open field tests. *Phytother Res* 1998;12:294.

[8] Kawaguchi K, et al. Colony stimulating factor-inducing activity of isoflavone C-glucosides from the bark of *Dalbergia monetaria*. *Planta Med* 1998;64 653.

[9] Asano T, et al. Oral compositions containing muira-puama for gastric mucosal lesions. 1999; Japanese Patent No. 11343244.

[10] Sudo D, et al. Evaluation of tonic effects of bioactive substances based on stress-induced change in blood calcium. 2000; Japanese Patent No. 2000009717.

[11] Vaz Z, et al. Analgesic effect of the herbal medicine catuama in thermal and chemical models of nociception in mice. *Phytother Res* 1997;11:101.

[12] Calixto J, et al. Herbal medicine catuama induces endothelium-dependent and -independent vasorelaxant action on isolated vessels from rats, guinea-pigs and rabbits. *Phytother Res* 1997;11:32.

[13] Waynberg J. Male sexual asthenia - interest in a traditional plant-derived medication. *J. Ethnopharmacol* 1995.

[14] Murray M. Yohimbine vs. muira puama in the treatment of erectile dysfunction. *Am J Nat Med* November 1994.

[15] Steinmetz E. Muira puama. *Quart J Crude Drug Res* 1971;11:1787.

Mullein

SCIENTIFIC NAME(S): *Verbascum thapsus* L., *V. phlomoides* L., *V. thapsiforme* Schrad. Family: Scrophulariaceae

COMMON NAME(S): American mullein, European or orange mullein, candleflower, candlewick, higtaper and longwort[1]

BOTANY: The common mullein, usually found throughout the United States, is a woolly-leafed biennial plant. During the first year of its growth, the large leaves form a low-lying basal rosette. In the spring of the second year, the plant develops a tall stem that can grow to 4 or more feet in height. The top portion of the stem develops yellow flowers consisting of a five-part corolla. This, along with the stamens, is what constitutes the active ingredient. The flowers bloom from June to September and have a faint, honey-like odor.[2] Electron microscopy performed on *V. thapsus* reveals distinctive pollen grains and trichomes, which may be helpful for identification purposes.[3]

HISTORY: Mullein boasts an illustrious history as a favored herbal remedy and, consequently, has found use in all manner of disorders. Its traditional uses have generally focused on the management of respiratory disorders where it was used to treat asthma, coughs, tuberculosis and related respiratory problems. However, in its various forms, the plant has been used to treat hemorrhoids, burns, bruises and gout. Preparations of the plant have been ingested, applied topically and smoked. The yellow flowers had once been used as a source of yellow hair dye. In Appalachia, the plant has been used to treat colds and the boiled root administered for croup. Leaves were applied topically to soften and protect the skin. An oil derived from the flowers has been used to soothe earaches.[4]

CHEMISTRY: Few compounds with known therapeutic effects have been identified in the plant. These contain saponins, mucilage and tannins.

In a report on the species *V. thapsus*, luteolin glycoside was identified for the first time.[5] Using spectroscopic methods and chemical evidence, five phenylethanoid glycosides and one lignan glycoside were found (in addition to three known phenylethanoid glycosides and four lignan glycosides).[6]

Saponins from *V. songaricum* were identified in European studies, reporting triterpene saponins from the aerial parts,[7] songarosaponin D based on spectral evidence[8] and songarosaponin E and F, the newest triterpenoid saponins.[9] Saponins from *V. nigrum*, a related species, are also reported.[10]

Also from European reports, iridoids from *V. sinuatum* and *V. olympicum* have been identified. New iridoid diglycosides have been isolated and described.[11,12,13,14]

A Czechoslovakian report on *V. pseudonobile* stoj. et stef., first identified (E)-cinnamamide.[15] A German study characterizes water-soluble polysaccharides from *V. phlomoides* L.[16] The content of verbacoside is reported in six *Verbascum* species growing in Poland.[17] Fatty acids from *V. phlomoides* and *V. thapsiforme* are reported in another Polish study,[18] along with sterols from the essential oils of these species.[19] Another related plant, *V. lasianthum*, yields hydrocarbons, ketone alcohols, beta-sitosterol and a triterpenic alcohol.[20]

PHARMACOLOGY: The flowers and leaves are used medicinally. The saponins, mucilage and tannins contained in the flowers and leaves likely contribute to the soothing topical effects of the plant. Similarly, some of these compounds have demulcent properties that may make them useful for the symptomatic treatment of sore throats.[21] The mild **expectorant** action of the saponins also supports use of mullein for the relief of coughs. It is included in many mixed teas for use as an **antitussive**.[2]

The **ganglionic-blocking effect** of *V. nobile* Vel. has been described.[22]

Antiviral activity of mullein has been reported in two studies. In the lyophilized infusion obtained from *Verbascum thapsiforme* Schrad. flowers, activity against herpes simplex type I virus was evaluated in vitro. A decrease in virus titer and inhibition of viral replication by mullein were demonstrated.[23] Another study confirms and evaluates antiviral activity in vitro against Fowl plague virus and influenza A and B strains.[24]

TOXICOLOGY: Plants from the genera *Verbascum* and *Senecio* have been given the common Spanish name senecio, and may cause some confusion. No adverse effects have been reported from the use of *Verbascum* or its extracts.[25]

SUMMARY: Mullein is a common plant with a long history of use in herbal medicine. There is little evidence to indicate that the plant can offer more than mild astringent and topical soothing effects. It may have mild demulcent properties when ingested. Antiviral activity of mullein has been reported against herpes and influenza. The plant has not been associated with toxicity.

PATIENT INFORMATION – Mullein

Uses: Mullein has expectorant and cough suppressant properties that make it useful for symptomatic treatment of sore throat and cough. Antiviral activity of mullein has been reported against herpes simplex type I virus and influenza A and B strains.

Side Effects: No adverse effects have been reported.

---

[1] Bianchini F, et al. Health Plants of the World, A Mondadori, Milan, 1975.
[2] Bisset N. Herbal Drugs and Phytopharmaceuticals. Stuttgart, Germany: CRC Press 1994;517-19.
[3] Fillippini R, et al. *International Journal of Crude Drug Research* 1990 Jun;28:129-33.
[4] Boyd EL, et al. Home Remedies and the Black Elderly. Univ. of Michigan, 1984.
[5] Mehrotra R, et al. *J Nat Prod* 1989 May-Jun;52:640–43.
[6] Warashina T, et al. *Phytochemistry* 1992;31(3):961-65.
[7] Seifert K, et al. *Phytochemistry* 1991;30(10):3395-400.
[8] Hartleb I, et al. *Phytochemistry* 1994;35(4):1009-11.
[9] Hartleb I, et al. *Phytochemistry* 1995;38(1):221-24.
[10] Klimek B, et al. *Phytochemistry* 1992;31(12):4368-70.
[11] Bianco A, et al. *Planta Med* 1981 Jan;41:75-79.
[12] Falsone G, et al. *Planta Med* 1982 Mar;44:150-53.
[13] Bianco A, et al. *J Nat Prod* 1984 Sep-Oct;47:901-2.
[14] Girabias B, et al. *Herba Polonica* 1989;35(1):3-8.
[15] Ninova P, et al. *Cesk Farm* 1984;33(2):66-67.
[16] Kraus J, et al. *Deutsche Apotheker Zeitung* 1987 Mar 26;127:665-69.
[17] Klimek B. *Acta Poloniae Pharmaceutica* 1991;48(3-4):51-54.
[18] Swiatek L. *Herba Polonica* 1984;30(3-4):173-81.
[19] Swiatek L. *Herba Polonica* 1985;31(1-2):29-33.
[20] Ulubelen A, et al. *Planta Med* 1975;27:14.
[21] Tyler VE. The New Honest Herbal, GF Stickley Co, 1987.
[22] Krushkov I, et al. *Nauchni Trudove Na Visshiia Meditsinski Institut*, Sofiia 1970;49(4):19-23.
[23] Slagowska A, et al. *Pol J Pharmacol Pharm* 1987;39(1):55-61.
[24] Zgorniak-Nowosielska I, et al. *Arch Immunol Ther Exp* 1991;39(1-2):103-8.
[25] Kay M. *Herbalgram* 1994;32:42-45, 57.

Musk

SCIENTIFIC NAME(S): *Moschus moschiferus* L. Family: Moschidae

COMMON NAME(S): Musk, Tonquin musk, deer musk

SOURCE: The musk deer (*M. moschiferus*) is a small, solitary animal that attains a stature of only 0.5 m. It is native to mountainous regions of Asia, including Tibet and northeastern China. Both the male and female lack antlers.[1]

Musk is an odiferous secretion derived from the musk gland under the abdomen near the pubis of the male musk deer. The glands weigh up to 30 g and contain about half their weight in musk.[2] According to Leung, there are two methods of obtaining musk.[1] In the first method, the trapped deer is killed in late winter or early spring and the gland is removed. The dried whole gland (known as the pod) or the dried glandular secretions inside (musk grains) are employed in commerce.

Alternately, musk is collected from deer raised in captivity. The musk is removed from the gland of immobilized animals by use of a special spoon. The musk is collected once or twice a year.

This material should not be confused with musk root (*Ferula sumbul* Hook, Family: Apiaceae), which is sometimes used as a substitute for musk in the perfume industry.[3]

HISTORY: The use of musk dates back more than 1300 years when it was used by rulers of early Chinese dynasties. Consequently, it has a broad historical tradition in Chinese herbal medicine. Today, it is used as a component of fragrances and as a fixative in perfumes.[1]

CHEMISTRY: The fresh musk secretion is a dark-brown viscous semi-solid that turns to brownish-yellow or purple-red granules when dried.[1] The term musk is used to describe other materials with a similar odor, although these preparations may be of synthetic or herbal origins.

When distilled, musk yields the principles muscone (muskone) (0.3% to 2%) and normuscone. Other compounds present in musk include steroids, paraffins, triglycerides, waxes, mucopyridine and other nitrogenous substances and fatty acids.[1,2]

Cyclopentadecanone is a synthetic compound that differs from muscone only in the absence of a methyl group.[2]

PHARMACOLOGY: Musk is reported to have anti-inflammatory and antihistaminic activity in animal models. Its anti-inflammatory activity has been reported to exceed that of phenylbutazone in rats with experimentally induced adjuvant arthritis.[1]

Musk has also been reported to have spasmolytic, CNS-depressant, stimulant and antibacterial activity.[1] In clinical studies, musk has been shown to have a beneficial effect in patients suffering from angina, with a therapeutic effect comparable to that observed with nitroglycerin.[1]

TOXICOLOGY: No significant reports of systemic toxicity have been associated with the use of musk.

As with many naturally derived compounds that are applied topically, there exists a potential for a dermal hypersensitivity reaction. Musk components are known to cause a variety of dermal reactions, including pigmented dermatitis following the application of musk-containing rouge[4] and photoallergic contact dermatitis following the use of musk-containing fragrances.[5] In a survey of dermatology clinics in Scandinavia, musk ambrette was among the leading topical photosensitizers reported.[6] This material was similarly cited as one of the most photosensitizing compounds reported by Mayo Clinic patients.[7]

SUMMARY: Musk is an odiferous material derived from a gland of the Asian musk deer. Its unique odor has made it an important component of perfumes. Although traditionally derived from deer that had been killed for the express purpose of musk collection, the material today is largely obtained from deer specifically raised for musk production.

PATIENT INFORMATION – Musk

Uses: Musk is used as a fragrance and component in herbal medicine. It reportedly shows anti-inflammatory and antihistaminic activity, and various other therapeutic effects as a stimulant, treatment for angina, etc.

Side Effects: Topical use may cause symptoms such as contact dermatitis, photosensitivity, etc.

[1] Leung AY. Encyclopedia of Common Natural Ingredients Used in Food, Drugs, and Cosmetics. New York, NY: J. Wiley and Sons, 1980.

[2] Evans WC. Trease and Evans' Pharmacognosy, 13th ed. Oxford, England: The Alden Press, 1989.

[3] Duke JA. Handbook of Medicinal Herbs. Boca Raton, FL: CRC Press, 1985.

[4] Hayakawa R, et al. Pigmented contact dermatitis due to musk moskene. J Dermatol 1991;18:420.

[5] Megahed M, et al. Persistent light reaction associated with photoallergic contact dermatitis to musk ambrette and allergic contact dermatitis to fragrance mix. Dermatologica 1991;182:199.

[6] Thune P, et al. The Scandinavian multicenter photopatch study 1980-1985 final report. Photo-Dermatology 1988;5:261.

[7] Menz J, et al. Photopatch testing: a six-year experience. J Am Acad Dermatol 1988;18:1044.

Mustard

COMMON NAME(S): Brown mustard: *Brassica juncea* (L.) Czern. et Cross. and *B. nigra* (L.) Koch. White mustard: *Sinapis alba* L. synonymous with *Brassica alba*. Family: Cruciferae or Brassicaceae. Other common names by which mustards are known include Chinese mustard (*S. juncea*), Indian mustard (*B. juncea*), yellow mustard (*S. alba*), and *black mustard* (B. nigra).

BOTANY: The mustards are annual or bienniel herbs that grow from 3 to 9 feet in height. All common mustards are cultivated worldwide. The dried ripe seed is used commercially.

Ground mustard, derived from the powdered mustard seed, is known as mustard flour. It may consist of a mixture of brown, black or white seeds. The more pungent mustards are derived from seeds from which the fixed oil has been removed.[1]

HISTORY: Mustard and its oil have been used for the topical treatment of rheumatisms and arthritis and as foot baths for aching feet. Internally, they have been used as appetite stimulants, emetics and diuretics.[1] When black mustard is prepared as a condiment with vinegar, salt and water, the product is properly termed German prepared mustard. Sinapis alba seeds, prepared in a similar manner but without spices, are known as English mustard.[4] Mustards are grown extensively as forage crops.

CHEMISTRY: The volatile mustard oil is derived from steam distillation or by expression. The fixed oil does not contribute to the pungency of the mustard, and ground mustard does not have a pungent aroma.

The pungency is produced when the mustard is mixed with water and the enzyme myrosin hydrolyzes sinigrin (a glucoside found in black and brown mustards) or sinalbin (found in white mustard), releasing allyl isothiocyanate or p-hydroxybenzyl isothiocyanate, which are responsible for the pungent aroma.[2] Depending on the variety of mustard, the yield of allyl isothiocyanate is approximately 1%.[1,5]

Other components of the oil include sinapic acid, sinapine, fixed oil, proteins and a mucilage.

PHARMACOLOGY/TOXICOLOGY: Allyl isothiocyanate is a powerful irritant and blistering agent. It has counterirritant properties and induces lacrimation. It is one of the most toxic essential oils and should not be tasted or inhaled undiluted.[1]

Isothiocyanate compounds such as those found in mustard and other Brassicaceae have been implicated in the development of endemic goiter and have been shown to produce goiter in laboratory animals.[1]

Derivatives of allyl isothiocyanate have formed the basis for toxic agents such as the "mustard gasses" and antineoplastic agents.

Because of its topical irritant effects, mustard has been used as a rubifacient and irritant; mustard plasters are prepared by mixing mustard with flour or other material to make a paste for topical application.[3]

SUMMARY: The pungent flavor of the mustard seeds has made it one of the most widely used spices in the Western world. The mustards have been used in traditional medicine, primarily as topical counterirritants and continue to find some use in a poultice (commonly but inappropriately described as a mustard plaster).[4] The oil is highly irritating and should be considered toxic.

PATIENT INFORMATION – Mustard

Uses: Mustard is used as food, flavoring, forage, emetic, diuretic, topical treatment for arthritis and rheumatism, etc. It contains antineoplastic agents.

Side Effects: The oil is highly irritating and should be considered toxic. Mustard compounds have been implicated in development of goiter.

---

[1] Leung AY. Encyclopedia of Common Natural Ingredients Used in Food, Drugs and Cosmetics. New York, NY: J Wiley and Sons, 1980.
[2] Simon JE. Herbs: An Indexed Bibliography, 1971-1980. Hamden, CT: Shoe String Press, 1984.
[3] Hoover JE, ed. Remington's Pharmaceutical Sciences, 14th ed. Easton, PA: Mack Publishing Co., 1970.
[4] Osol A, Farrar GE Jr, eds. The Dispensatory of the United States of America 25th ed. Philadelphia, PA: J.B. Lippincott, 1955.
[5] Tyler VE, Brady LR, Robbers JE. Pharmacognosy, 9th ed. Philadelphia, PA: Lea & Febiger, 1988.

Myrrh

SCIENTIFIC NAME(S): *Commiphora molmol* Engl. Synonymous with *C. myrrha*, *C. abyssinica* and other *Commiphora* species are used in commerce. Family: Burseraceae

COMMON NAME(S): African myrrh, Somali Myrrh (C. molmol), Arabian and Yemen myrrh (*C. abyssinica*), myrrha, gum myrrh[1], bola, bal, bol, heerabol[2]

BOTANY: The Commiphora species that serve as sources of myrrh are trees that grow to heights of 30 feet. They are native to Africa and are found in the Red Sea region. A pale yellow-white viscous liquid exudes from natural cracks in the bark or from fissures cut intentionally to harvest the material.[2] This exudate hardens into yellow-brown tears that weigh up to 250 g that form the basis of myrrh resin.[1,2]

HISTORY: Myrrh has been used for centuries[2] for diverse effects as an astringent, antiseptic, emmenagogue and antispasmodic. It also has been used to treat a variety of infectious diseases (including leprosy and syphilis), and to treat cancers.[1] Myrrh played a key role in the religious ceremonies of the ancient Egyptians.[3] It finds use in African, Middle Eastern and Chinese traditional medicine. Today, myrrh is used as a component of fragrances, and as an astringent in mouthwashes and gargles.[1,4] It is sometimes used to flavor beverages and foods.

CHEMISTRY: Myrrh is an oleo-gum-resin[2] that contains from 1.5% to 17% (typically about 8%) of a volatile oil composed of heerabolene, limonene, dipentene and more than a half-dozen additional fragrant compounds.[1] Up to 40% (average 20%) of the resin consists of commiphoric acids and about 60% of the product is a gum that yields a variety of sugars upon hydrolysis.[1] The gum has been reported to contain an oxidase enzyme.[2] The related *C. guidottii* contains the sesquiterpene (+)-T-cadinol.[5]

PHARMACOLOGY: Myrrh is reported to have mild astringent properties.[6] It has been reported to exert antimicrobial activity in vitro.[1]

Myrrh has been found to have a locally stimulating action on smooth muscle tissue and may stimulate peristalsis.[7,8] By contrast, T-cadinol has been shown to have a concentration-dependent smooth muscle relaxing effect on the isolated guinea pig ileum and a dose-dependent inhibitory effect on cholera toxin-induced intestinal hypersecretion in mice.[5]

In addition, extracts of C. mukul have been shown to inhibit the maximal edema response and total edema induced by carrageenan in the rat paw.[9]

A mixture of plant extracts that includes an extract of myrrh has been shown to reduce the rate of gluconeogenesis in rats and may be of interest in the management of diabetes mellitus.[10] An ethylacetate extract of C. mukul significantly prevented the rise in serum cholesterol and triglycerides caused by an atherogenic diet.[11]

TOXICOLOGY: Although myrrh is generally considered to be nonirritating, nonsensitizing and nonphototoxic to human and animal skins,[1] several cases of dermatitis due to myrrh have been reported.[12]

SUMMARY: Myrrh is a fragrant plant exudate that has been used in traditional medicine and as part of religious ceremonies for thousands of years. Today, myrrh is used in fragrances and as a food flavoring. Myrrh posseses potentially useful pharmacologic activity, although the components that exert these actions have not been well characterized.

PATIENT INFORMATION – Myrrh

Uses: Myrrh has been used as a fragrance, flavoring, astringent, antiseptic, emmenagogue, antispasmodic, and treatment for cancer and infectious diseases.

Side Effects: It has reportedly been associated with dermatitis.

---

[1] Leung AY. Encyclopedia of Common Natural Ingredients Used in Food, Drugs and Cosmetics. New York, NY: J. Wiley and Sons, 1980.

[2] Evans, WC. Trease and Evans' Pharmacognosy. 13th ed. London: Balliere Tindall, 1989.

[3] Dobelis IN. Magic and Medicine of Plants. Pleasantville, NY: Reader's Digest Association, 1986.

[4] Michie CA, Cooper E. Frankincense and myrrh as remedies in children. *J R Soc Med* 1991;84:602.

[5] Claeson P et al. T-cadinol: a pharmacologically active constituent of scented myrrh: introductory pharmacological characterization and high filed 1H and 13C-NMR data. *Planta Med* 1991;57:352.

[6] Tyler VE. The Honest Herbal: a sensible guide to the use of herbs and related remedies. Binghamton, NY: The Haworth Press, 1993.

[7] Spoerke DG. Herbal Medications. Santa Barbara, CA: Woodbridge Press, 1980.

[8] Morton JF. Major Medicinal Plants. Springfield, IL: Charles C. Thomas, 1977.

[9] Duwiejua M et al. Anti-inflammatory activity of resins from some species of the plant family Burseraceae. *Planta Med* 1993;59:12.

[10] al-Awadi F et al. The effect of a plants mixture extract on liver gluconeogenesis in streptozotocin induced diabetic rats. *Diabetes Res* 1991;18:163.

[11] Lata S et al. Beneficial effects of *Allium sativum*, *Allium cepa* and *Commiphora mukul* on experimental hyperlipidemia and atherosclerosis - a comparative evaluation. *J Postgrad Med* 1991;37:132.

[12] Lee TY, Lam TH. Allergic contact dermatitis due to a Chinese orthopaedic solution tieh ta yao gin. *Contact Derm* 1993;28:89.

Neem

SCIENTIFIC NAME(S): *Azadirachta indica* A. Juss. Formerly known as *Melia azadirachta* L. Family: Meliaceae. Often confused with *Melia azedarach* L. (the chinaberry or Persian lilac).

COMMON NAME(S): Neem, margosa, nim, nimba

BOTANY: The neem is a large evergreen tree that grows to 18 meters in height. The spreading branches of this tree form a broad crown. The plant is found commonly throughout India and the neighboring region, where it is often cultivated commercially.

HISTORY: Almost every part of the neem tree is used in traditional medicine in India, Sri Lanka, Burma, Indochina, Java and Thailand.[1] The stem, root bark and young fruits are used as a tonic and astringent and the bark has been used to treat malaria and cutaneous diseases. The tender leaves have been used in the treatment of worm infections, ulcers, cardiovascular diseases and for their pesticidal and insect-repellent actions.[2] The tree yields a high quality timber and a commercial gum.

CHEMISTRY: The seed kernels of neem yield about 10% of a fixed oil, comprised primarily of glycerides. The yellow bitter oil has a garlic-like odor and contains approximately 2% of bitter principles including nimbidin, nimbin, nimbinin, nimbidol and other related minor components.[3] All parts of the tree yield beta-sitosterol. Azadirachtin is the most active insecticidal component of neem, with a yield of about 5 g from 2 kg of seeds.[4]

PHARMACOLOGY: The variety of components in neem give the plant and its extracts a number of pharmacologic activities. Neem is being investigated for its potential as a contraceptive agent. The oil has been shown to inhibit sperm motility in vitro, and its intravaginal application to rabbits did not induce mucosal irritation.[5] Sodium nimbinate and nimbidinate have weak spermicidal activity in vitro, and the oil immobilizes human sperm within 30 seconds of contact.[6] In women, the intravaginal application of 1 ml of neem oil prior to intercourse did not affect cycle regularity, and provided effective contraception for ten couples over four cycles.[6] Initial acceptance problems due to the unpleasant smell of the oil were overcome by masking the odor with lemon grass scent.

When injected subcutaneously in rats, neem oil causes alterations in the luminal epithelium of the uterus, preventing pregnancy if administered for several days postcoitally; this appears to be a direct toxic effect and not hormonally dependent.[7] It has been suggested, therefore, that the lack of hormonal effect may offer a contraceptive alternative with fewer side effects than traditional steroidal contraceptives.[8] Neem oil exerts some contraceptive effect when administered orally to rats, but its efficacy by this route is insufficient to warrant further study.[9]

A 200 mg dose of seed oil administered orally to normoglycemic and diabetic rats produced reductions in mean glucose concentrations of up to 48% 6 hours after drug administration.[10] These preliminary results support the traditional use of neem in the management of diabetes.

Neem oil and azadirachtin are effective pesticides and insect repellents. Azadirachtin is one of the most potent insect antifeedant and ecdysis inhibitory compound known from a botanical source.[13] Because of the complex chemical structure of azadirachtin, only naturally derived products have been used commercially. This compound is effective in concentrations as low as 0.1 ppm and has been shown to be biodegradable, nonmutagenic and nontoxic to warm-blooded animals, fish and birds. The Environmental Protection Agency has approved the use of a neem formulation (Margosan-O) as a pesticide for limited use on nonfood crops.[12] Other insecticidal compounds from neem include deactyl-azadirachtinol and salannin.[11]

Gedunin and nimbolide, both isolated from neem, have shown antimalarial activity in vitro.[13] One survey of the in vitro antibacterial effect of neem oil against 200 clinical bacterial isolates resulted in 92% susceptibility.[14]

Neem oil has been used as a traditional dentifrice and the oil has been found to be anti-inflammatory, aseptic and healing in gingivitis. In toothpaste, the extract has low abrasiveness and good antimicrobial activity against oral flora.[15]

TOXICOLOGY: Neem oil is nonmutagenic in the Ames mutagenicity assay.[16]

Neem oil has traditionally been considered to be a relatively safe product in adults. The LD_{50} of neem oil is 14 ml/kg in rats and 24 ml/kg in rabbits. In rats, a dose of up to 80 ml/kg caused stupor, respiratory distress, depression of activity, diarrhea, convulsions and death.[17] Gross examination of all organs except the lungs was normal after acute dosing.

The seeds of neem, which are poisonous in large doses, resemble the more toxic drupes of *M. azadarach* and are sometimes confused. Severe poisoning in 13 infants who had received 5 ml to 30 ml doses of margosa (neem) oil has been reported. Toxicity was characterized by metabolic acidosis, drowsiness, seizures, loss of consciousness, coma and death in two infants.[1] These infants exhibited Reye's syndrome-like symptoms, with death from hepatoencephalopathy. Neem oil administered to mice can induce mitochrondrial injury, resulting in similar hepatic damage. The toxin has not been identified, but may be a long-chain monounsaturated free acid, to which infants and small children are particularly vulnerable.[18]

SUMMARY: Neem oil has been used in traditional Indian medicine for thousands of years, practically as a panacea. The oil and its extracts are insecticidal, can reduce blood sugar levels and may be the source of a contraceptive substance. Although the oil has not been generally associated with toxicity in adults, its use has resulted in Reye's syndrome-like symptoms and mortality in infants.

PATIENT INFORMATION – Neem

Uses: Neem has been used as an insecticide, insect repellent, oral dentifrice, and traditional medicine to treat malaria, diabetes, worms, and cardiovascular and skin diseases. It reportedly has contraceptive potential.

Side Effects: It is toxic in large doses. In infants, it can produce symptoms like those of Reye's syndrome.

---

[1] Sinniah D, Baskaran G. Margosa oil poisoning as a cause of Reye's syndrome. *Lancet* 1981;1:487.

[2] *Med and Aromat Plants Abstract* 1987;9:465.

[3] Windholz M, ed. The Merck Index, 10th ed. Rahway, NJ: Merck and Co., 1983.

[4] Schroeder DR, Nakanishi K. A simplified isolation procedure for azadirachtin. *J Nat Prod* 1987;50:241.

[5] Riar SS, et al. Volatile fraction of neem oil as a spermicide. *Contraception* 1990;42:479.

[6] Sinha KC, et al. Neem oil as a vaginal contraceptive. *Indian J Med Res* 1984;79:131.

[7] Tewari RK, et al. Biochemical and histological studies of reproductive organs in cyclic and ovariectomized rats supporting a non-hormonal action for neem oil. *J Ethnopharmacol* 1989;25:281.

[8] Prakash AO, et al. Non-hormonal post-coital contraceptive action of neem oil in rats. *J Ethnopharmacol* 1988;23:53.

[9] Lal R, et al. Antifertility effect of neem oil in female albino rats by the intravaginal and oral routes. *Indian J Med Res* 1986;83:89.

[10] Dixit VP, et al. Effect of neem seed oil on the blood glucose concentration of normal and alloxan diabetic rats. *J Ethnopharmacol* 1986;17:95.

[11] Kubo I, et al. New insect ecdysis inhibitory limonoid deacetylazadirachtinol isolated from *azadirachta indica* (meliaceae) oil. *Tetrahedron* 1986;42:489.

[12] Plants' natural defenses may be key to better pesticides. *Chem Eng News* 1985;63:47.

[13] Khalid SA, et al. Isolation and characterization of an antimalarial agent of the neem tree *azadirachta indica*. *J Nat Prod* 1989;52:922.

[14] Rao DVK, et al. In vitro antibacterial activity of neem oil. *Indian J Med Res* 1986;84:314.

[15] Patel VK, Venkatakrishna-Bhatt H. Folklore therapeutic indigenous plants in periodontal disorders in India (review, experimental and clinical approach). *Int J Clin Pharmacol Ther Toxicol* 1988;26:176.

[16] Polasa K, Rukmini C. Mutagenicity tests of cashew nut shell liquid, rice-bran oil and other vegetable oils using the *salmonella typhimurium*/microsome system. *Food Chem Toxicol* 1987;25:763.

[17] Gandhi M, et al. Acute toxicity study of the oil from *azadirachta indica* seed (neem oil). *J Ethnopharmacol* 1988;23:39.

[18] Sinniah R, et al. Animal model of margosa oil ingestion with Reye-like syndrome. Pathogenesis of microvesicular fatty liver. *J Pathol* 1989;159:255.

Nettles

SCIENTIFIC NAME(S): *Urtica dioica* L. Family: Urticaceae

COMMON NAME(S): Stinging nettle, nettle

BOTANY: Nettles are perennial plants native to Europe and found throughout the US and parts of Canada. This plant has an erect stalk and can stand up to 3 feet. It has dark green serrated leaves that grow opposite each other along the stalk. The plant flowers from June to September. The leaves contain bristles that transmit irritating principles upon contact. The nettle fruit is a small, oval seed about 1 mm wide. It is yellow-brown in color.[1]

HISTORY: This plant is known for its stinging properties. However, it has been used in traditional medicine as a diuretic, antispasmodic, expectorant and treatment for asthma. The juice has been purported to stimulate hair growth when applied to the scalp. Extracts of the leaves have been used topically for the treatment of rheumatic disorders. The tender tips of young nettles have been used as a cooked pot herb in salads.

CHEMISTRY: More than 24 chemical components have been identified in nettles. The primary structure of *Urtica dioica* agglutinin has been determined and found to be a two-domain member of the hevein family of proteins.[2] Compounds isolated from the roots and flowers include scopoletin, steryl derivatives, lignan glucosides and flavonol glycosides.[3] Sixteen free amino acids have been found in the leaves.[4] Nine flavonoid compounds have been isolated and identified.[5] Phenylpropanes and lignans from the roots have been isolated and described.[6] The plant also contains vitamins C, B-group and K, along with other various acids.[1] Mineral salts have also been found. Nitrate concentrations in nettle leaves have been reported.[7] Glucokinin (allegedly responsible for "antidiabetic activity") has been reported, but its presence in the plant is controversial.[1] In addition to sitosterol, at least six other related steroids have been identified.[8] The plant has been used as a commercial source of chlorophyll. The young shoots are rich in carotene and vitamin C. The stinging trichomes of nettle contain amines, such as histamine, serotonin and choline. Nettle fruit contains protein, mucilage and fixed oil.[1] Aqueous extracts of the plant have been studied.[10,11,12,13] Isolation and identification among nettles have been performed.[14] HPLC, GC and other methods have determined a specific lectin found only in *Urtica dioica* roots, which may help to standardize preparations.[15,16]

PHARMACOLOGY: Nettle herb is known to have mainly **diuretic** actions. Treatment over 14 days increases urine volume and decreases systolic blood pressure.[1] Nettle's "supposed" claims against diabetes, cancer, eczema, rheumatism, hair loss and aging have been reported[9,17] but are probably related to its "age-old" roles in folk medicine. Other folk medicine applications include wound healing, treatment of scalp seborrhea and greasy hair, and gastric juice secretion.[1] A combination product includes nettle to treat hyposecretory gastritis.[18]

Nettle in a combination product containing several other herbs has been tested in 22 patients for bladder irrigation. Post-operative blood loss, bacteriuria and inflammation were all reduced following prostatic adenomectomy.[19] *The German Commission E Monograph* supports this indication by its similar listing for "irrigation in inflammation of the urinary tract and in the prevention and treatment of kidney gravel."[1] Nettle's use in expelling bile has been studied.[20]

Urtica dioica in a combined extract to treat benign prostatic hyperplasia (BPH) in 134 patients was effective in reducing urine flow, noctura and residual urine. A 300 mg dose of the plant extract was as effective as 150 mg.[21] A possible mechanism may be caused by a hydrophobic constituent (eg, steroidal), which inhibits the sodium-potassium ATP-ase activity of the prostate, leading to suppressed cell growth in this area.[22] Another report explains a different mechanism but suggests the aqueous extract is the active component in BPH therapy to inhibit the sex hormone-binding globulin to its receptor.[23]

Freeze-dried nettle has been evaluated for allergic rhinitis. In a double-blind trial, 57% of 69 hay fever sufferers who completed the trial judged the nettle preparations to be moderately to highly effective in treatment vs placebo.[24]

CNS depressant effects of nettle extract in rats are described, suggesting diminished motor activity and reduced convulsions, along with hypothermic effects with its use.[27]

Animal reports on nettle pharmacology are available, including its dihydroergotamine-like effect on mouse uterine smooth muscle, probably caused by pyranocoumarin,[27] nettle's carbohydrate binding properties[28] and its ability *in vitro* to inhibit enzyme aromatase.[29] A study concerning a lectin present in nettle suggests a potent and selective inhibitor of HIV and cytomegalovirus replication *in vitro*. When evaluated for its anti-diabetic effect, *Urtica dioica* slightly increased glycemia, aggravating the condition in two reports.[25,26]

TOXICOLOGY: Nettles are known primarily for their ability to induce topical irritation following contact with exposed skin. This contact urticaria is accompanied by a stinging sensation lasting 12 hours or longer. A report closely associates mast cells and dermal dendritic cells. Immediate reaction to nettle stings is caused by histamine content, while the persistence of the sting may be caused by other substances directly toxic to nerves.[31]

The stinging hairs of the nettle plant comprise a fine capillary tube, a bladder-like base filled with the chemical irritant and a minute spherical tip, which breaks off on contact leaving a sharp-pointed tip that penetrates the skin. The irritants are forced into the skin as the hair bends and constricts the bladder at the base.

The topical irritation is treated by gently washing the affected area with mild soapy water. Treatment with systemic antihistamines and topical steroids may be of benefit. Other side effects of nettle are rare but include allergic effects such as edema, oliguria and gastric irritation.[1]

SUMMARY: Nettles have been part of our culture for thousands of years. They are more widely recognized for their irritation, but have been found to have many pharmacological benefits, proving some "folk remedies" to be effective. Its use in bladder irrigation, BPH treatment, hay fever relief and its CNS depressant effects have all been studied. Other than contact urticaria, side effects with plant ingestion are rare. The young herb (before stinging cells form) can be consumed as a pot vegetable.

PATIENT INFORMATION – Nettles

Uses: Prove as a diuretic, nettles are also being investigated as treatment for hay fever and irrigation of the urinary tract.

Side Effects: Internal side effects are rare and are allergic in nature. External side effects result from skin contact and take the form of burning and stinging that persist for 12 hours or more.

---

[1] Bisset N. *Herbal Drugs and Phytopharmaceuticals*, CRC Press, Stuttgart, Germay 1994;502–7.
[2] Beintema J, et al. *FEBS Letters* 1992;299(2):131–4.
[3] Chaurasia N, et al. *Deutsche Apotheker Zeitung* 1986;126(Jan 16):81–3.
[4] Adamski R, et al. *Herba Polonica* 1984;30(1):17–26.
[5] Ellnain-Wojtaszek M, et al. *Herba Polonica* 1986;32(3–4):131–7.
[6] Chaurasia N, et al. *Deutsche Apotheker Zeitung* 1986;126(Jul 17):1559–63.
[7] Peura P, et al. *ACTA Pharmaceutica Fennica* 1985;94(2):67–70.
[8] Chaurasia N,et al. *Journal of Natural Products* 1987;50(Sep-Oct):881–5.
[9] Atasu E, et al. *Farmasotik Bilimler Dergisi* 1984;9(2):73–81.
[10] Bakke I, et al. *Meddelelser Fra Norsk Farmaceutisk Selskap* 1978;40(3):181–8.
[11] Muraviev I, et al. *Farmatsiia* 1986;35(6):17–20.
[12] Beck E. *Deutsche Apotheker Zeitung* 1989;129(Oct 12):2169–72.
[13] Wagner H, et al. *Planta Medica* 1989;55(5):452–4.
[14] Shomakers J, et al. *Deutsche Apotheker Zeitung* 1995;135(Feb 16):40–44, 46.
[15] Schilcher H, et al. *Deutsche Apotheker Zeitung* 1986;126(Jan 16):79–81.
[16] Willer F, et al. *Deutsche Apotheker Zeitung* 1991;131(Jun 13):1217–21.
[17] Wichtl M. *Deutsche Apotheker Zeitung* 1992;132(Jul 23):1569–76.
[18] Krivenko V, et al. *Vrachebnoe Delo* 1989;(3):76–8.
[19] Davidov M, et al. *Urologiia I Nefrologiia* 1995;(5):19–20.
[20] Rossiiskaya G, et al. *Farmatsiia* 1985;34(1):38–41.
[21] Krzeski T, et al. *Clinical Therapeutics* 1993;15(6):1011–20.
[22] Hirano T, et al. *Planta Medica* 1994;60(1):30–3.
[23] Hryb D, et al. *Planta Medica* 1995;61(1):31–2.
[24] Mittman P. *Planta Medica* 1990;56(1):44–7.
[25] Swanston-Flatt S, et al. *Diabetes Research* 1989;10(2):69–73.
[26] Roman R, et al. *Archives of Medical Research* 1992;23(1):59–64.
[27] Broncano F, et al. *Anales De La Real Academia De Farmacia* 1987;53(1):69–75.
[28] Shibuya N, et al. *Archives of Biochemistry & Biophysics* 1986;249(1):215–24.
[29] Gansser D, et al. *Planta Medica* 1995;61(2):138–40.
[30] Balzarini J, et al. *Antiviral Research* 1992;l18(2):191–207.
[31] Oliver F, et al. *Clinical & Experimental Dermatology* 1991;16(1):1–7.

New Zealand Green-Lipped Mussel

SCIENTIFIC NAME(S): *Perna canaliculus*; *Mytilidae*

COMMON NAME(S): New Zealand Green-Lipped Mussel (NZGLM)The New Zealand green-lipped mussel (NZGLM) is freeze-dried and ground into a capsule preparation for human consumption. The gonad comprises > 70% of the weight of the mollusk, and some investigators use gonadal tissue selectively in their preparations.

HISTORY: Early reports suggested that the daily ingestion of NZGLM extract alleviates the symptoms of rheumatoid arthritis and osteoarthritis in humans. Supported by a worldwide media campaign, claims were made that the extract was safe and effective in treating rheumatic diseases. The Arthritis Foundation responded by calling the product unproven and feared that the campaign could delude arthritis sufferers and raise false hopes.[1] Although the FDA issued an "Import Alert" in 1980 to stop the importation of the extract, it persists in the marketplace.

CHEMISTRY: Virtually nothing is known about the chemistry of the components of *P. canaliculus*. Lipid fractions have been found to contain arachidonic acid and its sterol ester, other unidentified sterols and the compound phaeophytin-a. Freeze-dried mussel preparations contain 9% nitrogen, 9% lipid and 20% carbohydrate, with less than 4 ppm heavy metals. Glutamine and aspartate are the most prevalent amino acids.[2] An extract contains amino acids, fats, carbohydrates and minerals.[3]

PHARMACOLOGY: Evidence for the anti-inflammatory activity of NZGLM extract is believed to have originated in the US during the screening of marine mollusks for antitumor activity. Animal data describing its activity have been conflicting.

Oral administration of the lipid fraction to rats concomitantly with the anti-inflammatory agents aspirin, indomethacin, tolmetin or diclofenac was found to reduce gastric mucosal damage by these drugs in some instances by 100%. Oral administration of the crude mussel preparation and its lipid extracts slightly reduced carrageenan-induced rat footpad edema; however, the changes were not statistically significant.[2]

Other investigators found that *P. canaliculus* extract reduced carrageenan-induced rat footpad edema only following intraperitoneal injection. A 500 mg/kg dose of crude preparation was the lowest effective dose, and the effect was noted within 2 hours. Oral administration of the material had no effect on inflammation.[4] This effect was also reported by investigators at the Royal Melbourne Institute of Technology, Australia, who showed that rat paws injected with carrageenan had swelled by 3% two hours after injection with the extract compared with 26% after injection with aspirin, ibuprofen or indomethacin.[5]

The oral administration of a marketed preparation of NZGLM to pregnant rats retarded fetal development and delayed parturition (the action of giving birth), suggesting that the product contains an orally active prostaglandin inhibitor. Other inhibitors, such as aspirin, indomethacin and naproxen, are known to interfere with ovulation and prolong gestation periods in rats. This consistency of similar effects from NZGLM are shown in this study.[6] Contrary to earlier work by this group, this experiment indicated that pharmacologic activity could be obtained when the extract was administered orally.

The results of several human clinical trials using NZGLM have been reported. The studies have been generally small, some poorly designed and the data conflicting. A highly publicized study heralded the benefits of oral administration of NZGLM extract in patients with classical rheumatoid arthritis and osteoarthritis.[7] Patients took 3 capsules a day (350 mg NZGLM extract per capsule or placebo) under double-blind conditions for 3 months. Both groups were then given NZGLM during months 4 to 6. At the end of the first 3 months of treatment, 39% of the patients (13/33) taking NZGLM and 18% (6/33) of the placebo-treated patients showed improvement. Although additional patients improved during the second 3 months of treatment, the analysis of the data was insufficient to draw conclusions about the extent of clinical benefit. The FDA and the National Institute for Arthritis, Metabolism and Digestive Diseases found that the study was small and poorly described, and that the extract was no more effective than the placebo.[7] In a follow-up study, 30 patients with rheumatoid arthritis were given the compound (300 mg 3 times/day) for one month.[8] There were no significant differences between the NZGLM group and placebo for any measurement.[8] The authors of the *Practitioner* report objected to the conclusions of this study, indicating that a 1–month trial period was too short to detect efficacy with *Seatone*; even in their trial, improvement was not noted before 3 months of therapy. Further, this improvement was maintained for days to several months after discontinuing treatment. They emphasized that NZGLM was the "safest and most effective preparation for both rheumatoid arthritis and osteoarthritis that [we] have yet come across."[9]

In another study, patients with rheumatoid arthritis and osteoarthritis received naproxen (750 mg/day) concomitantly with either NZGLM extract (1050 mg/day) or placebo for 6 weeks. From weeks 7 to 12, naproxen was replaced with placebo in both groups. During the first 6 weeks, there were no significant differences between the groups in any measurement or any change in measurement. After withdrawing naproxen, 15 or 22 patients in the NZGLM group and 15 of 19 in the placebo group discontinued because of a lack of efficacy. The addition of the mussel extract was not superior to adding placebo for alleviating symptoms in patients already receiving naproxen, and neither placebo nor mussel extract alone provided adequate symptomatic relief in the majority of patients, despite 6 weeks of pretreatment.[12]

TOXICOLOGY: All studies with NZGLM and its extracts have reported a low incidence of adverse effects, which generally consisted of GI symptoms (eg, diarrhea, nausea, flatulence); no significant changes in laboratory test results have been noted.[13]

One case report describes granulomatous hepatitis, jaundice, colickly epigastric pain, anorexia and malaise in a 64-year-old woman taking NZGLM. Liver biopsy and eosinophil presence were suggestive of a drug reaction. Discontinuation of all medications yielded normal liver function tests after a 3–month period.[14]

SUMMARY: NZGLM extract is promoted for the relief of symptoms of rheumatoid arthritis and osteoarthritis. Some anti-inflammatory activity has been found in animal tests, but this effect is inconsistent. The results of several human trials indicate that the initial findings of effectiveness reported in 1980 have not been reproducible. NZGLM extract cannot be recommended at this time for the treatment of inflammatory disease. A low incidence of adverse effects has been reported primarily consisting of possible GI symptoms. NZGLM delays parturition in animals and, therefore, should be avoided in pregnancy. A case report of drug-induced granulomatous hepatitis also exists. Additional research is needed to determine efficacy with this product.

PATIENT INFORMATION – New Zealand Green-Lipped Mussel

Uses: This product is being investigated as a treatment for rheumatoid arthritis and osteoarthritis. Although anti-inflammatory activity has been reported, this has not been proven.

Side Effects: Gastrointestinal discomfort has been reported, but the incidence is low. Animal studies suggest that this product could be dangerous to a fetus. Do not take during pregnancy.

---

[1] *Drug Intell Clin Pharm* 1981;15:157.
[2] Rainsford KD, et al. *Arzneim Forsch* 1980;30:2129.
[3] Reynolds J, ed. *Martindale the Extra Pharmacopoeia* 31st ed., Royal Pharmaceutical Society, London, England 1996;1712–13.
[4] Miller T, et al. *New Zealand Medical Journal* 1980;92(667):187–93.
[5] *Scrip* 1986;1119:21.
[6] Miller T, et al. *New Zealand Medical Journal* 1984;97(757):355–7.
[7] Gibson RG, et al. *Practitioner* 1980;224:955.
[8] Huskisson EC, et al. *Br Med J* 1981;282:1358.
[9] Gibson RG, et al. *Br Med J* 1981;282:1975.
[10] Gibson R, et al. *New Zealand Medical Journal* 1981;94(688):67–8.
[11] Couch R, et al. Antiinflammatory activity in fractionated extracts of the green-lipped mussel. *New Zealand Medical Journal.* 1982; 95(720):803-6.
[12] Caughy D, et al. *European Journal of Rheumatology & Inflammation* 1983;6(2):197–200.
[13] *Lancet* 1981;1:85.
[14] Ahern M, et al. *Medical Journal of Australia* 1980;2(Aug 9):151–2.

Nigella Sativa

SCIENTIFIC NAME(S): *Nigella sativa* L. Family: Ranunculaceae

COMMON NAME(S): Black seed, black cumin, charnushka, "black caraway" (not true caraway), baraka (the blessed seed), fitch (Biblical), "love in the mist"

BOTANY: *Nigella sativa* (NS) is an annual herb with terminal, grayish-blue flowers reaching between 30 to 60 cm in height. The toothed seed pod contains the distinctive tiny (1 to 2 mm long), black, 3-sided seeds, that are the plant parts used for medicinal purposes.[1-3]

HISTORY: NS is said to have been used for 2000 years, with some recordings of traditional uses of the seed dating back 1400 years. Its use began in the Middle East and spread throughout Europe and Africa. NS was found in the tomb of King Tutankhamen. Ancient Egyptians believed that medicinal plants such as these played a role in the afterlife. In the 1st century AD, Greek physician Dioscorides documented that the seeds were taken for a variety of problems including headache, toothache, nasal congestion, and intestinal worms.[1,3]

CHEMISTRY: Active ingredients in the seeds include thymoquinone, nigellone, and 40% fixed oils. Nigellimine N-oxide, an isoquinoline alkaloid, has been isolated from the seeds, as well. Other constituents include 84% fatty acids (linoleic and oleic); volatile oils (1.4%); alkaloids; saponin (melantin); palmitic, glutamic, ascorbic and stearic acids; arginine; methionine; lysine; glycine; leucine; and phytosterols. Crude fiber, calcium, iron, sodium, and potassium are also present. Nutritional composition of the seeds breaks down to 21% protein, 35% carbohydrate, and 36% fat.[1,2,3,4,5]

PHARMACOLOGY: NS has been used to benefit the GI system, as it eases gas and colic.[1] It has been used for diarrhea (dysentery) and constipation (hemorrhoids).[2]

At least 2 references claim that the respiratory effects of NS make it beneficial for allergies, cough, bronchitis, emphysema, asthma, flu, and chest congestion.[2,3] Constituent nigellone, in low concentrations, inhibits the release of histamine from mast cells.[6] Another report discusses volatile oil of NS (with the thymoquinone component removed) to provide a centrally acting respiratory stimulant when tested in guinea pigs.[7]

There are many studies available discussing immune/protective or anticancer effects of certain preparations of

NS. One of these reports that a mixture of NS, including cysteine, vitamin E, and *Crocus sativus*, reduces cisplatin-induced side effects in rats, including nephrotoxicity.[8] In another report, NS protected against induced falls in hemoglobin levels and leukocyte counts.[9] NS also enhances production of certain human interleukins and alters macrophages, suggesting changes in immune response in vitro.[10] NS has inhibited stomach tumors in mice.[11] Antitumor activity against certain carcinoma cells in vitro has been shown. In vivo, Ehrlich ascites carcinoma was completely inhibited by NS.[12] Constituents thymoquinone and dithymoquinone have demonstrated cytotoxic actions in human cell lines, as well.[13] Thymoquinone protected against induced hepatotoxicity in mice in vivo,[14] and in rat hepatocytes.[15]

Traditional use (ground seeds in poultice form) for inflammatory ailments such as rheumatism, headache, and certain skin conditions is proven by modern studies. Topical application of an NS mixture delayed and reduced papilloma formation in mice.[16] A fixed oil preparation of NS demonstrated anti-eicosanoid and antioxidant activity, again supporting the seeds' use for anti-inflammatory actions.[17]

A mixture containing NS displayed hepatic gluconeogenesis in rats related to antidiabetic actions. This may be beneficial in non-insulin dependent diabetes mellitus patients.[18] However, NS was not proven to increase glucose tolerance as the other components of the investigational mixture.[19]

NS has been used as a vermifuge.[1] The essential oil of the seed has been reported as an effective antimicrobial and anthelmintic agent.[20] NS has eradicated staphlococcal infections in mice and has also displayed other gram negative and gram positive antimicrobial actions, some of which are synergistic with other antibiotics.[21] NS traditionally has been used for conjunctivitis,[2] abscesses, parasites, and other infections.[3]

NS also plays a role in women's health, stimulating menstruation and increasing milk flow.[1,3] One study reports NS to have an anti-oxytocic potential in rat uterine smooth muscle, inhibiting spontaneous contractions.[22] Another report discusses the use of a seed extract to prevent pregnancy in rats 1 to 10 days post-coitum.[23]

NS may also possess the ability to decrease arterial blood pressure as observed in rats, suggesting the possible use as an antihypertensive agent.[24]

NS has also been used as a flavoring or as a spice.[3]

TOXICOLOGY: One report discusses allergic contact dermatitis from topical use of the oil.[25]

SUMMARY: NS has a long history dating back to Biblical times. Its uses include therapy in digestive disorders, as a respiratory treatment, and for its immunological effects including anti-cancer properties, anti-inflammatory actions, and antimicrobial effects. Toxic effects include contact dermatitis. Use during pregnancy should be avoided.

PATIENT INFORMATION – Nigella Sativa

Uses: Nigella sativa has been used for GI disorders and respiratory problems. Studies have been performed researching its immune/protective or anticancer effects, anti-inflammatory actions, and antimicrobial and anthelmintic properties. More human studies are needed.

Side Effects: Contact allergic dermatitis can occur with topical use of the oil. Do not use NS during pregnancy.

[1] Chevallier A. Encyclopedia of Medicinal Plants. New York, NY: DK Publishing, 1996, 237.
[2] Ghazanfar S. Handbook of Arabian Medicinal Plants. Boca Raton, FL: CRC Press, 1994, 180-1.
[3] http://fisher.bio.umb.edu/pages/fatimah/fatimah.htm
[4] Al-Jassir. Food Chemistry 1992;45:239-42.
[5] Nergiz, et al. Food Chemistry 1993;48;259-61.
[6] Chakravarty N. Inhibition of histamine release from mast cells by nigellone. Ann Allergy 1993;70:237-42.
[7] el Tahir K, et al. The respiratory effects of the volatile oil of the black seed (Nigella sativa) in guinea-pigs: elucidation of the mechanism(s) of action. Gen Pharmacol 1993;24(5):1115-22.
[8] el Daly E. Protective effect of cysteine and vitamin E, Crocus sativus and Nigella sativa extracts on cisplatin-induced toxicity in rats. J Pharm Belg 1998;53(2):87-93.
[9] Nair S, et al. Modulatory effects of Crocus sativus and Nigella sativa extracts on cisplatin-induced toxicity in mice. J Ethnopharmacol 1991;31(1):75-83.
[10] Haq A, et al. Nigella sativa: effect on human lymphocytes and polymorphonuclear leukocyte phagocytic activity. Immunopharmacology 1995;30(2):147-55.
[11] Badary O, et al. Inhibition of benzo(a)pyrene-induced forestomach carcinogenesis in mice by thymoquinone. Eur J Cancer Prev 1999;8(5):435-40.
[12] Salomi N, et al. Antitumor principles from Nigella sativa seeds. Cancer Lett 1992;63(1):41-6.
[13] Worthen D, et al. The in vitro anti-tumor activity of some crude and purified components of blackseed, Nigella sativa L. Anticancer Res 1998;18(3A):1527-32.
[14] Nagi M, et al. Thymoquinone protects against carbon tetrachloride hepatotoxicity in mice via an antioxidant mechanism. Biochem Mol Biol Int 1999;47(1):153-9.
[15] Daba M, et al. Hepatoprotective activity of thymoquinone in isolated rat hepatocytes. Toxicol Lett 1998;95(1):23-9.
[16] Salomi M, et al. Inhibitory effects of Nigella sativa and saffron (Crocus sativus) on chemical carcinogenesis in mice. Nutr Cancer 1991;16(1):67-72.
[17] Houghton P, et al. Fixed oil of Nigella sativa and derived thymoquinone inhibit eicosanoid generation in leukocytes and membrane lipid peroxidation. Planta Med 1995;61(1):33-6.
[18] al-Awadi F, et al. The effect of a plants mixture extract on liver gluconeogenesis in streptozotocin induced diabetic rats. Diabetes Res 1991;18(4):163-8.
[19] al-Awadi F, et al. Studies on the activity of individual plants of an antidiabetic plant mixture. Acta Diabetol Lat 1987;24(1):37-41.
[20] Agarwal R, et al. Antimicrobial & anthelmintic activities of the essential oil of Nigella sativa Linn. Indian J Exp Biol 1979;17(11):1264-65.
[21] Hanafy M, et al. Studies on the antimicrobial activity of Nigella sativa seed (black cumin). J Ethnopharmacol 1991;34(2-3):275-78.
[22] Aqel M, et al. Effects of the volatile oil of Nigella sativa seeds on the uterine smooth muscle of rat and guinea pig. J Ethnopharmacol 1996;52(1):23-6.
[23] Keshri G, et al. Post-coital contraceptive efficacy of the seeds of Nigella sativa in rats. Indian J Physiol Pharmacol 1995;39(1):59-62.
[24] el Tahir K, et al. The cardiovascular actions of the volatile oil of the black seed (Nigella sativa) in rats: elucidation of the mechanism of action. Gen Pharmacol 1993;24(5):1123-31.
[25] Steinmann A, et al. Contact Dermatitis 1997;36(5):268-69.

Nutmeg

SCIENTIFIC NAME(S): *Myristica fragrans* Houtt. Family: Myristicaceae

COMMON NAME(S): Nutmeg, mace, nux moschata

BOTANY: The nutmeg tree is the source of the spices nutmeg and mace. This evergreen grows to over 60 feet. It is found in India, Ceylon, Malaysia and Granada. This slow-growing tree produces a fruit called a nutmeg apple, which is similar in appearance to a peach or apricot. When the fruit ripens, it splits to expose a bright-red, net-like aril wrapped around a shell, which contains the nut. The nut is removed and dried to produce nutmeg. The dried aril yields the spice mace, which possesses a flavor similar to that of nutmeg.[1,2]

HISTORY: Nutmeg is a widely used food spice that has received attention as an alternative hallucinogen. Both nutmeg and mace have been used in Indian cooking and folk medicine. The folk uses of nutmeg have included the treatment of gastric disorders and rheumatism, and it has been used as a hypnotic[3] and an aphrodisiac.[4]

Pliny, in the 1st century A.D., described a "comacum" tree with a fragrant nut and two perfumes. During the 6th century A.D., nutmeg and mace were imported by Arab traders. By the 12th century, these spices were well known in Europe. Chaucer writes of "nutmeg in ale" in *The Canterbury Tales* during the 14th century.[5]

At the turn of the 19th century, interest developed in the use of nutmeg as an abortifacient and a stimulant for menses. These properties have been largely discounted but remain a persistent cause of nutmeg intoxication in women with delayed menses.[6,7]

CHEMISTRY: Nutmeg seed contains 20% to 40% of a fixed oil called nutmeg butter, once used externally for sprains. Today, it has some commercial use in soaps and perfumes.[5] This oil contains myristic acid and glycerides of lauric, tridecanoic, stearic and palmitic acids. Nutmeg oil (also known as myristica oil) is produced from the steam distillation of the nut. Also present is starch, protein, saponin, catechins and others.[1]

The seed nut also contains 8% to 15% of an essential oil that is believed to be partially responsible for the effects associated with nutmeg intoxication. The aromatic oil contains d-camphene (60% to 80%), dipentene (8%),

myristicin (4% to 8%), elemicin (2%) and small amounts of iso-elemicin; d,l-pinene; geraniol; eugenol; isoeugenol; safrole; and limonene.[8,9] Also present in the oil is sabinene, cymene alpha-thujene, gamma-terpinene and monoterpene alcohols in smaller amounts. Mace and mace oil contain many of the same components of nutmeg and its oil, but mace appears to have a higher myristicin content, with less fixed oil.[1,3]

Nutmeg constituents have been identified by thin-layer chromatography.[10] Quantitative determination has been performed on its active constituents in the oil (eugenol and isoeugenol).[11] High-performance liquid chromatography (HPLC) has also been performed in the determination of safrole and myristicin in the nut and the aril.[12] Other recent reports are available concerning chemical composition.[13,14] Nutmeg and mace responded similarly to marijuana in a "simple field test for marijuana."[15]

PHARMACOLOGY: Nutmeg was known for its **psychoactive properties** as early as 1525 and has gained a reputation among inmates and drug cultists as a hallucinogen.[16] Doses of 5 to 20 g appear to be required for any pharmacologic activity to occur. This is equivalent to one to three whole nuts; 2 tablespoons of commercial ground nutmeg weight, about 14 g; or two grated nuts.[17]

Debate surrounds the issue of whether myristicin is the psychoactive component of nutmeg. It does not appear that myristicin alone can induce hallucinations.[18] Because synthetic myristicin does not imitate nutmeg intoxication, it has been suggested that the presence of other compounds (eugenol, geraniol) may be needed for the characteristic pharmacologic effect.[19] It has been proposed that the structural similarities of the allyl benzene components of nutmeg to those of amphetamine-like compounds may be responsible for the CNS activity of the spice. Alternately, it has been theorized that myristicin and elemicin may be metabolized to their amino derivatives following ingestion. The probable derivatives include the psychotomimetics MMDA (3-methoxy-4,5 dimethylenedioxyamphetamine) from myristicin and TMA (3,4,5-trimethoxyamphetamine) from elemicin.[20] A structural similarity exists among these metabolites, amphetamine and mescaline. One report suggests nutmeg oil to antagonize amphetamine stimulatory effects in chickens.[21]

The effects of nutmeg intoxication are variable, and the loss of the volatile oil from the ground spice results in part in the variability of the experience. Generally, nutmeg for intoxication is chewed or the powdered nut is suspended in a liquid and drunk. Geraniol is approximately three times as potent as ipecac in inducing emesis; hence, users may combine ground nutmeg with cola syrup to reduce the chances of emesis. This mixture is appropriately referred to as "brown slime."[22]

Nutmeg has received attention for the treatment of diarrhea in calves.[23] It has also been used in the **treatment of human diarrhea** secondary to thyroid medullary carcinoma[24] and in the treatment of human diarrhea in doses of 4 to 6 tablespoons of nutmeg per day. A fall in serum calcium levels was also noted in this case report, improving chronic hypercalcemia possibly related to this therapy.[25] The hexane-soluble fraction of nutmeg was found to be most active in inhibiting secretory activity against E coli toxins in an antidiarrheal report in animals.[26] **Inhibition** of the synthesis and activity **of prostaglandins** appears to be additionally responsible for this effect.[27] Another study on this effect reports dose-related inhibition of contraction in rat tissue. In human colon resections, nutmeg similarly reduced prostaglandin-like activity in doses from 0.1 to 500 mcg/ml (however, at 5 mcg/ml, an increase, not understood, was noted).[28] Eugenol appears to be the most potent antiprostaglandin component of nutmeg oil.[9] A later study confirms this fact by quantitative determination, reporting eugenol and isoeugenol to be the active principles. The mechanism is their capacity to inhibit platelet aggregation.[11] An earlier report on two subjects found no differences in aggregation using 1.5 to 4 grams of freshly ground nutmeg, 3 to 4 times a day for a 2-day period.[29] Ground nutmeg administered orally to rats decreased renal prostaglandin levels to a degree similar to that produced by indomethacin.[30] Other reported uses of nutmeg include use as a larvicidal agent, a flavoring agent in many foods and a fragrance component in soaps and perfumes.[1] Ethnopharmacology employs nutmeg for mouth sores and insomnia.[31] Traditional medicinal use is also discussed.[12]

TOXICOLOGY: Symptoms appear 3 to 8 hours after ingestion of large amounts of the spice. The episodes are characterized by weak pulse, hypothermia, disorientation, giddiness, nausea and vomiting and a feeling of pressure in the chest or lower abdomen. For up to 24 hours, an extended period of alternating delirium and stupor persists, ending in a heavy sleep. There is often a sensation of loss of limbs and a terrifying fear of impending death. Death has been reported following the ingestion of a very large dose.[32] A case report reviews a 25-year-old male expressing psychotic symptoms upon ingestion of 120 to 650 mg nutmeg. Haloperidol therapy was necessary to stabilize the patient.[33] Another case report discusses similar findings in a 23-year-old with acute psychotic break and anticholinergic toxic episode symptoms, such as hallucinations and palpitations.[34] In a similar case, an acute anticholinergic hyperstimulation occurred in a pregnant woman after excessive nutmeg ingestion.[35] Gastric lavage and supportive therapy have been recommended for nutmeg toxicity.[36] Recovery usually occurs within 24 hours but may extend for several days.[37] Additional reports discussing misuse of nutmeg are also available.[38,39]

Safrole, a minor component of the oil, has been shown to promote hepatocarcinomas in mice.[40] The oil is moderately irritating when applied to rabbit skin for 24 hours under occlusion but was found to be nonirritating and nonsensitizing to human skin.[32]

SUMMARY: Nutmeg is a common spice that is used widely in cooking. It has been used pharmacologically for diarrhea treatment and is being studied for its role in inhibition of prostaglandin synthesis and inhibition of platelet aggregation. The ingestion of several tablespoons of the spice can lead to a stuporous intoxication that may be severe in its presentation.

PATIENT INFORMATION – Nutmeg

Uses: Nutmeg is used as a flavoring agent and a fragrance. It has also been used as a larvicidal, a hallucinogen and treatment for diarrhea, mouth sores and insomnia.

Side Effects: Side effects include weak pulse, hypothermia, disorientation, giddiness, nausea, vomiting, a feeling of pressure in the chest or lower abdomen, a sensation of loss of limbs, a fear of impending death and, after a very large dose, death.

---

[1] Leung A, et al. Encyclopedia of Common Natural Ingredients. New York, NY: John Wiley and Sons, Inc. 1996;385-88.

[2] Dermarderosian A, et al. Natural Product Medicine. Philadelphia, PA: George F. Stickley Co. 1988;329-31.

[3] Forrest JE, Heacock RA. *Lloydia* 1972;35:44C.

[4] Weil AF. *J Psyc Drugs* 1971;3:72.

[5] Rosengarten F. The Book of Spices. Wynnewood, PA: Livingston Publishing Co. 1969;308-15.

[6] Green RC. *JAMA* 1959;171:1342.

[7] Painter JC, et al. *Clin Toxicol* 1971;4:1.

[8] Shulgin AT. *Nature* 1966;210:380.

[9] Rasheed A, et al. *N Engl J Med* 1984;310:50.

[10] Suzuki H, et al. *Eisei Shikenjo Hokoku* 1990;(108):98–100.

[11] Janssens J, et al. *J Ethnopharmacol* 1990;29(2):179-88.

[12] Archer A. *J Chromatogr* 1988;438(1):117-21.

[13] Briggs C. *Canadian Pharmaceutical Journal* 1991 Jul;124:349-50,52.

[14] Lawrence B. *Perfumer and Flavorist* 1990 Nov-Dec;15:45-6,48,51–3,55,56,58,60–2,64,66.

[15] Lau-Cam C, et al. *J Pharm Sci* 1979 Aug;68:976-78.

[16] Faguet RA, Rowland KF. *Am J Psychiatry* 1978;135:860.

[17] Mack RB. *N Carolina Med J* 1982 Jun;439.

[18] Farnsworth NR. *Am J Psychiatry* 1979;136:858.

[19] Truitt EB, et al. *J Neuropsych* 1961;2:205.

[20] Weil AT. *Economic Botany* 1965;19:194.

[21] Sherry C, et al. *International Journal of Crude Drug Research* 1982 Jun;20:89-92.

[22] Giannini AJ, et al. *Am Family Physician* 1986;33:207.

[23] Stamford JF, Bennett A. *Vet Record* 1980;106:389.

[24] Barrowman J, et al. *Br Med J* 1975 Jul 5;3:11-12.

[25] Shafran I, et al. *N Engl J Med* 1975 Dec 11;293:1266.

[26] Gupta S, et al. *Int J Pharmacognosy* 1992;30(3):179-83.

[27] Fawell W, et al. *N Engl J Med* 1973 Jul 12;289:108-9.

[28] Bennett A, et al. *N Engl J Med* 1974 Jan 10;290:110-11.

[29] Dietz W, et al. *N Engl J Med* 1976 Feb 26;294:503.

[30] Misra V, et al. *Indian J Med Res* 1978;67:482.

[31] Van Gils C. *J Ethnopharmacol* 1994;42(2):117-24.

[32] Updyke DLT. *Food Cosmet Toxicol* 1976;14:631.

[33] Brenner N, et al. *J R Soc Med* 1993 Mar;86:179-80.

[34] Abernethy N, et al. *Am J Emerg Med* 1992;10(5):429-30.

[35] Lavy G. *J Reprod Med* 1987;32(1):63-64.

[36] Harcin JW, Arena JM. Human Poisoning from Native and Cultivated Plants, Duke University Press, 1974.

[37] Brown JK, Malone MH. *Pacific Information Service on Street Drugs* 1977;5:20.

[38] Lewis P, et al. *J Drug Issues* 1974;4(2):162-75.

[39] Wills S. *Pharm J* 1993 Aug 14;251:227-29.

[40] Miller EC, et al. *Cancer Res* 1983;43:1124.

Oats

SCIENTIFIC NAME(S): *Avena sativa* L. Family: Gramineae

COMMON NAME(S): Oats

BOTANY: Oats probably originated in three geographic regions: Abyssinia, the Mediterranean and China. Today, the grain is grown primarily in the US, Canada, Russia and Germany. The oat is derived from wild grasses and evolved into today's cultivated plant, which adapted to climate and locality. The plant grows to be about 1 meter tall. Its linear leaves are long and narrow, and its flowers are gathered at the top of the plant, which contain two to three florets.[1]

HISTORY: Rich in fat and protein, oats, compared with other cereals, have one of the highest food values for humans.[2] The majority of oat stocks are used for feeding livestock, but recent interest in the fiber content of oats has resulted in an increased demand for human consumption. Oat extracts have been used for more than a century as soothing topical emollients. Since 100 B.C., the oat has been grown mainly in northern latitudes.[1]

CHEMISTRY: Aside from polyphenols, mono- and oligosaccharides, iron, manganese and zinc are also present in the plant. Concentration of these minerals is higher in oats than in other cereals. Other constituents include flavones, triterpenoid saponins in the leaves, carotenoids and chlorophyll derivatives.[3] Composition and physical behavior of oats have been evaluated in another report.[4]

PHARMACOLOGY: Oats are a good source of energy, protein and fat for humans, especially children.[5] Because of its gluten content, oat plant derivatives have been effective in **managing dry, itchy skin conditions.**[6] Bath products, including colloidal oatmeal mixtures, bath soaps and gels, and powders containing oat extracts are available commercially. An overview of oat use in cosmetics, including gels, balms and powders is available.[7]

An extract of oats is used in traditional Ayurvedic medicine to cure opium addiction. A case report shows six out of 10 opium addicts giving up the drug after a treatment period of 27 to 45 days using a decoction of green oats.[8] Oats may also reduce the desire to smoke cigarettes. In one poorly blinded study, 26 smokers received either an alcoholic extract of oats or placebo for 28 days. Mean cigarette use in the oat group was 20 per day at baseline, which decreased to six cigarettes/day after therapy (p < 0.001). Consumption in the control group remained constant (17 cigarettes/day). The difference between groups was statistically significant at the end of therapy. The reduction in consumption continued to be observed 2 months after terminating treatment.[9] However, these results could not be confirmed in another 12-week blinded study that showed no overall group effect on cigarette consumption during oat extract therapy.[10]

Oat bran, the ground inner husk of the grain, has become popular as a dietary means of **lowering blood lipids.** Oat bran and oatmeal are available in various breakfast foods, laxatives and baked goods. In general, water-soluble dietary fiber has a greater lipid-lowering effect than insoluble fiber. Soluble fiber may bind cholesterol and bile acids in the intestines, preventing absorption, or may be fermented to short chain fatty acids by colonic bacteria. Upon absorption, these compounds may inhibit cholesterol synthesis.[11] A serving of *Quaker Oat Bran* hot cereal provides 4.1 g of total dietary fiber, of which 1.9 g is soluble and 2.2 g is insoluble.

A large number of clinical studies have been conducted to evaluate the effect of oat bran supplementation on blood lipid levels.[11] Typically, the results of controlled clinical trials indicate that supplementation with oat bran products for 6 to 8 weeks results in a decrease in total cholesterol levels of approximately 6 mg/dl,[12] although the addition of 100 g of oat bran and dried beans daily for 3 weeks resulted in a 23% decrease in total cholesterol, a 23% decrease in LDL-cholesterol, a 21% decrease in triglycerides and a 20% decrease in HDL-cholesterol. Low cholesterol levels were maintained for up to 2 years of supplementation in this study.[13] However, at least one well-publicized study refutes the inherent value of dietary oat bran to lower serum cholesterol.[14] Swain, et al claim the value of oat bran ingestion is caused by basic diet manipulation, rather than a "pharmacologic" effect of the fiber itself. The study has been criticized for many methodologic flaws.[15] A later study evaluated the mechanism of oat bran in lowering serum lipids. Beta-glucan present in oats mediates an increase in bile acid secretion, explaining its effect in nine ileostomy patients.[16] Oat extract has also been studied in animals fed a high-fat diet. Results of one report suggest oat extract plays an appreciable role in atherosclerosis prophylaxis and management.[17]

Antibiotic and antifungal properties of oats have been evaluated.[18] In folk medicine, oat-herb tea is used as a sedative and to lower uric acid levels; neither use has been scientifically proven. The tea has also been used as a diuretic. Baths prepared from oat straw are used to treat arthritis, paralysis, liver and skin disorders.[1]

TOXICOLOGY: Oat bran increases the stool bulk, which may be uncomfortable to patients[19] and increased defecation frequency may result in perineal irritation. Fiber digestion by colonic bacteria may cause gaseous distention and flatulence. Although epidemiologic studies suggest that ingestion of large amounts of dietary fiber may reduce incidence of colonic cancer, one report provides evidence that the increase in fecal bile excretion that occurs in the presence of soluble fibers may promote chemically induced colonic cancer in animals fed oat bran.[20] As with any fiber product, oat bran products should be taken with plenty of water to ensure hydration and dispersion of the fiber in the GI tract.

Contact dermatitis from oat flour has been reported,[21] and the oat prolamine, avenin, has been shown to raise antibodies in rabbits.[22] Gluten should be avoided by patients with celiac disease. Oat gluten has been used as a stabilizer, emulsifier and food extender.[23]

While some fibers have been used successfully in the adjunctive management of glycemic control in diabetic patients, oat-based meals appear to have a smaller effect on blood glucose and insulin levels than most fiber sources.[24] A protease inhibitor has been identified in *Avena sativa*, but its clinical significance is not known.[25] A multimycotoxin detection method for "aflatoxins, ochratoxins, zearalenone, sterigmatocystin and patulin" has been developed to detect their presence in oats and other grains.[26]

SUMMARY: Oat and its extracts are commercially important as grains and dietary supplements. The ingestion of large amounts of fiber (40 g/day) may contribute to the reduction of blood cholesterol levels, an effect that is observed in as few as 2 to 3 weeks. Other effects of oat extract include possible cures for opium addiction or smoking and atherosclerosis prophylaxis. Oats are effective for itchy skin conditions, and its presence in bath and beauty products is well known. No significant toxicity has been associated with the ingestion of oat products.

PATIENT INFORMATION – Oats

Uses: Oats are used to manage dry, itchy skin conditions, to cure opium addiction, to reduce the desire to smoke cigarettes and to lower blood lipids.

Side Effects: Oat bran increases bulk of stool and frequency of defecation resulting in perineal irritation. Fiber may cause distention and flatulence.

---

[1] Bisset N. Herbal Drugs and Phytopharmaceuticals. Stuttgart, Germany: CRC Press 1994;96-98.
[2] Olmsted CE. The Story of Living Plants. Chicago: University of Knowledge, 1938.
[3] *Jagr Fd Chem* 1989;37:60.
[4] Paton D, et al. *Cosmetics and Toiletries* 1995 Mar;110:63,64,66,68,70.
[5] Graham GG, et al. *J Pediatr Gastroenterol Nutr* 1990;10:344.
[6] DerMarderosian AH, Liberti LE. *Natural Product Medicine*. Philadelphia, PA: G.F. Stickley Co., 1988.
[7] Lower E. Soap, *Perfumery and Cosmetics*. 1995 Oct;68:51,53.
[8] Anand C. *Br Med J* 1971 Sep 11;3:640.
[9] Anand CL. *Nature* 1971;233:496.
[10] Bye C, et al. *Nature* 1974;252:580.
[11] *Med Lett* 1988;30:111.
[12] Van Horn L, et al. *J Am Diet Assn* 1986;86:759.
[13] Anderson JW, et al. *J Can Diet Assn* 1984;45:140.
[14] Swain JF, et al. *N Engl J Med* 1990;322:147.
[15] Roubenoff RA, et al. *N Engl J Med* 1990;322:1746.
[16] Lia A, et al. *Am J Clin Nutr* 1995;62(6):1245-51.
[17] Juzwiak S, et al. *Herba Polonica* 1994;40(1–2):50-58.
[18] Gill S. *Farmacja Polska* 1985;41(10):592-94.
[19] Valle-Jones JC. *Curr Med Res Opin* 1985;9:716.
[20] Jacobs LR. *Proc Soc Exp Biol Med* 1986;183:299.
[21] Calzavara-Pinton PG, et al. *Giornale Ital Dermatol Venerol* 1989;124:289.
[22] van Twist-de Graaf MJ, et al. *Z Lebensm Unters Forsch* 1989;188:535.
[23] Anderson CR, Cerda JJ. *Compr Ther* 1989;15:62. <Review
[24] Heaton KW, et al. *Am J Clin Nutr* 1988;47:675.
[25] Liener IE. Toxic Constituents of Plant Foodstuffs. New York: Academic Press, 1980, 2nd ed.
[26] Stoloff L. *J Assoc Off Anal Chem* 1971 Jan;54:91-7.

Octacosanol

SCIENTIFIC NAME(S): 1-octacosanol, n-octacosanol, octacosyl alcohol

COMMON NAME(S): 24 to 36 carbon alcohols isolated from wheat germ oil or other plants.

HISTORY: Studies in the 1930s and 1940s suggested that athletes who were given daily or weekly doses of raw, unrefined wheat germ oil outperformed subjects who received only vitamin E supplements. The biologic value of wheat germ was reconfirmed in a 1951 study in which college students received wheat germ oil for 18 weeks. Treated subjects improved their "all-out" bicycle riding times by 47%, while the untreated controls increased their average riding times by only 4%. All of these studies suggested that some component of unrefined wheat germ oil increased physical endurance, and that vitamin E was not entirely responsible. Further investigations culminated in a patent for the combination of "physiologically active" components of raw wheat germ oil.[1] No published scientific studies were provided that evaluated the physiologic activity of these "active constituents."[2]

CHEMISTRY: Octacosanol is a constituent of vegetable waxes and has been isolated from wax on green blades of wheat.[3] The name octacosanol specifically pertains to a 28-carbon alcohol, but it is commonly used to denote a mixture of 24-, 26-, 28-, and 30-36-carbon alcohols, that are believed to possess most of the physiologic activity of wheat germ oil. These compounds are present as alcohols or acetates and can also be isolated from plants other than wheat.[2] A number of reports are available, isolating octacosanol as one of many components in certain plants. A brief listing follows, with references listed for those interested in these specific species: octacosanol from leaves of *Pithecolobium dulce* V.,[4] *Cymbopogon citratus* (Dc.) Stapf (Poaceae);[5] whole plant of *Euphorbia myrsinitis* L.,[6] *Euphorbia tinctoria* boiss,[7] *Daemia extensa* R. Br.;[8] stem bark of *Acacia modesta*;[9] Heart wood of *Cassia javanica*;[10] fruits of *Serenoa repens* Bartram,[11] *Poinsettia pulcherrima*,[12] *Citrullus colocynthis*;[13] roots of *Talinum paniculatum* Gaertner,[14] *Acanthus illicifolius*;[15] crude drug "jungle pepper" *Vitex pubescens*;[16] and octacosanol from *Eupolyphaga sinensis* Walker.[17]

PHARMACOLOGY: Specific biologic activity has been described for triacontanol (30-C alcohol); its application to seedlings and growing plants increases growth rate and fruit yield.[18] It is being investigated in humans for use as an antiviral for herpes and for the treatment of inflammatory skin diseases. The biologic activity of tetracosanol (24-C) and hexacosanol (26-C) are poorly understood.

To understand mechanisms such as increased physical exercise and improved motor endurance by octacosanol, its pharmacokinetic characteristics were evaluated. Octacosanol was found to distribute mainly to adipose tissue when administered orally in rats.[19] After ingestion of octacosanol in rats that were exercised, however, results showed significantly higher distribution to muscle tissue, supporting a theory of octacosanol muscle storage in response to exercise. A similar report by the same authors evaluates muscle storage of serially administered (orally through stomach tubs) radioactive octacosanol. At first, highest concentration is in the liver, but rapidly disappears (even when doses are increased). The muscle was able to store a considerable amount of octacosanol, which may help to explain increased muscle endurance in exercise.[20]

Also proposed is the possibility that octacosanol increases mobilization of free fatty acids from fat cells in the muscle, having "adipokinetic" activity affecting the muscle's lipolysis process.[21] In another report, lipid metabolism was evaluated in rats receiving octacosanol and a high-fat diet. Results suggest octacosanol to suppress lipid accumulation in adipose tissue. Additionally, it decreased serum triacylglycerol concentration and enhanced serum fatty acid concentration.[22]

Absorption of octacosanol was found to be low, with excretion mainly via feces. Metabolites of the alcohol were found to be present in urine.[19]

Orally administered combinations of octacosanol compounds were shown to produce a physiologic response characteristic of androgenic activity in the chick-comb test. 1-Octacosanol increased the size of the testes and seminal vesicles in rats, compared to those fed a cottonseed oil control diet. Further, guinea pigs fed a diet containing 2.2 mg/kg octacosanol for 28 days had a better swimming performance than animals fed rations without the alcohol. Animals that were fed a 2% wheat germ oil diet also swam longer than those fed the control diet. Patent 3,031,376 provided limited evidence that daily doses ranging from 0.05 to 150 mg of these compounds are well tolerated by humans; it indicated that the usual "maintenance dose" is 40 to 80 mg total alcohols daily.[2]

In one single-blind study, 12 men received 1-octacosanol daily in cottonseed oil (dose not specified) and 10 received placebo. Both treatment groups were tested before the study and again at a later, unspecified interval, for ECG R-wave changes, the mile run, 466-yard swim, pushups and six other athletic events. Significant ($p < 0.05$) improvements were noted for all test parameters in the octacosanol-treated group; however, statistically significant improvement was also noted in the placebo group for the mile run, 466-yard swim and step-up test. The maximum percent mean improvement for any test was 18%, and this was observed in both test groups. In another test using four matched groups of boys (population size not specified), subjects given an unspecified quantity of octacosanol for 8 weeks completed the 600-yard run an average of 10% faster than before starting the supplement. Boys who received wheat germ oil improved their times by 9%, those receiving wheat germ by 6% and those receiving placebo by 4%.[2]

A recent review article discusses efficacy of nutritional supplementation by athletes. Octacosanol is mentioned to have ergogenic qualities, but with little or no scientific evidence supporting this.[23]

The patent proposes that, theoretically, octacosanol improves stamina and vigor by improving oxygen utilization during anaerobic glycolysis. At the onset of exercise, when the circulation is increasing to meet muscle oxygen demand, a period of relative oxygen deficiency exists, and blood lactate levels rise. It is believed that octacosanol and related compounds may aid in the removal of lactic acid by increasing the efficiency of the tricarboxylic acid cycle, which operates through reactions connecting to the oxygen supply. This may also result in an increased oxygen uptake or a decreased oxygen requirement. However, no data exist to confirm this mechanism of action.

A small study suggests that octacosanol benefits patients with Parkinsonism. In a double-blind, placebo controlled trial, 10 patients received six weeks of treatment with 5 mg octacosanol in wheat germ oil or placebo, three times daily with meals. Three of the patients showed significant symptomatic improvement during the octacosanol phase of treatment. None of the patients showed worsening of their conditions during octacosanol treatment. Overall, the treated group showed a slight improvement in performance of activities of daily living.[24]

The promising results in Parkinson patients led to a double-blind, crossover study involving 11 patients with amyotropic lateral sclerosis. Patients received either 40 mg/day of each of the 28-C, 30-C, and 30-36-C alcohols or a placebo for 3 months. Although 3 patients in the drug phase and 3 in the placebo phase reported subjective improvement, neurological evaluations showed progression of the disease in all cases. Some patients showed some improvement in certain test scores, but there was no significant difference between the octacosanol and placebo groups.[25,26]

TOXICOLOGY: There are no data on the long-term toxicity of products containing octacosanol.[2] In the Parkinson's disease study, side effects were infrequent but included position-related nonrotational dizziness, mild increase in nervous tension, and worsening of carbidopa/levodopa-related dyskinesias. These effects suggested an interaction with levodopa.[25,26]

SUMMARY: Octacosanol commonly denotes a mixture of 24- to 36-carbon alcohols isolated from wheat germ oil. It is also found in many other plants. They have been touted as improving the stamina of athletes, but scientific proof of this is lacking. Animal studies on pharmacokinetic parameters may help to explain possible theories of increased muscle endurance and mobilization of free fatty acids from fat cells, but more research is needed for proof in the human population. There is preliminary evidence that octacosanol may benefit patients with Parkinsonism, but trials in patients with amyotropic lateral sclerosis have shown no therapeutic value. The long-term safety of octacosanol is not known.

PATIENT INFORMATION – Octacosanol

Uses: Octacosanol is being investigated as a herpes antiviral and as a treatment for inflammatory diseases of the skin. It has also demonstrated enhanced physical endurance in some studies.

Side Effects: There have been no reported side effects with the use of octacosanol except for a suggestion of interaction with levodopa/carbidopa in Parkinson's disease patients.

[1] US Pat 3,031,376;24 Apr 1962.

[2] DerMarderosian A, et al. *Natural Product Medicine.* George F. Stickley Co.: Philadelphia. 1988;331–3.

[3] Budavari S, ed. *The Merck Index*, 11th ed., Merck and Co., Inc.: Rahway, NJ. 1989;1069.

[4] Nigam S, et al. *Planta Med* 1970;18(Jan):44–50.

[5] De Matouschek B, et la. *Pharm Acta Helv* 1991;66(9–10):242–45.

[6] Aynehchi Y, et al. *J Pharm Sci* 1972;61(Feb):292–93.

[7] Aynehchi Y, et al. *Acata Pharmaceutica Suecica* 1974;11(May):185–90.

[8] Ravi J, et al. *Indian Drugs* 1993;30(Jun):292.

[9] Joshi K, et al. *Plant Med* 1975;27(May):281–83.

[10] Joshi K, et al. *Plant Med* 1975;28(Oct):190–92.

[11] Hatinguais P, et al. *Trav Soc Pharm Montpellier* 1981;41(4):253–62.

[12] Gupta D, et al. *J Nat Prod* 1983;46(Nov-Dec):937–38.

[13] Hatam N, et al. *Int J Crude Drug Res* 1990;28(Sep):183–84.

[14] Komatsu M, et al. *J Pharm Soc Japan* 1982;102(May):499–502.

[15] Kokpol U, et al. *J Nat Prod* 1986;49(Mar-Apr):355–56.

[16] Sukumar E, et al. *Indian J Pharm Sci* 1988;50(Jan-Feb):55–56.

[17] Lu Y, et al. *Chung Kuo Chung Yao Tsa Chih* 1992;17(8):487–89.

[18] Maugh TH. *Science* 1981;212:33.

[19] Kabir Y, et al. *Ann Nutr Metab* 1993;37(1):33–38.

[20] Kabir Y, et al. *Ann Nutr Metab* 1995;39(5):279–84.

[21] Kabir Y, et al. *Nahrung* 1994;38(4):373–77.

[22] Kato S, et al. *Br J Nutr* 1995;73(3):433–41.

[23] Belz S, et al. *Clin Pharm* 1993;12(12):900–08.

[24] Snider SR. *Ann Neurol* 1984;16:723.

[25] Norris F, et al. *Neurology* 1986;36(9):1263, 4.

[26] Norris FH, et al. *Adv Exp Biol* 1987;209:183.

Oleander

SCIENTIFIC NAME(S): *Nerium oleander* L. Synonymous with *N. indicum* Mill. Family: Apocyanaceae

COMMON NAME(S): Oleander, adelfa, laurier rose, rosa laurel, rose bay, rosa francesa.[1] Should not be confused with yellow oleander (Thevetia neriifolia), also a toxic plant.

BOTANY: The oleander is a shrub that grows to about 20 feet in height. It has long narrow leaves that attain almost a foot in length, and these are typically grouped in threes around the stem. The red, pink or white fluffy flowers form in small clusters. Cultivated plants rarely produce fruits.[1] Although native to the Mediterranean, the oleander is widely cultivated throughout warm climates.

HISTORY: Despite its well recognized toxic potential, the oleander has been used in traditional medicine for centuries. Its uses included the management of such diverse ailments as cardiac illnesses, asthma, corns, cancer and epilepsy.[2]

CHEMISTRY: The plant contains a number of related cardioactive glycosides similar in activity to digitalis.

PHARMACOLOGY: All parts of the plant contain the cardiac glycosides oleandrin and neriin, along with the cardenolides gentiobiosyloleandrin and odoroside A.[2] In addition, a variety of other pharmacologically active compounds, including folinerin, rosagenin, rutin and oleandomycin, have been identified in the plant.[2]

A water extract of oleander leaves yields approximately 2.3% of a crude polysaccharide. The structure of this compound has been characterized by NMR. The compound shows no in vivo antitumor activity, weak macrophage-mediated cell toxicity and weak mitogenic activity.[3]

The flavonol glycosides are reported to influence vascular permeability and to possess diuretic properties. Cornerine has been shown to be effective in the treatment of cardiac ailments in man, improving heart muscle function.[2]

TOXICOLOGY: The entire oleander plant is toxic. Smoke from the plant and water in which the plant has been immersed also can be toxic.[1]

In birds, as little as 0.12 to 0.7 g of the plant has been found to cause death.[4] A horse can be killed by as few as 15 to 20 g of fresh leaves and a sheep by 1 to 5 g.[2]

Deaths have been reported in children who ingested a handful of flowers and in adults who used the fresh twigs as meat skewers; the nectar makes honey toxic.[2,5]

Symptoms of oleander toxicity include pain in the oral cavity, nausea, emesis, abdominal pain, cramping and diarrhea. Special attention must be given to cardiac function. The cardioactive glycosides may induce conduction defects such as sinus bradycardia, and systemic hyperkalemia induced by the plant may worsen cardiac function.[1]

Oleander toxicity should be managed aggressively. Gastric lavage or induced emesis should be done, and activated charcoal may be administered orally. Saline cathartics have been reported to be of use. ECG monitoring for cardiac impairment and monitoring of serum potassium levels should be done frequently, and the conduction defects managed with atropine, phenytoin, transvenous pacing or other appropriate antiarrhythmic treatment, depending on the characteristics of the impairment.[1]

Assays for serum digoxin levels were reported to have been conducted in a patient who ingested oleander; the levels of the glycoside were high (4.4 ng/ml) and were associated with bradyarrhythmias and tachyarrhythmias, which decreased as the serum concentration of the toxin decreased.[6] Another patient who ingested seven oleander leaves in a suicide attempt demonstrated digoxin serum levels of 5.69 nmol/L using a digoxin radioimmunoassay. This assay confirmed the toxicity, but did not predict the severity of the toxicity.[7]

In dogs given a tincture of oleander IV, the administration of large doses of a digoxin-specific Fab resulted in the survival of all five treated dogs (3 of 5 untreated dogs died) with a conversion to normal sinus rhythm within 8 minutes of Fab infusion.[8] These antibodies have been used successfully to treat human oleander toxicity.[7,9]

SUMMARY: The oleander is an extremely toxic plant that is grown widely as an ornamental. Although it has been used in traditional medicine, its extreme toxicity precludes its use in any form.

PATIENT INFORMATION – Oleander

Uses: Oleander has been used in treatment of cardiac illness, asthma, corns, cancer, and epilepsy.

Side Effects: Oleander toxicity signs include pain in the oral cavity, nausea, emesis, abdominal pain, cramping, and diarrhea. Extreme toxicity precludes its use in any form.

[1] Lampe KE. AMA *Handbook of Poisonous and Injurious Plants*. Chicago, IL: Chicago Review Press, 1985.

[2] Duke JA. *Handbook of Medicinal Herbs*. Boca Raton, FL: CRC Press, 1985.

[3] Muller BM, et al. Polysaccharides from *Nerium oleander:* structure and biological activity. *Pharmazie* 1991;46:657.

[4] Arai M, et al. Evaluation of selected plants for their toxic effects in canaries. *J Am Vet Med Assn* 1992;200:1329.

[5] Osol A, Farrar GE Jr., eds. *The Dispensatory of the United States of America*, 25th ed. Philadelphia, PA: J.B. Lippincott, 1955.

[6] Mesa MD, et al. Digitalis poisoning from medicinal herbs. Two different mechanisms of production. *Rev Esp Cardiol* 1991;44:347.

[7] Romano GA, Monbelli G. Poisoning with oleander leaves. *Schweiz Med Wochenschr* 1990;120:596.

[8] Clark RF, et al. Digoxin-specific Fab fragments in the treatment of oleander toxicity in a canine model. *Ann Emerg Med* 1991;20:1073.

[9] Bayer MJ. Recognition and management of digitalis intoxication: implications for emergency medicine. *Am J Emerg Med* 1991;9(2 Suppl 1):29.

Olive Leaf

SCIENTIFIC NAME(S): *Olea europaea* L. Family: oleaceae.

COMMON NAME(S): Olive leaf

BOTANY: The olive tree is an evergreen, growing to approximately 10 m in height. Native to the Mediterranean regions, the trees are also cultivated in areas of similar climates in the Americas. The small, leathery leaves are gray-green on top, and the underside contains fine, white, scale-like hairs. The leaves are gathered throughout the year.[1,2,3]

HISTORY: The olive tree was cultivated in Crete as far back as 3500 BC, where the leaves had been used to clean wounds. Symbolically, the olive branch stands for peace. The leaves were worn by athletes in ancient Olympic games.[1] Medicinal properties of the plant in the 1800s include malaria treatment. In the 1900s, the leaf constituent oleuropein was found to resist disease. The plant has also been reported to possess some hypotensive properties.[2]

CHEMISTRY: Olive leaf contains the active constituent oleuropein (chief constituent 60 to 90 mg/g). This iridoid has been pharmacologically analyzed.[4] Other secoiridoids include 11–demethyloleuropein, 7,11–dimethyl ester of oleoside, ligustroside, oleuroside, and unconjugated secoiridoid-type aldehydes; triterpenes and flavonoids are also present, and include rutin, and glycosides of apigenin and luteolin.[3] Other sources list oleasterol, leine, and glycoside oleoside as being present in olive leaf.[1,2] A report on peroxidase and ethylene formation in olive leaves is available.[5] A comparison of organelles from young and mature olive leaves has been performed, finding no remarkable differences.[6]

PHARMACOLOGY: In animal experimentation, oleuropein has always produced a reproducible reduction in blood pressure.[2] It has been shown to increase coronary flow and left intraventricular pressure in rabbit myocardium.[3] A decoction of olive leaves caused relaxation of rat aorta preparations in another report.[7] Oleuropein exerts hypotensive action in cats and dogs as well. The hypotensive action of this iridoid depends on specific animal species.[4]

Also in animal experimentation, olive leaf has demonstrated antispasmodic, coronary dilator, and antiarrhythmic properties in addition to its hypotensive effects.[8] A proposed mechanism as to how oleuropein may exert its effects may be a result of its direct action on smooth muscle.[4] Oleuropeoside was found to be responsible for vasodilator activity in another report.[7]

Documentation regarding olive leaf's use as an antihypertensive in humans is insignificant.[8] Other sources state no definite proof of the therapeutic efficacy in this area.[3,9] In contrast, Italian folk medicine employs dried olive leaf as a remedy for high blood pressure.[9] Other sources state that olive leaves do lower pressure and help to improve circulatory function as well.[1] Another report mentions the hypotensive activity of olive leaves to be slight, but existent, and suggests their use only in mild cases of hypertension.[2]

Olive leaf has other documented properties. Hypoglycemic activity was demonstrated in animals. Mechanisms were stated as being potentiation of glucose-induced insulin release, and increased peripheral uptake of glucose.[10] Olive leaf is also said to be mildy diuretic. It enhances renal and digestive elimination functions, along with renal excretion of water.[3] It may be used to treat cystitis as well.[1] Oleuropein was also listed as a good antioxidant.[3] Many unsubstantiated claims and "cure-alls," except for "testimonial-type" proof, exist for olive leaf. Some of these claims include therapy for chronic fatigue syndrome, herpes and other viral infections, arthritis, yeast infection, skin conditions, and others. More research and clinical trials are necessary to validate these claims.

TOXICOLOGY: Potential toxicity of olive leaf is not well known.[3] Oleuropein in doses up to 1 g/kg body weight in albino mice did not provoke lethality in an analysis on olive leaf.[4] The German Commission E monographs list no known risks associated with the plant.[9] One source states the drug as causing gastric symptoms, and suggests that it be taken with meals because of this irritant effect.[2]

SUMMARY: The olive tree dates back to 3500 BC. The leaves possess hypotensive properties in animal experimentation, probably as a result of vasodilator activity. The leaves have been used in humans for hypertension, but the leaf's effects may only be useful in mild cases. Olive leaf also exhibits hypoglycemic, renal, and antimicrobial effects. Toxicity of the plant is not well known, but there seems to be little risk with its use.

PATIENT INFORMATION – Olive Leaf

Uses: The olive leaves possess hypotensive properties in animal experimentation and have been used in humans for hypertension (possibly only for mild cases). The olive leaves also have hypoglycemic, renal, and antimicrobial effects.

Side Effects: Toxicity is not well known, but the leaf may cause gastric symptoms. Use in diabetic patients should be followed carefully due to the hypoglycemic effects of olive leaf.

---

[1] Chevallier A. *Encyclopedia of Medicinal Plants*. New York, NY: DK Publishing. 1996;239.

[2] Weiss R. *Herbal Medicine*. Beaconsfield, England: Beaconsfield Publ. Ltd. 1988;160-1.

[3] Bruneton J. *Pharmacognosy, Phytochemistry, Medicinal Plants*. Paris, France: Lavoisier Publishing. 1995;487-89.

[4] Petkov V, et al. Pharmacological analysis of the iridoid oleuropein. *Arzneimittelforschung* 1972;22(9):1476-86.

[5] Vioque B, et al. Perioxidases and ethylene formation in olive tree leaves. *Rev Esp Fisiol* 1989;45(1):47-52.

[6] Daza L, et al. Isolation and characterization of subcellular organelles from young and mature leaves of olive tree. *Rev Esp Fisiol* 1980;36(1):7-12.

[7] Zarzuelo A. Vasodilator effect of olive leaf. *Planta Med* 1991;57(5):417-19.

[8] Blumenthal M, ed. *The Complete German Commission E Monographs* . Austin, TX: American Botanical Council. 1998;357.

[9] Schulz V, et al. *Rational Phytotherapy*. Verlin Heidelberg, Germany: Springer-Verlag. 1998;106.

[10] Gonzalez M, et al. Hypoglycemic activity of olive leaf. *Planta Med* 1992;58(6):513-15.

Olive Oil

SCIENTIFIC NAME(S): *Olea europaea* (fruit), *Oleum olivae* Family: Oleaceae

COMMON NAME(S): Olive oil, sweet oil, salad oil

BOTANY: The olive is technically a fruit, ellipsoid and drupaceous in character, measuring 2 to 3 cm in length. The fruits grow from an evergreen tree, which seldomly exceeds 10 or 12 m in height. The plants were first cultivated in Greece but are now widely grown in Mediterranean countries and the US. Many cultivated varieties are the result of its geographic diversity.

Olive oil is a fixed oil, expressed from ripe olive fruits. It is pale-yellow and may have a greenish tint, depending on the ratio of chlorophyll to carotene. Taste has been described as characteristic but slight or bland to faintly acrid. Olive oil is offered in several grades of purity, including "virgin" oil (initial unrefined oil from first fruit pressing) or "pure" (lower quality from subsequent pressings). Chemically, the difference between "extra virgin" and "virgin" oils involve the amount of free oleic acid (ie, virgin allows 4% free oleic acid, and extra virgin allows 1%).[1,2,3,4]

HISTORY: "Olea" comes from the Latin "oliva" meaning olive.[2] The fruit dates back to the 17th century BC and appears to be native to Palestine.[4] One source mentions that Ramses II, Egyptian ruler between 1300 and 1200 BC, used olive oil for every ailment.[5]

CHEMISTRY: Olive oils of different varieties and from varied climatic areas differ in composition. Oleic acid (a monounsaturated fatty acid) for example, can range from 65% to 86%. Linoleic acid can vary as well, from 0% to 15%. Palmitic and stearic acids range from 9% to 15%.[1,4,6,7] Oleuropein, a phenolic compound, is found in the fruits.[8,9]

TLC and GC analyses are employed to detect adulteration of the oil with foreign oils (eg, sesame, cottonseed, peanut oils). Certain percentage limits are set for the amounts of saturated fatty acid chain lengths and number of sterols.[4]

PHARMACOLOGY: Recent computer literature searches found > 1800 citations on olive oil, hence the following is only a brief outline of some main points.

Olive oil is classed as a pharmaceutic acid.[2] It is used as a vehicle for oily suspensions for injection.[3] Olive oil is also employed in the preparation of soaps, plasters, ointments, and liniments.[3,4] In addition, it is a good drug solvent.[3,6] Externally, olive oil is a demulcent and emollient. It is used to soften the skin in eczema and psoriasis.[3] It is useful as a lubricant for massage or for prevention of stretch marks. It also has been used as a wound dressing and for minor burns. In addition, olive oil softens ear wax and is helpful for ringing or pain in the ears. Effectiveness of certain applications is not documented.[10]

Olive oil is a nutrient, widely used as a salad oil and for cooking.[2] It is a common element in the Mediterranean diet.[11,12,13]

Olive oil is a mild laxative as an intestinal lubricant.[6] It is also claimed to be useful for gall bladder problems, including cholecystitis and cholelithiasis.[10]

A number of articles concerning olive oil's role against heart disease exist. Constituent oleic acid has been shown to lower blood cholesterol levels.[1] Monounsaturated fatty acids replacing saturated fatty acids in the diet decrease serum cholesterol as discussed in a review of population and clinical studies.[14] Olive oil supplementation in hypercholesterolemic patients was shown to reduce susceptibility of LDL to oxidation, which contributes to atherosclerotic processes.[15] Olive oil improves the good HDL-cholesterol ratios and combats arterial build-up of cholesterol as well. In middle-aged Americans, the oil decreased cholesterol by 13% and LDL-cholesterol by 21%. Four to five tablespoons per day of olive oil administered to heart surgery patients improved their blood profiles.[5] A comparative study of olive oil vs fish oil on blood lipids and atherosclerosis has been performed.[16]

Olive oil and cancer prevention have been correlated in experimental animals. In rats, olive oil had no colon tumor-enhancing effects as compared with other fatty-type diets.[17] A nutrition review of dietary fat and chronic disease risk finds monounsaturated oils, such as olive oil, to be a weak promoter of certain cancers (including breast and colon) as opposed to such strong promoters as n-6 polyunsaturated oils.[18] This author claims evidence for an enhancing effect of the latter strong promoters in increased breast cancers in western diets.

Other effects of olive oil include the following: Decreased tendency to develop spontaneous osteoarthritis in mice compared with other fats,[19] reduction of blood pressure,[5] and antimicrobial properties including gram-negative bacteria, fungi, and enterotoxin B production by *Staphylococcus aureus*.[8,9]

TOXICOLOGY: Ingestion of excessive amounts of olive oil has resulted in temporary mild diarrhea.[5] In rare cases, topical use of olive oil has caused allergic reactions.[10]

SUMMARY: Olive oil has been used for centuries as a food and pharmacological agent. It is an ingredient in certain preparations such as ointments. It is used to soften skin and ear wax. Olive oil is useful as a laxative and may be useful for gall bladder ailments. It also is beneficial as a nutrient, especially in the Mediterranean diet. It plays an important role against heart disease as it lowers cholesterol levels. Olive oil does not promote certain cancers compared with other fats. Toxicities from olive oil include mild diarrhea and rare skin reactions.

PATIENT INFORMATION – Olive Oil

Uses: Olive oil is used for cooking, as a salad oil, and as a vehicle for oily suspensions for injections. It is used to prepare soaps, plasters, ointments, and liniments and is used as a demulcent and emollient. It is a mild laxative, and it lowers cholesterol.

Side effects: Olive oil has caused temporary mild diarrhea and allergic reactions from external use.

---

[1] Murray M. *The Healing Power of Foods*. Rocklin, CA: Prima Publishing. 1993;188.

[2] Robbers J, et al. *Pharmacognosy and Pharmacobiotechnology*. Baltimore, MD: Williams & Wilkins. 1996;70-71.

[3] Reynolds J, ed. *Martindale-The Extra Pharmacopoeia 31st ed.* London, England: Royal Pharmaceutical Society. 1996;1734.

[4] Evans W. *Trease and Evans' Pharmacognosy, 14th ed.* London, England: WB Saunders Co. Ltd. 1996;185-86.

[5] Carper J. *The Food Pharmacy*. New York, NY: Bantam Books. 1989;242-45.

[6] Bruneton J. *Pharmacognosy, Phytochemistry, Medicinal Plants*. Paris, France: Lavoisier. 1995;127-29.

[7] Murray M. *Encyclopedia of Nutritional Supplements*. Rocklin, CA: Prima Publishing. 1996;243-48.

[8] Tranter H, et al. The effect of the olive phenolic compound, oleuropein, on growth and enterotoxin B production by *Staphylococcus aureus*. *J Applied Bacteriol* 1993;74:253-59.

[9] Fleming H, et al. Antimicrobial properties of oleuropein and products of its hydrolysis from green olives. *Applied Microbiol* 1973;26(5):777-82.

[10] Blumenthal M, ed. *The Complete German Commission E Monographs*. Austin, TX: American Botanical Council. 1998;358.

[11] Maiani G, et al. Vitamin nutritional status in Italy. *Eur J Cancer Prev* 1997;(6 suppl)1:S3-9.

[12] Haber B. The Mediterranean diet: a view from history. *Am J Clin Nutr* 1997;66(4 suppl):1053S-1057S.

[13] Haas C. Barley, the olive and wine, dietary and therapeutic triad of ancient Mediterranean people. *Ann Med Interne* 1998;149(5):275-79.

[14] Okolska G, et al. Recommendations concerning the rational consumption of fats. I. Population and clinical studies on the role of monounsaturated fatty acids. *Rocz Panstw Zakl Hig* 1989;40(2):89-99.

[15] Aviram M. Interaction of oxidized low density lipoprotein with macrophages in atherosclerosis, and the antiatherogenicity of antioxidants. *Eur J Clin Chem Clin Biochem* 1996;34(8):599-608.

[16] Mortensen A, et al. Comparison of the effects of fish oil and olive oil on blood lipids and aortic atherosclerosis in Watanabe heritable hyperlipidaemic rabbits. *Br J Nutr* 1998;80(6):565-73.

[17] Reddy B. Dietary fat and colon cancer: animal model studies. *Lipids* 1992;27(10):807-13.

[18] Weisburger J. Dietary fat and risk of chronic disease: mechanistic insights from experimental studies. *J Am Diet Assoc* 1997;97(7 suppl):S16-23.

[19] Wilhelmi G. Potential effects of nutrition including additives on healthy and arthrotic joints. I. Basic dietary constituents. *Z Rheumatol* 1993;52(3):174-79.

Onion

SCIENTIFIC NAME(S): *Allium cepa* Family: Liliaceae, Alliaceae.

COMMON NAME(S): Onion

BOTANY: The onion plant is a perennial herb growing to about 4 feet high, with 4 to 6 hollow cylindrical leaves. On top of the long stalk, greenish-white flowers are present in the form of solitary umbels growing up to 1-inch wide. The seeds of the plant are black and angular. The underground bulb, which is used medicinally, is made up of fleshy leaf sheaths forming a thin-skinned capsule. The onion is one of the leading vegetable crops in the world.[1,2,3,4]

HISTORY: Central Asia is believed to be the region of origin of the onion.[4] Onions were used as early as 5,000 years ago in Egypt, as seen on ancient monuments. Ancient Greek and Roman recordings also refer to the onion. During the Middle Ages, onions were consumed throughout Europe. They were later thought to guard against evil spirits and the plague, probably because of their strong odor. Onion "skin" dye has been used for egg and cloth coloring for many years in the Middle East and Europe. Columbus was said to have brought the onion to America. Folk healers used the onion to prevent infection. The combination of onions and garlic cooked in milk is a European folk remedy used to clear congestion. Onions are also used in homeopathic medicine.[1,2,5,6]

CHEMISTRY: Onions contain 89% water, 1.5% protein, and vitamins, including B_1, B_2, and C, along with potassium.[1,2] Polysaccharides such as fructosans, saccharose, and others are also present, as are peptides, flavonoids, and essential oil.[3,4] The alliums, like onion, contain alliin and similar sulfur compounds, including allylalliin and methyl and propyl compounds of cysteine sulfoxide.[3,4,6] Sulfur and other compounds of *A. cepa* have been analyzed.[7] The flavor components of onion have been evaluated by TLC.[8] Prostaglandins have also been identified in onion.[9] Onion cell wall analyses have also been performed.[10,11] The chemical analysis of onion seed oil is available.[12]

PHARMACOLOGY: The main properties of onion include antimicrobial activity, cardiovascular support, hypoglycemic action, antioxidant/anticancer effect, and asthma protection.

Antimicrobial effects: Onion has had antibacterial,[3] antiparasitic,[13] and antifungal actions.[14,15] *Salmonella typhimurium* mutagenicity was reduced in hamburger when onions were added.[16] Growth of oral pathogenic bacteria, including *Streptococcus mutans*, *S. subrinus*, *Porphyromonas gingivalis*, and *Prevotella intermedia*, the main causes of dental caries and periodontitis, was prevented by onion extracts.[17] Either onion juice or onion oil has also been shown to inhibit growth of other gram-positive bacteria and gram-negative bacteria *Klebsiella pneumoniae*.[14,15,18] Antifungal actions of onion include certain yeasts,[14] *Microsporum canis*, *M. gypseum*, *Trichophyton simi*, *Chrysosporium queenslandicum*, *T. mentagrophyes*, *Aspergillus flavus*, and *Penicillium rubrum*.[15] One source identifies thiosulfinate principle in the onion as one of the main antimicrobial agents.[4]

Cardiovascular disease: Onion may also be of benefit in cardiovascular disease. The hypolipidemic effects of sulfur-containing principles in onion, including s-methyl cysteine sulfoxide and allylpropyl disulfide, have been demonstrated in several studies in rats and rabbits.[19,20,21,22,23] Examples include onion's protective effects against diet-induced atherosclerosis[22] and onion's marked actions in controlling lipids[23] and triglycerides.[21] One report evaluates onion's hemostatic effects in humans,[24] but certain lipid-reducing and blood pressure-lowering effects in humans have not yet been clinically proven.[4] Cardiovascular disease risk factors also involve blood coagulability. Several reports confirm the onion's inhibitory effects on platelet formation. Raw onion (vs. cooked) demonstrated antithrombotic effects in rats.[25,26] Dose-dependent inhibitory effects on platelet aggregation were seen in rabbits also with raw onion.[27] Boiling onion may cause decomposition of the antithrombotic ingredient.[25] Certain onion genotypes containing higher contents of sulfur in the bulb correlated with greater antiplatelet activity.[28] Thiosulfinates dimethyl- and diphenylthiosulfinate, for example, are known to retard thrombocyte biosynthesis.[4,29] The least polar fraction of onion extract was associated with the most inhibitory activity toward platelet aggregation, thus a greater inhibition of thromboxane synthesis was reported.[30] Synthesis of thromboxanes and prostaglandins in vitro has been shown with onions, as well as with garlic and other liliaceae family members.[31] Onion's benefits relating to cardiovascular disease have been reviewed.[5,32]

Diabetes: Although more research is needed on the use of onion as a treatment for diabetes in humans, many articles describe onion's benefits in improving glucose levels.[33] Studies from 1965 to 1975 report antidiabetic activity, "hypoglycemic principles," and blood sugar level reduction in diabetic rabbits.[34,35,36] Recent reports confirm many of these claims, finding similar outcomes. Onion decreased the hyperglycemic peak in rabbits.[37] In addition, onion amino acid s-methyl cysteine sulfoxide (SMCS) contributed to antidiabetic effects in affected rats, controlling blood glucose and other diabetic effects comparable to insulin.[23,38]

Cancer: Onion has also proven to be an antioxidant and may be beneficial in certain cancers. The organosulfur compounds contained in onion exert chemopreventive effects on chemical carcinogenesis. The constituent diallyl disulfide possesses inhibitory properties against colon and renal cancers.[39] People consuming diets high in allium vegetables including onion suffer from fewer incidences of stomach cancer.[1,40] Onion's protective factors for breast cancer have been evaluated in a French case-control study.[41] Oil of onion is an effective antioxidant against nicotine-induced damage in rats.[42] Another report compares the antioxidant activity of onion polyphenols with those of other fruits and vegetables.[43] The quercetin component in onion, however, was found to be absorbed by humans from dietary sources but provided no direct protective effect during LDL oxidation.[44]

Respiratory problems: Folk medicine has used the onion for treatment of asthma, whooping cough, bronchitis, and similar ailments.[4,33] The onion is used in homeopathic medicine.[5] Onion juice administration protected guinea pigs from asthma attacks. An ethanol extract of onion reduced "allergy-induced" bronchial constriction in certain patients.[4] The thiosulfinates present in the onion are said to inhibit bronchoconstriction, but definite efficacy remains unproven in this area.[29]

Other uses: Onions have been used in the treatment of stingray wounds,[45] warts, acne,[2] appetite loss,[1,3] urinary tract disorders,[5] and indigestion.[1] Onion cell extract was ineffective in treating postsurgical scarring.[46] General reviews of therapeutic uses of onion are available.[47,48]

Dosage: The German Commission E Monographs lists the average daily dose as 50 g of fresh onion, the juice from 50 g of fresh onion, or 20 g dried onion. A maximum of 35 mg diphenylamine/day is recommended if onion preparations are used over several months.[3]

TOXICOLOGY: Certain sulfur compounds (eg, propanethial-s-oxide) escape from the onion in vapor form and hydrolyze to sulfuric acid when it is cut, causing the familiar eye irritation and lacrimation.[1,6] Corneal swelling from onion exposure has been reported.[49] Using a sharp knife also minimizes the crushing of onion tissue and liberation of volatiles, and cutting an onion under running water avoids lacrimation. Ingestion of onion seems relatively safe, as the German Commission E lists no contraindications, side effects, or interactions from the plant.[3] Onion can be taken frequently in low doses without any side effects as seen with rat experimentation.[25] Food colorant extracted from the tan onion bulb covering had no acute or subacute toxic effects in mice.[50] With large intake, the stomach may be affected, and frequent contact with onion rarely may cause allergic reaction.[4] The onion seeds have been reported as an occupational allergen.[51] Onion toxicity is only accociated with high intake.

A review of onion discussing ingestion of large amounts of the bulb finds toxicity unresolved.[32] Low doses of onion (50 mg/kg) given to rats had little effect on the lung and liver tissues. High doses (500 mg/kg) resulted in histological changes in these organs. IP administration was more damaging than oral, resulting in 25% mortality in rats.[52] Eighty-five young cattle were given 1000 kg of onions per day, affecting approximately 26%, with 1 fatality. New illnesses continued to occur for 5 days after the withdrawal of the onions, including lack of appetite, tachycardia, staggering, and collapse, all probably due to adverse red blood cell effects.[53]

SUMMARY: Onions have been used for thousands of years. The bulb contains certain sulfur compounds that are known to be antimicrobial. The onion may also be of benefit in cardiovascular disease, as it possesses hypolipidemic effects and has antiplatelet actions, retarding thrombosis. Some studies have been performed concerning diabetes treatment by onion with promising results in animal experimentation. The onion is also a proven antioxidant and may be helpful in treating certain cancers. More research is needed in the area of asthma treatment, although certain compounds are said to inhibit bronchoconstriction. Toxicology of onion is usually associated with high intake, but if taken properly it has few side effects. The proper dose for beneficial properties remains to be determined, particularly because newer, sweeter, and less potent varieties have been developed in recent years.

PATIENT INFORMATION – Onion

Uses: Onion is used as an antimicrobial, cardiovascular-supportive, hypoglycemic, antioxidant/anticancer, and asthma-protective agent. In folk medicine, onion has been used for asthma, whooping cough, bronchitis, and similar ailments. Other uses include the treatment of stingray wounds, warts, acne, appetite loss, urinary tract disorders, and indigestion. Onion skin dye has been used as an egg and cloth coloring.

Side Effects: The toxicity of large doses of onion has been unresolved, but the stomach may be affected. Frequent contact with onion seeds has been reported as an occupational allergen.

[1] Ensminger, A. et al. *Foods and Nutrition Encyclopedia*, 2nd ed. Vol. 2., CRC Press Inc., Boca Raton, FL. 1994;1684–88.

[2] Dwyer, J. Sr. Ed. et al. *Magic and Medicine of Plants*. The Reader's Digest Association, Inc. 1986;261.

[3] Blumenthal, M. Sr. Ed. et al. *The Complete German Commission E Monographs*, American Botanical Council, Austin, TX, 1998:176–7.

[4] Fleming, T. Ch. Ed. et al. *PDR for Herbal Medicines*. Medical Economics Company, Inc., Montvale, NJ. 1998;624–5.

[5] Reynolds J. ed. *Martindale, The Extra Pharmacopoeia*. Royal Pharmaceutical Society, London, England. 1996;1734.

[6] Schulz, V. et al. *Rational Phytotherapy*, Springer-Verlag Berlin. Heidelberg 1998;153.

[7] Breu W. *Phytomedicine*. 1996:3(3);293–306.

[8] Bandyopadhyav, C. et al. *J. Chromatogr.* 1970;47(3):400–7.

[9] Al-Nagdy, S. et al. *Comp Biochem Physiol C.* 1986;85(1):163–6.

[10] Haimmouril, M. et al. *Quim. Anal* 1997;16(Suppl. 1):S141–S145.

[11] Zeier, J. et al. *Planta*. 1998;206(3):349–61.

[12] Grujic-Injac, B. et al. *Hrana Ishrana*. 1985;25(7–10):167–9.

[13] Guarrera, P. *J Ethnopharmacol*. 1999;68(1–3):183–92.

[14] Dankert, J. et al. *Zentralbl Bakteriol [Orig A]*. 1979;245(1–2):229–39.

[15] Zohri, A. et al. *Microbial Res.* 1995;150(2):167–72.

[16] Kato, T. et al. *Mutat Res.* 1998;420(1-3):109–14.

[17] Kim, J. et al. *J Nihon Univ Sch Dent.* 1997;39(3):136–41.

[18] Elnima, E. et al. *Pharmazie*. 1983;38(11):747–8.

[19] Augusti, K. *Indian J Biochem Biophys.* 1974;11(3):264–5.

[20] Wilcox, B. et al. *Indian J Biochem Biophys.* 1984;21(3):214–6.

[21] Sebastian, K. et al. *Indian J. Physiol Pharmacol.* 1979;23(1):27–30.

[22] Lata, S. et al. *J. Postgrad Med.* 1991;37(3):132–5.

[23] Kumari, K. et al. *Indian J Biochem Biophys.* 1995;32(1):49–54.

[24] Doutremepuich, C. et al. *Ann Pharm Fr.* 1985;43(3):273–9.

[25] Bordia, T. et al. *Prostaglandins Leukot Essent Fatty Acids.* 1996;54(3):183–6.

[26] Chen, J. et al. *J Nutr.* 2000;130(1):34–7.

[27] Ali, M. et al. *Prostaglandins Leukot Essent Fatty Acids.* 1999;60(1):43–7.

[28] Goldman, I. et al. *Thromb Haemost.* 1996;76(3):450–2.

[29] Miller, L. et al. *Herbal Medicinals, A Clinician's Guide*. Pharmaceutical Products Press. Binghamton, NY. 1998;195–202.

[30] Makheja, A. et al. *Prostaglandins Med.* 1979;2(6):413–24.

[31] Ali, M. et al. *Gen Pharmacol.* 1990;21(3):273–6.

[32] Kendler, B. *Prev Med.* 1987;16(5):670–85.

[33] Bratman, S. et al. *Natural Health Bible*. Prima Publishing, 1999;62.

[34] Galal, E. et al. *J Egypt Med Assoc.* 1965;48Suppl:14–45.

[35] Augusti, K. et al. *Indian J Med Res.* 1973;61(7):1066–71.

[36] Matthew, P. et al. *Indian J Physiol Pharmacol.* 1975;19(4):213–17.

[37] Roman-Ramos, R. et al. *J Ethnopharmacol.* 1995;48(1)25–32.

[38] Sheela. C. et al. *Planta Med.* 1995;61(4):356–7.

[39] Fukushima, S. et al. *J Cell Biochem Suppl.* 1997;27:100–5.

[40] Winter, R. *Medicines in Food*. Crown Trade Paperbacks. New York, NY. 1995;61–3.

[41] Challier, B. et al. *Eur J Epidemiol.* 1998;14(8):737–47.

[42] Helen, A. et al. *Vet Hum Toxicol.* 1999;41(5):316–19.

[43] Paganga, G. et al. *Free Radic Res.* 1999;30(2):153–62.

[44] McAnlis, G. et al. *Eur J Clin Nutr.* 1999;53(2):92–6.

[45] Whiting, S. et al. *Med J Aust.* 1998;168(11):584.

[46] Jackson, B. et al. *Dermatol Surg.* 1999;25(4):267–69.

[47] Breu, W. et al. *Econ Med Plant Res.* 1994;6:115–47.

[48] Augusti, K. et al. *Indian J Exp Biol.* 1996;34(7):634–40.

[49] Chan, R. et al. *Am J Optom Arch Am Acad Optom.* 1972;49(9):713–5.

[50] Kojima, T. et al. *J Toxicol Environ Health.* 1993;38(1):89–101.

[51] Navarro, J. et al. *J Allergy Clin Immunol.* 1995;96(5 pt 1):690–3.

[52] Thomson, M. et al. *J Ethnopharmacol.* 1998;61(2):91–9.

[53] Verhoeff, J. et al. *Vet Rec.* 1985;117(19):497–8.

Ostrich Fern

SCIENTIFIC NAME(S): *Matteuccia struthiopteris* (L.) Tod. Family Aspleniaceae (Athyroideae)

COMMON NAME(S): Ostrich fern

BOTANY: The ostrich fern is a common fern that grows in the northeastern US and in large parts of Canada.

HISTORY: Fiddleheads (the young shoot tops) of the ostrich fern are a seasonal delicacy, harvested commercially throughout the northeastern US and coastal Canadian provinces. This spring vegetable had been a regular part of the diet of Canadian settlers by the early 1700s.[1] Unlike some ferns that have been considered carcinogenic or toxic, this fern had been considered to be nontoxic. Recent experience, however, indicates that it has the potential to induce severe food poisoning when not cooked properly. The ferns are available canned, frozen or fresh.

CHEMISTRY: Little is known about the chemistry of the ostrich fern. As described in the Toxicology section, poisonings due to this fern are believed to be caused by a heat-labile toxin that has not been characterized. The ostrich fern has been reported to accumulate heavy metals.[2]

A protein identified as matteuccin has been characterized in the fern. It is a small basic protein consisting of two small disulfide-linked polypeptides,[3] but there is no indication that this protein is responsible for the toxicity of the plant.

PHARMACOLOGY: The fiddleheads of the ostrich fern are generally considered to be edible following steaming.

One field guide indicates that wild greens may have laxative properties and recommends boiling them and discarding the first water, to limit this effect.[4] No other significant pharmacologic properties have been ascribed to the fern.

TOXICOLOGY: Boiling the yound fiddleheads of the fern is believed to deactivate the potentially toxic properties of the plant. Recently, several outbreaks of severe food poisoning were reported by the Centers for Disease Control and Prevention (CDC). Affected individuals had eaten raw or lightly cooked fiddleheads of the ostrich fern in New York and western Canada.[5] The ferns associated with toxicity had often been eaten in restaurants, where the fiddleheads had been blanched or sauteed for only two minutes or less. However, when the ferns had been boiled for ten minutes prior to being sauteed, no illness occurred at the same restaurants. Symptoms were repoted within 12 hours; nausea, vomiting and abdominal cramping were the most commonly reported adverse events. Consumption of fiddlehead soup was also associated with gastrointestinal illness.

SUMMARY: Fresh fiddlehead ferns have only recently become widely available in restaurants. Because many vegetables are now only lightly sauteed or blanched (rather than being fried or boiled), patrons may be at risk for developing severe gastrointestinal illness if they eat undercooked ostrich fern fiddleheads. The CDC recommends that they should be cooked thoroughly (eg, boiling for 10 minutes) before eating.

PATIENT INFORMATION – Ostrich Fern

Uses: Ostrich fern has been used as a seasonal delicacy.

Side Effects: Adverse effects due to undercooking ostrich ferns include nausea, vomiting, abdominal cramping, and GI illness.

---

[1] vonAderkas P. Economic history of ostrich fern, Matteuccia struthiopteris, the edible fiddlehead. *Economic Botany* 1984;38:14.

[2] Burns LV, Parker GH. Metal burdens in two species of fiddleheads growing near the ore smelters at Sudbury, Ontario, Canada. *Bull Environ Contam Toxicol* 1994;40:717.

[3] Rodin J, Rask L. Characterization of matteuccin, the 2.2S storage protein of the ostrich fern. Evolutionary relationship to angiosperm seed storage proteins. *Eur J Biochem* 1990;192:101.

[4] Tomikel J. Edible wild plants of Pennsylvania and New York. Pittsburgh: Allegheny Press, 1973.

[5] Bills D, et al. Ostrich fern poisoning-New York and Western Canada, 1994 *MMWR* 1994;43:67, 683.

Papaya

SCIENTIFIC NAME(S): *Carica papaya* L. Family: Caricaceae

COMMON NAME(S): Papaya, pawpaw, melon tree[1]

BOTANY: Papaya grow as small trees in the Americas and Africa. The common name pawpaw is sometimes given to an unrelated plant *Asimina triloba* (L.) Dunal. Family: Annonaceae.[2] The papaya produce large leaves and smooth-skinned edible melons.

HISTORY: *C. papaya* is cultivated for its milky juice which is the source of the proteolytic enzyme papain. The fruits are eaten fresh and are also the source of a flavoring used in candies and ice cream. Shallow cuts on the surface of fully grown but unripe fruits cause the exudation of a milky sap which is collected, dried and termed crude papain.[3] Papain has been used widely in folk medicine for the treatment of digestive disorders, particularly those associated with the ingestion of protein-rich foods. Teas brewed from fermented papaya leaves are said to produce a richer mixture of proteolytic enzymes than teas from fresh leaves. Papain has been used as a vermifuge and as a component of facial creams to soften skin. Papain is sold commercially as a meat tenderizer.[3]

CHEMISTRY: Papain (also known as vegetable pepsin) is found not only in the fruit latex but also in the leaves. Papain is a mixture of protein-degrading enzymes.[4] Other components of papain degrade carbohydrates and fats. The seeds contain a glycoside, caricin and myrosin, which, when combined, produce a mustard-like odor. The alkaloid carpaine has been identified in the leaves.[5]

Chymopapain has been fractioned into subcomponents designated "A" and "B."[6] It is very similar to papain in the spectrum of its proteolytic activity, although it is less potent with respect to protein degradation.[7]

PHARMACOLOGY: Papain is unstable in the presence of digestive juices, which may account for its general lack of efficacy as a vermifuge.[3]

Papain is used in digestive aids and in preparations to control edema and inflammation associated with surgical or accidental trauma.[7]

In the early 1980s, chymopapain (available as *Chymodiactin* from Boots-Flint[8]) was approved for intradiscal injection in patients with documented herniated lumbar intervertebral discs and who had not responded to conservative therapy. This procedure is effective but remains the focus of controversy, particularly regarding the safety of the administration of the enzyme.[9] Anaphylactic shock was initially reported in about 1% of those receiving the drug, and a number of fatalities were also reported.[10] More recently reported statistics, however, indicate that anaphylaxis occurs in less than 0.5% of patients,[8,11] and other adverse events such as neurological problems occur rarely.[8]

TOXICOLOGY: A 1978 report by Indian investigators suggested that papain was teratogenic and embryotoxic in rats;[3] however, these results have not been confirmed adequately. Ingestion of large amounts of papain or papaya has been associated with perforation of the esophagus.[5]

The enzyme may induce severe allergic responses in sensitive persons. The latex can be a severe irritant and vesicant. Internally, it may cause severe gastritis.[10]

Carpaine has been shown to cause paralysis, decrease heart rate and central nervous system activity[10] and may have some amebicidal activity.[5]

SUMMARY: Papain is a mixture of natural enzymes derived from the papaya fruit. Papain is used as a meat tenderizer and chymopapain is employed in the chemical degradation of herniated vertebral disks. The latex from the plant may induce dermatitis and allergic hypersensitivity reactions have been associated with the ingestion of the plant and its extracts.

PATIENT INFORMATION – Papaya

Uses: Papaya is used in digestive aids and in preparation to control edema and inflammation associated with surgical or accidental trauma.

Side Effects: Enzymes related to papaya have been associated with perforation of the esophagus, severe gastritis, paralysis, decreased heart rate and CNS activity, and may inhibit some amebicidal activity.

[1] Mabberley DJ. The Plant-Book. New York, NY: Cambridge University Press, 1987.
[2] Lampe KF. AMA Handbook of Poisonous and Injurious Plants. Chicago, IL: Chicago Review Press, 1985.
[3] Tyler VE. The New Honest Herbal. Philadelphia, PA: G.F. Stickley Co., 1987.
[4] Dubois T, et al. *Biol Chem Hoppe Seyler* 1988;369:741.
[5] Spoerke DG Jr. Herbal Medications. Santa Barbara, CA: Woodbridge Press, 1980.
[6] Barrett AJ, Buttle DJ. *Biochem J* 1985;228:527.
[7] Leung AY. Encyclopedia of Common Natural Ingredients Used In Food, Drugs, and Cosmetics. New York, NY: J. Wiley and Sons, 1980.
[8] Olin BR, Hebel SK, eds. Drug Facts and Comparisons. St. Louis, MO: Facts and Comparisons, 1989.
[9] Cole HM, ed. *JAMA* 1989;262(7):953.
[10] Duke JA. Handbook of Medicinal Herbs. Boca Raton, FL: CRC Press, 1985.
[11] Wright PH. *JAMA* (letter) 1990;263(7):948.

Parsley

SCIENTIFIC NAME(S): *Petroselinum crispum* (Mill.) Mansfield, *P. hartense* (Hoffman) and *P. sativum*. Family: Umbelliferae

COMMON NAME(S): Parsley, rock parsley, garden parsley

BOTANY: Parsley is an herb indigenous to the Mediterranean, but now cultivated worldwide.

Caution must be used when gathering wild parsley because of the general similarity of its leaves and flowers to those of three common poisonous plants. The first, *Aethusa cynapium* (dog poison, fool's parsley, small hemlock) can be distinguished from parsley by the shiny yellow-green underside of the leaves, which are dull in parsley, and the white flowers, which are yellowish in parsley. Similarly, collectors should be aware of *Conium maculatum* (poison hemlock, water hemlock, poison parsley) and *Cicuta maculata* (water hemlock). Poisonings have occurred when the leaves of *Conium* were mistaken for parsley and the seeds for anise. Symptoms of *Conium* and *Cicuta* poisoning include vomiting, diarrhea, weakness, paralysis, weak pulse, dilated pupils, convulsions and death.

HISTORY: Parsley leaves and roots are popular as condiments and garnish worldwide. In Lebanon, parsley is a major ingredient in a national dish called Tabbouleh. An average adult may consume as much as 50 g of parsley per meal.[1]

Parsley seeds were used traditionally as a carminative to decrease flatulence and colic pain. The root was used as a diuretic and the juice to treat kidney ailments. Parsley oil has also been used to regulate menstrual flow in the treatment of amenorrhea and dysmenorrhea, and is purported to be an abortifacient. Bruised leaves have been used to treat tumors, insect bites, lice and skin parasites, and contusions.[2,3] Parsley tea at one time was used to treat dysentery and gallstones.[2] Other traditional uses reported include the treatment of diseases of the prostate, liver and spleen, in the treatment of anemia, arthritis and cancers, and as an expectorant, antimicrobial, aphrodisiac, hypotensive, laxative and as a scalp lotion to stimulate hair growth.[2,4]

CHEMISTRY: Parsley oil comprises about 0.1% of the root, about 0.3% of the leaf and 2% to 7% of the fruit.[5] The oil contains two components, apiol and myristicin, which are pharmacologically active. Myristicin is chemically related to apiol and has been identified in nutmeg. More than 30 varieties of parsley are recognized and their relative content of apiol and myristicin vary. For example, "German" parsley oil contains about 60% to 80% apiol, whereas "French" parsley oil contains less apiol but more (50% to 60%) myristicin.[6]

Parsley contains psoralen and related compounds that can induce photosensitivity (see TOXICOLOGY); these include ficusin, bergapten, majudin and heraclin.[7]

PHARMACOLOGY: Parsley is a good natural source of vitamins and minerals including: Calcium, iron, carotene, ascorbic acid and vitamin A.[2,5]

Myristicin has been thought to be in part responsible for the hallucinogenic effect of nutmeg. It is not known whether parsley oil induces hallucinations, but the practice of smoking parsley as a cannabis substitute was well known during the 1960s. Parsley may have been smoked for a euphoric effect or as a carrier for more potent drugs such as phencyclidine.[8]

Apiol is an antipyretic and, like myristicin, is a uterine stimulant. Apiol was once available in capsules for use as an abortifacient. Although the effectiveness of this compound as uterotonics has not been quantitated, a Russian product called "Supetin" (which contains about 85% parsley juice) is used to stimulate uterine contractions during labor.[9] Data regarding the safety and efficacy of this drug are not readily available.

Apiol and myristicin may be responsible for the mild diuretic effect of the seeds and oil.[10] Parsley extracts have shown slight antibacterial and antifungal activity when tested in vitro,[11] but it is not known to what extent this activity is retained in vivo.

TOXICOLOGY: Adverse effects from the use of parsley are uncommon. Persons allergic to other members of the Umbelliferae (carrot, fennel, celery) may be sensitive to the constituents (especially in the flowers) of parsley. Because of the potential uterotonic effects, parsley oil, juice, and seeds should not be taken by pregnant women. Adverse effects from the ingestion of the oil have included headache, giddiness, loss of balance, convulsions and renal damage.

The psoralen compounds found in parsley have been linked to a photodermatitis reaction found among parsley cutters. This skin reaction is usually only evident if the areas that have contacted the juice are exposed to very strong sunlight; it can be minimized by the use of protective clothing and sunscreens.[12]

SUMMARY: The leaves, roots, seeds and oil of parsley have been used medicinally in the treatment of arthritis, diseases of the liver and spleen, and as expectorants. There is no good evidence to justify their use in these disorders. The use of parsley as a diuretic and for the control of dysmenorrhea stems from the presence of apiol and myristicin. The diuretic effect is small and variable. These compounds may stimulate the uterine muscles and, therefore, the seeds, juice and oil of parsley should not be administered to pregnant women. The safety of the herb seems limited primarily by potential allergic reactions.

PATIENT INFORMATION – Parsley

Uses: Parsley, in addition to being a source of certain vitamins and minerals, has been used in the treatment of prostrate, liver and spleen diseases, anemia, arthritis, and cancer.

Side Effects: Adverse effects from the ingestion of parsley oil include headache, giddiness, loss of balance, convulsions, and renal damage. Pregnant women should not take parsley because of its potential uterotonic effects.

---

[1] Zaynoun S, et al. *Clin Exp Dermatol* 1985;10:328.
[2] Duke JA. Handbook of Medicinal Herbs. Boca Raton, FL: CRC Press, 1985.
[3] Meyer J. The Herbalist. Hammond, IN: Hammond Book Co., 1934.
[4] Hoffman D. The Herbal Handbook. Rochester, VT: Healing Arts Press, 1988.
[5] Tyler VE, et al. Pharmacognosy, 9th ed. Philadelphia, PA: Lea & Febiger, 1988.
[6] Tyler VE. The Honest Herbal. Philadelphia, PA: G.F. Stickley Co., 1981.
[7] Pathak MA, et al. *J Invest Dermatol* 1962;39:225.
[8] Cook CE, et al. *Clin Pharm Ther* 1982;31:635.
[9] Chemical Abstracts 90:115465, 1979.
[10] Marczal G, et al. *Acta Agron Acad Sci Hung* 1977;26:7.
[11] Ross SA, et al. *Fitotherapia* 1980;51:303.
[12] Smith DA. *Practitioner* 1985;229:673.

Passion Flower

SCIENTIFIC NAME(S): *Passiflora* sp. Most often *P. incarnata* is used medicinally. Family: Passifloraceae

COMMON NAME(S): Passion flower; passion fruit, granadilla (species with edible fruit); water lemon; Maypop, apricot vine, wild passion flower (*P. incarnatus*); Jamaican honeysuckle (*P. laurifolia*).

BOTANY: The term "passion flower" connotes many of the ≈ 400 species of the genus *Passiflora*, which includes primarily vines. Some of the species are noted for their showy flowers, others for their edible fruit. Common species include *P. incarnata*, *P. edulis*, *P. alata*, *P. laurifolia*, and *P. quadrangularis*. Those with edible fruit include *P. incarnata*, *P. edulis*, and *P. quadrangularis*, the last being one of the major species grown for its fruit.[1] *Passiflora* species are native to tropical and subtropical areas of the Americas. In the US, *P. incarnata* is found from Virginia to Florida and as far west as Missouri and Texas. The flowers of *Passiflora* have 5 petals, sepals, and stamens, 3 stigmas, and a crown of filaments. The fruit is egg-shaped, has a pulpy consistency, and includes many small seeds.[1,2]

HISTORY: The passion flower was discovered in 1569 by Spanish explorers in Peru, who saw the flowers as symbolic of the passion of Christ, and therefore a sign of Christ's approval of their efforts. This is the origin of both the scientific and common names.[3] The folklore surrounding this plant possibly dates further into the past. The floral parts are thought to represent the elements of the crucifixion (3 styles represent 3 nails, 5 stamens for the 5 wounds, the ovary looks like a hammer, the corona is the crown of thorns, the petals represent the 10 true apostles, and the white and bluish purple colors are those of purity and heaven).[2,4] In Europe, passion flower has been used in homeopathic medicine to treat pain, insomnia related to neurasthenia or hysteria, and nervous exhaustion. Other indications have included bronchial disorders (particularly asthma), in compresses for burns, and for inflammation, inflamed hemorrhoids, climacteric complaints, pediatric attention disorders, and pediatric nervousness and excitability.[5]

CHEMISTRY: Researchers have identified a number of constituents in different passion flower species. "Official passion flower" is considered to be *P. incarnata*, which is the plant used for the drug.[6] Key constituents in *P. incarnata* generally include flavonoids, maltol, cyanogenic glycosides, and indole alkaloids (harmans).[2] Flavonoid content (2.5%) includes flavone di-C-glycosides shaftoside, isoshaftoside, isovitexin (found to be at highest concentration between pre-flowering and flowering stages in 1 report),[7] iso-orientin, vicenin, lucenin, saponarin, and passiflorine (similar to morphine).[8] Free flavonoids include apigenin, luteolin, quercetin, and campherol.[6] Another report confirms similar constituents above by mass spectral analysis.[9] Flavonoid determination by HPLC and other methods has been extensively reported.[10-17] The stability of dried extract also has been studied.[18] *P. incarnata* components also include phenolic, fatty, linoleic, linolenic, palmitic, oleic, and myristic acids, as well as formic and butyric acids,[5,19] coumarins, phytosterols, essential oil, maltol (0.05%;[6] which has been isolated and studied in 1 report),[20] and harman and its derivatives (0.03%). "Harmala" alkaloids include harmine, harmaline, and harmalol. Quantitative determination of harman and harmin in *P. incarnata* has also been performed.[21]

Other *Passiflora* species also have been studied in detail.

P. edulis: In this species, fatty acid from seed oil has been analyzed,[22] aroma precursors have been isolated from its fruits,[23] flavor analysis has been performed,[24] flavonoid and alkaloid compositions have been determined both by chromatographic and spectrometric methods,[25,26] and harman content of the leaf parts has been evaluated.[26,27]

P. bryonioides: Flavone compounds vitexin, quadrangularis, pulchella, and apigenin-7-monoglucosides have been identified.[28] Alkaloidal constituents also have been determined.[29]

P. palmeri: Isolation of 17 flavonoids and flavone tricetin 4'-methyl ether has been determined.[30]

P. coerulea: Constituent chrysin has been identified from this species and was found to be a ligand for benzodiazepine receptors.[31]

P. sexflora: Leaf parts of this Mexican species yield flavonoids luteolin, an aurone, and sulphuretin.[32]

P. pavonis: Flavonoids from this species have been isolated and identified.[33]

P. serratifolia: Five C-glycosylflavonoids have been isolated from this species' leaves.[34]

Comparative studies: C-glycoslyflavonoids from *Passiflora* species, *P. pittieri*, *P. alata*, *P. ambigua*,[35] *P. cyanea*, *P. oerstedii*, *P. menispermifolia*,[36] and *P. foetida*[37] have been reported. Thin layer chromatographic methods to differentiate *P. incarnata* from *P. edulis* and *P. caerulea* are described.[38] Quantitative analysis of different plant parts from *P. incarnata* and *P. edulis* indicate that *P. edulis* leaves have the highest alkaloid content, and that fruit rinds contain ≈ 0.25% alkaloids. Seeds and root tissue have the lowest alkaloid content. These findings may have economic importance. *P. edulis* fruit rinds, by-products of passion fruit juice production, may provide an economical source of alkaloids.[39] The cyclopentenoid cyanogenic compounds pasicapsin and linamarin have been isolated and identified from *P. capsularis* and *P. warmingii*.[40] Flavonoids from *P. trinervia* and *P. sanguinolenta* also have been reported.[41] A review of the chemical constitution of *Passiflora* species is available.[42]

PHARMACOLOGY: Animal studies have shown that *Passiflora* extracts have a complex action on the CNS, inducing dose-dependent stimulation and depression.[43] A report describes CNS-receptor binding sites of *P. incarnata*.[44]

Passion flower has been researched for its sedative and anxiolytic effects.[2,6,8] A 1986 survey of British herbal sedatives revealed passion flower as the most popular species (*P. incarnata*). Other popular species included *Valeriana officinalis*, *Humulus lupulus*, and *Scutellaria lateriflora*.[45,46] Martindale also lists many multi-ingredient preparations from other countries.[47]

The pharmacological activity of *Passiflora* is attributed primarily to the alkaloids and flavonoids. The harmala alkaloids have been found to inhibit monoamine oxidase and this may account for part of their pharmacologic effect.[20]

Passiflora species exhibit sedative activity in animals[48] and anxiolytic activity in mice.[49] The species *P. incarnata* when given to rats, showed diminished general activity when tested in a 1-arm, radial maze.[50] In mice, *P. incarnata*'s sedative and anxiolytic properties were confirmed to be caused by aqueous extracts of aerial plant parts.[51] The sedative effect of *Passiflora* may occur only when complexes of alkaloids and flavonoids are present.[39] Mice injected SC with 400 mg/kg of maltol and ethyl maltol showed reduced spontaneous activity, bradycardia, hypothermia, relaxation of skeletal muscle, and diminished pinna, corneal, and ipsilateral flexor reflexes.

An ethylene chloride-soluble fraction at 2 mg/ml significantly reduced brain oxygen consumption and the effect with the acid-soluble fraction was even greater. Both maltol and ethyl maltol potentiated the sleep-inducing effect of hexobarbital and counteracted the convulsive effects of pentylene or strychnine. These findings indicate that maltol and ethyl maltol may mask the stimulant effects of harmala alkaloids in *Passiflora*.[20]

Human studies in the sedative/anxiolytic areas of *Passiflora* species are reported. A case report using the plant in a combination natural product, "calmanervin," for successful sedation before surgery is discussed.[52] In 91 patients, *Passiflora* (in combination, "Euphytose") exhibited statistically significant differences when compared to placebo in the treatment of adjustment disorder with anxious mood, in a multicenter, double-blind trial.[53] *Passiflora* in the combination product *Compoz* contradicts these last 2 studies. It was not possible to differentiate from either aspirin or placebo when tested as a daytime sedative. However, this report was from the early 1970s and was only 2 weeks in duration.[54]

Other *Passiflora* species exhibit similar effects. *P. coerulea* has sedative actions.[31] Constituent chrysin, isolated from this same species (a central benzodiazepine [BDZ] ligand) has anxiolytic effects, due in part to this role as a partial agonist of central BDZ receptors.[55] Tranquilizing effects have been seen from alkaloids from the harman group in *P. edulis* species as well.[25]

Passion flower's ability to reduce anxiety makes it useful for asthma, palpitations, and other cardiac rhythm abnormalities, high blood pressure, insomnia, neurosis, nervousness, pain relief, and other related conditions.[2,6,8]

In vitro experiments have demonstrated that *Passiflora* kills a wide variety of molds, yeasts, and bacteria. Group A hemolytic streptococci are much more susceptible than *Staphylococcus aureus*, with *Candida albicans* being intermediate in susceptibility. The antimicrobial activity of *Passiflora* disappears rapidly from dried plant residues and fades gradually in aqueous extracts. Addition of dextran, milk, or milk products has a stabilizing effect on dry *Passiflora*.[56,57] A later report discusses *P. tetrandra* component, "4-hydroxy-2-cyclopentenone," to exhibit antipseudomonal actions. This consituent was also found to be cytotoxic to P388 murine leukemia cells.[58]

Other uses of passion flower include herbal treatment for menopausal complaints[59] and as a flavored syrup to mask drug taste.[60]

TOXICOLOGY: Little information is available on the clinical toxicity of *Passiflora*. Extracts produced no adverse effects in mice when administered intravenously.[56] Cyanogenesis from species *P. edulis* has been suggested.[61] The plant's known depressant actions may reduce arterial pressure affecting circulation and increasing respiratory rate.[8] There are no controlled human trials on single herb preparations of *Passiflora* extracts since the mid 1990s.[62] Some cases report vasculitis[63] and altered consciousness in 5 patients taking the herbal product *Relaxir*, produced mainly from *P. incarnata* fruits.[64] Induced occupational asthma and rhinitis may occur from the species *P. alata*, proven by skin testing and Western blot in vivo and in vitro studies.[65] *P. adenopoda* fruits may produce some toxic effect.[66]

Use of passion flower is contraindicated during pregnancy because of the uterine stimulant action of its alkaloids harman and harmaline, and the content of the cyanogenic glycoside gynocardin.[67]

SUMMARY: Passion flower denotes 1 of several species of the genus *Passiflora* that grow wild or are cultivated for their ornamental flowers and, in some species, for their edible fruit. In folk medicine, passion flower extracts have been used for their sedative and anxiolytic effects, which have been confirmed by animal and human studies. Edible passion fruit is used as food and in the production of juice. Some *Passiflora* species contain constituents that are active against molds, yeasts, and bacteria. No major clinical trials have been conducted to assess the plant's toxicities, although a few case reports are available.

PATIENT INFORMATION – Passion Flower

Uses: Passion flower has been used to treat sleep disorders and historically in homeopathic medicine to treat pain, insomnia related to neurasthenia or hysteria, and nervous exhaustion.

Drug Interactions: Passion flower may interact with MAOI therapy.[68]

Side Effects: Although no adverse effects of the passion flower have been reported, large doses may result in CNS depression.

---

[1] Seymour E. The Garden Encyclopedia. New York: Wm. H. Wise, 1940.

[2] Chevallier, A. Encyclopedia of Medicinal Plants. New York, NY: DK Publishing,1996;117.

[3] Encyclopedia Americana. Danbury, CT: Grolier, 1987.

[4] Tyler, V. The New Honest Herbal. Philadelphia, PA: G.F. Stickley Co, 1987.

[5] Lutomski J, et al. *Pharm Unserer Zeit* 1981;10:45.

[6] Bruneton, J. Pharmacognosy, Phytochemistry, Medicinal Plants. Paris, France: Lavoisier Publishing Inc., 1995:284-85.

[7] Menghini A, et al. TLC determination of flavonoid accumulation in clonal populations of *Passiflora incarnata* L. *Pharmacol Res Commun* 1988:(20 Suppl 5):113-16.

[8] Duke, J. CRC Handbook of Medicinal Herbs. Boca Raton, FL: CRC Press, 1989;347.

[9] Li Q, et al. Mass spectral characterization of C-glycosidic flavonoids isolated from a medicinal plant (*Passiflora incarnata*). *J Chromatogr* 1991;562(1-2):435-46.

[10] Bennati, E. Identification, by thin-layer chromatography, of liquid extract of *Passiflora incarnata*. *Boll Chim Farm* 1967;106(11):756-60.

[11] Glotzbach B, et al. Flavonoids from *Passiflora incarnata* L., *Passiflora quandrangularis* L., and *Passiflora pulchella* H.B.V.A. chromatographic study. *Planta Med* 1968;16(1):1-7.

[12] Bennati E, et al. Gas chromatography of fluid extract of *Passiflora incarnata*. *Boll Chim Farm* 1968;107(11):716-20.

[13] Lutomski J, et al. Pharmacochemical investigation of the raw materials from *Passiflora* genus. 1. New method of chromatographic separation and fluorometric-planimetric determination of alkaloids and flavonoids in harman raw materials. *Planta Med* 1974;26(4):311-17.

[14] Pietta P, et al. Isocratic liquid chromatographic method for the simultaneous determination of *Passiflora incarnata* L. and *Crataegus monogyna* flavonoids in drugs. *J Chromatogr* 1986;357(1):233-37.

[15] Schmidt P, et al. Passion flowers: assay of the total flavonoid contents in passiflorae herba. *Deutsche Apotheker Zeitung* 1993(Nov. 25);133:17-20, 23-26.

[16] Rehwald A, et al. Qualitative and quantitative reversed-phase high-performance liquid chromatography of flavonoids in *Passiflora incarnata* L. *Pharmaceutica Acta Helvetiae* 1994;69(3):153-58.

[17] Bokstaller S, et al. Comparative study on the content of passionflower flavonoids and sesquiterpenes from valerian root extracts in pharmaceutical preparations by HPLC. *Pharmazie* 1997(Jul);52:552-57.

[18] Ortega G, et al. Stability studies on dried extracts of passion flower (*Passiflora incarnata* L.) *STP Pharm Sciences* 1995;5(5):385-89.

[19] Brasseur T, Angenot L. *J Pharm Belg* 1984;39:15.

[20] Aoyagi N, et al. Studies on *Passiflora incarnata* dry extract. I. Isolation of maltol and pharmacological action of maltol and ethyl maltol. *Chem Pharm Bull* 1974;22(5):1008-13.

[21] Bennati E, et al. Quantitative determination of harman and harmin in extract of *Passiflora incarnata*. *Boll Chim Farma* 1971(Nov.);110:664-69.

[22] Zuniga, R. Oil seeds from the American tropics. *Arch Latinoam Nutr* 1981;31(2):350-70

[23] Chassagne D, et al. 6-O-alpha-L-Arabinopyranosyl-beta-D-glucopyranosides as aroma precursors from passion fruit. *Phytochemistry* 1996;41(6):1497-1500.

[24] George, G. Technique of negative ions and mass spectrometry. Use in flavor analysis problems. *Labo Pharma Probl Tech* 1984(Jun);32:479-81.

[25] Lutomski J, et al. Pharmacochemical investigations of the raw materials from *Passiflora* genus. *Planta Medica* 1975(Mar);27:112-21.

[26] Lutomski J, et al. Pharmacochemical investigations on raw materials genus *Passiflora*. 3. Phytochemical investigations on raw materials of *Passiflora edulis forma flavicarpa*. *Planta Medica* 1975(May);27:222-25.

[27] Lutomski J, et al. Pharmacological investigations on raw materials of the genus *Passiflora*. Part 4. Comparison of contents of alkaloids in some harman raw materials. *Planta Medica* 1975(Jun);27:381-84.

[28] Poethke W, et al. Constituents of *Passiflora bryonioides*. II. Flavone derivatives. *Planta Medica* 1970(Nov);19:177-88.

[29] Poethke W, et al. Constituents of *Passiflora bryonioides*. I. Alkaloids. *Planta Medica* 1970(Aug);18:303-14.

[30] Ulubelen A, et al. Flavonoids from *Passiflora palmeri*. *J Natural Products* 1984(Mar-Apr);47:384-85.

[31] Medina J, et al. Chrysin (5,7-di-OH-flavone), a naturally-occurring ligand for benzodiazepine receptors, with anticonvulsant properties. *Biochem Pharmacol* 1990;40(10):2227-31.

[32] McCormick S, et al. Flavonoids of *Passiflora sexflora*. *J Natural Products* 1982(Nov-Dec);45:782.

[33] McCormick S, et al. Flavonoids of *Passiflora pavonis*. *J Natural Products* 1981(Sep-Oct);44:623-24.

[34] Ulubelen A, et al. C-glycosylflavonoids of *Passiflora serratifolia*. *Lloydia* 1980(Jan-Feb);43:162-63.

[35] Ulubelen A, et al. C-glycosylflavonoids from *Passiflora pittieri, P. alata, P. ambigua, and Adenia mannii*. *J Natural Products* 1982(Nov-Dec);45:783.

[36] Ulubelen A, et al. C-glycosylflavonoids and other compounds from *Passiflora cyanea, P. oerstedii, and P. menispermifolia*. *J Natural Products* 1981(May-Jun);44:368-69.

[37] Ulubelen A, et al. C-glycosylflavonoids from *Passiflora foetida* var. Hispida and *P. foetida* var Hibiscifolia. *J Natural Products* 1982(Jan-Feb);45:103.

[38] Brasseur T, et al. Contribution to the pharmacognostical study of passion flower. *J de Pharmacie de Belgique* 1984(Jan-Feb);39:15-22.

[39] Lutomski J, Malek B. *Planta Med* 1975;27:381.

[40] Fischer F, et al. Cyanogenesis in *Passifloraceae*. Part 2. Cyanogenic compounds from *Passiflora capsularis, P. warmingii, and P. perfoliata*. *Planta Medica* 1982(May);45:42-45.

[41] Ulubelen A, et al. Flavonoids from *Passiflora trinervia* and *P. sanguinolenta*. *J Nat Prod* 1983(Jul-Aug);46:597.

[42] Turkoz, S. Chemical constitution and medical usage of *Passiflora* L. species. *Parmasotik Bilimler Dergisi* 1994;19(2):79-84.

[43] Speroni E, Minghetti A. Neuropharmacological activity of extracts from *Passiflora incarnata*. *Planta Med* 1988;54:488.

[44] Burkard W, et al. Receptor binding studies in the CNS with extracts of *Passiflora incarnata*. *Pharmaceutical & Pharmacological Letters* 1997;7(1):25-26.

[45] Tyler, V. Herbs of Choice, The Therapeutic Use of Phytomedicinals. Binghamton, NY: Pharmaceutical Products Press, 1994:119.

[46] Ross M, et al. Selection of plants for phytopharmacological study based on modern herbal practice. *International J Crude Drug Research* 1986(Mar);24:1-6.

[47] Reynolds J, ed. Martindale, The Extra Pharmacopoeia. London, England: Royal Pharmaceutical Society, 1996:1739.

[48] Geppert B, et al. Pharmacological evaluation of medicinal plant preparations for sedative action. *Herba Polonica* 1985;31(1-2):67-75.

[49] Della Loggia R, et al. Evaluation of the activity on the mouse CNS of several plant extracts and a combination of them. *Riv Neurol* 1981;51(5):297-310.

[50] Sopranzi N, et al. Biological and electroencephalographic parameters in rats in relation to *Passiflora incarnata* L. *Clin Ter* 1990;132(5):329-33.

[51] Soulimani R, et al. Behavioral effects of *Passiflora incarnata* L. and its indole alkaloid and flavonoid derivatives and maltol in the mouse. *J Ethnopharmacology* 1997;57(1):11-20.

[52] Yaniv R, et al. Natural premedication for mast cell proliferative disorders. *J Ethnopharmacology* 1995;46(1):71-72.

[53] Bourin M, et al. A combination of plant extracts in the treatment of outpatients with adjustment disorder with anxious mood: controlled study vs placebo. *Fundam Clin Pharmacol* 1997;11(2):127-32.

[54] Rickels K, et al. Over-the-counter daytime sedatives: a controlled study. *JAMA* 1973(Jan 1);223:29-33.

[55] Wolfman C, et al. Possible anxiolytic effects of chrysin, a central benzodiazepine receptor ligand isolated from *Passiflora coerulea*. *Pharmacol Biochem Behav* 1994;47(1):1-4.

[56] Nicolls J, et al. Passicol, an antibacterial and antifungal agent produced by *Passiflora* plant species: qualitative and quantitative range of activity. *Antimicrob Agents Chemother* 1973;3:110-17.

[57] Birner J, et al. Passicol, an antibacterial and antifungal agent produced by *Passiflora* plant species: preparation and physiocochemical characteristics. *Antimicrob Agents Chemother* 1973;3(1):105-09.

[58] Perry N, et al. 4-Hydroxy-2-cyclopentenone: and anti-psudomonas and cytotoxic component from *Passiflora tetrandra*. *Planta Med* 1981;57(2):129-31.

[59] Israel D, et al. Herbal therapies for perimenopausal and menopausal complaints. *Pharmacotherapy* 1997;17(5):970-84.

[60] Puffer H, et al. Comparison of pharmaceutical flavorants extracted from selected subtropical fruits. *Am J Hosp Pharm* 1971(Aug);28:633-35.

[61] Spencer K, et al. Cyanogenesis of *Passiflora edulis*. *J Agric Food Chem* 1983;31(4):794-96.

[62] Schulz V, et al. Rational Phytotherapy, 3rd edition. Berlin, Germany: Springer Verlag, 1998:83-84.

[63] Smith G, et al. Vasculitis associated with herbal preparation containing *Passiflora* extract. *Br J Rheumatol* 1993;32(1):87-88.

[64] Solbakken A, et al. Nature medicine as intoxicant. *Tidsskr nor Laegeforen* 1997;117(8):1140-41.

[65] Giavina-Bianchi Jr, P, et al. Occupational respiratory allergic disease induced by *Passiflora alata* and *Rhamnus purshiana*. *Ann Allergy Asthma Immunol* 1997;79(5):449-54.

[66] Saenz J, et al. Toxic effect of the fruit of *Passiflora adenopoda* D. C. on humans: phytochemical determination. *Rev Biol Trop* 1972;20(1):137-40.

[67] Brinker, F. Herb contraindications and drug interactions. Sandy, OR: Eclectic Medical Publications, 1998:109-10.

[68] Newall C, et al. Herbal Medicines: A Guide for Health Care Professionals. London, England: The Pharmaceutical Press, 1996:206.

Pawpaw

SCIENTIFIC NAME(S): *Asimina triloba* (L.) Dunal. Family: Annonaceae (Sometimes confused with *Carica Papaya*.)

COMMON NAME(S): Pawpaw, Custard apple, Poor man's banana

BOTANY: The pawpaw is a small, North American tree which grows from ≈ 3 to 12 meters high. It is common in the temperate woodlands of the eastern US. Its large leaves are "tropical looking" and droopy in nature. The dark brown, velvety flowers (≈ 5 cm across) grow in umbrella-like whorls, similar to some magnolia species, and can bloom for up to 6 weeks. Pawpaw fruit is smooth-skinned, yellow to greenish-brown in color, measuring from ≈ 8 to 15 cm long. It can reach up to 0.45 kg in weight. It resembles that of a short, thick banana, and is also similar in nutrient value. The yellow, soft, "custard-like" pulp is edible but sickly sweet in flavor and contains dark seeds.[1,2,3,4]

HISTORY: One source states that the pawpaw was introduced to the US in 1736.[3] It has been used as food for Native Americans. The thin, fibrous, inner bark has been used to make fish nets.[1,3] The bark was also used as medicine because it contains useful alkaloids.[3]

CHEMISTRY: The bark, roots, twigs, and seeds of the pawpaw plant contain the majority of acetogenins. Acetogenins are long-chain, aliphatic compounds with 35 to 39 carbon atoms ending with a gamma-lactone, cyclized in tetrahydrofuran rings.[5] They are polyketide-derived molecules and are unique to the Annonaceae family. Thus far, > 230 acetogenins from Asimina and other genera have been identified.[6] Acetogenins are known for their cytotoxic, antitumor (ie, asimicin, bullatacine), immunosuppressive antimalarial, pesticidal (ie, asimicin), antibacterial, and antifeedant properties.[5,6]

Known bioactive compounds from pawpaw bark include asimicin, bullatacin, bullatacinone, N-p-coumaroyltyramine, N-trans-feruloyltyramine, and (+)-syringaresinol. Trilobacin, a highly cytotoxic acetogenin, and trilobalicin and its ketolactones (2,4–cis and 2,4-trans-trilobacinone) have also been identified.[7,8] In addition, acetogenins cis- and trans-annonacin-a-one, cis- and trans-gigantetrocinone, trans-isoannonacin, and squamolone have been determined.[9] The acetogenins asimin, asiminacin, and asiminecin (all structural isomers) from pawpaw stem bark extracts were determined and also found to have highly cytotoxic properties.[10] Similar findings were described for acetogenins bis-tetrahydro-

furans,[11] asiminocin (-hydroxy-4–deoxyasimicin),[12] (2,4–cis)- and (2,4–trans)-asimicinone.[13] In addition, acetogenins asimilobin, cis- and trans-murisolinones, and cis- and trans-bullatacinones have been isolated from pawpaw seeds.[14] Asiminine and analobine alkaloids have also been found.[3] A variation of essential oils and other extracts from the plant has been reported.[15]

PHARMACOLOGY: The pawpaw acetogenins have consistently exhibited **cytotoxic** (antitumor) and **pesticidal** (antimicrobial) activities.

Brine shrimp lethality bioassay or "test" (BSLT) is a screening tool used to predict cytotoxic and pesticidal activity. Tiny shrimp, *Artemia salina*, are placed in brine where their eggs hatch within 48 hours. Extracts of test-plant material are then put in shrimp-containing vials where survivors are microscopically counted. LC_{50} values are then calculated to determine the potential killing activity of, in this case, pawpaw extracts.[16]

In several studies performed in this manner it was found that specific acetogenins exhibited potent cytotoxicities.[7,9,11,14] Examples include acetogenin's cytotoxic potential against lung carcinoma, breast carcinoma, and colon adenocarcinoma.[9] Certain seed extracts also possessed cytotoxic actions comparable with doxorubicin against 6 human solid tumor cell lines.[14]

Of all the acetogenins, the adjacent-bis-THF-ring compounds are the most potent, showing cytotoxic activity against human lung and breast tumor cell lines with up to a million times the potency of doxorubicin.[8] Compound asiminocin, a pawpaw acetogenin isolate from stem bark was highly inhibitory against 3 human cell lines, with over a billion times the potency of doxorubicin.[12] The mechanism of action is via potent inhibitors of mitochondrial NADH:ubiquinone oxidoreductase, thus causing a decrease in cellular ATP levels.[6,10]

Various pawpaw tree parts were tested for pesticidal potential. It was found that small twigs yielded the most potent extract, while the leaves were the least potent. Unripe fruits, seeds, root wood and bark, and stem bark were also notably potent.[17] A caterpillar-laden tree was sprayed with a pawpaw bark extract and 30 minutes later the majority of insects had died and fallen from the tree. Phlox plants infested with mildew fungus were also sprayed with pawpaw preparation and 10 days later improvement was markedly observed. Pawpaw tree samplings were collected, expressing monthly variation in pesticidal activity. All of these are examples of the plant's beneficial (and natural) properties. The pawpaw tree is usually insect- or disease-resistant because of its acetogenin content, which prevents the feeding of many organisms.[6]

TOXICOLOGY: Handling the fruit may produce a skin rash in sensitive individuals.[3] The sensitizing potential of the pawpaw was examined in guinea pigs; the crude extract of the stem bark was found to be a weak sensitizer and to elicit allergic contact dermatitis. This report also determined the active compound asimicin to be a weak irritant.[18]

SUMMARY: The pawpaw is a North American plant bearing an elongated fruit. The plant parts and seeds contain acetogenins that possess cytotoxic and pesticidal actions. Certain extracts are comparable to, or are a million or over a billion times more potent than, doxorubicin. The plant may cause contact dermatitis in certain individuals.

PATIENT INFORMATION – Pawpaw

Uses: Pawpaw has historically been used for food, fishing nets, and medicine. It exhibits cytotoxic and pesticidal activities.

Side Effects: May cause contact dermatitis in certain people.

---

[1] Hocking G. A Dictionary of Natural Products. Medford, NY: Plexus Publishing Inc., 1997;80.

[2] Davidson A. Fruit-A Connoisseur's Guide and Cookbook. NY, NY: Simon and Schuster, 1991;123-24.

[3] NNGA library. http://www.icserv.com/nnga/pawpaw.htm. Pawpaw and acetogenins.

[4] Univ. of Kentucky. http://www.pawpaw.kysu.edu. The return of the pawpaw.

[5] Bruneton J. Pharmacognosy, Phytochemistry, Medicinal Plants. Paris, France: Lavoisier, 1995;156.

[6] Johnson H, et al. Progress in New Crops. Arlington, VA: ASHS Press, 1996;609-14.

[7] Zhao G, et al. Additional bioactive compounds and trilobacin, a novel highly cytotoxic acetogenin, from the bark of Asimina triloba. J Nat Prod 1992;55(3):347-56.

[8] He K, et al. Additional bioactive annonanaceous acetogenins from Asimina triloba (Annonaceae). Bioorg Med Chem 1997;5(3):501-06.

[9] Zhao G, et al. Biologically active acetogenins from stem bark of Asimina triloba. Phytochemistry 1993;33(5):1065-73.

[10] Zhao G, et al. Asimin, asiminacin, and asiminecin: novel highly cytotoxic asimicin isomers from Asimina triloba. J Med Chem 1994;37(13):1971-76.

[11] He K, et al. Three new adjacent bis-tetrahydrofuran acetogenins with four hydroxyl groups from Asimina triloba. J Nat Prod 1996;59(11):1029-34.

[12] Zhao G, et al. The absolute configuration of adjacent bis-THF acetogenins and asiminocin, a novel highly potent asimicin isomer from Asimina. Bioorg Med Chem 1996;4(1):25-32.

[13] Zhao G, et al. (2,4–cis)-asimicinone and (2,4–trans)-asimicinone: two novel bioactive ketolactone acetogenins from Asimina triloba (Annonaceae). Nat Toxins 1996;4(3):128-34.

[14] Woo M, et al. Asimilobin and cis- and trans-murisolinones, novel bioactive Annonaceous acetogenins from the seeds of Asimina triloba. J Nat Prod 1995;58(10):1533-42.

[15] Derevinskaya T, et al. Some problems of the quality of drug-technical raw material of Asimina triloba. Farm Zh 1983;38(5):49-52.

[16] Colegate S, et al. Bioactive Natural Products. Boca Raton, FL: CRC Press, 1993;15-17.

[17] Ratnayake S, et al. Evaluation of various parts of the paw paw tree, Asimina triloba (Annonaceae), as commerical sources of the pesticidal annonaceous acetogenins. J Econ Entomol 1992;85(6):2353-56.

[18] Avalos J, et al. Guinea pig maximization test of the bark extract from pawpaw, Asimina triloba (Annonaceae). Contact Dermatitis 1993;29(1):33-35.

Pectin

SCIENTIFIC NAME(S): *Pectin*

COMMON NAME(S): Pectin

HISTORY: Pectin is found in the cell walls of all plant tissue where it acts as an intercellular "cement," giving the plant rigidity. The compound is found at concentrations of 15% to 30% in the fiber of fruits, vegetables, legumes and nuts.[1] Lemon and orange rinds are among the richest sources of the compound, containing up to 30% of this polysaccharide.[2] Pectin is also found in the roots of most plants.[3]

Pectin has been used in the food industry to add body and texture to jellies, jams, puddings and other gelatinous products. It has also been added to antidiarrheal products and has been particularly effective when combined with adsorbing clays such as kaolin.

CHEMISTRY: Pectin is a polysaccharide with a variable molecular weight ranging from 20,000 to 400,000 depending on the number of carbohydrate linkages.[2] The core of the molecule is formed by linked D-polygalacturonate and L-rhamnose residues. The neutral sugars D-galactose, L-arabinose, D-xylose and L-fucose form the side chains on the pectin molecule. Once extracted, pectin occurs as a coarse or fine yellowish powder that is highly water soluble and forms thick colloidal solutions. The parent compound, protopectin, is insoluble, but is readily converted by hydrolysis into pectinic acids (also known generically as pectins).[3]

PHARMACOLOGY: One of the best characterized effects of pectin supplementation is its ability to lower human blood lipoprotein levels.[4] Most studies have evaluated its ingestion in combination with other gums. For example, a mixture of guar and apple-pectin in combination with apple pomaces was evaluated in 15 diabetic women. Ingestion of the mixture before meals resulted in a significant decrease in total cholesterol level (an 11.3% to 12.6% drop) and triglycerides (a 15.5% to 19.2% drop), although HDL cholesterol levels remained relatively stable.[5]

Dietary fibers have been associated with a reduction in the risk of colon cancer, and this may also apply to pectin. Possible direct mechanisms include the binding of carcinogens to undegraded dietary fibers and the absorption of water by these fibers to increase stool bulk and to shorten gastrointestinal transit time.[6]

Pectin has also been investigated for its ability to reduce the consequence of exposure to radiation. Persons exposed to radiation after the Chernobyl accident were given pectin supplements which were found to have a beneficial effect on the antioxidant level of their hematologic systems, as well as normalizing their triglyceride and albumin levels.[7] Pectin supplements appear to act as "enteroabsorbents," protecting against the accumulation of ingested radioactivity.[8]

TOXICOLOGY: Pectin is a fermentable fiber that results in the production of short-chain fatty acids and methane.[9] Concomitant administration of pectin with beta-carotene containing foods or supplements can reduce the blood levels of beta-carotene by more than one-half.[10] There is some indication that concomitant ingestion of pectin with high energy diets may reduce the availability of these diets, as demonstrated in a controlled trial of undernourished children; urea production was also shown to be lower in children who ingested pectin with their caloric supplement.[11]

Occupational asthma associated with the inhalation of pectin dust is a well-recognized hazard.[12,13,14]

SUMMARY: Pectin is a natural polysaccharide that forms thick colloidal solutions in water. It is added to processed foods to create texture. Medicinally, the compound has been widely used in antidiarrheal products, serving as a stool-forming agent. It also appears to lower blood lipoprotein levels. Pectin is generally well tolerated, although it may interfere with the absorption of dietary nutrients.

PATIENT INFORMATION – Pectin

Uses: Pectin has been used to lower blood lipoprotein levels, in antidiarrheal products, and investigated for its ability to reduce the consequence of exposure to radiation.

Drug Interactions: Coadministration of pectin with beta-carotene containing foods or supplements can reduce the blood levels of beta-carotene by more than one-half.

Side Effects: Pectin is generally well tolerated when ingested. Occupational asthma has been associated with the inhalation of pectin dust.

---

[1] Marlett JA. *J Am Diet Assoc* 1992;92(2):175.
[2] Windholz M, ed. The Merck Index, ed. 10. Rahway, NJ: Merck & Co, 1983.
[3] Evans WC. Trease and Evans' Pharmacognosy, ed. 13. London: Balliére Tindall, 1989.
[4] Lewinska D, et al. *Artif Organs* 1994;18(3):217.
[5] Biesenbach G, et al. *Leber Magen Darm* 1993;23(5):204.
[6] Harris PJ, Ferguson LR. *Mutat Res* 1993;290(1):97.
[7] Bereza Vla, et al. *Vrach Delo* 1993;8:21.

[8] Trakhtenberg IM, et al. *Vrach Delo* 1992;5:29.
[9] Mortensen PB, Nordgaard-Andersen I. *Scand J Gastroenterol* 1993;28(5):418.
[10] Rock CL, Swendseid ME. *Am J Clin Nutr* 1992;55(1):96.
[11] Doherty J, Jackson AA. *Acta Paediatr* 1992;81(6–7):514.
[12] Baldwin JL, Shah AC. *Chest* 1992;102(5):1605.
[13] Cohen AJ, et al. *Chest* 1993;103(1):309.
[14] Kraut A, et al. *Chest* 1993;104(6):1936.

Pennyroyal

SCIENTIFIC NAME(S): *Hedeoma pulegeoides* (L) Persoom and *Mentha pulegium* L. Family: Labiatae

COMMON NAME(S): American pennyroyal, squawmint, mosquito plant, pudding grass

BOTANY: Both plants are members of the mint family and both are referred to as pennyroyal. *H. pulegeoides* (American pennyroyal) grows in woods through most of the northern and eastern United States and Canada while *M. pulegium* is found in parts of Europe. Pennyroyal is a perennial, creeping herb that possesses small, lilac flowers at the stem ends. It can grow to be 30 to 50 cm in height. The leaves are grayish green and, like other mint family members, are very aromatic.[1,2]

HISTORY: Pennyroyal has been recorded in history as far back as the 1st century AD, where it was mentioned by Roman naturalist Pliny and Greek physician Dioscorides. In the 17th century, English herbalist Nicholas Culpeper wrote about some uses for the plant including its role in women's ailments, venomous bites and digestion. European settlers used the plant for respiratory ailments, mouth sores and female disorders.[1] The plant's oil has been used as a flea-killing bath, hence the name *pulegeoides* (from the Latin word meaning flea), and has been used externally as a rubefacient. In addition, the oil has found frequent use among natural health advocates as an abortifacient and as a means of inducing delayed menses. The oil and infusions of the leaves have been used in the treatment of weakness and stomach pains.[3]

CHEMISTRY: The leaves and flowering tops are the source of pennyroyal oil, which is found in a concentration of 1% to 2% depending on the genus. The oil contains 80% to 92% of the cyclohexanone pulegone.[4,5] Other constituents include: Methone, iso-methone, octanol, piperitenone, pinene, limonene, dipentene and formic, acetic, butyric, salicylic and other acids.[6,7]

Quantitative determination of pulegone from Chilean *M. pulegium* oil has been performed.[8] Using mass spectrometry, biliary metabolites of pulegone, glucuronide, glutathione and conjugates have been detected.[9]

PHARMACOLOGY: Pennyroyal has been used as an **insect repellent** and **antiseptic**.[1,2,6,7] It has been employed as a flavoring agent for food and spice[7] and also as a fragrance in detergents, perfumes and soaps.[2,7]

The plant has been reported to be of use for female problems as an **emmenagogue** (to induce menstruation).

It has also been used as a **carminative, stimulant** and **antispasmodic**, and for **bowel disorders, skin eruptions, pneumonia** and other uses.[1,2,6,7]

TOXICOLOGY: Pennyroyal herb teas are generally used without reported side effects (presumably because of low concentration of the oil),[6] but toxicity for pennyroyal oil is well recognized, with many reports of adverse events and fatalities documented.

American or European pennyroyal can cause dermatitis and, in large doses, abortion, irreversible renal damage, severe liver damage and death. A teaspoonful of the oil can produce delirium, unconsciousness and shock.[7]

One case of pennyroyal oil ingestion resulted in generalized seizures and auditory and visual hallucinations following the ingestion of less than 1 teaspoonful (5 ml) of the oil; the patient recovered uneventfully.[10] Other symptoms of plant ingestion may also include: Abdominal pain, nausea, vomiting, lethargy, increased blood pressure and increased pulse rate.[6]

The major component, pulegone, is oxidized by hepatic cytochrome P450 to the hepatotoxic compound menthofuran.[11] Pulegone, or a metabolite, is also responsible for neurotoxicity and destruction of bronchiolar epithelial cells.[5, 2]

Pulegone extensively depletes glutathione in the liver, and its metabolites are detoxified by the presence of glutathione in the liver. Hepatic toxicity has been prevented by the early administration of acetylcysteine following ingestion of pennyroyal oil.[13] Various metabolite studies are available regarding hepatotoxicity.[14,15]

Pennyroyal toxicity in animals has been documented; intraperitoneal injections of pulegone in mice caused extensive liver injury.[16]

Rats given oral doses of pulegone for 28 days (80 or 160 mg/kg/day) developed encephalopathic changes characterized by cyst-like spaces in the cerebellum without concomitant demyelination. This resembles the neuropathy induced in rats by administration of hexachlorophene.[17] LD_{50} values for pennyroyal oil have been reported in rats and rabbits.[6] A dog treated for fleas with pennyroyal application suffered vomiting and, despite treatment, died within 48 hours.[18]

Case reports in humans are also widely reported: One woman who ingested up to 30 ml of the oil experienced abdominal cramps, nausea, vomiting and alternating lethargy and agitation. She later exhibited loss of renal function, hepatotoxicity and evidence of disseminated intravascular coagulation. She died 7 days after ingesting the oil. Another woman ingested 10 ml of the oil and only experienced dizziness.[19] Two infants (8 weeks of age and 6 months of age) who ingested mint tea containing pennyroyal oil developed hepatic and neurologic injury. One infant died, the other suffered hepatic dysfunction and severe epileptic encephalopathy.[20] A review of 18 previous cases reported moderate to severe toxicity in patients exposed to at least 10 ml of the oil, concluding

that pennyroyal continues to be an herbal toxin of concern to public health.[21] Another review concluded that pennyroyal oil is toxic as well.[22]

Pennyroyal is contraindicated in pregnancy. It possesses abortifacient actions (because of pulegone content) and irritates the genitourinary tract.[6] The abortifacient effect of the oil is thought to be caused by irritation of the uterus with subsequent uterine contraction. Its action is unpredictable and dangerous.[23] The dose at which the herb induces abortion is close to lethal, and in some cases it is lethal.[2,7] However, one letter does report a pregnancy unaffected by pennyroyal use.[24]

SUMMARY: Pennyroyal oil and teas made from the plant continue to find use in a variety of herbal self-treatment practices. Despite this use, these products are potentially toxic to both animal and man and should not be ingested. The principle toxic assaults appear to be on the central nervous system and the liver. The plant is contraindicated in pregnancy because of its abortifacient actions.

PATIENT INFORMATION – Pennyroyal

Uses: Pennyroyal may be used as an insect repellent, antiseptic, fragrance, flavoring, as an emmenagogue, carminative, stimulant, antispasmodic and for bowel disorders, skin eruptions and pneumonia.

Side Effects: Pennyroyal can cause abdominal pain, nausea, vomiting, lethargy, increased blood pressure and increased pulse rate, dermatitis and, in large portions, abortion, irreversible renal damage, severe liver damage and death. A small amount of oil can produce delirium, unconsciousness, shock, seizures and auditory and visual hallucinations.

---

[1] Low T, et al. eds. Pennyroyal. Magic and Medicine of Plants. Sydney, Australia: Reader's Digest, 1994;278.

[2] Lawless J. Pennyroyal. The Illustrated Encyclopedia of Essential Oils. Rockport, MA: Element Books, Inc., 1995;176.

[3] Da Legnano LP. The Medicinal Plants. Rome, Italy: Edizioni Mediterranee, 1973.

[4] Tyler VE. The New Honest Herbal. Philadelphia, PA: G.F. Stickley Co., 1987.

[5] Thomassen D, et al. *J Pharmacol Exp Ther* 1990;253(2):567.

[6] Newall C, et al. Pennyroyal. Herbal Medicines. London, England: Pharmaceutical Press, 1996;208.

[7] Duke J. *Hedeoma Pulegioides* CRC Handbook of Medicinal Herbs. Boca Raton, FL: CRC Press Inc., 1989;223,307–308.

[8] Montes M, et al. *Annales Pharmaceutiques Francaises* 1986;44(2):133–36.

[9] Thomassen D, et al. *Drug Metab Dispos* 1991;19(5):997–1003.

[10] Early DF. *Lancet* 1961;2:580.

[11] Gordon WP, et al. *Drug Metab Disp* 1987;15(5):589.

[12] Gordon WP, et al. *Toxicol Appl Pharmacol* 1982;65:413.

[13] Buechel DW, et al. *J Am Osteopath Assn* 1983;2:793.

[14] Thomassen D, et al. *J Pharmacol Exp Ther* 1988;244(3):825–29.

[15] Carmichael P. *Ann Intern Med* 1997;126(3):250–51.

[16] Mizutani T, et al. *Res Commun Chem Pathol Pharmacol* 1987;58(1):75–83.

[17] Olsen P, Thorup I. *Arch Toxicol* 1984;7(Suppl):408.

[18] Sudekum M, et al. *J Am Vet Med Assoc* 1992;200(6):817–18.

[19] Sullivan JB Jr., et al. *JAMA* 1979;242:2873.

[20] Bakerink J, et al. *Pediatrics* 1996(Nov);98:944–47.

[21] Anderson I, et al. *Ann Intern Med* 1996;124(8):726–34.

[22] Mack R. *NC Med J* 1997;58(6):456–57.

[23] Allen WT. *Lancet* 1897;2:1022.

[24] Black D. *J Am Osteopath Assoc* 1985;85(5):282.

Peppermint

SCIENTIFIC NAME(S): *Mentha x piperita* L. Peppermint is a hybrid of *M. spicata* L. (spearmint) and *M. aquatica* L. Family: Labiatae

COMMON NAME(S): Peppermint

BOTANY: This well-known perennial is a classical member of the mint family. It has a squarish purple-green stem with leaves of dark green or purple and lilac-colored flowers. The plant is generally sterile and spreads by means of stolons (basal branches). A variety of types of peppermint exist and these are cultivated worldwide.

HISTORY: Peppermint and its oil have been used in Eastern and Western traditional medicine as an aromatic, antispasmodic and antiseptic in treating indigestion, nausea, sore throat, colds, toothaches, cramps and cancers. Today, the oil is used widely as a flavoring and as an ingredient in cough and cold preparations. It is also found in numerous antiseptic and local anesthetic preparations.

CHEMISTRY: The chemistry of peppermint oil is complex. More than a hundred components have been found in the oil and their relative concentrations vary between cultivars and geographic location.[1,2] Peppermint yields 0.1% to 1% of a volatile oil that is composed primarily of menthol (29% to 48%), menthone (20% to 31%) and methyl acetate (3% to 10%).[3]

PHARMACOLOGY: As is observed with numerous other volatile oils, peppermint oil possesses antibacterial activity in vitro. However, this has not been of significant clinical benefit. Peppermint extracts have been reported to have antiviral activity against Newcastle disease, herpes simplex, vaccinia and other viruses in culture.[3]

Peppermint oil has been shown to exhibit spasmolytic activity on smooth muscles. Commercial preparations are available for use in the treatment of irritable bowel, abdominal pain and related symptoms. When administered orally, these peppermint-containing drugs appear to be effective.[4] Generally administered as enteric-coated capsules, these preparations release their contents in the large intestine and colon; peppermint, therefore, appears to act directly on this smooth muscle. The spasmolytic activity is related to menthol content and it has been demonstrated that this activity is due to the calcium antagonist effect of menthol.[5]

The flavonoids in peppermint leaves reportedly have choleretic (bile stimulating) effects in dogs.[3] A related effect was confirmed in one study in which guinea pigs were administered intravenous doses of the essential oil of peppermint in doses of 0.1 to 50 mg/kg. Prior to dosing, the sphincter of Oddi had been occluded by the administration of morphine. Following a single dose of 1 mg/kg of peppermint oil, a rapid and complete opening of the sphincter was observed. However, in doses of 25 or 50 mg/kg, peppermint oil again constricted the sphincter.[6]

Azulene, which is found in small quantities in peppermint oil, is known to have anti-inflammatory and antiulcerogenic effects in animals.

TOXICOLOGY: Peppermint is generally recognized as safe for human consumption as a seasoning or flavoring, as are other mints from which menthol is derived as a plant extract.

Menthol, the major component of peppermint oil, may cause allergic reactions (characterized by contact dermatitis, flushing and headache) in certain individuals.[3] The application of menthol-containing ointment to the nostrils of an infant for the treatment of cold symptoms has been reported to have caused instant collapse.[3]

Rats fed peppermint oil in daily doses of up to 100 mg/kg for 28 days developed dose-related brain lesions. These were similar in nature to the neuropathy induced by hexachlorophene.[7] However, one would only expect to observe doses of this magnitude ingested in a case of overdosage with the oil.

Because of the oil's ability to relax gastrointestinal smooth muscle, persons with hiatal hernia may experience worsening of symptoms while ingesting peppermint-containing preparations.

SUMMARY: Peppermint and its oil are used extensively in foods and drugs. The oil is a complex mixture of more than one hundred compounds. Menthol, which is found in the highest concentration, is pharmacologically active in relatively small doses. Extracts have been used with preliminary success in the treatment of certain gastrointestinal disorders.

PATIENT INFORMATION – Peppermint

Uses: In addition to being recognized as a seasoning and flavoring, peppermint has been used to treat irritable bowel and abdominal pain.

Side Effects: Peppermint oil may cause allergic reactions characterized by contact dermatitis, flushing and headache, and worsen the symptoms of hiatal hernias.

---

[1] Hoffmann BG, Lunder LT. *Planta Medica* 1984;50:361.
[2] Maffei M, Sacco T. *Planta Medica* 1987;53:214.
[3] Leung AY. Encyclopedia of Common Natural Ingredients Used in Food, Drugs, and Cosmetics. Wiley Interscience, 1980.

[4] Rees WDW, et al. *Brit Med J* 1979;2:835.
[5] Taylor BA, et al. Proceedings of the British Pharmacol Soc. April, 1985.
[6] Giachetti D, et al. *Planta Medica* 1988;54:389.
[7] Olsen P, Thorup I. *Arch Toxicol Suppl* 1984;7:408.

Perilla

SCIENTIFIC NAME(S): *Perilla frutescens* (L.) Britt. Family: Lamiaceae

COMMON NAME(S): Beefsteak plant, perilla, wild coleus

BOTANY: The broad oval leaves are reminiscent of the leaves of the common ornamental coleus. It is widely cultivated in the Orient.

HISTORY: The leaves and seeds of perilla are eaten in the orient and form part of the native Japanese dish known as "shisho."[1] Dried leaves are used as components of herbal teas. The seeds are expressed to yield an edible oil. This oil is also used in commercial manufacturing processes for the production of varnishes, dyes and inks. The leaf oil has a delicate fragrance and is used in food flavoring.

In oriental folk medicine, the plant has been used as an antispasmodic, to induce sweating, for asthma treatment, to quell nausea and to alleviate sunstroke, among other uses.[1]

CHEMISTRY: Apigenin and luteolin are the major flavones in the seeds. These also are found in the leaves together with many additional flavones, the primary one being shishonin. The leaves contain anthocyanin and perillanin chloride. Perillartine is reported to be 2000 times sweeter than sugar.[1] The oil is rich in citral, l-limonene and alpha-pinene.

PHARMACOLOGY: Perilla oil is receiving attention because it is high in alpha-linolenate, which may result in beneficial health effects. Serum cholesterol and triglyceride levels decreased in rats fed perilla oil. Similarly beneficial changes in the levels of eicosapentaenoic acid and arachidonic acid were observed[2] in these animals.

Perilla oil dietary supplementation to laboratory animals has been found to reduce the incidence of mammary tumor development compared to diets rich in safflower oil.[3] Perilla oil supplementation in animals also limits the development of colonic tumors.[4]

Perilla extracts may have an immunosuppressant effect that preferentially attenuates IgE production, and it has been postulated that this extract may be useful for the management of certain allergic disorders.[5]

TOXICOLOGY: The volatile perilla oil contains aldehyde antioxide, which has been used in the tobacco industry as a sweetener, however, this compound may be toxic.

Perilla ketone is a potent agent for the induction of pulmonary edema in laboratory animals.[6] Animals grazing on the plant have also developed pulmonary edema and respiratory distress. This ketone is chemically related to the toxic ipomeanols derived from moldy sweet potatoes. Intravenous doses of this compound can result in death secondary to pleural effusion and edema.[1] The ketone acts by increasing the permeability of endothelial cells and does not appear to require the presence of cytochrome P-450 to increase vascular permeability.[7]

Dermatitis has been reported in perilla oil workers and patch testing suggests that 1–perillaldehyde and perillalcohol contained in the oil are responsible for the effect.[1,8]

SUMMARY: Perilla oil is a valued product for both food flavoring and commercial applications. Preliminary evidence suggests that the oil may have beneficial antilipidemic effects and potential cancer-protective activity.

PATIENT INFORMATION – Perilla

Uses: Perilla has been used for food flavoring and may be useful for the management of certain allergic disorders. Preliminary research suggests that perilla may also have beneficial antilipemic effects and potential cancer-protective activity.

Side Effects: Perilla may cause dermatitis.

---

[1] Duke JA. Handbook of Medicinal Herbs. Boca Raton, FL: CRC Press, 1985.
[2] Sakono M, et al. *J Nutr Sci Vitaminol* 1993;39:335.
[3] Nakayama M, et al. *Anticancer Res* 1993;13:691.
[4] Narisawa T, et al. *Jpn J Cancer Res* 1991;82:1089.
[5] Imaoka K, et al. *Arerugi* 1993;42:74.
[6] Abernathy VJ, et al. *J Appl Physiol* 1992;72:505.
[7] Waters CM, et al. *J Appl Physiol* 1993;74:2493.
[8] Kanzaki T, Kimura S. *Contact Dermatitis* 1992;26:55.

Periwinkle

SCIENTIFIC NAME(S): *Catharanthus roseus* G. Don. Also referred to as *Lochnera rosea* Reichb., *Vinca rosea* L., and *Ammocallis rosea* Small. The related plant *Vinca minor* (common periwinkle, Myrtle) is used as a ground cover. Family: Apocyanaceae

COMMON NAME(S): Periwinkle, red periwinkle, Madagascar or Cape periwinkle, old maid, church-flower, ram-goat rose, "myrtle," magdalena[1]

BOTANY: Although the plant is said to be native to the West Indies, it was first described in Madagascar.[1] The periwinkle is a perennial herb that grows to about 2 feet.[2] It is highly branched and develops a woody base. The flowers can bloom throughout the year, depending on the climate. These are often bred for their unique colors ranging from white to green-yellow and lavender. The seed pod dries, splits and releases numerous tiny seeds, of which there are about 350,000/lb.[1]

HISTORY: The plant was introduced in Europe during the mid-1700s during which time it was cultivated as an ornamental. Today it grows throughout much of the world and plantations have been established on most continents in the warmer climates. The plant has been widely used in tropical folk medicine. Decoctions of the plant have been used for maladies ranging from ocular inflammation, diabetes and hemorrhage to treating insect stings and cancers.

CHEMISTRY: All parts of the plant contain alkaloids. By 1977, 73 unique alkaloids had been isolated and named, and today the number exceeds 100. The concentration of alkaloids varies with the part of the plant and the region of harvest. Roots collected in India have yielded up to 1.22% total alkaloids. The hypotensive alkaloids reserpine and alstonine have been isolated from the root in concentrations less than 0.03%.[1] The alkaloid designated ajmalicine, raubasine,[3] vinceine or vincaine appears to be structurally similar to yohimbine. The most well known of the "vinca" alkaloids derived from *C. roseus* are vinblastine (vincaleukoblastine) (eg, *Velban*)[4] and vincristine (leurocristine) (eg, *Oncovin*),[4] which are now widely used antineoplastic agents.

The leaves also contain a complex volatile oil.[1]

PHARMACOLOGY: A number of pharmacologic activities have been ascribed to the periwinkle plant. Injection of a concentrated aqueous extract was shown to lower blood sugar levels in cats and tended to moderate blood sugar levels in humans according to a treatise on African plant uses.[1]

Investigations by the Lilly company into the antidiabetic activity of the plant found no effect on blood sugar levels but uncovered the antineoplastic effects of plant extracts. Vincristine and vinblastine appear to bind to or crystallize important proteins in cellular microtubules, thus preventing proper polymerization, arresting cellular division and killing the cell. These drugs may also exert some immunosuppressant activity and may interfere with other components of the cell cycle to induce cellular death. These drugs are used for the treatment of leukemia, Hodgkin's disease, malignant lymphomas, neuroblastoma, Wilms tumor, Kaposi's sarcoma and mycosis fungoides, among others. An extensive body of literature exists on the clinical uses of the various purified alkaloids of *Catharanthus*.

Catharanthine has demonstrated diuretic properties.[3] Ajmalicine may improve cerebral blood flow and has been used to treat high blood pressure when given in combination with rauwolfia alkaloids.[3]

TOXICOLOGY: The periwinkle plant has been reported to have caused poisonings in grazing animals.[1] Severe systemic adverse events are associated with the prolonged use of vincristine and vinblastine, and fatalities have been associated with the use of these alkaloids. Acute dyspnea has been reported following antineoplastic treatment with the related alkaloids vindesine (*Eldisine*)[4] and vinorelbine (*Navelbine*).[4,5]

There has been at least one report of persons attempting to smoke periwinkle leaves as an hallucinogenic substitute for marijuana, but this appears to have passed in fancy because of a lack of any significant pharmacologic effect.[1]

The related *Vinca minor* has been declared "unsafe" for human consumption by the FDA.[2]

SUMMARY: Members of the periwinkle group are well known as ornamentals. The Madagascar periwinkle has a long history of folk use and today is an important source of antineoplastic alkaloids. The plant should not be ingested because of concerns of potential toxicity.

PATIENT INFORMATION – Periwinkle

Uses: Periwinkle has been used in the treatment of leukemia, Hodgkin's disease, malignant lymphomas, neuroblastoma, Wilms tumor, Kaposi's sarcoma, mycosis fungoides, to improve cerebral blood flow, and treat high blood pressure.

Side Effects: Periwinkle is potentially toxic and has been known to cause acute dyspnea.

---

[1] Morton JF. Major Medicinal Plants. Springfield, IL: Charles C. Thomas, 1977.
[2] Dobelis IN. Magic and Medicine of Plants. Pleasantville, NY: Reader's Digest Association, 1986.
[3] Duke JA. Handbook of Medicinal Herbs. Boca Raton, FL: CRC Press, 1985.

[4] Olin BR, Hebel SK, eds. Drug Facts and Comparisons. St. Louis, MO: Facts and Comparisons, 1994.
[5] Thomas P, et al. *Rev Mal Respir* 1993;10:268.

Peru Balsam

SCIENTIFIC NAME(S): *Myroxylon pereirae* (Royle) Klotzsch. Syn. with *M. balsamum* var. *pereirae*. Family: Leguminosae or Fabaceae

COMMON NAME(S): Peru balsam, Peruvian balsam, Indian balsam, black balsam, balsam Peru

BOTANY: Peru balsam is a large tree that grows 50 to 75 feet in height in Central America. It is often cultivated as a shade tree.[1] Crude Peru balsam is a dark brown, thick liquid with an aromatic smell of cinnamon and vanilla and bitter taste.[2,3] To remove it from the tree, the bark is alternately scorched and beaten. The balsam in the bark is obtained by boiling. Following removal of strips of bark from the tree, the exposed wood also secretes balsam. The material is soaked up by rags wrapped around the tree, which are then boiled in water. The balsam sinks to the bottom and is collected. Approximately two pounds is the annual yield per tree.

HISTORY: The drug was first imported from Spain through Peruvian ports, from which the material derives its name.[3] Peru balsam has been used for the treatment of topical wounds and infections and as a flavoring in the food industry. Indians used the material to stop bleeding and to promote wound healing. They also used the material as a diuretic and to expel worms.[1] Today, the material is in a number of pharmaceutical preparations and plays an important role in perfumery. The material has no use as an internal medication.

CHEMISTRY: The balsam contains 50% to 65% of a volatile oil called cinnamein along with about 25% resin. The volatile oil contains primarily benzyl cinnamate and benzoic and cinnamic acid esters, with small amounts of benzyl alcohol and related compounds. In addition, traces of styrene, vanillin and coumarin have been identified in the material. Oil distilled from the wood is about 70% nerolidol.[4] Considerable variations exist in the balsam based on the source of the material.[3]

PHARMACOLOGY: Peru balsam has mild antiseptic properties and is said to promote the growth of skin cells.[2] The balsam has been used in dentistry in the treatment of dry socket (postextraction alveolitis) and as a component of dental impression material. Topically it is included in preparations for the treatment of wounds and ulcers.[2] It was formerly used widely as a treatment for scabies, and it has been used in suppositories for hemorrhoids.[6]

TOXICOLOGY: Peru balsam is a contact allergen and contact dermatitis occurs frequently with the product. Systemic toxicity following application of Peru balsam to nipples of nursing mothers has been described.[5]

SUMMARY: Although Peru balsam is not used widely in American medicine, its use persists in topical applications and as a food flavoring. Its topical use is somewhat limited by contact dermatitis that occurs frequently with the product.

PATIENT INFORMATION – Peru Balsam

Uses: Peru balsam has been used in the treatment of dry socket, topically as a treatment of wounds and ulcers, and in suppositories for hemorrhoids.

Side Effects: Peru balsam may cause contact dermatitis.

---

[1] Dobelis IN, ed. Magic and Medicine of Plants. Pleasantville, NY: Reader's Digest Association, 1986.
[2] Leung AY. Encyclopedia of Common Natural Ingredients Used in Food, Drugs, and Cosmetics. New York, NY: J. Wiley and Sons, 1980.
[3] Evans WC. Trease and Evans' Pharmacognosy, ed. 13. London, England: Bailliere Tindall, 1989.

[4] Morton JF. Major Medicinal Plants. Springfield, IL: C.C. Thomas, 1977.
[5] Duke JA. Handbook of Medicinal Herbs. Boca Raton, FL: CRC Press, 1985.
[6] Osol A, Farrar GE Jr., eds. 25th ed. The Dispensatory of the United States of America. Philadelphia, PA: J.B. Lippincott, 1955:1023.

Pineapple

SCIENTIFIC NAME(S): *Ananas comosus* (L.) Merr. Family: Bromeliaceae

COMMON NAME(S): Pineapple

BOTANY: The plant grows to heights of 2 to 4 feet. The well-known fruit of the pineapple is actually a complex flowerhead that forms around the stem. The pineapple is the only cultivated fruit whose main stem runs completely through it.[1] Each of the eyes on the surface is the dried base of a small flower. The top crown of leaves contains a bud, which when mature, indicates the fruit is ready for cutting. Pineapples contain no seeds but are grown from their crowns.

HISTORY: Pineapples originated in South America and likely did not reach Hawaii until the 19th century.[2] Europeans spread the plant throughout much of the world. Because of rising labor costs, today the bulk of pineapple production no longer occurs in Hawaii, but in regions of South America and the Philippines.[1] The pineapple is cultivated for use as a fruit from which juices, syrups and candies are prepared.[3] The plant has a long history in traditional tropical medicine for the treatment of ailments ranging from constipation to jaundice.[3]

CHEMISTRY: The fruit is rich in citric acid, with some cultivars exceeding concentrations of 8%.[3] Malic acid also is found in significant quantities.[1] The ascorbic acid content also varies with the cultivar, but is generally in the low range.[1] The essential oil is rich in a variety of aromatic compounds. A steroidal component of the leaves possesses estrogenic activity.[3] The residue left after juice extraction is rich in vitamin A and is used as a component of livestock feed.

This residue, along with the juice and entire plant, also is used as a commercial source of the proteolytic enzyme bromelain. At least four proteolytic enzymes have been identified in pineapple, the most well studied of which is bromelain.[4] Bromelain is a mixture of protease and is used as a meat tenderizer, in the food and beverage industries, and has been used to treat edema and inflammation.[3] Slight differences in the composition of "stem" and "fruit" bromelain have been reported,[5] and the amino acid sequence has been identified.[6] Although products containing bromelain are available as nutritional supplements, therapeutic products are no longer available to the medical profession because the efficacy of these treatments could not be substantiated by well-designed trials.

PHARMACOLOGY: An antiedemic (diuretic) substance has been reported to be present in the rhizome, and the ripe fruit is said to have diuretic activity.[3] The juice from unripe pineapples can act as a violent purgative.[3]

Bromelain is a proteolytic enzyme that has been used to tenderize meat. Bromelain is absorbed unchanged from the intestine at a rate of about 40%. The product has been used for burn debridement and to reduce soft tissue inflammation and irritation. It also has been used to prevent ulcers and to enhance fat excretion as a component of some fad diets, but these effects have not been well substantiated.[3] The pharmacologic effects of bromelain are caused by an enhancement of serum fibrinolytic activity and inhibition of fibrinogen synthesis, as well as by direct degradation of fibrin and fibrinogen. Bromelain lowers kininogen and bradykinin serum tissue levels and has an influence on prostaglandin synthesis.[7] Topical application of pineapple-derived enzymes has been shown to enhance wound healing in animal models.[8] Bromelain is reported to have nematicidal activity.[3]

Ingestion of pineapple has been shown to result in the inhibition of endogenous nitrosation in human volunteers, suggesting that the ascorbic acid content of the fruit can limit the formation of potentially toxic digestive by-products.[9] Pineapple juice limits the mutagenic activity of carcinogens in the Ames' Salmonella/microsome assay test by approximately 50%.[10]

TOXICOLOGY: Repeated exposure of pineapple cutters to bromelain can result in the obliteration of fingerprints,[3] and the hooked margins of the leaves can cause painful injury. Ethyl acrylate, an aromatic component of the juice can produce dermal sensitization.

Angular stomatitis can result from eating large amounts of the fruit.[3] Large quantities of the juice have been reported to cause uterine contractions.

Bromelain ingestion has been associated with nausea, vomiting, diarrhea, skin rash and menorrhagia.[3]

SUMMARY: The pineapple is a widely cultivated fruit. It is the source of the proteolytic enzyme bromelain, which is used in commercial meat tenderizers, and which continues to be used in medical practice as a soft tissue anti-inflammatory and for topical debridement.

PATIENT INFORMATION – Pineapple

Uses: Pineapple has been used to prevent ulcers, enhance fat excretion, burn débridement, and to reduce soft tissue inflammation and irritation.

Side Effects: Pineapple extracts may produce dermal sensitization, uterine contractions, nausea, vomiting, diarrhea, skin rash, and menorrhagia.

---

[1] Morton JF. Major Medicinal Plants. Springfield, IL: C.C. Thomas, 1977.

[2] Dobelis IN, ed. Magic and Medicine of Plants. Pleasantville, NY: Readers Digest Association, Inc., 1986.

[3] Duke JA. Handbook of Medicinal Herbs. Boca Raton, FL: CRC Press, 1985.

[4] Rowan AD, et al. The cysteine proteinases of the pineapple plant. *Biochem J* 1990;266(3):869.

[5] Leung AY. Encyclopedia of Common Natural Ingredients Used in Food, Drugs, and Cosmetics. New York, NY: John Wiley & Sons, Inc., 1980.

[6] Lenarcic B, et al. Characterization and structure of pineapple stem inhibitor of cysteine proteinases. *Biol Chem Hoppe Seyler* 1992;373(7):459.

[7] Lotz-Winter H. On the pharmacology of bromelain: an update with special regard to animal studies on dose-dependent effects. *Planta Med* 1990;56:249.

[8] Rowan AD, et al. Debridement of experimental full-thickness skin burns of rats with enzyme fractions derived from pineapple stem. *Burns* 1990;16(4):243.

[9] Helser MA, et al. Influence of fruit and vegetable juices on the endogenous formation of N-nitrosoproline and N-nitrosthiozolidine-4-carboxylic acid in humans on controlled diets. *Carcinogenesis* 1992;13(12):2277.

[10] Edenharder R, et al. Antimutagenic activity of vegetable and fruit extracts against in vitro benzo(A)-pyrene. *Z Gesamte Hyg* 1990;36(3):144.

Plantain

SCIENTIFIC NAME(S): *Plantago lanceolata* L., P. major L., *P. psyllium* L., *P. arenaria* Waldst. & Kit. (*P. ramosa* Asch.) (Spanish or French psyllium seed), *P. ovata* Forsk. (Blond or Indian plantago seed) Family: Plantaginaceae. (Not to be confused with *Musa paradisiacae*, or edible plantain.)

COMMON NAME(S): Plantain, Spanish psyllium, French psyllium, blond plantago, Indian plantago, psyllium seed, flea seed, black psyllium.

BOTANY: Plantain is a perennial weed with almost worldwide distribution. There are about 250 species, of which 20 have wide geographic ranges, 9 have discontinuous ranges, 200 are limited to one region, and 9 have very narrow ranges. *P. lanceolata* and *P. major* are among the widest distributed.[1] Plantain species are herbs and shrubby plants characterized by basal leaves and inconspicuous flowers in heads or spikes. They grow aggressively. Plantain is wind-pollinated, facilitating its growth where there are no bees and few other plantain plants. It is very tolerant of viral infections. *P. major* produces 13,000 to 15,000 seeds per plant, and the seeds have been reported to remain viable in soil for up to 60 years. *P. lanceolata* produces 2500 to 10,000 seeds per plant and has a somewhat shorter seed viability. Plantain seeds can survive passage through the gut of birds and other animals, facilitating their distribution further.[1] Plantain, or psyllium seeds, are small (1.5 to 3.5 mm), oval, boat-shaped, dark reddish-brown, odorless and nearly tasteless. They are coated with mucilage, which aids in their transportation by allowing adhesion to various surfaces.[1,2]

HISTORY: Plantain has long been associated with man and with agriculture. Certain species have been spread by human colonization, particularly that of Europeans. As such, North American Indians and New Zealand Maori refer to plantain as "Englishman's foot," because it spread from areas of English settlement. *P. lanceolata* and *P. major* have been used in herbal remedies and were sometimes carried to colonies intentionally for that purpose. Psyllium seed has been found in malt refuse (formerly used as fertilizer) and wool imported to England. It has been commonly used in birdseed.[1] Pulverized seeds are mixed with oil and applied topically to inflamed sites; decoctions have been mixed with honey for sore throats. The seeds and refined colloid are used commonly in commercial bulk laxative preparations.[1,3]

CHEMISTRY: Plaintain constituents include acids (eg, benzoic, caffeic, chlorogenic, cinnamic, p-coumaric, fumaric, salicylic, ursolic, vanillic, ascorbic), alkaloids (boschniakine) and amino acids (eg, alanine, asparagine, histidine, lysine).[4] An analysis of 8 of 21 Egyptian species of plantain, including *P. major*, has identified a variety of sugar and polysaccharide components of the seed mucilage. These include galactose, glucose, xylose, arabinose, and rhamnose. In addition, galacturonic acid, planteose, plantiobiose, sucrose, fructose, and an unidentified sugar (in *P. ovata*) have been identified.[5] Other plant carbohydrates such as saccharose, stachyose, sorbitol and tyrosol have also been reported.[4] The mucilage of the seed's testa epidermis constitutes 20% to 30%.[2] Seed mucilage of one species, *P. ovata* was found to have better suspending and emulsifying power compared to tragacanth and methylcellulose.[6] Leaf mucilage has been reported as well and includes such polysaccharides as rhamnose, L-arabinose, mannose, galactose and dextrose.[7] The seeds also contain fixed oil, protein, iridoids and tannins.[2,3] The gel-forming fraction of the seed was found to be effective in prolonging release rates of tetracycline in vitro.[8]

Flavonoids found in plantain include apigenin, baicalein, scutellarein and others.[4] Isolation and identification of flavonoids and saponins from related species *P. tomentosa* have been reported.[9]

Iridoids found in plantain are aucubin, plantarenaloside and aucuboside.[4] The main iridoids (eg, aucubin) and catalpol, have been isolated from *P. lanceolata*, *P. major* and *P. media* leaves using HPLC analysis.[10] Iridoid glycosides and phenolic acids have been found in leaf extracts of *P. lanceolata* and *P. media*.[11]

Other components of the plant include choline, fat, resin, steroids and vitamins.[3,4]

Reports on related species *P. asiatica* list constituents as: A "new" phenylethanoid glycoside,[12] aucubin,[13] plantaginin and plantamajoside.[14]

PHARMACOLOGY: The pharmacology of plantain involves gastrointestinal tract therapy, hyperlipidemia treatment, anticancer effects, respiratory and other actions.

GI: Psyllium seed is classified as a bulk laxative. Mixed with water, it produces a mucilaginous mass. The indigestible seeds provide bulk for treatment of chronic constipation, while the mucilage serves as a mild laxative comparable to agar or mineral oil. The usual dose is 0.5 to 2 g of husk (5 to 15 g of seeds) mixed in 8 oz of water. A study of 10 healthy volunteers examined the effects of a 3 g ispaghula mixture (dried psyllium seed husks) given three times daily. It decreased intestinal transit time.[15] Effectiveness of psyllium seed on 78 subjects with irritable bowel syndrome (IBS) has been reported.[16] *P. ovata* fiber is also effective in regulating colon motility in a similar set of patients.[17] A postcholecystectomy patient with chronic diarrhea was given a 6.5 g dose of a 50% psyllium preparation, and symptoms resolved in 2 days.[18,19] Plantago seed as a cellulose/pectin mixture was as effective as a bulk laxative in 50 adult subjects.[20] The effects of different dietary fibers on colonic function, including plantago seed have been evaluated.[21] Gastroprotective action from plantago extract (polyholozidic substances) has also been reported.[22]

In a triple-blind, crossover study of 17 female patients, *P. ovata* seed preparation was investigated on appetite variables. The preparation was deemed useful in weight control diets where a feeling of fullness was desired. Total fat intake was also decreased, again, suggesting the product to be a beneficial weight control diet supplement.[23]

A trial involving 393 patients with anal fissures found conservative treatment with psyllium effective. After 5 years of follow-up, 44% of the patients were cured without surgery within 4 to 8 weeks. There were complications (abscesses and fistulas requiring surgery) in 8% of the cases. The recurrence rate was 27%, but about one third of these were fistulas that responded to further conservative management.[24]

A double-blind study of 51 patients with symptomatic hemorrhoids showed *Vi-Siblin*, a psyllium-containing preparation, to be effective in reducing bleeding and pain during defecation: 84% of the patients receiving the preparation reported improvement or elimination of symptoms, compared to 52% taking placebo.[25]

Hyperlipidemia: Many reports on psyllium have concluded that it can be helpful in treating various hyperlipidemias.[26,27]

In animal studies, plantain lowered total plasma lipids, cholesterol and triglycerides in arteriosclerotic rabbits.[4] Other animals may be less sensitive to psyllium's hypocholesterolemic actions.[28]

Attention has been focused on the cholesterol-lowering effects of psyllium preparations in human trials. Psyllium hydrophilic mucilloid (*Metamucil*, Procter & Gamble) was found to lower serum cholesterol in a study of 28 patients who took 3 doses (3.4 g/dose) per day compared with placebo for 8 weeks. After 4 weeks, the psyllium-treated patients showed decreases in total serum cholesterol levels compared with the placebo group. Decreases were also seen in LDL cholesterol and the LDL/HDL ratio. At the end of 8 weeks, values for total cholesterol, LDL cholesterol and the LDL/HDL ratio were 14%, 20% and 15%, respectively below baseline (all, $p < 0.01$). This study suggested that high cholesterol levels could be managed safely and easily by including psyllium preparations in the diet.[29]

Similar results of cholesterol reduction have been reported, including: Psyllium colloid administration for 2 to 29 months, reducing cholesterol levels by 16.9% and triglycerides by 52%,[30] a trial of 75 hypercholesterolemic patients, evaluating adjunct therapy of psyllium seed to a low cholesterol diet,[31] a 16–week, double-blind trial, proving plantago seed improved in both total and LDL cholesterol in 37 patients,[32] and increased tolerance of psyllium seed in combination with colestipol (rather than monotherapy alone) in 105 hyperlipidemic patients.[33]

Psyllium seed was found to be more effective than *P. ovata* husk in reducing serum cholesterol in normal and ileostomy patients.[34] A report on 20 hypercholesterolemic pediatric patients on low-fat diets, however, found psyllium seed to be ineffective in lowering cholesterol or LDL levels.[35]

Issues of cereal companies including plantago seed in their products and claims of "cholesterol reduction," have been addressed.[36]

A polyphenolic compound (from *P. major* leaves) was found to exhibit hypocholesterolemic activity,[37] but in addition, the mechanism by which plantago reduces cholesterol may also include enhancement of cholesterol elimination as fecal bile acids.[38]

Anticancer: The antitumor effects of plantain have been studied in animals. The isolate "plantagoside," from seeds of related species *P. asiatica*, has been found to suppress immune response in mouse tissue.[39] *P. major* has also inhibited carcinogen synthesis in induced toxic liver damage and has decreased tumor incidence in rats.[40] In mice given *P. major* subcutaneous injections, mammary cancer tumor formation frequency was 18%, as compared to 93% with placebo, suggesting prophylactic therapy for cancer of this type.[41] Immunotropic activity of *P. lan-*

ceolata extract on murine and human lymphatic cells in vivo and in vitro has also been demonstrated.[42]

Respiratory: An aqueous extract of plantain may possess bronchodilatory activity in guinea pigs; however, it is less active and of shorter duration than salbutamol or atropine.[4] In human studies, plantain has been effective for chronic bronchitis,[4] asthma, cough and cold.[3]

Other actions: A report by a physician described the topical use of crushed plantain leaves to treat poison ivy in 10 people. Although the trial was not conducted scientifically, the treatment eliminated itching and prevented spread of the dermatitis in all cases, one to four applications being required.[43] Fresh leaves of the plant have been poulticed onto herpes, sores, ulcers, boils and infections. Plantain has been used for insect bites and gout.[3] Leaf extracts have wound healing activity in rabbits, caused by chlorogenic and neochlorogenic acid content.[4]

Plantain oils may exhibit therapeutic action on chemical burns of rabbit eyes.[44]

Aqueous extracts of plantain leaves possess antimicrobial activity caused by aglycone and aucubigenin.[2]

Aerial parts of plantago have been used as an anti-inflammatory and as a diuretic in folk medicine.[45] A report on *P. lanceolata*'s phenylethanoids, acteoside and plantamajoside has been evaluated for inhibitory effects on arachidonic acid-induced mouse ear edema.[46] Plantain extract has decreased arterial blood pressure by 20 to 40 mm Hg in normotensive dogs.[4] Reports such as these and others may help support plantain's use in folk medicine.

Psyllium administration had no effect on postprandial plasma glucose in one report.[47]

TOXICOLOGY: Plantain pollen has been found to contain at least 16 antigens, of which 6 are potentially allergenic. The pollen contains allergenic glycoproteins that react with concanavalin A, as well as components that bind IgE.[48] Antigenic and allergenic analysis has been performed on psyllium seed. All three fractions, husk, endosperm and embryo, contained similar antigens.[49] Formation of IgE antibodies to psyllium laxative has been demonstrated.[50] In addition, IgE-mediated sensitization to plantain pollen has been performed, contributing to seasonal allergy.[51]

There are many reported incidences of varying degrees of psyllium allergy including: Nurses experiencing symptoms such as anaphylactoid reaction, chest congestion, sneezing and watery eyes (some of these reactions taking several years to acquire);[52,53] a case report describing severe anaphylactic shock following psyllium laxative ingestion, linked occupational respiratory allergies in pharmaceutical workers exposed to the substance;[54] consumption of plantago seed in cereal, responsible for anaphylaxis in a 60–year-old female (immunoglobulin E-mediated sensitization was documented, and patient was successfully treated with oral diphenhydramine);[55] and a report on workers in a psyllium processing plant evaluated for occupational asthma and IgE sensitization to psyllium.[56]

Another unusual adverse situation involves the occurrence of a giant phytobezoar composed of psyllium seed husks. The bezoar, located in the right colon, resulted in complete blockage of gastric emptying.[57] All psyllium preparations must be taken with adequate volumes of fluid. The seeds contain a pigment that may be toxic to the kidneys,[14] but this has been removed from most commercial preparations.[58]

Drug interactions reported with psyllium involve lithium and carbamazepine. Psyllium may inhibit absorption of lithium in the GI tract, decreasing blood levels of the lithium, as seen in a 47–year-old woman with schizoaffective disorder.[59] Plantago seed also has decreased the bioavailability of carbamazepine in 4 male subjects.[60]

Economic significance: As a weed, plantain is important because of its competition with commercial crops and small fruits. The presence of plantain seeds can make adequate cleaning of crop seed difficult, especially with small-seed legumes. Plantain, because of its tolerance of viral infection, can serve as a reservoir for economically important infections of crops including beets, potatoes, tomatoes, tobacco, turnips, cucumbers and celery. Commercially, plantain is grown for use in forage mixtures and, primarily, for use in bulk laxatives.[1]

SUMMARY: Plantain is an aggressive weed found almost worldwide. It can have negative agricultural effects by competing with crops, contaminating crop seeds, and serving as a reservoir for viral plant diseases. Medicinally, the plant is used in bulk laxatives for GI tract health, hyperlipidemia treatment, anticancer effects, respiratory actions, infections and edema. There are many antigenic components in the seed and the pollen; these may affect sensitive individuals. Drug interactions of psyllium with lithium and carbamazepine have been reported.

PATIENT INFORMATION – Plantain

Uses: The psyllium in plantain has been used as GI therapy, to treat hyperlipidemia, as a topical agent to treat some skin problems, as an anti-inflammatory and diuretic, for anticancer effects, and for respiratory treatment.

Side Effects: Adverse events include anaphylaxis, chest congestion, sneezing and watery eyes, occupational asthma, and a situation involving the occurence of a giant phytobezoar composed of psyllium seed husks.

Drug Interactions: Plantain may interact with lithium and carbamazepine, decreasing their plasma concentrations.

[1] Hammond J. *Adv Vir Res* 1982;27:103.

[2] Bisset N. Herbal Drugs and Phytopharmaceuticals. Stuttgart, Germany: CRC Press, Inc. 1994;378–83.

[3] Duke J. CRC Handbook of Medicinal Herbs. Boca Raton, FL: CRC Press, Inc. 1989;386.

[4] Newall C, et al. Herbal Medicines. London, England: Pharmaceutical Press. 1996;210–11.

[5] Ahmed ZF, et al. *J Pharm Sci* 1965;7:1060.

[6] Khanna M, et al. *Ind J Pharm Sci* 1988 Jul-Aug;50:238–40.

[7] Brautigam M, et al. *Dtsch Apoth Zeit* 1985 Jan 10;125:58–62.

[8] Singla A, et al. *Ind J Hosp Pharm* 1990 Jan-Feb;27:29–33.

[9] Jorge L, et al. *Rev Bras Farm* 1994 Jan-Mar;75:10–12.

[10] Long C, et al. *J Pharm Belg* 1995 Nov-Dec;50:484–88.

[11] Swiatek L. *Herba Polonica* 1977;23(3):201–9.

[12] Nishibe S, et al. *Phytochemistry* 1995;38(3):741–43.

[13] Guo Y, et al. *Chung Kuo Chung Yao Tsa Chih* 1991;16(12):743–44.

[14] Kamoda Y, et al. *Tokyo Ika Shika Daigaku Iyo Kizai Kenkyusho Hokoku* 1989;23:81–85.

[15] Connaughton J, McCarthy CF. *Ir Med J* 1982;75:93.

[16] Arthurs Y, Fielding JF. *Ir Med J* 1983;76:253.

[17] Soifer L, et al. *Acta Gastroenterol Latinoam* 1987;17(4):317–23.

[18] Dorworth T, et al. *ASHP Annual Meeting* 1989 Jun;46:P-57D.

[19] Strommen G, et al. *Clin Pharm* 1990 Mar;9:206–8.

[20] Spiller G, et al. *J Clin Pharmacol* 1979 May-Jun;19:313–20.

[21] Spiller R. *Pharmacol Ther* 1994;62(3):407–27.

[22] Hriscu A, et al. *Rev Med Chir Soc Med Nat Iasi* 1990;94(1):165–70.

[23] Turnbull W, et al. *Int J Obes Rel Metab Dis* 1995;19(5):338–42.

[24] Shub HA, et al. *Dis Colon Rectum* 1978;21:582.

[25] Moesgaard F, et al. *Dis Colon Rectum* 1982;25:454.

[26] Generali J. *US Pharmacist* 1989 Feb;14:16, 20–21.

[27] Chan E, et al. *Ann Pharmacother* 1995 Jun;29:625–27.

[28] Day C. *Artery* 1991;18(3):163–67.

[29] Anderson J, et al. *Arch Int Med* 1988 Feb;148:292–96.

[30] Danielsson A, et al. *Acta Hepatogastroenterol* 1979;26:148.

[31] Bell L, et al. *JAMA* 1989 Jun 16;261:3419–23.

[32] Sprecher D, et al. *Ann Int Med* 1993 Oct 1;119:545–54.

[33] Spence J, et al. *Ann Intern Med* 1995 Oct 1;123:493–99.

[34] Gelissen I, et al. *Am J Clin Nutr* 1994;59(2):395–400.

[35] Dennison B, et al. *J Pediatr* 1993 Jul;123:24–29.

[36] Gannon K. *Drug Topics* 1989 Oct 2;133:24.

[37] Maksyutina N, et al. *Farmat Zhurnal* 1978;33(4):56–61.

[38] Miettinen T, et al. *Clin Chim Acta* 1989;183(3):253–62.

[39] Yamada H, et al. *Biochem Biophys Res Comm* 1989;165(3):1292–98.

[40] Karpilovskaia E, et al. *Farmakol Toksikol* 1989;52(4):64–67.

[41] Lithander A. *Tumour Biol* 1992;13(3):138–41.

[42] Strzelecka H, et al. *Herba Polonica* 1995;41(1):23–32.

[43] Duckett S. *N Engl J Med* 1980;303:583.

[44] Nikulin A, et al. *Eksp Klin Farmakol* 1992;55(4):64–66.

[45] Tosun F. *Hacettepe U Eczacilik Fakultesi Dergisi* 1995;15(1):23–32.

[46] Murai M, et al. *Plant Med* 1995;61(5):479–80.

[47] Frape D, et al. *Brit J Nutr* 1995;73(5):733–51.

[48] Baldo BA, et al. *Int Arch Allergy Appl Immunol* 1982;68:295.

[49] Arlian L, et al. *J Allergy Clin Immunol* 1992;89(4):866–76.

[50] Rosenberg S, et al. *Ann Allergy* 1982;48:294.

[51] Mehta V, et al. *Int Arch Allergy Appl Immunol* 1991;96(3):211–17.

[52] Wray M. ASHP Midyear Clinical Meeting. 1989 Dec;24:P-90D.

[53] Ford M, et al. *Hosp Pharm* 1992 Dec;27:1061–62.

[54] Suhonen R, et al. *Allergy* 1983;38:363.

[55] Lantner R, et al. *JAMA* 1990;264:2534–36.

[56] Bardy J, et al. *Am Rev Respir Dis* 1987;135(5):1033–38.

[57] Agha FP, et al. *Am J Gastroenterol* 1984;79:319.

[58] Morton JF. Major Medicinal Plants. Springfield IL: C.C. Thomas, 1977.

[59] Perlman B. *Lancet* 1990 Feb 17;335:416.

[60] Etman M. *Drug Devel Indus Pharm* 1995;21(16):1901–6.

Podophyllum

SCIENTIFIC NAME(S): *Podophyllum peltatum* L., *P. hexandrum* Royle syn *P. emodi* Wall. Family: Podophyllaceae (formerly Berberidaceae)

COMMON NAME(S): Mayapple, mandrake, American podophyllum (*P. peltatum*), Indian podophyllum *P. hexandrum*). Other common names include wild or American mandrake, devil's apple, vegetable mercury and duck's foot. The plant should not be confused with the European mandrake (*Mandragora officinarum* L.) which contains the anticholinergics hyoscyamine, scopolamine and mandragorine.

BOTANY: A perennial plant with one or two large lobed leaves that grows in moist shaded areas throughout North America, *P. hexandrum* is found primarily in Tibet and Afghanistan.[1] A single white or cream-colored flower grows between the two leaves from May to August It bears a fruity berry that turns yellow when ripe.

HISTORY: Podophyllum resin was used by the American Indians and colonists as a cathartic and anthelmintic, as an antidote for snake bites and as a poison.[2] Podophyllum was a common ingredient in many proprietary medicines including Carter's Little Liver Pills.[1] It has been used for almost 40 years in the treatment of topical warts, especially condylomata. The resin had long been thought to possess anticancer activity; derivatives have been used successfully in controlled clinical trials. An FDA advisory panel has established that because of its drastic effect and great potential for toxicity, podophyllum resin is not considered a safe laxative.[3]

CHEMISTRY: Podophyllum resin is obtained from the dried roots and rhizomes of the plant. The major active constituents of podophyllum are the lignan derivatives, which occur in free or glycosidic form in the resin.[1] The resin constitutes 3% to 6% of *P. peltatum* and up to 12% of *P. hexandrum*. The resin is a mixture of more than a dozen compounds, including podophyllotoxin, picropodophyllum and podophyllic acid. Alpha- and beta-peltatin are the major lignans in American podophyllum.[4] Podophyllum tincture is often combined with benzoin for topical use.

PHARMACOLOGY: Podophyllum resin is a drastic cathartic used as a veterinary and human purgative. Its effects are believed to be due to colonic irritation attributed to the peltatins.[5] The activity depends on the presence of a lactone ring in the *trans* configuration.

Podophyllum is highly lipid soluble and is readily absorbed through the gastrointestinal tract. Topical administration to large areas can also result in significant absorption. Little is known about the distribution of the active compounds. A podophyllic acid preparation was eliminated predominantly in the urine with a half-life of 30 minutes; podophyllotoxin is eliminated in the bile with a half-life of 48 hours.[6]

Podophyllin acts as a spindle poison, blocking cell division in metaphase. It has a direct effect on mitochondria, reducing the activity of cytochrome oxidase and succinoxidase. Several components of podophyllin have tumor-inhibiting properties including the peltatins, podophyllotoxin and its derivatives. Several semisynthetic analogs have been investigated clinically.[7] Teniposide and etoposide are active orally and parenterally.[8] Etoposide is available commercially (*VP-16, VePesid* / Bristol-Myers Oncology) for the parenteral treatment of refractory testicular tumors and for the treatment of small cell cancers of the lung.[9,10] Teniposide is available under a treatment IND for use with cytarabine in the management of patients with acute lymphoblastic leukemia; it has also been used for a variety of lymphomas and other neoplastic diseases.[10]

The resin is used in the treatment of warts, especially condyloma. Alcoholic solutions (10% to 20%) of *P. peltatum* were as effective as those of *P. hexandrum* in the treatment of genital warts.[11] A topical solution of podophyllotoxin 0.5% twice daily for 3 days was more effective than repeated applications of topical podophyllin 20% ethanolic solution for the treatment of penile warts.[12] The use of these preparations should be restricted because of the potential for systemic toxicity from misapplication.[13] When used, the solutions should be washed off within 1 to 4 hours, and contact should not exceed more than 6 hours. Podophyllum ointment has been associated with severe toxicity.[13] There are several commercial preparations of podophyllum resin, generally as 25% solutions in tincture of benzoin for topical use.[10] There is also a purified topical product available for external genital warts, *Condylox* by Oclassen.[10]

A mixture of semisynthetic lignan glycosides termed CPH82 has been found to be more effective than placebo when given to patients with rheumatoid arthritis in ameliorating clinical and immunological variables.[14]

TOXICOLOGY: The ripe fruit pulp of the mayapple is edible, often being made into marmalades or jellies.[5] Podophyllin is potentially lethal when ingested. Great care must be taken in its external use. Chronic use of podophyllum resin as a cathartic has resulted in hypokalemia sometimes associated with metabolic alkalosis.[15] At least 3 deaths have been attributed to either oral ingestion or topical application.[16,17] Podophyllum toxicity is multisystemic with characteristic neurologic manifestations. Clinical signs appear within 12 hours and include altered mental states, tachypnea, peripheral neuropathy, nausea, hypotension, vomiting, and fever. Rapidly progressive neurologic deficit varying from confusion to coma is always observed. Muscle paralysis with respiratory failure, renal failure, hallucinations, and seizures have been reported. Bone marrow suppression has been noted in acute intoxication and in chronic laxative abusers.

Seven cases of podophyllin toxicity have resulted in severe peripheral neuropathies, from topical or oral administration. The onset of the neuropathies generally occurred within hours of application or ingestion and the duration ranged from months up to four years with some neurologic deficit still present. Exact doses that were used, as well as how long they were left in contact with the treated area are often not given.[18-24]

Emesis may be useful during the initial phases of toxicity.[25] Topically administered resin should be removed with petroleum jelly. Podophyllum is lipid soluble; hemodialysis is ineffective, while charcoal hemoperfusion has reversed acute symptoms within hours.[18]

Podophyllum is teratogenic in animals and humans. Limb deformities and septal heart defects have been associated with its ingestion by pregnant women.[26] Preauricular skin tags and a simian crease were noted in an infant born to a woman treated with topical podophyllum resin from the 23rd to 29th week of pregnancy. Total contact with the drug was 4 hours.[27] An intrauterine death has been reported in a woman treated with podophyllum for vulvar warts during week 32 of her pregnancy.[24]

SUMMARY: Podophyllum and its extracts have been used internally as drastic cathartics and externally in the treatment of venereal warts. Semisynthetic plant derivatives are used to manage a variety of neoplastic disorders. The resin is a mitotic poison, and its misuse can lead to significant toxicity. It should not be administered to children, and use in pregnant women has been associated with congenital abnormalities and fetal death.

PATIENT INFORMATION – Podophyllum

Uses: Podophyllum has been used to treat refractory testicular tumors, small cancer cells of the lung, a variety of lymphomas and other neoplastic diseases, warts, genital warts, and rheumatoid arthritis.

Side Effects: Podophyllm has resulted in hypokalemia, altered mental states, tachypnea, peripheral neuropathy, nausea, hypotension, vomiting, fever, and muscle paralysis with respiratory failure.

---

[1] Graham NA, Chandler RF. *Can Pharm J* 1990;123(7):330.
[2] Kelly ME, Hartwell JL. *J Nat Cancer Inst* 1954;14:967.
[3] Rosenstein G, et al. *Pediatrics* 1976;57:419.
[4] Jackson DE, Dewick PM. *J Pharm Pharmacol* 1982;(suppl):15P.
[5] Morton JF. Major Medicinal Plants. Springfield, IL: CC Thomas, 1977.
[6] Cassidy DE, et al. *J Toxicol Clin Toxicol* 1982;19(1):35.
[7] Canetta R, et al. *Cancer Chemother Pharmacol* 1982;7:93.
[8] Rozencweig M, et al. *Cancer* 1977;40:334.
[9] Abratt RP, Levin W. *Cancer Treat Rep* (letter) 1985;69(2):235.
[10] Olin BR, Hebel SK, eds. Drug Facts and Comparisons, St. Louis: Facts and Comparisons, 1991.
[11] von Krogh G. *Acta Dermatovener* 1978;58:163.
[12] Lassus A. *Lancet* (letter) 1987;2:512.
[13] White G, McFarlane A. *Australian Prescriber* 1990;13(2):36.
[14] Larsen A, et al. *Br J Rheumatol* 1989;28(2):124.
[15] Ramirez B, Marieb NJ. *Conn Med* 1970;34:169.
[16] Balucani M, Zellers DD. *JAMA* 1964 Aug 24;189:639.
[17] Ward JW, et al. *South Med J* 1954 Dec;47:1204.
[18] Slater GE, et al. *Obstet Gynecol* 1978;52(1):94.
[19] Clark ANG, Parsonage MJ. *Br Med J* 1957 Nov 16;4:1155.
[20] Campbell AN. *Lancet* 1980 Jan 26;1:206.
[21] Montaldi DH, et al. *Am J Obstet Gynecol* 1974 Aug 15;119:1130.
[22] Rate RG, et al. *Ann Intern Med* 1979;90:723.
[23] Moher LM, Maurer SA. *J Fam Pract* 1979;9:237.
[24] Chamberlain MJ, et al. *Br Med J* 1972;3:391.
[25] McFarland MF, McFarland J. *Clin Toxicol* 1981;18:973.
[26] Cullis JE. *Lancet* (letter) 1962;2:511.
[27] Karol MD, et al. *Clin Toxicol* 1980;16(3):283.

Poinsettia

SCIENTIFIC NAME(S): Varieties of *Euphorbia pulcherrima* Wild. ex Klotzsch Family: Euphorbiaceae. This plant has also been referred to as *E. poinsettia* Buist and *Poinsettia pulcherrima* Grah

COMMON NAME(S): Poinsettia, Christmas flower, Easter flower, papagallo, Mexican flame leaf, lobster flower plant

BOTANY: The Euphorbiaceae (spurge family) is a large family of more than 1000 herbs, shrubs, and trees. All members of this family are characterized by the presence of a milky latex emulsion found in lactiferous vessels. When damaged, the plants secrete this latex. The poinsettia is a perennial ornamental found throughout the warmer climates of the US, including Hawaii, and Mexico. The flowers are small and yellow; it is the showy red leaf (bract) that has resulted in the decorative popularity of this plant.

HISTORY: The plant was introduced from Mexico into the US by J. R. Poinsett in the early 1800s. Many members of the genus *Euphorbia* have been used in folk medicine. *E. pulcherrima* sap has been used as a depilatory, and extracts of the plant have been used as an antipyretic and to stimulate the flow of breast milk. The plant may have once been used as an abortifacient.[1] Folk uses include remedies for skin, warts and toothache.[3]

CHEMISTRY: The stems and leaves may contain small amounts of alkaloids; however, there is conflicting data regarding the presence of these compounds. The latex contains from 7% to 15% caoutchouc.[2] Compounds found in the leaves and stems include germanicol, beta-amyrin, pseudotaraxasterol, pulcherrol, octaeiccsanol, beta-sitosterol, rubber, caffeic acid and anthocyanin.[3] Epigermanicyl acetate, germanicyl acetate, germanicol, octacosanol and beta-sitosterol from poinsettia fruits have also been isolated.[4]

PHARMACOLOGY: Because this plant has often been associated with potential toxicity, a number of investigations have tried to establish the pharmacology of its components.

In rats fed 15 g/kg bracts or 5 g/kg leaf blades for 1 week, no change in behavior, body weight or adrenal weight was found.[5]

An increase in thyroid weight was observed among rats fed 15 g/kg of leaf material. No other pharmacologic activity was observed. Extracts of the plant have no antibiotic activity.[1]

The plant's latex has been used as a **depilatory**. Other reported uses include **pain relief**, **antibacterial**, and **emetic**. The latex contains 5% to 15% caoutchouc and some resin.[3]

TOXICOLOGY: Many published reports have warned of the toxicity of this plant; however, there appears to be little factual evidence for this claim. These reports seem to stem from a single case of death in a 2-year-old Hawaiian child after the ingestion of the leaves.[6] This poorly documented case remains the only known fatality and several authors have concluded that the report was based more on hearsay than fact.[1]

The results of an acute and a 1-week feeding study in rats found no changes in most parameters evaluated.[5] No deaths were found among 160 rats fed up to 22.5 g/kg of poinsettia, suggesting that the plant lacks oral toxicity.[7] Winek et al published the results of perhaps the most comprehensive evaluation of the toxicity of poinsettia. No rats died during an attempt to establish the oral LD-50; therefore, the LD-50 was considered to be greater than 25 g/kg body weight. Assuming no interspecies variation in toxicity, a 50 lb child would have to ingest about 1.25 lbs (500 to 600 leaves) to surpass the experimental LD-50. Vomiting would most likely preclude the ingestion of this amount of plant.[1]

Oral administration of poinsettia extracts in rats did not result in local toxicity (no erythema, edema, bleeding of the oral cavity) and instillation of the latex into the rabbit eye induced no corneal, iridal or conjunctival damage. No histologic abnormalities were found in rats fed high doses of the plant for 5 days. Repeated exposure to a water suspension of the plant induced mild skin irritation in albino rabbits, but this disappeared within 36 hours. Some photosensitivity was seen in albino rabbits.[7]

In mice, the intraperitoneal injection of 3 g of leaf extract per 100 g body weight resulted in one death in six animals tested; extracts of flowers and bracts, however, caused no deaths indicating a general lack of acute systemic toxicity. No alkaloids or glycosides were found in the plant.[8]

The National Clearinghouse for Poison Control Centers reported 228 cases of human ingestion of poinsettia in 1973; of these, only 14 cases had symptoms, the most serious being nausea and vomiting. A case report describes symptoms of local mucosa irritation and GI tract distress in an 8-month-old female who had chewed a poinsettia leaf.[9]

Some reports suggest that the milky latex of the poinsettia, like that of some other members of the Euphorbiaceae family (eg, pencil plant), may result in skin irritation in susceptible individuals,[10] or eye inflammation and temporary blindness.[3,11] However, animal studies and the lack of repeated documentation of topical irritation in humans indicates that this problem may not be widespread.

Suggested treatment of ingestion includes gastric lavage or emesis followed by symptomatic treatment,[12] in addition to demulcents, intestinal astringents and gastric sedatives. Give fluids to prevent dehydration.[11]

SUMMARY: The poinsettia is a popular ornamental most frequently seen around Christmas. Despite a legacy of severe toxicity, there is little published evidence to suggest that any part of the plant poses a great toxicologic danger. As a general precaution, this plant should be kept out of the reach of children and pets. If ingestion occurs, vomiting can be induced and the patient should be monitored. It is unlikely that a lethal or even pharmacologic dose could be ingested by a human. Topical irritation may occur in sensitive individuals, although the likelihood of this appears to be small.

PATIENT INFORMATION – Poinsettia

Uses: Poinsettias are used as Christmas ornamentation; their latex for a dipilatory; and for other uses such as pain relief, antibacterial and emetic. Folk uses include remedies for skin, warts, and toothache.

Side Effects: There is little published evidence to suggest that the plant poses a great toxicologic danger; however, the following side effects have occurred: Nausea, vomiting, local mucosa irritation, GI tract distress, skin irritation, eye inflammation, and temporary blindness.

---

[1] Winek CL, et al. *Clin Toxicol* 1978;13:27.
[2] Dominguez X, et al. *J Pharm Sci* 1967;59:1184.
[3] Duke J. *Euphorbia Pulcherrima Wild* CRC Handbook of Medicinal Herbs, Boca Raton, FL: CRC Press Inc. 1989;163-64.
[4] Gupta D, et al. *J Nat Prod* 1983 Nov-Dec;46:937–38.
[5] Runyon R. *Clin Tox* 1980;16:167.
[6] Rock JF. *Hawaiian Forest Agric* 1920;17:61.
[7] Stone and Collins. *Toxicon* 1971;9:301.
[8] DerMarderosian A, et al. *J Toxicol and Env Health* 1976;1:939.
[9] Edwards N. *J Pediatr* 1983 Mar;120:404–5.
[10] D'Arcy WG. *Arch Derm* 1974;109:909.
[11] DerMarderosian A. Common Poisonous Plants in Natural Product Medicine, Philadelphia, PA: George F. Stickley Co. 1988;153.
[12] Hardin JW, et al. Human Poisoning from Native and Cultivated Plants, 2nd ed. Durham NC: Duke University Press, 1974.

Poison Ivy

SCIENTIFIC NAME(S): *Tocicodendron diversilobum* (T & G); *T. quercifolium* (Michx.); *T. radicans* (L.) Kuntze; *T. vernix* (L.). Family: Anacardiaceae

COMMON NAME(S): Poison ivy; poison oak; poison sumac; markweed; poison elder; poison dogwood.

BOTANY: The contact sensitivities induced by poison ivy and several closely related species present a persistent public health problem. These dermatites affect from 50% to 70% of the general population.[1]

Poison ivy is a member of the sumac family (Anacardiaceae). Although originally classified as a member of the genus *Rhus*, it is now included in the genus *Toxicodendron*. Four related species are responsible for the majority of plant dermatites. These perennials are identified as:

T. diversilobum (T & G) Greene - Western poison oak

T. quercifolium (Michx.) Greene - Eastern poison oak

T. radicans (L.) Kuntze - Poison ivy, markweed, three-leaved ivy

T. vernix (L.) Kuntze - poison sumac, poison elder, poison dogwood

The nonpoisonous shrubby sumacs (*Rhus* spp.) also have long, pinnately divided leaves, but the flowers and fruits are in dense, terminal and erect clusters.[2]

T. diversilobum - The western poison oak is found along the Pacific coast from British Columbia to Mexico. It thrives in low places, thickets, and wooded slopes, usually below 5000 feet elevation. The 3-leaflet clusters are irregularly lobed and resemble oak leaves.

T. quercifolium - Eastern poison oak grows in the eastern and southern states from New Jersey to Missouri and North Florida. This erect, low, woody shrub is most frequently restricted to sandy soil, dry barrens and pine woods.

T. radicans - Poison ivy grows throughout the United States and Canada, with the exception of parts of the West Coast. The habit of this weed is extremely variable; it may grow as a nonclimbing woody shrub or as a vine along the ground, on low plants, or on high trees or poles. Only the presence of a cluster of 3 leaflets is a constant characteristic. The adage of "leaflets three, let it be; berries white, poison sight" remains a good rule of thumb.

The plant is odorless but has an acrid, slightly astringent taste.[3] The leaflets vary in color from green in spring to yellow and red in autumn. The waxy white to yellowish fruits may remain on the plant throughout the winter.

T. vernix - Poison sumac is native to bogs of the north (as a shrub) and to swamps and river bottoms of the south (as a small tree). Its distribution is widespread but is predominantly east of the Mississippi river. The 7- to 13-leaflet clusters are arranged in alternate pairs, with a single leaflet at the end of the midrib.

A major factor in poison plant dermatitis is the failure to recognize the plant. In general, all of the plants discussed here have 3-leaflet clusters (with the exception of poison sumac). They also have U- or V-shaped leaf scars (the scar remaining at the point that the leaf breaks from the stem), and flowers and fruits arising in the axillary position (in the angle between the leaf and the branch). Another helpful finding is a black deposit often present when *Toxicodendron* has been injured. Following trauma, the oleoresin exudes, darkens on exposure to air, and hardens. One source suggests crushing a few leaves of a suspected plant on a piece of white paper, releasing the sap from the petioles; the resulting stain will darken markedly within 10 minutes if it is from *Toxicodendron*. Although the test is not conclusive, it provides supportive evidence in making a positive identification.[4]

Other members of the family anacardiaceae include the tropical cashew nut tree (*Anacardium occidentale*), the tropical mango tree (*Mangifera indica*), the Indian marking nut tree (*Semecarpus anacardium*) and Japanese lacquer tree (*Rhus vernicifera*). Because of their chemically similar allergens, these also may cause allergic contact dermatitis in sensitive individuals.[5] For example, cashew ingestion has been associated with mouth blistering and perianal itching, if the antigens (cardol and anacardic acid) have not been properly removed.[6] Contact dermatitis can also result from mango ingestion without first removing the fruit skin, or from lacquer tree sap (from *Rhus* spp.) in furniture.[5]

CHEMISTRY: An oily phenolic resin called toxicodendrol (lobinol) is present in all poisonous *Toxicodendron* species and contains a complex active principle known as urushiol. The name "urushiol" is derived from the Japanese term "sap."[5] It is a mixture of antigenic catechols.[7] These antigens are closely related to 3-n-pentadecylcatechol (3- PDC, hydrourushiol) but differ in the degree of unsaturation at the 3n-alkyl side chains,[3,8] and in their side chain lengths sumac has 13 carbons, poison ivy 15 carbons and oak 17 carbons.[5] In general, the more unsaturated or longer the side chain is, the more antigenically reactive the catechol.[9] Urushiol is carried by resin canals found in the bark, stem, leaflets, and certain flower parts. The relative percentages of 3-PDC and related catechols varies among the species and may also be related to environmental conditions. The danger of toxicity is greatest in spring and summer, when the sap is abundant, the urushiol content is high, and the plant is bruised easily.

Chromatographic procedures have been developed for use in separation and characterization of urushiol in poison ivy and poison oak.[10,11]

PHARMACOLOGY: Extracts of poison oak have been used in homeopathic medicine to treat conditions such as osteoarthritis. Controlled studies have failed to substantiate the efficacy of such treatments,[12] but the methodology of these studies has been questioned.[13,14]

Urushiols are haptens that must bind with skin proteins to form complete antigens. This is thought to occur on the surface of Langerhans cells, where the urushiols are irreversibly bound.[3,5] Sensitization appears to require bonding of quinones derived from urushiol components with nucleophilic groups on the proteins.[15] A later report suggests free radicals, and not quinones, to be the haptenic species derived from urushiol.[16] Blocking the C5–position on the catechol ring seems to suppress sensitivity.[15] Mouse data suggest that contact sensitivity to urushiol is mediated by serum factors.[17] In vitro studies with human lymphocytes, however, indicate that urushiol reacts initially with T cells. Interaction with a non-T accessory lymphocyte is necessary for reactivity.[18] A recent report describes processing or urushiol hapten by both endogenous and exogenous pathways for presentation to T-cells.[19] After the previously sensitized T-lymphocytes have been activated, the allergy cascade is locally initiated.[5]

Many more recent immunological studies continue, including: Isolation of urushiol triggered T-cells;[20] T-cell clone generation from blood;[20,21,22] enrichment and function of urushiol-specific T-lymphocytes;[23] role of keratinocytes in allergic contact dermatitis;[24,25] increased levels of telomerase activity in poison ivy dermatitis;[26] UL-8 enhanced expression;[27] and modulation;[28] and poison ivy analog sensitization.[29,30,31,32]

TOXICOLOGY: Toxicodendrol does not enter the blood. Minute quantities (0.001 mg) applied to the skin can cause dermatitis. The sensitivity may persist for years. Infants are not as readily sensitized as adults, and with intermittent exposure, the sensitivity decreases with age. After contact, the first symptoms of itching, burning and redness may appear in a few hours or may take up to 5 days, depending on the sensitivity of the individual. The rash is characterized by linear streaks of erythematous lesions where the plant has "brushed" the skin.[5] Urticarial plaques and bullae may develop, filled with fluid. Contrary to popular belief, this blister fluid does not contain urushiol, and therefore, cannot spread infection by fluid contact. Continued spreading of infection actually results from variation in time of onset of clinical reaction ("delayed reaction"), antigen load and individual sensitivity.[1] Secondary changes include the blisters oozing until a crust is formed. Intense itching may last for up to 7 days. Rare complications include hematologic changes, renal damage and psychological reactions. Barring complications, the dermatitis is self-limiting, lasting from 1 to 3 weeks. The skin usually recovers unblemished, because only the epidermal layer is involved; however, excessive scratching and infection may result in permanent scarring.[3]

Other means of exposure from the plant include inhaling resin droplets carried in smoke from burning poison ivy, which can cause fever, major lung infection and even death from the throat swelling shut.[32] Exposure to urushiol can also come about by contact through animal fur, contaminated clothing, garden tools and sports equipment. Urushiol is so long-lasting, (if not properly washed away), that dermatitis can occur years later if these still contaminated items are touched again.[3,32] Soaking contaminated clothing in a 1% solution of hypochlorite for 15 minutes, followed by laundering, should remove the resin (caution: may discolor clothing). Avoidance, however, remains the best approach to preventing *Toxicodendron* dermatitis.

If ingested, poison ivy can produce severe gastrointestinal effects.[3] Some individuals, however, can consume poison ivy without effect, apparently because of a lack of reactivity in the digestive mucosa.[33]

The choice of an appropriate treatment is dependent upon the severity of the episode. Treatment objectives include protecting the damaged skin until the acute reaction has subsided, preventing accumulation of epidermal debris, relieving the intense itching, and avoiding excoriation. Affected areas should be cleaned immediately with soapy water, however, oils from certain soaps may spread the sap. According to the American Academy of Dermatology in a recent report, water alone is best to use when contact with the plant is known. Urushiol is neutralized by water, and if the exposed area is washed with water within 5 to 10 minutes after contact, the reaction may be avoided.[34] Swabbing with alcohol may not halt the allergic reaction but may limit its spread. Wet compresses (Burow's solution, normal saline, potassium permanganate, 10% tannic solution), cornstarch, or oatmeal baths may provide symptomatic relief. Astringent soaks should not be used on the skin of the face or genitals. Other over-the-counter therapies include local anesthetics, antipruritics, antiseptics and counterirritants (eg, menthol).[5,35-40]

Calamine lotion has long been the drug of choice in poison ivy dermatitis. Its astringent action may also provide relief of itching, pain and discomfort of poison ivy.[41,42] Oral antihistamines can provide transient symptomatic improvement of pruritis (eg, hydroxyzine 10–25 mg 4 times/day as needed).[1,5] Topical antihistamines should be discouraged, because their use has been associated with skin sensitization; further, their use here is irrational, because these dermatites are not dependent on the release of histamine.[43] Two to three times per day application of topical corticosteroids such as betamethasone valerate 0.1% (*Valisone*), betamethasone dipropionate 0.05% (*Diprolene*), flucinolone acetonide 0.01%-0.25% (*Synalar*) and triamcinolone acetonide 0.1% (*Aristocort, Kenalog*) are all frequently prescribed and may slightly reduce erythema and pruritis, but they hardly alter the natural overall course of the lesions, unless applied early in the course.[1,44] Some systemic absorption may occur so application to the sensitive areas (eg, face), pregnant/nursing mothers, diabetics, etc, should be avoided. Occlusive dressings should not be placed over these creams because increased absorption will occur as well.[38] Low-dose otc topical steroids haven't been proven effective, except in the most mild cases.[1] In cases of extensive dermatitis, systemic steroids (for adult patients) are indicated. Oral prednisone 1 mg/kg/day tapered over 14 to 21 days is standard, and can dramatically improve the condition.[1] A common mistake is to taper the steroid dosages too quickly, resulting in rebound flares. Complications can result from prepackaged "dosepaks," because initial dosage here is approximately ½ the recommended dosage. Other problems with this treatment

include rapid tapering and too short a course of therapy. The manufacturer of this methylprednisolone dosepak does, however, include such a warning on its product.[1] A case report describes an example of this type of treatment failure and how it was resolved.[45]

Other treatment options include use of poultices prepared from narrow and broad leaf plantain to control the itching[46] and acupuncture, both with clinically unsubstantiated but variable results. A report of four cases has noted success with acupuncture in relieving the itching of the dermatites within a few hours to 2 days and promoting healing of skin lesions within 2 to 4 days.[47]

Desensitization by the administration of plant extracts is not regularly attained. In general, hyposensitization procedures require large doses and months of treatment, and the sensitivity is regained rapidly upon cessation of therapy.[48] Oral ingestion of antigens (bypassing Langerhans cells) may allow suppressor T-cell populations to develop, that can inhibit the response to skin contacting the plant.[1] Oral administration in inducing tolerance and desensitization to poison ivy dermatitis in Guinea pigs has been reported.[1,49] The three most widely used agents for hyposensitization are crude plant extract, alum-precipitated pyridine extracts, and synthetic 3-PDC. Commercial products vary in antigen content. The preparations are taken in gradually increasing daily doses for at least 4 weeks with maintenance doses several times a week during the growing season. Intramuscular preparations are usually given at weekly or biweekly intervals.[50] No well-controlled studies have established the efficacy of these preparations, although studies with a purified urushiol extract have demonstrated good hyposensitization compared with placebo.[51] A double-blind, placebo-controlled study of a 1:1 oral mixture of 3-PDC and heptadecylcatechol failed to demonstrate any decrease in sensitivity to poison ivy or poison oak in 44 subjects.[52] Animal studies, however, suggest that topical application of 5-methyl-3-n-pentadecylcathechol or a related compound could be effective in inducing tolerance to 3-PDC.[53] At best, hyposensitization reduces the duration and severity of the dermatitis, while inducing numerous side effects, including gastrointestinal disturbances, itching, and inflammation. There still remains no US Food and Drug Administration (FDA)-approved or reliable oral regimen for desensitization.[1]

Topical application may provide an alternative to systemic administration of agents to protect against poison-plant dermatitis. Clinical patch tests have identified several polyamide salts of a linoleic acid dimer that prevented dermatitis in 70% of subjects tested. The salts were particularly effective when both the preparation and the plant antigen were washed off the skin within 8 to 12 hours of antigen exposure.[54] The effectiveness of this, and other barrier preparations to prevent dermatitis has been evaluated in another report. The percent reductions in dermatitis severity per day in order of effectiveness were: *Stokogard* (Stockhausen, Greensboro, NC) which contains PPG-3 diamine dilinoleate; *Hollister Moisture Barrier* (Hollister, Inc., Libertyville, IL) containing a propylparaben, BHA mixture; *Hydropel* (C & M Pharmacal, Inc., Hazel Park, MI) with 30% silicone; *Ivy Shield* (Interpro, Inc., Haverhill, MA) a tea stearate mixture; *Shield Skin* (Mentor Corp., Minneapolis, MN) with plasticized ethyl cellulose; *Dermofilm* (Innovetec, Brussels, Belgium); and *Uniderm* (Smith & Nephew, Inc., Largo, FL) with lanolin, benzethonium chloride, quaternium-15 and others.[55]

Organoclay, an ingredient of antiperspirants, is the most recent, effective barrier cream studied thus far. This agent has reduced or totally prevented experimental dermatitis.[56] The oranoclay, quaternium-18 bentonite, has the ability to "bind" with urushiol. This product, recently approved by the FDA, contains 5% quaternium-18 bentonite in the form of a lotion, called *Ivyblock* (Enviroderm Pharmaceuticals, Inc.). When applied, the product lays down an active barrier on skin, blocking potential contact with the allergan, thus, offering protection from poison ivy, poison oak and poison sumac rash.[57] *Ivyblock* should be be available as of late 1996, and should be of great help in "high risk" individuals, including firefighters, utility and lumber workers, armed forces and certain medical professionals.

SUMMARY: The dermatites induced by poison ivy and closely related plant species remain a persistent problem for more than half of the US population. The oily resin, urushiol, causes the contact dermatitis. This binds with skin proteins, causing an allergic reaction. The rash is characterized by linear streaks of erythematous and pustular lesions, which may last several weeks. Treatment depends on the severity of the episodes, but systemic steroids have the most dramatic therapeutic effects. Desensitization by plant extracts is not reliable. New barrier creams are effective in preventing the dermatitis if applied before contact, especially products like *Ivyblock*. Avoidance remains the best approach to reducing the incidence of dermatitis.

PATIENT INFORMATION – Poison Ivy

Uses: There are **unsubstantiated** claims of usefulness in the treatment of conditions such as osteoarthritis.

Side Effects: Dermatitis in severity ranging from mild to fatal, depending upon point of contact and individual resistance.

---

[1] Williford P, et al. *Arch Fam Med* 1994;3(2):184–8.
[2] Hardin JW, Arena JM. Human Poisoning from Native and Cultivated Plants, 2nd Ed. Durham: Duke Univ. Press, 1975.
[3] DerMarderosian AH. *Drug Therapy* 1977;7:57.
[4] Guin JD. *J Am Acad Dermatol* 1980;2(4):332–3.
[5] Guay D. *J Prac Nurs* 1993;43(4):24–31.
[6] *MMWR* 1983;32:129.
[7] Dawson CR. *Recent Chem Prog* 1954;15:39.
[8] Corbett M, Billets D. *J Pharm Sci* 1975;64:1715.
[9] El Sohly MA, et al. *J Med Chem* 1986;29:606.
[10] El Sohly MA, et al. *J Pharm Sci* 1980;69(May):587–9.
[11] El Sohly MA, et al. *J Nat Prod* 1982;45(Sep-Oct):532–8.
[12] Shipley M, et al. *Lancet* 1983;8316:97.
[13] Kennedy CO. *Lancet* 1983;8332:482.
[14] Ghosh A. *Lancet* 1983;8319:304.
[15] Dunn IS, et al. *Cell Immunol* 1986;97:189.
[16] Schmidt R, et al. *Arch Dermatol Res* 1990;282(1):56–64.
[17] Dunn IS, et al. *J Invest Dermatol* 1987;89:296.
[18] Byers VS, et al. *J Clin Invest* 1979;64:1437.
[19] Kalish R, et al. *J Clin Invest* 1994;93(5):2039-47.
[20] Kalish R, et al. *J Invest Dermatol* 1989;92(1):46–52.
[21] Kalish R, et al. *J Clin Invest* 1988;82(3):825–32.
[22] Kalish R, et al. *J Invest Dermatol* 1990;94(6–Suppl):108S-111S.
[23] Kalish R, et al. *J Immunol* 1990;145(11):3706–13.
[24] Griffiths C, et al. *Am J Pathol* 1989;135(6):1045–53.
[25] Barker J. *Contact Dermatitis* 1992;26(3):145–8.
[26] Taylor R, et al. *J Invest Dermatol* 1996;106(4):759–65.
[27] Mohamadzadeh M, et al. *Exp Dermatol* 1994;3(6):298–303.
[28] Griffiths C, et al. *J Dermatol* 1991;124(6):519–26.
[29] Roberts D, et al. *Contact Dermatitis* 1993;29(2):78–83.
[30] Haas J, et al. *Exp Dermatol* 1992;1(2):76–83.
[31] Fraginals R, et al. *J Med Chem* 1991;34(3):1024–7.
[32] Vietmeyer N. *Smithsonian Magazine* 1995.
[33] Heald P, et al. *N Carolina Med J* 1983;44:437.
[34] Lane L. *Austin American Statesman* 1995;June 16;F1–2.
[35] Witkowski J, et al. *Drug Ther* 1984;14(Jun):81–3, 87–8.
[36] Bagley J. *Am Druggist* 1986;193(Feb):114, 116.
[37] Levine H. *Am Druggist* 1988;197(Apr):47–8.
[38] Praw W. *US Pharmacist* 1991;16(Aug):16, 19, 20, 24.
[39] Anonymous. *Drug Store News for Pharmacists* 1994;4(Jun 13):55–61.
[40] Praw W. *US Pharmacist* 1994;19(Jun):99–100.
[41] Desimone E. *Am Pharm* 1983;NS23(Jun):8–13.
[42] Olin B, ed. Facts and Comparisons. St Louis, MO: Facts and Comparisons, Inc. May 1992 Update: 564.
[43] Reynolds H. Poison Ivy Dermatitis, Current Therapy. Philadelphia: W.B. Saunders, 1972.
[44] Beyea S. *RN* 1989;52(8):23–5.
[45] Ives T, et al. *JAMA* 1991;266(Sep 11):1362.
[46] Duckett S. *N Engl J Med* 1980;303(Sep 4):583.
[47] Liao SJ. *Electrother Res* 1988;13:31.
[48] Watson ES, et al. *J Pharm Sci* 1981;70:785.
[49] El Sohly M, et al. *J Pharm Sci* 1983;72(Jul):792–5.
[50] *Medical Letter* 1981;23:40.
[51] Epstein WL, et al. *Arch Dermatol* 1974;109:356.
[52] Marks JG, et al. *Arch Dermatol* 1987;123:476.
[53] Stampf JL, et al. *J Invest Dermatol* 1986;86:535.
[54] Orchard S, et al. *Arch Dermatol* 1986;122:783.
[55] Grevelink S, et al. *J Am Acad Dermatol* 1992;27:182–8.
[56] Marks J, et al. *J Am Acad Dermatol* 1995;33:212–6.
[57] Anonymous. Fact Sheet from Product Info. Packet, EnviroDerm Pharmaceuticals, 929 S. 3rd St., Louisville, KY 40203 (502) 634–7700.

Pokeweed

SCIENTIFIC NAME(S): Several species of *Phytolacca* are common throughout the United States, with the most common being *P. americana* L., *P. decandra* L. and *P. rigida*. Family: Phytolaccaceae

COMMON NAME(S): The plant goes by a long list of synonyms, some of which are American nightshade, cancer jalap, cancerroot, chongras, coakum, pokeberry, crowberry garget, inkberry, pigeonberry, poke, red ink plant and scoke.

BOTANY: Pokeweed is an ubiquitous plant found in fields, along fences, in damp woods and in other undisturbed areas. Pokeweed is indigenous to eastern North America, California and Hawaii. This vigorous shrub-like perennial can grow to 12 feet. The reddish stem has large pointed leaves which taper at both ends.[1] The flowers are numerous, small and greenish-white which develop into juicy purple berries that mature from July to September.

HISTORY: The folk uses of pokeweed leaves have included the treatment of chronic rheumatisms and arthritis, and as an emetic and purgative.[2] The plant has also been used to treat edema,[3] skin cancers, rheumatism, catarrh, dysmenorrhea, mumps, ringworm, scabies, tonsillitis and syphilis. Poke greens, the young immature leaves, are commercially canned and sold under the name "poke salet." The juice of the berries has been employed as an ink, dye and coloring agent in wine.[4]

CHEMISTRY: The toxic components of the plant are triterpene saponins which include phytolaccigenin, aligonic acid and phytolaccagenic acid (also called phytolaccinic acid),[5] esculenic acid and the minor component pokeberrygenin.[3] A tannin and resin are present in all portions of the plant. In addition, a toxic protein called pokeweed mitogen (PWM) has also been isolated. This mitogen has been shown to induce blood cell abnormalities. For this reason, protective gloves should be worn when handling the plant.[4]

PHARMACOLOGY: The pharmacologic activity of the plant has not been well defined. Small doses of all parts of the plant can cause adverse reactions (see Toxicology), but the mechanisms of these actions are generally unknown. Extracts of the plant that contain PWM can cause "transformation" of T and B lymphocytes, most likely through an immune-mediated mechanism.[6] PWM is used as a "cellular probe" in pharmacologic experiments. Several anti-inflammatory saponins have been isolated from the root;[7] the root, however, has no known medicinal value.

TOXICOLOGY: Pokeweed poisonings were common in eastern North America during the 19th century, especially from the use of tinctures as antirheumatic preparations, and from eating berries and roots collected in error for parsnip, Jerusalem artichoke or horseradish.[8]

All parts of pokeweed are toxic except the above-ground leaves that grow in the early spring. The poisonous principles are in highest concentration in the rootstock, less in the mature leaves and stems and least in the fruits. Young leaves collected before acquiring a red color are edible if boiled for 5 minutes, rinsed and reboiled. Berries are toxic when raw but are edible when cooked.

Ingestion of poisonous parts of the plant causes severe stomach cramping, nausea with persistent diarrhea and vomiting, slow and difficult breathing, weakness, spasms, hypotension, severe convulsions and death.[9] Less than 10 uncooked berries are generally harmless to adults. Several investigators have reported deaths in children following the ingestion of uncooked berries or pokeberry juice.[9,10]

Severe poisonings have been reported in adults who ingested mature pokeweed leaves[11] and following the ingestion of a cup of tea brewed from one-half teaspoonful of powdered pokeroot.[8]

In addition, a case of toxicity in campers who ingested properly cooked young shoots has been reported by the CDC. Sixteen of the 51 cases exhibited case-definitive symptoms (vomiting followed by any three of the following: Nausea, diarrhea, stomach cramps, dizziness, headache). These symptoms persisted for up to 48 hours (mean, 24 hr).[12]

Poisoning may also occur when the toxic components enter the circulatory system through cuts and abrasions in the skin.

Symptoms of mild poisoning generally last 24 hours. In severe cases, gastric lavage, emesis and symptomatic and supportive treatment have been suggested.[9]

In an attempt to curb potential poisonings from the use of this commercially available plant, the Herb Trade Association (HTA) formulated a policy stressing that the poke root is toxic and "should not be sold as an herbal beverage or food, or in any other form which could threaten the health of the uninformed consumer." Further, the HTA recommended that products containing pokeroot should be labeled clearly as to their toxicity.[13]

The FDA classifies pokeweed as an herb of undefined safety which has demonstrated narcotic effects.

SUMMARY: Pokeweed is a common plant found throughout parts of the United States. The young leaves may be eaten and the berries used for food, both only after being cooked properly. Mature leaves and all other parts of the plant are toxic (primarily gastrointestinal and central) if ingested.

PATIENT INFORMATION – Pokeweed

Uses: The young pokeweed leaves may be eaten and the berries used for food, both only after being cooked properly.

Side Effects: Ingestion of poisonous parts of the plant causes severe stomach cramping, nausea with persistent diarrhea and vomiting, slow and difficult breathing, weakness, spasms, hypotension, severe convulsions, and death.

---

[1] Dobelis IN, ed. Magic and Medicine of Plants. Pleasantville, NY: Reader's Digest Association, Inc., 1986.

[2] Bianchini F, Corbetta F. Health Plants of the World. New York, NY: Newsweek Books, 1975.

[3] Kang SS, Woo SS. *J Nat Prod* 1980;43:510.

[4] Duke JA. CRC Handbook of Medicinal Herbs. Boca Raton, FL: CRC Press, 1985.

[5] Johnson A, Shimizu Y. *Tetrahedron* 1974;30:2033.

[6] Barker BE, et al. *Pediatrics* 1966;38:490.

[7] Woo WS, et al. *Planta Medica* 1978;34:87.

[8] Lewis WH, Smith PR. *JAMA* (letter) 1975;242:2759.

[9] Hardin JW, Arena JM. Human Poisoning from Native and Cultivated Plants, 2nd ed. Durham, NC: Duke University Press, 1974.

[10] Toxic reactions to plant products sold in health food stores. *Medical Letter* 1979;21:29.

[11] Stein ZLG. *Am J Hosp Pharm* 1979;36:1303.

[12] Plant poisonings - New Jersey. *MMWR* 1981;30:65.

[13] Herb Trade Association Policy Statement #2. May 1979.

Poppy

SCIENTIFIC NAME(S): Although a variety of members of the genus *Papaver* are called poppies, *P. somniferum* L. and *P. bracteatum* Lindl. are important commercially and medicinally.[1] Family: Papaveraceae

COMMON NAME(S): *P. somniferum*: Opium poppy, poppyseed poppy. *P. bracteatum*: Thebaine poppy, great scarlet poppy.

BOTANY: The opium poppy is a small annual. The bright showy flowers of the genus *Papaver* range in color from white to deep reds and purples. The seeds of the plants vary in color from light cream to blue-black.

HISTORY: The earliest accounts of the use of poppy derivatives date to the Sumerians in Mesopotamia, where the plant was used medicinally and was known as *hul gil* (the plant of joy).[2] The medicinal uses of poppy were described by the Ancient Greeks, and opium, as an addictive agent, was described by the Arabs more than 900 years ago. Because of the wide distribution of the opium poppy, its use has been recognized by most major cultures. Opium has been used in the United States since its birth and was used widely during the Civil War. Morphine was isolated from crude opium in 1803, and in 1874, morphine was boiled with acetic anhydride to yield diacetylmorphine (heroin). This compound was developed by Bayer and Company for cough, chest pain and pneumonia. It was later recognized as having a high addiction potential. Derivatives of opium continue to play a major role as antitussives, antidiarrheals and analgesics. Their abuse potential remains high and strict efforts to curtail the illicit cultivation of the opium poppy have met with limited success. Poppy seeds are used in the preparation of confections and breads.

CHEMISTRY: The chemistry of the *Papaver* is well known. Upon scoring the unripened seed capsule, a milky latex exudes and is collected.[3] This material is known as opium. Purification of opium results in the isolation of more than 30 alkaloids.[4] The most important of these alkaloids are morphine (20%), codeine (2%), papaverine (2%), noscapine (5%, once called narcotine) and thebaine (1%). Codeine is the most widely used opium alkaloid and is obtained from natural sources or through the methylation of morphine or modification of thebaine. About 90% of morphine isolated from opium is converted synthetically to codeine.

Because of the medicinal importance of morphine derivatives, efforts have been underway to identify a species of *Papaver* that contains high levels of a suitable starting compound for the commercial synthesis of codeine, yet which contains low levels of abusable morphine (which can be readily converted illicitly to heroin). In some varieties of *P. bracteatum*, thebaine constitutes 98% of the total alkaloid content.[5] Commercially, thebaine may be readily converted to codeine, oxycodone, hydrocodone or dihydrocodeine. Its conversion to morphine and subsequently to heroin requires advanced chemical skills and equipment, which makes such procedures less likely to be used illicitly.[6] Consequently, *P. bracteatum* may become the species of choice as a legal source of alkaloid precursors.

The alleged presence of morphine in hops has never been confirmed. The sedative alkaloid hopeine, purported to have been isolated from hops, was actually a material prepared from morphine and cocaine and sold as a hoax in Europe at the end of the 19th century.[6]

PHARMACOLOGY: The pharmacologic effects of the morphine alkaloids differ widely. Codeine and morphine are sedative analgesics and can relax smooth muscle tone, making them useful in the treatment of diarrhea and abdominal cramping. Codeine and its derivatives are antitussives. Papaverine relaxes involuntary smooth muscle and increases cerebral blood flow. Although large doses of thebaine can induce convulsions, no case of human thebaine abuse has been reported.[6] The addictive characteristics of the opium alkaloids have been recognized for millenia.

TOXICOLOGY: The abuse potential of opium has had an enormous impact on most societies. Deaths due to respiratory depression have been reported and heroin-induced deaths are reported commonly. As little as 300 mg of opium can be fatal to humans, although addicts tolerate 2000 mg over 4 hours. Death from circulatory and respiratory collapse is accompanied by cold, clammy skin, pulmonary edema, cyanosis and pupillary constriction. Thebaine has an LD_{50} of 20 mg/kg in mice.[4]

Significant attention has been focused on the fact that morphine and codeine can be detected in significant amounts in urine following the ingestion of foods prepared with poppy seeds. After the ingestion of three poppy-seed bagels, urinary codeine and morphine levels were 214 ng/ml and 2797 ng/ml, respectively after 3 hours. Analysis of poppy seeds indicated that an individual consuming a single poppy-seed bagel could ingest up to 1.5 mg of morphine and 0.1 mg of codeine.[7] Opiates have been detected in urine more than 48 hours after the ingestion of culinary poppy seeds.[8] These results confirm that a positive finding of morphine or codeine in urine may not always be due to the ingestion of drugs of abuse.

The Mexican poppy (*Argemone mexicana*) L. has been associated with poisoning, demonstrating symptoms of sedation, sluggishness and abdominal contractions in rats fed its seeds.[9]

SUMMARY: The opium poppy continues to represent one of the most commercially important plants worldwide. Its use in medicine dates to antiquity as does its harmful addictive effects. Although an important commercial source of morphine, *P. somniferum* may be supplanted by *P. bracteatum*, a related plant high in thebaine, a compound which can be readily converted commercially to codeine, but only with extreme difficulty to morphine and heroin.

PATIENT INFORMATION – Poppy

Uses: Poppy has been used to relax smooth muscle tone, making it useful in the treatment of diarrhea and abdominal cramping, and used as sedative analgesics and antitussives.

Side Effects: Poppy is known for its highly addictive qualities and has been associated with poisoning and demonstrating symptoms of sedation and sluggishness, and abdominal contractions.

---

[1] Duke JA. *Economic Botany* 1973;27:390.
[2] Hoffmann JP. *J Psychoactive Drugs* 1990;22:53.
[3] Simon JE. Herbs: An indexed bibliography. Hamden, CT: Shoe String Press, 1984.
[4] Duke JA. Handbook of Medicinal Herbs. Boca Raton, FL: CRC Press, 1985.
[5] Nyman U, Bruhn JG. *Planta Medica* 1979;35:97.
[6] Theuns HG, et al. *Economic Botany* 1986;40:485.
[7] Struempler RE. *J Analytical Toxicol* 1987;11:97.
[8] Hayes LW, et al. *Clin Chem* 1987;33:806.
[9] Pahwa R, et al. *Vet Human Toxicol* 1989;31:555.

Potato

SCIENTIFIC NAME(S): *Solanum tuberosum* L.

COMMON NAME(S): Potato, white potato

BOTANY: The potato is a weedy plant recognized for its tuberous growth and valued as a commercial foodstuff. Potatoes are propagated vegetatively from the underground runners of the plant from the "eyes" of the potato.[1]

HISTORY: Potatoes have been cultivated since 500 BC; the Central and South American Indians were probably among the first to select hardy cultivators of the potato as a food staple.[1,2] Despite the Spaniard introduction of the plant into Europe in the late 1500s, the tubers did not become a popular food source until the 17th century because of church and mythological concerns about the toxicity of the plant. Once accepted, potatoes were widely disseminated to Germany, other parts of Europe and Russia.

By the 17th and 18th centuries, potatoes formed such a significant part of the Irish diet that intake for adults exceeded 8 lbs/day. However, the potato blight destroyed more than 80% of the crop, resulting in the starvation of more than 3 million Irish.[2]

Traditional uses of the potato include: Using raw potato poultices for arthritis, infections, boils, burns and sore eyes; brewing potato peel tea to soothe edema or bodily swelling; and drinking raw potato juice to soothe gastritis or stomach disorders.[3] (No clinical data exist to support these uses.)

Today, the potato remains an important food with over 200 metric tons being harvested annually worldwide; surpassed only by wheat.[2] Potatoes are also used as a source of starch[4] and alcohol.

CHEMISTRY: Potatoes are a poor source of protein, with only about 5% of the composition being protein. They are, however, reasonable sources of iron, riboflavin and vitamin C,[1] which are found primarily in the thick periderm of the skin.[2] The potato contains a variety of steroidal alkaloids chemically related to the cholestane ring structure. Examples of these compounds include solasodine and solanidine.[5] Potatoes are rich in starch, and potato maltodextrin may be used in the preparation of commercial foods.[6]

PHARMACOLOGY: Over 2000 species of *Solanum* are potentially toxic; *S. tuberosum* is one of only six of these species that produces a tuber.[2] Crop residues from the potato are often implicated in animal/livestock toxicoses.

TOXICOLOGY: The toxicity is related to the presence of the steroidal solanum alkaloids. The solanum glycosides, such as solanine, produce gastrointestinal disturbances including nausea, vomiting, diarrhea and hemolytic and hemorrhagic damage to the gastrointestinal tract.[5] Solanine may also cause an exanthemous syndrome which, together with gastrointestinal and neurological symptoms, may be severe enough to be fatal.[7] Solanine is not destroyed in the cooking process.[8] Ingested solanine is relatively less toxic than that administered parenterally.[7] The biological half-life of solanine is 11 hours.[9]

Even though human fatalities due to the consumption of green potatoes have been reported periodically, proof that solanine was the causal agent has not been firmly established.[8] Concentrations of 38 to 45 mg/100 g solanine have been found in potatoes implicated in human fatalities, compared to 3 to 66 mg/100 g in fresh, healthy potatoes.[8] A level of 20 mg/100 g is generally considered the upper limit of safety.[8]

Solanine has been specifically implicated in the development of fetal malformation in livestock.[5] Solasodine is teratogenic in hamsters when given orally; in some experiments in which pregnant hamsters were fed potato extracts, more than one-quarter of the pups exhibited malformations.[5] Other studies have found that neural tube defects in hamsters may be caused by the solanidine triglycosides, alpha-chaconine and high-dose solanine.[10]

The association between the ingestion of blighted potatoes by pregnant women and subsequent fetal deformities in offspring has not been well established, but remains a growing concern. Anencephaly may have been associated with the ingestion of potatoes infected with Phytophora infestans in women in the Congo.[11]

Potatoes also contain contain a variety of compounds that may potentially interfere with biological systems. These include cholinesterase inhibitors, invertase inhibitors and protease inhibitors;[8] all may have evolved as part of a defense mechanism toward invading microbes.

Because potatoes may be high in bacteria and fungi counts, persons exposed to potato dust have demonstrated a high incidence of work-related respiratory and general symptoms;[12,13] in one survey, 46% of those assessed had respiratory symptoms secondary to exposure to potato dust.[12]

Potatoes may affect glycemic control[14] and insulin levels; therefore, diabetic persons may eat the vegetables as appropriate starch equivalents.

SUMMARY: The potato remains an economically and socially important food product. While its ingestion is safe, persons should refrain from eating damaged or green potatoes which may have elevated levels of solanum alkaloids that have been associated with a variety of types of toxicity.

PATIENT INFORMATION – Potato

Uses: Potatoes are rich in starch and may affect glycemic control and insulin levels of diabetic persons.

Side Effects: Ingestion of damaged or green potatoes can result in GI and neurological disturbances. Exposure to potato dust has demonstrated a high incidence of work-related respiratory and general symptoms.

---

[1] Mabberley DJ. The plant-book. Cambridge, England: Cambridge University Press, 1987.
[2] Spoerke D. *Vet Human Toxicol* 1994;36:324.
[3] Boyd E, et al. Home Remedies and the Black Elderly: A Reference Manual for Health Care Providers. Levittown, PA: Pharmaceutical Information Associates, Ltd., 1991.
[4] Evans, WC. Trease and Evans' Pharmacognosy, ed. 13. London: Bailliére Tindall, 1989.
[5] Kinghorn D, ed. Toxic Plants. New York: Columbia University Press, 1979.
[6] Specter SE, Setser CS. *J Dairy Sci* 1994;77:708.
[7] Dalvi RR, Bowie WC. *Vet Human Toxicol* 1983;25:13.
[8] Liener IE, ed. Toxic Constituents of Plant Foodstuffs, ed. 2. New York: Academic Press, 1980.
[9] Hellenas KE, et al. *J Chromatogr* 1992;573:69.
[10] Renwick JH, et al. *Teratology* 1984;30:371.
[11] Iioki LH, et al. *J Gynecol Obstet Biol Reprod* 1993;22:621.
[12] Dutkiewicz J. *Am J Ind Med* 1994;25:43.
[13] Hollander A, et al. *Occup Environ Med* 1994;51:73.
[14] Gannon MC, et al. *Diabetes Care* 1993;16:874.

Precatory Bean

SCIENTIFIC NAME(S): *Abrus precatorius* L. Family: Leguminosae (Fabaceae)

COMMON NAME(S): Precatory bean, love bean, rosary pea, crab's eye, jequirity seed, bead vine, black-eyed Susan, prayer beads and numerous other locally used common names.

BOTANY: The plant originated in southeast Asia and is now found in other tropical and subtropical regions. It is found commonly in Florida and Hawaii where it grows as a slender vine generally supported by other plants or a fence. The leaves are sensitive to light, drooping at night and on cloudy days. The fruit splits open as it dries to reveal three to five hard coated, brilliant scarlet seeds with a small black spot at the point of attachment. This spot helps identify the seeds, which are sometimes confused with *Rhynchosia*, in which the black and red colors are reversed.[1] Seeds of *A. precatorius* may also be confused with those of *Ormosia*, also a toxic member of the Leguminosae.

HISTORY: The rosary pea has found widespread use as an art object and ornament. The colorful, hard beans have been used as pendants, rosaries, necklaces and in toys such as noise shakers. All parts of the plant have been used in traditional medicine. Dilute infusions have been used in South American and African folk medicine for the treatment of ophthalmic inflammations. They have been used to hasten labor, stimulate abortion and have also found some use as an oral contraceptive in traditional medicine.[2] Because of the great potential for toxicity, the use of this plant should not be recommended.

CHEMISTRY: Several indole alkaloids (abrine, hyaphorine, precatorine) have been isolated from the plant.[2] Most importantly, the toxic protein abrin has been isolated from the seed. It has been described as a single glycoprotein of molecular weight 60,000 to 65,000.[3] Two proteins of differing amino acid composition have been purified from jequirity beans. Designated Abrin A and C, Abrin C exhibits more potent hemoagglutination activity than Abrin A.[4] Both Abrin A and C may be subdivided into smaller units of molecular weight of about 30,000.

Another lectin, abrus agglutinin, which is nontoxic to animal cells and exhibits potent agglutinating activity toward erythrocytes, has been described. Abrus seeds also contain a potent proteinase inhibitor.[5]

PHARMACOLOGY: According to current theories, the toxin is composed of two chains (A and B), with a separate function having been assigned to each unit. The B chain (the haptomere) binds to cell surfaces. This function was based on studies which showed that the B chain binds to galactose units of surface carbohydrates.[6]

The A chain (effectomere) is responsible for the toxic activity. Once inside the cell, the A chain migrates to the 60S unit of the ribosome, acting to inhibit further protein synthesis. Abrin has a strong inhibitory effect on protein synthesis, moderate inhibitory effect on DNA synthesis and little effect on RNA synthesis.[7]

Abrin has been used as a "molecular probe" to investigate cellular function. It has also been evaluated in the treatment of experimental cancers. Although effective when given IP to mice pretreated with L1210 leukemia, no increase in lifespan was noted when the compound was administered intravenously.[8] Abrin has been used with some clinical success as an analgesic in terminally ill patients.[9]

Ethanolic extracts of the leaves of *Abrus* possess d-tubocurarine-like neuromuscular blocking activity.[10]

TOXICOLOGY: Fatal poisoning in children has been reported after the thorough chewing of one seed.[1] Ingestion of jequirity seeds causes severe stomach cramping accompanied by nausea, severe diarrhea, cold sweat, fast pulse, coma and circulatory collapse.[11] The onset of toxicity usually occurs in 1 to 3 days. The seeds must be chewed thoroughly; unchewed or intact seeds remain impervious to gastric fluid and pose less of a toxicologic potential.[12] Gastric lavage or emesis should be followed by measures to maintain circulation including the correction of hypovolemia and electrolyte disturbances.[1] Alkalinization of the urine to control uremia and enhance toxin excretion has been recommended.[11] Necklaces made of the pierced seeds have been reported to induce dermatitis.[13]

A radioimmunoassay has been developed for abrin.[14]

The LD_{50} of abrin given IP to mice is 0.04 mcg;[3] 5 mg of the alkaloid abrine is reported to be toxic to humans.[13] In goats, ground seeds administered at a dose of 1 and 2 g/kg/day caused death in 2 to 5 days.[15]

SUMMARY: Phytotoxin poisoning from *Abrus* represents a rare but extremely dangerous and potentially fatal hazard, especially to the young. Prompt emesis followed by supportive therapy may result in uncomplicated recovery from poisoning. While rosary peas generally have little exposure in American culture, health professionals should remain aware of their potential danger.

PATIENT INFORMATION – Precatory Bean

Uses: The precatory bean has experienced some success as an analgesic in terminally ill patients and evaluated in the treatment of experimental cancers.

Side Effects: The precatory bean is highly toxic and has been known to cause severe stomach cramping, nausea, severe diarrhea, cold sweat, fast pulse, coma, and circulatory collapse.

---

[1] Lampe KF. AMA Handbook of Poisonous and Injurious Plants. Chicago, IL: Chicago Review Press, 1985.

[2] Evans WC. Trease and Evans' Pharmacognosy, ed 13. London, England: Bailliere Tindall, 1989.

[3] Olsnes S, et al. *Nature* 1974;249:627.

[4] Wei CH, et al. *J Biol Chem* 1974;249:3061.

[5] Joubert FJ. *Int J Biochem* 1983;15(8):1033.

[6] Sandvig K, et al. *J Biol Chem* 1976;251:3977.

[7] Lin JY, et al. *Toxicon* 1973;11:379.

[8] Fodstad O, Pihl A. *Int J Cancer* 1978;22:558.

[9] Chen CC, et al. *Taiwan I Hsueh Hui Tsa Chih* 1976;75:239.

[10] Wambebe C, Amosun SL. *J Ethnopharmacol* 1984;11:49.

[11] Hardin JW, Arena JM. Human Poisoning from Native and Cultivated Plants, ed 2. Durham, NC: Duke University Press, 1974.

[12] Sullivan G, Chavez PI. *Vet Hum Toxicol* 1981;23:259.

[13] Duke JA. Handbook of Medicinal Herbs. Boca Raton, FL: CRC Press, 1985.

[14] Godal A, et al. *J Toxicol Environ Health* 1981;8:409.

[15] Barri MES, et al. *Vet Hum Toxicol* 1990;32(6):541.

Prickly Pear

SCIENTIFIC NAME(S): *Opuntia tuna mill* (tuna) and *Opuntia ficus-indica* (barbary fig, Indian fig). Other species include: *Opuntia fragilis* (brittle prickly pear), *Opuntia streptacantha*.

COMMON NAME(S): Prickly pear, Nopal

BOTANY: Prickly pear is a perennial cactus native to tropical America and Mexico, preferring a dry habitat and rocky soil. It can grow to approximately 3 m high. The round stems (pads) have a thorny skin covered in spines. Prickly pear flowers are yellow. The oval, pear-shaped, purplish fruit has prickly outer skin with a sweet inner pulp.[1,2,3,4]

HISTORY: Prickly pear has been used as a food source (conserves) and for alcoholic drinks in Mexico for hundreds of years. Native Americans have applied the pads to wounds and bruises.[2,5]

CHEMISTRY: Older studies concerning certain enzyme studies from *Opuntia* species are available.[6,7,8,9] Constituents of *O. fragilis* have been identified.[10] Later studies discuss the chemistry of various *Opuntia* species, including isolation of albumin from *O. ficus-indica*,[11] amino acid composition (including taurine) in *O. ficus-indica* fruits,[12] and fatty acid evaluation in 3 varieties from *O. ficus-indica* seeds.[13] Prickly pear fruit is high in nutritional value. Analysis of pulp, skin, and seeds reveals high amounts of calcium, potassium, and carbohydrates.[14] Other reported nutrients include vitamin C, iron, and phosphorus.[4,15] Mucilage, sugars, and other fruit acids are also found in the fruit.[2] Flavonoids, isorhamnetin-glucoside, kaempferol, luteolin, penduletin, piscidic acids, quercetrin, rutin, and beta-sitosterol have been found in *O. ficus-indica* flowers.[3]

PHARMACOLOGY:

Nutrition: Prickly pear fruit is nutritious.[2,14] The cactus pads are used in a variety of cooking preparations, including soups and salads. The taste has been compared with green beans or asparagus, with the sticky mucilage similar to okra.[5] Prickly pear fruit liquid has been studied as a natural sweetener.[16]

Dermatologic effects: Prickly pear cactus flowers have been used as an astringent for wounds and for their healing effects on the skin.[3] The cactus pads have been used for medicinal purposes (mainly by Indian tribes in Mexico and the southwestern US) as a poultice for rash, sunburn, burns, insect bites, minor wounds, hemorrhoids, earaches, and asthmatic symptoms.[17]

GI effects: The pectins and mucilage from the plant are beneficial to the digestive system. The flowers are used for GI problems such as diarrhea, colitis, and irritable bowel syndrome.[2] *Opuntia* has been studied as a dietary fiber source.[18] *O. ficus-indica* species extracts exhibit protective effects on gastric mucosa and exert an anti-inflammatory action.[19] Anti-inflammatory actions have also been demonstrated in species *O. dillenii* in induced rat paw edema.[20]

Lipid effects: Raw *O. ficus-indica* plant had potentially beneficial effects in hypercholesterolemic parameters in rats.[21] A pectin isolate from *Opuntia* decreased LDL metabolism in guinea pigs.[22,23,24] However, *Opuntia* in capsule form in a human trial had only a marginal beneficial effect on cholesterol and glucose levels.[25]

Hypoglycemic effects: *Opuntia* species have been studied for these effects.[26,27,28] Several reports demonstrate specifically species *O. streptacantha* as having hypoglycemic actions in animal and human studies.[29,30,31,32] *O. fuliginosa* extract has controlled induced diabetes in rats.[33] *O. megacantha* has reduced blood glucose levels in rats but was also shown to be nephrotoxic.[34]

Antiviral actions: One study reports *O. streptacantha* as having antiviral actions in animals and humans.[35]

TOXICOLOGY: Dermatitis from the plant was the most common toxicity found in current literature searches on prickly pear. A case report of cactus dermatitis in a 2-year-old child was described after contact with *O. microdasys*.[36] Two other patients were affected by this same species, both experiencing dermatitis, and one developing severe keratoconjunctivitis in the right eye.[37] A case of cactus granuloma in a 24-year-old male is described from contact with *O. bieglovii* thorns.[38] Granuloma formation has also been seen from *O. acanthocarpa* spines embedded in the dermis with onset occurring within several days and lasting several months. Treatment with topical corticosteroids has been recommended.[39]

Side effects may include exacerbation of hypoglycemia if combined with oral hypoglycemic agents.

Other toxicities include the following: *O. streptacantha* is nontoxic in mice, horses, and humans in oral and IV preparations;[35] *O. megacantha* is nephrotoxic, as described in 1 report in rats.[34]

SUMMARY: Prickly pear is a cactus native to tropical America and Mexico. It has been a source of food and drink for hundreds of years by Native Americans. The fruit is high in nutritional value. The flowers have been used to treat wounds, as have the cactus pads. Application of the pads to rashes, burns, and other wounds appears to be beneficial. Certain *Opuntia* species may also be of use in GI disorders and to lower cholesterol and glucose levels. Dermatitis is the most common toxicity associated with the plant and its spines.

PATIENT INFORMATION – Prickly Pear

Uses: Prickly pear has been used to treat wounds, GI complaints, lipid disorders, and diabetes.

Side Effects: Dermatitis may be the most common side effect from prickly pear. *O. megacantha* has been shown to be nephrotoxic in rat studies. Side effects may include exacerbation of hypoglycemia if combined with oral hypoglycemic agents.

---

[1] Hocking G. A Dictionary of Natural Products. Medford, NJ: Plexis Publishing, Inc., 1997:546-47.

[2] Chevallier A. The Encyclopedia of Medicinal Plants. New York, NY: DK Publishing, 1996:240.

[3] D'Amelio F. Botanicals (A Phytocosmetic Desk Reference). Boca Raton, FL: CRC Press, 1999:71.

[4] Ensminger A, et al. Foods & Nutrition Encyclopedia. Boca Raton, FL: CRC Press, 1994, 2nd ed, vol 2:1856.

[5] http://www.desertusa.com/magdec97/eating/nopales.html

[6] Mukerji S, et al. Malate dehydrogenase (decarboxylating) (NADP) isoenzymes of *Opuntia* stem tissue. Mitochondrial, chloroplast, and soluble forms. *Biochim Biophys Acta* 1968;167(2):239-49.

[7] Mukerji S, et al. Malic dehydrogenase isoenzymes in green stem tissue of *Opuntia* isolation and characterization. *Arch Biochem Biophys* 1969;131(2):336-51.

[8] Sisini A. [On glucose-6-phosphate isomerase in *Opuntia ficus indica*.] *Boll Soc Ital Biol Sper* 1969;45(12):794-96.

[9] Bhatia D, et al. Histochemical studies in stomatal apparatus of *Phaseolus mungo* Linn, *Lathyrus sativus* Linn and *Opuntia elatior* Mill. *Folia Histochem Cytochem (Krakow)* 1977;15(4):315-32.

[10] Abramovitch R, et al. Identification of constituents of *Opuntia fragilis*. *Planta Med* 1968;16(2):147-57.

[11] Uchoa A, et al. Isolation and characterization of a reserve protein from the seeds of *Opuntia ficus-indica* (Cactaceae). *Braz J Med Biol Res* 1998;31(6):757-61.

[12] Stintzing F, et al. Amino acid composition and betaxanthin formation in fruits from *Opuntia ficus-indica*. *Planta Med* 1999;65(7):632-35.

[13] Barbagallo R, et al. Determination of fatty acids in oil from seeds of *Opuntia ficus-indica* L. (Miller). *Ind Aliment* 1999;38(383):815-17.

[14] El Kossori R, et al. Composition of pulp, skin and seeds of prickly pears fruit (*Opuntia ficus indica* sp.). *Plant Foods Hum Nutr* 1998;52(3):263-70.

[15] http://oac3.uth.tmc.edu/pub_affairs/mm/cactus.html.

[16] Saenz C, et al. Cactus pear fruit: A new source for a natural sweetner. *Plant Foods Hum Nutr* 1998;52(2):141-49.

[17] http://www.arizonacactus.com/medicine.htm

[18] Rosado J, et al. [Physico-chemical properties related to gastrointestinal function of 6 sources of dietary fiber.] *Rev Invest Clin* 1995;47(4):283-99.

[19] Park E, et al. Studies on the pharmacological action of cactus: Identification of its anti-inflammatory effect. *Arch Pharm Res* 1998;21(1):30-34.

[20] Loro J, et al. Preliminary studies of analgesic and anti-inflammatory properties of *Opuntia dillenii* aqueous extract. *J Ethnopharmacol* 1999;67(2):213-18.

[21] Cardenas M, et al. [Effect of raw and cooked nopal (*Opuntia ficus indica*) ingestion on growth and profile of total cholesterol, lipoproteins, and blood glucose in rats.] *Arch Latinoam Nutr* 1998;48(4):316-23.

[22] Fernandez M, et al. Pectin isolated from prickly pear (*Opuntia* sp.) modifies low density lipoprotein metabolism in cholesterol-fed guinea pigs. *J Nutr* 1990;120(11):1283-90.

[23] Fernandez M, et al. Prickly pear (*Opuntia* sp.) pectin alters hepatic cholesterol metabolism without affecting cholesterol absorption in guinea pigs fed a hypercholesterolemic diet. *J Nutr* 1994;124(6):817-24.

[24] Fernandez M, et al. Prickly pear (*Opuntia* sp.) pectin reverses low density lipoprotein receptor suppression induced by a hypercholesterolemic diet in guinea pigs. *J Nutr* 1992;122(12):2330-40.

[25] Frati Munari A, et al. [Evaluation of nopal capsules in diabetes mellitus.] *Gac Med Mex* 1992;128(4):431-36.

[26] Roman-Ramos R, et al. Experimental study of the hypoglycemic effect of some antidiabetic plants. *Arch Invest Med (Mex)* 1991;22(1):87-93.

[27] Ibanez-Camacho R, et al. Hypoglycemic effect of *Opuntia* cactus. *Arch Invest Med (Mex)* 1979;10(4):223-30.

[28] Frati-Munari A, et al. Decreased blood glucose and insulin by nopal (*Opuntia* sp.). *Arch Invest Med (Mex)* 1983;14(3):269-74.

[29] Frati A, et al. Acute hypoglycemic effect of *Opuntia streptacantha* Lemaire in NIDDM. *Diabetes Care* 1990;13(4):455-56.

[30] Frati-Munari A, et al. [Activity of *Opuntia streptacantha* in healthy individuals with induced hyperglycemia.] *Arch Invest Med (Mex)* 1990;21(2):99-102.

[31] Frati A, et al. The effect of two sequential doses of *Opuntia streptacantha* upon glycemia. *Arch Invest Med (Mex)* 1991;22(3-4):333-36.

[32] Roman-Ramos R, et al. Anti-hyperglycemic effect of some edible plants. *J Ethnopharmacol* 1995;48(1):25-32.

[33] Trejo-Gonzalez A, et al. A purified extract from prickly pear cactus (*Opuntia fuliginosa*) controls experimentally induced diabetes in rats. *J Ethnopharmacol* 1996;55(1):27-33.

[34] Bwititi P, et al. Effects of *Opuntia megacantha* on blood glucose and kidney function in streptozotocin diabetic rats. *J Ethnopharmacol* 2000;69(3):247-52.

[35] Ahmad A, et al. Antiviral properties of extract of *Opuntia streptacantha*. *Antiviral Res* 1996;30(2-3):75-85.

[36] Vakilzadeh F, et al. [Cactus dermatitis.] *Z Hautkr* 1981;56(19):1299-301.

[37] Whiting D, et al. Dermatitis and keratoconjunctivitis caused by a prickly pear (*Opuntia microdasys*). *S Afr Med J* 1975;49(35):1445-48.

[38] Suzuki H, et al. Cactus granuloma of the skin. *J Dermatol* 1993;20(7):424-7.

[39] Spoerke D, et al. Granuloma formation induced by spines of the cactus, *Opuntia acanthocarpa*. *Vet Hum Toxicol* 1991;33(4):342-44.

Propolis

SCIENTIFIC NAME(S): *Propolis balsam, propolis resin, propolis wax*

COMMON NAME(S): Propolis, bee glue, hive dross

BOTANY: Propolis is a natural resinous product collected from the buds of conifers and used by honeybees to fill cracks in their hives.[1] It is a sticky mass that is greenish brown in color with a slight aromatic odor and is important in the defense of the hive.[2]

HISTORY: Propolis displays strong antimicrobial activity and has been used as a chemotherapeutic agent since ancient times.[3] Its use was found in folk medicine as early as 300 B.C. for medical and cosmetic purposes, as well as an anti-inflammatory drug and wound healing agent.[4,5,6] More recently, it has been reported to possess versatile biologic activity as an antibacterial, antiviral, fungicidal, local anesthetic, anti-ulcer, anti-inflammatory, immunostimulant, hypotensive and cytostatic properties in vitro.[7,8] Proponents of the use of propolis suggest that it stimulates the immune system, thereby raising the body's natural resistance to infection.[1] It has been advocated for both internal and external use.

CHEMISTRY: The composition of propolis continues to be elucidated and appears to vary with its vegetation source. The alcohol extract of the resin is called propolis wax; the residue is called propolis resin. Extraction of the resin with hot petroleum ether is called propolis balsam. Propolis contains 50% resin and vegetable balsam, 30% wax, 10% essential and aromatic oils, 5% pollen and 5% other substances (minerals).[9] Several flavonoids have been isolated and may be responsible for its antibacterial and fungicidal effects.[8] The flavonoids pinocembrin, galangin and pinobanksin, in addition to p-coumaric acid benzyl ester and caffeic acid phenethyl ester (CAPE), demonstrate antimicrobial activity.[1] The extract contains amino acids, flavonoids, terpenes and cinnamic acid derivatives.[10] The water extract also contains lectin.[11] Propolis balsam is described as having a hyacinth-like odor due to its cinnamyl alcohol content.

PHARMACOLOGY: Romanian and other Eastern European researchers have published numerous reports of successful clinical trials in which propolis was given to aid wound healing and to treat tuberculosis, fungal and bacterial infections.[12] More recently, Western researchers have investigated the antibacterial properties of this material. Propolis was active in vitro against some gram-positive bacterial and tubercle bacillus; it also demonstrated limited activity against gram-negative bacilli. Some propolis flavonoids have demonstrated antiviral activity in vitro.[13] Propolis inhibits bacterial growth of *Streptococcus agalactiae* by preventing cell division as well as disorganizing the cytoplasm, cytoplamsic membrane and the cell wall. It also causes a partial bacteriolysis and inhibits protein synthesis.[14] None of the chemical constituents, however, are as effective as anti-infective agents in vitro as streptomycin, chloramphenicol, oxytetracycline, nystatin and griseofulvin.[15,16] No antibacterial activity was observed in the urine of three volunteers who ingested propolis 500 mg 3 times a day for 3 days.[16]

Ethanolic and aqueous extracts of propolis indicate anti-inflammatory and antibiotic activities in vitro and in vivo. The exact mechanism for these effects is not clear. An aqueous extract of propolis has been shown to inhibit the enzyme dihydrofolate reductase. This activity may be partially due to the content of caffeic acid in propolis. This may explain some of the protective functions of propolis, similar to those shown for several nonsteroidal anti-inflammatory drugs (NSAIDs).[17]

A 13% aqueous extract of propolis was tested orally in three doses (1, 5 and 10 ml/kg) on the carrageenan rat paw edema model and on adjuvant-induced arthritis in rats. The extract showed potent dose-related anti-inflammatory activity comparable to diclofenac (as the reference standard).[10] Diethyl ether extracts of propolis were shown to possess cytostatic activity against cultured human KB (nasopharynx carcinoma) and HeLa (carcinoma cervicis uteri) cells in vitro.[7] Ethanolic extracts resulted in a 55% survival rate for mice bearing Ehrlich carcinoma and compared well with a 40% survival rate after bleomycin therapy. The investigators noted; however, an interaction between the agents that resulted in a reduction in survival rate when used as a combination therapy.[18] The ethanolic extracts have also been shown to accerlerate bone formation, regenerate tissue and induce some enzyme systems in vitro.[1]

The effect of the active component of propolis, caffeic acid phenethyl ester (CAPE), was studied on the growth and antigenic phenotype of a human melanoma cell line (HO-1) and a human glioblastoma multiforme cell line (GBM-18). The growth of both cell lines was suppressed by CAPE in a dose-dependent way, with HO-1 cells being more sensitive than GBM-1 cells. The results suggest a potential role for CAPE as an antitumor agent.[19]

Another study explored whether CAPE inhibits the tumor promoter processes associated with carcinogenesis. The treatment of SENCAR mice with very low doses of CAPE (0.1–6.5 nmol/topical treatment) strongly inhibits the oxidative processes that are essential for tumor promotion. The findings show CAPE as a potent chemopreventive agent, which may be useful in combating diseases with strong inflammatory or oxidative stress components.[6]

Propolis extracts also possess weak free radical scavenging characteristics.[20] This activity has been associated with an extended longevity among mice that had been pretreated with propolis and exposed to high doses of radiation.[21]

Propolis was studied in albino rats of various ages with toxic liver damage of various duration. The drug was found to have moderate antioxidative properties (30% to 60%) and showed improvements in the hepatic secretion of bile, cholic acids and cholesterol. However, the membrane-stabilizing effect of the drug was not exerted in all models.[22]

Ethanolic extracts of two propolis types showed a similar scavenging action against the different species of generated oxygen radicals. The antioxidative properties of propolis may be attributed to their free radical scavenging activity against alkoxy radicals.[23]

Activity tests prove the high antioxidative and inhibitory capacities of propolis in vitro. Experiments documented the photodynamic quenching properties of propolis extracts.[4] Topical application of propolis extract to dental sockets have been shown to enhance epithelial growth.[24] Propolis decreases dental caries of rats infected with *Streptococcus sobrinus* 6715.[2] Propolis prepared as a mouth rinse aids repair of intra-buccal surgical wounds and exerts a small pain-killing and anti-inflammatory effect on patients who underwent sulcoplasty.[25]

TOXICOLOGY: While reports of toxicity are rare, propolis has long been recognized by apiary workers as being a potent skin sensitizer. Several cases of propolis-induced dermatitis have been reported. These have occurred after the topical use of cosmetics containing propolis and, in one case, after the application of a 10% alcoholic propolis solution for the treatment of genital herpes.[26] Acute oral mucositis with ulceration following the use of propolis-containing lozenges has also been reported.[27]

SUMMARY: Propolis is employed in a variety of topical and systemic preparations. Claims range from the treatment of wounds to improvement of the immune response. A number of in vitro investigations have found a variety of activities to be associated with propolis. Significant studies have shown the anti-inflammatory, antitumor and antioxidant effects of propolis. These three capacities of the drug may contribute significantly to the medical field in the future. However, more studies are needed to confirm these effects.

PATIENT INFORMATION – Propolis

Uses: Studies have shown that propolis has anti-inflammatory, antitumor, and antioxidant effects.

Side Effects: Propolis has been reported to cause propolis-induced dermatitis and acute oral mucositis with ulceration.

---

[1] Tyler VE. The New Honest Herbal. Philadelphia: G.F. Stickley Co., 1987.
[2] Ikeno K, et al. *Caries Res* 1991;25(5):347.
[3] Higashi KO, de Castro SL. *J Ethnopharmacol* 1994;43(2):149.
[4] Volpert R, Elstner EF. *Z Naturforsch* 1993;48(11–12):858.
[5] Volpert R, Elstner EF. *Z Naturforsch* 1993;48(11–12):851.
[6] Frenkel K, et al. *Cancer Res* 1993;53(6):1255.
[7] Hladon B, et al. *Arzneim-Forsch* 1980;30(11):1847.
[8] Bankova VS, et al. *J Nat Prod* 1983;46(4):471.
[9] Metzner J, Schneidewind EM. *Pharmazie* 1978;33(7):465.
[10] Khayyal MT, et al. *Drugs Exp Clin Res* 1993;19(5):197.
[11] Dumitrescu M, et al. *Rev Roum Virol* 1993;44(1–2):49.
[12] New Research in Apitherapy. Second International Symposium of Apitherapy. September 2–7, 1976; Bucharest, Romania. Bucharest, Romania: Apimondia Press, 1976.
[13] Debiaggi M, et al. *Microbiologica* 1990;13(3):207.
[14] Takaisi-Kikuni NB, Schilcher H. *Planta Medica* 1994;60(3):222.
[15] Metzner J, et al. *Pharmazie* 1979;34:97.
[16] Brumfitt W, et al. *Microbios* 1990;62(250):19.
[17] Strehl E, et al. *Z Naturforsch* 1994;49(1–2):39.
[18] Scheller S, et al. *Z Naturforsch* 1989;44:(11–12):1063.
[19] Guarini L, et al. *Cell Mol Biol* 1992;38(5):513.
[20] Scheller S, et al. *Int J Radiat Biol* 1990;57(3):461.
[21] Scheller S, et al. *Z Naturforsch* 1989;44(11–12):1049.
[22] Drogovoz SM, et al. *Eksperi Klin Farmakologiia* 1994;57(4):39.
[23] Pascual C, et al. *J Ethnopharmacol* 1994;41(1–2):9.
[24] Magro-Filho O, de Carvalho AC. *J Nihon Univ Sch Dent* 1990;32(1):4.
[25] Magro-Filho O, de Carvalho AC. *J Nihon Univ Sch Dent* 1994;36(2):102.
[26] Pincelli C, et al. *Contact Derm* 1984;11(1):49.
[27] Hay KD, Greig DE. *Oral Surg Oral Med Oral Pathol* 1990;70(5):584.

Pycnogenol

SOURCE: The name "pycnogenol" is in itself a source of confusion. In product literature, this term is a trademark of a British company for a proprietary mixture of water-soluble bioflavonoids, presumably derived from the bark of the European coastal pine, *Pinus maritima* (also known as *P. nigra* var. maritima, a widely planted variety of pine in Europe).

However, pycnogenol has also been assigned to a group of flavonoids termed the flavan-3-ol derivatives.[1] Numerous plants have been found to be sources for the class of compounds generally termed the flavonoids, and the chemical condensation of flavonoid precursors results in the formation of compounds known as condensed tannins. The broader term, bioflavonoid, has been used to designate those flavonoids with biologic activity.

HISTORY: Pycnogenol is now available commercially over the counter in the United States in health-food stores and pharmacies. Product literature indicates that pycnogenol, when taken as a dietary supplement, is a powerful free radical scavenger. The compound may improve circulation, reduce inflammation and protect collagen from natural degradation. Pycnogenol has been available in Europe for some time, where it is taken as a supplement or incorporated into topical "anti-aging" creams.

CHEMISTRY: Pycnogenol appears to be a mixture of bioflavonoids designated proanthocyanidins. In some studies, pycnogenol-related compounds are designated procyanidol oligomers (PCO).[2]

PHARMACOLOGY: A US patent for this material describes a mixture of proanthocyanidins that are effective in combating the deleterious effects of free radicals. The compound is said to assist in the treatment of hypoxia following atherosclerosis, cardiac or cerebral infarction, and to reduce tumor promotion, inflammation, ischemia, alterations of synovial fluid and collagen degradation.

Several studies have been conducted in Europe to evaluate the pharmacologic activity of pycnogenol. In one study, daily oral doses of pycnogenol were given for 30 days to patients with a variety of peripheral circulatory disorders. Pain, limb heaviness and feeling of swelling decreased significantly during therapy in most patients.[3] Similar results have been reported by other investigators.[4]

PCO has been shown to bind to skin elastic fibers when injected intradermally to young rabbits. As a result, these connective fibers became highly resistant to degradation by elastases injected into the same tissue. These preliminary data suggest that some connective tissues may be protected from enzymatic degradation by procyanidol oligomers.[2]

TOXICOLOGY: No significant reports of adverse effects from pycnogenol specifically have been published.

SUMMARY: Pycnogenol appears to be a mixture of water-soluble bioflavonoids derived from a European species of pine. Preliminary animal and clinical data suggest that the oral ingestion of pycnogenol may be beneficial in the management of peripheral vascular diseases and inflammatory collagen diseases.

PATIENT INFORMATION – Pycnogenol

Uses: Pycnogenol is said to assist in the treatment of hypoxia following atherosclerosis, cardiac or cerebral infarction, reduce tumor promotion, inflammation, ischemia, alteration of synovial fluid and collagen degradation.

Side Effects: There are no reported side effects.

---

[1] Masquelier J, et al. Flavonoids and pycnogerols. *Int J Vitam Nutr Res* 1979;49:307.
[2] Tixier JM, et al. *Biochem Pharmacol* 1984;33:3933.
[3] Sarrat L. *Bordeaux Medical* 1981;14:685.
[4] Mollmann H, Rohdewald P. *Therapiewoche* 1983;33:4967.

Pygeum

SCIENTIFIC NAME(S): *Pygeum africanum* Hook. f., or *Prunus africana* (Hook. f.) Kalkm. (Rosaceae)

COMMON NAME(S): Pygeum, African plum tree

BOTANY: Pygeum is an evergreen tree native to African forest regions. It can grow to 150 feet in height. The thick leaves are oblong in shape; the flowers are small and white. Pygeum fruit is a red berry, resembling a cherry when ripe. The bark (red, brown or gray) is the part of the plant used for medicinal purposes. It has a "hydrocyanic acid"-like odor.[1,2,3]

HISTORY: The hard wood of pygeum is valued in Africa and is often used to make wagons.[1] Powdered pygeum bark is used by African natives to treat urinary problems.[1,3]

CHEMISTRY: The major bark components are fat soluble compounds. Triterpenes are present (14%), including ursolic, oleanolic and crataegolic acids. The lipid fraction contains fatty acids, which are 12 to 24 carbons in length. The ferulic acid esters are those bound to n-tetracosanol and n-docosanol.[3] N-docosanol has been used in some patent medicines.[4] Phytosterols present in pygeum include beta-sitosterol, beta-sitosterone and campesterol.[1,2,3,5] Tannins have also been found in the plant.[1]

PHARMACOLOGY: In France, *Pygeum africanum* extract (PAE) has become the primary course of **treatment for enlarged prostate**. In contrast, surgery is the main option in other Western countries.[1] Drugs used to alleviate symptoms of benign prostatic hypertrophy (BPH) (or hyperplasia) include anticholinergics, muscle relaxants, calcium antagonists, prostaglandin inhibitors, beta-agonists, tricyclic antidepressants and alpha blockers.[6] Pygeum clinical trials (mostly European), are encouraging, but more research is needed in the United States. Usual dosage of PAE is 100 mg/day in 6- to 8-week cycles.[2] The highest activity is found in the lipophilic extracts of the plant. Dosage of these extracts are standardized to contain 14% triterpenes and 0.5% n-docosanol.[3]

Most trial results report improvement of BPH symptoms. Reduction in gland size and other parameters occur, but are not as profound.[3] Pygeum is also therapeutic as an **anti-inflammatory**, to **increase prostatic secretions** and to **decrease certain hormones** in the glandular area, which reduces the hypertrophy. Other actions of pygeum include **increase in bladder elasticity** and **histological modifications** of glandular cells.[2]

PAE has had positive results in animal "hypophyseo-genito-adrenal axis" and prostatic adenoma.[7,8] Pretreatment of rabbits with pygeum reduces partial outlet obstruction in bladder dysfunction secondary to BPH.[9]

In human trials, symptomatic relief from BPH using PAE has been documented.[10-17] The extract, in combination with mepartricin, was successful in treating urinary symptomatology in 22 subjects with varying stages of prostatic adenoma.[12] In a 74-patient study, extracts of both pygeum and testosterone alleviated obstructive bladder symptoms caused by BPH.[13] Using PAE, nocturnal frequency, difficulty in initiation of urination and bladder fullness were three parameters improved over placebo in 60 patients.[14] In a placebo controlled, double-blind, multicenter evaluation, pygeum capsules (50 mg) were given twice daily for 60 days. Out of 263 patients in eight locations, 66% (vs 31% placebo) showed marked clinical improvement in micturitional disorders.[15] High dose PAE (200 mg/day) administered to 18 patients for 60 days improved both urinary symptoms and sexual behavior in another report.[16] PAE in combination with *Urtica dioica* in half doses was found to be as safe and effective as full doses (300 mg urtica and 25 mg PAE) in treating urine flow, residual urine and nycturia.[17]

Gland size reduction has also been reported for pygeum. PAE was found to be a potent inhibitor of rat prostatic fiberblast proliferation.[18] The extract also displays anti-inflammatory activity, which may affect gland size. It has been demonstrated that macrophages (inflammatory cells) produce chemotactic mediators that worsen BPH development. In one recent report, the proposed mechanism is that pygeum antagonizes 5-lipoxygenase metabolite production (in vitro), which decreases inflammation.[19]

Pygeum may help reverse sterility, which can be caused by insufficient prostatic secretions.[1] PAE has increased prostate secretions in both rats and humans.[20] It has also been shown to improve seminal fluid composition.[1] By improving an underlying problem, PAE may improve sexual function.[3,16]

When compared with saw palmetto in a double-blind trial, it was demonstrated that saw palmetto produced greater reduction of symptoms and was better tolerated; however, PAE may have greater effects on prostate secretion.[3]

The ferulic acid ester components are responsible for pygeum's endocrine system activity. N-docosanol reduces LH, testosterone and prolactin levels. This is important because accumulation of testosterone within the prostate (and subsequent conversion to the more potent form) is believed to be a major factor in prostatic hyperplasia. PAE's "phyto-estrogenic" action markedly reduces volume of prostatic hypertrophy.[21] Fat soluble components reduce cholesterol content within the prostate as well, decreasing accumulation of cholesterol metabolites.[3]

TOXICOLOGY: In human trials, a low incidence of toxicity has been demonstrated as well. No side effects were reported in 18 patients taking 200 mg/day of pygeum for 60 days.[16] Gastrointestinal irritation ranging from nausea to severe stomach pain has been documented but with only a small percentage discontinuing therapy.[3] In 263 patients, GI adverse effects occurred in five patients with only three patients having to stop treatment.[15] It is recommended that pygeum be taken only under professional supervision.[1]

SUMMARY: Pygeum bark has been used by African natives to treat urinary problems. In France, it is the main course of treatment for BPH. Most activity from the plant is found in the lipophilic extracts. Pygeum extract has decreased the incidence of many clinical symptoms of BPH including urine flow, difficulty in starting micturition and other bladder symptomatology. Pygeum may also play a role in anti-inflammation and cell proliferation inhibition in the gland area. Pygeum has increased prostate secretions and may improve sexual function. The extract also acts on the endocrine system, reducing certain hormones known to enlarge the gland. Pygeum has a low toxicity profile.

PATIENT INFORMATION – Pygeum

Uses: Pygeum has been used to improve symptoms of benign prostatic hypertrophy and to improve sexual function. Usual dosage is 100 mg/day in 6- to 8-week cycles.

Side Effects: GI irritation has been reported with the use of pygeum.

---

[1] Chevallier A. Encyclopedia of Medicinal Plants. New York, NY: DK Publishing 1996;257.
[2] Bruneton J. Pharmacognosy, Phytochemistry. Medicinal Plants Paris, France: Lavoisier Publishing 1995;142.
[3] Murray M. The Healing Power of Herbs. Rocklin, CA: Prima Publishing 1995;286-93
[4] Pierini N, et al. Boll Chim Farm 1982;121(1):27-34.
[5] Longo R, et al. Farmaco 1983;38(7):287-92.
[6] Dagues F, et al. Rev Prat 1995;45(3):337-41.
[7] Thieblot L, et al. Therapie 1971;26(3):575-80.
[8] Thieblot L, et al. Therapie 1977;32(1):99-110
[9] Levin R, et al. Eur Urol 1997;32 (Suppl 1):15-21.
[10] Bassi P, et al. Minerva Urol Nefrol 1987;39(1):45-50.
[11] Menchini-Fabris G, et al. Arch Ital Urol Nefrol Androl 1988;60(3):313-22.
[12] Casella G, et al. Arch Sci Med 1978;135(1):95-98.
[13] Flamm J, et al. Wien Klin Wochenschr 1979;91(18):622-27.
[14] DuFour B, et al. Ann Urol 1984;18(3):193-95.
[15] Barlet A, et al. Wien Klin Wochenschr 1990;102(22):667-73.
[16] Carani C, et al. Arch Ital Urol Nefrol Androl 1991;63(3):341-45.
[17] Krzeski T, et al. Clin Ther 1993;15(6):1011-20.
[18] Yablonsky F, et al. J Urol 1997;157(6):2381-87.
[19] Paubert-Braquet M. et al. J Lipid Mediat Cell Signal 1994;9(3):285-90.
[20] Clavert A, et al. Ann Urol 1986;20(5):341-43.
[21] Mathe G, et al. Biomed Pharmacother 1995;49(7-8):339-43.

Quassia

SCIENTIFIC NAME(S): Quassia is a collective term for two herbs: *Picrasma excelsa* and *Quassia amara* L. Family: Simaroubaceae.

COMMON NAME(S): Bitter wood, picrasma, Jamaican quassia (*Picrasma excelsa*), Surinam quassia, *Quassia amara*, Amara species, Amargo, Surinam wood, and ruda.

BOTANY: Surinam quassia is a 2-to-5 meter tall shrub or small tree native to northern South America, specifically Guyana, Colombia, Panama, and Argentina. Jamaican quassia is a taller tree, reaching 25 meters, native to the Caribbean Islands, Jamaica, West Indies, and northern Venezuela. The pale yellow wood parts are used medicinally. Leaves are also used.[1,2,3]

HISTORY: Quassia has been used for malaria in the Amazon. It has also been used topically for measles, and orally or rectally for intestinal parasites, diarrhea, and fever. The plants at one time were also used as anthelmintics and insecticides. Central Americans have been known to build boxes to store clothing out of the quassia wood, which acts as a natural repellent.[1,3,4]

CHEMISTRY: Both quassia species have similar constituents. These include alkaloids (0.25%) such as canthin-6-one, 5-methoxycanthin-6-one, and carboline alkaloids. Terpenoids in one or both plants include isoquassin, mixtures of bitter principles (said to be 50 times more bitter than quinine), including quassin, neo-quassin, and 18-hydroxyquassin. Dihydronorneoquassin and simalikalactone D are also present. Other constituents include coumarins (*Q. amara*), thiamine (*P. excelsa*), B-sitosterol, and B-sitostenone.[1,2,3,4] From *Q. amara*, quassinoid quassimarin has been reported[5] and amarid 18-oxyquaxine has been isolated.[6] Nucleotide sequences of certain genes in *Q. amara* have been obtained.[7]

PHARMACOLOGY: Quassia has been used as an insecticide. Traditional use includes remedies for infestations of lice or worms, anorexia, and dyspepsia.[3] Certain tribes have used the plants for measles, fever, and as a mouthwash.[8,9,10]

Quassin demonstrates antilarval activity as well, being effective at concentrations of 6 ppm.[11] A mechanism of this larvicidal activity may be due to inhibition of cuticle development, as suggested in one report.[12] Quassia, as a tincture, has been used to successfully treat head lice in 454 patients. Canthin-6-one possesses antibacterial and antifungal activity.[3]

Quassimarin has been reported to have antileukemic properties when tested in animals. Antitumor activity in mice has been demonstrated, as has in vitro testing of quassin against human nasopharynx carcinoma.[3]

Quassin also displays antifertility effects, inhibiting testosterone secretion in rat Leydig cells.[13] Other changes include reduction in testis, epididymis, and seminal vesicle weight, reduction in sperm count, and decreased LH and FSH levels.[14]

The B-carboline alkaloids exhibit positive inotropic activity in animals.[3]

The extracts and purified mixtures of bitter principles ("quassin") have been used to give a bitter taste to various food products, especially alcoholic (eg, liqueurs and bitters) and nonalcoholic beverages, desserts, candy, baked goods, and puddings.[14]

TOXICOLOGY: Quassia is listed as generally regarded as safe (GRAS) by the FDA. No side effects were reported upon topical application of the scalp preparation in the 454 patients in the head lice study.[3] In doses of 250 to 1000 mg/kg, no signs of acute toxicity were observed in rats given quassia extract.[15] Large amounts, however, have been known to irritate the mucus membrane in the stomach and may lead to vomiting.[1] Excessive use may also interfere with existing cardiac and anticoagulant regimens. Due to the plant's cytotoxic and emetic properties, its use during pregnancy is best avoided.[3] Parenteral administration of quassin is toxic, leading to cardiac problems, tremors, and paralysis.[1]

SUMMARY: Quassia is a collective term for both *Picrasma excelsa* and *Quassia amara*. The plants have been used traditionally as anthelmintics, insecticides, and for malaria. They have been effective in treating head lice and also demonstrate antibacterial and antifungal actions. Quassia also possesses antifertility and antitumor actions. It is listed as a safe drug by the FDA, but in large doses may irritate the GI tract and cause vomiting. Use in pregnancy is not recommended. Low concentrations (about 0.007%) are used in bitter food and beverage formulations and sometimes as a flavoring substitute for quinine.

PATIENT INFORMATION – Quassia

Uses: Quassia has a variety of uses including treatment for measles, diarrhea, fever, and lice. Quassia has antibacterial, antifungal, antifertility, antitumor, antileukemic, and insecticidal actions as well.

Side Effects: Quassia is used in a number of food products and is considered to be safe by the FDA. If taken in large doses, this product can irritate the GI tract and cause vomiting. It is not recommended for women who are pregnant.

---

[1] Bisset NG. *Herbal Drugs and Phytopharmaceuticals.* Stuttgart: CRC Press, 1994;400-1.

[2] Schulz V, et al. *Rational Phytotherapy.* Berlin: Springer, 1998;171.

[3] Newall CA, et al. *Herbal Medicines.* London: Pharmaceutical Press, 1996;223-4.

[4] Duke JA. *CRC Handbook of Medicinal Herbs.* Boca Raton, FL: CRC Press, Inc., 1989;399.

[5] Kupchan SM, et al. Quassimarin, a new antileukemic quassinoid from *Quassia amara. J Org Chem* 1976; 41(21):3481-2.

[6] Casinovi C,. et al. A new amarid 18-oxyquaxine, isolated from *Quassia amara. Ann Ist Super Sanita* 1966;2(2):414-6.

[7] Fernando ES, et al. Rosid affinities of *Surianaceae*: molecular evidence. *Mol Phylogenet Evol* 1993;2(4):344–50.

[8] Rutter R. *Catalogo de Plantas Utiles de la Amazonia Peruana.* Yarinacocha, Peru: Instituto Linguistico de Verano, 1990.

[9] Branch L, et al. *Folk Medicine of Alter do Chao.* Para, Brazil: Acta Amazonica 1983; 13(5/6):737–97.

[10] Duke JA, et al. *Amazonian Ethnobotanical Dictionary.* Boca Raton, FL: CRC Press, Inc., 1994.

[11] Evans DA, et al. Larvicidal efficacy of Quassin against *Culex quinquefasciatus. Indian J Med Res* 1991; 93:324–7.

[12] Evans D, et al. Effect of quassin on the metabolism of catecholamines in different life cycle stages of *Culex quinquefasciatus. Indian J Biochem Biosphys* 1992; 29(4):360–63.

[13] Njar V, et al. Antifertility activity of *Quassia amara*: quassin inhibits the steroidogenesis in rat Leydig cells in vitro. *Planta Med* 1995; 61(2):180–2.

[14] Raji Y, et al. Antifertility activity of *Quassia amara* in male rats — in vivo study. *Life Sci* 1997; 61(11):1067–74

[15] Garcia Gonzales M, et al. Pharmacologic activity of the aqueous wood extract from *Quassia amara (Simarubaceae)* on albino rats and mice. *Rev Biol Trop* 1997; Mar.44-45;47-50. Spanish.

Quillaia

SCIENTIFIC NAME(S): *Quillaja saponaria* Molina. Family: Rosaceae

COMMON NAME(S): Quillaia, soapbark, soap tree, murillo bark, quillaja, Panama bark, China bark[1]

BOTANY: Quillaia is a large evergreen tree with shiny thick leaves. The generic name is derived from the Chilean word quillean, to wash, from the use made of the bark.[2] Although it is native to Chile and Peru, it is now widely cultivated in southern California. The inner bark is separated from the cork and collected for commercial use. It has an acrid, astringent taste.[2]

HISTORY: Quillaia has been used in traditional medicine to relieve cough and bronchitis, and topically to relieve scalp itchiness and dandruff.[1,3] The bark has been used by South Americans to aid in washing clothes.[3] Quillaia extracts are approved for food use and are used as foaming agents in some carbonated beverages and cocktail mixes. They are typically used in concentrations of about 0.01%.[1]

CHEMISTRY: Quillaia contains about 10% saponins.[2] These consist primarily of glycosides of quillaic acid (quillaja sapogenin, hydroxygypsogenin).[1,2] Quillaia saponin has been shown to be a mixture of acetylated triterpenoid oligoglycosides.[2] In addition, the bark contains tannin, calcium oxalate and numerous additional components.[1]

A highly purified saponin, designated QS-21, has been used as an adjuvant to enhance the activity of viral vaccines.[4] This saponin has been found to be a combination of two structural isomers.[5]

PHARMACOLOGY: The saponins derived from quillaia or its powdered bark can induce localized irritation and are also strong sneeze inducers.[1] Although the saponin is too irritating to the stomach and too strongly hemolytic to be ingested, it nevertheless has been shown to possess expectorant effects. The saponin depresses cardiac and respiratory activity.[1]

As noted above, a number of saponins have been derived from quillaia that serve as adjuvants when coadministered with certain vaccines. These saponins have been shown to boost antibody levels by 100-fold or more when used in the mouse.[6]

TOXICOLOGY: The effects of chronic low-low ingestion of quillaia are not well-defined. However, a short-term study in rats and long-term study in mice indicate that quillaia saponins are nontoxic.[1]

Quillaia saponin (sapotoxin) is reported to be highly toxic.[3] Severe toxic effects following the ingestion of large doses of the bark include liver damage, gastric pain, diarrhea, hemolysis, respiratory failure, convulsions and coma.[1] Digitalis may stabilize cardiac involvement.[3]

SUMMARY: Quillaia extracts are widely used to induce foaming in beverages. The saponins are responsible for this effect. However, quillaia saponins are generally considered to be highly toxic in high doses. Consequently, the traditional medical uses of quillaia have focused on its external application. Purified quillaia saponins have been shown to enhance the activity of certain vaccines in animals.

PATIENT INFORMATION – Quillaia

Uses: Reports show that quillaia can depress cardiac and respiratory activity and induce localized irritation and sneezing.

Side Effects: The ingestion of the quillaia bark results in liver damage, gastric pain, diarrhea, hemolysis, respiratory failure, convulsions, and coma.

---

[1] Leung AY. *Encyclopedia of Common Natural Ingredients Used in Food, Drugs and Cosmetics.* New York, NY: J. Wiley and Sons, 1980.
[2] Evans WC. *Trease and Evans' Pharmacognosy*, 13th ed. London: Balliere Tindall, 1989.
[3] Duke JA. *Handbook of Medicinal Herbs.* Boca Raton, FL: CRC Press, 1985.
[4] Kensil CR, et al. *J Am Vet Med Assoc* 1991;199:1423.
[5] Soltysik S, et al. *Ann N Y Acad Sci* 1993;690:392.
[6] Kensil CR, et al. *J Immunol* 1991;146:431.

Quinine

SCIENTIFIC NAME(S): *Cinchona succirubra* Pav. ex Klotsch (red cinchona), *C. calisya* Wedd. and *C. ledgeriana* Moens ex Trim. (yellow cinchona). Family: Rubiaceae

COMMON NAME(S): Red bark, Peruvian bark, Jesuit's bark, China bark, cinchona bark, quina-quina, fever tree

BOTANY: The cinchonas are evergreen shrubs and trees that grow to heights of 50 to 100 feet.[1] They are native to the mountainous areas of tropical Central and South America, including regions of Bolivia, Costa Rica and Peru. The oblong seed capsule is about 3 cm long and, when ripe, splits open at the base. Each capsule contains from 40 to 50 slender seeds that are so light that approximately 75,000 seeds equal one ounce.[2] In addition, these trees are found in Africa, South America and Southeast Asia.[1,3] At least one other genus (Remijia) of the same family has been reported to contain quinidine.[4]

HISTORY: The dried ground bark of the cinchona plant has been used for centuries for the treatment of malaria, fever, indigestion, mouth and throat diseases, and cancer.[1,2,3] The name cinchona is said to be derived from the Countess of Chinchon, the wife of a viceroy of Peru, who it was long believed was cured in 1638 from a fever by the use of the bark;[4] however, the story has been widely disputed. Formal use of the bark to treat malaria was established in the mid–1800s when the British began the worldwide cultivation of the plant[2] in order to assure the continuing availability, which was in danger of extinction in some regions due to overcultivation.[4]

Extracts of the bark have been used to treat hemorrhoids, to stimulate hair growth and to manage varicose veins. Quinine has been used as an abortifacient.[2] Extracts of cinchona have a bitter, astringent taste and have been used as flavoring for foods and beverages. Although the use of quinine for the treatment of malaria has been largely supplanted by treatment with semisynthetic anti-infectives, its use persists in some regions of the world.

CHEMISTRY: The typical cinchona bark contains about 16% of quinoline alkaloids consisting mainly of quinine, quinidine, cinchonine and cinchonidine. The primary component of this mixture is quinine. Quinidine is the dextrorotatory isomer of quinine. Approximately 35 additional minor compounds related to quinine have been identified in the plant.[1,2] As a rule the yellow cinchona has a higher alkaloid content than other varieties.

The cinchona alkaloids are extremely bitter tasting and concentrations in the 100 to 300 ppm range are used to flavor beverages such as tonic (quinine) water.

PHARMACOLOGY: Quinine is among the most potent of the cinchona alkaloids with respect to antimalarial activity,[1] although resistant strains of the pathogen have been identified. A second common use of quinine is for the treatment of leg cramps caused by vascular spasm.

Quinine is bacteriostatic, highly active in vitro against protozoa, and it inhibits the fermentation of yeast.[2] Both quinine and the related quinidine have cardiodepressant activity and the latter compound in particular is used for its anti-arrhythmic activity. Both quinine and quinidine are available as commercial products.[5] Quinine also has analgesic and antipyretic actions.[5]

A mixture of quinine and urea hydrochloride is injected as a sclerosing agent in the treatment of internal hemorrhoids, varicose veins and pleural cavities after thoracoplasty.[2]

TOXICOLOGY: Ground cinchona bark and quinine have been reported to cause urticaria, contact dermatitis and other hypersensitivity reactions in humans. These reactions also may occur in persons using topical preparations containing cinchona extracts or quinine.[2] The ingestion of these alkaloids can result in the clinical syndrome known as "cinchonism." Persons who are hypersensitive to these alkaloids also may develop the syndrome, which is characterized by severe headache, abdominal pain, convulsions, visual disturbances and blindness, auditory disturbances such as ringing in the ears, paralysis and collapse.[1]

Therapeutic doses of quinine have resulted in acute hemolytic anemia,[3] a limitation for its use in a small but significant portion of the population who are glucose-6-phosphate dehydrogenase (G-6-PD) deficient.[5]

Quinidine and related alkaloids are rapidly absorbed from the gastrointestinal tract, and a single 2 to 8 g oral dose of quinine may be fatal to an adult.[1,2,5]

Quinine use is discouraged during pregnancy due to fetal and abortifacient effects.[5] Treatment of overdose is generally supportive. Urinary acidification and renal dialysis can be employed if necessary.[5]

SUMMARY: Quinine and its related alkaloids have been used for more than 100 years for the treatment of malaria and associated febrile states. Other alkaloids possess antiarrhythmic activity. Chronic ingestion may lead to cinchonism, and hypersensitivity reactions have been observed.

PATIENT INFORMATION – Quinine

Uses: Quinine has been used for the treatment of leg cramps caused by vascular spasm, internal hemorrhoids, varicose veins and pleural cavities after thoracoplasty, malaria, and associated febrile states.

Side Effects: Quinine has been known to cause urticaria, contact dermatitis, and other hypersensitivity reactions.

---

[1] Leung AY. *Encyclopedia of Common Natural Ingredients Used in Food, Drugs, and Cosmetics.* New York, NY: J. Wiley and Sons, 1980.

[2] Morton JF. *Major Medicinal Plants.* Springfield, IL: C.C. Thomas Publisher, 1977.

[3] Duke JA. *Handbook of Medicinal Herbs.* Boca Raton, FL: CRC Press, 1985.

[4] Evans WC. *Trease and Evans' Pharmacognosy*, ed. 13. Philadelphia, PA: W.B. Saunders, 1989.

[5] Olin BR, Hebel SK, eds. *Drug Facts and Comparisons.* St. Louis, MO: Facts and Comparisons, 1993.

Raspberry

SCIENTIFIC NAME(S): *Rubus idaeus* L. and *Rubus strigosus* Michx. Family: Rosaceae (roses)

COMMON NAME(S): Red raspberry

BOTANY: The cultivated red raspberries *Rubus idaeus* (Eurasian) or *R. strigosus* (North American, also known as *R. idaeus* var. *strigosus*) are two of many *Rubus* species worldwide. While the berries are cultivated as food items, it is the leaves that have been used medicinally. Raspberries grow as brambles with thorny canes bearing three-toothed leaflets and stalked white flowers with five petals. The red berries detach easily from their cores when ripe. While some species of *Rubus* primarily reproduce clonally and commercial red raspberries are propagated as clones, DNA fingerprinting has indicated that wild *R. idaeus* populations exhibit substantial genetic diversity.[1]

HISTORY: The leaves of red raspberry were used for their astringent properties to treat diarrhea in the 19th century. A strong tea of raspberry leaves was used in painful or profuse menstruation and to regulate labor pains in childbirth.[2] The Eclectics used a decoction of the leaves to suppress nausea and vomiting. A gargle of raspberry leaf infusion has been used for sore throats and mouths and to wash wounds and ulcers.[3]

CHEMISTRY: While substantial effort has been devoted to the chemistry of raspberry fruit as a food item, relatively less has been published on the chemistry of the leaves. The principal compounds isolated from red raspberry leaves are hydrolyzable tannins. Simple compounds such as 1,2,6-tri-*O*-galloyl-glucose and penta-*O*-galloyl glucose[4] are oxidatively coupled through galloyl groups to form more complex compounds such as casuarictin, pendunculagin, sanguin H-6,[5] and lambertianin A,[6] with as many as 15 galloyl groups coupled to 3 glucose units.[7]

Common flavonoids have also been isolated from the leaves of raspberry. Rutin was isolated,[8] as were kaempferol, quercitin, quijaverin, and kaempferol-3-*O*-β-D-glucuronopyranoside.[9] Major leaf volatiles studied by GC-MS include the monoterpenes geraniol and linalool as well as 1-octane-3-ol and decanal.[10] Phenolic acids common to the Rosaceae family have also been identified.[11]

PHARMACOLOGY: The tannin components of the leaves have a definite astringent action,[12] which may be helpful in diarrhea or as a mouthwash; however, there is little pharmacologic evidence at present to support the use of raspberry leaf tea in pregnancy, menstruation, or childbirth. A preliminary study found fractions of raspberry leaf extract that stimulated and relaxed uterine muscle in pregnant rats, but this must be confirmed.[13] Blackberry (*R. strigosus*) leaves, which have similar chemistry to raspberry leaves, have been found to have a slight hypoglycemic activity in rabbit models; however, the chemistry responsible for this effect was not elucidated.[14,15]

TOXICOLOGY: There is no evidence that raspberry leaf tea is toxic.

A raspberry leaf monograph is included in the *British Herbal Pharmacopeia*, vol. 2.[16] It is listed as unapproved in the *German Commission E Monographs*.[17]

SUMMARY: Raspberry leaf tea is a source of hydrolyzable tannins, which have an astringent action. There is little pharmacology to support its wide use in pregnancy; however, it appears to be safe under normal conditions of use.

PATIENT INFORMATION – Raspberry

Uses: Raspberry leaves may be helpful for diarrhea or as a mouthwash because of their astringent action. They have been used historically in painful or profuse menstruation and to regulate labor pains in childbirth, but there is little evidence to support this use.

Side effects: There is no evidence that raspberry leaf tea is toxic.

[1] Antonius K, et al. DNA fingerprinting reveals significant amounts of genetic variation in a wild raspberry *Rubus idaeus* population. *Mol Ecol* 1994;3(2):177.

[2] Erichsen-Brown C. *Medicinal and Other Uses of North American Plants.* Dover, NY. 1989:471-73.

[3] Grieve M. *A Modern Herbal.* London, England: Jonathan Cape, 1931:671-72.

[4] Haddock E, et al. The metabolism of gallic acid and hexahydroxydiphenic acid in plants. Part I. Introduction. Naturally occurring galloyl esters. *J Chem Soc* 1982;11:2515.

[5] Nonaka G, et al. A dimeric hydrolyzable tannin, Sanguin H-6 from *Sanguisorba officinalis* L. *Chem Pharm Bull* 1982;30(6):2255.

[6] Tanaka T, et al. Tannins and related compounds. CXXII. New dimeric, trimeric and tetrameric ellagitannins, lambertianins A-D, from *Rubus lambertianus* Seringe. *Chem Pharm Bull* 1993;41(7):1214.

[7] Gupta R, et al. The metabolism of gallic acid and hexahydroxydiphenic acid in plants. Part 2. Esters of (S)-hexahydroxydiphenic acid with D-glucopyranose ($^4C_1$). *J Chem Soc* 1982;11:2525.

[8] Khabibullaeva L, et al. Phytochemical study of raspberry leaves. *Mater Yubileinoi Resp Nauchn Konf Farm* 1972;98. *Chem Abs* 1972;83:4960z.

[9] Gudej J, et al. Flavonoid compounds from the leaves of *Rubus idaeus* L. *Herba Pol* 1996;42(4):257.

[10] Maga J, et al. Bramble leaf volatiles. *Dev Food Sci* 1992;29:145.

[11] Krzaczek T. Phenolic acids in some tannin drugs from the Rosaceae family. *Farm Pol* 1984;40(8):475. CA 102:146198s.

[12] Haslam E, et al. Traditional herbal medicines — the role of polyphenols. *Planta Med* 1989;55:1.

[13] Briggs CJ, et al. Title unknown. *Can Pharm J* 1997:41.

[14] Alonso R, et al. A preliminary study of hypoglycemic activity of *Rubus fruticosus.* *Planta Med* 1980;(Suppl):102.

[15] Swanston-Flatt S, et al. Traditional plant treatments for diabetes. Studies in normal and streptozotocin diabetic mice. *Diabetologia* 1990;33(8):462.

[16] *British Herbal Pharmacopoeia.* Bournemouth, Dorset: British Herbal Medicine Association, 1990.

[17] Blumenthal M, et al. *The Complete German Commission E Monographs.* Austin, TX: American Botanical Council, 1998.

Red Bush Tea

SCIENTIFIC NAME(S): *Aspalathus linearis* (Burm. f.) R. Dahlgr. This plant is also referred to as *Borbonia pinifolia* Marloth or *Aspalathus contaminata* (Thunb.) Druce. Family: Leguminosae

COMMON NAME(S): Red bush tea, rooibos tea

BOTANY: Red bush grows as a low bush, attaining a height of 4 to 5 feet. It has long, needle-like leaves and small colorful flowers. The plant is native to South Africa and is cultivated extensively for its commercial value as a substitute for common tea. The leaves and twigs are collected, washed, bruised, fermented, dried, cut and packaged for use in preparing teas. During this procedure, the leaves change from green to brick red due to the release of a red pigment found in the leaves and stems.[1]

HISTORY: "Bush teas" are common throughout Africa and are frequently used as substitutes for common tea. Red bush tea has been popular in South Africa for decades, and commercial preparations are sometimes found in Europe and the US. One reason for the popularity of this tea is its almost total lack of physiologically active compounds. Consequently, red bush tea is selected as a fragrant, nonstimulating beverage.[2]

CHEMISTRY: Red bush tea is devoid of significantly active compounds. It contains no caffeine and is low in tannins (less than 5%). It contains a relatively high level of vitamin C (approximately 9.4%).[1,3]

PHARMACOLOGY: Red bush tea and its **protective** and **suppressive effects** have been studied. Suppression of mutagenic activity of "certain potent mutagens" has been performed in mice.[4] Oncogenic transformation of mouse cells induced by x-rays was suppressed in the presence of the tea extract. Suppression variability was dependent upon extract concentration and length of treatment time.[5] Prevention of age-related accumulation of lipid peroxides in rat brain has also been reported. Red bush tea's protective effects against CNS damage in certain brain areas have been additionally demonstrated.[6] Flavonoids contained in the tea show antioxidative qualities both in vitro and in vivo. Red bush tea's radioprotective effects may be due to a "free radical scavenging" mechanism.[7,8]

TOXICOLOGY: No reports have been identified regarding toxicity with this plant or its teas. A single article reports salmonella contamination from rooibos tea, possibly from lizard origin.[9]

SUMMARY: Red bush tea is a native African beverage that is also sold in Europe and the United States. It was found to have both protective and suppressive effects in animal studies. The mechanism may be due to the plant's ability to scavenge free radicals. More research is needed to further prove red bush tea's antimutagenic and CNS-protective effects. The plant appears to have a low toxicity profile, and the tea is a good option for those who wish to drink a mild, nonstimulating or sedating tea.

PATIENT INFORMATION – Red Bush Tea

Uses: Although no significantly active compounds exist in the leaves, red bush tea has a high vitamin C content. It is being investigated as an anti-cancer drug and as a prevention for brain damage caused by aging.

Side Effects: No reports have been identified regarding toxicity with red bush tea. There is one report of salmonella contamination from rooibos tea, possibly from lizard origin.

---

[1] Cheney RH, Scholtz E. *Economic Botany* 1963;17:186.
[2] Watt J, et al. *Medicinal and Poisonous Plants of Southern and Eastern Africa,* 2nd ed. London: E & S Livingstone Ltd, 1962.
[3] Tyler VA. *The New Honest Herbal.* Philadelphia, PA: GF Stickley Co., 1987.
[4] Sasaki Y, et al. *Mutation Research* 1993;286(2):221–32.
[5] Komatsu K, et al. *Cancer Letters* 1994;77(1):33–8.
[6] Inanamni O, et al. *Neuroscience Letters* 1995;196(1–2):85–8.
[7] Shimoi K, et al. *Mutation Research* 1996;350(1):153–61.
[8] Yoshikawa T, et al. *Adv Exp Med Biol* 1990;264:171–4.
[9] Swanepoel ML. *S African Med J* 1987 Mar 21;71(6):369-70.

Reishi Mushroom

SCIENTIFIC NAME(S): *Ganoderma lucidum* (Leysser ex Fr.) Karst. Family: Polyporaceae

COMMON NAME(S): Reishi, ling chih, ling zhi, "spirit plant"

BOTANY: The reishi mushroom is a purplish-brown fungus with a long stalk and fan-shaped cap. It has a shiny, "varnish"-coated appearance, with spores resembling brown powder that can sometimes be seen. The reishi grows on decaying wood or tree stumps. It prefers the Japanese plum tree but also grows on oak. The fruiting body is the part of the plant used for medicinal purposes. This mushroom grows in China, Japan, and North America and is cultivated throughout other Asian countries. Cultivation of reishi is a long, complicated process. The reishi grows in 6 colors, each having its own characteristics: *Aoshiba* (blue reishi), *Akashiba* (red reishi), *Kishiba* (yellow reishi), *Shiroshiba* (white reishi), *Kuroshiba* (black reishi), and *Murasakishiba* (purple reishi).[1]

HISTORY: Reishi has been used in traditional Chinese medicine for over 4000 years for treating problems such as fatigue, asthma, cough, and liver ailments, and to promote longevity.[1] The Chinese name *ling zhi* means "herb of spiritual potency."[1] A Japanese name for the reishi is *mannentake*, meaning "10,000-year-old mushroom." Reishi's use is documented in what is said to be the oldest Chinese medical text, which is over 2000 years old. This book contains information on about 400 medicines but lists the reishi as the most superior.[2] Cultivation of reishi began in the 1980s.[3]

CHEMISTRY: The reishi mushroom is known to be high in polysaccharide content, including beta-d-glucan and GL-1.[1,4] Triterpene constituents of the plant also have been analyzed.[5] Triterpene antioxidants including ganoderic acids (A, B, C, and D), lucidenic acid B, and ganodermanontriol have been found in reishi.[1,6] Terpenoids 1, 2, and 3, and terpenes lucidenic acid O and lucidenic lactone also exist in the plant.[7] One report discusses peptidoglycan from reishi containing $\approx$ 7% protein and 76% carbohydrate.[8] Certain enzymes from reishi have also been reported.[9] The reishi mushroom contains minerals including calcium, magnesium, and potassium. Germanium, lanostan, coumarins, ergosterol, and cerevisterol are also found in reishi.[1,7]

PHARMACOLOGY:

Anticancer immunostimulant effects: Older texts make mention of reishi's immunostimulatory and anticancer effects.[2] Modern research confirms these indications, attributing the polysaccharide components to be responsible for these properties. Polysaccharides beta-d-glucan and GL-1 have been found to inhibit sarcoma.[4] Reishi has been shown to be of benefit in myeloblastic leukemia and nasopharyngeal carcinoma in combination with other chemotherapeutic agents, demonstrating tumor shrinkage, significant changes in hemoglobin counts, and overall quality-of-life markers.[3] In vitro studies find reishi (and other plant) polysaccharides to be antigenotoxic and antitumor promoting.[10] Extract of reishi shows radioprotective ability and protective ability against hydroxyl radical-induced DNA strand breaks in another report.[11] Reishi has demonstrated positive effects on cytokine release from human macrophages and T-lymphocytes, confirming its role in immunopotentiation.[12] Reishi's anticancer properties are almost certainly "host-mediated" through stimulation of the immune system.

Hepatitis: The reishi mushroom also has been beneficial in the treatment of hepatitis.[12] One report describes how it minimized experimental liver damage when studied in rats.[13] Another report shows improvement in 92% of 355 hepatitis patients taking reishi.[14]

Cardiovascular effects: Positive effects on the cardiovascular system also have been demonstrated by reishi. Decreases in high blood pressure have been affected by the ganoderic acids.[1,3] ACE-inhibiting triterpenes from reishi have also been discussed.[15] The risk of coronary artery disease may also be decreased by reishi, which was found to decrease platelet adhesion.[1] In one report, ganodermic acid was found to exert inhibitory effects on platelets, leading to decreased thromboxane formation.[16] Reduction of cholesterol from reishi has been addressed, including decreases in triglycerides and LDL.[1]

Antiviral effects: Certain polysaccharides isolated from reishi have been proven effective against herpes simplex virus types 1 and 2.[17] Certain reishi isolates also have been tested against other viral strains including influenza A and demonstrated effectiveness against their growth.[18]

Other effects: There are numerous claims for reishi (some unconfirmed) including the following: Decrease in blood glucose levels in mice, treatment of diabetic ulcers,[3] altitude sickness,[1] and headaches.[3]

TOXICOLOGY:

Side Effects: Side effects from reishi may include dizziness, dry mouth, stomach upset, nose bleed, sore bones, irritated skin, diarrhea, or constipation from initial use, which may disappear with continued use or may develop from use over 3 to 6 months.[1] Because reishi may increase bleeding time, it is not recommended for use with anticoagulants. Pregnant or lactating women should consider these issues and consult a doctor before taking reishi.[1]

SUMMARY: The reishi mushroom has been used in traditional Chinese medicine for over 4000 years. It is high in polysaccharide content, which is mainly responsible for anticancer and immunostimulatory effects. It has liver protectant actions, beneficial effects on the cardiovascular system, antiviral actions, and other effects. Side effects are mild and may include dizziness, GI upset, or irritated skin. The use of reishi with anticoagulants or in pregnant or lactating women is not recommended.

PATIENT INFORMATION – Reishi Mushroom

Uses: Reishi is high in polysaccharide content, which is mainly responsible for possible anticancer and immunostimulatory effects. It also may have liver protectant actions, beneficial effects on the cardiovascular system, antiviral actions, and other effects.

Drug Interactions: Do not take with anticoagulants.

Side Effects: Side effects are mild and may include dizziness, GI upset, or irritated skin. Do not use reishi with pregnant or lactating women.

---

[1] Lininger S, et al, eds. *The Natural Pharmacy*. Rocklin, CA: Prima Publishing, 1998;303-04.

[2] Matsumoto, K. *The Mysterious Reishi Mushroom*. Santa Barbara, CA: Woodbridge Press Publishing, 1979.

[3] http://www.kyotan.com/lectures/lectures/lecture6.html

[4] Miyazaki T, et al. Studies on fungal polysaccharides. XXVII. Structural examination of a water-soluble, antitumor polysaccharide of *Ganoderma lucidum*. *Chem Pharma Bull* (Tokyo) 1981;29:3611-16.

[5] Khoda H, et al. The biologically active constituents of *Ganoderma lucidum* (Fr.) Karst. Histamine release-inhibitory triterpenes. *Chem Pharm Bull* (Tokyo) 1985;33:1367-74.

[6] Zhu M, et al. Triterpene antioxidants from *Ganoderma lucidum*. *Phytother Res* 1999;13(6):529-31.

[7] Mizushina Y, et al. Lucidenic acid O and lactone, new terpene inhibitors of eukaryotic DNA polymerases from a basidiomycete, *Ganoderma lucidum*. *Bioorg Med Chem* 1999;7(9):2047-52.

[8] Cheong J, et al. Characterization of an alkali-extracted peptidoglycan from Korean *Ganoderma lucidum*. *Arch Pharm Res* 1999;22(5):515-19.

[9] D'Souza T, et al. Lignin-modifying enzymes of the white rot basidiomycete *Ganoderma lucidum*. *Appl Environ Microbiol* 1999;65(12):5307-13.

[10] Kim H, et al. In vitro chemopreventive effects of plant polysaccharides (*Aloe barbadensis* Miller, *Lentinus edodes*, *Ganoderma lucidum*, and *Coriolus versicolor*). *Carcinogenesis* 1999;20(8):1637-40.

[11] Kim K, et al. *Ganoderma lucidum* extract protects DNA from strand breakage caused by hydroxyl radical and UV irradiation. *Int J Mol Med* 1999;4(3):273-77.

[12] Wang S, et al. The role of *Ganoderma lucidum* in immunopotentiation: Effect on cytokine release from human macrophages and T-lymphocytes. In: Program and Abstracts of the 1994 International Symposium on Ganoderm Research.

[13] Byun S, et al. Studies on the concurrent administration of *Ganoderma lucidum* extract and glutathione on liver damage induced by carbon tetrachloride in rats. *J Pharm Boo* 1987;31:133-39.

[14] Chang H, et al. *Pharmacology and Applications of Chinese Materia Medica*. Vol. 1 Singapore: World Scientific, 1986.

[15] Morigiwa A, et al. Angiotensin converting enzyme-inhibiting triterpenes from *Ganoderma lucidum*. *Chem Pharm Bull* (Tokyo) 1986;34:3025-28.

[16] Su C, et al. Differential effects of ganodermic acid S on the thromboxane A2-signaling pathways in human platelets. *Biochem Pharmacol* 1999;58(4):587-95.

[17] Eo S, et al. Antiherpetic activities of various protein bound polysaccharides isolated from *Ganoderma lucidum*. *J Ethnopharmacol* 1999;68(1-3):175-81.

[18] Eo S, et al. Antiviral activities of various water and methanol soluble substances isolated from *Ganoderma lucidum*. *J Ethnopharmacol* 1999;68(1-3):129-36.

Rose Hips

SCIENTIFIC NAME(S): Commonly derived from *Rosa canina* L., *R. rugosa* Thunb., *R. acicularis* Lindl. or *R. cinnamomea* L. Numerous other species of rose have been used for the preparation of rose hips. Family: Rosaceae

COMMON NAME(S): Rose hips, "heps," dog rose (R. canina)

BOTANY: Rose hips grow from a perennial plant, which can grow 3 to 5 meters in height. Their thorny branches give way to pink and white flowers and scarlet fruits, called "hips."[1,2] These rose hips are the ripe ovaries or seeded fruit of roses forming on branches after the flower.[3] They are approximately 1 to 2 cm long by 0.5 to 1.5 cm thick; oval in shape; and fleshy, shrunken, and wrinkled. Inside the hips are 3 or more small (3 to 5 mm), angular, yellow-brown seeds.[2] *R. canina* is native to Europe, North Africa, and temperate areas of Asia. The fruits (hips) are picked in autumn and used for the "drug."

HISTORY: Once used as a folk remedy for chest ailments, *R. canina* hips were popular in the Middle Ages.[1] They are a natural source of vitamin C, which has led to their widespread use in natural vitamin supplements, teas, and various other preparations including soups and marmalades.[4] Although these products have been used historically as nutritional supplements, they have also been used as mild laxatives and diuretics.[5] Rose hip syrup was used as a nourishing drink for children.[1] It was also used to flavor teas and jams.[2]

CHEMISTRY: Fresh rose hips contain 0.5% to 1.7% vitamin C,[4] usually determined as a combination of l-dehydroascorbic acid and l-ascorbic acid.[6] However, the content of dried, commercially available rose hips products varies considerably. One report evaluates stability of vitamin C, using photometry and thin layer chromatography (TLC). Results showed that loss of vitamin C was dependent on "degree of coarseness" of rose hips. Fruits cut in half lost less than 50% vitamin C in 18 months storage, while ground drug lost 100% in 6 months.[7]

While some accounts suggest that rose hips are the richest natural source of vitamin C, a number of more concentrated sources have been identified. Citrus fruits contain approximately 50 mg vitamin C per 100 g; uncooked broccoli, kale, and kiwi fruit, approximately 100 mg; black currants, guavas, and some tropical vegetables, 200 to 300 mg; rose hips (*Rosa canina*), 1250 mg; acerola or Barbados cherry (*Malpighia punicifolia*), 1000 to 2330 mg; and *Terminalia ferdinandiana*, up to 3150 mg.[8]

Rose hips also contain vitamins A, B_1, B_2, B_3, and K. Other ingredients include pectin (11%), tannins (2% to 3%), malic and citric acids, flavonoids, red and yellow pigments, especially carotenoids, polyphenols, invert sugar, volatile oil, vanillin, and a variety of minor components.

PHARMACOLOGY: Vitamin C is used as a nutritional supplement for its antiscorbutic properties. Use of rose hips for their vitamin C content, in supportive therapy for cases of this vitamin deficiency is rational.[2] Because a significant amount of the natural vitamin C in rose hips may be destroyed during drying and processing, many "natural vitamin supplements" have some form of vitamin C added to them. One must read the label carefully to determine what proportion of the vitamin C is derived from rose hips vs other sources. Unfortunately, this information is not always available on the package label. However, when freshly consumed, rose hips have extremely high levels of vitamins in a form readily absorbed by the body.

A small pediatric population with osteogenesis imperfecta received ascorbic acid from rose hips, 250 to 600 mg/day for 10 to 42 months. Eight of 13 patients showed a decrease in number of fractures vs control, suggesting a positive outcome of vitamin C supplementation in this specific disease.[9]

Rose hips' effects have been evaluated on blood glucose levels in rabbits. No significant changes in levels were reported.[10]

The laxative activity of rose hips may be related to the presence of malic and citric acids, to purgative glycosides (multiflorin A and B),[11] or to pectin content in the plant.[2] Rose hips have also been used for diuretic actions, to reduce thirst, and to alleviate gastric inflammation.[1] Its diuretic action has been disputed.[2]

TOXICOLOGY: Rose hips ingestion is not generally associated with toxicity. More than 100 g of plant material would have to be ingested to obtain a 1200 mg dose of vitamin C, an impractical amount to ingest. Most people do not have any side effects from ingesting small quantities of the plant. Adverse effects associated with the long-term ingestion of multi-gram doses of vitamin C (ie, oxalate stone formation) have not been reported with rose hips.[12] *The German Commission E Monographs* lists risks of rose hips as "none known."[2] However, production workers exposed to rose hips dust have developed severe respiratory allergies, with mild-to-moderate anaphylaxis.[3] One report describes a German ground rose hips product sold as "itching powder" in novelty shops. The fibers of the plant seem to provoke itch and prickle sensations not by allergic means, but by mechanical irritation, similar to those of wool.[13]

SUMMARY: Rose hips are a pleasant-tasting source of natural vitamin C. Because the concentration of the vitamin is relatively low, one must ingest large amounts of the product to serve as a nutritional supplement. Many natural rose hips products are fortified with ascorbic acid. Rose hips also contain other vitamins and may be used as supplementation for deficiencies. Rose hips are not generally associated with toxicity.

PATIENT INFORMATION – Rose Hips

Uses: Rose hips provide vitamin C supplements. Rose hips have been used for diuretic actions, to reduce thirst, to alleviate gastric inflammation, and to flavor teas and jams.

Side Effects: There have been no reported side effects except in those exposed to rose hips dust who have developed severe respiratory allergies.

---

[1] Chevallier A. *Herbal Medicines.* London, England: Pharmaceutical Press, 1996;261.
[2] Bisset N. *Herbal drugs and phytopharmaceuticals.* Stuttgart, Germany: CRC Press, 1994;424-27.
[3] Kwaselow A, et al. *J Allergy Clin Immunol* 1990;85(4):704.
[4] Tyler VE. *The New Honest Herbal.* Philadelphia, PA: G.F. Stickley Co., 1987.
[5] Duke JA. *Handbook of Medicinal Herbs.* Boca Raton, FL: CRC Press, 1985.
[6] Ziegler SJ, et al. *J Chromatogr* 1987;391:419.
[7] Lander C, et al. *Pharmazeutische Zeitung* 1986 Jun 19;131:1441-43.
[8] Brand JC, et al. *Lancet* 1982;2:873.
[9] Kurz D, et al. *Pediatrics* 1974 Jul;54:56-61.
[10] Can A, et al. *Acta Pharmaceutica Turcica* 1992;34(1):17-22.
[11] Leung AY. *Encyclopedia of Common Natural Ingredients Used In Food, Drugs and Cosmetics.* New York, NY: J Wiley and Sons, 1980.
[12] Roth DA, Breitenfield RV. *JAMA* (letter) 1977;237(8):768.
[13] Albert M. *Australas J Dermatol* 1998;39(3):188-89.

Rosemary

SCIENTIFIC NAME(S): *Rosmarinus officinalis* L. Family: Labiatae or Lamiaceae.

COMMON NAME(S): Rosemary, Old Man

BOTANY: Rosemary grows as a small evergreen shrub with thick aromatic leaves.[1] The plant has small pale-blue flowers that bloom in late winter and early spring. Although rosemary is native to the Mediterranean, it is now cultivated worldwide.[2,3] Other types of rosemary include bog rosemary (*Andromeda* species) and wild or marsh rosemary (*Ledum palustre* L.).

HISTORY: Rosemary is a widely used culinary spice. Tradition holds that rosemary will grow only in gardens of households where the "mistress" is truly the "master."[4] The plant has been used in traditional medicine for its astringent, tonic, carminative, antispasmodic, and diaphoretic properties. Extracts and the volatile oil have been used to promote menstrual flow and as abortifacients.[4,5] Rosemary extracts are commonly found as cosmetic ingredients and a lotion of the plant is said to stimulate hair growth and prevent baldness.[6]

Historical reports regarding the therapeutic use of rosemary as a medicinal plant are available.[7,8] Rosemary is one of the oldest known medicinal herbs, having been used centuries ago to enhance mental function and memory.[9]

CHEMISTRY: The leaves contain 0.5% to 2.5% of volatile oil. The major components of the oil include monoterpene hydrocarbons (alpha and beta-pinene), camphene, limonene, camphor (10% to 20%), borneol, cineole, linalool, and verbinol. Rosemary contains a wide variety of volatile and aromatic components. Flavonoids in the plant include diosmetin, diosmin, genkwanin, luteolin, hispidulin, and apigenin.[1,4,10] One analysis reports 3 new flavonoid glucuronides, also found in the leaves.[11] Other terpenoid constituents in rosemary include triterpenes oleanolic and ursolic acids and diterpene carnosol.[10] The concentration of phenolic diterpenes in certain commercial rosemary extracts has been determined by HPLC.[12] Phenols in rosemary include caffeic, chlorogenic, labiatic, neochlorogenic, and rosmarinic acids.[10] Rosemary contains high amounts of salicylates.[13]

PHARMACOLOGY: Rosemary is a known antimicrobial agent. The powdered leaves are used as an effective natural flea and tick repellent.[14] Rosemary oil possesses marked antibacterial, antifungal, antimold, and antiviral properties.[9,10] Activity against certain bacteria including *Staphylcoccus aureus*, *S. albus*, *Vibrio cholerae*, *Escherichia coli*, and *Corynebacteria* has been observed.[10] Rosemary oil was found to be most active against "meat spoiling" gram-negative (eg, *Pseudomonas*) and gram-positive (eg, *Lactobacillus*) bacteria in 1 report.[15] The effect of rosemary on *Candida albicans* has been described.[16] Another report discusses growth inhibition of *Aspergillus parasiticus* by rosemary oil.[17] However, a report on the use of rosemary to treat head lice found it to be ineffective.[18]

There are numerous reports available evaluating rosemary's anticancer effects. The extract contains properties that induce quinone reductase, an anticarcinogenic enzyme.[19] Other anticancer mechanisms include polyphenol constituents that inhibit metabolic activation of procarcinogens by Phase I enzymes (P450), and induction of the detoxification pathway caused by Phase II enzymes (glutathione S-transferase).[20] Dietary supplementation of laboratory animals with 1% rosemary extract resulted in a 47% decrease in the incidence of experimentally-induced mammary tumors compared to controls.[21,22] This extract was found to enhance activities of enzymes that detoxify reactive substances in mouse liver and stomach.[23] Skin tumors in mice have been inhibited by application of rosemary extract to the area.[24] Rosemary increased detoxification of carcinogens in human bronchial epithelial cells as well.[25] Rosemary diterpene, carnosic acid, exhibited strong inhibitory effects against HIV-protease.[26]

Several reports exist concerning rosemary's antioxidative actions.[27,28,29,30,31] Carnosol and carnosic acid have been reported to account for more than 90% of the antioxidant properties of rosemary extract. Both are powerful inhibitors of lipid peroxidation and are good scavengers of peroxyl radicals.[32,33] Antioxidant activity depends directly on concentration of diterpenes such as these.[12] Rosemary antioxidants have less scavenging potential than green tea polyphenols but have more potential than vitamin E.[34]

Various reports involving other actions of rosemary include spasmolytic actions in smooth and cardiac muscle, alteration of complement activation,[10] liver effects,[35] immune effects,[36] aromatherapy for chronic pain treatment,[37] inhibition of adult respiratory distress syndrome in rabbits,[10] reduction of capillary permeability,[4] and antigonadotrophic activity in mice.[10] Rosemary may also reverse headaches, reduce stress, and aid in asthma and bronchitis treatment.[9] Rosemary inhibits uterotropic actions of estradiol and estrone by 35% to 50% vs controls.[38] Rosemary's pharmacology has been reviewed.[39]

TOXICOLOGY: Although the oil is used safely as a food flavoring and the whole leaves are used as a potherb and spice, ingestion of large quantities of the oil can be associated with toxicity.[40] Toxicity from the oil is characterized by stomach and intestinal irritation and kidney damage.[4] Although rosemary oil is irritating to rabbit skin, it is not generally considered to be a sensitizer for human skin. However, preparations containing the oil may cause erythema, and toiletries can cause dermatitis in sensitive individuals.[1,6,10] Allergic contact dermatitis from rosemary has been reported.[41] A case report discusses contact dermatitis in a 56-year-old man reacting to carnosol, the main constituent in a rosemary preparation.[42]

At least 3 case reports concerning toxic seizures associated with rosemary exist. The plant's monoterpene ketones are powerful convulsants with known epileptogenic properties.[43]

Certain molds may grow on rosemary.[44]

A case of occupational asthma caused by rosemary has been reported.[45]

Rosemary extract may possess an anti-implantation effect as seen in rat experimentation.[46] The plant is a reported abortifacient, and also affects the menstrual cycle.[10]

SUMMARY: Rosemary is a popular herb and widely used culinary spice. It has antimicrobial actions against a variety of bacteria, fungi, mold, and viruses. Its anticancer effects have been numerously reported and include inhibition of skin tumors, mammary tumors, and others. Rosemary has antioxidative actions. Certain constituents scavenge peroxyl radicals and detoxify harmful products. Other effects of rosemary include spasmolytic actions, liver and immune effects, and various actions from asthma treatment to aromatherapy. Allergic contact dermatitis has been associated with the plant, but rosemary is not generally considered to be a human skin sensitizer. Rosemary's constituents, monoterpene ketones, are convulsants, and have caused seizures in large doses. Rosemary is also an abortifacient.

PATIENT INFORMATION – Rosemary

Uses: Rosemary has been reported to decrease capillary permeability and fragility. Extracts have been used in insect repellents. The plant may have anticancer properties and has spasmolytic actions, liver and immune effects, and other various actions from asthma treatment to aromatherapy. It has antimicrobial actions against a variety of bacteria, fungi, mold, and viruses.

Side Effects: Ingestion of large quantities of rosemary can result in stomach and intestinal irritation and kidney damage. Allergic contact dermatitis has been associated with the plant, but rosemary is not generally considered to be a human skin sensitizer. Rosemary's constituents, monoterpene ketones, are convulsants, and have caused seizures in large doses. Rosemary is also an abortifacient.

---

[1] Leung A. *Encyclopedia of Common Natural Ingredients Used in Food, Drugs and Cosmetics.* NY: Wiley, 1980.

[2] Simon J. *Herbs: An Indexed Bibliography, 1971-1980.* Hamden, CT: Archon Books, 1984.

[3] Osol A, Farrar G Jr, eds. *The Dispensatory of the United States of America.* 25th ed. Philadelphia: Lippincott, 1955.

[4] Tyler V. *The New Honest Herbal.* Philadelphia, PA: G.F. Stickley Co., 1987.

[5] *Magic and Medicine of Plants.* Pleasantville, NY: Reader's Digest, 1986.

[6] Duke J. *Handbook of Medicinal Herbs.* Boca Raton, FL: CRC Press, 1935.

[7] Selmi, G. Therapeutic use of rosemary through the centuries. *Policlinico* 1967;74(13):439-41. Italian.

[8] Zimmermann, V. Rosemary as a medicinal plant and wonder-drug. A report on the medieval drug monographs. *Sudhoffs Arch Z Wissenschaftsgesch* 1980;64(4):351-70. German.

[9] http://www.droregano.com/orosemary.html

[10] Newall C, et al. *Herbal Medicines: A Guide for Health Care Professionals.* London: Pharmaceutical Press, 1996;229-30.

[11] Okamura N, et al. Flavonoids in *Rosmarinus officianalis* leaves. *Phytochemistry* 1994;37(5):1463-66.

[12] Schwarz K, et al. Antioxidative constituents of *Rosmarinus officinalis* and *Salvia officinalis.* III. Stability of phenolic diterpenes of rosemary extracts under thermal stress as required for technological processes. *Z Lebensm Unters Forsch* 1992;195(2):104-07.

[13] Swain A, et al. Salicylates in foods. *J Am Diet Assoc* 1985;85(8):950-60.

[14] http://www.rexseedco.com/pest.htm

[15] Ouattara B, et al. Antibacterial activity of selected fatty acids and essential oils against six meat spoilage organisms. *Int J Food Microbiology* 1997;37(2-3):155-62.

[16] Steinmetz M, et al. Transmission and scanning electronmiscroscopy study of the action of sage and rosemary essential oils and eucalyptol on *Candida albicans.* *Mycoses*1988;31(1):40-51.

[17] Tantaoui-Elaraki A, et al. Inhibition of growth and aflatoxin production in *Aspergillus parasiticus* by essential oils of selected plant materials. *J Environ Pathol Toxicol Oncol* 1994;13(1):67-72.

[18] Veal, L. The potential effectiveness of essential oils as a treatment for head-lice, Pediculus humanus capitis. *Complement Ther Nurs Midwifery* 1996;2(4):97-101.

[19] Tawfiq N, et al. Induction of the anticarcinogenic enzyme quinone reductase by food extracts using murine hepatoma cells. *Eur J Cancer Prev* 1994;3(3):285-92.

[20] Offord E, et al. Mechanisms involved in the chemoprotective effects of rosemary extract studied in human liver and bronchial cells. *Cancer Lett* 1997;114(1-2):275-81.

[21] Singletary K, et al. Inhibition of 7,12-dimethylbenzanthracene (DMBA)-induced mammary tumorigenesis and of in vivo formation of mammary DMBA-DNA adducts by rosemary extract. *Cancer Lett* 1991;60(2):169-75.

[22] Singletary K, et al. Inhibition by rosemary of 7,12-dimethylbenzanthracene (DMBA)-induced rat mammary tumorigenesis and in vivo DMBA-DNA adduct formation. *Cancer Lett* 1996;104(1):43-48.

[23] Singletary K, et al. Tissue-specific enhancement of xenobiotic detoxification enzymes in mice by dietary rosemary extract. *Plant Foods Hum Nutr* 1997;50(1):47-53.

[24] Huang M, et al. Inhibition of skin tumorigenesis by rosemary and its constituents carnosol and ursolic acid. *Cancer Research* 1994;54(3):701-08.

[25] Offord E, et al. Rosemary components inhibit benzopyrene-induced genotoxicity in human bronchial cells. *Carcinogenesis* 1995;16(9):2057-62.

[26] Paris A, et al. Inhibitory effect of carnosic acid on HIV-1 protease in cell-free assays. *J Nat Prod* 1993;56(8):1426-30.

[27] Minnunni M, et al. Natural antioxidants as inhibitors of oxygen species-induced mutagenicity. *Mutation Research* 1992;269(2):193-200.

[28] Kim S, et al. Measurement of superoxide dismutase-like activity of natural antioxidants. *Biosci Biotechnol Biochem* 1995;59(5):822-26.

[29] Aruoma O, et al. An evaluation of the anioxidant and antiviral action of extracts of rosemary and Provencal herbs. *Food Chem Toxicol* 1996;34(5):449-56.

[30] Lopez-Bote C, et al. Effect of dietary administration of oil extracts from rosemary and sage on lipid oxidation in broiler meat. *Br Poult Sci* 1998;39(2):235-40.

[31] Aruoma, O. Antioxidant actions of plant foods; use of oxidative DNA damage as a tool for studying antioxidant efficacy. *Free Radical Research* 1999;30(6):419-27.

[32] Aruoma O, et al. Antioxidant and pro-oxidant properties of active rosemary constituents: carnosol and carnosic acid. *Xenobiotica* 1992;22(2):257-68.

[33] Geoffroy M, et al. Radical intermediates and antioxidants: an ESR study of radicals formed on carnosic acid in the presence of oxidized lipids. *Free Radical Research* 1994;21(4):247-58.

[34] Zhao B, et al. Scavenging effect of extracts of green tea and natural antioxidants on active oxygen radicals. *Cell Biophys* 1989;14(2):175-85.

[35] Singletary, K. Rosemary extract and carnosol stimulate rat liver glutathione-S-trasferase and quinone reductase activities. *Cancer Lett* 1996;100(1-2):139-44.

[36] Babu U, et al. Effect of dietary rosemary extract on cell-mediated immunity. *Plant Food Hum Nutr* 1999;53(2):169-74.

[37] Buckle, J. Use of aromatherapy as a complementary treatment for chronic pain. *Altern Ther Health Med* 1999;5(5):42-51. Review.

[38] Zhu B, et al. Dietary administration of an extract from rosemary leaves enhances the liver microsomal metabolism of endogenous estrogens and decreases their uterotropic action in CD-1 mice. *Carcinogenesis* 1998;19(10):1821-27.

[39] al-Sereiti M, et al. Pharmacology of rosemary (*Rosmarinus officinalis* Linn.) and its therapeutic potentials. *Indian J Exp Biol* 1999;37(2):124-30.

[40] Spoerke D. *Herbal Medications*. Santa Barbara, CA: Woodbridge Press, 1980.

[41] Fernandez L, et al. Allergic contact dermatitis from rosemary (*Rosmarinus officinalis* L.). *Contact Dermatitis* 1997;37(5):248-49.

[42] Hjorther A, et al. Occupational allergic contact dermatitis from carnosol, a naturally-occurring compound present in rosemary. *Contact Dermatitis* 1997;37(3):99-100.

[43] Burkhard P, et al. Plant-induced seizures: reappearance of an old problem. *J Neurol* 1999;246(8):667-70.

[44] Llewellyn G, et al. Potential mold growth, aflatoxin production, and antimycotic activity of selected natural spices and herbs. *J Assoc Off Anal Chem* 1981;64(4):955-60.

[45] Lemiere C, et al. Occupational asthma caused by aromatic herbs. *Allergy* 1996;51(9):647-49.

[46] Lemonica I, et al. Study of the embryotoxic effects of an extract of rosemary (*Rosmarinus officinalis* L.). *Braz J Med Biol Res* 1996;29(2):223-27.

Royal Jelly

SOURCE: Royal jelly is a milky-white secretion produced by worker bees of the species *Apis mellifers* L. to induce differentiated growth and the development of the queen bee. Queen bees are fed mostly royal jelly. Because of this specialized nutrition, queen bees differ from workers in several ways; the queens are about twice the size, they lay about 2000 eggs a day (female worker bees are infertile) and they live 5 to 8 years (about 40 times longer than worker bees).

HISTORY: These differences have led to the marketable assumption that ingestion of this product will do as much for humans as it does for bees; that is, increase size, improve fertility and enhance longevity. Royal jelly has also been sold as a skin tonic and hair growth stimulant.[1]

CHEMISTRY: Royal jelly is a complex mixture of proteins (12%), sugar (12%), fats (6%) and variable amounts of minerals, vitamins[2] and pheromones. About 15% of royal jelly is 10-hydroxy-trans-(2)-decanoic acid (HDA),[3] which is thought to play an important role in bee growth regulation. The product is rich in B vitamins, the most abundant of which is pantothenic acid.[1]

PHARMACOLOGY: The jelly has been found to possess antitumor activity in experimental mouse leukemias.[4] HDA has slight, pH-dependent antimicrobial activity; the compound is 25% less active than penicillin and 20% less active than chlortetracycline.[5]

There is no evidence that royal jelly has estrogenic activity or that it affects growth, longevity or fertility in animals.[6] In terms of revitalizing dried skin, the results from one 3-month study of 24 women noted that 10 showed improvement, 10 had no change and 4 showed symptoms of skin irritation.[1]

Despite these pharmacologic actions, there is little strong clinical evidence for any beneficial effects in man.[7]

TOXICOLOGY: Other than skin irritation, there are no reports of toxicity. Because some persons have reported allergic reactions to other bee products such as bee pollen, the potential for these events with royal jelly should be kept in mind. However, there have not been significant reports of allergic reactions with this product.

SUMMARY: Lyophilized royal jelly is sold in 100 mg capsules (50 capsules for more than $10) and is incorporated into topical creams and ointments. It is an adequate but expensive source of certain B vitamins. It does not possess recognizable preventive, therapeutic or rejuvenatory characteristics.

PATIENT INFORMATION – Royal Jelly

Uses: Royal jelly has been used in topical creams and ointments.

Side Effects: Royal jelly has caused some allergic reactions.

---

[1] Tyler VE. *The New Honest Herbal.* Philadelphia, PA: G.F. Stickley Co., 1987.
[2] Dixit PK. *Nature* 1964;202:189.
[3] Barker S. *Nature* 1959;183:996.
[4] Townsend GF, et al. *Nature* 1959;183:1270.
[5] Blum MS, et al. *Science* 1959;130:452.
[6] Dayan AD. *J Pharm Pharmacol* 1960;12:377.
[7] Worthinton-Roberts B, Breskin MA. *Am Pharm* 1983;23(8):30.

Rue

SCIENTIFIC NAME(S): *Ruta graveolens* L., *R. montana* L. and *R. bracteosa* L. have also been reported to be used medicinally. Family: Rutaceae

COMMON NAME(S): Rue, common rue, garden rue, German rue. Not to be confused with meadow rue (*Thalictrum* spp.)

BOTANY: Rue is native to Europe but is now cultivated worldwide. It is often found growing along roadsides and in waste areas. It is an herbaceous evergreen half-shrub that grows to 2 or 3 feet tall. The leaves have three fleshy lobes and are "teardrop"-shaped. It blooms greenish-yellow flowers from June to August. The flowers have a characteristically disagreeable odor. The aerial parts, which are gathered in the summer, are used. The plant is both ornamental and medicinal.[1]

HISTORY: The leaves, other parts, and extracts of rue have been used for hundreds of years as insect repellents and, in folk medicine, as antispasmodics, sedatives and stimulants for the onset of menses. Depending on the local culture, rue extracts have been used as abortifacients.[2]

In New Mexico, rue is used traditionally as a tisane for ailments such as stiff neck, dizziness, headache, tightness in the stomach and inner ear problems. The oil has a strong bitter taste and was once used for the treatment of intestinal worms.

Roman naturalist Pliny the Elder (23 to 79 AD) mentions 84 remedies containing rue.[3] In ancient Greece and Egypt, aside from its use as an abortifacient, rue was also used to strengthen eyesight.[1]

CHEMISTRY: Rue has been studied extensively and has been found to contain a large number of chemical components.[4] Common rue contains a mixture of furoquinoline alkaloids in a concentration of approximately 1.5%, the most important of which appear to be arborine, arborinine and gamma fagarine.[5,6]

The acridone alkaloids (rutacridone epoxide, hydroxyrutacridone epoxide) are found in greatest concentration in the roots.[7] Other alkaloids include graveoline, graveolinine, kokusaginine, rutacridone and skimmianine. Flavonoid rutin is also present in the plant and is said to support and strengthen blood vessels, reducing pressure.[1,3]

A volatile oil is present in a concentration of approximately 0.1%. The oil is 90% methyl-nonylketone with the balance composed of related ketones, esters and phenols.[8]

The plant and its oil are rich in coumarin derivatives that appear to contribute significantly to the pharmacologic activity of the plant. These furocoumarins include bergapten, psoralen, xanthoxanthin, xanthotoxin, isopimpinellin and rutamarin.[1,3,9] Isolation of such furocoumarins has been performed using an improved extraction technique.[10] A new coumarin, "exo-dehydrochalepin" has been synthesized from rutamarin.[11] Other reports have described: Isolation of alkaloid isogravacridonchlorine from rue roots;[12] identification of dihydropyrano and dihydrofuro;[2,3,4,5,6] quinolinium alkaloids;[13] and purification of acridone synthase from rue cell cultures.[14]

PHARMACOLOGY: The rue plant and its extracts, in particular the tea and oil, have been reported to have antispasmodic effects on smooth muscles. This pharmacologic action has been attributed to the alkaloids arborine and arborinine and to the coumarins, in particular rutamarin. One study found the spasmolytic effect of arborinine on pig coronary muscle to be as potent as that of papaverine, while rutamarin was 20-fold more potent than papaverine. The antispasmodic effects of these compounds were reversible. While the pharmacologic half-life of arborinine was about the same as for papaverine, that of rutamarin was approximately 20 times longer. These spasmolytic effects were also observed in isolated gastrointestinal smooth muscle.[4]

A report studies *R. graveolens* extract as a potential potassium channel blocker on ionic currents in myelinated nerve cells.[15] Rue has been used to treat many ailments including epilepsy, eye strain, multiple sclerosis, Bell's palsy, heart conditions and as a uterine stimulant to encourage onset of menstruation.[1,3]

There are many references to the abortifacient effects of rue teas and oil. The abortifacient effect may be due to an anti-implantation action[2] or to a generalized state of systemic toxicity resulting in fetal death.[8] Antifertility action of *R. graveolens* has been reported in rats.[16,17] In one report, Chalepensin was found to be the active component, acting at early stages of pregnancy.[16]

More than 15 compounds have been identified that have significant in vitro antibacterial and antifungal activity.[6]

The acridone alkaloids are the most potent antimicrobial compounds; the coumarins resulted in growth inhibition only at higher doses. The essential oil and flavonoids tested did not show significant activity. Other researchers have found that a number of components of rue interact directly with DNA replication, thereby preventing the propagation of some viruses.[18] The leaf of rue is said to alleviate cancer of the mouth, tumors and warts. In Chinese medicine, rue is used as a vermifuge and for insect bites.[1,3]

TOXICOLOGY: Because the antispasmodic effect of this plant occurs at relatively small doses, rue should only be taken with caution, if at all. The safety of the plant in pregnant women has not been established and most of the literature describing its potential abortifacient effects indicate that the plant should never be ingested by women of childbearing potential.[1,3]

Extracts of rue have been found to be mutagenic in experimental mutagenicity screens, but the clinical importance of these findings has not been established.[19,20]

The furocoumarins have been associated with photosensitization, resulting in skin blistering following contact and exposure to sunlight. This occurs in people who collect fresh rue and has been reported in those who rubbed fresh rue on themselves as an insect repellent. The toxicity of the dried leaves is most likely less than for fresh leaves because of the loss of volatile oil.[21,22] A tincture of *R. graveolens* L. exhibited marked photomutagenicity of varying degrees based on different alkaloid concentrations present in the compound.[23]

The volatile oil has an irritant quality and may result in kidney damage and hepatic degeneration if ingested.[8]

Large doses (more than 100 ml of the oil or about 120 g of the leaves in one dose) can cause violent gastric pain, vomiting and systemic complications including death. A single oral dose of 400 mg/kg given to guinea pigs has been reported to be fatal because of hemorrhages of the adrenal gland, liver and kidney. However, an oral daily dose of 30 mg given to human subjects for 3 months did not result in abnormal hepatic function.[24]

SUMMARY: Rue is an odiferous herb that has been used in traditional medicine and noted in folklore for hundreds of years. It has been used as an antispasmodic, and recent studies indicate that several of its components are similar to or more potent spasmolytics than papaverine in their effects on gastrointestinal and cardiac smooth muscle. The oil has been used as a folkloric abortifacient, and the plant should not be ingested, especially by pregnant women. Many compounds present in the plant possess antibacterial and antifungal properties. Rue has been used to treat intestinal worms and to repel insects. The furocoumarins contained in the plant are photosensitizers, and the topical application of the plant should be avoided. Although rue continues to be found in some herbal remedies, its use should be avoided.

PATIENT INFORMATION – Rue

Uses: Rue extract is useful as a potential potassium channel blocker. It has been used to treat many neuromuscular problems and to stimulate menstruation onset. Because rue has an antispasmodic effect at relatively small dose, take with caution, if at all.

Side effects: Rue extracts are found to be mutagenic and furocoumains have been associated with photosensitization. If ingested, the rue oil may result in kidney damage and hepatic degeneration. Large doses can cause violent gastric pain, vomiting and systemic complications including death. Because of possible abortifacient effects, the plant should never be ingested by women of childbearing potential.

---

[1] Chevallier A. *Encyclopedia of Medicinal Plants.* New York, NY: DK Publishing Inc., 1996;262-3.
[2] Conway GA, Slocumb JC. *J Ethnopharmacol* 1979;1:241.
[3] Duke J. *CRC Handbook of Medicinal Herbs,* Boca Raton, FL: CRC Press Inc., 1989;417-18.
[4] Minker E, et al. *Acta Pharm Hung* 1980;50:7.
[5] Tyler VE. *The New Honest Herbal.* Philadelphia: GF Stickley Co., 1987.
[6] Wolters B, Eilert U. *Planta Med* 1981;43:166.
[7] Verzar-Petri VG, et al. *Planta Med* 1976;29:372.
[8] Spoerke DG. *Herbal Medications.* Santa Barbara, CA: Wood-bridge Press Publishing Co, 1980.
[9] Haesen JP, et al. *Planta Med* 1971;19:285.
[10] Zobel A, et al. *J Nat Prod* 1988;51(Sep-Oct):941-6.
[11] Reisch J, et al. *Sci Pharm* 1988;56(Sep):171-4.
[12] Paulini H, et al. *Planta Med* 1991;57(1):59-61.
[13] Montagu M, et al. *Pharmazie* 1989;44(May):342-4.
[14] Baumert A, et al. *Z Naturforsch [C]* 1994;49(1-2):26-32.
[15] Bethge E, et al. *Gen Physiol Biophys* 1991;10(3):225-44.
[16] Kong Y, et al. *Planta Med* 1989;55(2):176-8.
[17] Gandhi M, et al. *J Ethnopharmacol* 1991;31(1):49-59.
[18] Istvan N, et al. *Acta Pharm Hung* 1967;37:130.
[19] Paulini H, et al. *Mutagenesis* 1987;2:271.
[20] Paulini H, et al. *Mutagenesis* 1989;4(1):45-50.
[21] Tyler, Heskel NS, et al. *Contact Dermatitis* 1983;9:278.
[22] Ortiz-Frutos F, et al. *Contact Dermatitis* 1995;33(4):284.
[23] Schimmer O, et al. *Mutant Res* 1990;243(1):57-62.
[24] Leung AY. *Encyclopedia of Common Natural Ingredients Used in Food, Drugs and Cosmetics.* New York: J Wiley and Sons, 1980.

Safflower

SCIENTIFIC NAME(S): *Carthamus tinctorius* L. Family: Compositae

COMMON NAME(S): Safflower, American saffron, zafran, bastard saffron, false saffron, dyer's-saffron

BOTANY: Safflower is native to the Middle East and today is widely cultivated throughout Europe and the United States. This annual reaches heights of about 3 feet with a single, smooth, upright stem. Its shiny oval, spiny-edged leaves alternate around the stem. The plant produces profuse flowers of yellow to deep red color. Seeds are produced in August and are enclosed in a mass of down.

HISTORY: Although safflower is today recognized primarily as a source of a healthful edible oil, its traditional uses had not focused on the oil. Rather, safflower was originally valued for the yellow and red dyes yielded by its flowers. These dyes had been used for centuries to color cosmetics and fabrics. The use of safflower extract to dye the wrappings of mummies has been reported.[1] Safflower had been used as a replacement for saffron, but because of its lack of taste, lost its popularity. Traditional uses of safflower tea included inducing sweating and reducing fever. The oil has been used as a solvent in paints.

CHEMISTRY: Safflower oil is characterized by the presence of a high proportion of unsaturated fatty acids. These fatty acids include linoleic (76% to 79%), oleic (13%), palmitic (6%), stearic (3%) and other minor straight-chained fatty acids.[2,3]

PHARMACOLOGY: There is a significant body of evidence that indicates that diets high in unsaturated and polyunsaturated fatty acids can reduce cholesterol levels, particularly those fractions associated with the development of atherosclerosis and cardiovascular disease. However, the degree to which this benefit accrues is subject to dispute.

Dietary supplementation for 8 weeks with safflower oil resulted in a significant increase in platelet linoleic acid levels that was also associated with an acute change in thromboxane B_2 levels. Another 8-week study found that dietary modification with safflower oil reduced total serum cholesterol levels significantly from baseline by 9% to 15%, low-density lipoprotein cholesterol by 12% to 20% and apolipoprotein B levels by 21% to 24%. However, there were no significant changes from baseline in serum triglyceride levels, high-density lipoprotein cholesterol levels or apolipoprotein A-I levels.[4]

There is some suggestion from animal studies that a moderate dietary intake of the essential fatty acids of the type found in safflower oil may be required to maintain the integrity of central nervous system function.[5] Low levels of essential polyunsaturated oils may be associated with the development of cardiovascular disease.

Although safflower oil is a rich source of linoleic acid, it requires the activity of delta 6-desaturate for its conversion to dihomo-gamma-linolenic acid (DHGA) and arachidonic acid. By contrast, evening primrose oil appears to be a more physiologic source of fatty acids for the production of DHGA than safflower oil.[6]

Apart from its effectiveness in modifying lipid profiles, safflower has had limited medical uses, having been employed as a laxative and to treat fevers.[1]

TOXICOLOGY: No significant toxicity has been associated with the ingestion of safflower oil.

SUMMARY: Safflower had been widely recognized as a source of dye. However, more recently, the beneficial properties of the high unsaturated fat content of its oil has resulted in the worldwide consumption of the oil in place of saturated fats. Although the results of clinical studies generally indicate that dietary supplementation with this oil can reduce serum cholesterol levels, the changes in lipid profiles may not be as important as previously suggested in terms of reducing the risk of cardiovascular disease.

PATIENT INFORMATION – Safflower

Uses: Safflower has been used as a dietary supplement to modify lipid profiles and has been used to treat fevers and as a laxative.

Side Effects: There are no known side effects.

[1] Dobelis IN, ed. Magic and Medicine of Plants. Pleasantville, NY: Reader's Digest Association, 1986.

[2] Kwon JS, et al. Effects of diets high on saturated fatty acids, canola oil or safflower oil on platelet function, thromboxane B_2 formation, and fatty acid composition of platelet phospholipids. *Am J Clin Nutr* 1991;54:351.

[3] Windolz M, ed. The Merck Index, ed. 10. Rahway, NJ: Merck & Co., 1983.

[4] Wardlaw GM, et al. Serum lipid and apolipoprotein concentrations in healthy men on diets enriched in either canola oil or safflower oil. *Am J Clin Nutr* 1991;54:104.

[5] Okuyama H. Minimum requirements of n-3 and n-6 essential fatty acids for the function of the central nervous system and for the prevention of chronic disease. *Proc Soc Exp Biol Med* 1992; 200(2):174.

[6] Abraham RD, et al. Effects of safflower oil and evening primrose oil in men with a low dihomo-gamma-linolenic level. *Atherosclerosis* 1990;81(3):199.

Saffron

SCIENTIFIC NAME(S): *Crocus sativus* L. Family: Iridaceae

COMMON NAME(S): Saffron

BOTANY: True saffron is native to Asia Minor and southern Europe. Its blue-violet, lily-shaped flowers contain the orange stigmas (part of the pistil), which are collected to produce the spice saffron. The plant is a bulbous perennial, growing 6 to 8 inches in height. Mature stigmas are collected by hand during a short blooming season. Over 200,000 dried stigmas, obtained from about 70,000 flowers, yield one pound of true saffron.[1] Saffron commands as much as $30 per ounce in the American market.

True saffron should not be confused with American saffron (safflower, Indian safflower) *Carthamus tinctorius* L. (family Compositae) that is produced from the tubular florets and is lighter red than true saffron. The two often are used for the same purposes, and less expensive American saffron is sometimes used to adulterate true saffron.

HISTORY: Saffron has been widely used for flavoring food and as a dye for cloth where it continues to find use in underdeveloped countries and among back-to-basics artisans. Folkloric uses of saffron have included its use as a sedative, expectorant, aphrodisiac and diaphoretic. Anecdotal reports from the tropical regions of Asia describe the use of a paste composed of sandalwood and saffron as a soothing balm for dry skin.

CHEMISTRY: The stigmas of *C. sativus* are rich in riboflavin, a yellow pigment and vitamins. In addition, saffron contains crocin, the major source of yellowish-red pigment. A hypothetical protocrocin of the fresh plant is decomposed on drying into one molecule of crocin (a colored glycoside) and two molecules of picrocrocin (a colorless bitter glycoside).[2] Crocin is a mixture of glycosides: crocetin, a dicarboxylic terpene lipid, and alpha-crocin, a digentiobiose ester of crocetin. In addition, cis- and trans- crocetin dimethylesters have been identified. Similar compounds have been isolated from other members of the Iridaceae. A compound named gardenidin, obtained from gardenias, has been shown to be identical with crocetin. The characteristic taste of the spice is attributed to the glycoside picrocrocin. Following hydrolysis, the compound yielded glucose and safranal, the main odiferous constituent. The essential oil derived from saffron is a complex mixture of more than 30 components, mainly terpenes and their derivatives.[2]

PHARMACOLOGY: United States patents have been issued for the proposed use of crocetin in the treatment of skin papillomas, spinal cord injuries, hypertension and cerebral edema in cats. It also has been used to increase fermentation yields. In vitro, a concentrated saffron extract has been shown to limit the growth of experimental tumor colony cells by inhibiting cellular nucleic acid synthesis.[3] Orally administered saffron (200 mg/kg) has been shown to increase the lifespan of mice with a variety of intraperitoneally transplanted and topical cancers,[4,5] suggesting that the product may have the potential to act as an anticancer agent.

A German patent has been granted for a preparation that contains a mixture of opium, quinine and saffron, which is used in the prevention of premature ejaculation. An aqueous extract of the corm (underground bulb) in combination with salicylic acid and vegetable oils is said to restore hair growth in baldness and has been granted an Australian patent.

Perhaps the most poorly understood of saffron's actions is its ability to increase oxygen diffusion. Atherosclerosis may be initiated by hypoxia at the vascular wall, and this hypoxia may be due to a decreased rate of oxygen diffusion from the red blood cells.[6] A way to counteract such diffusion decreases would be to use a drug that increases oxygen diffusion in plasma. Although few compounds appear to do this, crocetin has been found to bring about an 80% increase in the oxygen diffusivity of plasma.[7] A patent has been issued for the use of crocetin to increase oxygen diffusion into solutions such as plasma (US Patent No. 3,788,468 Jan. 29, 1974). Crocetin binds strongly to serum albumin.[8]

Injections of crocetin in rabbits fed 1% cholesterol diets for four to five months have been found to decrease cholesterol and triglyceride levels.[6,7] Serum cholesterol levels were 50% lower in the crocetin-treated animals than in the controls. The triglyceride level of the crocetin group remained in the normal range while the controls increased by 2000%. Vascular (aortic) damage was much less severe in the rabbits that received crocetin. The mechanism for these effects is poorly understood.

Epidemiologic evidence suggests that the low incidence of cardiovascular disease in parts of Spain may be related to the liberal, almost daily consumption of saffron. Algae in Japanese diets may have a similar protective effect.[9] Limited data make it difficult to correlate the effects observed following crocetin injections in animals with the oral consumption of saffron in humans.

TOXICOLOGY: There is no evidence to support saffron's reported emmenagogue (induces or increases menstruation) or abortifacient effects. Large doses of the stigmas have been reported to act as sedatives,[1] and Duke cites fatalities that have occurred from the use of saffron as an abortifacient.[10] The saponin-containing corm is toxic to young animals. Nevertheless, saffron is not generally associated with toxicity when ingested in culinary amounts.

SUMMARY: Saffron is a widely used spice. It is one of the few natural compounds that increases oxygen diffusion in vivo. An association between a reduced incidence of cardiovascular disease and chronic saffron injection has been suggested, but well-designed demographic studies must be conducted to confirm this relationship. Other data suggest that saffron may possess antineoplastic activity.

PATIENT INFORMATION – Saffron

Uses: Saffron increases oxygen diffusion in vivo and may possess antineoplastic activity.

Side Effects: Saffron is generally not associated with toxicity when ingested in culinary amounts.

---

[1] Bricklin Mark, Der Marderosian AH contributor. The Practical Encyclopedia of Natural Healing. Emmaus, PA: Rodale Press, Inc., 1976.

[2] Evans WC. Trease and Evans' Pharmacognosy, ed. 13. London: Balliere Tindall, 1989.

[3] Abdullaev FI, Frenkel GD. Effect of saffron on cell colony formation and cellular nucleic acid and protein synthesis. *Biofactors* 1992;3:201.

[4] Nair SC, et al. Antitumor activity of saffron (*Crocus sativus*). *Cancer Lett* 1991;57:109.

[5] Salomi MJ, et al. Inhibitory effects of *Nigella sativa* and saffron (*Crocus sativus*) on chemical carcinogenesis in mice. *Nutr Cancer* 1991;16:67.

[6] Gainer JL, Jones JR. The Use of Crocetin in Experimental Atherosclerosis. *Experientia* 1975;31:548.

[7] Gainer JL, Chisolm III GM. Oxygen Diffusion and Atherosclerosis. *Atherosclerosis* 1974;19:135.

[8] Miller TL, et al. Binding of Crocetin to Plasma Albumin. *J Pharm Sci* 1982;71:173.

[9] Grisolia S. Hypoxia, Saffron, and Cardiovascular Disease. *Lancet* 1974;7871:41.

[10] Duke JA. Handbook of Medicinal Herbs. Boca Raton, FL: CRC Press, 1985.

Sage

SCIENTIFIC NAME(S): *Salvia officinalis* L. (Dalmatian sage), *S. lavandulaefolia* Vahl. (Spanish sage). Although a large number of other species of Salvia have been cultivated, these two represent the most commercially important species. Family: Labiatae or Lamiaceae

COMMON NAME(S): Garden sage, true sage, scarlet sage, meadow sage

BOTANY: Sage is a small, evergreen perennial plant with short woody stems that branches extensively and can attain heights of 2 to 3 feet.[1] Its violet-blue flowers bloom from June to September. The plant is native to the Mediterranean region and grows throughout much of the world. This plant should not be confused with red sage or the brush sage of the desert.

HISTORY: Dried sage leaf is used as a culinary spice and as a source of sage oil, which is obtained by steam distillation. Traditionally, sage and its oil have been used for the treatment of a wide range of illnesses; the name *Salvia* derives from the Latin word meaning "healthy" or "to heal."[2,3] Extracts and teas have been used to treat digestive disorders, as a tonic and antispasmodic. The plant has been employed topically as an antiseptic and astringent, and has been used to manage excessive sweating.[4] Sage has been used internally as a tea for the treatment of dysmenorrhea, diarrhea, gastritis and sore throat. The dried leaves have been smoked to treat asthma. Despite these varied uses, there is little evidence that the plant exerts any significant pharmacologic activity. The fragrance of the plant is said to suppress the odor of fish. Sage oil is used as a fragrance in soaps and perfumes. It is a widely used food flavoring, and sage oleoresin is also used in the culinary industry.

CHEMISTRY: *S. officinalis* contains 1% to 2.8% of a volatile oil. The highly aromatic plant contains a wide variety of minor chemical constituents including picrosalvin, carnosol, salvin and related ethers, flavonoids, phenolic acids and salviatannin (a tannin that undergoes degradation to phlobaphenes upon storage). Sage oil contains alpha- and beta-thujones, which account for about half of the composition of the oil.[1]

The composition of Spanish sage oil differs somewhat, with variable amounts of camphor, cineol, limonene, camphene and pinene.[1,4] Sage oil is often adulterated by the addition of thujone derived from the leaves of *Juniperus virginiana* (red cedar).

PHARMACOLOGY: Sage extracts have been shown to have strong antioxidative activities, with labiatic acid and carnosic acid reported to be the active compounds.[1]

The phenolic acid salvin and its monomethyl ether have antimicrobial activity, especially against *Staphylococcus aureus*.[1]

Sage oil has antispasmodic effects in laboratory animals and this is likely related to its effect as a gastrointestinal antispasmodic. There is some evidence that sage oil may exert a centrally mediated antisecretory action; the carminative effect is likely due to the irritating effects of the volatile oil.[5]

TOXICOLOGY: Although sage oil contains thujone, the oil does not have a reputation for toxicity. The oil has been found to be nonirritating and nonsensitizing when applied topically to human skin in diluted concentrations. Spanish sage oil was also nonphototoxic when applied to mice and pigs.[1]

Cheilitis and stomatitis, however, have been reported in some cases following the ingestion of sage tea.[4] Others have reported that ingestion of large amounts of the plant extract may cause dry mouth or local irritation.

SUMMARY: Sage is a widely used, popular spice and sage oil is used in a variety of culinary applications. Although the plant has a long history of use in traditional medicine, there is little evidence that it provides any unique effects beyond those typically associated with other volatile oils (ie, antispasmodic, carminative). Although the oil contains thujone, there is no evidence of direct toxicity.

PATIENT INFORMATION – Sage

Uses: Sage has no proven medical effects, but may be antispasmodic and carminative.

Side Effects: The only side effects reported with the ingestion of sage include cheilitis, stomatitis, dry mouth, or local irritation.

[1] Leung AY. Encyclopedia of Common Natural Ingredients Used in Food, Drugs, and Cosmetics. New York, NY: J. Wiley and Sons, 1980.

[2] Dobelis IN, ed. Magic and Medicine of Plants. Pleasantville, NY: Reader's Digest Association, Inc., 1986.

[3] Simon JE. Herbs: an indexed bibliography, 1971-1980. Hamden, CT: Shoe String Press, 1984.

[4] Duke, JA. Handbook of Medicinal Herbs. Boca Raton, FL: CRC Press, 1985.

[5] Spoerke DG, Jr. Herbal Medications. Santa Barbara, CA: Woodbridge Press, 1980.

SAMe

SCIENTIFIC NAME(S): *S-adenosylmethionine*, *S-adenosyl-L-methionine*, *ademetionine*, *ademetionine 1,4-butanedisulfonate*, *ADE-SD4*.

COMMON NAME(S): SAMe, SAM

BOTANY/SOURCE SAMe is found in all living cells. It is a naturally occurring molecule produced by a reaction between the amino acid methionine and ATP. SAMe acts as a substrate in many biological reactions and is the precursor of certain essential amino acids.[1,2] The commercial product is not a botanical, but a supplement or biochemical compound produced in yeast cell cultures. One manufacturing process describes its preparation through fermentation of yeast *Saccharomyces cerevisiae*, enriched by the Schlenk method in the presence of methionine.[1]

HISTORY: SAMe was discovered in Italy in 1952. Since that time, numerous clinical studies have been performed on its efficacy.[3] SAMe has been used in Europe, where it has been available by prescription since 1975, to treat arthritis and depression. It is available in the US as a supplement by several companies (eg, Natural Made, Pharmavite, GNC).[2,3]

CHEMISTRY: SAMe is involved in a number of biochemical reactions involving enzymatic transmethylation. It is a precursor of certain compounds, including the amino acids cysteine, taurine, and glutathione. SAMe is an initiator of 3 metabolic pathways in the human body: Transmethylation, transsulfuration, and polyamine synthesis. Transmethylation involves methyl-group transfer to other molecules, enabling them to proceed to certain anabolic or catabolic reactions. Transsulfuration involves a pathway resulting in sulfates and reduced glutathione, an important antioxidant, which provides sulfhydryl groups to bind to and detoxify certain compounds. Eighty-five percent of all transmethylation reactions occur in the liver. SAMe, after donating the methyl group, is converted to cysteine, which is important for synthesis of glutathione and other sulfur-containing compounds.[1,4]

Determination of SAMe using high performance liquid chromatographic (HPLC) has been reported.[5]

PHARMACOLOGY: The properties of SAMe have been studied in a variety of areas including the CNS, osteoarthritis, fibromyalgia, liver disorders, and others.

CNS: SAMe's uses in depressive disorders were first seen in the early 1970s. Shortcomings from trials around this time (varied dosages of SAMe, small number of patients enrolled, severity of depression variation, etc) eventually led to improvement in consistency, specifically the Hamilton rating scale, grouping similar patients.[4]

Studies indicate the importance of the methylation process in the brain. SAMe is known to be an important methyl donor for a wide range of substrates (eg, proteins, lipids, hormones, nucleic acids). SAMe has shown some value in psychiatry, particularly in depressive disorders. A meta-analysis of all studies comparing SAMe with either placebo or standard tricyclic antidepressants has shown SAMe to have greater efficacy than placebo and efficacy comparable to that of tricyclics.[6] An adequate supply of SAMe must be attained for normal CNS function. Vitamin B_{12} or folate deficiency decreases the levels of SAMe, which lowers serotonin levels associated with depression.[7] Low SAMe levels in the cerebrospinal fluid (CSF) of patients with neurological and psychiatric disorders (eg, Alzheimer's disease, spinal cord degeneration, HIV-type neuropathies) suggest that supplementation with this compound may be beneficial in treating these disorders.[8,9] Similarly, increased plasma concentrations of SAMe were associated with mood improvement in depressed patients.[10] In another report, disruption of methylation by low SAMe levels was found to cause structural and functional abnormalities including myelopathy and depression.[11] Nerve regeneration requires the presence of SAMe.[12]

These findings support the hypothesis that in the CNS, SAMe has modulating effects on mood, with adequate amounts needed to maintain normal mood and remission of symptoms in patients with major depressive disorders. Dosage ranges for depression have been reported as 400 mg 3 to 4 times daily. If nausea and GI upset occur, the dosage can be tapered.[2]

Osteoarthritis: Animal studies have shown SAMe to prevent induced osteoarthritis in rabbits.[13] Higher chondrocyte counts and increased cartilage thickness were observed in rabbits administered SAMe vs placebo.[14]

SAMe appears to enhance native proteoglycan synthesis and secretion in human chondrocyte cultures in the cartilage of patients with osteoarthritis.[15] It possesses analgesic properties similar to NSAIDs but with no or minimal GI side effects.[16] SAMe has demonstrated gastric cytoprotective actions in animals.[17] Another problem with NSAID use involves in vitro suppression of articular cartilage proteoglycans synthesis which suggests that NSAIDs may even accelerate cartilage damage.[18]

Clinical trials involving a total of greater than 21,000 patients who received SAMe treatment, 458 patients who were given different NSAIDs (ibuprofen, indomethacin, naproxen, and piroxicam), and 279 who received placebo. The periods of treatment ranged from 3 weeks to 2 years. These controlled clinical trials demonstrated that SAMe improved both subjective and objective symptoms of osteoarthritis more than placebo and showed the same efficacy as the NSAIDs.[1,19,20] Maintenance dosage of SAMe for osteoarthritis is 200 mg twice daily.[2]

Fibromyalgia: Fibromyalgia is a disorder that is a common cause of chronic musculoskeletal pain and fatigue. At least 3 clinical trials found SAMe to be beneficial. Subjects given 200 mg SAMe per day parenterally demonstrated reductions in certain trigger points and painful areas, as well as mood improvements. The other reports confirmed SAMe's benefits in pain relief, morning stiffness, and mood enhancement.[2]

Liver disorders: Through methylation, SAMe regulates liver cell membrane lipid composition and fluidity, and by activation of the transsulfuration pathway, promotes endogenous detoxification processes in the liver. Further, it is the main source of glutathione, a major compound involved in several detoxification reactions in this organ.[21] SAMe restores normal hepatic function in conditions such as cirrhosis and cholestasis and aids in reversing hepatotoxicity.[4] Its liver-protectant actions are apparent in several studies, including actions against membrane alterations in rabbits fed high-cholesterol diets,[22] and in experimentation where high concentrations of SAMe were associated with reduced liver injury.[23,24,25,26,27] SAMe can be considered an important nutrient in alcoholic subjects.[28]

Others: Other beneficial effects of SAMe include treatment of migraine headaches (200 to 400 mg twice daily),[29] alteration of the aging process,[30,31,32] and sleep modulation.[33]

TOXICOLOGY: Other than occasional nausea and GI disturbances, no side effects, drug interactions, or disease contraindications have been found in recent literature reviews. Patients with bipolar disorder should not take SAMe, as it may lead to the manic phase.[2] In a field trial involving greater than 20,000 patients, the overall withdrawal rate caused by adverse effects was $\approx$ 5%, mainly during the first 2 weeks of treatment when the oral dose of SAMe was the highest (800 to 1200 mg daily).[4]

Toxicological studies of SAMe by parenteral and oral administration performed in different animal species recommended and commonly utilized in preclinical research labs included mutagenicity and carcinogenicity studies. They concluded that SAMe is completely safe even at the highest dosages.[1]

SUMMARY: SAMe is a naturally occurring molecule found in all living cells. It has been used in Europe, by prescription only, for depressive illness and arthritis since the mid-1970s. In the US, it is sold as a nutritional supplement. SAMe is useful in the treatment of depressive disorders, osteoarthritis, fibromyalgia, liver disorders, migraine headaches, and for sleep modulation. SAMe appears to have no significant side effects associated with its use.

PATIENT INFORMATION – SAMe

Uses: SAMe has been used in the treatment of depressive disorders, osteoarthritis, fibromyalgia, liver disorders, migraine headaches, and for sleep modulation.

Side Effects: Other than occasional nausea and GI disturbances, no side effects have been reported. Bipolar disorder patients should not use SAMe.

---

[1] Proceedings of a symposium in SAMe (Osteoarthritis: The clinical picture, pathogenesis, and management with studies on a new therapeutic agent S-adenosylmethionine. *Am J Med* 1987;Nov 20 83(5A):1-110.

[2] Murry M. Encyclopedia of Nutritional Supplements. Rocklin, CA: Prima Pub., 1996;365-73.

[3] http://www.mothernature.com/articles/sam-e/about_sam-e.stm

[4] Focus on s-adenosylmethionine. *Drugs* 1989;38(3):390-416.

[5] Luippold G, et al. Simultaneous determination of adenosine, S-adenosylhomocysteine and S-adenosylmethionine in biological samples using solid-phase extraction and high-performance liquid chromatography. *J Chromatogr B Biomed Sci Appl* 1999;724(2):231-38.

[6] Bressa G, S-adenosyl-l-methicnine (SAM-e) as antidepressant: meta-analysis of clinical studies. *Acta Neurol Scand* 1994(Suppl. 154):7-14.

[7] Young S. The use of diet and dietary components in the study of factors controlling affect in humans: a review. *J Psychiatry Neurosci* 1993;18(5):235-44.

[8] Bottigueri T, et al. S-adenosylmethionine levels in psychiatric and neurological disorders: a review. *Acta Neurol Scand* 1994(Suppl. 154):19-26.

[9] Lesley D, et al. Brain S-Adenosylmethionine Levels Are Severely Decreased in Alzheimer's Disease. *J Neurochem* 1999;67(3):1328.

[10] Bell K, et al. S-adenosylmethionine blood levels in major depression: changes with drug treatment. *Acta Neurol Scand* 1994;(Suppl. 154):15-18.

[11] Scott J, et al. Effects of the disruption of transmethylation in the central nervous system: an animal model. *Acta Neurol Scand* 1994;(Suppl. 154):27-31.

[12] Cestaro B. Effects of arginine, S-adenosylmethionine and polyamines on nerve regeneration. *Acta Neurol Scand* 1994;(Suppl. 154):32-41.

[13] Moskowitz R, et al. Experimentally induced degenerative joint lesions following partial meniscectomy in the rabbit. *Arthritis Rheum* 1973;16:397-405.

[14] Barceló H, et al. Effects of s-adenosylmethionine on experimental osteoarthritis in rabbits. *Am J Med* 1987;83(5A):55-59.

[15] Harmand, et al. Effects of s-adenosylmethionine on human articular chondrocyte differentiation and in vitro study. *Am J Med* 1987;83(5A):48-54.

[16] Di Padova C. S-Adenosylmethionine in the treatment of osteoarthritis. *Am J Med* 1987;83(5A):60-65.

[17] Laudanno O. Cytoprotective effect of S-Adenosylmethionine compared with that of misoprostol against ethanol-, aspirin-, and stress-induced gastric damage. *Am J Med* 1987;83(5A):43-47.

[18] Brandt K. Effects of nonsteroidal anti-inflammatory drugs on chonodrocyte metabolism in vitro and in vivo. *Am J Med* 1987;83(5A):29-34.

[19] Montrone F, et al. Double blind study of s-adenosylmethionine versus placebo in hip and knee arthrosis. *Clin Rheumatol* 1985;4:484-85.

[20] Caruso I, et al. Italian double-blind multicenter study comparing s-adenosylmethionine, naproxen, and placebo in the treatment of degenerative joint disease. *Am J Med* 1987;83(5A):66-71.

[21] Kaplowitz N. The importance and regulation of hepatic glutathione. *Yale J Biol Med* 1981;54:407-502.

[22] Pezzoli C, et al. S-adenosylmethionine protects against erythrocyte membrane alterations induced in rabbits by cholesterol-rich diets. *Pharmacol Res Commun* 1983;15(9):785-95.

[23] Shivapurkar N, et al. Decreased levels of S-adenosylmethionine in the livers of rats fed phenobarbital and DDT. *Carcinogenesis* 1982;3(5):589-91.

[24] Poirier L. The role of methionine in carcinogenesis in vivo. *Adv Exp Med Biol* 1986;206:269-82.

[25] Barak A, et al. Dietary betaine promotes generation of hepatic S-adenosylmethionine and protects the liver from ethanol-induced fatty infiltration. *Alcohol Clin Exp Res* 1993;17(3):552-55.

[26] Dausch J, et al. Increased levels of S-adenosylmethionine in the livers of rats fed various forms of selenium. *Nutr Cancer* 1993;20(1):31-39.

[27] Barak A, et al. S-adenosylmethionine generation and prevention of alcoholic fatty liver by betaine. *Alcohol* 1994;11(6):501-03.

[28] Chawla R, et al. Effect of ethanol consumption of metabolism of S-adenosyl-L-methionine in rat liver. *Drug Invest* 1992;4(4):41-45.

[29] Gatto G, et al. Analgesizing effect of a methyl donor (S-adenosylmethionine) in migraine: an open clinical trial. *Int J Clin Pharmacol Res* 1986;6:15-17.

[30] Baldessarini R, et al. S-adenosylmethionine in brain and other tissues. *J Neurochem* 1966;13;769-77.

[31] Stramentinoli G, et al. Tissue levels of S-Adenosylmethionine in aging rats. *J Gerontology* 1977;32(4):392-94.

[32] Bohuon C, et al. S-Adenosylmethionine in human blood. *Clinica Chimica Acta* 1971;33:256.

[33] Stramentinoli G. Ademetionine, a new candidate for nutraceutical. *Scandinavica* 1994;(Suppl. 154), vol. 59:5-41.

Sandalwood

SCIENTIFIC NAME(S): *Santalum album* L. Family: Santalaceae

COMMON NAME(S): Sandalwood, santal oil, white saunders oil, white or yellow sandalwood oil, East Indian sandalwood oil[1]

BOTANY: Indigenous to India, the Malay Archipelago, and Indonesia, the sandalwood is an evergreen tree that grows to 8 to 12 meters in height.[2] Australian sandalwood oil is prepared by distillation of the wood of *Eucarya spicata*, a small tree native to western Australia that contains sesquiterpene alcohols known as fusanols.[2] This oil is similar to the native Indian sandalwood oil in odor, although its topnotes are characteristically different.[1]

HISTORY: Sandalwood oil commonly is used as a fragrance in incense, cosmetics, perfumes and soaps. It also is used as a flavor for foods and beverages.[3] The wood has been valued in carving because of its dense character.

In traditional medicine, sandalwood oil has been used for a wide variety of conditions ranging from an antiseptic and astringent to the treatment of headache, stomach ache and urogenital disorders.

CHEMISTRY: Sandalwood oil is obtained from the heartwood of the plant. This volatile oil contains about 90% alpha- and beta-santalols with a variety of minor components including sesquiterpene hydrocarbons (about 6%).[3] The santalols are responsible for the pleasant odor of sandalwood although 2-furfuryl pyrrole also may contribute an effect.[3]

The seeds yield about 50% of a viscid, dark red, fixed oil. This oil contains stearolic acid and santalbic acid. Gas chromatography fingerprinting of sandalwood oils has been used successfully in light of the complex nature of the components of the oils.[4]

PHARMACOLOGY: Good clinical studies are lacking in support of the effects of sandalwood oil. The oil has been reported to have diuretic and urinary antiseptic properties.[1]

TOXICOLOGY: The oil has been found to be irritating in both mouse and rabbit skin test models. Santalol can cause dermatitis in sensitive persons[3] although it is generally considered to be nonirritating to human skin.[1] The santalols and related compounds have been identified in the blood of mice that inhaled sandalwood fumes under experimental conditions, indicating that systemic absorption of these compounds can occur.[5]

SUMMARY: Sandalwood is a fragrant wood from which an oil is derived for use in foods and cosmetics. The oil has been used widely in traditional Asian medicine and had been official in the United States at the turn of the century. Today, the oil finds little medicinal use but its widespread use as a popular fragrance continues.

PATIENT INFORMATION – Sandalwood

Uses: Sandalwood has been reported to have diuretic and urinary antiseptic properties, but mainly the oil extracted from the wood has been used as a fragrance enhancer.

Side Effects: Sandalwood can cause dermatitis in sensitive persons.

---

[1] Leung AY. Encyclopedia of Common Natural Ingredients Used in Food, Drugs and Cosmetics. New York, NY: J. Wiley and Sons, 1980.
[2] Evans WC. Trease and Evans' Pharmacognosy, ed. 13. London, England: Balliere Tindall, 1989.
[3] Duke JA. Handbook of Medicinal Herbs. Boca Raton, FL: CRC Press, 1985.
[4] Wang Z, Hong X. Comparative GC analysis of essential oil in imported sandalwood. *Chung Kuo Chung Yao Tsa Chih* 1991;16:40.
[5] Jirovetz L et al. Analysis of fragrance compounds in blood samples of mice by gas chromatography, mass spectrometry, GC/FTIR and GC/AES after inhalation of sandalwood oil. *Biomed Chromatogr* 1992;6:133.

Sarsaparilla

SCIENTIFIC NAME(S): *Smilax* species including *Smilax aristolochiifolia* Mill. (Mexican sarsaparilla), *S. officinalis* Kunth (Honduras sarsaparilla), *Smilax regelii* Killip et Morton (Honduras, Jamaican sarsaparilla), *Smilax febrifuga* (Ecuadorian sarsaparilla), *Smilax sarsaparilla*, *Smilax ornata*. Family: Liliaceae.

COMMON NAME(S): Sarsaparilla, smilax, smilace, sarsa, khao yen

BOTANY: Sarsaparilla is a woody, trailing vine, which can grow to 50 meters in length. It is grown in the areas listed above. Many *Smilax* species are very similar in appearance regardless of origin. The part of the plant used for medicinal purposes is the root. Although this root has a pleasant fragrance and spicy sweet taste, and has been used as a natural flavoring agent in medicines, foods, and non-alcoholic beverages, it should not be confused with the sassafras tree, which has the distinctive flavoring of American root beer.[1,2]

HISTORY: The French physician Monardes described using sarsaparilla to treat syphilis in 1574. In 1812, Portuguese soldiers suffering from syphilis recovered faster if sarsaparilla was taken to treat the disease versus mercury, the standard treatment at the time.[3] Sarsaparilla has been used by many cultures for other ailments as well, including skin problems, arthritis, fever, digestive disorders, leprosy, and cancer.[1,3] Late 15th century accounts explaining the identification and the first descriptions of American drugs include sarsaparilla.[4] Sarsaparilla's role as a medicinal plant in American and European remedies in the 16th century is also evident.[5]

CHEMISTRY: Many *Smilax* species contain a number of steroidal saponins. *S. sarsaparilla* contains approximately 2% steroidal saponins, including sarsaponin, smilasaponin (smilacin), sarsaparilloside and its aglycones sarsasaponin (parillin), sarsasapogenin (parigenin), and smilagenin.[1,3] Other saponins include diosgenin, tigogenin, and asperagenin.[1] Phytosterols listed are sitosterol, stigmasterol, and pollinastanol.[1,2] One report lists three new steroidal saponins from *S. officinalis*.[6] Various saponins from other *Smilex* species exist as well, from *S. menispermoidea*,[7] *S. sieboldii*,[8,9] *S. lebrunii*,[10] *S. riparia*, and *S. china*.[11]

Other constiuents present in sarsaparilla include starch (50%), resin, cetyl alcohol, volatile oil,[1,2] caffeoylshikimic acid, shikimic acid, ferulic acid,[1] sarsapic acid,[12] kaempferol, and quercetin.[1] Minerals reported in the genus include aluminum, chromium, iron, magnesium, selenium, calcium, zinc, and others.[12] A related species, *S. glabra*, contains flavonol glycosides such as isoastilbin, isoengetitin, and astilbin.[13,14]

PHARMACOLOGY: Sarsaparilla has been used for treating **syphilis** and other sexually transmitted diseases (STDs) throughout the world for 40 years and was documented as an adjuvant for **leprosy** treatment in 1959.[15]

The ability of sarsaparilla to bind to endotoxins may be a probable mechanism of action as to how the plant exerts its effects. Problems associated with high endotoxin levels circulating in the blood stream such as liver disease, psoriasis, fevers, and inflammatory processes, all seem to improve with sarsaparilla.[3] Sarsaparilla has also displayed hepatoprotective properties in rats.[16]

Antibiotic actions of sarsaparilla are also seen but are probably secondary to its endotoxin-binding effects.[3] Antibiotic properties of the plant[1] are shown by its treatment of leprosy and its actions against leptosirosis, a rare disease transmitted by rats, as proven by Chinese studies.[12]

Other positive effects of sarsaparilla on the skin have been demonstrated. The endotoxin-binding sarsaponin from the plant has improved psoriasis in 62% of patients and has completely cleared the disease in 18%, as seen in a 1940s study.[17] Antidermatophyte activity from the species *S. regelii* has been demonstrated in a later report.[18] In addition, sarsaparilla has been used as an herbal or folk remedy for other skin conditions including eczema, pruritus, rashes, and wound care.[2,12]

Sarsaparilla's anti-inflammatory actions have made the plant useful for treating arthritis, rheumatism, and gout.[3,12] *S. sarsaparilla* inhibited carrageenan-induced paw inflammation in rats, as well as cotton pellet-induced exudation.[19]

The saponin sarsasapogenin can be synthetically transformed into testosterone in-vitro, for example, but it is unlikely that this can happen in-vivo. Some advertising claims of sarsaparilla being a "rich source of testosterone," are unsubstantiated as there is no testosterone present in the plant.[3] However, some sources state that sarsaparilla exhibits testosterogenic actions on the body, increasing muscle bulk and estrogenic actions as well to help alleviate female problems. In Mexico, the root is still used for its alleged aphrodisiac properties.[12] A recent review addresses smilax compounds (among others) present in bodybuilding supplements said to "enhance performance." Results of the study of over 600 commercially available supplements determined that there was no research to validate these claims.[20]

Other documented uses of sarsaparilla include the following: Improvement in appetite and digestion,[1] adaptogenic effects from *S. regelii*,[21] sarsaparilla in combination as an herbal remedy and mineral supplement,[22] and haemolytic activity of steroidic saponins from *S. officinalis*.[23] An overview of medicinal uses of sarsaparilla is available.[24] One report evaluating fracture healing finds sarsaparilla to have insignificant effects on tensile strength and collagen deposition.[25] Other species of smilax have been evaluated for antimutagenic actions (*S. china*),[26] GI disorders (*S. lundelii*),[27] and actions on hyperuricemic and hyperuricosuric rats (*S. macrophylla*).[28] The species *S. glabra* exhibits wormicidal effects,[29] improves hepatitis B in combination,[30] had marked therapeutic effects (in combination) in the treatment of intestinal metaplasia and atypical hyperplasia,[31] and hypoglycemic effects in mice,[32] and has hepatoprotective effects.[33]

TOXICOLOGY: No major contraindications, warnings, or toxicity data have been documented with sarsaparilla use. No known probelms have been seen regarding its use in pregnancy or lactation either; however, excessive ingestion should be avoided.[1] In unusually high doses, the saponins present in the plant could possibly be harmful, resulting in GI irriation.[2] The fact that sarsaparilla binds bacterial endotoxins in the gut, making them unabsorbable, greatly reduces stress on the liver and other organs.[3] Sarsaparilla has inhibited induced hepatocellular damage in rats, without any significant adverse reactions reported.[16]

One report describing occupational asthma caused by sarsaparilla root dust exists in the literature.[34]

SUMMARY: Sarsaparilla root has been used for many centuries and by many cultures for syphilis, inflammatory disorders, digestve problems, and skin diseases. The plant is rich in saponins, which may bind to endotoxins to exert its "blood purifying" and other related effects. The steroid structures present in sarsaparilla have been erroneously advertised as muscle bulk and performance enhancers, but no research thus far has validated these claims. Related species to sarsaparilla have their own documented effects as well. No major toxicity problems have been associated with the plant. Excessive dosing may cause gastric irritation.

PATIENT INFORMATION – Sarsaparilla

Uses: Sarsaparilla has been used for treating syphiis, leprosy, psoriasis, and other ailments.

Side effects: No major contraindications, warnings or side effects have been documented; avoid excessive ingestion. In unusually high doses, the plant possibly could be harmful, including GI irritation.

---

[1] Newall C, et al. Herbal Medicines. London, England: Pharmaceutical Press, 1996;233-34.

[2] Duke J. CRC Handbook of Medicinal Herbs. Boca Raton, FL: CRC Press, Inc., 1989;446.

[3] Murray M. The Healing Power of Herbs, 2nd Ed. Rocklin, CA: Prima Publishing, 1995;302-5.

[4] Estes J. European reception of the first drugs from the new world. *Pharmacy in History* 1995;37(1):3-23.

[5] Elferink J. Significance of pre-Columbian pharmaceutical knowledge for European medicine in the XVIth century. *Pharmaceutica Acta Helvitiae* 1979;54(9-10):299-302.

[6] Bernardo R, et al. Steroidal saponins from *Smilax officinalis*. *Phytochemistry* 1996;43(2):465-69.

[7] Ju Y, et al. Steroidal saponins from the rhizomes of *Smilax menispermoidea*. *Phytochemistry* 1992;31(4):1349-51.

[8] Kubo S, et al. Steroidal saponins from the rhizomes of *Smilax sieboldii*. *Phytochemistry* 1992;31(7):2445-50.

[9] Okanishi T, et al. Studies on the steroidal components of domestic plants. XLVII. Constiuents of the stem of *Smilax sieboldi* Miq. (1). The structure of laxogenin. *Chem Pharm Bull* 1965;13(5):545-50.

[10] Jia Z, et al. Steroidal saponins from *Smilax lebrunii*. *Phytochemistry* 1992;31(9):3173-75.

[11] Sashida Y, et al. Steroidal saponins from *Smilax riparia* and *S. china*. *Phytochemistry* 1992;31(7) 2439-43.

[12] Chevallier A. Encyclopedia of Medicinal Plants. New York, NY: DK Publishing 1996;268.

[13] Chen G, et al. Flavanonol glucosides of *Smilax glabra* Roxb. *Chung Kuo Chung Yao Tsa Chih* 1996;21(6):355-57,383.

[14] Li Y, et al. Studies on the structure of isoastilbin. *Yao Hsueh Hsueh Pao* 1996;31(10):761-63.

[15] Rollier R. *Int J Leprosy* 1959;27:328-40.

[16] Rafatullah S, et al. Hepatoprotective and safety evaluation studies on sarsaparilla. *Int J Pharmacognosy* 1991;29(4):296-301.

[17] Thurman F. *New Engl J Med* 1942;227:128-33.

[18] Caceres A, et al. Plants used in Guatemala for the treatment of dermatophytic infections. 1. Screening for antimycotic activity of 44 plant extracts. *J Ethnopharmcol* 1991 Mar;31(3):263-76.

[19] Ageel A, et al. Experimental studies on antirheumatic crude drugs used in Saudi traditional medicine. *Drugs Exp Clin Res* 1989;15(8):369-72.

[20] Grunewald K, et al. Commercially marketed supplements for bodybuilding athletes. *Sports Med* 1993;15(2):90-103.

[21] Di Pasquale M. Stimulants and adaptogens. Part 2. *Drugs in Sports* 1993 Feb;2:2-4.

[22] Hamlin T. Matol. *Can J Hosp Pharm* 1991;44(1):39-40.

[23] Santos W, et al. Haemolytic activities of plant saponins and adjuvants. Effect of *Periandra mediterranea* saponin on the humoral response to the FML antigen of *Leishmania donovani. Vaccine* 1997;15(9):1024-29.

[24] Osborne F, et al. Sarsaparilla. *Can Pharm J* 1996 Jun;129:48-51.

[25] Ahsan S, et al. Studies on some herbal drugs used in fracture healing. *Int J Crude Drug Res* 1989 Dec;27:235-39.

[26] Lee H, et al. Antimutagenic activity of extracts from anticancer drugs in Chinese medicine. *Mutat Res* 1988;204(2):229-34.

[27] Caceres A, et al. Plants used in Guatemala for the treatment of gastrointestinal disorders. 1. Screening of 84 plants against enterobacteria. *J Ethnopharmacol* 1990;30(1):55-73.

[28] Giachetti D, et al. Effects of *Smilax macrophylla* Vers. in normal or hyperuricemic and hyperuricosuric rats. *Pharmacol Res Commun* 1988;20 Suppl 5:59-62.

[29] Rhee J, et al. Screening of the wormicidal Chinese raw drugs on *Clonorchis sinensis. Am J Chin Med* 1981;9(4):277-84.

[30] Chen Z. Clinical study of 96 cases with chronic hepatitis B treated with jiedu yanggan gao by a double-blind method. *Chung Hsi I chieh Ho Tsa Chih* 1990;10(2):71-74, 67.

[31] Liu X, et al.Treatment of intestinal metaplasia and atypical hyperplasia of gastric mucosa with xiao wei yan powder. *Chung Kuo Chung Hsi I chieh Ho Tsa Chih* 1992;12(10):602-3, 580.

[32] Fukunaga T, et al. Hypoglycemic effect of the rhizomes of *Smilax glabra* in normal and diabetic mice. *Biol Pharm Bull* 1997;20(1):44-46.

[33] Chen T, et al. A new flavanone isolated from rhizoma smilacis glabrae and the structural requirements of its derivatives for preventing immunological hepatocyte damage. *Planta Med* 1999;65(1):56-59.

[34] Vandenplas O, et al. Occupational asthma caused by sarsaparilla root dust. *J Allergy Clin Immunol* 1996;97(6):1416-18.

Sassafras

SCIENTIFIC NAME(S): *Sassafras albidum* (Nuttal) Nees, synonymous with *S. officinale* Nees et Erbem. and *S. variifolium* Kuntze. Family: Lauraceae

COMMON NAME(S): Sassafras, saxifras, ague tree, cinnamon wood, saloop

BOTANY: Sassafras is the name applied to three species of trees, two native to eastern Asia and one native to eastern North America. Fossils show that sassafras was once widespread in Europe, North America and Greenland. The trees grow up to 100 feet in height and 6 feet in diameter, though they are usually smaller. Sassafras bears leaves 10 to 15 cm long that are oval on older branches but mitten-shaped or three-lobed on younger shoots and twigs. All parts of the tree are strongly aromatic. The drug is from the peeled root of the plant (root wood).[1]

HISTORY: Native Americans have used sassafras for centuries and told early settlers that it would cure a variety of ills. The settlers then exported it to Europe, where it was found to be ineffective.[2] A report on experiences of explorers and doctors finding, identifying and describing sassafras bark and other drugs during the late 15th century is available.[3]

Over the years the oil obtained from the roots and wood has been used as a scent in perfumes and soaps. The leaves and pith, when dried and powdered, have been used as a thickener in soups. The roots are often dried and steeped for tea, and sassafras was formerly used as a flavoring in root beer. Its use as a drug or food product has been banned by the US Food and Drug Administration (FDA) as carcinogenic; however, its use and sale persist throughout the United States. Medicinally, sassafras has been applied to insect bites and stings to relieve symptoms.[2]

CHEMISTRY: The pleasant-tasting oil of sassafras consists of approximately 2% of the roots and 6% to 9% of the root bark. The main constituent of the oil is safrole, which chemically is p-allyl-methylenedioxybenzene, which comprises up to 80% of the oil. Volatile oil also contains anethole, pinene apiole, camphor, eugenol and myristicin.[4,5]

The plant contains less than 0.2% total alkaloids (primarily boldine and its derivatives and reticuline) along with tanins, resins, mucilage and wax.[4,5,6] Six alkaloids, apor-

phine and benzylsoquinoline derivatives, have been found in root bark.[1] Two antimicrobial neolignans, magnolol and its related isomer (isomagnolol), from related species *S. randaiensis* have been isolated.[1] Analysis has also been performed on sassafras teas, using supercritical fluid extraction (SFE) with gas chromatographic-mass spectrometric (GC-MS) methods, commonly reporting 1% safrole levels.[8]

PHARMACOLOGY: Sassafras has been used as a sudorific agent,[9] a flavoring agent for dentifrices, root beers and tobaccos, and for treatment of eye inflammation.[4] Extracts of the roots and bark have been found to mimic insect juvenile hormone in *Oncopeltus fasciatus*.[10] The oil has been applied externally for relief of inset bites and stings and for pediculicides. Other external uses include treatment of rheumatism, gout, sprains, swelling and cutaneous eruptions.[4,5] A recent report compares safrole (the main constituent from sassafras oil), to indomethacin for anti-inflammatory activity and pain treatment in mice.[11]

The plant has been reported to have antineoplastic activity[12] and to induce cytochrome P-488 and P-450 enzymes.[5] Sassafras is said to be antagonistic to certain alcohol effects.[4] Alcohol extracts of the related *S. randaiense* Rehder exhibit antimicrobial and antifungal activity in vitro, and this activity appears to be due to the presence of magnolol and isomagnolol.[7]

TOXICOLOGY: Sassafras oil and safrole have been banned for use as flavors and food additives by the FDA because of their carcinogenic potential. Safrole and its metabolite, 1'-hydroxysafrole, act as nerve poisons and have caused malignant hepatic tumors in animals. Based on animal data and a margin-of-safety factor of 100, a dose of 0.66 mg safrole per kg body weight is considered hazardous for humans; the dose obtained from sassafras tea may be as high as 200 mg (3 mg/kg).[1,13] One study showed that even a safrole-free extract produced malignant mesenchymal tumors n more than 50% of black rats treated. These tumors corresponded to malignant fibrous histiocytomas in humans.[15]

Oil of sassafras is toxic in doses as small as 5 ml in adults.[16] Ingestion of 1 tsp (5 ml) produced shakes, vomiting, high blood pressure and pulse in a 47-year-old female.[17] Another case of a 1 tsp dose of sassafras oil in a young man also caused vomiting, along with dilated pupils, stupor and collapse.[4] There have been additional reports of the oil being fatal,[5] causing abortion[4] and causing liver cancer.[1,4,5] Safrole is a potent inhibitor of liver microsome hydroxylating enzymes; this effect may result in toxicity caused by altered drug metabolism.[13] Aqueous and alcoholic extracts of root bark can cause a range of effects in mice, inducing ataxia, ptosis, hypersensitivity to touch, CNS depression and hypothermia. Symptoms of sassafras oil poisoning in humans may include vomiting, stupor, lowering of body temperature, exhaustion, tachycardia, spasm, hallucinations, paralysis and collapse.[1,5]

Additionally, sassafras can cause diaphoresis[18] and contact dermatitis in certain individuals.[4] A case study reported oil of sassafras in combination as a teething preparation, which resulted in false positive blood tests for diphenylhydantoin, in a 4-month-old child.[19]

SUMMARY: Sassafras is an aromatic tree that has long served as a source for scents and flavorings. Considerable evidence indicates that sassafras, the principal component of oil of sassafras, and other components are carcinogenic in animals. Other toxic effects of sassafras include vomiting, stupor and hallucinations. It has also been associated with causing abortion, liver cancer, diaphoresis and dermatitis. Because there is no documented therapeutic benefit to ingesting sassafras or any of its extracts, the ingestion of this plant cannot be recommended.

PATIENT INFORMATION – Sassafras

Uses: Sassafras has been used historically for a variety of illnesses, and is now banned in the US, even for use as a flavoring or fragrance.

Side Effects: Besides being a cancer-causing agent, sassafras can induce vomiting, stupor and hallucinations. It can also cause abortion, diaphoresis and dermatitis.

---

[1] Bisset N. Sassafras lignum. Herbal Drugs and Phytopharmaceuticals. Stuttgart, Germany: CRC Press, 1994;455–56.
[2] Winter R. The People's Handbook of Allergies and Allergens. Chicago: Contemporary Books, 1984.
[3] Estes J. *Pharmacy in History* 1995;37(1):3–23.
[4] Duke J. *Sassafras albidum* (Nutt.). CRC Handbook of Medicinal Herbs. Boca Raton, FL: CRC Press, Inc., 1989;430–31.
[5] Newall C, et al. Sassafras. Herbal Medicine. London: Pharmaceutical Press, 1996;235–36.
[6] Chowdhury BK, et al. *Phytochem* 1976;15:1803.
[7] El-Feraly F, et al. *J Nat Prod* 1983;46(Jul-Aug):493–98.
[8] Heikes D. *J Chromatogr Sci* 1994;32(7):253–58.
[9] Merck Index, 10th ed. Rahway, NJ: Merck and Co., 1983.
[10] Jacobson M, et al. *Lloydia* 1975;38:455.
[11] Pereira E, et al. *Braz J Med Biol Res* 1989;22(11):1415–19.
[12] Hartwell JL. *Lloydia* 1969;32:247.
[13] Segelman AB. *JAMA* 1976;236:477.
[14] Kapadia GJ, et al. *J Natl Cancer Inst* 1978;60:683.
[15] Benedetti MS, et al. *Toxicology* 1977;7:69.
[16] Spoerke DG. *Herbal Medications* Santa Barbara, CA: Woodridge Press Publishing Co., 1980.
[17] Grande G, et al. *Vet Hum Toxicol* 1987;29(dec):447.
[18] Haines J. *Postgrad Med* 1991;90(4):75-76.
[19] Jones M, et al. *Am J Dis Child* 1971;122(Sep):259–60.

Savory

SCIENTIFIC NAME(S): Summer savory: *Satureja hortensis* L., syn. with *Calamintha hortensis* Hort. Winter savory: *Satureja montana* L., syn. with *S. obovata* Lag. and *Calamintha montana* Family: Labiatae

BOTANY: Summer savory is an annual herb that grows to about 2 feet in height featuring oblong leaves. Although it is native to Europe, it is now found throughout many parts of the world. Winter savory is a perennial shrub that grows to about the same height as summer savory, the leaves of which share some common characteristics with summer savory. Flowers of both species are pink to blue-white[1] and flower from June to September.[2]

HISTORY: The savories have been used for centuries as cooking herbs and have flavors reminiscent of oregano and thyme.[3] Because the flavor of the summer savory is somewhat sweeter than that of the winter savory, summer savory is used almost exclusively in commerce.[1] The green leaves and stems, both fresh and dried, along with extracts, are used as flavors in the baking and foods industries. Both summer and winter savory have a history of use in traditional medicine as tonics, carminatives, astringents and expectorants, and for the treatment of intestinal problems such as diarrhea and nausea. Summer savory is said to be an aphrodisiac[2] while winter savory has been said to decrease libido.[4]

CHEMISTRY: Dried summer savory contains approximately 1% of a volatile oil which is composed primarily of carvacrol, thymol and monoterpene hydrocarbons such as beta-pinene, p-cymene, limonene, camphene, etc.[1,5] The leaves contain a variety of minor components including minerals and vitamins. Winter savory contains about 1.6% of a volatile oil composed primarily of carvacrol (up to 65%), p-cymene and thymol. It also contains triterpenic acids including ursolic and oleanolic acids.[3,5] The relative composition of the volatile oil varies with location of cultivation, the species and the strain.

PHARMACOLOGY: The volatile oil of summer savory, as with many other volatile oils, possesses antifungal and antibacterial activity.[1,5] Summer savory has been reported to have a spasmolytic effect on isolated smooth muscle[5] and may have an antidiarrheal effect due to the phenolic compounds in the oil[1] and the tannins contained in the plant.[4]

The oil has been reported to possess an antidiuretic effect due to the carvacrol.[3] Teas of savory have been used traditionally in Europe to treat excessive thirst in diabetic patients, a use that may have some pharmacologic basis.[4]

TOXICOLOGY: Savory is generally recognized as safe for use as a condiment and flavor. When applied undiluted to the backs of hairless mice, summer savory oil was lethal to half of the animals within 48 hours. The oil is strongly irritating to other animal skin models, but is not phototoxic.[5] In diluted form the oil is not irritating to human skin.

SUMMARY: Summer and winter savory have been used for centuries as condiments. Their use in traditional medicine centers primarily on the antispasmodic and antibacterial effects of the volatile oil. Savory is not associated with significant toxicity and should be investigated for its antidiuretic properties.

PATIENT INFORMATION – Savory

Uses: Savory has antifungal, antibacterial, and antidiuretic effects, in addition to being widely used as a condiment.

Side Effects: Savory is not associated with any significant toxicity.

---

[1] Simon JE. Herbs: An Indexed Bibliography, 1971-1980. Hamden, CT: Shoe String Press, 1984.

[2] Schauenberg P, Paris F. Guide To Medicinal Plants. New Canaan, CT: Keats Publishing, 1977.

[3] Duke JA. Handbook of Medicinal Herbs. Boca Raton, FL: CRC Press, 1985.

[4] Tyler VE. The New Honest Herbal. Philadelphia, PA: G.F. Stickley Co., 1987.

[5] Leung AY. Encyclopedia of Common Natural Ingredients Used In Food, Drugs, and Cosmetics. New York, NY: J. Wiley and Sons, 1980.

Saw Palmetto

SCIENTIFIC NAME(S): *Serenoa repens* (Bartram) Small. Also referred to as *Sabal serrulata* (Michx.) Nicholson or *Sabal serrulatum* Schult. Family: Palmae (Palms)

COMMON NAME(S): Saw palmetto, sabal, American dwarf palm tree, cabbage palm, fan palm, scrub palm

BOTANY: The saw palmetto is a low, scrubby palm that grows in the coastal plain of Florida and other southeastern states. Its fan-shaped leaves have sharp saw-toothed edges that give the plant its name. Dense clumps of saw palmetto can form an impenetrable thicket. The abundant 2 cm long berries are harvested from the wild in the fall and are dried for medicinal use. They also serve as a source of nutrition for deer, bears, and wild pigs.[1]

HISTORY: Native tribes of Florida relied on saw palmetto berries for food; however, Europeans often found the taste of the berries objectionable.[1] While native medicinal use of saw palmetto is not recorded, it was introduced into Western medical practice in the 1870s and was a favorite of Eclectic medical practitioners for prostate and other urologic conditions. Saw palmetto berries were official in the US Pharmacopeia in 1906 and 1916, and in the National Formulary from 1926 to 1950. While use in the US declined after that time, saw palmetto has long been a staple phytomedicine in Europe. Recent interest has been rekindled, and saw palmetto is currently ranked in the top 10 herbal products in the US.[2] It is primarily used for its activity in benign prostatic hyperplasia (BPH).

CHEMISTRY: Saw palmetto berries contain large quantities of beta-sitosterol and other plant sterols,[3] as well as free and esterified fatty acids.[4] Most standardized commercial preparations are "liposterolic" extracts containing nonpolar constituents such as fatty acids and sterols, produced either by conventional hexane extraction or by supercritical carbon dioxide extraction. The fatty acid components have been quantitated by gas chromatography[5] and supercritical fluid chromatography,[6] while the alcohols and sterols have been analyzed by TLC and electrospray mass spectrometry of ferrocenyl derivatives.[7] An acidic polysaccharide has been isolated from saw palmetto fruit that had anti-inflammatory activity.[8,9]

PHARMACOLOGY:

BPH: Saw palmetto's mechanism of action in suppressing the symptoms of BPH is poorly understood. The leading hypothesis involves the inhibition of testosterone 5-alpha reductase, an enzyme that converts testosterone to 5-alpha-testosterone in the prostate. Hexane extracts of saw palmetto were found to inhibit the enzyme from human foreskin fibroblasts, while they had no direct effect on androgen receptor binding.[10] Investigators found various saw palmetto extracts to be much weaker 5-alpha reductase inhibitors in vitro than the synthetic drug finasteride.[11] Similarly, in humans, serum levels of dihydrotestosterone (DHT) were reduced markedly by finasteride, but not by saw palmetto.[12] Further studies using both known 5-alpha reductase isozymes found that finasteride inhibited only type 1 reductase, while saw palmetto inhibited formation of all testosterone metabolites in both cultured prostate epithelial cells and fibroblasts.[13] A different saw palmetto extract, IDS 89, dose dependently inhibited 5-alpha reductase in both the stroma and epithelium of human BPH tissue. This inhibition was related to the free fatty acids present in the extract.[14] A tracer study found that radiolabeled oleic acid in saw palmetto extract was taken up preferentially by rat prostate compared with other tissues.[15] Studies in a coculture model of human prostate epithelial cells and fibroblasts found that saw palmetto inhibited both type 1 and type 2 isoforms of 5-alpha reductase without altering the secretion of prostate-specific antigen.[16] Other recent work has shown that saw palmetto extract inhibits trophic as well as androgenic effects of prolactin in a rat model of prostatic hyperplasia.[17] Structure-activity studies of pure fatty acid inhibition of steroid 5-alpha reductase have found gamma-linolenic acid to be the most potent and specific inhibitor of the enzyme.[18] It is possible that the C_{18} monounsaturated fatty oleic acid found in saw palmetto is partly responsible for the observed effects on 5-alpha reductase, though more extensive analysis of saw palmetto fatty acids is required.

There is less support for other hormonal mechanisms. One study found 5-alpha reductase inhibition and inhibition of DHT binding to androgen receptors,[19] and another study demonstrated inhibition of DHT and testosterone receptor binding.[20] Administration of saw palmetto extract over 30 days led to no changes in plasma levels of testosterone, follicle stimulating hormone, or luteinizing hormone.[21] Hormonal pathways were invoked to explain reduced prostate weights in castrated rats treated with estradiol, testosterone, and saw palmetto extract as opposed to estradiol and testosterone alone.[22] In the human prostate cancer line LNCaP, saw palmetto induced a mixed proliferative/differentiative effect that was not seen in the nonhormone-responsive PC3 human prostate cancer cell line.[23] Treatment of patients for 3 months with saw palmetto preceding prostatectomy caused a reduction in DHT levels in BPH tissue along with a corresponding rise in testosterone levels. A marked reduction in epidermal growth factor concentration was also observed in the periurethral region of the prostate.[24]

Although the mechanism of action of saw palmetto is not completely understood, clinical trials in BPH have shown convincing evidence of moderate efficacy. A 6-month, double-blind, head-to-head study vs finasteride in 1098 men found equivalent efficacy and a better side effect profile for saw palmetto.[29] Likewise, a 3-year study of IDS 89 in 435 BPH patients found clear superiority to placebo in reduction of BPH symptoms.[30] A 1-year study of 132 patients comparing 2 dose levels of saw palmetto demonstrated efficacy in symptom reduction but little difference between dose levels.[31] The general consensus has been that saw palmetto extracts reduce BPH symptoms without reducing prostate size, therefore delaying surgical intervention.[32] A meta-analysis that included a total of 18 clinical trials in BPH concluded that saw palmetto was better tolerated than finasteride and equivalent in efficacy.[33] A clinical trial in BPH of the saw palmetto constituent beta-sitosterol showed similar efficacy to that seen with saw palmetto itself.[34]

Other observations of saw palmetto extracts include a spasmolytic effect on rat uterus which was suggested to be because of effects on cyclic AMP and calcium mobilization,[25] an inhibition of smooth muscle contraction in rat deferens, guinea pig ileum, and bladder postulated as alpha-adrenoreceptor antagonistic,[26] shown by others to be noncompetitive in nature,[27] and interference with 5-lipoxygenase metabolites in neutrophils.[28]

INTERACTIONS: Because of well-documented antiandrogen and antiestrogenic activity, avoid taking with any hormone therapy including oral contraceptive and hormone replacement therapy. Saw palmetto also has shown immunostimulant and anti-inflammatory activity; hence, watch for patients taking drugs that may increase or decrease these effects. For reproducible effects, it is recommended that the fat-soluble saw palmetto extracts standardized to contain 85% to 95% fatty acids and sterols be taken at the recommended dosage of 160 mg twice daily. Effects occur in 4 to 6 weeks. There have been no demonstrated effect on serum prostate-specific antigen levels.

TOXICOLOGY: Saw palmetto products are generally well tolerated, with occasional reports of adverse GI effects. Its antiandrogenic activity suggests that it should not be used in pregnancy.

SUMMARY: Saw palmetto extracts are effective in the treatment of benign prostatic hyperplasia, reducing frequency of urination, increasing urinary flow, and decreasing nocturia. It is generally well-tolerated and may delay the need for prostate surgery.

Saw palmetto is approved by the German Commission E, and is monographed by WHO (vol 2), the British Herbal Pharmacopeia (vol 2), and in supplement 9 of the National Formulary. An American Herbal Pharmacopeia monograph is forthcoming.

PATIENT INFORMATION – Saw Palmetto

Uses: Saw palmetto is used to treat symptoms of benign prostatic hyperplasia, including reduction of urinary frequency, increase of urinary flow, and decrease of nocturia. Saw palmetto may delay the need for prostate surgery.

Side Effects: Saw palmetto is generally well tolerated, with occasional reports of adverse GI effects; do not use in pregnancy.

---

[1] Bennett B, et al. Uses of saw palmetto (*Serenoa repens, Arecaceae*) in Florida. *Econ Bot* 1998;52:381.

[2] Winston, D. *Saw Palmetto for Men & Women*. Pownal,VT: Storey Books, 1999.

[3] Elghamry M, et al. Activity and isolated phytoestrogen of shrub palmetto fruits (*Serenoa repens* Small), a new estrogenic plant. *Experientia* 1969;25:828-29.

[4] Shimada H, et al. Biologically active acylglycerides from the berries of saw-palmetto (*Serenoa repens*). *J Nat Prod* 1997;60:417-18.

[5] De Swaef S, et al. Simultaneous quantitation of lauric acid and ethyl laureate in *Sabal serrulata* by capillary gas chromatography and derivatisation with trimethyl sulphoniumhydroxide. *J Chromatogr* 1996;719:479.

[6] De Swaef S, et al. Supercritical fluid chromatography of free fatty acids and ethyl esters in ethanolic extracts of *Sabal serrulata*. *Phytochem Anal* 1996;7:223.

[7] Van Berkel G, et al. Derivatization for electrospray ionization mass spectrometry. 3. Electrochemically ionizable derivatives. *Anal Chem* 1998;70:1544.

[8] Wagner H, et al. A new antiphlogistic principle from *Sabal serrulata* I. *Planta Med* 1981;41:244-51. German.

[9] Wagner H, et al. Über ein neues antiphlogistisches wirkprinzip aus *Sabal serrulata* II. *Planta Med* 1981;41:252.

[10] Düker E, et al. Inhibition of 5α-reductase activity by extracts from *Sabal serrulata*. *Planta Med* 1989;55:587.

[11] Rhodes L, et al. Comparison of finasteride (*Proscar*), a 5-alpha reductase inhibitor, and various commercial plant extracts in in-vitro and in-vivo 5-alpha-reductase inhibition. *Prostate* 1993;22:43-51.

[12] Strauch G, et al. Comparison of finasteride (*Proscar*) and *Serenoa repens* (*Permixon*) in the inhibition of 5-alpha reductase in healthy male volunteers. *Eur Urol* 1994;26:247-52.

[13] Délos S, et al. Testosterone metabolism in primary cultures of human prostate epithelial cells and fibroblasts. *J Steroid Biochem Mol Biol* 1995;55:375.

[14] Weisser H, et al. Effects of the *Sabal serrulata* extract IDS 89 and its subfractions on 5-alpha reductase activity in human benign prostatic hyperplasia. *Prostate* 1996;28:300-06.

[15] Chevalier G, et al. Distribution study of radioactivity in rats after oral administration of the lipido/sterolic extract of *Serenoa repens* (*Permixon*) supplemented with [1-14C]-lauric acid, [1-14C]-oleic acid or [4-14C]-beta-sitosterol. *Eur J Drug Metab Pharmacokinet* 1997;22:73-83.

[16] Bayne C, et al. *Serenoa repens* (*Permixon*): a 5-alpha reductase types I and II inhibitor-new evidence in a coculture model of BPH. *Prostate* 1999;40:232-46.

[17] Van Coppenolle F, et al. Pharmacological effects of the liposterolic extract of *Serenoa repens* (*Permixon*) on rat prostate hyperplasia induced by hyperprolactinemia: Comparison with finasteride. *Prostate* 2000;43:49-58.

[18] Liang T, et al. Inhibition of steroid 5-alpha reductase by specific aliphatic unsaturated fatty acids. *Biochem J* 1992;285:557-62.

[19] Sultan C, et al. Inhibition of androgen metabolism and binding by a liposterolic extract of "*Serenoa repens* B" in human foreskin fibroblasts. *J Steroid Biochem* 1984;20:515-19.

[20] el-Sheikh M, et al. The effect of *Permixon* on androgen receptors. *Acta Obstet Gynecol Scand* 1988;67:397-99.

[21] Casarosa C, et al. Lack of effects of a lyposterolic extract of *Serenoa repens* on plasma levels of testosterone, follicle-stimulating hormone, and luteinizing hormone. *Clin Ther* 1988;10:585-88.

[22] Paubert-Braquet M, et al. Effect of Serenoa repens extract (*Permixon*) on estradiol/testosterone-induced experimental prostate enlargement in the rat. *Pharmacol Res* 1996;34:171-79.

[23] Ravenna L, et al. Effects of the lipidosterolic extract of *Serenoa repens* (*Permixon*) on human prostatic cell lines. *Prostate* 1996;29:219-30.

[24] Di Silverio F, et al. Effects of long-term treatment with *Serenoa repens* (*Permixon*) on the concentrations and regional distribution of androgens and epidermal growth factor in benign prostatic hyperplasia. *Prostate* 1998;37:77-83.

[25] Gutiérrez M, et al. Spasmolytic activity of a lipidic extract from *Sabal serrulata* fruits. Further study of the mechanisms underlying this activity. *Planta Med* 1996;62:507-11.

[26] Odenthal, K. Phytotherapy of benign prostatic hyperplasia (BPH) with *Cucurbita*, *Hypoxis*, *Pygeum*, *Urtica* and *Sabal serrulata* (*Serenoa repens*). *Phytother Res* 1996;10:S141.

[27] Goepel M, et al. Saw palmetto extracts potently and noncompetitively inhibit human alpha-1-adrenoceptors in vitro. *Prostate* 1999;38:208-15.

[28] Paubert-Braquet M, et al. Effect of the lipidic lipidosterolic extract of *Serenoa repens* (*Permixon*) on the ionophore A23187-stimulated production of leukotriene B4 (LTB4) from human polymorphonuclear neutrophils. *Prostaglandins Leukot Essent Fatty Acids* 1997;57:299-304.

[29] Carraro J, et al. Comparison of phytotherapy (*Permixon*) with finasteride in the treatment of benign prostatic hyperplasia: A randomized international study of 1,098 patients. *Prostate* 1996;29:231-40.

[30] Bach D, et al. Long-term drug treatment of benign prostatic hyperplasia. Results of a prospective 3-year multicenter study using Sabal extract IDS 89. *Phytomedicine* 1996;3:105.

[31] Braeckman J, et al. Efficacy and safety of the extract of *Serenoa repens* in the treatment of benign prostatic hyperplasia: Therapeutic equivalence between twice and once daily dosage forms. *Phytother Res* 1997;11:558.

[32] Marandola P, et al. Main phytoderivatives in the management of benign prostatic hyperplasia. *Fitoterapia* 1997;68:195.

[33] Wilt T, et al. Saw palmetto extracts for treatment of benign prostatic hyperplasia. *JAMA* 1998;280:1604-09.

[34] Berges R, et al. Randomised, placebo-controlled, double-blind clinical trial of beta-sitosterol in patients with benign prostatic hyperplasia. *Lancet* 1995;345:1529-32.

Schisandra

SCIENTIFIC NAME(S): *Schisandra chinensis* Baillon, *S. arisanensis*, *S. sphenanthera* Rehd, *S. rubriflora* franch. Family: Schizandraceae

COMMON NAME(S): Schisandra, schizandra; gomishi, hoku-gomishi, kita-gomishi (Japanese); *wu-wei-zu* (Chinese)

BOTANY: The family schizandraceae (schisandraceae) comprises two genera (*Schisandra* and *Kadsura*). *Schisandra* spp. are climbing, aromatic trees, with white, pink, yellow or reddish male or female flowers. The fruits are globular and red with several kidney-shaped seeds. The fruit is harvested in autumn when fully ripened.[1] *S. chinensis* is native to northeastern and north central China and is found in eastern Russia.

HISTORY: Schisandra is one of the many traditional Chinese materia medica that are recommended for coughs and various nonspecific pulmonary diseases.[2] It has been studied extensively in the Chinese and Japanese literature. Schisandra had been used for healing purposes for over 2,000 years. It is often used as an ethanolic tincture. The Chinese name for the plant, "wu-wei-zu," means "5–flavored herb," because of the flavor of the 5 main "elemental energies" of the plant. The fruit have a salty, sour taste.[1]

CHEMISTRY: This plant's chemistry has been studied extensively. The fruit contains reducing sugars and up to 10% organic acids (carboxylic, malic, citric, tartaric). The seeds contain reducing sugars, alkaloids and fatty esters. No flavones, glycosides or tannins are in the seeds or fruit.[3] About 2% of the fruit by weight is composed of lignins with a dibenzocyclooctane skeleton (eg, schizandrin, deoxyschizandrin and related compounds such as schizandrol, and schizanderer). In some specimens, the lignin content can approach 19% in the seeds and 10% in the stems.[4] More than 30 lignins have been identified in the seed,[2] including gomisins A, B, C, D, F and G;[5] tigloylgomisin P and angeloylgomisin.[6] Other plant constituents include phytosterols, volatile oil and vitamins C and E.[1] Determination methods have been performed for processing and standardization purposes.[7,8,9]

PHARMACOLOGY: Besides serving as a tonic and restorative, schisandra has other reported uses, such as liver protection, nervous system effects, respiratory treatment, GI therapy, adaptogenic properties and others.

Liver: The lignin components in schisandra possess pronounced liver protectant effects. The active principles appear to be the lignins such as wu-wei-zu C, shisan- therin D, deoxygomisin A, gomisin N and gomisin C. The presence of one or two methylene dioxy groups appear to play an important role in hepatoprotection.[2,10] Animal studies on gomisin A offer convincing evidence of liver protection, including protective actions against: Halothane-induced hepatitis;[11] carbon tetrachloride; d-galactosamine and dl-ethionine toxicities;[12,13] hepatic failure induced by bacterium;[14] and preneoplastic hepatic lesions.[15,16,17,18] Gomisin A's mechanism for tumor inhibition may be a result of its ability to improve bile acid metabolism.[19] Gomisin A causes hepatic cell proliferation, improves liver regeneration, hepatic blood flow and liver function recovery in rats.[20] These effects are caused by protection of hepatocyte plasma membrane.[21] Ethanol extracts of schisandra have been found to increase liver weight in rats and mice. This action has been attributed to schizandrin B and schizandrol B. In a mouse study, extract added to a semipurified basal diet over a 14-day period increased the enzymatic metabolism of the mutagens benzopyrene (BaP) and aflatoxin B (AFB) and increased cytochrome P450 activity. Despite this increased level of metabolism, schisandra extract increased the in vitro mutagenicity of AFB. However, chemicals inducing similar patterns of enzymes have been found to reduce the in vivo binding of AFB to DNA.[22] It is also recognized that the schizandrins and about one-half dozen related compounds may temporarily inhibit or lower the activity of hepatic ALT. This has been observed in animals pretreated with hepatotoxins.[23,24,25]

Nervous System: Schisandra is a nervous system stimulant, increasing reflex responses and improving mental alertness. In China, the berries are used to treat mental illnesses such as depression. It is also used for irritability and memory loss.[1] Schisandra in combination with other herbs has improved memory retention disorder and facilitated memory retention deficit in animal testing. This suggests a possible use in treating age-related memory deficits in humans.[26] Schisandra, (also in combination with *Zizyphus spinosa* and *Angelica sinensis*) has accelerated neurocyte growth and may prevent atrophy of neurocyte process branches.[27]

Schisandra has been evaluated for its inhibitory effects on the CNS as well. In Chinese medicine, it is used as a sedative for insomnia.[1] This inhibition mechanism has been evaluated and may be related to the effects on dopaminergic receptors.[28] Gomisin A has also inhibited spontaneous and methamphetamine-induced motor activity in animals.[29]

Respiratory: Schisandra is used to treat respiratory ailments such as shortness of breath, wheezing and cough.[1] Gomisin A exerted antitussive effects when evaluated in guinea pigs.[29]

GI: In the rat intestine, schisandra extract reduces BaP metabolism, which is the opposite effect from that in the liver. Experiments show that it increases the activity of glutathione S-transferase. In the intestine, schisandra shifts BaP metabolism in favor of diols and 3-hydroxybenzopyrene and away from BaP- 4,5-epoxide and the mutagenic BaP quinones. Schisandra does not increase intestinal cytochrome P450 activity.[30] Schisandra has been used for treatment of diarrhea and dysentery.[1] One report found schisandra extract to have no significant effects on gastric secretory volume, gastric pH and acid output,[31] while another study found schisandra to have inhibitory effects on gastric contraction and stress-induced gastric ulceration when administered IV and orally in rats.[29] Metabolism of schisandra has been

reported.[32,33,34] The plant helps the body "adapt" to stress. It has been used to balance fluid levels, improve sexual stamina, treat rash, stimulate uterine contractions and improve failing senses.[1] One report found antibacterial effects in alcohol and acetone extracts of the fruit.[3]

TOXICOLOGY: Schisandra has the capability to produce profound CNS depression. Because of its documented effects on hepatic and gastric enzyme activity, it is possible that schisandra may interfere with the metabolism of other concurrently administered drugs. The full spectrum of the clinical effects of the plant on the liver are not well-documented and the safety of the plant has not been established scientifically. However, research does not report any incidence of side effects.

SUMMARY: Schisandra is a traditional Chinese medicinal plant; the fruit is used most frequently in herbal medicine. The lignin content in the plant, the component responsible for pronounced hepatoprotectant effects, has been extensively studied. The plant may also help improve mental alertness, treat respiratory and GI problems, and help the body adapt to stress. Little information is available on side effects.

PATIENT INFORMATION – Schisandra

Uses: Schisandra has been used as a tonic and restorative, as well as for liver protection, nervous system effects, respiratory treatment, GI therapy and others.

Side Effects: Research indicates that side effects are infrequent, although schisandra has the ability to produce profound CNS depression and may interfere with the metabolism of other concurrently administered drugs.

---

[1] Chevallier A. Encyclopedia of Medicinal Plants. New York, NY: DK Publishing, 1996.
[2] Hikino H, et al. *Planta Medica* 1984;50:213.
[3] Ma TS, Roper R. *Mikrochemica Acta* 1968;1:167.
[4] Song WZ, et al. *Acta Pharm Sin* 1983;18:138.
[5] Ikeya Y, et al. *Chem Pharm Bull* 1979;27:1383, 1395.
[6] Ikeya Y. *Chem Pharm Bull* 1980;28:3357.
[7] Suprunov N, et al. *Farmatsiia* 1975;24(2):35–37.
[8] Rao W, et al. *Chung Yao Tung Pao Bulletin of Chinese Materia Medica* 1986;11(Mar):154–55.
[9] Zhu Y, et al. *Chin J Pharm Anal* 1988;8(Mar):71–73.
[10] Maeda S, et al. *Yakugaku Zasshi* 1982;102(6):579–88.
[11] Jiaxiang N, et al. *J Appl Toxicol* 1993;13(6):385–88.
[12] Ko K, et al. *Planta Medica* 1995;61(2):134–37.
[13] Takeda S, et al. *Nippon Yakurigaku Zasshi* 1986;87(2):169–87.
[14] Mizoguchi Y, et al. *Planta Medica* 1991;57(4):320–24.
[15] Nomura M, et al. *Cancer Letters* 1994;76(1):11–18.
[16] Ohtaki Y, et al. *Biol Pharm Bull* 1994;17(6):808–14.
[17] Nomura M, et al. *Anticancer Res* 1994;14(5A):1967–71.
[18] Miyamoto K, et al. *Biol Pharm Bull* 1995;18(10):1443–45.
[19] Ohtaki Y, et al. *Anticancer Res* 1996;16(2):751–55.
[20] Takeda S, et al. *Nippon Yakurigaku Zasshi* 1986;88(4):321–30.
[21] Nagai H, et al. *Planta Medica* 1989;55(1):13–17.
[22] Hendrich S, Bjeldanes LF. *Food Chem Toxicol* 1986;24:903.
[23] Tiangtong B, et al. *Chin Med J* 1980;93:41.
[24] Maeda S, et al. *Japan J Pharmacol* 1985;38:347.
[25] Pao T, et al. *Chung Hua I Hsueh Tsa Chih* 1974;54(May):275–77.
[26] Nishiyama N, et al. *Biol Pharm Bull* 1996;19(3):388–93.
[27] Hu G, etal. *Chin Pharm J* 1994;29(Jun):333–36.
[28] Zhang L, et al. *Chung Kuo I Hsueh Ko Hsueh Yuan Hsueh Pao* 1991;13(1):13–16.
[29] Maeda S, et al. *Yakugaku Zasshi* 1981;101(Nov):1030–41.
[30] Salbe AD, Bjeldanes LF. *Food Chem Toxicol* 1985;23:57.
[31] Hernandez D, et al. *J Ethnopharmacol* 1988;23(May/Jun):109–14.
[32] Hendrich S, et al. *Food Chem Toxicol* 1936;24(9):903–12.
[33] Chi Y, et al. *Yao Hsueh Hsueh Pao* 1992;27(1):57–63.
[34] Chi Y, et al. *Eur J Drug Metab Pharmacokinet* 1993;18(2):155–60.

Scullcap

SCIENTIFIC NAME(S): *Scutellaria laterifolia* L. Family: Labiatae

COMMON NAME(S): Scullcap, skullcap, helmetflower, hoodwort, mad-dog weed

BOTANY: Scullcap (*S. laterifolia*), a member of the mint family, is native to the United States where it grows in moist woods. Although it is widely distributed throughout large regions of North America, the plant has related species found as far away as China. Scullcap is an erect perennial that grows to 2 to 3 feet in height. Its bluish flowers bloom from July to September. Official compendia (eg, NF VI) recognized only the dried overground portion of the plant as useful; however, some herbal texts listed all parts as medicinal.[1] The aerial parts of the plant are collected during the flowering period, typically August and September. A number of species have been used medicinally, and the most common European variety has been *S. baicalensis* Georgii, a native of East Asia.

HISTORY: Scullcap appears to have been introduced into traditional American medicine toward the end of the 1700s, when it was promoted as an effective treatment for the management of hydrophobia (hence the derivation of one of its common names). It was later used as a tonic, particularly in proprietary remedies for "female weakness."[2] The plant had been reputed to be an herbal tranquilizer, particularly in combination with Valerian, but has fallen into disuse.

CHEMISTRY: The various species of *Scutellaria* contain several flavonoid glycoside pigments. These include scutellarein, wogonin, isoscutellarein and baicalin. A diterpenoid (scuterivulactone) has also been identified.[3]

PHARMACOLOGY: At the turn of the century, interest in scullcap grew and the pharmacologic properties of an extract were investigated. The extract was evaluated for its effect on the contractility of the guinea pig uterus in vitro and was found to have only a slight depressant effect in high doses and no effect in vivo when given in "normal" doses.[2]

Extracts of two other species also were found to be devoid of effects on the central nervous or circulatory systems in cats or rabbits. A more recent report using a tincture of the plant found a long-lasting decline in blood pressure in dogs.

Over the past 15 years, Japanese researchers have investigated the activity of the related plant *S. baicalensis*, which is more readily available in Japan. Animal studies indicate that extracts of the plant have a demonstrable anti-inflammatory effect. Although the mechanism of action is not well understood, it is believed that hot water extracts of *Scutellaria* and the active metabolites of the flavonoids baicalin and wogonin glucuronide (baicalein and wogonin, respectively) are potent inhibitors of the enzyme sialidase.[4] In another study, isoscutellarein-8-o-glucuronide from the leaf was found to be a potent inhibitor of the enzyme.[5]

Sialic acids are widely distributed in tissues where they occur as constituents of glycolipids and glycoproteins. They are present in mucus secretions and cell membranes where they are thought to be the sites at which viruses and other compounds attach and penetrate the cell wall. Serum sialic acid is known to increase in certain disease states (cancers, rheumatic diseases, infections, inflammations), and it has been postulated that an inhibitor of sialidase, such as scullcap extract, may have a therapeutic application.

A preliminary animal report suggests that the coadministration of scullcap with cyclophosphamide and 5–fluorouracil may decrease tumor cell viability and improve the tolerability of the cytostatic agents.[6]

Teas prepared from *Scutellaria* species have demonstrable in vitro antibacterial and antifungal activity.[7]

TOXICOLOGY: There is no evidence to indicate that *Scutellaria* is toxic when ingested at "normal" doses. According to the FDA, however, overdose of the tincture causes giddiness, stupor, confusion, twitching of the limbs, intermission of the pulse and other symptoms indicative of epilepsy.[8]

SUMMARY: *Scutellaria* has been employed in traditional American medicine for more than 200 years. It is generally recognized as being devoid of therapeutic activity although early claims suggested that the plant had potentially useful antibacterial and sedative effects. Recent studies indicate that it may possess anti-inflammatory activity related to its ability to inhibit the enzyme sialidase. The plant continues to be found in some herbal teas.

PATIENT INFORMATION – Scullcap

Uses: Scullcap is not recognized as having therapeutic activity, although recent studies suggest that it might have anti-inflammatory activity.

Side Effects: If taken in a normal dose, scullcap does not seem to exhibit any adverse effects.

---

[1] Meyer JE. The Herbalist. Hammond, IN: Hammond Book Co., 1934.
[2] Tyler VE. The New Honest Herbal. Philadelphia, PA: G.F. Stickley Co., 1987.
[3] Kizu H, et al. *Chem Pharm Bull* 1987;35:1656.
[4] Nagai T, et al. *Planta Medica* 1989;55:27.
[5] Nagai T, et al. *Biochem Biophys Res Comm* 1989;163:25.
[6] Razina TG, et al. *Vopr Onkol* 1987;33:80.
[7] Franzblau SG, Cross C. *J Ethnopharmacol* 1986;15:279.
[8] Duke JA. Handbook of Medicinal Herbs. Boca Raton, FL: CRC Press, 1985.

Senega Root

SCIENTIFIC NAME(S): *Polygala senega* L. Family Polygalaceae (Milkworts)

COMMON NAME(S): Seneca snakeroot, Rattlesnake root, Milkwort, Mountain flax

BOTANY: Senega root is an uncommon perennial herb about 1 foot high that grows throughout eastern North America. The leaves are small, alternate, and narrowly lanceolate. Numerous pinkish-white or greenish-white flowers are crowded on a terminal spike. The root is twisted and has an irregular, knotty crown with a distinctive ridge. The variety *P. senega* var. *latifolia* Torr. & Gray has been distinguished, but occurs throughout the same habitat and differs from *P. senega* only in the size of leaves and flowers and in having a slightly later flowering period. The related species *P. tenuifolia* Willd., *P. reinii* Franch., *P. glomerata* Lour., and *P. japonica* Houtt. are used in Asia for similar purposes.

HISTORY: Senega root was used by eastern Native American tribes including the Seneca, from whom its name is derived. Snakeroot refers to the purported use in snakebite. However, even the early European observers gave little credence to this use. Senega root found use among the colonists and in Europe as an emetic, cathartic, diuretic and diaphroetic in a variety of pulmonary diseases such as pneumonia, asthma, and pertussis, and also in gout and rheumatism.[1] Its main use in the 19th century was as an expectorant cough remedy. It was official in the US Pharmacopeia from 1820 to 1936, and in the National Formulary from 1936 to 1960.

CHEMISTRY: Seneca snakeroot contains a series of saponins constructed from the 2,3,27–trihydroxy-oleanane 23,28–dioic acid triterpene skeleton (presenegenin), having a single sugar attached at position 3 and a 4 to 6 sugar chain appended at position 28. A variety of methoxy-cinnamate esters are attached at the internal sugar of the C-28 chain.[2-9] These saponins have been named senegins I-IV and senegasaponins A-C. The senegins can be analyzed by HPLC.[10] Several other species of *Polygala* (see Botany) contain distinct but very similar saponins based on the same sapogenin.[11] An extensive series of ester oligosaccharides, senegoses A-O, have been isolated from *P. senega* var. *latifolia*.[12,13,14] The root also contains a small amount of methyl salicylate, which gives it a characteristic wintergreen odor.

PHARMACOLOGY: The **antitussive** effect of senega root has generally been attributed to the saponin content of the plant, which is consistent with the general detergent property of saponins in breaking up phlegm. In addition, senega is thought to act by irritation of the gastric mucosa, leading by reflex to an increase in bronchial mucous gland secretion.

The senega saponins have been shown to possess **hypoglycemic activity** in normal and diabetic mice, but not in streptozotocin-treated mice.[7-9,15-17] Thus, these compounds have activity relevant to non-insulin-dependent diabetes. This activity is quite potent when the saponins are injected intraperitoneally, but can also be detected with higher oral doses. The same saponins have also been found to substantially reduce alcohol absorption when given orally 1 hour before alcohol.[7,8,9]

The aqueous extract of the related species *P. tenuifolia* has been shown to have a potent effect in blocking inflammatory processes in cultured mouse astrocytes. Substance P and lipopolysaccharide-induced production of tumor necrosis factor and interleukin-1 was blocked by the saponin-containing extract at low concentration.[18] It is possible that a systemic anti-inflammatory effect may be the result of a similar mechanism.

No biological activity has been reported for the oligosaccharides. Senegose A was found to be inactive in the hypoglycemia model cited above.[17]

TOXICOLOGY: High doses of powdered senega root (> 1 g) or tincture have been reported to be emeteogenic and irritating to the GI tract. The use of senega root is contraindicated in pregnancy and in patients with peptic ulcer disease or inflammatory bowel disease.[19]

SUMMARY: Senega root is an antitussive herb with additional potential for use in non-insulin-dependent diabetes and in reducing alcohol absorption. While toxic at high doses, its emetic action makes further toxicity self-limiting.

Senega snakeroot is approved in the German Commission E monographs for catarrh of the respiratory tract. It is also monographed in ESCOP F-3, WHO volume 2, BHP volume 1.

PATIENT INFORMATION – Senega Root

Uses: Senega has been used as an antitussive.

Side Effects: High doses of powdered senega root or tincture are emetogenic and irritating to the GI tract.

[1] Erichsen-Brown C. Medicinal and other uses of North American plants. Dover, NY. 1979;359–362.

[2] Shoji J, et al. Constituents of Senegae radix. I. Isolation and qualitative analysis of the glycosides. *Yakugaku Zasshi* 1971;91(2):198.

[3] Akada Y, et al. Glycon moiety of Senega saponins. I. Isolation and purification of the Senega saponins. *Yakugaku Zasshi* 1971;91(11):1178.

[4] Shoji J, et al. Structure of senegin-II of Senegae Radix. *Chem Pharm Bull* (Tokyo) 1971;19(8):1740.

[5] Shoji J, et al. Structure of senegin-III of Polygala senega root. *Chem Pharm Bull* 1972;20(2):424.

[6] Tsukitani Y, et al. Constituents of Senegae Radix. III. Structures of senegin-III and -IV, saponins from *Polygala senega* var. latifolia. *Chem Pharm Bull* (Tokyo) 1973;21(7):1564.

[7] Yoshikawa M, et al. Bioactive saponins and glycosides. I. Senegae radix. (1): E-senegasaponins a and b and Z-senegasaponins a and b, their inhibitory effect on alcohol absorption and hypoglycemic activity. *Chem Pharm Bull* (Tokyo) 1995;43(12):2115.

[8] Yoshikawa M, et al. Bioactive saponins and glycosides. II. Senegae Radix. (2): Chemical structures, hypoglycemic activity, and ethanol absorption-inhibitory effect of E-senegasaponin c, Z-senegasaponin c, and Z-senegins II, III, IV. *Chem Pharm Bull* (Tokyo) 1996;44(7):1305.

[9] Yoshikawa M, et al. E-senegasaponins A and B, Z-senegasaponins A and B, Z-senegins II and III, new type inhibitors of ethanol absorption in rats from senegae radix, the roots of *Polygala senega* L. var. latifolia Torr. et Gray. *Chem Pharm Bull* (Tokyo) 1995;43(2):350.

[10] Kanazawa H, et al. Determination of acidic saponins in crude drugs by high-performance liquid chromatography on octadecylsilica porous glass. *J Chromatogr* 1993;630(1/2):408.

[11] Zhang D, et al. Polygalasaponins XLII-XLVI from roots of *Polygala glomerata*. *Phytochemistry* 1998;47(3):459.

[12] Saitoh H, et al. Senegoses A-E, oligosaccharide multi-esters from *Polygala senega* var. latifolia Torr. et Gray. *Chem Pharm Bull* (Tokyo) 1993;41(6):1127.

[13] Saitoh H, et al. Senegoses F-I, oligosaccharide multi-esters from the roots of *Polygala senega* var. latifolia Torr. et Gray. *Chem Pharm Bull* (Tokyo) 1993;41(12):2125.

[14] Saitoh H, et al. Senegoses J-O, oligosaccharide multi-esters from the roots of *Polygala senega* L. *Chem Pharm Bull* (Tokyo) 1994;42(3):641.

[15] Kako M, et al. Effect of senegin-II on blood glucose in normal and NIDDM mice. *Biol Pharm Bull* 1995;18(8):1159.

[16] Kako M, et al. Hypoglycemic effect of the rhizomes of *Polygala senega* in normal and diabetic mice and its main component, the triterpenoid glycoside senegin-II. *Planta Med* 1996;62(5):440.

[17] Kako M, et al. Hypoglycemic activity of some triterpenoid glycosides. *J Nat Prod* 1997;60(6):604.

[18] Kim HM, et al. Effect of *Polygala tenuifolia* root extract on the tumor necrosis factor- alpha secretion from mouse astrocytes. *J Ethnopharmacol* 1998;61(3):201.

[19] Grieve M. A Modern Herbal. London: Jonathan Cape. 1931;733–734.

Senna

SCIENTIFIC NAME(S): *Cassia acutifolia* Delile, syn. with *Cassia senna* L. Also includes references to *C. angustifolia* Vahl. Family: Caesalpinaceae

BOTANY: *C. acutifolia* is native to Egypt and the Sudan while *C. angustifolia* is native to Somalia and Arabia. Plants known as "wild sennas" (*C. hebecarpa* Fern. and *C. marilandica* L.) grow on moist banks and woods in the eastern US. This plant should not be confused with "cassia," a common name for cinnamon. Senna is a ow branching shrub, growing to about 3 feet in height. It has a straight woody stem and yellow flowers.[1] The top parts are harvested, dried and graded. The hand-collected senna is known as Tinnevally senna. Leaves that have been harvested and graded mechanically are known as Alexandria senna. There are over 400 known species of cassia.[1]

HISTORY: Senna was first used medicinally by Arabian physicians as far back as the 9th century A.D.[1] It has long found use in traditional Arabic and European medicine as well, primarily as a cathartic. The leaves have been brewed and the tea administered for its strong laxative effect. Because it is often difficult to control the concentration of the active ingredients in the tea, an unpredictable effect may be obtained. Therefore, standardized commercial dosage forms have been developed, and these concentrates are available as liquids, powders and tablets in over-the-counter laxatives. The plant derives its name from the Arabic "sena" and from the Hebrew word "cassia," which means "peeled back," a reference to its peelable bark.

CHEMISTRY: Senna contains anthraquinones including dianthrone glycosides (1.5% to 3%), sennosides A and B (rhein dianthrones), sennosides C and D (rhein aloe-emodin heterodianthrones). Other numerous minor sennosides have been identified, and all appear to contribute to the laxative effect. The plant also contains free anthroquinones in small amounts including rhein, aloe-emodin, chrysophanol and their glycosides.[2,3]

Senna pods also contain the same rhein dianthrone glycosides as the leaves.

Carbohydrates in the plant include 2% polysaccharides, and ± 10% mucilage consisting of galactose, arabinose, rhamnose and galacturonic acid.[2,3] Other carbohydrates include mannose, fructose, glucose, pinitol and sucrose.[2]

Flavonols present include isorhamnetin and kaempferol. Glycosides 6-hydroxymusizin and tinnevellin are also found.

Other constituents in senna include chrysophanic acid, salicylic acid, saponin, resin, mannitol, sodium potassium tartrate and trace amounts of volatile oil.[2,4]

PHARMACOLOGY: Senna is a potent **laxative**. Its cathartic effects can be obtained from a tea prepared from one or two teaspoonfuls of dried leaves.

Senna's use in treating constipation is well documented. It is one of the most popular laxatives, especially in the elderly.[5] Many reports are available discussing senna's role in constipation,[6,7] its use in the elderly,[8-12] in psychiatric patients,[13] in spinal cord injury patients[14] and in pregnancy, where it is the stimulant laxative of choice.[15] In cancer treatment protocols, senna has also been noted to reverse the constipating effects of narcotics, and may prevent constipation if given with the narcotic.[16] It may, however, cause more adverse effects than other laxatives, primarily abdominal pain.[17] Castor oil was superior to senna for chronic constipation sufferers in another report.[18]

Senna may affect influence on intestinal transit time.[19-21] Its effectiveness as part of a cleansing regimen to evacuate the bowels in preparation for such tests as colonoscopies or barium enemas is documented.[22-32] Results from these studies include reduced ingestion of commercial *Golytely* solution and simethicone when given with senna,[27] and more effective colon cleansing with senna in combination with polyethylene glycol electrolyte lavage solution, compared to the solution alone.[28] Senna has also been studied in chronic constipation,[33] and for long-term laxative treatment.[34] Several mechanisms are postulated as to how senna acts as an effective laxative. The anthraquinone glycosides are hydrolyzed by intestinal bacteria to yield the active, freed anthraquinones. Alternately, it has been suggested that anthraquinones are absorbed in small quantities from the small intestine and hydrolyzed in the liver. The resultant anthraquinones are secreted into the colon.[35] One report using human intestinal flora finds sennoside A to eventually be converted to rheinanthrone, which is the active principle causing peristalsis of the large intestines. Sennosides A and B also play a role in inducing fluid secretion in the colon. Sennosides irritate the lining of the large intestine, causing contraction, which results in a bowel movement approximately 10 hours after the dose is taken.[1]

Prostaglandins may also be involved in the laxative actions.[2] One report suggests prostaglandin-mediated action of sennosides.[36] Indomethacin can partly inhibit the actions of sennosides A and B.[2] However, conflicting reports suggest that prostaglandins do not contribute to the laxative effect.[37,38] In addition, studies on the rat colon suggest that the laxative effect produced by senna may involve histamine formation.[39]

Metabolism of anthranoid laxatives has been reported,[40,41] as has the metabolism of sennosides.[42-44] The kinetics of senna constituents rhein and aloe-emodin have been investigated in man.[45]

The senna constituents, aloe-emodin and beta-sitosterol, possess inhibitory activity against cancer cells in mice.[2,4]

Senna was not found to have antidiabetic activity when tested in diabetic mice.[46]

TOXICOLOGY: Chronic use of any laxative, in particular irritant laxatives such as senna, often results in a "laxative-dependency syndrome" characterized by poor gastric motility in the absence of repeated laxative administration. Other reports of laxative abuse include laxative-induced diarrhea,[47,48] and osteomalacia and arthropathy associated with prolonged use of the product.[49]

The chronic use of anthroquinone glycosides has been associated with pigmentation of the colon (melanosis coli). Several cases of reversible finger clubbing (enlargement of the ends of the fingers and toes) have been reported following long-term abuse of senna-containing laxatives.[50-52] One report described a woman who developed finger clubbing following ingestion of from 4 to 40 *Senokot* tablets per day for about 15 years.[53] Clubbing reversed after the laxative was discontinued. The mechanism has been postulated to be related to either increased vascularity of the nail beds or a systemic metabolic abnormality secondary to chronic laxative ingestion.

Senna abuse has been associated with the development of cachexia and reduced serum globulin levels after chronic ingestion.[54]

Risk assessment for senna's use during pregnancy has been addressed.[55] One review suggests senna to be the "stimulant laxative" of choice during pregnancy and lactation.[15] Uterine motility was not stimulated by sennosides in one report in pregnant ewes.[56] None of the breast-fed infants experienced abnormal stool consistency from their mothers' ingestion of senna laxatives. The constituent rhein, taken from milk samples varied in concentration from 0 to 27 mg/ml, with between 89% to 94% of values $\leq$ 10 mg/ml.[57,58] Nonstandardized laxatives are not recommended during pregnancy.[2]

Myenteric neurons in the rat colon are not destroyed by sennosides, as had been earlier suggested.[59,60,61] Anthraquinone purgatives in excess were said to have caused degeneration of neurons. Toxicity studies separating toxic components of senna's anthraquinone derivatives have been performed.[62]

Generally, senna may cause mild abdominal discomfort such as cramping. Prolonged use may alter electrolytes. Patients with intestinal obstruction should avoid senna.[2]

Various case reports of senna toxicity are available, and include coma and neuropathy after ingestion of a senna-combination laxative,[63] hepatitis after chronic use of the plant,[64] occupational asthma and rhinoconjunctivitis from a factory worker exposed to senna-containing hair dyes,[65] and asthma and allergy symptoms from workers in a bulk laxative manufacturing facility.[66]

SUMMARY: Senna has been used for many years as an effective laxative. It is used to treat constipation and to cleanse bowels in preparation for certain procedures. It has many mechanisms of action including bowel irritation, increased peristaltic action, and fluid secretion. Toxicity includes laxative abuse and abdominal discomfort. Caution is advised for long-term use of "dietary teas" containing laxatives.

PATIENT INFORMATION – Senna

Uses: Senna is most commonly used as a laxative.

Side Effects: The chronic use of senna has resulted in pigmentation of the colon, reversible finger clubbing, cachexia and a dependency on the laxative.

[1] Chevallier A. Encyclopedia of Medicinal Plants. New York, NY: DK Publishing, 1996;72.
[2] Newall C, et al. Herbal Medicines. London, England: Pharmaceutical Press, 1996;243-44.
[3] Bisset N. Herbal Drugs and Phytopharmaceuticals. Stuttgart, Germany: CRC Press Inc., 1994;463-66.
[4] Duke J. CRC Handbook of Medicinal Herbs. Boca Raton, FL: CRC Press Inc., 1989;102-3.
[5] Heaton K, et al. Dig Dis Sci 1993;38(6):1004-8.
[6] Marlett J, et al. Am J Gastroenterol 1987;82(4):333-37.
[7] Godding E. Pharmacology 1988;36(Suppl)1:230-36.
[8] Maddi V. J Am Geriatr Soc 1979 Oct;27:464-68.
[9] Passmore A, et al. BMJ 1993;307(6907):769-71.
[10] Kinnunen O, et al. Pharmacology 1993;47(Suppl)1:253-55.
[11] Passmore A, et al. Pharmacology 1993;47(Suppl)1:249-52.
[12] Pahor M, et al. Aging 1995;7(2):128-35.
[13] Georgia E. Curr Ther Res 1983 Jun;33(Sec 1):1018-22.
[14] Cornell S, et al. Nurs Res 1973 Jul-Aug;22:321-28.
[15] Gattuso J, et al. Drug Saf 1994;10(1):47-65.
[16] Cameron J. Cancer Nurs 1992;15(5):372-77.
[17] Sykes N. J Pain Sympt Manage 1996; 11(6):363-69.
[18] Pawlik A, et al. Herba Polonica 1994;40(1-2):64-67.
[19] Rogers H, et al. Br J Clin Pharmacol 1978 Dec;6:493-97.
[20] Sogni P, et al. Gastroenterol Clin Biol 1992;16(1):21-24.
[21] Ewe K, et al. Pharmacology 1993;47(Suppl)1:242-48.
[22] Staumont G, et al. Pharmacology 1988;36(Suppl).1:49-56.
[23] Han R. Chung Hua Hu Li Tsa Chih 1989;24(5):273-75.
[24] Hangartner P, et al. Endoscopy 1989;21(6):272-75.
[25] Labenz J, et al. Med Klin 1990;85(10):581-85.
[26] Borkje B, et al. Scand J Gastroenterol 1991;26(2):162-66.
[27] Wildgrube H, et al. Bildgebung 1991;58(2):63-66.
[28] Ziegenhagen D, et al. Gastrointest Endosc 1991;37(5):547-49.
[29] Bailey S, et al Clin Radiol 1991;44(5):335-37.
[30] Fernandez S, et al. Rev Esp Enferm Dig 1995;87(11):785-91.
[31] Tooson J, et al. Postgrad Med 1996;100(2):203-4;207-12, 214.
[32] Ziegenhagen D, et al. Z. Gastroenterol 1992;30(1):17-19.
[33] Mishalany H. J Pediatr Surg 1989;24(4):360-62.
[34] Ralevic V, et al. Gastroenterology 1990;99(5):1352-57.
[35] Bowman WC, Rand MJ. Textbook of Pharmacology, 2nd ed., Blackwell Scientific Publications 1980.
[36] Beubler E, et al. Pharmacology 1988;36(Suppl)1:85-91.
[37] Mascolo N, et al. Pharmacology 1988;36(Suppl)1:92-97.
[38] Mascolo N, et al. J Pharm Pharmacol 1988;40(12):882-84.
[39] Autore G, et al. Eur J Pharmacol 1990;191(1):97-99.
[40] deWitte P, et al. Hepatogastroenterology 1990;37(6):601-5.
[41] deWitte P. Pharmacology 1993;47(Suppl)1:86-97.
[42] Lemli J. Pharmacology 1988;36(Suppl)1:126-28.
[43] Hietala P, et al. Pharmacology 1988;36(Suppl)1:138-43.
[44] Lemli J. Ann Gastroenterol Hepatol (Paris) 1996;32(2):109-12.
[45] Krumbiegel G, et al. Pharmacology 47(Suppl)1:120-24.
[46] Swanston-Flatt S, et al. Acta Diabetol Lat 1989;26(1):51-55.
[47] Cummings J, et al. BMJ 1974 Mar 23;1:537-41.
[48] Morris A, et al. Gastroenterology 1979 Oct;77:780-86.
[49] Frier B, et al. Br J Clin Pract 1977 Jan-Feb-Mar;31:17-19.
[50] Prior J, White I. Lancet i ;1978,947.
[51] Malmquist J, et al. Postgrad Med 1980 Dec;56:862-64.
[52] Armstrong R, et al. BMJ 1981 Jun 6;282:1836.
[53] FitzGerald O, Redmond J. Irish J Med Sci 1983:152:246.
[54] Levin D, et al. Lancet 1981;1:919.
[55] Anonymous. Pharmacology 1992;44(Suppl)1:20-22.
[56] Garcia-Villar R. Pharmacology 1988;36(Suppl)1:203-11.
[57] Faber P, et al. Pharmacology 1988;36(Suppl)1:212-20.
[58] Faber P, et al. Geburtshilfe Frauenheilkd 1989;49(11):958-62.
[59] Kiernan J, et al. Neuroscience 1989;30(3):837-42.
[60] Heinicke E, et al. J Pharm Pharmacol 1990;42(2):123-25.
[61] Milner P, et al. J Pharm Pharmacol 1992;44(9):777-79.
[62] Hietala P, et al. Pharmacol Toxicol 1987;61(2):153-56.
[63] Dobb G, et al. Med J Aust 1984 Apr 14;140:495-96.
[64] Beuers U, et al. Lancet 1991;337(8737):372-73.
[65] Helin T, et al. Allergy 1996;51(3):181-84.
[66] Marks G. Am Rev Respir Dis 1991;144(5):1065-69.

Shark Derivatives

SCIENTIFIC NAME(S): *Squalus acanthias* (spiny dogfish shark), *Sphyrna lewini* (Hammerhead Shark) and other shark species

COMMON NAME(S): Spiny dogfish shark, hammerhead shark and other species

HISTORY: Shark cartilage is prepared from the cartilage of freshly caught sharks in the Pacific Ocean. The cartilage is cut from the shark, cleaned, shredded, and dried. One of the main processing plants for dogfish shark is in Costa Rica. The finely ground cartilage is uniformly pulverized (in a 200 mesh screen), sterilized, and encapsulated. Gelatin capsules contain 740 mg, usually without additives or fillers, and are claimed to be "all natural." The 100% pure shark cartilage is also available in 200 g and 500 g capsules in safety-sealed bottles (eg, *Cartilade©*).[1,2]

Squalamine was originally isolated from shark stomachs, but has subsequently been synthesized.[1] This compound is still in the experimental stage and is not yet commercially available.

CHEMISTRY: Early claims were made that extracts of shark cartilage inhibited tumor angiogenesis when implanted in rabbit corneas. The active principle(s) has not been found, although some believe it might be a protein.[1,2] Several studies have been done on various sharks. Pettit and Ode[3] isolated and characterized sphyrnastatin 1 and 2 from the hammerhead shark. Neame et al[4] recently reported on the isolation of a protein from reef shark (*Carcharhinus springeri*) cartilage which bears a striking resemblance to human tetranectin. Moore et al[5] discovered a broad-spectrum steroidal antibiotic from the dogfish shark which they nemed squalamine; chemically it is 3–beta-N-1–(N--1,3–diamino-propane)-7 alpha, 24 zeta-dihydroxy-5 alpha-cholestane 24–sulfate.

PHARMACOLOGY: Many claims have been made that shark cartilage can cure cancer. The rationale includes the fact that sharks rarely get cancer, that sharks are cartilaginous fish and that cartilage is avascular and contains agents that inhibit vascularization (angiogenesis). The reasoning then follows that sharks do not get cancer because the inhibited vascularization prevents the formation of tumors; hence, giving it to humans may inhibit tumor angiogenesis and thus cure cancer.[1]

In late 1992, incomplete and since nonreplicated clinical studies (unpublished) in Havana, Cuba, purported to show some progress in terminally ill cancer patients. The National Cancer Institute reviewed these studies and decided against researching shark cartilage.[1] Recently, however, the FDA granted an IND application for a shark cartilage product, *Benefin*, by Lane Labs-USA, Inc. to investigate benefits in prostate cancer and AIDS-associated Kaposi's sarcoma.[6]

Certainly, future work should continue to focus on the isolation of the responsible proteins or small molecules. The tetranectin-like protein from the reef shark is important since, in man, tetranectin enhances plasminogen activation catalyzed by the tissue plasminogen activator. It may also play a role in cancer metastasis. Research along these lines by Moore et al[5] has demonstrated the presence of a broad-spectrum aminosterol antibiotic in the dogfish shark which they named squalamine. It shows significant bactericidal activity against both Gram-negative and Gram-positive bacteria. It is also fungicidal and induces activity against protozoa.[5] This discovery implicates a unique steroid acting as a potential host-defense agent in vertebrates and provides unique concepts of chemical design for a new family of much needed broad-spectrum antibiotics.

TOXICOLOGY: No toxicity data has appeared in current literature on either shark cartilage or squalamine.

SUMMARY: Initial interest on the purported anticancer effects of cartilage from dogfish shark has waned since the National Cancer Institute decided against supporting studies on it. A few studies on related species show interesting active protein substances that may be useful as cancer control agents. However, the only active small molecule with promise is the aminosterol called squalamine. Its major experimental activity has been as a unique and potent antibiotic with fungicidal and antiprotozoal activity. Clinical data should be forthcoming.

PATIENT INFORMATION – Shark Derivatives

Uses: The shark cartilage was thought to be a cancer control agent, but no studies have proven this theory. Squalamine has been used as a potent antibiotic with fungicidal and antiprotozoal activity.

Side Effects: No adverse effects have appeared on either substance.

[1] Masslo Anderson J. Biotech Discovers the Shark. *MD Magazine* 1993;37:43.

[2] Moss RW. Cancer Therapy: The Independent Consumers Guide to Non-Toxic Treatment & Prevention. New York: Equinox Press, 1992.

[3] Pettit GR, Ode RH. Antineoplastic agents L: isolation and characterization of sphyrnastatins 1 and 2 from the hammerhead *shark* Sphyrna lewini. *J Pharm Sci* 1977:66:757.

[4] Neame PJ, et al. Primary structure of a protein isolated from reef shark (Carcharhinus springeri) cartilage that is similar to the mammalian C-type lectin homolog, tetranectin. *Protein Sci* 1992:1(1):161.

[5] Moore KS, et al. Squalamine: an aminosterol antibiotic from the shark. *Proc Nat Acad Sci USA* 1993;90(4):1354.

[6] Hunt TJ, Connelly JF. Shark cartilage for cancer treatment. *Am J Health-Syst Pharm* 1995;52:1756.

Shark Liver Oil

SCIENTIFIC NAME(S): Shark liver oil may be obtained from several species of sharks, including the deep sea shark (*Centrophorus Squamosus*), the dogfish shark (*Squalus Acanthias*), and the basking shark (*Cetorhinus Maximus*).

SOURCE: Shark liver oil (SLO) is commercially produced from several species of deep sea sharks' liver oil. The liver constitutes about 25% of the total shark body weight. SLO is a major natural source of squalene and alkyglycerols.[1]

HISTORY: SLO has been used for over 40 years for its therapeutic benefits. Initially, it was employed by Scandinavian fishermen to treat skin conditions and certain cancers. The active components, alkylglycerols, have been studied in a number of areas, including use as an immune system stimulant.[2]

CHEMISTRY: SLO contains alkylglycerols, squalene, pristane, vitamins A and D, esters of fatty acids, glycerol ethers, triglycerides, cholesterol, and fatty acids.[1] Alkylglycerols are a group of ether-linked glycerols and have been found in a number of shark species. For example, 1-O-(2-hydroxyalkyl) glycerols have been isolated from Greenland SLO.[3] Dogfish shark contains 40% to 70% SLO, containing 30% to 40% 1-O-alkyl diacylglycerol ethers.[4] Purification and characterization of deep sea shark, liver oil 1-O-alkylglycerols have been performed. The oil contained glycerol esters, 60% unsaponifiable matter, including squalene (45%) and cholesterol (4.5%).[5] Between ≈ 60% to 90% of liver weight in the *Centrophorus* species is oil, containing squalene that increases in concentration with the age of the shark. More than 50 fatty acids were identified, as well.[6]

Analyses concerning shark liver components from the late 1960s through the early 1970s include the following: Oil composition of the basking shark including sterols and glyceryl esters,[7,8] separation of neutral lipids from shark liver,[9] and hydrocarbon and fatty acid research.[10,11]

PHARMACOLOGY: SLO has been classified as a topical protectant.[1] An early use of alkylglycerols from SLO was to treat leukemia and to prevent radiation sickness from cancer X-ray therapy.[2] A Danish study reports less cases of irradiation damage in alkoxyglycerol-treated uterine cancer patients.[12] Another report suggests alkylglycerols' radioprotective effects may operate by a mechanism that may incorporate the substance into a pool of platelet-activating factors, increasing their biosynthesis.[13] Alkoxyglycerol also may increase leukocyte and thrombocyte counts in specific dosages.[12] The natural alkylglycerol level rises within tumor cells, apparently an attempt in controlling cell growth. An essential step in cell proliferation involves activating protein kinase C, which can be inhibited by alkylglycerols. SLO demonstrates inhibitory actions against cutaneous angiogenesis in certain cancer cells in mice, human kidney cancer, and human urinary bladder cancer cells including sarcoma L-1 syngeneic.[14] However, a conflicting report finds no documentation regarding inhibition of tumor growth in alkoxyglycerol-treated cancer patients, even though it is used in Denmark as a supplementary agent in cancer treatment.[12]

Another effect of alkylglycerols include the ability to stimulate the immune system. One mechanism involved may include activation of macrophages.[2]

Dietary SLO also has been studied for its effects on lipid and fatty acid composition in guinea pig hearts.[15] A glycerol monoether mixture from SLO was found to be an effective skin penetration enhancer when studied in mice.[16]

TOXICOLOGY: It has been stated that SLO has no side effects in dosages of 100 mg three times daily.[2] However, in Sweden, a SLO product (*Ecomer*) was prohibited by the National Board of Health and Welfare.[17] A report on SLO-induced pneumonia in pigs is described,[18] as well as a case report concerning shark oil pneumonia.[19]

SUMMARY: SLO has been used therapeutically for the past 40 years in the areas of skin conditions, cancer treatment, and prevention of radiation sickness. Few toxic effects from SLO use have been reported, although caution regarding SLO-induced pneumonia is advised.

PATIENT INFORMATION – Shark Liver Oil

Uses: SLO has been used to prevent radiation sickness, to treat skin conditions, and as a cancer treatment. Alkylglycerols have been studied as an immune system stimulant.

Side Effects: Few toxic effects have been reported; advise caution with SLO concerning SLO-induced pneumonia.

[1] Budavari S, et al, eds. The Merck Index, 11th ed. Rahway NJ:Merck and Co., 1989.

[2] Pugliese P, et al. Some biological actions of alkylglycerols from shark liver oil. *J Altern Complement Med* 1998;4(1):87-99. Review.

[3] Hallgren B, et al. 1-O-(2–hydroxyalkyl) glycerols isolated from Greenland shark liver oil. *Acta Chem Scand B* 1974;28(9):1074-76.

[4] Kang S, et al. Digestion of the 1-O-alkyl diacylglycerol ethers of Atlantic dogfish liver oils by Atlantic salmon Salmo salar. *Lipids* 1997;32(1):19-30.

[5] Bordier C, et al. Purification and characterization of deep sea shark Centrophorus squamosus liver oil 1-O-alkylglycerol ether lipids. *Lipids* 1996;31(5):521-28.

[6] Peyronel D, et al. Fatty acid and squalene compositions of Mediterranean Centrophorus SPP egg and liver oil in relation to age. *Lipids* 1984;19(9):643-48.

[7] Lombardi R, et al. Analysis of ointments, oils, and waxes. X. Study of the composition of oil of basking-shark, *Cetorhinus maximus* Gunner. *Ann Pharm Fr* 1971;29(7):429-36. French.

[8] Nevenzel J. Basking shark liver oil sterols and glyceryl ethers. UCLA-12-636. *UCLA Rep* 1968;Jun 30:16-18.

[9] Casey A. Separation of neutral lipids of shark liver by "dry-column" chromatography. *J Lipid Res* 1969;10(4):456-59.

[10] Gelpi E, et al. Gas chromatographic-mass spectrometric analysis of isoprenoid hydrocarbons and fatty acids in shark liver oil products. *J Am Oil Chem Soc* 1968;45(3):144-47.

[11] Blumer M. Hydrocarbons in digestive tract and liver of a basking shark. *Science* 1967;156(773):390-91.

[12] Hasle H, et al. Shark liver oil (alkoxyglycerol) and cancer treatment. *Ugeskr Laeger* 1991;153(5):343-46. Danish.

[13] Hichami A, et al. Modulation of platelet-activating-factor production by incorporation of naturally occurring 1-O-alkylglycerls in phospholipids of human leukemic monocyte-like THP-1 cells. *Eur J Biochem* 1997;250(2):242-48.

[14] Skopinska-Rozewska E, et al. Inhibitory effect of shark liver oil on cutaneous angiogenesis induced in Balb/c mice by syngeneic sarcoma L-1, human urinary bladder and human kidney tumour cells. *Oncol Rep* 1999;6(6):1341-44.

[15] Murphy M, et al. Diets enriched in menhaden fish oil, seal oil, or shark liver oil have distinct effects on the lipid and fatty-acid composition of guinea pig heart. *Mol Cell Biochem* 1997;177(1–2):257–69.

[16] Loftsson T, et al. Unsaturated glycerol monoethers as novel skin penetration enhancers. *Pharmazie* 1997; 52(6):463–65.

[17] The National Board of Health and Welfare prohibits Ecomer. Shark liver oil is suspected of adverse effects. *Lakartidningen* 1990;87(7):473. Swedish.

[18] Seo J, et al. Shark liver oil-induced lipoid pneumonia in pigs: Correlation of thin-section CT and histopathologic findings. *Radiology* 1999;212(1):88–96.

[19] Asnis D, et al. Shark oil pneumonia. An overlooked entity. *Chest* 1993;103(3):976-77.

Shellac

SCIENTIFIC NAME(S): Family: Coccidae

COMMON NAME(S): Shellac, lac, gommelaque, lacca

SOURCE: Shellac is the purified product of lac, the red, hardened secretion of the insect *Laccifer (Tachardia) lacca* Kerr. This tiny insect sucks the sap of selected trees and bushes, and secretes lac as a protective covering. The name lac is said to derive from *lakh*, the Sanskrit word for one hundred thousand, a reference to the very large number of insects involved in producing appreciable amounts of the product.[1]

Lac is cultivated in India, Thailand, and Burma.

The whitest lac is produced by insects infesting the kusum tree (*Schleichera trijuga*). The harvester cuts twigs coated with lac into small pieces called sticklac. The crude material is ground and soaked in water to remove debris and insect bodies. The remaining material is soaked in sodium carbonate, which removes laccaic acid, a complex mixture of at least four structurally related pigments. The resulting granules retain the yellow pigment erythrolaccin and are dried to form seedlac. Further treatment by melting, evaporating, or filtering yields shellac.[2]

CHEMISTRY: The National Formulary XV of the USA recognizes four grades of shellac: Orange, dewaxed orange, regular bleached and refined wax-free bleached. The grades differ in the manner in which the seedlac is treated. Orange shellac is obtained by the evaporation of filtered ethanolic solutions of seedlac. It may be dewaxed by further filtration. Regular bleached shellac is obtained by dissolving the seedlac in aqueous sodium carbonate at a high temperature. After filtration, a bleaching agent (such as sodium hypochlorite) is added. The resin is removed by sulfuric acid precipitation. Refined wax-free bleached shellac adds another filtration step to remove the waxes.[3]

The exact chemical composition of shellac is unknown. It appears to be composed of a network of hydroxy fatty acid esters and sesquiterpene acid esters with a molecular weight of about 1000. Aleuretic acid, r-butolic acid, shellolic acid, and jalaric acid are the major constituents. The composition is a function of the source and time of harvest of the sticklac. Variability in the product may be a problem for commercial users of shellac. The physical properties of shellac also vary. For example, the reported melting point ranges from 77° to 120°C. Shellac is soluble in ethanol, methanol, glycols, glycol ethers, and alkaline water.[1]

PHARMACOLOGY: Shellac is most often used as a finish for fine furnitures. Further, the material has been used for almost 100 years by the pharmaceutical industry. Examples of shellac's role in this field include: Tablet coating formulations,[4,5,6,7] microencapsulation,[8-12] matrix formation,[13] enteric coating,[14] humidity tolerance,[15] and binding ability.[16] However, shellac undergoes an "aging effect" upon storage and thus has fallen into disfavor as an ingredient in some preparations.[2]

Dentistry has also used shellac in various ways.[17,18] Reported uses include binding agents for dentures, restorations, and mouldings and as a constituent in "artificial calculus" for training purposes in dental schools.[19-23]

Shellac has also been used as an ingredient in hair spray[24] and in other cosmetics[25] and as pretreatment against mushroom toxins in mice.[26]

TOXICOLOGY: Little data are available regarding toxicity. One study investigated the short-term inhalation toxicity in rabbits of a hair spray-containing shellac; the product did not induce any significant toxicologic problems.[27] Shellac NF is food grade and is listed as Generally Recognized as Safe (GRAS) by the FDA. One report discusses contact cheilitis to shellac.[28] Another report reviews bezoars (accumulations of foreign material in the stomach) such as shellac. This unusual collection in the GI tract, if untreated, may lead to anorexia, weight loss, bleeding, or perforation.[29]

SUMMARY: Shellac is a crude natural material composed of variable constituents. It is produced from insect *Laccifer* secretions, then treated to form the final product. Shellac is used in furniture finishing, tablet coatings and matrices, dentistry, and cosmetics. The crude product poses little health hazard, although commercial products that dilute shellac in solvents may pose a health problem.

PATIENT INFORMATION – Shellac

Uses: The most common use is as a furniture finish, but it has also been used in the pharmaceutical industry, in dentistry, and in cosmetics.

Side effects: Little data are available. One report discusses contact cheilitis.

---

[1] Yates P, Field GF. Tetrahedron. 1970;26:3135.
[2] Dermarderosian A. Natural Product Medicine. Philadelphia, PA: George F Stickley Co. 1988;356–57.
[3] Pharmaceutical Glazes, Bulletin 70-09-01, William Zinsser and Co.
[4] Pancula E, et al. *Acta Pharm Hung* 1970 Jan;40:25–28.
[5] Alam A, et al. *J Pharm Sci* 1972 Feb;61:265–68.
[6] Tuerck P, et al. *J Pharm Sci* 1973 Sep;62:1534–37.
[7] Shecrey D, et al. *Indian J Pharm Sci* 1992;54(5):169–73.
[8] El Banna H, et al. *Pharm Indus* 1932;44(6):641–45.
[9] Labhasetwar V, et al. *J Microencapsul* 1989;6(1):115–18.
[10] Labhasetwar V, et al. *J Microencapsul* 1990;7(4):553–54.
[11] Sheorey D, et al. *Int J Pharm* 1991 Feb 1;68:19–23.
[12] Sheorey D, et al. *J Microencapsul* 1991;8(3):375–80.
[13] Serajuddin A, et al. *J Pharm Sci* 1984 Sep;73:1203–8.
[14] Chang R, et al. *Int J Pharm* 1990 Apr 30;60;171–73.
[15] Gursoy A, et al. *Pharmazie* 1986;41(8):575–78.
[16] Labhasetwar V, et al. *Indian J Pharm Sci* 1988 Nov-Dec:50:343–45.
[17] Azouka A, et al. *J Oral Rehabil* 1993;20(4):393–400.
[18] Harrison A, et al. *J Oral Rehabil* 1995;22(7):509–13.
[19] Lie T, et al. *J Clin Periodontal* 1987;14(3):149–55.
[20] Escoe R. *Int J Prosthodon* 1989;2(3):243–44.
[21] Hitge M, et al. *Ned Tijdschr Tandheelkd* 1989;96(8):372–77.
[22] Lee C, et al. *J Pros Dent* 1991;66(5):623–30.
[23] Heath J, et al. *J Oral Rehabil* 1993;20(4):363–72.
[24] Tannert U. *Seifen, Oele, Fette, Wachse* 1992 Oct 30;118:1079–80.
[25] Penning M. *Seifen, Oele, Fette, Wachse* 1990 Apr 5;116:221–24.
[26] Adams W, et al. *J Pharmacol Exp Ther* 1989;249(2):552–56.
[27] Monograph on Shellac, Informatics Inc., Rockville MD, 1978, PB-287-765.
[28] Rademaker M, et al. *Contact Dermatitis* 1986;15(5):307–8.
[29] Andrus C, et al. *Am J Gastroenterol* 1988;83(5):476–78.

Slippery Elm

SCIENTIFIC NAME(S): *Ulmus rubra* Muhl. Also known as *U. fulva* Michx. Family: Ulmaceae

COMMON NAME(S): Slippery elm, red elm, Indian elm, moose elm, sweet elm

BOTANY: The genus *Ulmus* contains 18 species of deciduous shrubs and trees.[1]

The slippery elm tree is native to eastern Canada and eastern and central United States, where it is found most commonly in the Appalachian mountains. The trunk is reddish brown with gray-white bark on the branches. The bark is rough, with vertical ridging. The slippery elm can grow to 18 to 20 meters in height.[2] In the spring, dark brown floral buds appear and open into small, clustered flowers at the branch tips.[3] White elm (*U. americana*) is 1 related species and is used in a similar manner.[2]

HISTORY: North American Indians and early settlers used the inner bark of the slippery elm not only to build canoes, shelter, and baskets, but as a poultice or as a soothing drink.[2,4,5] Upon contact with water, the inner bark, collected in spring, yields a thick mucilage or demulcent that was used as an ointment or salve to treat urinary tract inflammation and applied topically for cold sores and boils. A decoction of the leaves was used as a poultice to remove discoloration around blackened or bruised eyes. Surgeons during the American Revolution treated gun-shot wounds in this manner.[3] Early settlers boiled bear fat with the bark to prevent rancidity.[1,4] Late in the 19th century, a preparation of elm mucilage had been recognized as an official product by the United States Pharmacopoeia.[6]

CHEMISTRY: Slippery elm contains carbohydrates including starches with mucilage being the major constituent. It contains hexoses, pentoses, and polyuronides.[2,7] The plant also has phytosterols, sesquiterpenes, calcium oxalate, cholesterol, and tannins (3% to 6.5%) as constituents.[2,4,7] Isolation and structure of a cyanidanol glycoside has been reported from related species *U. americana*.[8]

PHARMACOLOGY: Slippery elm prepared as a poultice coats and protects irritated tissues such as skin or intestinal membranes. The powdered bark has been used in this manner for local application to treat **gout, rheumatism, cold sores, wounds, abscesses, ulcers**, and **toothaches**.[4,7] It has also been known to "draw out" toxins, boils, splinters, or other irritants.[2]

Powdered bark is incorporated into lozenges to provide demulcent action (soothing to mucous membranes) in the treatment of throat irritation.[9] It is also used for its emollient and antitussive actions, to treat bronchitis and other lung afflictions, and to relieve thirst.[1-3,5,7]

When slippery elm preparations are taken internally, they cause reflex stimulation of nerve endings in the GI tract, leading to mucus secretion.[2] This may be the reason they are effective for protection against stomach ulcers, colitis, diverticulitis, gut inflammation, and acidity. Slippery elm is also useful for diarrhea, constipation, hemorrhoids, irritable bowel syndrome, and to expel tapeworms. It also has been used to treat cystitis and urinary inflammations.[2,3,4,7]

The plant is also used as a lubricant to ease labor,[3,4] as a source of nutrition for convalescence or baby food preparations,[2] and for its activity against herpes and syphilis.[4] The tannins present are known to possess astringent actions.[7]

TOXICOLOGY: The FDA has declared slippery elm to be a safe and effective oral demulcent.[5] An oleoresin from several *Ulmus* species has been reported to cause contact dermatitis[6] and the pollen is allergenic.[4] Preparations of slippery elm had been used as abortifacients, a practice that has not remained popular.[1,7] Generally, there are no known problems regarding toxicity of slippery elm or its constituents.[7]

SUMMARY: Slippery elm has been used for more than 100 years in traditional American medicine. The plant contains mucilage as its major component, which can be therapeutic in a variety of conditions. It has been used to protect irritated skin or mucous membranes in wounds, GI irritations, and respiratory ailments. It is also a good nutrient and possesses antiherpetic and antisyphilitic activity. Slippery elm is usually nontoxic but may cause dermatitis or an allergic reaction.

PATIENT INFORMATION – Slippery Elm

Uses: Parts of slippery elm have been used as an emollient and in lozenges. It protects irritated skin and intestinal membranes in such conditions as gout, rheumatism, cold sores, wounds, abscesses, ulcers, and toothaches.

Side Effects: Extracts from slippery elm have caused contact dermatitis, and the pollen has been reported to be allergenic. The FDA has declared slippery elm to be a safe and effective oral demulcent.

[1] Hocking G. A Dictionary of Natural Products. Medford, NJ: Plexus Publishing Inc. 1997;826-27.

[2] Chevallier A. Encyclopedia of Medicinal Plants. New York, NY: DK Publishing. 1996;144.

[3] Low T, et al, eds. Magic and Medicine of Plants. Surry Hils, NSW:Reader's Digest Assoc. Inc. 1994;385.

[4] Duke J. CRC Handbook or Medicinal Herbs. Boca Raton, FL: CRC Press, Inc. 1989;495-96.

[5] Tyler V. Herbs of Choice, The Therapeutic Use of Phytomedicinals. Binghamton, NY: Pharmaceutical Products Press. 1994;93,94.

[6] Lewis W, Elvin-Lewis MPF. Medical Botany. New York, NY: J. Wiley and Sons, 1977.

[7] Newall C, et al. Herbal Medicines. London, England: Pharmaceutical Press. 1996;248.

[8] Langhammer I. Isolation and structure of a rarely occurring cyanidanol glycoside from *Cortex betulae*. *Planta Medica* 1983 Nov;49:181-82.

[9] Morton J. Major Medicinal Plants. Springfield, IL: C.C. Thomas, 1977.

Smokeless Tobacco

BOTANY: Smokeless tobacco (ST) products are derived from the same botanical source as smoking tobacco (*Nicotiana* species). Smokeless tobaccos are often flavored with sugar or artificial sweeteners.

HISTORY: Smokeless tobaccos have been used by men and women of all levels of society. In Europe, snuffing involves placing a small pinch of tobacco in the nostrils while inhaling slightly. In the United States and many other parts of the world, "snuff dipping" is the more common practice. In this case, the user places a "quid" of powdered tobacco in the buccal area between the gum and cheek and retains the material for a period of time, usually swallowing the resultant saliva. Quids are taken as loose portions or as small prepackaged bags of tobacco. In many parts of the world, the quid is mixed with other stimulants such as betel nut. Lastly, some users chew a "chaw" of ST.

Recent national data compiled from several large-scale studies indicate that 10 to 12 million Americans use some form of ST.[1] The use of ST is prevalent throughout the United States and users often begin at very early ages. From the responses of 3,725 high school students in the southeastern United States, 20% reported trying ST products at some time. Of these users, 44% reported a first use of ST before age 13. Family influences and peer pressure were major factors in initiating use. Of concern was the indication that 8.4% of the users felt they were addicted to the substance.[2] Another survey of children in grades 3 to 12 in a Pennsylvania school district found that experimentation with ST had begun as early as the third grade, with the prevalence of use increasing with age. Nearly half of the boys in grades 7 to 12 did not believe ST products to be harmful.[3]

Children are strongly influenced by role models regarding the use of ST. To this end a survey was conducted of major league baseball personnel during the 1987 season to determine their use and understanding of the hazards of ST. Twenty-five of 26 teams participated. The players (46%) "dipped" or "chewed," more than the managers (35%), followed by the trainers (30%). Although the users recognize the harmful potential of ST, its use remains high among baseball personnel.[4] ST use is generally more prevalent among males. It should be noted that in one study, the prevalence of snuff use by women in the general population of central North Carolina was 30% (compared to 1.3% of women and 2.5% of men in the general US population).[5]

Analysis of the personality characteristics of 289 college-age users of ST found them to be significantly more reserved, less socially outgoing, less sentimental, more conforming, and more group-dependent than non-ST users.[6]

PHARMACOLOGY: As with smoking tobacco, the pharmacologic effect of ST is related to its nicotine content. Blood nicotine levels are achieved rapidly (within 5 minutes) and reach 40 ng/ml, comparable to peak levels found in heavy cigarette smokers (who average approximately 35 ng/ml).[7] The use of ST, therefore, carries many of the risks and dangers of smoking tobacco. Although there does not appear to be an increased risk of lung cancer or pulmonary disease with its use.

Oropharyngeal risks: The oral problems associated with ST use include bad breath, discolored teeth and restorative materials, excessive tooth surface wear from abrasion, decreased ability to taste and smell, gingival recession, advanced periodontal soft and hard tissue destruction, tooth loss and soft tissue erythema.[1] A common pathologic change observed in ST users is oral leukoplakia. In a study of Navajo Indians (ages 14 to 19), 25% of the users compared with 4% of non-users had leukoplakia.[8] One in 20 cases of leukoplakia will undergo malignant transformation into an epidermoid carcinoma. Nitrosamines found in ST have been shown to be tumorogenic in animals.[9]

An increased incidence of cancers of the mouth and gums, pharynx, and salivary glands have also been reported in ST users.[10] Case-controlled analyses of chronic female snuff users in North Carolina found an exceptionally high mortality from oropharyngeal cancers. The relative risk associated with snuff dipping among nonsmokers was 4.2%; among chronic users the risk approached 50–fold for cancers of the gum and buccal mucosa.[11] Users of loose portion snuff exhibit increased thickening of the oral mucosa epithelium while portion bag users show variable thickened surface layers with evidence of keratinization.[12] In an analysis of more than 2000 patients with oropharyngeal cancers, chewing, smoking, or both accounted for 70% of the cancers of the oral cavity, 84% of the oropharynx, and 75% of the hypopharynx.[9]

Tooth loss and periodontal softening occurs with chronic snuff use. Extracts of ST have served as a growth substrate for three species of oral streptococci frequently associated with human dental caries.[13]

Other risks: Thromboangitis obliterans, a distinct clinical entity characterized by segmental inflammatory and proliferative lesions of the walls of small arteries and veins has been observed frequently in heavy cigarette smokers. At least one case has also been attributed to chronic snuff use.[14]

Approximately one-third of ST users swallow the salivary juices. Persistent hyperglycemia was observed in diabetic patients who used "candified" chewing tobacco and regularly swallowed the juice. Analysis of several brands found 50 to 150 mg of glucose per gram of tobacco. Blood sugar levels returned to normal once snuff use was discontinued.[15] Other investigators suggest that saccharin added to flavor some snuffs may pose an increased risk of bladder cancer.[16]

Nicotine per se is toxic. Its cardiovascular effects include vasoconstriction, hypertension, and tachycardia. Nausea and dizziness are often experienced by novice snuff users.[17]

SUMMARY: The use of ST is increasing in the United States and remains prevalent throughout the world. Flavored tobaccos are used orally or nasally. ST preparations deliver as much nicotine as cigarettes. The use of ST is associated with a constellation of side effects. The risk of oral leukoplakia is more than 5 times greater among snuff users, and the use of ST is a major determinant of most oropharyngeal cancers. Public Law 99–252 (the Comprehensive Smokeless Tobacco Health Education Act of 1986) was developed as a federal platform for disease prevention and health promotion with respect to ST use.

PATIENT INFORMATION – Smokeless Tobacco

Uses: Smokeless tobacco has not been used medically. Its recreational use carries many of the risks and dangers of smoking tobacco.

Side Effects: Smokeless tobacco has caused bad breath, discolored teeth, excessive tooth surface wear, decreased ability to taste and smell, gingival recession, advanced periodontal soft and hard tissue destruction, tooth loss, oral leukoplakia, and increased risk of cancers in the mouth and gums.

---

[1] Christen AG, et al. *Pediatrician* 1989;16:170.
[2] Riley WT, et al. *J Adolesc Health Care* 1989;10:357.
[3] Cohen RY, et al. *AM J Publ Health* 1987;77:1454.
[4] Wisniewski JF, Bartolucci AA. *J Oral Path Med* 1989;18:322.
[5] Schottenfeld D. *N Engl J Med* 1981;304:778.
[6] Edmundson EW, et al. *Int J Addict* 1987;22:671.
[7] Russell MAH, et al. *Lancet* 1980;1:474.
[8] Wolfe MD, Carlos JP. *Comm Dent Oral Epidem* 1987;15:230.
[9] Blum A. *JAMA* 1980; 244:192.
[10] Stockwell, HG, Lyman GH. *Head Neck Surg* 1986;9:104.
[11] Winn DM, et al. *N Engl J Med* 1981;304:745.
[12] Andersson G, et al. *J Oral Path Med* 1989;18:491.
[13] Falker WA, et al. *Arch Oral Biol* 1987;32:221.
[14] O'Dell JR, et al. *Arthritis Rheum* 1987;30:1054.
[15] Pyles ST, et al. *N Engl J Med* 1981;304:365.
[16] Goldsmith DF, Winn DM. *Lancet* 1980;1:825.
[17] Gonzalez ER. *JAMA* 1980;244:112.

Soapwort

SCIENTIFIC NAME(S): *Saponaria officinalis* L. Family: Caryophyllaceae

COMMON NAME(S): Bruisewort, Bouncing Bet, Dog Cloves, Fuller's Herb, Latherwort, Lady's-Washbowl, Old-Maid's-Pink

BOTANY: Common to pastures and roadsides from coast to coast, soapwort is a perennial herbaceous plant growing to a height of 1 to 2 feet, with a single smooth stem and lanceolate leaves. Its five-petaled flowers appear during late July through September in the form of fragrant clusters varying from white to pale lavender in color.[1]

HISTORY: Soapwort was originally native to northern Europe and was introduced to England during the Middle Ages by Franciscan and Dominican monks who brought it as "a gift of God intended to keep them clean."[2] By the end of the 16th century the herb had become widespread in England, where it was used as a soap for cleansing dishes and laundry. John Gerard's Herbal (1597) recommended it as a topical disinfectant for "green wounds" and "filthy diseases."[2] Soapwort also has been administered topically for the treatment of acne, psoriasis, eczema and boils. An extract of the roots is still a popular remedy for poison ivy. While an exact time of its arrival in North America cannot be established, there is little doubt that the Puritans brought it with them to the New World. Once established, the herb spread and can now be found wild throughout the United States and southern Canada. The herb was used extensively in the early textile industry as a cleaning and sizing agent. This process, known as fulling, accounts for the name "Fuller's Herb." Another use for the product was found by the Pennsylvania Dutch who used it to impart a foamy head to the beer they brewed. To this day some beer makers use saponins, a component of the plant, to provide and maintain that foamy head.[1]

CHEMISTRY: Soapwort contains a natural source of water-soluble steroidal saponins, which allow it to form a soaplike lather. These active principles are found in all parts of the plant[1] and act as surface active agents to facilitate cleaning.

TOXICOLOGY: Saponins tend to be highly toxic (usually hemolytic) only if injected. Most are relatively inocuous when ingested orally, unless there is an underlying disease of the mucosa (ie, ulcers). Ingestion of soapwort has led to severe vomiting and diarrhea.[3] For this reason, ingestion is to be avoided.

SUMMARY: While once used internally as a diuretic, laxative, and expectorant, soapwort lacks these pharmacological actions once attributed to it by herbalists or pharmacologists.[3] Its chief use today is as a source of natural saponins to be used in making "natural" soaps and shampoos. These soaps are extracted from the rhizomes and leaves of the plant and find their chief use in brightening and cleaning delicate fabrics.

PATIENT INFORMATION – Soapwort

Uses: Soapwort is generally used to make "natural" soaps and in brightening and cleaning delicate fabrics.

Side Effects: Soapwort adverse effects are usually experienced only if taken internally, causing severe vomiting and diarrhea.

---

[1] Meyer JE. The Herbalist. Hammond, IN: Hammond Book Co., 1934.
[2] Sculley FX. God's gift, nature's soap. *The Herb Quarterly* 1989;Spring:7.
[3] Dobelis IN, ed. Magic and Medicine of Plants. Pleasantville, NY: Reader's Digest Association, 1986.

SOD

SCIENTIFIC NAME(S): Superoxide dismutase, orgotein

Superoxide dismutase (SOD, orgotein) is an ubiquitous enzyme that has received attention because of its therapeutic activity and because of claims that its ingestion may improve health and lengthen the human lifespan.

PHARMACOLOGY: A highly reactive superoxide free radical is generated as a toxic metabolite in a wide range of normal biological reactions that reduce oxygen. Since the superoxide radical is toxic to normal living cells, the enzyme superoxide dismutase which is present in all cells catalyzes the conversion of superoxide to the harmless components oxygen and hydrogen peroxide.[1]

At least three distinct types of the compound are found in humans and other mammals.[2] In mammals, SOD s usually confined to intracellular areas; only traces of the enzyme are found extracellularly.[3]

White blood cells involved in the acute inflammatory response release large amounts of superoxide, which appears to contribute to the destruction of bacteria. Similarly, the amount of superoxide released at the site of an inflamed joint has been shown to cause extensive and rapid degradation of synovial fluid. SOD generally protects the fluid against this degradation. Furthermore, it protects the leucocytes themselves from free radical damage.[4]

Low levels of SOD at birth appear to be related to the development of infant respiratory distress syndrome.[2] Furthermore, alterations in the superoxide level and the activity of SOD have been implicated in the development of a wide variety of chronic disorders, including diabetes and renal diseases.[5]

Although intravenous infusion of SOD has little anti-inflammatory activity due to its rapid renal clearance, the local injection of SOD has proven to be an effective treatment for a variety of inflammatory disorders. SOD's mechanism of action remains speculative. It protects leukocytes and macrophages against lysis induced by phagocytosis, probably by stabilizing membranes involved in the inflammatory events. In turn this reduces the spillage of cellular inflammants, thereby interrupting the cycle that maintains inflammation.[6]

VETERINARY USES: Parenteral SOD is approved for the treatment of soft tissue inflammation in horses and dogs. The compound has been used successfully in a variety of veterinary disorders including canine allergic dermatitis, canine lick granuloma, and upper respiratory infections in cats.

CLINICAL USES: Similarly, superoxide has been successfully used to treat human inflammatory diseases. In West Germany, where orgotein has been in general medical use for some years, the drug is injected locally for the management of osteoarthritis, sports injuries,[7] and knee joint osteoarthritis.[8]

In a placebo-controlled study in patients with osteoarthritis of the knee, intra-articular orgotein, given as two 16 mg doses, was effective in reducing symptoms for up to 3 months after treatment.[9] One double-blind study showed that intra-articular (IA) orgotein was superior to IA aspirin (a nontraditional route of administration) in the treatment of rheumatoid arthritis of the knee.[10] The anti-inflammatory effectiveness of IM orgotein is good but less effective than that of IM gold in the treatment of active rheumatoid arthritis (52% improvement with orgotein vs 86% with gold after 6 months of treatment); the investigators concluded that SOD is a safe and effective drug for the short-term treatment of rheumatoid arthritis.[11]

In some countries, the drug has also been approved for local use in the treatment of chronic bladder inflammations including radiation-induced and interstitial cystitis.[12,13] SOD therapy has also been suggested for the treatment of hyperuricemic syndromes[14] and the management of acute paraquat poisoning.[15] Studies are underway to evaluate the effects of orgotein therapy in aiding cancer patients to tolerate radiation therapy.

SOD is currently in Phase III clinical trials to improve rejection rates after kidney transplantation and has been thought to be of use in the managment of "reperfusion injury" following an acute myocardial infarction. A recent study, however, found no clinical benefit for the intravenous administration of SOD to patients with acute myocardial infarction who underwent percutaneous transluminal angioplasty; no improvement in left ventricular function was observed in these patients, suggesting that the effects of SOD in this population may be limited.[16]

SOD has been investigated for the treatment of infant

respiratory distress syndrome. While initial studies were criticized because the SOD preparation could not effectively penetrate into pulmonary cells, subsequent experiments with SOD encapsulated in liposomes and SOD complexed with polyethylene glycol have enhanced the effectiveness of this treatment. In addition, transgenic mouse cells that express superoxide may be administered by inhalation in the near future; this "gene therapy" would increase the SOD-producing capacity of pulmonary epithelial cells in patients at risk for developing oxygen-associated lung disorders.[2]

Other studies are currently underway to investigate the effectiveness of SOD in reducing oxygen radical damage following myocardial infarction or surgery where perfusion is reduced, including renal transplants.[2,17]

The superoxide radical has been implicated in the development of hepatic cirrhosis, and a reduction in the concentration of this radical by SOD treatment could be a theoretical way to limit the progression of this disease.[18]

SOD is obtained for clinical use through genetically engineered biotechnology sources.

HEALTH FOOD CLAIMS: Several reports have described an association between free radicals and aging. One researcher suggested that lifespans could be increased by 5-10 years by reducing body weight and increasing the levels of free-radical scavengers such as ascorbic acid, selenium and alpha-tocopherol.[19] Some data indicate that longer-lived animal species have a higher internal degree of protection against free radicals.[20]

Based on such reports, some health food manufacturers have promoted products containing SOD as a nutritional supplement. These oral supplements have been said to remove wrinkles and age lines, slow the aging process, and give a longer, healthier life.

There is no published data to support these claims. SOD is a labile enzyme that is rapidly degraded by gastric acids when ingested. It is essentially unabsorbed after oral administration even when enteric coated, and confers no pharmacologic activity when taken orally. While many foods (red meats, vegetables) are rich in SOD, their SOD is degraded when ingested and is rendered enzymatically inactive. The inactivity of oral SOD supplementation has been confirmed by at least one team that examined the

effect of an oral SOD supplement on tissue SOD levels in mice. The animals received a diet containing 0.004% SOD, equivalent to 10 times the "recommended" intake for humans. No differences were found in the levels (activity) of two forms of SOD in tissue or blood between the control and treated groups.[21] Additionally, the analysis of 12 brands of SOD tablets purchased from health food stores indicated that one product contained zero activity and ten contained less than 20% of the labeled activity claim.[22]

TOXICOLOGY: The safety of SOD has been investigated in numerous animal models using doses up to 40,000 times the average human clinical dose of 0.1 mg/kg/day. Abnormalities were noted rarely following acute or chronic parenteral administration in mice, rats, dogs and monkeys. SOD did not induce embryonic or teratogenic changes in rats or rabbits. Parenteral administration resulted in occasional allergic sensitization in guinea pigs, but did not cause allergic reactions in horses treated for up to 6 months.[23] No immune suppression was noted after doses of up to 50 mg/kg. SOD has not been found to cause drug interactions with a variety of antibacterial agents or steroidal and nonsteroidal anti-inflammatory drugs in animals and man.[6] Pain at the injection site is usually the most common clinical complaint.

The minimal lethal dose in animals was greater than 40,000 times the anticipated human clinical dose.[24]

SUMMARY: SOD is a common enzyme found in essentially all living cells. It scavenges the toxic superoxide radical, preventing cellular damage. When administered parenterally, SOD has a local anti-inflammatory effect that has been used clinically in the management of arthritic disorders. SOD may be effective in the management of a variety of oxygen-related disorders, but significant additional research will be needed to verify its activity. To date, SOD has only shown clinical activity following parenteral and not oral administration.

Although claims have been made that the ingestion of SOD can improve health and extend life, there is no evidence that SOD is absorbed orally or that it can result in any of the claimed benefits. Even following parenteral administration, SOD is a remarkably nontoxic compound.

PATIENT INFORMATION – SOD

Uses: Sod has been used for the treatment of soft tissue inflammation in horses and dogs, human inflammatory diseases, and chronic bladder inflammations.

Side Effects: Sod has been recognized as a remarkably nontoxic compound, whereas the main complaint seems to be pain at the injection site.

1. McCord JM, Fridovich I. Superoxide dismutase. An enzymic function for erythrocuprein (hemocuprein). *J Biol Chem* 1969;244:6049.
2. Koppa SD. Superoxide Dismutase: A Scavenger for Health. *Drug Therapy* 1993;23(4):47.
3. McCord JM. Free Radicals and Inflammation: Protection of Synovial Fluid by Superoxide Dismutase. *Science* 1974;185:529.
4. Salin ML, McCord JM. Free Radicals and Inflammation: Protection of phagocytosing leukocytes by superoxide dismutase. *J Clin Invest* 1975;56:1319.
5. Adachi T, et al. Quantitative and qualitative changes of extracellular-superoxide dismutase in patients with various diseases. *Clin Chim Acta* 1994;229(1–2):123.
6. Michelson AM, et al. Superoxide and Superoxide Dismutases. London: Academic Press, 1977.
7. Huber W, Menander-Huber KB. Orgotein. *Clin Rheum Dis* 1980;6(3):1.
8. Huskisson EC, Scott J. Orgotein in osteoarthritis of the knee joint. *Eur J Rheum* 1981;4:212.
9. McIlwain H, et al. Intra-articular orgotein in osteoarthritis of the knee: a placebo-controlled efficacy, safety, and dosage comparison. *Am J Med* 1989;87:295.
10. Goebel KM, et al. Intrasynovial orgotein therapy in rheumatoid arthritis. *Lancet* 1981;1:1015.
11. Walravens M, Dequeker J. Comparison of gold and orgotein treatment in rheumatoid arthritis. *Curr Ther Res* 1976;20:62.
12. Kadrnka F. [Results of a multicenter orgotein study in radiation induced and interstitial cystitis.] *Eur J Rheum* 1981;4:237.
13. Marberger H, et al. Orgotein: a new drug for the treatment of radiation cystitis. *Curr Ther Res* 1975;18:466.
14. Proctor PH, et al. Superoxide-dismutase therapy in hyperuricaemic syndromes. *Lancet* 1978;2:95.
15. Patterson CE, Rhodes ML. The effect of superoxide dismutase on paraquat mortality in mice and rats. *Toxicol and Appl Pharmacol* 1982;62:65.
16. Flaherty JT, et al. Recombinant human superoxide dismutase (h-SOD) fails to improve recovery of ventricular function in patients undergoing coronary angioplasty for acute myocardial infarction. *Circulation* 1994;89(5):1982.
17. FDC Reports, December 12, 1984.
18. Lewis KO, Paton A. Could superoxide cause cirrhosis? *Lancet* 1982;2(8291):188.
19. Harman D. The aging process. *Proc Soc Nat Acad Sci* 1981;78:7124.
20. Tolmasoff JM, et al. Superoxide dismutase: correlation with life-span and specific metabolic rate in primate species. *Proc Soc Nat Acad Sci* 1980;77:2777.
21. Zidenberg-Cherr S, et al. Dietary superoxide dismutase does not affect tissue levels. *Am J Clin Nutrit* 1983;37:5.
22. DD (Diagnostic Data, Inc.), Annual Stockholder Report. October 1981.
23. Carson S, et al. Safety tests of orgotein, an anti-inflammatory protein. *Toxicol Applied Pharmacol* 1973;26:184.
24. Lund-Olesen K, Menander KB. Orgotein: a new antiinflammatory metalloprotein drug: preliminary evaluation of clinical efficacy and safety in degenerative joint disease. *Curr Ther Res* 1974;16:706.

Sour Cherry

SCIENTIFIC NAME(S): *Prunus cerasus* L. (*Cerasus vulgaris* Mill.) Family: Rosaceae.

COMMON NAME(S): Sour cherry, morello cherry, tart cherry, pie cherry, red cherry

BOTANY: There are ≈ 270 varieties of sour cherries, a handful of which are of commercial importance (eg, Montmorency, Richmond, English morello). The sour cherry tree is smaller than the sweet cherry tree (*Prunus avium*) and is more tolerant of extremes in temperature.[1] The sour cherry originated in Europe, but is widely cultivated in America. The trees may reach ≈ 13 yards in height, with a trunk diameter of 30 to 45 cm. The bark is a grayish-brown, flowers are white to pale pink, and leaves are ovate with serrated edging.[2,3] Sour cherry fruits can grow to 20 mm in length and 18 mm in width. They are cordate drupes by nature, with color ranging from light to dark red. This fruit envelops a light brown seed.[4]

HISTORY: The Greek botanist Theophrastus described the cherry circa 300 BC; although it is believed to have been cultivated even earlier than this time. In 70 AD, Pliny indicated locations of cherry trees to be in Rome, Germany, England, and France. By the mid-1800s, cherries were being cultivated in Oregon. The first commercial cherry orchard was planted in the late 1800s. By the early 1900s, the sour cherry industry was flourishing. As of the late 1900s, 100,000 tons of sour cherries are produced in the US each year.[1,5]

CHEMISTRY: Cherries contain 80% to 85% water. Sour cherries have 58 calories per 100 grams, which contain 1000 IU vitamin A (per 100 g) as compared to 110 IU in sweet cherries.[1] Nutrients and other constituents found per 100 g of dried tart cherries include potassium, vitamin A, vitamin C, calcium, iron, phosphorus, sugars, fiber, and carbohydrates.[5] Citric acid, amygdalin, malic acid, tannin, dextrose, sucrose, quercetin, and anthocyanin are all present in juice preparations of the fruit.[3] The antioxidants kaempferol and quercetin are found in the fruits, as are ≈ 15 other compounds with antioxidant properties.[5]

Older studies have determined the presence of coumarin derivatives,[6] glycoside 2,3-dihydro-wogonin-7-mono-beta-D-glucoside,[7] and flavonoids in tart cherries.[8]

More recent studies have determined other compounds. The pigment cyanidin-3-glycoside has been isolated from the tart cherry.[9] Polyprenol patterns have been found in the leaves of the plant.[10] Chlorogenic acid methyl ester and the new compounds 2-hydroxy-3-(0-hydroxyphenol) propanoic acid, 1-(3′,4′-dihydroxycinnamoyl)-cyclopenta-2,3-diol and 1-(3′,4′-dihydroxycinnamoyl)-cyclopenta-2,3-diol have also been identified by spectral data.[11]

PHARMACOLOGY: Cherries were traditionally used by Cherokee Indians as a remedy for arthritis and gout. Today, we are finding components of the plant responsible for this anti-inflammatory and antioxidant activity.[11] Michigan State University studies indicate tart cherry compounds (eg, cyanidin) to be 10 times more active than aspirin, without the side effects. Antioxidant activity has been studied as well. Tart cherry's anthocyanins have the potential to inhibit tumor growth, slow cardiovascular disease, and possibly retard the aging process.[5]

The juice of tart cherries is used in the formulation of cherry syrup, USP, as a vehicle for unpleasant-tasting drugs.[3,4]

TOXICOLOGY: Little information concerning the toxicology of tart cherry was found in recent literature searches. One document reports in an analysis of fruits and vegetables, the contamination percentages of the mycotoxin, patulin, in sour cherry.[12]

SUMMARY: There are ≈ 270 varieties of sour cherries. They originated in Europe, but are widely cultivated in America. Sour cherries contain more vitamin A than sweet cherries. Other nutrients include potassium, vitamin C, and carbohydrates. Sour cherries contain compounds that have both anti-inflammatory and antioxidant activities; studies are continuing in these areas. Tart cherry juice is used in the popular pharmaceutical vehicle, cherry syrup. Few reports of tart cherry toxicity exist.

PATIENT INFORMATION – Sour Cherry

Uses: A study has been done on the anti-inflammatory and antioxidant properties of sour cherries. Tart cherry's anthocyanins have the potential to inhibit tumor growth, slow cardiovascular disease, and possibly retard the aging process. Tart cherry juice is used to mask the unpleasant taste of some drugs.

Side Effects: Little information exists; one document reports the contamination percentages of the mycotoxin, patulin, in sour cherry.[12]

[1] Ensminger A, et al. Foods and Nutrition Encyclopedia, 2nd ed. Boca Raton, FL: CRC Press, 1994;386-89.

[2] http://www.gypsymoth.ento.vt.edu/[]ravlin/Treeimages/cherry.html

[3] Youngken, H. Textbook of Pharmacognosy, 6th ed. Philadelphia, PA: The Blakiston Co., 1950;414-15.

[4] Osol A, et al. The Dispensatory of the United States of America, 25th ed. Philadelphia, PA: JB Lippincott Co., 1960;272-73.

[5] http://www.cherrymkt.org/mediinfo.html

[6] Shcherbanovskii, L. On the presence of cumarin derivatives in sour cherry and prune leaves. *Ukr Biokhim Zh* 1965;37(6):915-19.

[7] Wagner H, et al. Synthesis of 2,3-dihydro-wogonin-7-mono-beta-D-glucoside, a new gylcoside from *Prunus cerasus* L. *Tetrahedron Lett* 1969;19:1471-73

[8] Nagarajan G, et al. Flavonoids of *prunus cerasus*. *Planta Med* 1977;32(1):50-53.

[9] Hansmann, C. Synthesis and characterisation of methyl 2-O-(beta-D-glucopyranosyl)-6-O-(alpha-L-rhamnopyranosyl)-alpha-D-glucop. *Carbohydr Res* 1990;204:221-26.

[10] Wanke M, et al. The diversity of polyprenol pattern in leaves of fruit trees belonging to Rosaceae and Cornaceae. *Acta Biochim Pol* 1998;45(3):811-18.

[11] Wang H, et al. Novel antioxidant compounds from tart cherries (*prunus cerasus*). *J Nat Prod* 1999;62(1):86-88.

[12] Thurm V, et al. Hygienic significance of patulin in food. 2. Occurrence of patulin in fruit and vegetables. *Nahrung* 1979;23(2):131-34.

Soy

SCIENTIFIC NAME(S): Glycine Max

COMMON NAME(S): Soy, Soybean, Soya

BOTANY: The soybean plant belongs to the "pea" family, Leguminosae. Legumes are able to transform free nitrogen from the air into a form they can use to grow, providing the bacteria *Rhizobium Japonicum* is available. The soybean is an annual plant that grows from 1 to 5 feet tall. The bean pods are covered with short, fine hairs, as are the stems and leaves of the plant. The pods contain up to 4 oval seeds, which can be yellow to brownish in color. The cotyledons account for most of the seed's weight, and contain nearly all the oil and protein.[1]

HISTORY: Soybeans were cultivated in China as far back as the 11th Century BC. Described by Chinese Emperor Shung Nang in 2838 BC, they were said to have been China's most important crop. Cultivation of the plant went to Japan, then Europe, and eventually to the US (in the early 1800s). The US now produces 49% of the world's soybeans. Soybeans possess a number of health benefits, including anticarcinogenic effects, improvement in cardiovascular and intestinal problems, and relief of menopausal symptoms. Soybeans are also an important source of nutrition.[1,2,3]

CHEMISTRY: Soybeans are high in nutritional value and can contain up to 25% oil, up to 24% carbohydrate, and up to 50% protein.[1] Isolation of certain proteins and protein determination methods may be used to characterize soybeans and their products.[5] Fatty acids in beans include linoleic (55%), palmitic (9%), stearic (67%), and others. The soybean is also rich in minerals including calcium, iron, and potassium, amino acids, and vitamins. It is also a good fiber source.[1,2] Soybeans also contain compounds known as isoflavones, structures molecularly similar to natural body estrogens (phytoestrogens). Isoflavonoid analysis has been performed using HPLC-mass spectrometry methods and has proven to be helpful in phytoestrogen and pharmacokinetic research.[6,7] Constituents genistein, the most abundant isoflavone in soybeans, and daidzein are the focus of most isoflavone research.[4] Radioimmunoassay for daidzein has been recently established.[8] Soybeans, as well as other legumes, are excellent food sources for both of these anticancer metabolites.[9] Glycitein and equol are other isoflavones found in the plant. Isoflavones behave not only as "estrogen mimics," but have other non-hormonal roles as well.[4]

PHARMACOLOGY:

Food use: Soy is an important food source and has been used in Asian cultures for thousands of years. These cultures consume 2 to 3 ounces of soy per day, as compared to Western diets that contain about 1/10 of that amount.[3] Soybeans products are numerous and include soybean milk, soybean flour, soybean curd, sufu, tofu (cheese-like cake high in protein and calcium), tempeh (Indonesian main dish), fermented soybean paste (miso), soybeans sprouts, soy sauce, soybean oil, textured soy proteins (in meat extenders), soy protein drinks, and livestock feeds. Because of its low cost, good nutritional value, and versatility, soy protein is also used as part of food programs in less developed countries. It is also used in infant formulas (most often if milk protein allergy exists).[1]

Pharmacologic use: Over 7000 citations are available (circa '97–'98) concerning different pharmacologic aspects of soy. A summary of the main topic follows.

Isoflavones, the phytoestrogens from the soybean, are similar in structure to the main female hormone estradiol; hence, they have similar effects in the two, including hormonal as well as non-hormonal actions. Hydrolysis of these isoflavones that become hydrolyzed by intestinal glucosidases, yields genistein, daidzein, and glycitein. These may also become further metabolized to additional metabolites including equol and p-ethyl phenol. This metabolism is highly individualistic and can vary, for example, with carbohydrate intake altering intestinal fermentation. Isoflavones undergo enterohepatic circulation and are secreted into bile. Plasma half-life of genistein and daidzein is approximately 8 hours, with peak concentration being achieved in 6 to 8 hours in adults. Elimination is via urine, primarily as glucuronide conjugates.[4]

Dietary phytoestrogens may play important roles in cancer prevention, menopausal symptoms, osteoporosis, cardiovascular disease, and gastrointestinal disorders.

Proposed mechanisms of the phytoestrogens include estrogenic and antiestrogenic effects, induction of cancer cell differentiation, inhibition of tyrosine kinase and DNA topoisomerase activity, angiogenesis suppression, and antioxidant effects.[10]

Anticancer: Soybeans are one of the foods highest in anticancer activity.[11] Inhibition of early cancer markers in human epithelial cells has been demonstrated by genistein.[12] Another report found genistein retards growth of implanted tumors both in vivo (mice) and in vitro.[13] The anticancer effects of genistein may be related to its ability to reduce expression of stress response related genes. Induction of stress proteins in tumor cells protects them against cell death, so inhibition of this stress response by the isoflavone is beneficial.[14]

When foods with weak estrogen-like compounds such as soy, are consumed by women, their blood estrogen levels drop, reducing one of the risk factors for breast cancer (high estrogen blood levels).[2] Soy has also been found to lengthen the menstrual cycle, decreasing the number of cycles in a woman's lifetime. This reduces the incidence of each estrogen surge, which occurs early in each cycle. This reduction in estrogen may play another important role in fighting breast cancer as well. Menstrual cycles in Asian women are 2 to 3 days longer than those of western women.[2] Soy protein delayed menstruation by 1 to 5 days in one report. The mitotic rate for breast tissue is 4 times as great in the luteal phase as during the follicular phase. With longer cycles, longer follicular phases are present, which in addition, protects against breast cancer. Breast cancer rates are 0.2% in England, but only 0.05% in Japan.[15] Genistein-treated rats exhibited chemopreventative properties in carcinogenic-induced breast cancer, as a result of its estrogenic effects. It also exhibited anti-proliferative effects against human breast cancer cell growth.[16] Asian women experience lower breast cancer incidence, which may be related to the high content of soy products in their diet. Soy supplementation as adjuvant treatment in early breast cancer patients may decrease risk of cancer recurrence.[17] A diet rich in legumes, especially soybeans, has been associated with a reduction of risk in endometrial cancer in a Hawaiian, case-controlled study in 332 diagnosed endometrial cancer patients.[18]

Male cancer preventative effects have also been documented from soy, genistein has decreased growth of BPH and prostate cancer in vitro, suggesting the isoflavone to be of potential therapeutic benefit.[19] Asian men consuming low-fat, high-fiber, soy-based diets, have been observed to have a lower incidence of prostate cancer than European or North American men. Isoflavonoids present in prostatic fluid, and the metabolic data on these males has been reported.[20]

Isoflavone daidzein is also biologically active and in high doses enhances immune functions in mice, including the increase of phagocytic response of macrophages.[21]

Menopausal symptoms/osteoporosis: Women of menopausal age suffering from symptoms of decreased estrogen production may warrant the need to replace this important hormone. In standard hormone replacement therapy (HRT), a combination of estrogen and progesterone is commonly prescribed. This combination not only helps to alleviate menopausal symptoms, but the progesterone component prevents osteoporosis and reduces uterine cancer risk compared to using estrogens alone. HRT has also been shown to reduce risk of coronary heart disease.[22] However, HRT is less effective than estrogens alone in protection against heart disease and may increase the risk of breast cancer.[4] In addition, HRT regimens have low acceptance rates among postmenopausal women.[22] Soy products, then, may offer a favorable but not necessarily safer alternative to conventional HRT.

Hot flashes and postmenopausal symptoms, including bone mineral loss, can be reduced by 45 g of soyflour.[2] Hot flashes were decreased by 45% in one report in postmenopausal women given soy powder, as compared to 30% reduction with placebo powder.[4] Soy phytochemical consumption may even prevent osteoporosis.[23]

A mechanism that may help explain isoflavones' role in bone loss prevention is as follows. Estrogens attach to estrogen receptor (ER) sites in certain areas of the body, "ER alpha," and the more recently found "ER beta." ER alpha is mostly present in the female reproductive system, where ER beta predominates in other estrogen-responsive tissue such as bladder and bone. This may help explain why estrogen has beneficial actions in bone and elsewhere. Genistein, the primary isoflavone from soy binds to ER alpha (weakly), but complexes ER beta as well as estrogen does. This bound portion then exerts its beneficial actions.[4] Studies that may support this model include genistein's ability to prevent bone loss in ovariectomized rats,[24] and a randomized, double-blind, human clinical trial demonstrating symptomatic efficacy (vs placebo) when avacado and soybean unsaponifiables were administered to 164 osteoarthritis patients.[25]

Cardiovascular disease/lipid alterations: Increased consumption of soy in Asian populations is associated with decreased rates in cardiovascular disease.[23] A vegetarian diet, consisting of soy-based products was given to 32 coronary heart disease patients who discontinued their conventional hyperlipidemic medications. The diet resulted in normalization of serum lipids, with the best results associated with the group who maintained this diet for the longest period of time.[26] In another report, although arterial elasticity was improved 26% by soy isoflavone intake (80 mg/day) in 21 women, plasma lipids in this trial were unaffected.[27] Another study also concludes no differences in serum lipids from isoflavonoid supplementation. However, these effects were evaluated in patients with average serum cholesterol levels.[28] A review concerning effects of soy phytoestrogens on cardiovascular risk factors is available.[22]

GI benefits: Beneficial effects on large bowel function were found in rats given a mixture of soybean and cereals vs a standard diet. In addition, lower glycemic response was observed.[29] Soybean fiber can prevent constipation, reducing the incidence of bowel diseases.[2] The use of fiber-supplemented soy formula in one report reduced the duration of diarrhea in 44 infants.[30] Soy can have an important role in GI health.

TOXICOLOGY: Tolerance to soy preparations in a 164-patient study was good to excellent for most patients.[25]

The effects of phytoestrogens in soy-base infant formulas is of concern and may have some biological impact.[31,32] Daily exposure of infants to the isoflavones in soy-based formula, in one report, was found to be 13,000 to 22,000 times higher than estradiol concentrations in early life.[33] Effects of these soy isoflavones on steroid-dependent developmental processes in human babies should be studied. Carefully controlled, large-scale clinical trials in this infant population should be a priority.[34,35]

Inhalation of soy dust caused an asthma epidemic in 26 patients exposed to an unloading of the product. This incident was confined only to a specific area, Barcelona. Skin prick tests confirmed exposure to soy in all cases.[36] Specific immunoglobulins such as IgE, are associated with this type of "soy bean asthma."[37]

Soybeans treated with the appropriate proteases reduces allergenicity of the soybeans themselves.[38] Another report describes how fatal allergic reactions from soy can be prevented.[39]

Soybean isoflavones may inhibit thyroid synthesis, which can induce goiter and thyroid neoplasia in animals. Effects in humans consuming soy products has yet to be addressed.[40]

SUMMARY: The soybean is a versatile legume and has been used in Asian populations for thousands of years. They are high in nutritional value and are an excellent source of proteins, vitamins, and minerals. Soybeans contain compounds known as isoflavones, molecularly similar to natural body estrogens. The effects of these "phytoestrogens" are both hormonal and non-hormonal. They may have effects against cancer, may alleviate menopausal symptoms, may prevent osteoporosis, and may combat cardiovascular disease and GI problems. Soy is usually safe, except in individuals who are allergic to it. More research is needed in the areas of its actions on infants consuming soy-based formulas and how it alters thyroid synthesis.

PATIENT INFORMATION – Soy

Uses: Soy is commonly used as a source of fiber, protein, and minerals. The isoflavone compounds in soybeans may have anticancer affects, alleviate menopausal symptoms, prevent osteoporosis, and combat cardiovascular and GI problems.

Side Effects: Overall tolerance to soybeans is good to excellent for most patients. Although there are no strong studies, the effects on developmental processes of phytoestrogens in soy-based infant formulas is of concern. Soy dust has caused an asthma epidemic.

---

[1] Ensminger A, et al. Foods and Nutrition Encyclopedia, 2nd ed. Boca Raton, FL: CRC Press, 1994;2017-35.
[2] Polunin M. Healing Foods, 1st ed. New York, NY: DK Publishing, 1997;70.
[3] Craig S, et al. The Complete Book of Alternative Nutrition. Emmaus, PA: Rodale Press, 278-79.
[4] Anonymous. The Soy Connection, United Soybean Board. Chesterfield, MO. Vol. 6, #2, Spring 1998.
[5] Garcia M, et al. Crit Rev Food Sci Nutr 1997;37(4):361-91.
[6] Barnes S, et al. Proc Soc Exp Biol Med 1998;217(3):254-62.
[7] Franke A, et al. Proc Soc Exp Biol Med 1998;217(3):263-73.
[8] Lapcik O, et al. Steroids 1997;62(3):315-20.
[9] Kaufman P, et al. J Altern Complement Med 1997;3(1):7-12.
[10] Kurzer M, et al. Annu Rev Nutr 1997;17:353-81.
[11] Craig W. J Am Diet Assoc 1997;97(10 Suppl 2):S199-S204.

[12] Katdare M, et al. Oncol Rep 1998;5(2):311-15.
[13] Record I, et al. Int J Cancer 1997;72(5):860-64.
[14] Zhou Y, et al. J Natl Cancer Inst 1998;90(5):381-88.
[15] Cassidy A, et al. Am J Clin Nutr 1994;60:333-40.
[16] Barnes S. Breast Cancer Res Treat 1997;46(2-3):169-79.
[17] Stoll B. Ann Oncol 1997;8(3)223-25.
[18] Goodman M, et al. Am J Epidemiol 1997;146(4):294-306.
[19] Geller J, et al. Prostate 1998;34(2):75-79.
[20] Morton M, et al. Cancer Lett 1997;114(1-2):145-51.
[21] Zhang R, et al. Nutr Cancer 1997;29(1):24-28.
[22] Clarkson T, et al. Proc Soc Exp Biol Med 1998;217(3):365-68.
[23] Barnes S. Proc Soc Exp Biol Med 1998;217(3):386-92.
[24] Blair H, et al. J Cell Biochem 1996;61:629-37.
[25] Maheu E, et al. Arthritis Rheum 1998;41(1):81-91.

[26] Medkova I, et al. *Ter Arkh* 1997;69(9):52-55.
[27] Nestel P, et al. *Arterioscler Thromb Vasc Biol* 1997;17(12):3392-98.
[28] Hodgson J, et al. *J Nutr* 1998;128(4):728-32.
[29] Olguin M, et al. *Arch Latinoam Nutr* 1995,45(3):187-92.
[30] Vanderhoof J, et al. *Clin Pediatr* 1997;36(3):135-39.
[31] Bluck L, et al. *Clin Chem* 1997;43(5):851-52.
[32] Huggett A, et al. *Lancet* 1997;350(9080):815-16.
[33] Setchell K, et al. *Lancet* 1997;350(9070):23-27.

[34] Sheehan D. *Proc Soc Exp Biol Med* 1998;217(3):379-85.
[35] Irvine C, et al. *Proc Soc Exp Biol Med* 1998;217(3):247-53.
[36] Pont F, et al. *Arch Bronconeumol* 1997;33(9):453-56.
[37] Codina R, et al. *Chest* 1997;111(1):75-80.
[38] Yamanishi R, et al. *J Nutr Sci Vitaminol* 1996;42(6):581-87.
[39] Kjellman N, et al. *Lakartidningen* 1997;94(30-31):2633-34.
[40] Divi R, et al. *Biochem Pharmacol* 1997;54(10):1087-96.

Spirulina

SCIENTIFIC NAME(S): *Spirulina* spp. Family: Oscillatoriaceae

COMMON NAME(S): Spirulina, dihe, tecuitlatl, blue-green algae

BIOLOGY: The term spirulina encompasses several thousand species of cyanophyta (blue-green algae), a few of which have been used by humans. These organisms, which take the form of microscopic, corkscrew-shaped filaments, can be found around the world. In some locations they impart a dark-green color to bodies of water. They are noted for their characteristic behavior in carbonated water and their energetic growth in laboratory cultures.[1]

HISTORY: Spirulina has been known at least since the 16th century. Spanish explorers found the Aztecs harvesting a "blue mud" that probably consisted of spirulina. The mud, which was dried to form chips or formed into cheese-like loaves, was obtained from Lake Texcoco, in what is now Mexico. Spirulina was similarily harvested by natives of the Sahara Desert, where it was known by the name *dihe*. Spirulina has been sold in the United States as a health food or food supplement since about 1979. It is available as a fine powder or tablets. Some authors have suggested the use of spirulina as a source of protein.[2]

CHEMISTRY: Spirulina consists of approximately 65% crude protein and high levels of B-complex vitamins. The protein content includes all 22 amino acids, but the balance of these is not as desirable as that in many types of animal protein. Spirulina preparations contain iron at levels of 300 to 400 ppm dry weight. Unlike many forms of plant iron, this iron has a high bioavailability when ingested by humans. A dosage of 10 g/day can contain 1.5 to 2 mg absorbable iron. Trace elements present at high levels include manganese, selenium, and zinc. Also concentrated in the organisms are calcium, potassium, and magnesium.[3] Spirulina is the first prokaryote found to contain a ferredoxin.[4] Ferredoxin obtained from *S. maxima* is a stable, easily extractable plant type. A superoxide dismutase has been isolated from *S. platensis*.[5]

PHARMACOLOGY: Promoters of spirulina have claimed that the product can be used as a diet pill. The theory is that high levels of phenylalanine act to inhibit the appetite. However, an FDA review found no evidence to support this claim.[6,7]

Spirulina's role as a nutritional supplement has been well documented in animal studies. A study in rats found that *S. maxima* is a good protein source, as indicated by weight gain, but the rats showed no sign of reduction of total caloric intake.[8] The nutritional value of spirulina depends on the method of processing: Protein in concentrates prepared from disintegrated cellular material has greater bioavailability than preparations of whole cells.[9,10] An examination of three commercial preparations of spirulina indicated that more than 80% of what is thought to be vitamin B12 may actually be analogs that have little or no nutritional value for humans.[11] *S. fusiformis* is a valuable source of vitamin A in rats.[12] Spirulina as a beta-carotene source is questionable compared with standard sources, but the spirulina-fed rats exhibited better growth patterns than standard.[13] *S. maxima*'s effects to alter vitamins A and E storage and utilization have been reported in rats.[14] Availability of iron from spirulina fed to rats is comparable to rats being fed standard ferrous sulfate.[15] Spirulina alone or in combination is a good dietary supplement during pregnancy in animals as well.[16]

Extract of spirulina and dunaliella algae injected into induced oral carcinoma in animals resulted in 70% partial tumor regression.[17] A similar study reported the absence of gross tumors in experimental oral cancer in hamsters.[18] Tumor regression is accompanied by significant induction of tumor necrosis factor, suggesting a possible mechanism of tumor destruction.[19] A later evaluation confirms spirulina's chemopreventative effects in human oral leukoplakia in tobacco chewers in India (45% lesion regression vs 7% placebo).[20]

S. platensis and its constituent polysaccharide "calcium spirulan" were found to inhibit replication of several enveloped viruses. These include herpes simplex I, cytomegalovirus, mumps and measles viruses, influenza A virus, and HIV-1. Inhibition of virus entry into host cells appears to be the mechanism.[21]

Spirulina has been reported to enhance antibody production,[22] improve dietary hyperlipidemia,[23] reduce gastric secretory activity,[24] exert a preventative effect on liver triglycerides,[25,26] and provide radioprotection (against gamma radiation) in mouse bone marrow cells.[27]

COSTS: Spirulina has been touted as a food source. Cost is therefore a significant consideration in choosing it as a food. Studies have shown the protein content of spirulina to be no better than protein from sources such as meat or milk. The cost of spirulina protein is about 17 cents per gram, compared with only a half-cent per gram of beef. Dietary iron of spirulina is highly bioavailable but could be costly as well.[28]

TOXICOLOGY: Nutritional tests have established spirulina as nontoxic to humans.[2] However, spirulina can contain amounts of mercury as high as 10 ppm. Consumption of 20 g of spirulina per day could produce a mercury consumption above the maximum 180 mcg considered prudent for safety.[3] Reported mean heavy metal levels include arsenic 0.42 ppm, cadmium 0.1 ppm, lead 0.4 ppm, and mercury 0.24 ppm. Microbial contamination may occur if spirulina is grown on the effluent of fermented animal wastes.[29] Spirulina can concentrate radioactive di- and trivalent metallic ions.[30] Some spirulina manufacturers report that microbiological data for standard plate counts, fungi, yeasts and coliforms conform to US standards for spray-dried powdered milk.

At least two reports evaluate spirulina toxicity in animals.[31,32]

SUMMARY: Spirulina is a blue-green algae that is used as a food and food supplement. It contains high levels of protein and B-complex vitamins; the nutritional value, particularly of the latter, has been questioned. Spirulina represents an expensive source of dietary protein and iron. Reports find spirulina effective in tumor regression, chemo- and radioprotection, virus inhibition, and enhancing antibody production. Spirulina seems to be nontoxic in humans but may harbor some contaminants such as heavy metals or microbes.

PATIENT INFORMATION – Spirulina

Uses: Spirulina is sold in the US as a health food or health food supplement and has also been reported to enhance antibody production, improve dietary hyperlipidemia, reduce gastric secretory activity, exert a preventative effect on liver triglycerides, and cause tumor regression.

Side Effects: Spirulina is nontoxic in humans.

---

[1] Guerin-Dumartrait E, et al. *Ann Nutr Aliment* 1975;29:489.
[2] Clement G. In Tannenbaum SR & Wang DI, eds. Single-Cell Proteins II. Cambridge, MA: MIT Press, 1975.
[3] Johnson PE, Shubert LE. *Nutr Res* 1986;6:85.
[4] Tanaka M, et al. *Biochemistry* 1975;14:5535.
[5] Lumsden J, Hall DO. *Biochem Biophys Res Comm* 1974;58:35.
[6] FDA Consumer Sept. 1981, p. 3.
[7] ACSH News & Views, April 1982, p. 3
[8] Maranesi M, et al. *Acta Vitaminol Enzymol* 1984;6:295.
[9] Omstedt P, et al. In Tannenbaum SR & Wang DI, eds. Single-Cell Proteins II. Cambridge, MA: MIT Press, 1975.
[10] Ciferri O. *Microbiol Rev* 1983;47:551.
[11] Herbert V, Drivas G. *JAMA* 1982;248:3096.
[12] Annapurna V, et al. *Plant Foods Hum Nutr* 1991;41(2):125–34.
[13] Kapoor R, et al. *Plant Foods Hum Nutr* 1993;43(1):1–7.
[14] Mitchell G, et al. *J Nutr* 1990;120(10):1235–40.
[15] Kapoor R, et al. *Plant Foods Hum Nutr* 1993;44(1):29–34.
[16] Kapoor R, et al. *Plant Foods Hum Nutr* 1993;43(1):29–35.
[17] Schwartz J, et al. *J Oral Maxillofac Surg* 1987;45(6):510–15.
[18] Schwartz J, et al. *Nutr Cancer* 1988;11(2):127–34.
[19] Shklar G, et al. *Eur J Cancer Clin Oncol* 1988;24(5):839–50.
[20] Mathew B, et al. *Nutr Cancer* 1995;24(2):197–202.
[21] Hayashi T, et al. *J Nat Prod* 1996;59(1):83–87.
[22] Hayashi O, et al. *J Nutr Sci Vitaminol* 1994;40(5):431–41.
[23] Iwata K, et al. *J Nutr Sci Vitaminol* 1990;36(2):165–71.
[24] Cristea E, et al. *Farmacia* 1992 Jan-Dec;40:73–82.
[25] Michele D, et al. *Farmacia* 1992 Jan-Dec;40:119–26.
[26] Gonzalez de Rivera C, et al. *Life Sci* 1993;53(1):57–61.
[27] Qishen P, et al. *Toxicol Letter* 1989;48(2):165–69.
[28] Tyler VE. The New Honest Herbal. Philadelphia: G. F. Stickley, 1987.
[29] Wu JF, Pond WG. *Bull Environ Contam Toxicol* 1981;27:151.
[30] Tseng CL, et al. *Radioisotopes (Japan)* 1986;35:540.
[31] Chamorro G, et al. *J Pharm Belg* 1988;43(1):29–36.
[32] Chamorro G, et al. *J Toxicol Clin Exp* 1988;8(3):163–67.

Squill

SCIENTIFIC NAME(S): European or white squill (*Urginea maritima* L. Baker); Indian squill (*U. indica* Kunth.). Commercial samples of Indian squill are often mixtures of *U. indica* and *Scilla indica* Roxb. Red squill (*U. maritima* var. *pancratium* Stein Baker). Referred to in some texts as *U. scilla* Steinh. Family: Liliaceae

COMMON NAME(S): European squill, Mediterranean squill, white squill, Indian squill, red squill, sea onion, sea squill

BOTANY: Squill is a perennial herb that is native to the Mediterranean. It often grows in sandy soil. The bulbous portion of the base is harvested and the dried inner scales of the bulb are used. White squill has sometimes been adulterated by the inclusion of Indian squill.

HISTORY: Some varieties of squill have been known for more than a thousand years to be effective rodenticides. In man, extracts of the bulb have been used as a cardiotonic for the treatment of edema, as an expectorant, and as an emetic. Today it continues to find use as an expectorant in some commercial cold preparations.[1] Due to the popularity of the digitalis glycosides, squill components are rarely used as cardioactive agents.

CHEMISTRY: Squill contains several related steroidal cardioactive glycosides. Those found in the greatest concentration in the bulb include scillaren A and proscillaridin A (the aglycone of both is scillarenin). In addition, glucoscillaren A, scillaridin A, and scilliroside have been characterized. In one study, the most common components identified in dried bulbs were scilliroside (appr. 45 ppm) and scillaren A (appr. 38 ppm);[2] others have found proscillaridin A in the greatest concentration.[3] Scillaren B has been used to describe a mixture of squill glycosides as opposed to pure scillaren A.[4] Squill bulbs contain more than a dozen unique flavonoids. Components of squill tissue cultures appear to vary significantly in quantitative composition from whole bulb extracts.[5] Further, the extracts from fresh bulbs can vary significantly by season.

PHARMACOLOGY: Squill extracts cause peripheral vasodilation and bradycardia in anesthetized rabbits.[5]

Squill glycosides have cardiotonic properties similar to digitalis. However, squill components are generally poorly absorbed from the gastrointestinal tract and are less potent than digitalis. Some preparations do exist for oral administration and these are enteric coated to prevent degradation by gastric acidity. A semisynthetic derivative, meproscillaren derived from proscillaridin, is absorbed orally and may be effective in some patients.

The strength of squill preparations and extracts may vary and therefore must be used with caution. An analysis of the comparative potencies of extracts of *U. maritima* and *U. indica* based on a British Pharmacopoeial assay for digitalis found no significant differences between the species when activity was expressed as ml tincture/kg of guinea pig weight.[6]

Squill induces vomiting by both a central action and local gastric irritation. Vomiting may be preceded by a generalized increase in the flow of secretions, and therefore these compounds appear to exert an expectorant effect in sub-emetic or near-emetic doses.

Methanolic extracts of red squill have been said to be effective as hair tonics in treating seborrhea and dandruff, the activity being ascribed to scilliroside.[4] In general, red squill is not employed medicinally. The powdered dried bulbs of red squill find their main use as rodenticides. Death is due to the centrally-induced convulsant action of scilliroside rather than direct cardiotoxicity. Rats lack the vomit reflex and are insensitive to the emetic action of these glycosides. Because squill-laced bait is vomited by domestic animals before a lethal dose can be absorbed, it is often considered to be a rat-specific agent.

Squill has been used traditionally as a cancer remedy, and silliglaucosidin has shown activity in an experimental cancer cell line.[7]

TOXICOLOGY: Although white squill and its extracts have the potential to induce life-threatening cardiac effects in relatively low doses, they have not generally been associated with human toxicity. Vomiting is often induced as a reflex in cases of overdosage, minimizing the absorbed dose. The toxic dose of squill soft mass (a galenical extract form used to make certain squill preparations) in guinea pigs is 270 mg/kg; tinctures made from Indian squill caused death at a dose of 36 mg/kg.[8] Red squill may induce central nervous system effects resulting in convulsions. Fresh bulbs contain a vesicant.[7]

SUMMARY: Squill and its extracts have been used for centuries in medicine and as a rat poison. White squill continues to find use in some traditional medicine preparations for its digitalis-like cardiotonic effects, although this use is almost extinct. Squill extracts do continue to find some use in low doses as expectorants. Red squill is used as a rodenticide, causing death via a centrally-induced convulsant action.

PATIENT INFORMATION – Squill

Uses: Squill has been used in hair tonics treating seborrhea and dandruff, as a cancer remedy, and as a rodenticide.

Side Effects: Side effects related to squill include vomiting and convulsions.

---

[1] Morton JF. Major Medicinal Plants. Springfield, IL: C.C. Thomas, 1977.
[2] Balbaa SI, et al. TLC-spectrophotometric assay of the main glycosides of red squill, a specific rodenticide. *J Nat Prod* 1979;42:522.
[3] Garcia Casado P, et al. Proscillaridin a yield from squill bulbs. *Pharm Acta Helv* 1977;52:218
[4] Leung AY. Encyclopedia of Common Natural Ingredients Used In Food, Drugs, and Cosmetics. New York, NY: J. Wiley and Sons, 1980.
[5] Shyr SE, Staba EJ. Examination of squill tissue cultures for bufadienolides and anthocyanins. *Planta Medica* 1976;29:86.
[6] Hakim FS, et al. Comparative potencies of European and Indian squill. *J Pharm Pharmacol* 1976;28:81.
[7] Duke JA. Handbook of Medicinal Herbs. Boca Raton, FL: CRC Press, 1985.
[8] Hakin FS, Evans FJ. The potency and phytochemistry of Indian squill soft extract. *Pharm Acta Helv* 1976;51:117.

St. John's Wort

SCIENTIFIC NAME(S): *Hypericum perforatum* L. Family: Hypericaceae

COMMON NAME(S): St. John's wort, klamath weed, John's wort, amber touch-and-heal, goatweed, rosin rose, and millepertuis

BOTANY: St. John's wort is a perennial native to Europe but is now found throughout the US and parts of Canada. The plant is an aggressive weed found in the dry ground of roadsides, meadows, woods, and hedges. It generally grows to a height of 1 to 2 feet, except on the Pacific coast where it has been known to reach heights of 5 feet.[1] The plant has oval-shaped leaves and yields golden-yellow flowers, which bloom from June to September. The petals contain black or yellow glandular dots and lines. Some sources say that the blooms are at their brightest coincidental with the birthday of John the Baptist (June 24).[2] There are ≈ 370 species in the genus *Hypericum*, which is derived from the Greek words, *hyper* and *eikon* meaning "over an apparition," alluding to the plant's ancient use to "ward off" evil spirits. *Perforatum* refers to the leaf's appearance; when held up to light, the translucent leaf glands resemble perforations.[4,5] Harvest of the plant for medicinal purposes must occur in July and August; the plant must be dried immediately to avoid loss of potency.[3] The dried herb consists of the plant's flowering tops.[4]

HISTORY: This plant has been used as an herbal remedy for its anti-inflammatory and healing properties since the Middle Ages.[2,3] Many noteworthy ancient herbalists, including Hippocrates and Pliny, recorded the medicinal properties of St. John's wort. It was noted for its wound-healing and diuretic properties as well as for the treatment of neuralgic conditions such as back pain. In 1633, Gerard recorded the plant's use as a balm for burns. The oil of the plant was also popular during this time.[4] An olive oil extract of the fresh flowers that acquires a reddish color after standing in the sunlight for several weeks has been taken internally for the treatment of anxiety but has also been applied externally to relieve inflammation and promote healing. Its topical application is believed to be particularly useful in the management of hemorrhoids. Although it is often listed as a folk treatment for cancer, there is no scientific evidence to document an antineoplastic effect.[2,3]

Although it fell into disuse, a renewed interest in St. John's wort occurred during the past decade, and it is now a component of numerous herbal preparations for the treatment of anxiety and depression. The plant has been used in traditional medicine as an antidepressant and diuretic and for the treatment of gastritis and insomnia. Since 1995, St. John's wort has become the most prescribed antidepressant in Germany. Sales have increased from $10 million to over $200 million in the past 8 years in the US. Since 1997, St. John's wort has been one of the leading herbal products; estimated sales of St. John's wort worldwide total $570 million.[6]

CHEMISTRY: Several reports regarding the chemical components in St. John's wort are available.[7,8,9] The most commonly described constituents are naphthodianthrones, flavonoids, phloroglucinols, and essential oils.

Naphthodianthrones occur in St. John's wort in concentrations of < 0.1 to 0.15%. The anthraquinone derivatives hypericin and pseudohypericin (also emodin-anthranol and cyclo-pseudohypericin) are the best known components of the plant. Isohypericin and protohypericin are also present. The reddish dianthrone pigment hypericin (hypericum red) is found in a concentration ranging from 0.02% to 2.5%,[2] depending on harvesting period, drying process, and storage.[3,10] Hypericin content also varies widely among growing regions.[11] Hypericin concentration varies among plant parts: Flowers, buds, top leaves, and secondary stems yielding the highest amount.[4] Microscopic evaluation finds hypericin to accumulate in secretory cell globules within these plant structures.[12] Several reports concerning determination and analysis (ie, HPLC) of hypericin in St. John's wort exist.[13-20] Liposoluble pigments from the plant, including hypericin, carotenoids, and chlorophylls, have also been reported.[21]

Flavonoid concentrations in St. John's wort occur at < 12% in flowers and ≈ 7% in leaves/stalks.[4] Flavonoids include kaempferol, quercetin, quercitrin, isoquercitrin, amentoflavone, luteolin, myricetin, hyperin, hyperoside, and rutin.[3,4,10] The proanthocyanidins (≈ 12% of aerial parts) are certain forms of catechin and epicatechin.[4] Other flavonoids found are miquelianin and astilbin.[22]

Hyperforin and adhyperforin are in the phloroglucinol class of compounds.[4,5,23] Hyperforin appears in St.

John's wort in concentrations of 2% to 4%. Isolation, purity, and stability of this compound have been reported.[24] Recovery of hyperforin in plasma has been measured.[25] Related structure furohyperforin, an oxygenated analog of hyperforin has been isolated from the plant,[26] as have other hyperforin analogs.[27]

The essential oil component of St. John's wort is reported to be between 0.05% and 0.9%.[4,5] It consists of mono- and sesquiterpines, mainly 2-methyl-octane (16 to > 30%), n-nonane, alpha- and beta-pinene, alpha-terpineol, geraniol, and traces of myrecene, limonene, caryophyllene, and others.[3,4,10]

Other compounds present in St. John's wort include xanthones (1.28 mg/100 g) and tannins (3% to 16%). One study reports that tannin content (in extracts) is influenced by parameters such as temperature of maceration.[28] Phenol constituents include caffeic, chlorogenic, and p-coumaric acids, and hyperfolin. Other plant constituents include acids (eg, nicotinic, myristic, palmitic, stearic), carotenoids, choline, pectin, hydrocarbons, and long-chain alcohols. Amino acids include cysteine, GABA, glutamine, leucine, lysine, and others.[3,4,5,10]

Because St. John's wort products are classified as dietary supplements, they are not regulated by the FDA.[29] Several reports evaluating commercial preparations of St. John's wort have found inconsistencies in active ingredients such as variations from 47% to 165% of labeled hypericin concentrations,[30] different concentrations of major components between brands,[31] and marked deviations in hyperforin (and adhyperforin) amounts in certain St. John's wort preparations.[32] Several reports are available addressing these issues, with various proposed standardization methods.[33,34,35,36] One such method has been developed by Paracelsian Inc., a private biotechnology company (www.paracelsian.com/biofit.html). Their *Biofit* (bio functional integrity tested) quality assurance method has tested several St. John's wort products for structure and function claims of mood support on *otc* labeling. This testing process evaluated the product's ability to inhibit reuptake of serotonin and dopamine.

PHARMACOLOGY:

Depression: Early research focused on the hypericin constituents in St. John's wort. Originally, hypericin was thought to exert its tranquilizing effect by increasing capillary blood flow. Later studies in rats found hypericin to be a strong inhibitor of the enzyme monoamine oxidase

(MAO).[37] However, in the mid-1990s, two studies examined *H. perforatum* fractions in vitro and ex vivo and reported no evidence of any relevant MAO inhibition, concluding that St. John's wort's antidepressant effects cannot be explained by this mechanism alone.[38,39]

Many reports have postulated certain mechanisms and behavioral characteristics of *H. perforatum*, concentrating mostly on hypericin as the active ingredient. The following are major findings: Inhibition of serotonin uptake by postsynaptic receptors has been confirmed in a number of reports; in rat synaptosomes, *H. perforatum* caused a 50% inhibition of serotonin uptake;[40] neuroblastoma cells treated with the extract demonstrated reduced expression of serotonin receptors;[41] *H. perforatum* extract inhibited both serotonin and norepinephrine uptake in astrocytes, the cells surrounding synaptic terminals that regulate neurotransmission by their uptake systems;[42] and *H. perforatum* has also increased brain dopamine function in humans.[43] St. John's wort extract has been found to modulate interleukin-6 (IL-6) activity, linking the immune system with mood. IL-6 is involved in cell communication within the immune system and in modulating the hypothalamic-pituitary-adrenal (HPA) axis. St. John's wort has the ability to reduce IL-6 levels, which reduce HPA axis elevations and certain hormones, which if elevated, are associated with depression.[39] Sigma receptor binding of hypericin has been demonstrated.[44] *H. perforatum* does not act as a classical serotonin inhibitor but resembles reserpine's properties. Its antidepressant effects are unlikely to be associated with serotonin, benzodiazepine, or GABA receptors.[45] In addition, *H. perforatum* differs from other selective serotonin reuptake inhibitors (SSRIs) by failing to enhance natural killer cell activity (NKCA).[46] Other effects on neurotransmitters from hypericin include inhibition of dopamine-beta-hydroxylase[47] and inhibition of metekephaline and tyrosine dimerization.

Hyperforin is the major lipophilic constituent in the plant and is also a potent inhibitor of serotonin, noradrenaline, and dopamine uptake, increasing their concentrations in the synaptic cleft. Some identify it as the major active principle for its efficacy as an antidepressant.[48,49,50,51] Antidepressant activity was found in rodent models given extracts containing hyperforin (< 39%) but devoid of hypericines. Hyperforin's spectrum of central activity, however, is affected by other constituents, as proven by alteration of serotonergic effects using different extracts of the plant.[52,53] Hyperforin is confirmed to be a major neuroactive component of *H. perforatum* extracts; modulating neuronal ionic conductances is only one of many mechanisms of action it possesses.[54] Hyperforin inhibits serotonin uptake by elevating free intracellular sodium, not seen with conventional SSRIs.[55] In a clinical trial involving 147 patients with mild-to-moderate depression, subjects given *H. perforatum* extract containing greater concentrations of hyperforin exhibited the largest Hamilton Rating Scale for Depression (HAMD) reduction compared with those given lower concentrations or placebo, confirming that the therapeutic effects of St. John's wort depend on its hyperforin content.[56]

St. John's wort continues to be a topic of interest because of its antidepressant effects.[57,58] Reports from 1994 to 1996, including a study using the HAMD, evaluate St. John's wort as clinically effective in the treatment of depression,[59,60,61] rating close to 70% in treatment response.[62] A meta-analysis evaluating 23 randomized trials, including 1757 mildly or moderately depressed patients, was conducted to investigate St. John's wort (vs placebo and other conventional antidepressants). Results found St. John's wort to be superior to placebo. Side effects occurred in ≈ 20% of patients on *H. perforatum* and 53% of patients on standard antidepressants.[63] Other reviews described similar outcomes; lower doses of standard antidepressants were used.[3,59,64]

Review articles and meta-analyses concerning *H. perforatum*'s antidepressive effects have become available from 1998 to 2000,[65-73] of which the most notable are the following: Question and answer format in common language containing tables summarizing clinical trials;[74] a review of clinical studies, most commonly using 300 mg 3 times daily of 0.3% hypericin (600 mg in severe depression); a review of *H. perforatum*'s equivalence in efficacy to numerous antidepressants with fewer incidences of side effects;[75] meta-analyses on *H. perforatum* finding a response rate of 60% to 70% (estimate of pooled data) in patients with mild-to-moderate depression,[76] and its use resulting in 1.5 times the likelihood to observe antidepressant response than placebo, along with equivalence in efficacy to tricyclic antidepressants (TCAs);[77] a clinical trial review confirming greater efficacy vs placebo and equal efficacy to TCAs, MAO inhibitors, and SSRIs, with superior side-effect profile;[71] a review of 20 clinical trials including 1787 patients, describing similar outcomes;[78] and a broad-based literature search from 1980 to 1998, yielding ≈ 1300 records confirming St. John's wort's increased efficacy over placebo in treating mild-to-moderate depressive disorders.[79] Some opposing views mention a lack of information regarding long-term effects, use in other depressive states, the use of different preparations,[80] and the exact mechanism of action being unknown with more definitive data being needed.[81] Mechanisms of action similar to SSRIs or MAO inhibitors are

seen in *H. perforatum*, but its clinical efficacy is probably attributable to the combined contribution of several mechanisms.[82]

Other literature concerning the antidepressant effects of St. John's wort includes the following: Ongoing confirmation of *H. perforatum*'s benefits for depression; dose-dependent response rates were seen using 3 different standardized extracts;[83] different population-type trials, including adolescents with psychiatric problems,[84] elderly patients experiencing dementia such as Alzheimer's disease,[85] and mild-to-moderate depression;[86] *H. perforatum* compared with conventional antidepressant medications was found to have effects similar to the antidepressant properties of TCAs, imipramine, and fluoxetine;[87] 800 mg of a certain St. John's wort extract compared with 20 mg fluoxetine proved to be equally effective in ≈ 150 depressed elderly patients (both groups experiencing adverse reactions, however);[88] certain dosages of St. John's wort significantly increased latency to REM sleep without affecting other sleep patterns, consistent with other antidepressants' mechanisms of action;[89] and seasonal affective disorder (SAD), a type of depression in which symptoms occur in fall/winter and resolve in spring/summer, benefited from St. John's wort, in combination with light therapy.[90]

There are a few overall limitations to the studies that make drawing conclusions about St. John's wort's efficacy in treating depression difficult. In most of the studies, the antidepressant doses used were low, the diagnosis of depression was not uniformly documented, and the trials were of short duration (average: 4 to 6 weeks). In addition, the studies standardized St. John's wort to hypericin that varied widely among studies, and there is evidence that hyperforin might be the active ingredient, which was not quantified in the studies.[56]

Pharmacokinetic studies of hypericin and pseudohypericin performed in humans found that, while similar in structure, they possess substantial pharmacokinetic differences.[91] Single-dose and steady-state pharmacokinetics have also been evaluated.[92] A daily dose of *H. perforatum*, as determined by trials and studies, is 200 to 900 mg of alcohol extract,[3] or 300 mg 3 times daily of a 0.3% hypericin-containing, standardized extract.[74]

HIV: Hypericin is still in the early stages of clinical trials investigating its effects against certain viruses, including HIV. One study found 16 of 18 patients had improved CD4 cell counts over a 40-month period. CD4/CD8 ratios also improved in the majority of patients. Hypericin and pseudohypericin inhibit a variety of encapsulated viruses, including HIV.[4]

The FDA sanctioned hypericin as an investigational new drug, making it eligible to be tested on humans. It is in Phase 1/Phase 2 clinical trial testing and is being developed under the name *VIMRxyn*. In late 1996, its developers (VIMRx Pharmaceuticals, Inc.) announced "a well tolerated oral dose with no untoward toxicity or cutaneous photosensitivity." Viral load measured in a 12-patient population ranged from no change to 97% reduction.[93,94] Another report in 1999 of a Phase 1 study evaluating hypericin's effects concluded hypericin had no antiretroviral activity (in a 30-patient trial), with phototoxicity being observed.[95]

Antiviral: Hypericin and pseudohypericin exert effects against a wide spectrum of other viruses, including influenza virus, herpes simplex virus types 1 and 2, Sindbis virus, poliovirus, retrovirus infection in vitro and in vivo, murine cytomegalovirus, and hepatitis C.[3,4,10,96] Hypericin and pseudohypericin have been found to exert unique and uncommonly effective antiviral actions, possibly due to nonspecific association with cellular and viral membranes. It has been reported more than once that the antiviral activity involves a photoactivation process.[4] Recent reports find that exposure of hypericin to fluorescent light markedly increases its antiviral activity.[3] *H. perforatum* has been considered as a photodynamic agent and may be helpful in future therapeutics and diagnostics.[97]

Antibacterial: Extracts of the plant have been active against gram-negative and gram-positive bacteria in vitro.[98] Reports have documented antimicrobial effects against such organisms as *S. equinus, K. pneumoniae, E. coli, B. lichteniforms,* and *S. flexneri.*[99] Antibacterial activity of constituent hyperforin against *S. aureus* and other gram-positive bacteria has also been reported.[100] In another study, *H. perforatum* extract showed bacteriostatic activity at a dilution of 1:200,000 and bactericidal action at 1:20,000.[3] St. John's wort has also been used in a 20% tincture form to treat otitis. The tannin component of the plant probably exerts an astringent action that contributes to the plant's traditional use as a wound-healing agent.[5]

Other uses: Other uses of the plant include the following: Wound-healing effects, including burn treatment;[3,4,101] oral and topical administration of hypericin for treatment of vitiligo (failure of skin to form melanin)[102] and other skin diseases;[103] anti-inflammatory and anti-ulcerogenic properties from the component amentoflavone (a biapigenin derivative);[5,104] treatment for hemorrhoids,[3] alcoholism,[87] bedwetting,[5] glioblastoma brain cancer,[105] and menopausal symptoms of psychological origin.[106] St. John's wort is capable of increasing and suppressing

immunity.[107] Hypericin has been shown to inhibit T-type calcium channel activity.[108] *H. perforatum* enhances coronary flow and also may be useful in treating certain headaches.[4] Fibromyalgia, causing chronic musculoskeletal pain and fatigue, may also benefit from St. John's wort extracts by keeping serotonin levels high and decreasing pain sensations. Other neuralgias may also benefit from the plant.[5,74]

INTERACTIONS: Several recent articles concerning drug interactions with *H. perforatum* include the following: A meta-analysis of St. John's wort and other herbs possessing potentially unsafe effects;[109] reviews regarding similar issues;[110,111,112,135] and a letter.[113] More specific reports include drug interactions with St. John's wort and theophylline,[114] digoxin[115] (decreasing bioavailability in both), and indinavir. St. John's wort reduced the AUC of this HIV-1 protease inhibitor 57% in 16 patients, indicating possible treatment failure or drug resistance issues.[116] An interaction between St. John's wort and cyclosporine caused acute rejection in 2 heart transplant patients.[117] At least 7 cases of a decrease in the anticoagulant effects of warfarin have been reported.[136] Central serotonergic syndrome was reported among elderly patients combining St. John's wort with other prescription antidepressants.[118] The use of St. John's wort along with SSRIs, venlafaxine HCl, and various TCAs (with close monitoring of symptoms) has been successfully undertaken. Avoidance of tyramine-containing foods during coadministration of St. John's wort and MAO inhibitors has been recommended; recent information proving lack of MAO inhibition does not justify this.[74]

Since St. John's wort may induce the isozymes cytochrome P450 1A2, 2C9, and 3A4 in addition to inducing p-glycoprotein transporter, numerous other drug interactions with St. John's wort are possible.[135] Research is needed to determine the magnitude and clinical importance of these potential drug interactions.

Women taking oral contraceptives and St. John's wort have experienced breakthrough bleeding.[137]

TOXICOLOGY: When ingested, hypericin can induce photosensitization characterized by inflammation of the skin and mucous membranes following exposure to light, which was recognized in animals grazing on the plant.[119,120] Mice given 0.2 to 0.5 mg of herb also developed severe photodynamic effects.[10] Phototoxic activity by *H. perforatum* has been observed when tested on human keratinocytes.[121] A review of the chemistry of phenanthroperylene quinones from hypericin reveals photosensory pigments.[122] After oral administration, concentrations of hypericin in human serum and blister fluid have been detected.[123] Most reports of photosensitivity, however, have been limited to those taking excessive quantities of *H. perforatum*, primarily to treat HIV.[74] For example, both IV (eg, 0.5 mg/kg twice weekly) and oral dosing (eg, 0.5 mg/kg/day) of *H. perforatum* caused significant phototoxicity in 30 HIV patients tested, with 16 of 30 discontinuing treatment for this reason.[95]

A number of studies report no serious adverse effects. In a 22-patient study evaluating St. John's wort, 50% reported no side effects. Those reported include jitteriness, insomnia, change in bowel habits, or headache.[124] In a study of 3250 patients taking St. John's wort for 1 month, fewer than 3% suffered from dry mouth, GI distress, or dizziness.[125] In another review of clinical trials, St. John's wort was associated with fewer and milder adverse reactions as compared with any other conventional antidepressant. Adverse effects from *H. perforatum* were "rare and mild." No information on overdose was found.[126] A case report describes acute neuropathy after sun exposure in a patient using St. John's wort.[127] A review on photodermatitis in general is available, discussing mechanisms, clinical features, and treatment options.[128] Various other reports regarding other adverse effect studies concerning St. John's wort are available. A 7-patient evaluation reports St. John's wort to be unlikely to inhibit cytochrome P-450 enzymes 2D6 and 3A4 activity.[129] Reports of mania induction have been associated with St. John's wort.[130,131] Uterotonic actions also have been reported.[132] A letter discussing St. John's wort's use during pregnancy has been published.[133] Due to lack of toxicity data in this area, St. John's wort is best avoided during pregnancy.[10] Potent inhibition of sperm motility was observed from in vitro experimentation of St. John's wort.[134] The volatile oil of St. John's wort is an irritant.[10]

SUMMARY: St. John's wort has been used traditionally as an herbal treatment in the management of anxiety and depression. Several constituents acting by different mechanisms may contribute to its potent antidepressant activity. Clinical trials concerning use of St. John's wort to treat AIDS and certain cancers are ongoing. *H. perforatum* possesses antiviral and antibacterial actions, making it potentially useful in treating skin diseases and in wound healing. Side effects from St. John's wort are rare in standard dosing. With higher dosing, photosensitivity is observed. Drug-drug interactions have been documented with theophylline, digoxin, indinavir, cyclosporine, and SSRIs. Hyperforin appears to be a major active antidepressive agent.

PATIENT INFORMATION – St. John's Wort

Uses: St. John's wort has been primarily studied for its potential antidepressant and antiviral effects. There is information to show that St. John's wort is more effective than placebo, but evidence is still lacking regarding its efficacy compared to the standard antidepressants, partially due to ineffective dosing. In addition, at least 3 studies have shown that commercially available St. John's wort products vary considerably in content and may be standardized to the wrong component (hypericin instead of hyperforin). St. John's wort is still in the early stages of clinical trials investigating its effects against certain viruses, including HIV.

Drug Interactions: St. John's wort has been reported to decrease the efficacy of theophylline, warfarin, and digoxin and reduce AUC of indinavir (and potentially other protease inhibitors). Known interactions to cyclosporine have occurred. Concomitant use with prescription antidepressants is not recommended. Use with oral contraceptives may cause breakthrough bleeding but has not been reported to result in unexpected pregnancy.

Side Effects: Side effects are usually mild. Potential side effects include the following: Dry mouth, dizziness, constipation, other GI symptoms, and confusion. Photosensitization may also occur. In clinical trials, side effects and medication discontinuation with St. John's wort were usually less than that observed with standard antidepressants. Other possible rare side effects include induction of mania and effects on male and female reproductive capabilities.

Dose: The majority of clinical trials for the treatment of depression administered St. John's wort 300 mg tid standardized to 0.3% hypericin, but research has shown that products should contain ≥ 2% to 4% hyperforin.

---

[1] Awang D. St. John's wort. *CPJ-RPC* 1991 Jan:33.
[2] Tyler V. The New Honest Herbal. Philadelphia, PA: G.F. Stickley Co., 1987.
[3] Bombardelli E, et al. Hypericum perforatum. *Fitoterapia* 1995;66(1):43-68.
[4] Upton R, ed. St. John's wort Hypericum perforatum. Austin TX: American Herbal Pharmacopoeia and Therapeutic Compendium, 1997.
[5] Hahn G. Hypericum perforatum (St. John's wort)—a medicinal herb used in antiquity and still of interest today. *J Naturopathic Med* 1992;3(1):94-6.
[6] Gruenwald J. The world market for hypericum products. *Nutraceuticals World* 1999;May/June:22–25.
[7] Reuter H. Chemistry and biology of Hypericum perforatum (St. John's wort). *ACS Symp Ser* 1998;691:287–98.
[8] Hansen S, et al. High-performance liquid chromatography on-line coupled to high-field NMR and mass spectrometry for structure elucidation of constituents of Hypericum perforatum L. *Anal Chem* 1999;71(22):5235–5241.

[9] Mauri P, et al. High performance liquid chromatography/electrospray mass spectometry of *Hypericum perforatum* extracts. *Rapid Commun Mass Spectrom* 2000;14(2):95–9.

[10] Newall C, et al. St. John's wort. *Herbal Medicines*. London, England: Pharmaceutical Press 1996;250-52.

[11] Melikian E, et al. Hypericin content in St. John's wort (*Hypericum perforatum*) growing in Armenia. *Pharm Pharmacol Lett* 1998;8(3):101–2.

[12] Liu W, et al. The secretory structure of *Hypericum perforatum* and its relation to hypericin accumulation. *Zhiwu Xuebao* 1999;41(4):369–72.

[13] Tateo F, et al. Hypericin and hypericin-like substances: analytical problems. *Dev Food Sci* 1998;40:143–157.

[14] Stochmal A, et al. Solid phase extraction and HPLC determination of hypericin in *Hypericum perforatum* *Herba Pol* 1998;44(4):315–23.

[15] Chi J, et al. Determination of hypericin in plasma by high-performance liquid chromatography. *J Chromatogr B Biomed Sci App* 1999;724(11):195–8.

[16] Mulinacci N, et al. HPLC-DAD and TLC-densitometry for quantification of hypericin in *Hypericum perforatum* extracts. *Chromatographia* 1999;49(3/4):197–201.

[17] Balogh M, et al. HPLC analysis of hypericin with photodiode-array and MS detection: the advantages of multispectral techniques. *LC-GC* 1999;17(6):556,558,560–2.

[18] Michelitsch A, et al. Determination of hypericin in herbal medicine products by different pulse polarography. *Phytochem Anal* 2000;11(1):41–4.

[19] Sirvent T, et al. Rapid isocratic HPLC analysis of hypericins. *J Liq Chromatogr Relat Technol* 2000;23(2):251–259.

[20] Fourneron J, et al. Pseudohypericin and hypericin in St. John's wort extracts. *Acad Sci Chim* 1999;2(3):127–31.

[21] Omarova M, et al. Liposoluble pigments from the herb *Hypericum perforatum*. *Chem Nat Compd* 1998;Volume Date 1997;33(6):691-92.

[22] Butterweck V, et al. Flavonoids from *Hypericum perforatum* show antidepressant activity in the forced swimming test. *Planta Med* 2000;66(1):3–6.

[23] Erdelmeier C, et al. Hyperforin, possible the major non-nitrogenous secondary metabolite of *Hypericum perforatum* L. *Pharmacopsychiatry* 1998;31(suppl):2–6.

[24] Orth H, et al. Isolation, purity analysis and stability of hyperforin as a standard material from *Hypericum perforatum* L. *J Pharm Pharmacol* 1999;51(2):193–200.

[25] Chi J, et al. Measurement of hyperforin a constituent of St. John's wort in plasma by high-performance liquid chromatography. *J Chromatogr B Biomed Sci App* 1999;735(2):285–8.

[26] Verotta L, et al. Furohyperforin, a prenylated phloroglucinol from St. John's wort. *J Nat Prod* 1999;62(5):770–72.

[27] Verotta L, et al. Hyperforin analogues from St. John's wort (*Hypericum perforatum*). *J Nat Prod* 2000;63(3):412–15.

[28] Rafajlovska V, et al. Influence of some factors on tannin contents in extracts of St. John's wort (*Hypericum perforatum* L.). *Herba Pol* 1998;44(4):307–14.

[29] Dietary Supplement Health and Education Act of 1994, 103rd Congress, S784.

[30] Constantine G, et al. Variations in hypericin concentrations in *Hypericum perforatum* L. and commercial products. *Pharm Biol* 1998;36(5):365–7.

[31] Liu F, et al. High-performance liquid chromatography determination of biologically active components in extracts of St. John's wort leaves and dietary supplements. Book of Abstracts, 217th ACS National Meeting, Anaheim, CA March 21–25, 1999. AGFD-102.

[32] Melzer M, et al. Hyperforin in St. John's wort. *Dtsch Apoth Ztg* 1998;138(49),4754,57–60.

[33] Schempp C, et al. Biochemical activities of extracts from *Hypericum perforatum* L. 3rd communication: modulation of peroxidase activity as a simple method for standardization. *Arzneimittelforschung* 1999;49(2):115–9.

[34] Khwaja T, et al. Pharmaceutical grade St. John's wort. *PCT Int Appl* 1999:104.

[35] Mason D, et al. The quantity and isolation of hypericin and pseudohypericin from over-the-counter preparations. Book of Abstracts, 217th ACS National Meeting, Anaheim, CA, March 21–25, 1999. CHED–454.

[36] Kurth H, et al. Phytochemical characterization of various St. John's wort extracts. *Adv Ther* 1998;15(2):117–28.

[37] Suzuki O, et al. Inhibition of monoamine oxidase by hypericin. *Planta Med* 1984;2:272.

[38] Bladt S, et al. Inhibition of MAO by fractions and constituents of *Hypericum* extract. *J Geriatr Psychiatry Neurol* 1994;7(suppl. 1):S57-S59.

[39] Thiede H, et al. Inhibition of MAO and COMT by *Hypericum* extracts and hypericin. *J Geriatr Psychiatry Neurol* 1994;7(suppl. 1):S54–6.

[40] Perovic S, et al. Pharmacological profile of *Hypericum* extract. Effect on serotonin uptake by postsynaptic receptors. *Arzneimittelforschung* 1995;45(11):1145-48.

[41] Muller W, et al. Effects of *Hypericum* extract on the expression of serotonin receptors. *J Geriatr Psychiatry Neurol* 1994;7(suppl. 1):S63–4.

[42] Neary J, et al. *Hypericum* LI 160 inhibits uptake of serotonin and norepiniphrine in astrocytes. *Brain Res* 1999;816(2):358–63.

[43] Franklin M, et al. Neuroendocrine evidence for dopaminergic actions of *Hypericum* extract (LI 160) in healthy volunteers. *Biol Psychiatry* 1999;46(4):581–4.

[44] Raffa R. Screen of receptor and uptake-site activity of hypericin component of St. John's wort reveals sigma receptor binding. *Life Sci* 1998;62(16):PL265–70.

[45] Gobbi M, et al. *Hypericum perforatum* L. extract does not inhibit 5–HT transporter in rat brain cortex. *Arch Pharmacol* 1999;360(3)262–9.

[46] Helgason C, et al. The effects of St. John's wort (*Hypericum perforatum*) on NK cell activity in vitro. *Immunopharmacology* 2000;46(3):247–51.

[47] Kleber E, et al. Biochemical activities of extracts from *Hypericum perforatum* L. 1st communication: inhibition of dopamine-beta-hydroxylase. *Arzneimittelforschung* 1999;49(2):106–9.

[48] Chatterjee S, et al. Hyperforin as a possible antidepressant component of *Hypericum* extracts. *Life Sci* 1998;63(6):499–510.

[49] Chatterjee S, et al. Antidepressant activity of *Hypericum perforatum* and hyperforin: the neglected possibility. *Pharmacopsychiatry* 1998;31(suppl):7–15.

[50] Muller W, et al. Hyperforin represents the neurotransmitter reuptake inhibiting constituent of *Hypericum* extract. *Pharmacopsychiatry* 1998;31(suppl):16–21.

[51] Kaehler S, et al. Hyperforin enhances the extracellular concentrations of catecholamines, serotonin, and glutamate in the rat locus coeruleus. *Neurosci Lett* 1999;262(3):199–202.

[52] Bhattacharya S, et al. Activity profiles of two hyperforin-containing *Hypericum* extracts in behavioral models. *Pharmacopsychiatry* 1998;31(suppl):22–29.

[53] Dimpfel W, et al. Effects of a methanolic extract and a hyperforin-enriched CO_2 extract of St. John's wort (*Hypericum perforatum*) on intracerebral field potentials in the freely moving rat (Tele-Stereo-EEG). *Pharmacopsychiatry* 1998;31(suppl):30–5.

[54] Chatterjee S, et al. Hyperforin accentuates various ionic conductance mechanisms in the isolated hippocampal neurons of rat. *Life Sci* 1999;65(22):2395–2405.

[55] Singer A, et al. Hyperforin, a major antidepressant constituent of St. John's wort, inhibits serotonin uptake by elevating free intracellular Na^{+1}. *J Pharmacol Exp Ther* 1999;290(3):1363–8.

[56] Laakmann G, et al. St. John's wort in mild to moderate depression: the relevance of hyperforin for the clinical efficacy. *Pharmacopsychiatry* 1998;31(suppl. 1):54–9.

[57] Okpanyi V, et al. Animal experiments on the psychotropic action of *Hypericum* extract. *Arzneimittelforschung* 1987;37:10.

[58] Muldner V, et al. Antidepressive effect of a *Hypericum* extract standardized to the active hypericine complex. *Arzneimittelforschung* 1984;34:918.

[59] Ernst E. St. John's wort as antidepressive therapy. *Fortschr Med* 1995;113(25):354-55.

[60] Mueller W, et al. St. John's wort: in vitro studies of *Hypericum* extract, hypericin, and camphor oil as antidepressants. *Deutsche Apotheker Zeitung* 1996 Mar 28;136:17-22,24.

[61] DeSmet P, et al. St. John's wort as an antidepressant. *Br Med J* 1996 Aug 3;313:241-42.

[62] Harrer G, et al. Treatment of mild/moderate depressions with *Hypericum*. *Phytomedicine* 1994;1:3-8.

[63] Linde K, et al. St. John's wort for depression—an overview and meta-analysis of randomised clinical trials. *Br Med J* 1996;313(7052):253-58.

[64] Witte B, et al. Treatment of depressive symptoms with a high concentration *Hypericum* preparation. A multicenter placebo-controlled double-blind study. *Fortschritte Der Medizin* 1995;113(28):404-8.

[65] Heiligenstein E, et al. Over-the-counter psychotropics: a review of melatonin, St. John's wort, valerian, and kava-kava. *J Am Coll Health* 1998;46(6):271–6.

[66] Cott J, et al. Is St. John's wort (*Hypericum perforatum*) an effective antidepressant? *J Nerv Ment Dis* 1988;186(8):500–1.

[67] Rey J, et al. *Hypericum perforatum* (St. John's wort) in depression: pest or blessing? *Med J Aust* 1998;169(11–12):583–6.

[68] Nordfors M, et al. New discoveries on St. John's wort can improve pharmacotherapy in depression. *Lakartidningen* 1999;96(1–2):12–13.

[69] Clark C. St. John's wort latest results. *Nurs Spectr* (Wash. DC) 1999;9(4):19.

[70] Meier B. The science behind *Hypericum*. *Adv Ther* 1999;16(3):135–47.

[71] Josey E, et al. St. John's wort: a new alternative for depression? *Int J Clin Pharmacol Ther* 1999;37(3):111–19.

[72] Muller W, et al. *Hypericum* extract. From a tea for calming nerves to a modern anti-depressant. *Dtsch Apoth Ztg* 1999;139(17):1741–6, 1748–50.

[73] Gaster B, et al. St. John's wort for depression: a systematic review. *Arch Intern Med* 2000;160(2):152–6.

[74] Murray M. Common questions about St. John's wort extract. *Am J Nat Med* 1997;4(7):14–19.

[75] Miller A. St. John's wort *Hypericum perforatum*: clinical effects on depression and other conditions. *Altern Med Rev* 1998;3(1):18–26.

[76] Hippius H. St. John's wort *Hypericum perforatum* —a herbal antidepressant. *Curr Med Res Opin* 1998;14(3):171–84.

[77] Kim H, et al. St. John's wort for depression: a meta-analysis of well-defined clinical trials. *J Nerv Ment Dis* 1999;187(9):532–8.

[78] Kasper S, et al. High dose St. John's wort as a phytogenic antidepressant. *Wien Med Wochenschr* 1999;149(8–10):191–6.

[79] Mulrow C, et al.Treatment of depression—newer pharmacotherapies. *Psychopharmacol Bull* 1998;34(4):409–795.

[80] Stevinson C, et al. *Hypericum* for depression. An update of the clinical evidence. *Eur Neuropsychopharmacol* 1999;9(6):501–5.

[81] Deltito J, et al. The scientific, quasi-scientific, and popular literature on the use of St. John's wort in the treatment of depression. *J Affect Disord* 1998;51(3):345–51.

[82] Bennet D, et al. Neuropharmacology of St. John's wort (*Hypericum*). *Ann Pharmacother* 1998;32(11):1201–8.

[83] Lenoir S, et al. A double-blind randomized trial to investigate 3 different concentrations of a standardized fresh plant extract obtained from the shoot tips of *Hypericum perforatum*. *Phytomedicine* 1999;6(3):141–6.

[84] Walter G, et al. Use of St. John's wort by adolescents with a psychiatric disorder. *J Child Adolesc Psychopharmacol* 1999;9(4):307–11.

[85] Chatterjee S, et al. Use of hyperforin and hyperforin-containing extracts in the treatment and prophylaxis of dementia. *Pct Int Appl* 1999.

[86] Ernst E. Herbal medications for common ailments in the elderly. *Drugs Aging* 1999;15(6):423–28.

[87] DeVry J, et al. Comparison of *Hypericum* extracts with imipramine and fluoxetine in animal models of depression and alcoholism. *Eur Neuropsychopharmacol* 1999;9(6):461–8.

[88] Harrer G, et al. Comparison of equivalence between the St. John's wort extract LoHyp-57 and fluoxetine. *Arzneimittelforschung* 1999;49(4):289–96.

[89] Sharpley A, et al. Antidepressant-like effect of *Hypericum perforatum* (St. John's wort) on the sleep polysomnogram. *Psychopharmacology* 1998;139(3):286–7.

[90] Martinez B, et al. *Hypericum* in the treatment of seasonal affective disorders. *J Geriatr Psychiatry Neurol* 1994;7(suppl. 1):S29–33.

[91] Staffeldt B, et al. Pharmacokinetics of hypericin and pseudohypericin after oral intake of the *Hypericum perforatum* extract LI 160 in healthy volunteers. *J Geriatr Psychiatry Neurol* 1994 Oct 7;Suppl 1:S47-53.

[92] Kerb R, et al. Single-dose and steady-state pharmacokinetics of hypericin and pseudohypericin. *Antimicrob Agents Chemother* 1996;40(9):2087-93.

[93] Hebel SK, Burnham TH, eds. Drug Facts and Comparisons. St. Louis, MO: Facts and Comparisons, 1998.

[94] *VimRxyn* press release taken from the Internet, dated 10/19/96.

[95] Gulick R, et al. Phase I studies of hypericin, the active compound in St. John's wort, as an antiretroviral agent in HIV-infected adults. AIDS Clinical Trials Group Protocols 150 and 258. *Ann Intern Med* 1999;130(6):510–14.

[96] Taylor R, et al. Antiviral activities of Nepalese medicinal plants. *J Ethnopharmacol* 1996;52(3):157-63.

[97] Diwu Z. Novel therapeutic and diagnostic applications of hypocrellins and hypericins. *Photochem Photobiol* 1995;61(6):529-39.

[98] Barbagallo C, et al. *Fitoterapia* 1987;58:175.

[99] Ang C, et al. Antimicrobial activities of St. John's wort extracts. Book of Abstracts, 217th ACS National Meeting, Anaheim, CA, March 21–25, 1999.

[100] Schempp C, et al. Antibacterial activity of hyperforin from St. John's wort, against multiresistant *Staphylococcus aureus* and gram-positive bacteria. *Lancet* 1999;353(9170):2129.

[101] Hayakawa A. The wound-healing effect St. John's wort herb (*Hypericum perforatum*). *Food Style* 21 1999;3(4):74–77.

[102] Duke J. Handbook of Medicinal Herbs. Boca Raton, FL: CRC Press, 1985.

[103] VIMRx Successfully Completes Phase I Clinical Studies for VIMRxyn-R—Synthetic Hypericin—as Topical Phototherapy for Skin Disease. *Business Wire* April 25, 1997.

[104] Berghofer R, et al. Isolation of 13′, II8-biapigenin (amentoflavone) from *Hypericum perforatum*. *Planta Med* 1989;55:91.

[105] VIMRx Successfully Completes Phase I/II Clinical Study of VIMRxyn—Synthetic Hypericin—for the Treatment of Glioblastoma Brain Cancer. *Business Wire* Oct. 28, 1998.

[106] Grube B, et al. St. John's wort extract: efficacy for menopausal symptoms of psychological origin. *Adv Ther* 1999;16(4):117–86.

[107] Evstifeeva T, et al. The immunotropic properties of biologically active products obtained from Klamath weed *Hypericum perforatum* L. *Eksperimentalnaia I Klinicheskaia Farmakologiia* 1996;59(1):51-54.

[108] Shan J, et al. Hypericin, hypericin derivatives, and *Hypericum* extract as specific T-type calcium channel blockers, and their use as T-type calcium channel targeted therapeutics. *Pct Int Appl* 2000.

[109] Klepser T, et al. Unsafe and potentially safe herbal therapies. *Am J Health Syst Pharm* 1999;56(2):125–38.

[110] Duncan M. The effects of nutritional supplements on the treatment of depression, diabetes, and hypercholesterolemia in the renal patient. *J Ren Nutr* 1999;9(2):58–62.

[111] Fugh-Berman A. Herb-drug interactions. *Lancet* 2000;355(9198):134–38.

[112] Cupp M. Herbal remedies: Adverse effects and drug interactions. *Am Fam Physician* 1999;59(5):1239–45.

[113] Ciordia R. Beware "St. John's wort," potential herbal danger. *J Clin Monit Comput* 1998;14(3):215.

[114] Nebel A, et al. Potential metabolic interaction between St. John's wort and theophylline. *Ann Pharmacother* 1999;33(4):502.

[115] Johne A, et al. Pharmacokinetic interaction of digoxin with an herbal extract from St. John's wort (*Hypericum perforatum*). *Clin Pharm Ther* 1999;66(4):338–45.

[116] Piscitelli S, et al. Indinavir concentrations and St. John's wort. *Lancet* 2000; 355 (9203):547–8.

[117] Ruschitzka F, et al. Acute heart transplant rejection due to St. John's wort. *Lancet* 2000;355 (9203):548–9.

[118] Lantz M, et al. St. John's wort and antidepressant drug interactions in the elderly. *J Geriatr Psychiatry Neurol* 1999;12(1):7–10.

[119] Araya O, et al. An investigation of the type of photosensitization caused by the ingestion of St. John's wort (*Hypericum perforatum*) by calves. *J Comp Pathol* 1981;91(1):135–41.

[120] Kumper H. *Hypericum* poisoning in sheep. *Tierarztl Prax* 1989;17(3):257–61.

[121] Bernd A, et al. Phototoxic effects of *Hypericum* extract in cultures of human keratinocytes compared with those of psoralen. *Photochem Photobiol* 1999;69(2):218–21.

[122] Falk H. From the photosensitizer hypericin to the photoreceptor stentorin-the chemistry of phenanthroperylene quinones. *Angew Chem* Int. Ed. 1999;38(21):3117–3136.

[123] Schempp C, et al. Hypericin levels in human serum interstitial skin blister fluid after oral single-dose and steady-state administration of *Hypericum perforatum* extract. *Skin Pharmacol Appl Skin Physiol* 1999;12(5):299–304.

[124] Carey B. The sunshine supplement. *Health* 1998;Jan/Feb:52–5.

[125] Wagner P, et al. Taking the edge off: Why patients choose St. John's wort. *J Pharm Pract* 1999;48:615–19.

[126] Stevinson C, et al. Safety of *Hypericum* in patients with depression: a comparison with conventional antidepressants. *CNS Drugs* 1999;11(2):125–32.

[127] Bove G. Acute neuropathy after exposure to sun in a patient treated with St. John's wort. *Lancet* 1998;352(9134):1121–2.

[128] Bowers A. Phytodermatitis. *Am J Contact Dermat* 1999;10(2):89–93.

[129] Markowitz J, et al. Effect of St. John's wort *Hypericum perforatum* on cytochrome P-450 2D6 and 3A4 activity in healthy volunteers. *Life Sci* 2000;66(9):PL133-9.

[130] Nierenberg A, et al. Mania associated with St. John's wort. *Biol Psychiatry* 1999;46(12):1707–8.

[131] Moses E, et al. St. John's wort: Three cases of possible mania induction. *J Clin Psychopharmacol* 2000;20(1):115–17.

[132] Shipochliev T. Uterotonic action of extracts from a group of medicinal plants. *Vet Med Nauki* 1981;18(4):94–8.

[133] Grush L, et al. St. John's wort during pregnancy. *JAMA* 1998;28(18):1566.

[134] Ondrizek R, et al. Inhibition of human sperm motility by specific herbs used in alternative medicine. *J Assist Reprod Genet* 1999;16(2):87–91.

[135] Tatro D. Drug Interactions with St. John's wort. *Drug Link* 2000;4(5):34.

[136] Yue Q-Y, et al. Safety of St. John's wort (*Hypericum perforatum*). *Lancet* 2000;355:576.

[137] Ernst E. Second thoughts about safety of St. John's wort. *Lancet* 1999 Dec 11;354:2014–16.

[138] Shiplochliev T. Extracts from a group of medicinal plants enhancing uterine tonus. *Vet Med Nauki* 1981;18:94.

Stevia

SCIENTIFIC NAME(S): *Stevia rebaudiana* Bertoni. Family: Asteraceae

COMMON NAME(S): Stevia, Sweet Leaf of Paraguay, Caa-he-é, Ca-a-yupi, Eira-caa, Capim doce

BOTANY: Stevia is a perennial shrub indigenous to northern South America, but commercially grown in areas such as Central America, Israel, Thailand, and China. The plant can grow to 1 m in height, with 2-to-3 cm long leaves. The leaves are the parts of the plant used.[1]

HISTORY: Stevia has been used to sweeten tea for centuries, dating back to the Guarani Indians of South America. For hundreds of years, native Brazilians and Paraguayans have also employed the leaves of the plant as a sweetening agent. Europeans learned about stevia in the 16th century, whereas North American interest in the plant began in the 20th century when researchers heard of its sweetening properties. Paraguayan botanist Moises Bertoni documented stevia in the early 1900s. Glycosides responsible for the plant's sweeteners were discovered in 1931. Stevia extracts are used today as food additives by the Japanese and Brazilians as a non-caloric sweetener. In the US, however, use is limited to supplement status only.[1,2]

CHEMISTRY: Eight of stevia's glycosides were discovered and named in 1931.[3] Recently, the glycosides have been analyzed by capillary electrophoresis. Rebaudioside A and steviobioside have been isolated by HPLC methods.[4] Glycoside stevioside determination has been reported.[5] The main glycosides of stevia include stevioside and rebaudioside. Two glucosyl transferases acting on steviol and its glycosides have been isolated.[6] Stevioside (6 to 18% in leaves) is the sweetest glycoside and was tested and found to be 300 times sweeter than saccharose in one report.[7] Steviol hydroxylation has been reported.[8] Sterols in stevia include stigmasterol, beta-sitosterol, and campesterol.[9] Isolation of the principal sugars of stevia has also been studied.[10]

Also found in stevia are certain vitamins (C, B, A), minerals (iron, zinc, calcium), electrolytes (sodium, potassium), protein and others.[1]

Cultivation studies have been performed on the plant,[11,12] as has tissue culture experimentation.[13]

PHARMACOLOGY: Stevia has been used for centuries as a natural sweetener.[1] The plant contains sweet ent-

kaurene glycosides,[14] with the most intense sweetness belonging to the *S. rebaudina* species.[15] Stevia has been evaluated for sweetness in animal response testing.[16] In humans, stevia as a sweetening agent works well in weight-loss programs to satisfy "sugar cravings," and it is low in calories. The Japanese are the largest consumers of stevia leaves and employ the plant to sweeten foods (as a replacement for aspartame and saccharin) such as soy sauce, confections, and soft drinks.[1]

Stevia may be helpful in treating diabetes. Steviol, isosteviol, and glucosilsteviol decreased glucose production in rat renal cortical tubules.[17] Oral use of stevia extract in combination with chrysanthemum to manage hyperglycemia has been discussed.[18] Aqueous extracts of the plant increased glucose tolerance in 16 healthy volunteers, as well as markedly decreasing plasma glucose levels.[19]

Stevia's effects on blood pressure have been reported. The plant displayed vasodilatory actions in both normo- and hypertensive animals.[20] Stevia has also produced decreases in blood pressure, and has increased diuretic and natriuretic effects in rats.[21,22] The plant has cardiotonic actions, which normalize blood pressure and regulate heartbeat.[1]

Stevia extract has exhibited strong bactericidal activity against a wide range of pathogenic bacteria, including certain *E. coli* strains.[23] Steviol, stevia's aglycone, is mutagenic toward salmonella and other bacterial strains, under various conditions and toward certain cell lines.[24,25,26,27] Stevia may also be effective against *Candida albicans*.[1] One report addresses stevia's role against dental plaque.[28]

Certain metabolic aspects of stevioside have been described, including rat liver effects,[29,30,31] and cell membrane transport.[32]

TOXICOLOGY: Stevia has been shown not to be mutagenic or genotoxic.[1] One report indicates that constituents of stevioside and steviol are not mutagenic in vitro.[33] Stevioside was found to be nontoxic in acute toxicity studies in a variety of laboratory animals.[1] Chronic administration of stevia to male rats had no effect in fertility vs. controls.[34] Another report concludes that stevioside in high doses affected neither growth nor reproduction in hamsters of both sexes.[35]

SUMMARY: The use of stevia as a sweetening agent is centuries old and it is still used today as a natural sweetener. Other effects of the plant include hypoglycemic, hypotensive, and bactericidal. Stevia is not mutagenic and was found to be nontoxic, having no effect on growth reproduction or fertility in animal experimentation. More studies are needed to determine if it is an acceptable sweetening agent, as well as an effective agent against dental plaque.

PATIENT INFORMATION – Stevia

Uses: Stevia is used as a sweetening agent. It has also been found to have hypotensive, hypoglycemic, and bactericidal properties.

Side Effects: No major contraindications, warnings, or side effects have been documented.

---

[1] Sousa M. Constituintes Quimicos Ativos De Planta Medicinais Brasileiras. Fortaleza, Brasil: Laboratorio de Produtos Naturais.

[2] Blumenthal M. Perspectives of FDA's new Stevia Policy. After four years, the agency lifts its ban — but only partially. *Whole Foods* Feb. 1996.

[3] Bridel M, et al. *J Pharm Chim* 1931; 14:99.

[4] Mauri P, et al. Analysis of Stevia glycosides by capillary electrophoresis. *Electrophoresis* 1996; 17(2):367–71.

[5] Mitsuhashi H, et al. Studies on the cultivation of Stevia rebaudiana Bertoni. Determination of stevioside. *Yakugaku Zasshi* 1975; 95(1):127–30.

[6] Shibata H, et al. Steviol and steviol-glycoside: glucosyltransferase activities in Stevia rebaudiana Bertoni — purification and partial characterization. *Arch Biochem Biophys* 1995; 321(2):390–96.

[7] Samuelsson G. *Drugs of Natural Origin* Stockholm, Sweden: Swedish Pharmaceutical Press; 1992.

[8] Kim K, et al. Hydroxylation of ent-kaurenoic acid to steviol in Stevia rebaudiana Bertoni — purification and partial characterization of the enzyme. *Arch Biochem Biophys* 1996; 332(2):223–30.

[9] D'Agostino M, et al. Sterol in Stevia rebaudiana Bertoni. *Boll Soc Ital Biol Sper* 1984; 60(12):2237–40. Italian.

[10] Aquino RP, et al. Isolation of the principal sugars of Stevia rebaudiana. *Boll Soc Ital Biol Sper* 1985; 61(9):1247–52. Italian.

[11] Mitsuhashi H, et al. Studies on the cultivation of Stevia rebaudiana Bertoni. Determination of stevioside. II. *Yakugaku Zasshi* 1975; 95(12):1501–03.

[12] Miyazaki Y, et al. Studies on the cultivation of Stevia rebaudiana Bertoni. III. Yield and stevioside content of 2–year old plants. *Eisei Shikenjo Hokoku* 1978; (96):86–89.

[13] Handro W, et al. Tissue culture of Stevia rebaudiana, a sweetening plant. *Planta Med* 1977; 32(2):115–17.

[14] Kinghorn A, et al. A phytochemical screening procedure for sweet ent-kaurene glycosides in the genus Stevia. *J Nat Prod* 1984; 47(3):439–44.

[15] Soejarto D, et al. Potential sweetening agents of plant origin. III. Organoleptic evaluation of Stevia leaf herbarium samples for sweetness. *J Nat Prod* 1982; 45(5):590–99.

[16] Jakinovich W, et al. Evaluation of plant extracts for sweetness using the Mongolain gerbil. *J Nat Prod* 1990; 53(1):190–95.

[17] Yamamoto N, et al. Effect of steviol and its structural analogues on glucose production and oxygen uptake in rat renal tubules. *Experientia* 1985; 41(1):55–57.

[18] White J, et al. Oral use of a topical preparation containing an extract of Stevia rebaudiana and the chrysanthemum flower int he management of hyperglycemia. *Diabetes Care* 1994; 17(8):940.

[19] Curi R, et al. Effect of Stevia rebaudiana on glucose tolerance in normal adult humans. *Braz J Med Biol Res* 1986; 19(6):771–74.

[20] Melis MS. A crude extract of Stevia rebaudiana increases the renal plasma flow of normal and hypertensive rats. *Braz J Med Biol Res* 1996; 29(5):669–75.

[21] Melis MS, et al. Effect of calcium and verapamil on renal function of rats during treatment with stevioside. *J Ethnopharmacol* 1991; 33(3):257–62.

[22] Melis MS. Chronic administration of aqueous extract of Stevia rebaudiana in rats: renal effects. *J Ethnopharmacol* 1995; 47(3):129–34.

[23] Tomita T, et al. Bactericidal activity of a fermented hot-water extract from Stevia rebaudiana Bertoni towards enterohemorrhagic *Escherichia coli* O157:H7 and other food-borne pathogenic bacteria. *Microbiol Immunol* 1997; 41(12):1005–9.

[24] Pezzuto J, et al. Metabolically activated steviol, the aglycone of stevioside, is mutagenic. *Proc Natl Acad Sci* 1985; 82(8):2478–82.

[25] Pezzuto J, et al. Characterization of bacterial mutagenicity mediated by 13–hydroxy-ent-kaurenoic acid (steviol) and several structurally-related derivatives and evaluation of potential to induce glutathione S-transferase in mice. *Mutat Res* 1986; 169(3):93–103.

[26] Matsui M, et al. Evaluation of the genotoxicity of stevioside and steviol using six in vitro and one in vivo mutagenicity assays. *Mutagenesis* 1996; 11(6):573–79.

[27] Klongpanichpak S, et al. Lack of mutagenicity of steviodside and steviol in *Salmonella typhimurium* TA 98 and TA 100. *J Med Assoc* 1997; 80 Suppl 1: S121–28.

[28] Pinheiro C, et al. Effect of guarana and Stevia rebaudiana Bertoni (leaves) extracts, and stevioside, on the fermentation and synthesis of extracellular insoluble polysaccharides of dental plaque. *Rev Odontol Univ Sao Paulo* 1987; 1(4):9–13.

[29] Kelmer-Bracht A, et al. Effects of Stevia rebaudiana natural products on rat liver mitochondria. *Biochem Pharmacol* 1985; 34(6):873–82.

[30] Ishii E, et al. Stevioside, the sweet glycoside of Stevia rebaudiana, inhibits the action of atractyloside in the isolated perfused rat liver. *Res Commun Chem Pathol Pharmacol* 1986; 53(1):79–91.

[31] Ishii-Iwamoto EL, et al. Stevioside is not metabolized in the isolated perfused rat liver. *Res Commun Mol Pathol Pharmacol* 1995; 87(2):167–75.

[32] Constantin J, et al. Sensitivity of ketogenesis and citric acid cycle to steviosdie inhibition of palmitate transport across the cell membrane. *Braz J Med Biol Res* 1991; 24(8):767–71.

[33] Suttajit M, et al. Mutagenicity and human chromosomal effect of stevioside, a sweetener from Stevia rebaudiana Bertoni. *Environ Health Perspect* 1993; 101 Suppl 3:53–56.

[34] Oliveira-Filho RM, et al. Chronic administration of aqueous extract of Stevia rebaudiana (Bert.) Bertoni in rats: endocrine effects. *Gen Pharmacol* 1989; 20(2):187–91.

[35] Yodyingyuad V, et al. Effect of stevioside on growth and reproduction. *Hum Reprod* 1991; 6(1):158–65.

Storax

SCIENTIFIC NAME(S): *Liquidambar orientalis, L. styraciflua* Family: Hamamelidaceae

BOTANY: Levant storax (*L. orientalis* Mill.) is obtained from a small tree native to Turkey. American storax is obtained from *L. styraciflua* L., a large tree found near the Atlantic coast from New England to as far south as Central America.[1] Also known as the sweet gum tree, red gum, bilsted, star-leaved gum, styrax, and the alligator tree.[2,3,5]

HISTORY: The bark of the tree is mechanically ruptured in early summer, then stripped as late as autumn. The bark is then pressed in cold water alternating with boiling water, and crude liquid storax obtained from this process is collected. The crude balsam is then dissolved in alcohol, filtered, and collected in a manner so as not to lose the volatile constituents.

Storax has been used as an expectorant, especially in inhalation with warm air vaporizers. It has also been used to treat parasitic infections. The leaves are rich in tannins and have been used to treat diarrhea and to relieve sore throat.[2] In Latin America, the gum is used to promote sweating and as a diuretic. It is also applied topically to sores and wounds.[2] Storax had been used in the US as a component of hemorrhoid preparations, but today its only official use is as an ingredient in compound tincture of benzoin,[2] where it is used as a topical protectant.[3] Resins derived from storax have been used in perfumes, incense and as food flavors.

The reddish-brown wood of the tree, called satin walnut, is used in furniture making.

CHEMISTRY: Crude storax is a gray, thick liquid with a pleasing odor but a bitter taste. About 85% of the crude material is alcohol soluble.[1] Purified storax forms a brown semi-solid mass that is completely soluble in alcohol. Storax is high in free and combined cinnamic acid. Purified storax yields up to 47% total balsamic acids.[1] Its major components include phenylethylene (styrene), cinnamic esters, and vanillin.[1]

Upon steam distillation, the leaf yields an oily liquid containing about three dozen components, the major ones being terpinen-4-ol, alpha-pinene, and sabinene.[4] Benzaldehyde is produced from certain chemical reactions with the cinnamic acid in storax. Storax also contains an aromatic liquid (styrocamphene).[2]

PHARMACOLOGY: The leaf oil is rich in terpinen-4-ol, and the oil has a composition that is similar to that of the essential oil of *Melaleuca alternifolia* (Australian tea tree oil, see monograph), which has been investigated clinically as a topical antiseptic. Although the leaf oil of *Liquidambar styraciflua* has not yet been bioassayed, its similarity in composition indicates that it may demonstrate similar antibacterial and protectant properties to tea tree oil.[4]

TOXICOLOGY: No significant toxicity has been reported following the use of storax, although some persons may display sensitivity to compound tincture of benzoin.

SUMMARY: Storax has been used in traditional medicine for many years and continues to be used topically as a skin protectant. It is also widely used as a flavor and in perfumes.

PATIENT INFORMATION – Storax

Uses: Although not yet proven, storax may demonstrate similar antibacterial and protectant properties such as those of tea tree oil. Presently it is used topically as a skin protectant, as a flavor, and in perfumes.

Side Effects: There have been no demonstrated adverse effects.

---

[1] Evans, WC. Trease and Evans' Pharmacognosy. 13th ed. London: Balliere Tindall, 1989.
[2] Morton JF. Major Medicinal Plants. Springfield, IL: Charles C. Thomas, 1977.
[3] Dobelis IN. Magic and Medicine of Plants. Pleasantville, NY: Reader's Digest Association, 1986.
[4] Wyllie SG, Brophy JJ. The Leaf Oil of *Liquidambar styraciflua*. Planta Medica 1989;55:316.
[5] Osol A, Farrar GE Jr, ed. The Dispensatory of the United States of America. 25th ed. Philadelphia: JB Lippincott, 1955:1315.

Sweet Vernal Grass

SCIENTIFIC NAME(S): *Anthoxanthum odoratum* L., Family: Graminae

COMMON NAME(S): Grass, spring grass, sweet vernal grass

BOTANY: Sweet vernal grass is a fragrant plant in the grass family that has flat leaves and narrow spike-like panicles of proterogynous flowers. It grows perennially in tufts, without stolons or basal scaly offshoots. The culms are slender, erect, and 2 to 10 dm high. Its spikelets are brownish-green, 8 to 10 mm long, and spread at the time of flowering. The grass is originally native to Eurasia and Africa, but is common in American fields, pastures, and waste places as far north as southern Ontario and as far south as Louisiana.[1]

HISTORY: Like many aromatic plants, sweet vernal grass has been used historically as a flavoring agent because of its vanilla-like aroma. In Russia and related countries, it was used in the manufacture of special brandy.[2]

CHEMISTRY: Except where veterinary poisoning has shown the presence of dicoumarol in its hay, very few chemical studies have been carried out directly on sweet vernal grass.[3]

PHARMACOLOGY: An outbreak of a hemorrhagic diathesis has been reported in cattle fed home-produced sweet vernal grass hay. The same syndrome was later reproduced experimentally in calves fed the same hay.[3] The poisoning is characterized by increased prothrombin and partial thromboplastin times, while the leukocyte and erythrocyte counts stayed normal until the terminal hemorrhage was evidenced. Symptoms include rapid onset of progressive weakness, mucosal pallor, stiff gait, tachypnea, tachycardia, and hematomata, quickly ending in death. Necropsy revealed no blood coagulation, but petechial, ecchymotic, and free hemorrhages were observed in most organs. Most striking were the massive ecchymotic hemorrhages on the peritoneal rumen surface. Each kidney was enveloped by a bloody gelatinous mass. A second feeding trial was undertaken to see if vitamins K_1 and K_3 were antidotal. No trichothecene mycotoxins were found in the hay.

A multi-allergen dipstick IgE assay to skin-prick test and RAST tests have been compared. Generally, immunological sensitivity to sweet vernal grass is low.[4]

Based on the current warnings about the use of natural sources of coumarin and dicoumarol, and their known anticoagulant properties, use of *A. odoratum* for flavoring should be discouraged. Coumarin is widely distributed in plants, and the FDA has banned its use for flavoring purposes.[5]

Other than historical reference to the use of sweet vernal grass as a flavoring, no other pharmacological or toxicological studies are found in the recent literature.

SUMMARY: Historically, sweet vernal grass has been used as a flavoring. However, recent veterinary experiences on its anticoagulant principle (dicoumarol) should discourage its use for this purpose. The FDA has banned coumarin for flavoring purposes.

PATIENT INFORMATION – Sweet Vernal Grass

Uses: Sweet vernal grass is used as a flavoring and sometimes in the manufacture of brandy. Recent veterinary poisonings show reason to discourage its use in humans.

Side Effects: In cattle, hay made from sweet vernal grass has caused progressive weakness, stiff gait, breathing difficulties and hemorrhage followed by quick death. This reaction has been attributed to the dicoumarol content of the hay and makes human consumption dangerous.

---

[1] Fernald ML. Gray's Manual of Botany, ed. 8. New York: American Book Co., 1950.
[2] Hocking GM. Dictionary of Terms in Pharmacognosy. Springfield, IL: Charles C. Thomas Publ. 1955.
[3] Pritchard DG, et al. *Vet Rec* 1983;113(4):78.
[4] Iwamoto I, et al. *Clin Expt Allergy* 1990;20(2):175.
[5] Leung AY, Foster S. Encyclopedia of Common Natural Ingredients Used in Food, Drugs and Cosmetics, ed. 2. New York: John Wiley & Sons, 1996.

Taheebo

SCIENTIFIC NAME(S): *Tabebuia avellanedae* Lorentz ex Griseb. Family: Bignoniaceae (Trumpet creepers). This species is synonymous with *T. impetiginosa* Mart. ex DC., *T. heptaphylla* Vell. Toledo, and *T. ipé* Mart. ex Schum. The distinct related species *Tecoma curialis* Solhanha da Gama is sometimes marketed under the same names.

COMMON NAME(S): Taheebo, Pau d'Arco, Lapacho morado, Lapacho colorado, Ipé Roxo

BOTANY: *Tabebuia* is a large genus of tropical trees that grows worldwide. According to one source, the correct name for the source species is *T. impetiginosa*;[1] however, the majority of biological and chemical studies of the plant refer to *T. avellaneda*. The commercial product is derived from the inner bark. The tree grows widely throughout tropical South America, including Brazil, Paraguay, and northern Argentina. It has a hard, durable, and attractive wood that is extremely resistant to insect and fungal attack.

HISTORY: Taheebo has been promoted for many years as an anticancer herb, and lay reports have claimed efficacy in a variety of cancers.[2] Antifungal and antibiotic properties are also claimed in promotional literature, with both topical and oral dosing for candidiasis.

CHEMISTRY: The naphthoquinone lapachol was isolated from the heartwood of the species in 1882,[3] and other related naphthoquinones (lapachones) have also been found in the wood.[4] Their structures were elucidated by Hooker[5] and others[6] and lapachol was synthesized by Fieser in 1927.[7] The inner bark has a distinct group of furanonaphthoquinones not found in the wood,[8,9,10] and these compounds are more likely to be responsible for the bioactivity observed in commercial samples of taheebo than lapachol and lapachones.[11,12] Analysis of commercial samples has found only trace amounts of lapachol and lapachones.[8] HPLC methods have been published about the analysis of taheebo bark[13] and wood.[14] The furanonaphthoquinones have been produced in good yield in callus and cell suspension cultures of *T. avellanedae*.[15] They are found in a number of species of *Tabebuia* and related Bignoniaceae.[16,17,18]

Other constituents of taheebo bark include 3 iridoid glycosides[19] and a number of simple benzoic acid derivatives.[9] A series of anthraquinones was also isolated from the wood.[20]

PHARMACOLOGY: Lapachol was extensively evaluated as an **anticancer** agent by the US National Cancer Institute and the Pfizer Co. in the 1960s.[21,22] It showed reproducible activity in mouse cancer models.[22] While oral absorption in humans was relatively poor, peak blood levels of 14 to 31 mcg/ml were attained with doses of 30 to 50 mg/kg.[21] Extensive modifications of the lapachol structure have been performed in pursuit of better antitumor activity,[23] in the search for **antimalarial** drugs,[24] and for **antipsoriatic** drugs.[25] Lapachol has also been reported to have modest **antifungal** and **antibacterial** activity,[26] as well as **anti-inflammatory** activity[27] and weak estrogenic action.[28]

Active β-lapachone has been found in tumor models.[29] It inhibits both murine leukemia virus reverse transcriptase and DNA polymerase-α, but not DNA polymerase-β and several other related enzymes.[30]

While having apparent potential for drug development, the biological activity of lapachol and β-lapachone is not relevant to the use of taheebo bark, because the bark contains little of these constituents. Instead, the furanonaphthoquinones are the important constituents, having cytotoxic,[16,17] antifungal, antibacterial,[11,18] and rather potent immunomodulatory activity.[12] Stimulation of host response to cancer cells or microbial infection may be responsible, at least in part, for the activity of the bark extract in vivo.

Despite the promising activity shown by the furanonaphthoquinone constituents, there do not appear to be clinical studies to support the use of taheebo for any of the indications mentioned.

TOXICOLOGY: The toxicology of lapachol was studied in detail by Morrison et al.,[31] who found hemolytic anemia to be the principle limiting toxicity in dogs, monkeys, rats, and mice. Human toxicity because of lapachol was seen at doses > 1.5 g/day, with an elevated prothrombin time that was reversed by administration of vitamin K.[21] Because lapachol is not a major constituent of taheebo bark, these studies are not entirely relevant to the commercial product. No toxicology has been reported for either the bark extract or its main constituents.

SUMMARY: Taheebo, also known as Pau d'Arco and Ipé Roxo, is derived from the inner bark of *Tabebuia avellanedae* and related species. Lapachol has been mistakenly identified as the active constituent, whereas the furanonaphthoquinones appear to be responsible for the biological activity of the product. Widely used in alternative cancer therapy without sufficient scientific proof, it may be more useful in antifungal applications, although no clinical trials appear to have been conducted for any indication. There are no reports of serious adverse effects; however, it should not be used with anticoagulants.

PATIENT INFORMATION – Taheebo

Uses: Taheebo is widely used in alternative cancer therapy without sufficient scientific proof. It may be more useful in antifungal applications, although no clinical trials have been conducted for any indication.

Drug Interactions: Do not use taheebo with anticoagulants.

Side Effects: There are no reported serious side effects.

---

[1] Woodson R, et al. Flora of Panama: IX. Family 172: Bignoniaceae. *Ann Missouri Bot Gard* 1973;60:45.

[2] Hartwell J. Plants used against cancer. A survey. *Lloydia* 1968;31:71.

[3] Paterno E. Ricerche sull'acido lapico. *Gazz Chim Ital* 1882;12:337.

[4] Gonçalves de Lima O, et al. Antibiotic substances in higher plants. XX. Antimicrobial activity of some derivatives of lapachol as compared with xyloidone, a new natural o-naphthoquinone isolated from extracts of heartwood of *Tabebuia avellanedae*. *Rev Inst Antibiot, Univ Fed Pernambuco, Recife* 1962;4:3.

[5] Hooker S. Constitution of lapachol and its derivatives. The structure of the amylene chain. *J Chem Soc* 1896;69:1356.

[6] Casinovi C, et al. Quinones from *Tabebuia avellanedae*. *Ann Chim (Italy)* 1962;52:1184.

[7] Fieser L. Alkylation of hydroxynaphthoquinone. A synthesis of lapachol. *J Amer Chem Soc* 1927;49:857.

[8] Girard M, et al. Naphthoquinone constituents of *Tabebuia* spp. *J Nat Prod* 1988;51:1023.

[9] Wagner H, et al. Structure determination of new isomeric naphthofuran-4,9-diones from *Tabebuia avellanedae* by the selective-INEPT technique. *Helv Chim Acta* 1989;72:659.

[10] Fujimoto Y, et al. Studies on the structure and stereochemistry of cytotoxic furanonaphthoquinones from *Tabebuia impetiginosa*: 5- and 8-hydroxy-2-(1-hydroxyethyl)naphthofuran-4,9-diones. *J Chem Soc Perkin Trans I* 1991;2323.

[11] Binutu O, et al. Antibacterial and antifungal compounds from *Kigelia pinnata*. *Planta Med* 1996;62:352.

[12] Kreher B, et al. New furanonaphthoquinones and other constituents of *Tabebuia avellanedae* and their immunomodulating activities in vitro. *Planta Med* 1988;54:562.

[13] Steinert J, et al. HPLC separation and determination of naphthofuran-4,9-diones and related compounds in extracts of *Tabebuia avellanedae* (Bignoniaceae). *J Chromatogr A* 1995;693:281.

[14] Steinert J, et al. High-performance liquid chromatographic separation of some naturally occurring naphthoquinones and anthraquinones. *J Chromatogr A* 1996;723:206.

[15] Ueda S, et al. Production of anti-tumour-promoting furanonaphthoquinones in *Tabebuia avellanedae* cell cultures. *Phytochemistry* 1994;36:323.

[16] Diaz F, et al. Furanonaphthoquinones from *Tabebuia ochracea* ssp. *neochrysanta*. *J Nat Prod* 1996;59:423.

[17] Rao M, et al. Plant anticancer agents. XII. Isolation and structure elucidation of new cytotoxic quinones from *Tabebuia cassinoides*. *J Nat Prod* 1982;45:600.

[18] Gafner S, et al. Antifungal and antibacterial naphthoquinones from *Newbouldia laevis* roots. *Phytochemistry* 1996;42:1315.

[19] Nakano K, et al. Iridoids from *Tabebuia avellanedae*. *Phytochemistry* 1993;32:371.

[20] Burnett A, et al. Naturally occurring quinones. Part X. The quinonoid constituents of *Tabebuia avellenedae* (Bignoniaceae). *J Chem Soc (C)* 1967;2100.

[21] Block J, et al. Early clinical studies with lapachol (NSC-11905). *Cancer Chemother Repts* 1974;4:27.

[22] Rao K, et al. Recognition and evaluation of lapachol as an antitumor agent. *Cancer Res* 1968;28:1952.

[23] Linardi M, et al. A lapachol derivative active against mouse lymphocytic leukemia P-388. *J Med Chem* 1975;18:1159.

[24] Fieser L, et al. Naphthoquinone antimalarials: general survey. *J Amer Chem Soc* 1948;70:3151.

[25] Müller K, et al. Potential antipsoriatic agents: Lapacho compounds as potent inhibitors of HaCaT cell growth. *J Nat Prod* 1999;62:1134.

[26] Guirard P, et al. Comparison of antibacterial and antifungal activities of lapachol and β-lapachone. *Planta Med* 1994;60:373.

[27] De Almeida E, et al. Antiinflammatory actions of lapachol. *J Ethnopharmacol* 1990;29:239.

[28] Sareen V, et al. Evaluation of oestrogenicity and pregnancy interceptory efficacy of lapachol. *Phytotherapy Res* 1995;9:139.

[29] Schaffner-Sabba K, et al. β-Lapachone: Synthesis of derivatives and activities in tumor models. *J Med Chem* 1984;27:990.

[30] Schürch A, et al. β-Lapachone, an inhibitor of oncornovirus reverse transcriptase and eukaryotic DNA polymerase-α. *Eur J Biochem* 1978;84:197.

[31] Morrison R, et al. Oral toxicology studies with lapachol. *Toxicol Appl Pharmacol* 1970;17:1.

Tanning Tablets

HISTORY: A variety of over-the-counter tablets and capsules containing the pigments beta-carotene and canthaxanthin have been available for more than a decade and have been promoted to give the user a natural-looking skin tan. These products have long been available in Europe and Canada, and "tan" by systemically pigmenting the skin. Today, they can be found in many tanning salons throughout the US.

CHEMISTRY: The natural pigments beta-carotene and canthaxanthin (beta-carotene-4,4'-dione) form the basis for orally administered tanning products.[1] The majority of these products contain synthetic versions of these carotenoid pigments, which are responsible for much of the yellow, orange, and red coloration in plants.[2] Canthaxanthin, a highly lipid soluble, deep red-orange pigment, is often the only color in these tanning preparations; it is sometimes referred to as Food Orange 8,[3] carophyll red or roxanthin red 10.[4]

NONCLINICAL USES: In the US, these pigments are approved as color additives for use in food and drugs, but are unapproved for use as ingested agents intended to color the body. The typical dietary intake of beta-carotene and canthaxanthin added during food manufacturing is 0.3 mg and 5.6 mg, respectively.[2] A recommended maximum daily intake of canthaxanthin is 25 mg/kg.[1] In monkeys, canthaxanthin concentrates preferentially in the liver and spleen.[5]

CLINICAL USES: Antineoplastic effects: Epidemiologic evidence suggests that the incidence of cancers may be slightly lower among individuals with an above-average intake of beta-carotene and other carotenoids. These compounds may deactivate reactive chemical species such as singlet oxygen and free radicals.[6] They may also have some slight pro-vitamin A effect that may contribute to the neoplastic protectant effect.[7] Mice supplemented with beta-carotene for 5 weeks prior to and 26 weeks after the administration of a nitrosamine derivative to induce bladder cancer developed significantly fewer tumors than did unsupplemented mice. Mice receiving canthaxanthin showed no protection.[8] Mice receiving canthaxanthin, retinyl palmitate or a combination developed fewer cutaneous tumors following exposure to ultraviolet irradiation.[9] Dietary supplementation of canthaxanthin inhibited the initiation of experimental breast tumors in mice, but did not slow their spread.[10]

Porphyrias: Beta-carotene and canthaxanthin administration help prevent photosensitivity in people with inherited erythropoietic protoporphyria. This skin disorder is characterized by burning, itching skin often with ulceration, following exposure to sunlight. Beta-carotene effectively protects against photosensitivity but does not protect from ultraviolet-induced sunburn.[2,11]

Dermatologic uses: Canthaxanthin has been used for the treatment of vitiligo, a disorder in which the melanocytes cease to synthesize melanin and disappear from the involved areas. When given orally to 48 patients with vitiligo, self-rating showed that 54% were not satisfied, 35% were satisfied and 10% were very satisfied with the results of canthaxanthin pigmentation.[1]

Tanning effects: Labeling for over-the-counter products recommends taking several tablets a day for 2 to 3 weeks, then smaller periodic doses to maintain the coloration. The skin color accumulates over a 2-week period, then fades in about as much time when the product is stopped. Ingestion of too much pigment can make the palms of the hands turn orange.[1] One brand of tablets contains 4 mg of beta-carotene and 36 mg of canthaxanthin per dose; the resulting daily intake of beta-carotene and canthaxanthin would be 12 to 16 mg and 108 to 144 mg, respectively.[2] Ingestion of these large amounts of pigment results in the accumulation of dyes in adipose tissue with a resultant yellow discoloration of the skin. The "tan" has a distinct orange tinge and affords no protection against sunburn.[1]

TOXICOLOGY: Both beta-carotene and canthaxanthin are classified as "Generally Recognized As Safe (GRAS)" substances by the FDA.[12] The conversion of beta-carotene to vitamin A is limited by physiologic requirements and, therefore, the ingestion of these tablets does not pose a threat of hypervitaminosis A. Canthaxanthin is not metabolized to vitamin A in humans, and some question exists as to whether it may interfere with the conversion of carotene to vitamin A.[2]

In short- and long-term animal studies, the LD $_{50}$ for canthaxanthin in mice, rats, and dogs has been found to be greater than 10,000 mg/kg.[1]

A small amount of the drug is absorbed and large quantities are excreted, imparting a brick-red color to the stool, a side effect that may mask the presence of rectal bleeding.[1]

There have been no reports of teratogenicity, carcinogenicity, or histotoxicity.[1] No toxicity was noted in volunteers who ingested 180 mg/day of beta-carotene for 10 weeks.[13] These dyes afford no protection to sunburn and patients should be instructed to take adequate precautions against exposure. Severe orange discoloration of plasma has been noted by blood collection agencies in blood samples obtained from subjects who ingested tanning tablets, although toxic levels of vitamin A were not found in the samples.[14]

The most common non-dermatologic adverse effects include nausea, cramps and diarrhea, which occurred in about one-third of patients receiving these pigments as treatment for photosensitivity. The Food and Drug Administration has received reports of a drug-induced hepatitis and a case of severe itching and welts, which may have been related to oral tanning products.[2]

Amenorrhea has been reported among women receiving carotenoid therapy, although with a very low prevalence.[15] A survey of 50 patients who took more than 200 tanning tablets over a period of time found golden crystalline deposits in the inner layers of the retina and around the macula in 12%.[16] No alterations in visual acuity were observed, but the long-term implications of these deposits are not understood. Retinopathy does not appear to develop in patients taking beta-carotene alone.[12] A recent report described a 20-year-old woman who died secondary to developing aplastic anemia after ingesting a course of high-dose canthaxanthin-containing tanning tablets. Although supportive measures may have saved the patient, her religious beliefs precluded the use of these interventions.[17]

SUMMARY: Tanning tablets containing a combination of beta-carotene and canthaxanthin are available over the counter to promote the development of a "suntan." This is accomplished by pigmenting the skin with an orange-red color accumulated in subcutaneous fat deposits. Side effects include discoloration of the stool, gastrointestinal discomfort and at least one case of aplastic anemia. These products cannot be recommended for use as tanning agents because of the unknown safety associated with their long-term use. Carotenoids such as these may impart a cancer-protective effect, although they offer no protection against the development of sunburn.

PATIENT INFORMATION – Tanning Tablets

Uses: Tanning tablets have been used to give a natural-looking skin tan, prevent photosensitivity in people with inherited erythropoietic protoporphyria, and in the treatment of vitiligo.

Side Effects: Some adverse effects reported with tanning tablets include discoloration of the stool, GI discomfort, and at least one case of aplastic anemia.

---

1 Gupta AK, et al. Canthaxanthin. *Int J Dermatol* 1985;24(8):528.
2 Fenner L. The tanning pill, a questionable inside dye job. *FDA Consumer* 1982;16(1):23.
3 Levit F. Availability of canthaxanthin in the United States. *J Am Acad Dermatol* (letter) 1985;12(1):129.
4 Windholz M, ed. *Merck Index*, ed. 10. Rahway NJ: Merck and Co., Inc., 1983.
5 Mathews-Roth MM, et al. Distribution of [14C] canthaxanthin and [14C] lycopene in rats and monkeys. *J Nutr* 1990;120(10):1205.
6 Burton GW, Ingold KU. β-Carotene: An unusual type of lipid antioxidant. *Science* 1984;224(4649):569.
7 Bertram JS, et al. Diverse carotenoids protect against chemically induced neoplastic transformation. *Carcinogenesis* 1991;12(4):671.
8 Mathews-Roth MM, et al. Effects of carotenoid administration on bladder cancer prevention. *Oncology* 1991;48(3):177.
9 Gensler HL, et al. Cumulative reduction of primary skin tumor growth in UV-irradiated mice by the combination of retinyl palmitate and canthaxanthin. *Cancer Lett* 1990;53(1):27.

10 Grubbs CJ, et al. Effect of canthaxanthin on chemically induced mammary carcinogenesis. *Oncology* 1991;48(3):239.
11 Wilson JD, et al. *Harrison's Principles of Internal Medicine.* New York, NY: McGraw-Hill, Inc., 1991.
12 Mathews-Roth MM. Reply to V. Herbert. *Am J Clin Nutr* (letter) 1991;53(2):573.
13 Mathews-Roth MM. Plasma concentrations of carotenoids after large doses of β-carotene. *Am J Clin Nutr* 1990;52(3):500.
14 Rock GA, et al. Orange plasma from tanning capsules. *Lancet* (letter) 1981;1:1419.
15 Mathews-Roth MM. Amenorrhea associated with carotenemia. *JAMA* (letter) 1983;250:731.
16 Rousseau A. Canthaxanthine deposits in the eye. *J Am Acad Dermatol* (letter) 1983;8(1):123.
17 Bluhm R, et al. Aplastic anemia associated with canthaxanthin ingested for 'tanning' purposes. *JAMA* 1990;264(9):1141.

Tansy

SCIENTIFIC NAME(S): *Tanacetum vulgare* L. also referred to as *Chrysanthemum vulgare* (L.) Bernh. Family: Compositae

COMMON NAME(S): Tansy, scented fern, stinking willie, bitter buttons[1], parsley fern.[1] Not to be confused with other plants referred to as "tansy" such as the tansy ragworts (Senecio sp).

BOTANY: The tansy is a popular plant which grows throughout Europe, Canada, and the United States. This hardy, aromatic, perennial plant grows erect to about 3 feet. It has feathery, dark-green, narrow lance-shaped leaves that grow alternately around the stem. The top blooms as a dense cluster of small yellow flowers from July to October.[2] Patches of the plant may continue growing for years and the name tansy is said to be derived from the Greek word for immortality, "athanasia." Thought to impart immortality, the herb was used for embalming.

HISTORY: The tansy has been used extensively in traditional medicine and as a popular herb for centuries, this despite its recognized potential toxicity. The dried leaves are said to be an effective insect repellent. Extracts of the plant and the seeds have been used as a vermifuge, an emmenagogue (to bring on menses), and an antispasmodic. The leaves have been used to prepare teas and as a food flavoring. Extracts have been used in perfumery and are a source of green dye.

CHEMISTRY: Analysis of the composition of tansy plant extracts has found that a wide variety of genotypes of the plant exists, and these are distinguished by the varying composition of their essential oil. The herb contains about 0.2% to 0.6% of an essential oil. In some strains, the essential oil is composed almost exclusively of thujone, with a variety of minor sesquiterpene and flavone components present.[3] By contrast, some varieties of the plant are almost thujone-free;[4] in these plants, compounds such as artemisia ketone, chrysanthenyl acetate, beta-caryophyllene and germacrene-D account for the major components of the oil.[5]

PHARMACOLOGY: There is little evidence to support the use of tansy for any pharmacologic indication. As with many other essential oils, tansy oil is said to be an antispasmodic.[2]

The oil has demonstrated some in vitro activity against gram-positive bacteria, but was not active against tested gram-negative strains;[6] however, the activity of the various phenotypes of the plant was determined by the relative chemical composition of the oil. Aqueous extracts of the plant partially inactivate tick-borne encephalitis virus in vitro, but have been found to induce resistance to the virus in infected mice.[7]

TOXICOLOGY: Ingestion of tansy and its extracts has been reported to cause serious systemic toxicity in animals and humans. As little as ten drops of the oil may be lethal, but recovery has been reported after ingestion of one-half fluid ounce.[4,8] The tea has also been fatal.[8] Thujone is likely responsible for much of the toxicity associated with the plant. Symptoms of internal tansy poisoning include rapid and feeble pulse, severe gastritis, violent spasms, and convulsions; gastric lavage or emesis has been suggested followed by symptomatic treatment.[9]

Tansy has also been associated with the development of often severe dermatitis following contact with the plant or extracts. An allergic contact dermatitis may be due to the presence of allergenic sesquiterpene lactones, arbusculin-A and tanacetin.[4] This dermatitis has been recognized as an occupational hazard among individuals working with cultivated chrysanthemums and tansy.[10] A cross-allergenicity with other members of the Family Compositae (eg, arnica, sunflower, yarrow) may occur in some individuals.

SUMMARY: Tansy is a common plant having no role in herbal medicine. Although used as an antispasmodic and vermifuge, the potential toxicity of the plant outweighs its benefits. Some strains of the plant contain the toxic component thujone. Allergic dermatitis is common with this plant. While the plant has been used to prepare teas and to flavor foods, its use should be discouraged.

PATIENT INFORMATION – Tansy

Uses: Although tansy has no role in herbal medicine, it has been used as an antispasmodic and vermifuge.

Side Effects: Because of the toxicity of the plant, tansy may cause allergic dermatitis and internal poisoning with symptoms of rapid and feeble pulse, severe gastritis, violent spasms, and convulsions.

[1] Meyer JE. *The Herbalist.* Hammond, IN: Hammond Book Co., 1934.

[2] Dobelis IN, ed. *Magic and Medicine of Plants.* Pleasantville, NY: Reader's Digest Association, 1986.

[3] Gallino M. Essential oil from *Tanacetum vulgare* growing spontaneously in "Tierra del Fuego" (Argentina). *Planta Medica* 1988;54:182.

[4] Duke JA. *Handbook of Medicinal Herbs.* Boca Raton, FL: CRC Press, 1985.

[5] Hendricks H, et al. The essential oil of *Tanacetum vulgare. Planta Medica* 1989;55:212.

[6] Holopainen M, Kaupinnen V. Antimicrobial activity of different chemotypes of Finnish tansy. *Planta Medica* 1989;55:102.

[7] Fokina GI, et al. Experimental phytotherapy of tick-borne encephalitis. *Vopr Virusol* 1991;36(1):18.

[8] Osol A, Farrar GE Jr., eds. The Dispensatory of the United States of America, ed. 25. Philadelphia, PA: J.B. Lippincott, 1955.

[9] Hardin JW, Arena JM. *Human Poisoning from Native and Cultivated Plants.* Durham, NC: Duke University Press, 1974.

[10] Hausen BM, Oestmann G. The incidence of occupationally-induced allergic skin diseases in a large flower market. *Occupational & Environmental Dermatoses* 1988;36(4):117.

Tea Tree Oil

SCIENTIFIC NAME(S): *Melaleuca alternifolia* (Cheel)

COMMON NAME(S): Tea tree oil

BOTANY: There are many plants known as "tea trees," but species *melaleuca alternifolia* is responsible for the "tea tree oil," which has recently gained popularity. Native to Australia, the tea tree is found in coastal areas. It is an evergreen shrub that can grow to 6 meters tall. Its narrow, 4 cm, "needle-like" leaves release a distinctive aroma when crushed. The fruits grow in clusters, and its white flowers bloom in the summer.[1]

Other related species include *M. quinquenervia* (Cav.) S.T. Blake (*M. viridiflora* sol.) from the Caledonian evergreen tree yielding "niaouli oil" and *M. leucaden* L. and *M. cajuputi* Powell (= *M. minor* sm.) yielding "oil of cajuput." These oils contain similar constituents resembling camphor and peppermint and are used in aromatherapy.[2,3]

HISTORY: Tea tree oil (TTO) was first used in surgery and dentistry in the mid-1920s. Its healing properties were also used during World War II for skin injuries to those working in munition factories. Tea tree oil's popularity has resurfaced within the last few years with help from promotional campaigns and may be present in soaps, shampoos, and lotions.[1]

CHEMISTRY: The essential oil is normally obtained by steam distillation of the leaves.[2] The main constituent is tea tree's essential oil, terpin-4-ol, present in concentrations of 40% or more.[1,2] The related species contain eucalyptol, cineole, nerolidol, viridiflorol, or phenylpropanoids.[2,3] Listings of chemical compositions of tea tree oils have been reported.[4,5] An essential oil overview, use and purity issues are also available on this topic.[6]

PHARMACOLOGY: Tea tree oil has been used mainly for its **antimicrobial** effects without irritating sensitive tissues. It has been applied to cuts, stings, acne, and burns. In hospitals, TTO has been used in soap form and soaked in blankets to make an **antibacterial** covering for burn victims. When run through air-conditioning ducts, TTO has been shown to exert bactericidal effects.[1] A considerable amount of literature has become available on this topic.

Disc diffusion and broth microdilution methods have been used to determine antimicrobial effects against eight TTO constituents. Terpin-4-ol was active against all test organisms including *Candida albicans*, *Escherichia coli*, *Staphylococcus aureus* and *Pseudomonas aeruginosa*. Other constituents of the oil (such as linalool and alpha-terpineol) had some antimicrobial activity as well.[7,8] In addition, constituents terpin-4-ol, alpha-terpineol, and alpha-pinene were found to possess antimicrobial effects against *Staphylococcus epidermidis* and *Propionibacterium acnes*.[9]

TTO may be useful in removing "transient skin flora while suppressing but maintaining resident flora."[10] TTO was also shown to be an effective topical treatment of monilial and fungal dermatoses and superficial skin infections in 50 human subjects over a 6-month period with minimal or no side effects reported.[11] A report suggests TTO to be useful in treatment of "methicillin-resistant *S. aureus* (MRSA) carriage." In this evaluation, all 66 isolates of *S. aureus* were susceptible to the essential oil (64 isolates being MRSA, 33 being mupirocin-resistant).[12]

TTO's activity against anaerobic oral bacteria has been surveyed.[13] A case report exists, discussing antibacterial efficacy of TTO in a 40-year-old woman with anaerobic vaginosis.[14]

In a randomized, double-blind study comparing the efficacy of 10% (w/w) tea tree oil cream with 1% tolnaftate (and placebo creams) against **tinea pedis** (athlete's foot), TTO was found to be as effective as tolnaftate in reducing symptoms but no more effective than placebo in achieving mycological cure.[15] In a report on **onychomycosis** (nail fungus), TTO (100%) vs clotrimazole solution (1%) application yielded similar results in treatment. Both therapies, however, had high recurrence rates.[16]

TTO can be added to baths or vaporizers to help treat **respiratory disorders**. Related species oil has been used for **nasal antiseptic** purposes, **pulmonary anti-inflammatory** use, and for **coughs**.[1,2,3] TTO is also used in **perfumery** and **aromatherapy**.[2]

TOXICOLOGY: Allergic contact eczema was found to be caused primarily by the α-limonene constituent (in TTO) in 7 patients tested. In this same report, alpha-terpinene and aromadendrene additionally caused dermatitis in 5 of the patients.[17] Eucalyptol was found to be the contact allergan in a Dutch report.[18] Contact allergy due to TTO may be related to cross-sensitization to colophony.[19] A case report describes a petechial body rash and marked neutrophil leukocytosis in a 60–year-old man who ingested ± ½ teaspoonful of the oil (for common cold symptoms). He recovered 1 week later.[20]

TTO in comparison to conifer resin acids was found to exhibit no cytotoxic activity in vitro using human epithelial and fibroblast cells.[21]

Another case report describes ataxia and drowsiness as a result of oral TTO ingestion (< 10 ml) by a 17-month-old male. He was treated with activated charcoal, which was only paritally successful, but after a short time appeared normal and was discharged 7 hours after ingestion.[22]

Various additional reports on TTO toxicity can be referenced.[23,24,25]

SUMMARY: Tea tree oil from species *Melaleuca alternifolia* native to Australia has recently gained popularity. Since the mid-1920s, its remarkable healing properties have been known. TTO's antimicrobial effects have been well documented, and its therapeutic use has been beneficial for skin infection treatment, respiratory disorders, and aromatherapy. Possibility of contact dermatitis exists. Do not ingest the oil. Adverse effects have been reported.

PATIENT INFORMATION – Tea Tree Oil

Uses: Tea tree oil has been used mainly for its antimicrobial effects. TTO should be applied topically. Do not ingest orally.

Side Effects: Use of tea tree oil has resulted in allergic contact eczema and dermatitis.

---

[1] Low T, et al. (contributing editors). Reader's Digest (Aust) Magic and Medicines of Plants. Surry Hills, NSW, 2010 Australia: PTY Limited 1994;349.
[2] Bruneton J. *Medicinal Plants*. Seacaus, NY: Lavoisier Publ. Inc. 1995;461.
[3] Osol et al, eds. The Dispensatory of the United States of America. Philadelphia, PA: J.B. Lippincott Co. 1960;1750.
[4] Altman, P. *Aust J Pharm* 1988 Apr;69:276-78.
[5] Lawrence B. *Perfumer and Flavorist* 1990 May-Jun;15:63-69.
[6] "Anon." *Manufacturing Chemist* 1993 Mar;64:20–21,23.
[7] Carson C, et al. *J Appl Bacteriol* 1995;78(3):264–69.
[8] Carson C, et al. *Microbios* 1995;82(332):181–85.
[9] Raman A, et al. *Letters in Applied Microbiology* 1995;21(4):242–45.
[10] Hammer K, et al. *Am J Infect Control* 1996;24(3):186-89.
[11] Shemesh A, et al. *Aust J Pharm* 1991 Sep;72:802-3.
[12] Carson C, et al. *J Antimicrob Chemother* 1995;35(3):421-24.
[13] Shapiro S, et al. *Oral Microbiology and Immunology* 1994;9(4):202-8.
[14] Blackwell A. *Lancet* 1991;337(Feb 2):300.
[15] Tong M, et al. *Australas J Dermatol* 1992;33(3):145-49.
[16] Buck D, et al. *J F Pract* 1994;38(6):601-5.
[17] Knight T, et al. *J Am Acad Dermatol* 1994;30(3):423-27.
[18] Van der Valk P, et al. *Ned Tijdschr Geneeskd* 1994;138(16):823-25.
[19] Selvaag E, et al. *Contact Dermatitis* 1994;31(2):124–25.
[20] Elliott C. *Med J Aust* 1993 Dec 6;159:830-31.
[21] Soderberg T, et al. *Toxicology* 1996;107(2):99-109.
[22] Del Beccaro M. *Vet Hum Toxicol* 1995;37(6):557–58.
[23] de Groot A, et al. *Contact Dermatitis* 1993;28(5):309.
[24] Moss A. *Med J Aust* 1994;160(4):236.
[25] Carson, et al. *J Toxicol Clin Toxicol* 1995;33(2):193-94.

Terminalia

SCIENTIFIC NAME(S): *Terminalia arjuna*, *Terminalia bellirica* (*T. belerica*), *Terminalia chebula*.

COMMON NAME(S): Arjuna, Axjun, Argun (T. arjuna); Behada, Bahera (Bahira), Balera (T. belerica); Hara, Harada, Hirala, Myrobalan, Haritaki (T. chebula); Bala harade (T. chebula black variety). Family: Combretaceae.[1,2,3,4,5]

BOTANY: The *Terminalia* species are evergreen trees. *T. arjuna* reaches ≈ 30 meters, has light-yellow flowers, and cone-shaped leaves. *T. belerica* has clustered oval leaves, and greenish, foul-smelling flowers with brown, hairy fruit about the size of walnuts. *T. chebula* grows ≈ 21 meters in height with white flowers and small, ribbed fruits.[2]

T. arjuna is used for its bark. In other *Terminalia* species, the fruit is the plant part used.[1] For example, in India, 100,000 metric tons of *T. chebula* fruit was produced in 1 year.[6]

A traditional Ayurvedic herbal combination dating back 5000 years is a mixture of 3 herbs, 2 of which are terminalia species: *T. belerica* (for health-harmonizing qualities), *T. chebula* (to normalize body balance), and *Emblica officinalis* (for vitamin C content; see separate monograph).[3]

HISTORY: Arjuna bark has been used in Indian medicine for at least 3000 years as a remedy for heart ailments. *T. chebula* also has been used by this culture as a digestive aid.[2] This species, referred to as "King of Medicine" by Tibetans is often depicted in the extended palm of Buddha. The *Emblica officinalis /T. chebula /T. belerica* herbal combination product is said to have been formulated by Ayurvedic physicians thousands of years ago.[3]

CHEMISTRY: *T. chebula* contains tannins, anthraquinones, chebulic acid, resin, and fixed oil.[2] Other constituents include amino acids, fructose, succinic acid, and beta sitosterol.[3] This specific species is an important source for industrial tannins.[6] One source lists *T. chebula* as having 32% tannin content.[1]

T. arjuna contains tannins, flavonoids, and sterols. *T. belerica* contains tannins and anthraquinones.[2] Gallic acid also has been isolated from this species.[7]

PHARMACOLOGY: Some similarity in pharmacologic actions exist among the 3 species. *T. arjuna's* traditional use as a cardiotonic has been confirmed by modern research. Although some results of these studies (performed since the 1930s) appear conflicting, (eg, increases and decreases in heart rate or blood pressure), the herb seems to work best when blood supply to the heart is compromised as in ischemic heart disease or angina.[2] Ayurvedic medicine employs *T. arjuna* to restore balance of the "3 humors."[3] *T. arjuna* also has been used as an aphrodisiac, diuretic, and for earaches.[1,2] This species has reduced cholesterol levels, as well.[2] Studies done on *T. arjuna* combinations find the herb to be the most potent hypolipidemic agent compared with *T. belerica* and *T. chebula*. *T. arjuna* may also play a role as an anti-atherogenic.[8]

T. belerica has been studied for its effects on similar disease states. In combination with *E. officinalis* and *T. chebula*, *T. belerica* has reduced cholesterol-induced atherosclerosis in rabbits.[5] In another report, *T. belerica* reduced lipid levels in hypercholesterolemic animals.[9] The herb has also exhibited protective effects against myocardial necrosis in rats.[10] *T. belerica's* role in treating liver disorders is also apparent.[1] Constituent gallic acid displays significant hepatoprotective effects. Marked reversal of most altered parameters was shown including lipid peroxidation, drug metabolizing enzymes, and others.[7] *T. belerica* has also been used as primary treatment for digestive and respiratory (eg, cough, sore throat) problems.[2] Other uses include the following: As an astringent, laxative,[2,11] lotion for sore eyes,[2] and retroviral reverse transcriptase inhibitory activity in murine leukemia enzymes.[12]

T. chebula is used in Indian medicine to treat digestive problems. It improves bowel regularity, thus making it possibly useful as a laxative and to treat diarrhea and dysentery.[1,2] Other uses include as a mouthwash/gargle, astringent, and douche for vaginitis.[2]

T. chebula and *T. belerica* have demonstrated antimicrobial properties.[13,14] *T. chebula* has also been evaluated for activity against methicillin-resistant *Staphylococcus aureus*.[15]

Certain *Terminalia* species demonstrate antifungal[16] and antiviral[17,18,19,20] activities, as well.

TOXICOLOGY: Few reports were found from recent literature searches regarding *Terminalia* species and toxicity. One source warns against taking *T. belerica* and *T. chebula* during pregnancy.[2]

SUMMARY: *Terminalia* species have been used in Indian medicine for thousands of years. Certain species are used for cardiac effects, anti-atherogenic and hypolipidemic actions, hepatoprotection, GI problems, and as antimicrobials. Little information on toxicity is available.

PATIENT INFORMATION – Terminalia

Uses: *T. arjuna's* traditional use as a cardiotonic has been confirmed by modern research. It has also been used as an aphrodisiac, diuretic, and for earaches,[1,2] it may play a role as an anti-atherogenic,[8] and has reduced cholesterol. *T. belerica* has been used in treating liver disorder[1] and as a primary treatment for digestive and respiratory (eg, cough, sore throat) problems.[2] Other uses include the following: As an astringent, laxative,[2,11] lotion for sore eyes,[2] and retroviral reverse transcriptase inhibitory activity in murine leukemia enzymes[12] *T. chebula* is used in Indian medicine to treat digestive problems. Other uses include as a mouthwash/gargle, astringent, and douche for vaginitis.[2] *T. chebula* and *T. belerica* have demonstrated antimicrobial properties.[13,14] Certain *Terminalia* species demonstrate antifungal[16] and antiviral[17,18,19,20] activities.

Side Effects: Few toxicity reports exist; do not use during pregnancy.

---

[1] Evans W. *Trease and Evans' Pharmacognosy*, 14th ed. WB Saunders Co. Ltd, 1996;493.

[2] Chevallier A. *Encyclopedia of Medicinal Plants*. New York, NY: DK Publishing, 1996;141,273.

[3] Khorana M, et al. *Indian J Pharm* 1959;21:331.

[4] Rukmini C, et al. Chemical and nutritional studies on *Terminalia chebula* Retz. *J Am Oil Chem Soc* 1986;63(3):360-63.

[5] Thakur C, et al. The Ayurvedic medicines Haritaki, Amala, and Bahira reduce cholesterol-induced atherosclerosis in rabbits. *Int J Cardiol* 1988;21(2):167-75.

[6] Bruneton J. *Pharmacognosy, Phytochemistry, Medicinal Plants*. Paris, France: Lavoisier Publishing, 1995;333.

[7] Anand K, et al. 3,4,5-Trihydroxy benzoic acid (gallic acid), the hepatoprotective principle in the fruits of *Terminalia belerica* -bioassay guided activity. *Pharmacol Res* 1997;36(4):315-21.

[8] Shaila H, et al. Hypolipidemic activity of three indigenous drugs in experimentally induced atherosclerosis. *Int J Cardiol* 1998;67(2):119-24.

[9] Shaila H, et al. Preventive actions of *Terminalia belerica* in experimentally induced atherosclerosis. *Int J Cardiol* 1995;49(2):101-06.

[10] Tariq M, et al. Protective effect of fruit extracts of *Emblica officinalis* (Gaertn.) and *Terminalia belerica* (Roxb.) in experimental myocardial necrosis in rats. *Indian J Exp Biol* 1997;15(6):485-86.

[11] Dhar H, et al. Studies on purgative action of an oil obtained from *Terminalia berlerica*. *Indian J Med Res* 1969;57(1):103-05.

[12] Suthienkul O, et al. Retroviral reverse transcriptase inhibitory activity in Thai herbs and spices: Screening with Moloney murine leukemia viral enzyme. *Southeast Asian J Trop Med Public Health* 1993;24(4):751-55.

[13] Ahmad I, et al. Screening of some Indian medicinal plants for their antimicrobial properties. *J Ethnopharmacol* 1998;62(2):183-93.

[14] Phadke S, et al. Screening of in vitro antibacterial activity of *Terminalia chebula*, *Eclapta alba*, and *Ocimum sanctum*. *Indian J Med Sci* 1989;43(5):113-17.

[15] Sato Y, et al. Extraction and purification of effective antimicrobial constituents of *Terminalia chebula* RETS against methicillin-resistant *Staphylococcus aureus*. *Biol Pharm Bull* 1997;20(4):401-04.

[16] Dutta B, et al. Antifungal activity of Indian plant extracts. *Mycoses* 1998;41(11-12):535-36.

[17] Shiraki K, et al. Cytomegalovirus infection and its possible treatment with herbal medicines. *Nippon Rinsho* 1998;56(1):156-60.

[18] Yukawa T, et al. Prophylactic treatment of cytomegalovirus infection with traditional herbs. *Antiviral Res* 1996;32(2):63-70.

[19] Kurokawa M, et al. Efficacy of traditional herbal medicines in combination with acyclovir against herpes simplex virus type I infection in vitro and in vivo. *Antiviral Res* 1995;27(1-2):19-37.

[20] el-Mekkawy S, et al. Inhibitory effects of Egyptian folk medicines on human immunodeficiency virus (HIV) reverse transcriptase. *Chem Pharm Bull* 1995;43(4):641-48.

Thunder God Vine

SCIENTIFIC NAME(S): *Tripterygium wilfordii* Hook.

COMMON NAME(S): Lei-kung t'eng, lei gong teng (Chinese), thunder god vine, huang-t'eng ken (yellow vine root), tsao-ho-hua (early rice flower)

BOTANY: *Tripterygium* is a perennial twining vine that grows in southern China, usually close to water sources. It is native to the Hunan province. It has reddish-brown branches with oval leaves. In the summer, small white terminal flowers bloom.[1]

HISTORY: The thunder god vine has been used for centuries in traditional Chinese medicine to treat fever, boils, abscesses, and inflammation. It has also been put to use as an insecticide to kill maggots or larvae and as a rat and bird poison.[1]

CHEMISTRY: Triterpene compounds (eg, tripterygone) have been isolated from thunder god vine roots.[2] Also found in the plant's roots are diterpenoid triepoxices, triptolide, and tripdiolide.[3] A new diterpene triepoxide, 16-hydroxytriptolide, has been isolated from the leaves of the plant.[4] A nortriterpenoid has also been isolated.[5] An anti-HIV constituent, neotripteriferdin, has been recently identified.[6] Six diterpene epoxides have been identified, and listed as triptolide, tripdiolide, triptolidenol, tripchlorolide, 16-hydroxytriptolide, and one other unpublished structure.[7]

PHARMACOLOGY: Pharmacology of thunder god vine includes reports in the areas of **antifertility**, **autoimmune disease**, **antiviral**, **antitumor**, and other effects.

Antifertility: During the late 1980s and early 1990s, human studies evaluating thunder god vine for rheumatoid arthritis and psoriasis treatment revealed an unexpected side effect in male subjects. It was discovered that thunder god vine had reversible effects on sperm, producing fewer of them and making them less mobile. This suggested the plant's use as a possible "male antifertility" drug.[1] A number of thunder god vine constituents are responsible for these potent antifertility actions, including triptolide and tripdiolide.[8] One report suggests 6 compounds of the plant to show antifertility effect in mice.[9] A later report confirms the 6 antifertility compounds in both rats and man. These compounds act primarily on sperm development (eg, sperm head-tail separation), other than affecting testosterone levels.[1,7] Fertility is reversible after termination of thunder god vine preparations. Sperm returned to normal 6 weeks later.[7] A review of thunder god vine's fertility regulatory effects is available.[10]

The effective antifertility dose is 1/3 the recommended dose for treatment of arthritis or skin diseases, which may be associated with less adverse effects when thunder god vine is taken for antifertility.[10]

One report compared 1 thunder god vine constituent to gossypol, finding inhibition of spermatogenesis, "turnover of basic nuclear protein in late elongated spermatids" and head-tail separation (among other antifertility effects) to be more pronounced in the thunder god vine constituent than in gossypol.[11]

Autoimmune disease: Thunder god vine has been reported to be effective in treating autoimmune diseases in in vitro models and in animal and human studies.

In vitro, immunosuppressive activity was shown to be caused by the constituents tripchlorolide and tribromolide.[12] Another report analyzes T2 (a chloroform methanol extract of the plant) and an ethyl acetate extract, both of which contained triptolide and tripdiolide as the major immunosuppressive diterpenoids.[13] A new immunosuppressive component has been determined and was found to be phenolic nortriterpene demethylzeylasteral.[14]

n vitro analysis indicates thunder god vine to inhibit transcription of cytokine genes IL2 and gamma interferon.[15] The plant is also capable of inhibiting several other immune functions in vitro, including response of human mononuclear cells and generation of cytotoxic T-cells.[16] Another report measures ability of thunder god vine to affect cytokine secretion from monocytes or T-cells, prostaglandin E2 secretion from monocytes and other parameters of immune response. Results confirmed powerful suppressive effects in vitro, suggesting its use in rheumatic disease.[17] A similar study examining the mechanism of thunder god vine's effectiveness in rheumatoid arthritis isolates human peripheral blood mononuclear cells, then separates them into monocytes, T-cells, and B-cells. Thunder god vine alcoholic extract inhibited T-cell and B-cell proliferation, IL2 production by T-cells, and immunoglobulin production by B-cells.[18] Peripheral blood mononuclear cells from rheumatoid arthritic patients and control patients were studied for effects of thunder god vine polyglycosides. The thunder god vine preparation was found to act on both monocytes and lymphocytes, again confirming the immunosuppressive activity of the plant.[19]

In mice, thunder god vine isolate triterene inhibited antibody response and inhibited granuloma growth in rats.[20] Also in rodents, results of another report indicated six diterpenes (triptolide, tripchlorolide, triptonide, tripdiolide, triptolidenol, and 16–hydroxytriptolide) all to possess anti-inflammatory and immunosuppressive actions in vivo. The constituent triptriolide had anti-inflammatory activity only.[21] A thunder god vine isolate in different concentrations was studied for its anti-inflammatory effects. It markedly inhibited increased vascular permeability in mice, inhibited hind paw edema and also inhibited proliferation of granuloma, suggesting the isolate's ability to stimulate pituitary-adrenal axis.[22] In another report, it was suggested that the suppressive effect of thunder god vine may be mediated by substance P, when studied in rat spinal dorsal horn.[23]

Human clinical trials evaluating the beneficial effects of thunder god vine preparations to treat autoimmune diseases are very promising. An analysis of 165 cases of thunder god vine's actions on rheumatoid arthritis is available.[24] Later reports confirm the plant's efficacy, as well. In a prospective, controlled double-blind crossover study in 70 rheumatoid arthritis patients, polyglycoside constituent "T2" from thunder god vine had "impressive, curative effects."[25] Multi-glycosides of TGV, 30 mg/day, in 32 rheumatoid arthritis patients, resulted in "significant improvements in clinical and laboratory variables."[26] Oral tablets containing thunder god vine had obvious "anti-inflammatory, analgesia and immunosuppressive actions" in both standard and sustained release forms, when evaluated in a 226-patient, prospective, multi-center study.[27]

Antiviral: Neotripterifordin has been found to show potent anti-HIV replication activity in vitro.[6,28] Triptofordin C-2 and other sesquiterpene components of thunder god vine, have been evaluated for their antiviral activity including human cytomegalovirus.[29]

Antitumor: It has been demonstrated that low doses of the diterpene triptolide isolate from thunder god vine possesses antileukemic activities in rodents[30] Additionally, it shows marked antitumor activity in mice.[30,31] Demethylzeylasteral (a nortriterpenoid isolate of thunder god vine) inhibits proliferation of vascular endothelial cells 30 times more effectively than for the proliferation of human tumor cells, suggesting the isolate to be useful in treating highly vascularized and metastatic tumors.[5] Effects of thunder god vine on tumor necrosis factor have been reported.[32]

Other: Other effects studied on thunder god vine include therapeutic actions in 12 cases of menorrhagia[33] and as treatment for multiple sclerosis.[34] A review is available on clinical uses of thunder god vine.[35]

TOXICOLOGY: The triptolide constituent of thunder god vine exhibited non-specific cytotoxicity in cultured mammalian cell lines. Treatments of 50 mcg/mouse 3 times weekly in one preparation were lethal.[30]

Gastrointestinal upset, infertility and suppression of lymphocyte proliferation are the usual side effects of thunder god vine.[36] Rash symptoms and alimentary canal incidences were experienced in one report, more so with a higher dose of the drug than with a lower dose.[26] Similarly, adverse reactions from a sustained release formulation of thunder god vine was approximately 20% in 226 rheumatoid arthritis patients, as opposed to a 70% side effect rate from standard release tablets.[27]

Fourteen female rheumatoid arthritis patients developed amenorrhea after treatment with "T2" (thunder god vine constituent), suggesting its site of action to be the ovary. These effects were reversible after discontinuation of the drug.[37]

Little information about lethal toxicities has been reported; however, one case report describes an incidence of death (in a seemingly young and healthy male) 3 days post-ingestion of the drug. Later investigation found some incidence of coexisting cardiac damage. Prior to death, the patient experienced profuse vomiting, diarrhea, leukopenia, renal failure, hypotension, and shock.[36]

SUMMARY: The thunder god vine has been used in ancient Chinese medicine for centuries. Most studies evaluate its role in autoimmune diseases such as arthritis, but recently its antifertility effects in men have been of interest. The plant also possesses antiviral and antitumor actions. Side effects of the drug include GI upset and lymphocyte proliferation. Amenorrhea and at least one death have been reported from ingestion.

PATIENT INFORMATION – Thunder God Vine

Uses: Thunder god vine has antifertility properties. In clinical trials it has been effective in treating autoimmune disease. Thunder god vine has shown antiviral and antitumor activity.

Side Effects: Side effects include gastrointestinal upset, infertility suppression of white blood cells, amenorrhea, and one incidence of death.

---

[1] Jones C. *Herbs for Health* 1998 Jan/Feb:25.
[2] Zhang D, et al. *Yao Hsueh Hsueh Pao* 1991;26(5):341–44.
[3] Gu W, et al. *Int J Immunopharmacol* 1995;17(5):351–56.
[4] Ma P, et al. *Yao Hsueh Hsueh Pao* 1991;26(10):759–63.
[5] Ushiro S, et al. *Int J Cancer* 1997;72(4):657–63.
[6] Chen K, et al. *Bioorg Med Chem* 1995;3(10):1345–48.
[7] Zhen Q, et al. *Contraception* 1995;51(2):121–29.
[8] Matlin S, et al. *Contraception* 1993;47(4):387–400.
[9] Zheng J. *Chung Kuo I Hsueh Ko Hsueh Yuan Hsueh Pao* 1991;13(6):398–403.
[10] Qian S. *Contraception* 1987;36(3):335–45.
[11] Lu Q. *Chung Kuo I Hsueh Ko Hsueh Yuan Hsueh Pao* 1990;12(6):440–44.
[12] Yu D, et al. *Yao Hsueh Hsueh Pao* 1992;27(11):830–36.
[13] Tao X, et al. *J Pharmacol Exp Ther* 1995;272(3):1305–12.
[14] Tamaki T, et al. *Transplant Proc* 1996;28(3):1379–80.
[15] Lipsky P, et al. *Semin Arthritis Rheum* 1997;26(5):713–23.
[16] Li X, et al. *Transplantation* 1990;50(1):82–86.
[17] Chang D, et al. *J Rheumatol* 1997;24(3):436–41.
[18] Tao X, et al. *Arthritis Rheum* 1991;34(10):1274–81.
[19] Ye W. *Chung Kuo I Hsueh Ko Hsueh Yuan Hsueh Pao* 1990;12(3):217–22.
[20] Zhang L, et al. *Yao Hsueh Hsueh Pao* 1990;25(8):573–77.

[21] Zheng J. *Chung Kuo I Hsueh Ko Hsueh Yuan Hsueh Pao* 1991;13(6):391–97.
[22] Zheng Y, et al. *Chung Kuo Yao Li Hsueh Pao* 1994;15(6):540–43.
[23] Liu Y, et al. *Chung Kuo I Hsueh Ko Hsueh Yuan Hsueh Pao* 1995;17(4):269–73.
[24] Yan B. *Chung Hsi I Chieh Ho Tsa Chih* 1985;5(5):280–83.
[25] Tao X, et al. *Chin Med J* 1989;102(5):327–32.
[26] Tao X, et al. *Chung Hsi I Chieh Ho Tsa Chih* 1990;10(5):289–91.
[27] Li R, et al. *Chung Kuo Chung Hsi I Chieh Ho Tsa Chih* 1996;16(1):10–13.
[28] Chen K, et al. *J Nat Prod* 1992;55(1):88–92.
[29] Hayashi K, et al. *J Antimicrob Chemother* 1996;37(4):759–68.
[30] Shamon L, et al. *Cancer Lett* 1997;112(1):113–17.
[31] Xu J, et al. *Chung Kuo Chung Hsi I Chieh Ho Tsa Chih* 1992;12(3):161–64.
[32] Zeng X, et al. *Chung Kuo I Hsueh Ko Hsueh Yuan Hsueh Pao* 1996;18(2):138–42.
[33] Shu H, et al. *J Tradit Chin Med* 1984;4(3):237–40.
[34] Sun J. *Chung Hsi I Chieh Ho Tsa Chih* 1988;8(2):87–89.
[35] Chu W. *Chung Hsi I Chieh Ho Tsa Chih* 1988;8(7):443–45.
[36] Chou W, et al. *Int J Cardiol* 1995;49(2):173–77.
[37] Gu C. *Chung Kuo I Hsueh Ko Hsueh Yuan Hsueh Pao* 1989;11(2):151–53.

Tolu Balsam

SCIENTIFIC NAME(S): Derived from *Toluifera balsamum* L. which is synonymous with *Myroxylon toluiferum* HBK and *M. balsamamum* (L.) Harms. Family: Leguminosae[1,2,3]

COMMON NAME(S): Opobalsam, resin tolu, Thomas balsam, tolu balsam,[3] balsamum tolutanum, balsam of Tolu, resina tolutana

BOTANY: *T. balsamum* is a tall tree native to South America and grows abundantly on the high plains and mountains of Venezuela, Columbia, and Peru. It is also cultivated in the West Indies. The balsam is collected from incisions made in the tree trunk. The tree differs little from that yielding Balsam of Peru.[4]

HISTORY: Tolu balsam has been used for centuries as a fragrance in perfumes, candies, and chewing gums. Today, it remains in use in pharmaceutical preparations, in the form of a syrup, as an expectorant and as a fragrant vehicle for other compounds.[1,2] It is an ingredient in compound benzoin tincture[2] that is used for the treatment of bedsores, cracked skin, and minor cuts. It has been reported to have been used in the folk treatment of cancer.[3]

CHEMISTRY: Tolu balsam is a yellow-brown semifluid or near solid material with an aromatic vanilla-like odor and taste. On drying it becomes hard and brittle. It is insoluble in water but soluble in pharmaceutical solvents such as alcohol, ether, sodium hydroxide solution, and chloro-form. The balsam contains up to 80% resin, approximately 15% free cinnamic acid and benzoic acid, and about 40% of the benzyl and related esters of these free acids. A volatile oil is present in small amounts (from 1.5% to 7%)[1,2] as is a small amount of vanillin (0.05%).[2] A wide variety of additional minor components have been identified in the balsam.[5] The concentrations of these components vary widely in commercial products because of a lack of international standards for tolu balsam.[3]

PHARMACOLOGY: Tolu balsam has mild antiseptic and expectorant properties.[3]

TOXICOLOGY: Allergic reactions to tolu balsam have been reported to occur in some individuals.[3]

SUMMARY: Tolu balsam is an aromatic plant extract that finds widespread use as a fragrance and in flavoring pharmaceutical products. It is not generally used for any unique pharmacologic action, although it is a component of compound tincture of benzoin, which is used to speed wound healing.

PATIENT INFORMATION – Tolu Balsam

Uses: Tolu balsam is most known for its fragrance and flavoring in pharmaceutical products, although it does have mild antiseptic and expectorant properties.

Side Effects: Allergic reactions have been reported in conjunction with tolu balsam.

---

[1] Windholz M, ed. *The Merck Index*, 10th edition. Rahway NJ: Merck and Co., 1983.
[2] Hoover JE, ed. *Remington's Pharmaceutical Sciences*, 145th edition. Easton, PA: Mack Publishing Co., 1970.
[3] Leung AY. *Encyclopedia of Common Natural Ingredients Used in Food, Drugs and Cosmetics*. New York, NY: J. Wiley and Sons, 1980.
[4] Evans WC. *Trease and Evans' Pharmacognosy*. 13th ed. London: Balliere Tindall, 1989.
[5] Wahlberg I, Enzell CR. 20R, 24 epsilon-2–ocotillone, a triterpenoid from commercial tolu balsam. *Acta Chem Scand* 1970;25:352.
[6] Osol A, Farrar GE Jr, eds. The Dispensatory of the United States of America. 25th ed. Philadelphia: JB Lippincott, 1955:1439.

Tonka Bean

SCIENTIFIC NAME(S): *Dipteryx odorata* (Aubl.) Willd. Also *D. oppositifolia* may be used. Family: Fabaceae (Leguminosae)

COMMON NAME(S): Tonka bean, tonga bean, tongo bean, tonco seed, tonquin bean, torquin bean, cumaru, tonco bean

BOTANY: Members of the genus *Dipteryx* are native to South America (Venezuela, Guyana, and Brazil), and are typically large trees bearing single-seeded fruits about 3 to 5 cm in length. The fruit is dried with the seed removed. If not processed further, the fruit is known as "black beans." The beans are macerated in rum and then air-dried. This treatment results in the formation of a crystalline deposit of coumarin and the seeds appear to be frosted.

Tonka beans are rounded at one end and bluntly pointed at the other. The bean is black and deeply wrinkled longitudinally. The bean has a very fragrant odor and an aromatic, bitter taste.[1]

HISTORY: Tonka beans contain the chemical coumarin. Coumarin is used in the food, cosmetic and related industries to impart a pleasant fragrance to cakes, preserves, tobacco, soaps and liqueurs.[2,3] The seeds are sometimes cured in rum.[4] However, according to the FDA Code of Federal Regulations Section 189.130, food containing any coumarin as a constituent of tonka beans or tonka extracts is deemed to be impure.[5] Synthetic coumarin has, to some extent, replaced the natural product.

South American natives mix the seed paste with milk to make a thick nutty flavored beverage. Extracts of the plant have been used in traditional medicine to treat cramps and nausea, as well as a tonic. Seed extracts are administered rectally for schistosomiasis in China. The fruit has been said to have aphrodisiac properties.

CHEMISTRY: Coumarin is present in 1% to 3% (by weight) of the fermented seed, but some strains may contain up to 10%.[2,3,6] Tonka beans also contain 25% fat (containing unsaponifiable sitosterin and stigmasterin)

and a larger amount of starch.[1] Coumarin has an odor reminiscent of vanillin. Umbelliferone (7–hydroxycoumarin) has been isolated from the seed. A number of related isoflavones have been isolated from the heartwood, including odoratin and dipteryxin. The bark exudes a resin that contains lupeol, betulin, and other minor components.

PHARMACOLOGY: There are no well-controlled studies describing the pharmacologic effects of Tonka beans or their components. As noted below, coumarin is toxic when ingested in high doses.

Synthetic coumarin has been developed to replace the natural product in some cases. A related compound, warfarin (eg, *Coumadin*) is a potent anticoagulant used in human therapeutics as well as rodenticides.[7,8] Further literature reviews from 1966–1995 yielded no new studies on Tonka bean.

TOXICOLOGY: Dietary feeding of coumarin to rats and dogs has been associated with extensive hepatic damage, growth retardation, and testicular atrophy.[2] It is said that large oral doses of the fluid extract can result in cardiac paralysis.[2] The LD50 (Oral) is 680 mg/kg in rats and 202 mg/kg in guinea pigs.[9]

SUMMARY: Tonka beans contain the chemical coumarin. Coumarin is used as a flavoring in foods and tobacco, as well as a fragrance in cosmetics. Coumarin is safe when ingested in normal food-level amounts, but may cause severe hepatic damage when ingested in large amounts. According to the FDA Code of Federal Regulations Section 189.130, food containing any coumarin as a constituent of tonka beans or tonka extracts is deemed to be impure.[5]

PATIENT INFORMATION – Tonka Bean

Uses: Tonka bean contains the element coumarin that is used as a flavoring in foods and tobacco, as well as a fragrance in cosmetics. Otherwise, tonka beans have no proven pharmacological effects.

Side Effects: If ingested in safe amounts, tonka beans do not have any potent side effects. When ingested in animals, ingredients in the tonka bean have caused severe hepatic damage, growth retardation, and testicular atrophy. Large doses of the fluid extract can result in cardiac paralysis.

---

[1] Evans WC. *Pharmacognosy.* London: Bailliere Tindall, 1989.

[2] Duke JA. *Handbook of Medicinal Herbs.* Boca Raton, FL: CRC Press, 1985.

[3] Lewis WH, Elvin-Lewis MPF. *Medical Botany.* Plants affecting man's health. New York: John Wiley & Sons, 1977.

[4] Mabberley DJ. *The Plant-Book.* Cambridge: Cambridge University Press, 1987.

[5] Food and Drug Administration: Coumarin. 21 CFR 4–1–94 Edition. Ch. 1, Section 189.130.

[6] Osol A, Farrar GE Jr, eds. The Dispensatory of the United States of America, ed. 25. Philadelphia: JB Lippincott, 1955.

[7] Olin BR, Hebel SK, eds. Drug Facts and Comparisons. St. Louis: Facts and Comparisons, July 1992.

[8] Claus EP, et al. *Pharmacognosy,* ed. 6. Philadelphia: Lea & Fegiber, 1970.

[9] Windholz M, ed. *Merck Index,* ed. 10. Rahway, NJ: Merck and Co., 1983.

Tragacanth

SCIENTIFIC NAME(S): A wide variety of *Astragalus* species, but most commonly *A. gummifera*, are used in commerce. Family: Leguminosae or Fabaceae.

COMMON NAME(S): Goat's thorn, green dragon, gum dragon, gum tragacanth, gummi tragacanthae, hog gum, Syrian tragacanth, tragacanth[1,2,10]

BOTANY: The tragacanth species are generally characterized as low-growing, thorny shrubs that are native to the mountainous regions of the Middle East.[1] Gum tragacanth is obtained by tapping the branches and tap roots. The gum dries as it exudes and is collected rapidly. The word tragacanth is said to derive from the Greek meaning "goat's horn," which may describe the appearance and texture of the crude gum.[1]

HISTORY: Tragacanth has been used since ancient times as an emulsifier, thickening agent, and suspending agent.[1,3] Today it is used extensively in foods and dressings and to thicken ice cream.

CHEMISTRY: Tragacanth contains from 20% to 30% of a water-soluble fraction called tragacanthin (composed of tragacanthic acid and arabinogalactan). It also contains from 60% to 70% of a water-insoluble fraction called bassorin. Tragacanthic acid is composed of D-galacturonic acid, D-xylose, L-fructose, D-galactose, and other sugars. Tragacanthin is composed of uronic acid and arabinose and dissolves in water to form a viscous colloidal solution (sol), while bassorin swells to form a thick gel.[1,2]

Tragacanthin partially dissolves and partially swells in water yielding a viscous colloid. The maximal viscosity is attained only after 24 hours at room temperature or after heating for 8 hours at high temperatures. The viscosity of these solutions is generally considered to be the highest among the plant gums.[1] The solutions are heat stable and stable under a wide range of pH levels.

PHARMACOLOGY: Tragacanth has been used as a demulcent in cough and cold preparations and to manage diarrhea.[2] As with other water-soluble gums, there is some preliminary evidence that concomitant ingestion of tragacanth with a high sugar load can moderate the blood sugar levels in patients with diabetes,[4] although this effect has not been demonstrated consistently[5] and requires much more detailed investigation. Although gum tragacanth swells to increase stool weight and decrease GI transit time, it appears to have no effect on serum cholesterol, triglyceride or phospholipid levels after a 21–day supplementation period as do other soluble fibers.[5,6]

Tragacanth has been reported to inhibit the growth of cancer cells in vitro and in vivo.[1,2]

Because of its mucilaginous adhesive properties, tragacanth is used as a component of some denture adhesives.[7]

TOXICOLOGY: Tragacanth is Generally Recognized as Safe (GRAS) in the US for food use.[8] There is no indication that dietary supplementation for up to 21 days has any significant adverse effects in man.[5]

Tragacanth is highly susceptible to bacterial degradation, and preparations contaminated with enterobacteria have been reported to have caused fetal deaths when administered intraperitoneally to pregnant mice.[1] A cross-sensitivity to the asthma-induced effects of quillaja bark has been observed for gum tragacanth.[9]

SUMMARY: Gum tragacanth is widely used throughout the world as a thickener and suspending agent in foods and pharmaceuticals. It is characterized by a very safe use profile. It does not appear to have any beneficial influence on serum lipid or glucose levels as do other soluble gums.

PATIENT INFORMATION – Tragacanth

Uses: Tragacanth has been used as a demulcent in cough and cold preparations and to manage diarrhea. It also has been shown to moderate the blood sugar level, but this has not been demonstrated consistently.

Side Effects: Presently, tragacanth is not recognized as having any adverse effects.

---

[1] Leung Ay. *Encyclopedia of Common Natural Ingredients Used in Food, Drugs and Cosmetics*. New York, NY: J. Wiley and Sons, 1980.

[2] Morton JF. *Major Medicinal Plants*. Springfield, IL: Charles C. Thomas, 1977.

[3] Evans WC. *Trease and Evans' Pharmacognosy*. 13th ed. London: Balliere Tindall, 1989.

[4] Nuttall FQ. Dietary fiber in the management of diabetes. *Diabetes* 1993;42:503.

[5] Eastwood MA, et al. The effects of dietary gum tragacanth in man. *Toxicol Lett* 1984;21:73.

[6] Eastwood MA, et al. The effect of polysaccharide composition and structure of dietary fibers on cecal fermentation and fecal excretion. *Am J Clin Nut* 1986;44:51.

[7] Berg E. A clinical comparison of four denture adhesives. *Int J Prosthodont.* 1991;4:449.

[8] Anderson DM. Evidence for the safety of gum tragacanth (*Asiatic Astragalus* spp.) and modern criteria for the evaluation of food additive. *Food Addit Contam* 1989;6:1.

[9] Raghuprasad PK, et al. Quillaja bark (soapbark)-induced asthma. *J Allergy Clin Immunol* 1980;65:285.

[10] Onsol A, Farrar GE Jr, eds. The Dispensatory of the United States of America, 25th ed. Philadelphia: J.B. Lippincott, 1955:1442.

Trillium

SCIENTIFIC NAME(S): *Trillium erectum* L. Family: Liliaceae (Trilliaceae). *T. grandiflorum* (Michaux) Salisb. has also been used medicinally in American traditional medicine.

COMMON NAME(S): Trillium, birthroot, bethroot, Indian balm, purple trillium, stinking Benjamin, wake-robin, trillium pendulum, ground lily, cough root, jewsharp, snake bite[1,2]

BOTANY: Trillium grows abundantly in the southern Appalachians. *T. erectum* is a low-growing perennial that reaches a height of about 18 inches. It has 3 dark green diamond-shaped leaves, each about 7 inches long. From April to June it produces a solitary odiferous, reddish brown flower. The smell is the reason for the name stinking Benjamin. The flower produces an oval reddish berry.

HISTORY: Birthroot is a popular folk remedy for bleeding, snakebites, and skin irritations. Teas made from the plant had been used traditionally to stop bleeding following childbirth, hence the name birthroot. The Indians applied topical preparations to relieve insect bites and skin irritations. The leaves have been used as a potherb or salad green.

CHEMISTRY: Little is known about the chemistry of this plant. *Trillium* species have been reported to contain a fixed and volatile oil, a saponin (trillarin, which is a diglycoside of diosgenin), a glycoside resembling convallamarin, tannic acid, and considerable starch.[3]

PHARMACOLOGY: Although trillium has been used for many years as an herbal means of controlling postpartum bleeding as well as other uterine bleeding problems, a clear mechanism for this systemic effect has not been identified.[1,4] The plant may have astringent properties that account for its ability to limit topical bleeding and irritation. This action was also the basis for its historic use in diarrhea.[2,4] The plant has been used traditionally as an expectorant, but no chemical basis has been identified for this action. There is not evidence to support the use of trillium for the treatment of snoring. Extracts of trillium have been used as molecular probes in chromosome studies.[5] The saponin glycosides have been shown to have significant antifungal activity.[6]

TOXICOLOGY: Although the leaves of the plant have been considered to be edible by some, there remains the possibility of toxicity from the plant. The saponin could have potential membrane-irritating effects and the convallamarin-like glycoside could induce some cardiac activity, although neither of these events have been observed clinically.[3]

SUMMARY: Trillium has a long history of use in traditional medicine for the management of bleeding particularly following childbirth. There are no studies to support this use. The chemistry of trillium is not well defined, but the tannin content may play a role in the topical control of bleeding and the relief from insect bites that the plant is said to afford.

PATIENT INFORMATION – Trillium

Uses: Trillium has been used to stop postpartum bleeding, although there are no studies to support this use. It may also play a role in the topical control of bleeding and relief from insect bites.

Side Effects: Although not yet clinically observed, trillium could have potential membrane-irritating effects and induce some cardiac activity.

---

[1] Dobelis IN, ed. *Magic and Medicine of Plants.* Pleasantville, NY: Reader's Digest Association, 1986.
[2] Meyer JE. *The Herbalist.* Hammond, IN: Hammond Book Co., 1934.
[3] Spoerke DG, Jr. *Herbal Medications.* Santa Barbara, CA: Woodbridge Press, 1980.
[4] Osol A, Farrar GE Jr, eds. *The Dispensatory of the United States of America,* ed. 25. Philadelphia, PA: J.B. Lippincott, 1955.
[5] Mabberley DJ. *The Plant-Book.* Cambridge, England: Cambridge University Press, 1987.
[6] Hufford CD, et al. Antifungal activity of *Trillium grandiflorum* constituents. *J Nat Prod* 1988;51(1):94.

Tung Seed

SCIENTIFIC NAME(S): *Aleurites moluccana* (L.) Willd or *A. cordata* Steud. Family: Euphorbiaceae

COMMON NAME(S): Tung, candlenut, candleberry, varnish tree, balucanat, otaheite walnut, China-wood oil

BOTANY: The tung is indigenous to China and Japan but now grows in many warm regions, including Florida.

HISTORY: The seed is the source of an oil that has been widely used as a wood preservative. It dries faster than linseed oil, making it a near perfect drying oil. The oil is incorporated into paints and varnishes, soaps, rubber substitutes, linoleum, and insulation.[1] The seed cake is used as a fertilizer, but the seeds can be poisonous. The roasted kernels, however, are said to be edible.[1] An extract of the bark is used to treat tumors in Japanese traditional medicine. The oil is a purgative. Tung seed is used in Hawaiian traditional medicine for the treatment of asthma.[2]

CHEMISTRY: The seed is the source of an inedible, semi-drying oil. The pale yellow oil contains eleostearic acid, linolenic, linoleic, and oleic acids. It is high in protein. The presence of a toxalbumin and HCN have been suggested.[1]

PHARMACOLOGY: There are no good studies to assess the human pharmacology of tung seed.

TOXICOLOGY: The various species of *Aleurites* vary in their potential toxicity. *A. fordii* is said to be about twice as toxic as *A. trisperma*, with *A. montana* and *A. moluccana* demonstrating intermediate toxicity. Ingesting the seeds can result in severe stomach pain, vomiting, diarrhea, slowed reflexes, and possibly death. The seeds are thrown into fishing areas to stupefy fish in some remote regions, which reflects the potential human toxicity of this plant.[1] Contact with the latex can result in dermatitis; this appears to be related to the presence of a saponin and phytotoxin.

SUMMARY: The tung plant is the source of commercially important tung oil, which is used as a wood finish and a component of paints and varnishes. The tung seed is generally considered to be toxic.

PATIENT INFORMATION – Tung Seed

Uses: Tung seed is commonly used as a wood finish and a component of paints and varnishes. No studies assess the human pharmacology of tung seed.

Side Effects: The tung seed is considered to be toxic, resulting in stomach pain, vomiting, diarrhea, slowed reflexes, and possibly death.

---

[1] Duke JA. *Handbook of Medicinal Herbs*. Boca Raton, FL: CRC Press, 1985.

[2] Hope BE, et al. Hawaiian materia medica for asthma. *Hawaii Med J* 1993;52:160.

Turmeric

SCIENTIFIC NAME(S): *Curcuma longa* L. Synonymous with *C. domestica* Val. Family: Zingiberaceae

COMMON NAME(S): Turmeric, curcuma, Indian saffron

BOTANY: Turmeric is a perennial member of the ginger family characterized by a thick rhizome. The plant grows to a height of 3 to 5 feet and has large (1.5' x 8") oblong leaves. It bears funnel-shaped yellow flowers.[1] The plant is cultivated widely throughout Asia, India, China, and tropical countries. The primary (bulb) and secondary (lateral) rhizomes are collected, cleaned, boiled, and dried; and lateral rhizomes contain more yellow coloring material than the bulb.[2] The dried rhizome forms the basis for the culinary spice.

HISTORY: Turmeric has a warm, bitter taste and is a primary component of curry powders and some mustards. The powder and its oleoresins are also used extensively as food flavorings in the culinary industry. The spice has a long history of traditional use in Asian medicine. In Chinese medicine, it has been used to treat problems as diverse as flatulence and hemorrhage. It also has been used topically as a poultice, as an analgesic and to treat ringworms.[3] The spice has been used for the management of jaundice and hepatitis.[2] The oil is sometimes used as a perfume component.

CHEMISTRY: Turmeric rhizome contains up to 7% of an orange-yellow volatile oil composed primarily of tumerone (60%), isomers of atlantone and zingiberene (25%). More than a half-dozen minor components have been identified in the oil.

Turmeric contains about 5% diaryl heptanoids known as curcuminoids (curcumin and related compounds) that impart the yellow color.[2]

PHARMACOLOGY: A number of soluble fractions of turmeric, including curcumin, have been reported to have antioxidant properties. Turmeric inhibits the degradation of polyunsaturated fatty acids.[4] Dietary administration of this compound at a level of 2% to mice reduced the incidence of experimentally-induced colonic hyperplasia, indicating that the antioxidant effects are active in vivo.[5] The curcumins inhibit cancer at initiation, promotion, and progression stages of development.[6]

Tumor-preventing activity has been reported in hamsters given turmeric, and the effect was additive to that ob-served during treatment with betel leaf extract.[7] In smokers, turmeric given at a daily dose of 1.5 g for 30 days significantly reduced the urinary excretion of mutagens compared with controls; turmeric had no effect on hepatic enzyme levels or lipid profiles suggesting that the spice may be an effective antimutagen useful in chemoprevention.[3]

Ukonan-A, a polysaccharide with phagocytosis-activating activity has been isolated from *C. longa*[9] and Ukonan-D has demonostrated strong reticuloendothelial system-potentiating activity.[10] Aqueous extract of *C. longa* has recently been shown to have cytoprotective effects that inhibit chemically-induced carcinogenesis, and this activity may form a basis for the traditional use of turmeric as an anticancer treatment.[11]

A fraction of curcuma oil has been shown to have anti-inflammatory and antiarthritic activity in a rat model.[3] A combination of turmeric and neem (*Azadirachta indica*) applied topically has been shown to effectively eradicate scabies in 97% of 814 people treated within 3 to 15 days.[12] Curcumin has a slight antiedemic effect in rats; other pharmacologic properties of turmeric include choleretic, hypotensive, antibacterial, and insecticidal activity.

The choleretic (bile stimulating) activity of curcumin has been recognized for almost 40 years, and these compounds have been shown to possess strong antihepatotoxic properties.[13]

TOXICOLOGY: Acute and chronic (100 mg/kg/day for 90 days) evaluation of *C. longa* ethanolic extracts in mice found the material to be relatively devoid of serious side effects. No reports of significant toxicity have been reported following the ingestion of turmeric. No significant change in weight was observed following chronic treatment, although significant changes in heart and lung weights were observed; a significant decrease in white and red blood cell levels were observed. Although a gain in weight of sexual organs and an increase in sperm motility was observed, no spermatotoxic effects were found.[14]

SUMMARY: Turmeric is a widely used spice that is a major component of curry powder. The spice has a long history of use in traditional Asian medicine. Recent investigations indicate that the strong antioxidant effects of several components of turmeric result in an inhibition of carcinogenesis, and extracts of the spice may play a role as chemoprotectants, which limit the development of cancers.

PATIENT INFORMATION – Turmeric

Uses: Turmeric is used as a spice. Recent investigations indicate that the strong antioxidant effects of several components of turmeric result in an inhibiton of carcinogenesis and may play a role in limiting the development of cancers.

Side Effects: There are no known side effects.

---

[1] Dobelis IN, ed. *Magic and Medicine of Plants.* Pleasantville, NY: Reader's Digest Association, Inc., 1986.

[2] Evans WC. *Trease and Evans' Pharmacognosy,* ed. 13. London, England: Balliere Tindall, 1989.

[3] Leung AY. *Encyclopedia of Common Natural Ingredients Used in Food, Drugs and Cosmetics.* New York, NY: J. Wiley and Sons, 1980.

[4] Reddy AC, Lokesh BR. Studies on spice principles as antioxidants in the inhibition of lipid peroxidation of rat liver microsomes. *Mol Cell Biochem* 1992;111:117.

[5] Huang MT, et al. Effect of dietary curcumin and ascorbyl palmitate on azoxymethanol-induced colonic epithelial cell proliferation and focal areas of dysplasia. *Cancer Lett* 1992;64:117.

[6] Nagabhushan M, Bhide SV. Curcumin as an inhibitor of cancer. *J Am Coll Nutr* 1992;11:192.

[7] Azuine MA, Bhide SV. Protective single/combined treatment with betel leaf and turmeric against methyl (acetoxymethyl) nitrosamine-induced hamster oral carcinogenesis. *Int J Cancer* 1992;51:412.

[8] Polasa K, et al. Effect of turmeric on urinary mutagens in smokers. *Mutagenesis* 1992;7:107.

[9] Gonda R, et al. The core structure of ukonan A, a phagocytosis-activating polysaccharide from the rhizome of curcumin longa, and immunological activities of degredation products. *Chem Pharm Bull* 1992;40:990.

[10] Ibid. 1992;40:185.

[11] Azuine MA, et al. Protective role of aqueous turmeric extract against mutagenicity of direct-acting carcinogens as well as benzo [alpha] Pyrene-induced genotoxicity and carcinogenicity. *J Cancer Res Clin Oncol* 1992;118:447.

[12] Charles V, Charles SX. The use and efficacy of Azadirachta indica ADR ("Neem") and curcuma longa ("Turmeric") in scabies. *Trop Geogr Med* 1992;44:178.

[13] Kiso Y, et al. *Phytochemistry* 1983;49:185.

[14] Qureshi S, et al. Toxicity studies on Alpinia galanga and curcuma longa. *Planta Med* 1992;58:124.

Turpentine

SCIENTIFIC NAME(S): *Pinus palustris* Mill. and several other species and varieties of *Pinus*. Family: Pinaceae

COMMON NAME(S): Turpentine, gum turpentine, gum thus, turpentine oil, turpentine balsam

HISTORY: The primary use of turpentine has been as a solvent in paints. During the last century, it became an important starting material for the commercial synthesis of many widely used compounds, including camphor and menthol. Various products derived from turpentine have been used in chewing gums, and steam-distilled turpentine oil has been used as a food and beverage flavoring in very small quantities (typically about 20 ppm). Turpentine and its related products have a long history of medicinal use, where they have been employed primarily as topical counterirritants for the treatment of rheumatic disorders and muscle pain. A gum derived from turpentine was used in traditional Chinese medicine to relieve the pain of toothaches.

Other extracts (including the semi-synthetic derivative terpin hydrate) have been used for the treatment of cough and cold symptoms;[1] the cis-form of terpin hydrate is used as an expectorant.[2]

A variety of gum and resin products had been derived from pines for use in the early naval industry as tars and pitches. Consequently the terms "wood naval stores" and "gum naval stores" came to be associated with these pine-derived products.[3]

SOURCE AND COMPOSITION: Research suggests that the term "turpentine" is used imprecisely to describe either the oleoresin obtained from the longleaf pine (*Pinus palustris* Mill.) or the slash pine (*P. elliottii* Engelm.) along with other *Pinus* species that yield exclusively terpene oils, or the essential oil obtained from the above oleoresin.[4] More than a half-dozen additional *Pinus* species have been used in the production of turpentine.[3] The oleoresin is sometimes referred to as ''gum turpentine'' while turpentine or its oil (also known as spirits of turpentine) are terms for the essential oil. Following steam distillation, gum turpentine yields turpentine oil and a resin called colophony (also known as rosin). Alternately, rosin is collected by scarring the tree trunk, and various grades of material are then refined.[3] Turpentine and rosin also are obtained by the steam distillation of wood chips of pine that are by-products of the lumber and paper industries, and these sources account for the bulk of the production of these compounds. In terms of volume,

turpentine is the largest volume essential oil product in the world, with the bulk of production occurring in the United States. The labor-intensive production of rosin, however, occurs to a greater extent in Spain, Greece, India, and Morocco.

Turpentine is composed primarily of monoterpene hydrocarbons, the most prevalent of which are the pinenes, camphene, and 3-carene. Rosin contains mostly diterpene resin acids such as abietic acid, dehydroabietic acid palustric acid and isopimaric acid. Numerous other compounds are present in small quantities in all turpentine products.

Canada turpentine or Canada balsam is an oleoresin obtained from the stems of the balsam fir, *Abies balsamae* (Family Pinaceae).

PHARMACOLOGY: When applied topically, turpentine causes skin irritation and, therefore, has been shown to exert rubefacient and counterirritant actions.

Turpentine possesses antibacterial activity in vitro[4] and has been applied topically to debride severe wounds infested with fly larvae.[5] Preliminary reports from Russia suggest that turpentine baths may assist in the treatment of disseminated sclerosis,[6] but the safety of this treatment has not been established.

Turpentine is now being injected in animals as part of experimental models of inflammation to induce a systemic inflammatory immune response.[7]

TOXICOLOGY: The contact allergenic activity of turpentine is believed to be due primarily to the pinenes, 3-carene, and dipentene.[4,8] The resin also has irritant potential. In one survey of persons involved in the manufacture of tires, patch testing indicated that 2.6% of those tested developed hypersensitivity reactions to turpentine. Benign skin tumors have been observed in animal models following chronic topical application of turpentine.

Turpentine has been used for traditional self-medication in the United States, and fatal poisonings have been reported in children who have ingested as little as 15 ml of the material.[9] Turpentine is among the most commonly ingested poisons among childhood cases reported to poison control centers.[10] Toxic effects of turpentine ingestion include headache, insomnia, coughing, vomiting, hematuria, albuminuria, and coma.[4]

SUMMARY: Turpentine and its related products (the oil and rosin) are important in commerce and traditional medicine. These products can pose a toxicity problem, and should be handled and stored carefully.

PATIENT INFORMATION – Turpentine

Uses: Turpentine has been used experimentally in a bath for the treatment of disseminated sclerosis, and is presently being injected into animals as experimental models of inflammation to induce a systemic inflammatory immune response.

Side Effects: If ingested, turpentine is highly toxic.

---

[1] Ziment I. History of the treatment of chronic bronchitis. *Respiration* 1991;58:37.

[2] Morton JF. *Major Medicinal Plants*. Springfield, IL: Thomas Books, 1977.

[3] Evans WC. *Trease and Evans' Pharmacognosy*, ed. 13. London, England: Balliere Tindall, 1989.

[4] Leung AY. *Encyclopedia of Common Natural Ingredients Used in Food, Drugs, and Cosmetics*. New York, NY: John Wiley & Sons, Inc., 1980.

[5] Agarwal DC, Singh B. Orbital myiasis a case report. *Indian J Ophthalmol* 1990;38:187.

[6] Ludianskii EA. The extension of the use of physical methods of treatment to patients with disseminated sclerosis. *Vopr Kurortol Fizioter Lech Fiz Kult* 1992;3:34.

[7] Pous C, et al. Recombinant human interleukin 1 beta and tumor necrosis factor affect glycosylation of serum alpha 1-acid glycoprotein in rats. *Inflammation* 1992;16:197.

[8] Rudzki E, et al. Contact allergy to oil of turpentine: a 10-year retrospective view. *Contact Dermatitis* 1991;24:317.

[9] Boyd EL, et al. *Home Remedies and the Black Elderly: A reference manual for health care providers*. Levittown, PA: Pharmaceutical Information Associates, Ltd., 1991.

[10] Melis K, et al. Chemical pneumonia in children. *Ned Tijdschr Geneeskd* 1990;134:811.

Ubiquinone

SCIENTIFIC NAME(S): Coenzyme Q-10, Ubidecarenone, mitoquinone

COMMON NAME(S): Adelir, Heartcin, Inokiton, Neuquinone, Taidecanone, Udekinon, Ubiquinone

HISTORY: The first ubiquinone was isolated in 1957. Since that time, ubiquinones have been extensively studied in Japan, Russia, and Europe with research in the US having begun more recently. Lay press accounts claim that roughly 12 million Japanese now use ubiquinones as the medication of choice for management of cardiovascular diseases supplying the demand for more than 250 commercially available preparations. Ubiquinone is touted as an effective treatment of congestive heart failure (CHF), cardiac arrhythmias and hypertension, and in the reduction of hypoxic injury to the myocardium. Other claimed effects include the increase of exercise tolerance, stimulation of the immune system, and counteracting of the aging process. Clinical uses have included the treatment of diabetes, obesity, and periodontal disease. Ubiquinone has not been approved for therapeutic use in the US, but it is available as a food supplement.[1]

CHEMISTRY: Ubiquinones are a class of lipid-soluble benzoquinones that are involved in mitochondrial electron transport. They are found in the majority of aerobic organisms, from bacteria to mammals, hence the name "ubiquinone" ("quinone found everywhere"). Studies in rats have shown that levels of ubiquinone and cytochrome C reductase increase adaptively during endurance exercise training. This increase occurs in red quadriceps and soleus muscle but not in white cardiac or quadriceps muscle. The increase in red muscle levels represents a positive adaptation to training.[2] Experiments have shown that ubiquinones participate in oxidation-reduction reactions in the mitochondrial respiratory chain. They also have properties of hydrogen carriers, thus providing a coupling of proton translocation to respiration by means of a chemiosmotic mechanism.[3]

Structurally ubiquinones are analogous to vitamin K. The basic molecule is 2,3-dimethoxy-5-methylbenzoquinone, to which are attached variable terpenoid side chairs containing 1 to 10 monounsaturated trans-isoprenoid units. The 6- to 10-unit chain forms (Q-6 to Q-10) are found in animals, with Q-10 being exclusive to humans. All of the ubiquinones have been synthesized in the laboratory.[4] Studies with deuterated analogs of Q-10 have demonstrated that Q-10 occurs in a mobile environment within the cell, physically separate from the orientational constraints of bilayer lipid chains. This suggests that the bulk of the long-chain ubiquinones are not directly involved functionally in electron transport. Q-10 may represent only a small fraction of total ubiquinone.[5]

HPLC of ubiquinone-10 has been performed,[6] as has sodium lauryl sulfate use in hexane extraction of ubiquinone-10 from plasma samples.[7]

PHARMACOLOGY: Biomedical evidence provides the rationale for the use of ubiquinone in cardiovascular diseases. Endogenous forms function as essential cofactors in several metabolic pathways, especially in oxidative respiration. Supraphysiologic doses of ubiquinone may benefit tissues that have been rendered ischemic and then reperfused. Ubiquinone appears to function in such tissues as a free-radical scavenger, membrane stabilizer, or both.[8] Ubiquinone as a mobile component in mitochondrial membrane and its role in electron transfer has been reported.[9] It may have applications in treating ischemic heart disease, CHF, toxin-induced cardiopathy and possibly hypertension. It protects ischemic myocardium during surgery.[8]

Experiments with rabbit hearts measured the effects of Q-10 during hypoxia and following reoxygenation. In untreated hearts, reoxygenation was followed by a release of ATP metabolites and creatine phosphokinase. Pretreatment of the hearts with Q-10 eliminated these releases. This suggests that Q-10 retards the breakdown of ATP metabolites, providing a pool from which ATP can be constructed by a salvage process during reoxygenation.[10,11] Coenzyme Q-10 also provides a protective effect when used on rat mitochondria.[12]

Q-10 has also been shown to eliminate biochemical derangements (reductions of norepinephrine and ATP) in thyrotoxic rabbit hearts.[13] In beef hearts, Q-10 protected mitochondria from oxidative damage to lipid membranes induced by treatment with an adriamycin-iron complex. In these experiments, it reduced the inactivation of NADPH and succinate oxidases.[14] In transplantation experiments, rats receiving livers subjected to prior warm ischemic damage did not survive more than 2 days. Pretreatment of the donors with Q-10 significantly increased the duration of survival, decreased AST and ALT levels and increased total protein to the normal range without affecting total bilirubin or hepatic histology. Thus, ubiquinone had a protective effect on donated livers subjected to heat-induced ischemia before transplantation.[15]

Ubiquinone's role in cardiac treatment using human subjects is promising. In geriatric patients, Q-10 treatment improved both symptoms and clinical conditions of all 34 patients with CHF.[16] It was also effective for symptomatic mitral valve prolapse and improved stress-induced cardiac dysfunction in 400 pediatric patients.[17] Activity tolerance improvements were observed in a double-blind study of 19 patients with chronic myocardial disease given oral ubiquinone-10.[18] In advanced heart failure, 12 patients given 100 mg daily of the drug showed marked clinical improvement.[19] Immune system effects were enhanced in myocardial failure in another report, when Q-10 was used in conjunction with other drugs.[20] Aiding defective myocardial supply, ubiquinone's role in oxidative phosphorylation offers positive results in adjunctive treatment, clinical outcomes, symptoms, and quality of life in these cardiac patients.[21]

Q-10 actions on lipids have also been reported. The mechanism may be membrane phospholipid protection against phospholipase attack.[22] In its reduced form, ubiquinone's presence in all cellular membrane, blood serum, and serum lipoproteins, allows protection from lipid peroxidation.[23] Its ability to remain stable in hypercholesterolemia patients has been studied.[24,25] Ubiquinol

can also sustain vitamin E's antioxidant effects by regenerating the vitamin from its oxidized form.[23,26]

One report describes ubiquinone and its role in human nutrition.[27] A case report uses ubiquinone to treat drug-induced rhabdomyolysis and hepatotoxicity.[28]

TOXICOLOGY: No serious side effects have been associated with the use of ubiquinone. Use of the substance is contraindicated in people with demonstrated hypersensitivity. Use during pregnancy or lactation is not recommended, because studies have not demonstrated the safety of ubiquinone for fetuses and infants. Rare side effects have included epigastric discomfort, loss of appetite, nausea and diarrhea, affecting fewer than 1% of more than 5000 individuals in one study.[1]

SUMMARY: Ubiquinones, particularly Q-10, are naturally occurring compounds found in aerobic organisms. Q-10 has been widely used in Japan, Russia, and Europe for a variety of indications, notably cardiovascular diseases. Studies using ubiquinone offer mainly positive outcomes in CHF therapy. Reports on ubiquinone's effects on lipid disorders and antioxidant effects have also been promising. This research indicates that Q-10 may have value for some of the purposes claimed by proponents, and toxicity appears to be minimal. No doses have been established for the treatment of any human disorder and no RDA has been established for this compound. This compound appears to possess important pharmacologic activity and warrants further investigation in disease states.

PATIENT INFORMATION – Ubiquinone

Uses: Ubiquinone may have applications in treating ischemic heart disease, congestive heart failure, toxin-induced cardiopathy and hypertension, and protects ischemic myocardium during surgery.

Side effects: Rare side effects include epigastric discomfort, loss of appetite, nausea and diarrhea. Use is not recommended in pregnancy and lactation and in people with demonstrated hypersensitivity.

---

[1] Lay press accounts and promotional brochures.
[2] Gohil K, et al. *J Appl Physiol* 1987;63:1638.
[3] Trumbower BL. *J Bioenerg Biomembr* 1981;13:1.
[4] Windholz M, ed. Merck Index. Rahway:Merck, 1983.
[5] Cornell BA, et al. *Biochemistry* 1987;26:7702.
[6] Yamano Y, et al. *Yakugaku Zasshi* 1977;97(May):486–94.
[7] Hirota K, et al. *J Chromatogr* 1984;310(Sep14):204–7.
[8] Greenberg SM, et al. *Med Clin North Am* 1987;72:243.
[9] Lenaz G, et al. *Drugs Exp Clin Res* 1985;11(8):547–56.
[10] Takeo S, et al. *J Pharmacol Exp Ther* 1987;243:1131.
[11] Yoshikawa Y, et al. *Arch Int Pharmacodyn Ther* 1987;287:96.
[12] Solani G, et al. *Drugs Exp Clin Res* 1985;11(8):533–7.
[13] Kotake C, et al. *Heart Vessels* 1987;3:84.
[14] Solani G, et al. *Biochem Biophys Res Comm* 1987;147:572.

[15] Sumimoto K, et al. *Surgery* 1987;102:821.
[16] Cascone A, et al. *Boll Chim Farm* 1985;124(May):435–525.
[17] Oda T. *Drugs Exp Clin Res* 1985;11(8):557–76.
[18] Langsjoen P, et al. *Drugs Exp Clin Res* 1985;11(8):577–9.
[19] Mortensen S, et al. *Drugs Exp Clin Res* 1985;11(8):581–3.
[20] Folkers K, et al. *Drugs Exp Clin Res* 1985;11(8):539–45.
[21] Mortensen S. *Clin Investigator* 1993;71(8 Suppl):S116–23.
[22] Sugiyama S, et al. *Arzneimittelforschung* 1985;35(1):23–5.
[23] Ernster L, et al. *Biochem Biophys Acta* 1995;1271(1):195–204.
[24] Mabuchi H, et al. *N Engl J Med* 1981;305(Aug 27):478–82.
[25] Laaksonen R, et al. *Clin Pharmacol Ther* 1995;57(Jan):62–6.
[26] Ernster L, et al. *Clin Investigator* 1993;71(8 Suppl):S60–5.
[27] Hotzel D. *Dtsch Apothek Zeit* 1995;135(Jul 6):27–8, 31–2, 35–6.
[28] Lees R, et al. *N Engl J Med* 1995;333(Sept 7):664–5.

Uva Ursi

SCIENTIFIC NAME(S): *Arctostaphylos uva ursi* L. Sprengel. (Also referred to as *Arbutus uva ursi* L.). The related plants *A. adenotricha* and *A. coactylis* Fern et Macbr. have also been termed uva ursi by some authors. Family: Ericaceae

COMMON NAME(S): Uva ursi, bearberry, kinnikinnik, hogberry, rockberry, beargrape, manzanita.

BOTANY: Uva ursi is a low-growing evergreen shrub with creeping stems that form a dark green carpet of leaves. It can grow to 20 inches in height. The plant has small, dark, fleshy, leathery leaves and clusters of small white or pink bell-shaped flowers. It blooms from April to May and produces a dull orange berry. The plant grows abundantly throughout the northern hemisphere from Asia to the United States.[1,2]

HISTORY: "Uva ursi" means "bear's grape" in Latin, probably because bears are fond of the fruit. Uva ursi was first documented in a 13th century Welsh herbal.[2] Teas and extracts of the leaves have been used as urinary tract antiseptics and diuretics for centuries. The plant has been used as a laxative and the leaves have been smoked.[3] Bearberry teas and extracts have been used as vehicles for pharmaceutical preparations. In homeopathy, a tincture of the leaves is believed to be effective in the treatment of cystitis, urethritis, and urinary tract inflammations. The berries are not used medicinally. They are juicy but have an insipid flavor that improves upon cooking.[4]

CHEMISTRY: The leaves contain hydroquinone derivatives, mainly arbutin and methyl-arbutin in concentrations ranging from 5% to 15%. HPLC determination of these substances has been evaluated.[5] Tannins are also present (6% to 40%) including hydrolysable types, ellagic and gallic acid tannins. Because of this high concentration of tannin, teas prepared from this plant are generally made by soaking the leaves in cold water overnight. This minimizes extraction of the bitter tannins. A report on tannin isolation from uva ursi leaves is available.[6]

Flavonoids including hyperoside, myricetin, quercetin, and glycosides such as hyperin, isoquercitrin, myricitrin, and quercitrin are also found.

Triterpenes, monotropein, piceoside, phenol-carboxylic acids such as gallic and p-coumaric, and syringic acids can be found. Terpenoids such as alpha-amyrin and ursolic acids are present in the plant, as well as other constituents, including malic acid, allantoin, resin, volatile oil, and wax.[1,2,7]

Reports are available, including: Isolation of 14 phenolic acids from uva ursi leaves using GLC;[8] isolation of 8 triterpenoids from uva ursi roots;[9] isolation and identification of free and bonded saccharides in the plant leaves;[10] and differentiation of adulterated uva ursi leaf samples.[11]

PHARMACOLOGY:

Antimicrobial effects: Arbutin is hydrolyzed in gastric fluid to hydroquinone. In alkaline urine, hydroquinone is mildly astringent and is an effective antimicrobial agent. Despite this activity, in practice, large amounts of uva ursi must be consumed for any significant effect to occur and the urine must be alkalinized.[12] Evidence suggests that arbutin itself may contribute to the antiseptic activity of the plant, because both arbutin and crude leaf extracts have been shown to possess mild antimicrobial activity in vitro.[13] A report discusses liquid concentration of uva ursi possessing antiseptic and diuretic properties.[14] Uva ursi aerial part extracts were found to be most active against *Escherichia coli* and *Proteus vulgaris*.[15]

Urinary tract effects: Antibacterial activity of arbutin causing urinary tract infection is caused by beta-glucosidase activity of the infective organism.[13] Uva ursi is one of the best natural urinary antiseptics and has been extensively used in herbal medicine.[2] The German Commission E monograph lists its use as "for inflammatory disorders of the lower urinary tract." An herbal remedy including uva ursi is used to treat "compulsive strangury, enuresis, and painful micturition."[1] One report discusses metabolite production of uva ursi,[16] other reports discuss bile expelling/lowering effects of the plant[17] and its beneficial effects on treatment of kidney stone formation.[18]

Several plant compounds (ursolic acid and isoquercetin) are mild diuretics and contribute to the plant's diuretic effect. Uva ursi is a constituent in many over-the-counter herbal diuretic preparations. A report on bearberry reviews diuretic effects and other plant properties.[19]

Other effects: Arbutin may increase inhibitory action of prednisolone and dexamethasone on induced contact dermatitis, allergic reaction-type hypersensitivity, and arthritis, suggesting uva ursi's therapeutic effects against immuno-inflammation.[20,21,22,23] Another study reports reduced hyperphagia, reduced polydipsia and reduced loss of weight in diabetes-induced mice given bearberry. There was no effect on glucose or insulin plasma concentrations, but it may be of some benefit in these diabetes symptoms.[24] Therapy of experimentally induced hepatitis in rats with extract of *A. uva ursi* has been reported.[18,25] Bearberry leaf was also found to be effective in inhibiting melanin production in vitro.[26]

TOXICOLOGY: Hydroquinone is toxic in large doses (oral LD-50 in rats is 320 mg/kg).[27] Ingestion of 1 g of the compound resulted in ringing of the ears, nausea, vomiting, cyanosis, convulsions and collapse. Death followed the ingestion of 5 g of hydroquinone.[7] These symptoms are rare; most commercial products have less than 1 g of crude uva ursi per dose. Doses up to 20 g of uva ursi have not caused pharmacologic responses in healthy individuals.[28] Products containing uva ursi may turn urine green.

The plant's astringent tannin content may cause gastric discomfort and usually limits the dose ingested.

The published report of the Expert Advisory Committee in Herbs and Botanical Preparations to the Canadian Health Protection Branch (January 1986) recommended that food preparations containing uva ursi provide labeling contraindicating their use during pregnancy and lactation because large doses of uva ursi are oxytocic.[7]

Do not use uva ursi if suffering from kidney disease. Do not take the plant for more than 7 to 10 days at a time.[2]

SUMMARY: Uva ursi has been used for urinary tract ailments; however, the urine must be alkaline for its antimicrobial effects. Studies have been done on the plant's effects against inflammation, diabetes symptoms and other effects. Hydroquinone, a plant constituent, is toxic in large doses. Use is contraindicated in pregnancy.

PATIENT INFORMATION – Uva Ursi

Uses: Uva ursi is useful in treating urinary tract infections; as a diuretic; to treat induced contact dermatitis, allergic reaction-type hypersensitivity, and arthritis in conjuction with prednisolone and dexamethasone.

Side effects: Ingestion of uva ursi in large doses has resulted in ringing of the ears, nausea, vomiting, cyanosis, convulsions, collapse, and death. The product may also impart a green color to the urine and cause gastric discomfort.

---

[1] Bisset N. *Herbal Drugs and Phytopharmaceuticals*. Stuttgart, Germany: CRC Press, 1994.
[2] Chevallier A. *Encyclopedia of Medicinal Plants*. New York, NY: DK Publishing Inc., 1996.
[3] Spoerke DG. *Herbal Medications*. Santa Barbara, CA: Woodbridge Press Publishing Co., 1980.
[4] *Wild Edible and Poisonous Plants of Alaska*, Univ. of Alaska Cooperative Extension Service: 1985.
[5] Stambergova A, et al. *Cesk Farm* 1985;34(5):179–82.
[6] Ostrowska B, et al. *Herba Polonica* 1988;34(1–2):21–5.
[7] Newall C, et al. Herbal Medicine. London: Pharmaceutical Press, 1996.
[8] Dombrowicz E, et al. *Pharmazie* 1991;46(Sep):680–1.
[9] Jahodar L, et al. *Pharmazie* 1988;43(Jun):442–3.
[10] Leifertova I, et al. *Farmaceut Obzor* 1989;58(Nov):507–11.
[11] Schier W, et al. *Dtsch Apoth Zeitung* 1990;130(Mar):463–5.
[12] Frohne D. *Planta Med* 1970;18:1.
[13] Jahodar L, et al. *Cesk Farm* 1985;34:174.
[14] Zaits K, et al. *Farmatsiia* 1975;24(1):40–2.
[15] Holopainen M, et al. *Acta Pharm Fenn* 1988;97(Apr): 197–202.
[16] Duskova J, et al. *Cesk Farm* 1991;40(Feb):83–5.
[17] Azhunova T, et al. *Farmatsiia* 1988;37(2):41–3.
[18] Grases F, et al. *Int Urol Nephrol* 1994;26(5):507–11.
[19] Houghton P, et al. *Pharm J* 1995;255(Aug):272–3.
[20] Kubo M, et al. *Yakugaku Zasshi* 1990;110(1):59–67.
[21] Matsuda H, et al. *Yakugaku Zasshi* 1990;110(1):68–76.
[22] Matsuda H, et al. *Yakugaku Zasshi* 1991;111(4–5):253–8.
[23] Matsuda H, et al. *Yakugaku Zasshi* 1992;112(9):673–7.
[24] Swanston-Flatt S, et al. *Acta Diabetol Lat* 1989;26(1):51–5.
[25] Sambueva Z, et al. *Farmatsiia* 1987;36(2):40–5.
[26] Matsuda H, et al. *Yakugaku Zasshi* 1992;112(4):276–82.
[27] Woodard T, et al. *Fed Proc* 1949;8:348.
[28] Tyler VE. *The Honest Herbal*. Philadelphia, PA: G. F. Stickley Co., 1981.

Valerian

SCIENTIFIC NAME(S): *Valeriana officinalis* L. Family: Valerianaceae. A number of other species have been used medicinally, including *V. wallichi* DC, *V. sambucifolia* Mik., and the related *Centranthus ruber* L.

COMMON NAME(S): Valerian, baldrian, radix valerianae, Indian valerian (*V. wallichii*), red valerian (*C. ruber*)

BOTANY: Members of the genus *Valeriana* are herbaceous perennials widely distributed in the temperate regions of North America, Europe, and Asia. Of the approximately 200 known species, the Eurasian *V. officinalis* is the species most often cultivated for medicinal use. The dried rhizome contains a volatile oil with a distinctive, unpleasant odor.[1] The fresh drug has no appreciable smell; however, drying liberates the odiferous constituent isovaleric acid.[2]

HISTORY: Despite its odor, valerian was considered a perfume in 16th century Europe. The tincture has been used for its sedative properties for centuries; it is still widely used in France, Germany, and Switzerland as a sleep aid. About 50 tons of valerian are sold each year in France.[2]

CHEMISTRY: Three distinct classes of compounds have been associated with the sedative properties of valerian: 1) mono- and sesquiterpenes, 2) iridoid triesters (valepotriates), and 3) pyridine alkaloids. The composition of the volatile oil varies markedly between cultivars and species, as does the amount and relative proportion of valepotriates, making chemical standardization difficult but highly desirable.

The most important sesquiterpenes include valerenic acid and its congeners, although in the Japanese *V. officinalis* var. latifolia, kessyl alcohols and esters predominate. Valtrate, acevaltrate, and didrovaltrate are the most important iridoids; European valerian extracts were formerly standardized on these rather unstable compounds, which have a short shelf-life in the tincture. The alkaloid concentration in roots and rhizomes is low, usually less than 0.2%. The aqueous extract of valerian has been found to contain substantial quantities of GABA; however, it is doubtful whether GABA penetrates the blood-brain barrier with oral administration.[3]

Many analytical high performance liquid chromatographic (HPLC) methods have been developed for the sesquiterpenes and valepotriates.[4] The seasonal variation in valerenic acids and valepotriates has been studied.[5] Tissue culture of valerian species has focused on production of valepotriates.[6]

PHARMACOLOGY: While there is substantial debate over the constituents responsible for valerian's sedative activity, it is undeniable that valerian preparations have sedative effects. Human studies have documented valerian's effectiveness as a sleep aid.

Aqueous and hydroalcoholic extracts of valerian induced release of [3H]GABA from synaptosomal preparations, which was interpreted as an effect on the GABA transporter. The in vitro effect was correlated with the content of GABA itself in the extract. Thus GABA may be responsible for some of the peripheral effects of valerian, while glutamine, another free amino acid in the extract, can cross the blood-brain barrier and be metabolized to GABA in situ, thereby producing central sedation.[3]

An ethanol extract containing no valepotriates antagonized picrotoxin convulsions in mice but had no effect on metrazol- or harman-induced convulsions. The same extract prolonged barbiturate sleeping time, but did not affect spontaneous motility, pain perception, or body temperature. The effects were traced to valerenic acid.[7] A commercial aqueous alkaline extract of valerian (*Valdispert*), standardized on valerenic acid given orally to mice, reduced spontaneous motility and increased barbiturate sleeping time, but had no effect on metrazol-induced convulsions.[8] Cerebral metabolism was examined in rats with PET scanning, and an effect consistent with a GABAergic mechanism was reported with the methylene chloride extract of valerian; however, valepotriates and valerenic acids were not responsible for the effect. The active compounds were not identified.[9]

Valerenic acid has been found to inhibit GABA transaminase, the principle enzyme that catabolizes GABA. GABA-T inhibition increases the inhibitory effect of GABA in the CNS, and can therefore contribute to valerian's sedative properties.[10] Valerenic acid given intraperitoneally had CNS depressant effects in mice, including potentiating barbiturate sleeping time and decreasing spontaneous motor activity and rotorod performance.[11,12] The valepotriates isovaltrate and valtrate, along with valerenone, were found to have antispasmodic effects in isolated guinea pig ileum, as well as other smooth muscle preparations.[13]

Clinical trials: There is abundant evidence that valerian is effective as a sleep aid and as a mild antianxiety agent, although the effect appears to be weaker in healthy subjects than in poor sleepers. An aqueous extract of the root (400 mg extract) improved sleep quality in a number of subjective parameters in 128 healthy volunteers using a crossover design.[2] Elderly patients with nervous disorders responded positively to a commercial valerian preparation in a placebo-controlled study, as measured by both subjective and objective parameters.[14] Sleep latency was decreased in a group of 8 poor sleepers given an aqueous extract of valerian in a double-blind, placebo-controlled study.[15] A sleep laboratory study found minor sedative effects in healthy volunteers.[16] An uncontrolled multicenter study of > 11,000 patients suffering from sleep-related disorders found subjective improvements in 94% of those treated.[17] Another multicenter trial of the same preparation in a younger study population found progressive symptomatic improvement over 10 days of treatment.[18] Valerian was found to increase slow-wave sleep in a pilot study of poor sleepers.[19] In contrast to previous studies that demonstrated a prompt decrease in symptoms, one study found that 2 to 4 weeks was required to see improvement in 121 patients with serious insomnia.[20] These studies have been reviewed.[21]

Combination studies: Valerian is often combined with other herbs such as hops, St. John's wort, or balm in commercial products. A number of these combinations have been evaluated in clinical studies. A combination of Hyperion and valerian was evaluated for antidepressant activity in a double-blind study of 93 patients treated for 6 weeks. All psychometric scales showed statistically significant improvement.[22] A second study of the same combination in the treatment of anxiety reached similar positive conclusions.[23] A combination of valerian and *Hibiscus syriacus* (rose of sharron) was active in 130 depressed patients over 6 weeks.[24] A valerian combination preparation containing valerenic acid sesquiterpenes, but not valepotriates, improved sleep quality in a small crossover study of poor sleepers.[25] Valerian and *Melissa officinalis* (balm) were effective in combination in

a study (20 patients) of poor sleepers.[26] The same combination was found to be tolerated in healthy volunteers, and increased the quality of sleep.[27] A complex product made up of 6 herbs (*Crataegus, Ballota, Passiflora, Valeriana, Cola*, and *Paullinia*) was used to treat generalized anxiety (n = 91), producing progressive decreases in the Hamilton Anxiety Scale that were significantly greater than with placebo.[28]

TOXICOLOGY: Concern was raised over the discovery that valepotriates are mutagenic in the Ames assay; however, their poor bioavailability makes them a dubious source of toxicity for patients.[29] Mice have tolerated > 1 g/kg doses of valerian by oral and intraperitoneal routes, showing ataxia, muscle relaxation, and hypothermia.[30]

Clinical studies have generally found valerian to have fewer side effects than positive control drugs such as diazepam, producing little hangover effect when used as a sleep aid. An intentional overdose has been reported in which 20 times the recommended dose was ingested; the patient experienced mild symptoms that resolved within 24 hours.[31] A case of withdrawal after chronic use of valerian has been reported; however, the complex nature of the patient's medical history provides weak support for valerian's role.[32]

Valerian has been classified as GRAS (generally recognized as safe) in the US for food use; extracts and the root oil are used as flavorings in foods and beverages.

SUMMARY: Valerian root was approved by the German Commission E for restlessness and sleep disorders based on nervous conditions, and is official in the European Pharmacopoeia. A USP supplemental monograph on valerian was completed. ESCOP (F-4), BHP (vol.1) and WHO (vol.1) have also produced valerian monographs. While it appears to be safe and efficacious as a sleep aid, further research is required to elucidate the compounds responsible for its activity.

PATIENT INFORMATION – Valerian

Uses: Valerian has been used for the treatment of restlessness and sleep disorders. Valerian is classified as GRAS in the US for food use.

Side Effects: Studies have generally found valerian to have fewer side effects than other positive control drugs.

---

[1] Houghton P. The scientific basis for the reputed activity of valerian. *J Pharm Pharmacol* 1999;51(5):505-12.
[2] Leathwood P, et al. Aqueous extract of valerian root (Valeriana officinalis L.) improves sleep quality in man. *Pharmacol Biochem Behav* 1982;17(1):65-71.
[3] Santos M, et al. The amount of GABA present in aqueous extracts of valerian is sufficient to account for [3H]GABA release in synaptosomes. *Planta Med* 1994;60(5):475-76.

[4] Bos R, et al. Analytical aspects of phytotherapeutic valerian preparations. *Phytochem Anal* 1996;7(3):143-51.

[5] Bos R, et al. Seasonal variation of the essential oil, valerenic acid and derivatives, and valepotriates in *Valeriana officinalis* roots and rhizomes, and the selection of plants suitable for phytomedicines. *Planta Med* 1998;64(2):143-47.

[6] Granicher F, et al. Rapid high performance liquid chromatographic quantification of valepotriates in hairy root cultures of *Valeriana officinalis* L. var. *sambucifolia* Mikan. *Phytochem Anal* 1994;5(6):297-301.

[7] Hiller K, et al. Neuropharmacological studies on ethanol extracts of *Valeriana officinalis* L: behavioural and anticonvulsant properties. *Phytother Res* 1996;10:145-51.

[8] Leuschner J, et al. Characterization of the central nervous depressant activity of a commercially available valerian root extract. *Arzneimittelforschung* 1993;43(6):638-41.

[9] Krieglstein J, et al. Central depressant constituents in Valeriana, valepotriate, valerenic acid, valeranone and volatile oil are ineffective after all. *Dtsch Apoth Ztg* 1988;128(40):2041.

[10] Riedel E, et al. Inhibition of gamma-aminobutyric acid catabolism by valerenic acid derivatives. *Planta Med* 1982;46:219-20.

[11] Hendriks H, et al. Pharmacological screening of valerenal and some other components of essential oil of Valeriana officinalis. *Planta Med* 1981;42(1):62-68.

[12] Hendriks H, et al. Central nervous depressant activity of valerenic acid in the mouse. *Planta Med* 1985;51(1):28.

[13] Hazelhoff B, et al. Antispasmodic effects of valeriana compounds: an in-vivo and in-vitro study on the guinea-pig ileum. *Arch Int Pharmacodyn Ther* 1982;257(2):274-87.

[14] Kamm-Kohl A, et al. Modern valerian therapy of nervous disorders in elderly patients. *Med Welt* 1984;35:1450.

[15] Leathwood P, et al. Aqueous extract of valerian reduces latency to fall asleep in man. *Planta Med* 1985;Apr(2):144-48.

[16] Balderer G, et al. Effect of valerian on human sleep. *Psychopharmacology (Berl)* 1985;87(4):406-09.

[17] Schmidt-Vogt J. Treatment of nervous sleep disturbances and inner restlessness with a purely herbal sedative. *Therapiewoche* 1986;36:663-67.

[18] Seifert T. Therapeutische effekte von baldrian bei nervösen störungen. *Therapeutikon* 1988;2:94-98.

[19] Schulz H, et al. The effect of valerian extract on sleep polygraphy in poor sleepers: a pilot study. *Pharmacopsychiatry* 1994;27(4):147-51.

[20] Vorbach E, et al. Therapie von insomnien: wirksamkeit und verträglichkeit eines baldrian-präparates. *Psychopharmakotherapie* 1996;3109.

[21] Schulz V, et al. Clinical trials with phyto-psychopharmacological agents. *Phytomedicine* 1997;4(4):379-87.

[22] Steger W. Depressions: A randomized double blind study to compare the efficaciousness of a combination of plant derived extracts with a synthetic antidepressant. *Therapeutisches Erfahrungen* 1985;61:914-18.

[23] Panijel M. Therapy of symptoms of anxiety. *Therapiewoche* 1985;414659.

[24] Kniebel R, et al. Therapy of depression in the clinic. A multicenter double-blind comparison of herbal extracts from valerian roots and roses of sharron with the standard antidepressant amitryptiline. *Therapeutisches Erfahrungen* 1988;64:689-96.

[25] Lindahl O, et al. Double blind study of a valerian preparation. *Pharmacol Biochem Behav* 1989;32(4):1065-66.

[23] DreBing H, et al. Insomnia: Are valerian/balm combinations of equal value to benzodiazepine? *Therapiewoche* 1992;42:726-36.

[27] Cerny A, et al. Tolerability and efficacy of valerian/lemon balm in healthy volunteers (a double-blind, placebo-controlled, multicentre study). *Fitoterapia* 1999;70:221-28.

[23] Bourin M, et al. A combination of plant extracts in the treatment of outpatients with adjustment disorder with anxious mood: controlled study vs placebo. *Fundam Clin Pharmacol* 1997;11:127-32.

[23] von der Hude W, et al. Bacterial mutagenicity of the tranquilizing constituents of Valerianaceae roots. *Mutat Res* 1986;169:23-27.

[30] Hobbs C. Valerian: a literature review. *Herbalgram* 1989;(21):19.

[31] Willey L, et al. Valerian overdose: a case report. *Vet Hum Toxicol* 1995;37(4):364.

[32] Garges H, et al. Cardiac complications and delirium associated with valerian root withdrawal. *JAMA* 1998;280(18):1566-67.

Vanilla

SCIENTIFIC NAME(S): *Vanilla planifolia* Andr. (synonymous with *V. fragrans* and *V. tahitensis*). Family: Orchidaceae

COMMON NAME(S): Vanilla, Bourbon vanilla, Mexican vanilla, Tahiti vanilla.

BOTANY: The vanilla plant is a perennial herbaceous vine that grows to heights of 25 m in the wild and can produce fruit for 30 to 40 years.[3] It is native to tropical America and grows abundantly in Mexico. It is now cultivated throughout the tropics, including Reunion (Bourbon);[3] Madagascar produces approximately 80% of the world's supply.[4] The fully-grown unripe fruit (called the bean or pod) is collected and subjected to a complicated and labor-intensive fermentation process; together with the drying stage, this curing process requires from 5 to 6 months to complete.[1] During this time, vanillin is produced by the enzymatic conversion of glucovanillin[3] within the bean and vanillin may accumulate as white crystal on the bean surface giving it a frosted appearance.

HISTORY: Vanilla has a long history of use as a food flavoring and fragrance. Westerners were likely introduced to vanilla by the Aztec emperor Montezuma II, who prepared a vanilla-flavored chocolate drink for Hernando Cortez in the early 1500s.[4] Although vanillin is often used in bulk food preparation, it cannot be readily substituted for the natural extract where the delicate fragrance of the pure extractive is desired. Traditional uses of vanilla have included its use as an aphrodisiac, carminative, antipyretic, and stimulant. It has been added to foods to reduce the amount of sugar needed for sweetening and has been said to curb the development of dental caries.[2]

CHEMISTRY: The quality of the vanilla bean is not dependent on the vanillin content even though vanillin is associated with the characteristic fragrance of the plant. Numerous other constituents characterize the flavor and quality of vanilla and its extracts.[1]

Vanilla extracts are prepared by percolating ground vanilla bean with an alcohol/water mixture. Vanilla has been reported to contain up to approximately 3% vanillin, the major flavoring component. However, more than 150 other minor components contribute to the full-bodied fragrance of natural vanilla. The vanillin content differs with the variety of the bean, with Bourbon beans containing generally higher amounts than Mexican and Tahiti beans.[1]

Because synthetically-produced vanillin can be obtained inexpensively, it is often used as a substitute or adulterant for natural vanilla extract. Extracts of Mexican origin have been adulterated with coumarin, presumably arising from the use of tonka beans.[3] These products do not meet FDA food safety standards. The FDA has prohibited use of coumarin in food since 1954, due to its potential hazards. Unfortunately, there is no simple method to distinguish if a vanilla extract is authentic, although more sophisticated chromatographic methods can assist in defining the quality of an extract.[3] Only about 6% of the market for vanilla flavoring is held by pure vanilla extract.[4] Vanilla extract produced by biotechnological methods of plant culturing have yielded good grades of natural vanilla.[4]

PHARMACOLOGY: The anti-caries effects of vanilla have not been well documented but are believed to be related to the catechin content of the plant.[2]

Meals flavored with vanilla have been shown in controlled studies to provide a greater degree of satiety relative to nutritionally-identical unflavored meals.[6]

TOXICOLOGY: Although allergenic properties have been associated with vanilla, they do not appear to be related to the vanillin component of the plant.[1] Rather, the dermatitis may be caused by the calcium oxalate crystal in the plant.[2] Workers preparing vanilla have reported headache, dermatitis, and insomnia, which together have been characterized as a syndrome known as "vanillism."[2]

In a recent survey of ingredients of prescription and OTC health care products, vanilla was the second most common flavoring, superseded only by cherry, suggesting that persons with a known hypersensitivity to vanilla extract should be vigilant to the wide-spread use of this flavoring in pharmaceuticals.[5]

SUMMARY: Vanilla and its extract are widely used as food and perfume components. The fragrance of vanilla is the result of the combined characteristics of more than 150 volatile components, although vanillin accounts for the majority of the flavor.

PATIENT INFORMATION – Vanilla

Uses: Vanilla has been used widely as a food, flavoring, and in perfume components.

Side Effects: Some allergenic properties have been associated with vanilla.

[1] Leung AY. *Encyclopedia of Common Natural Ingredients used in Food, Drugs, and Cosmetics.* New York, NY: J. Wiley and Sons, 1980.

[2] Duke JA. *Handbook of Medicinal Herbs.* Boca Raton, FL: CRC Press, 1985

[3] vans WC. *Trease and Evans' Pharmacognosy,* 13th edition. London: Balliere-Tindall, 1989.

[4] King J. Plain Vanilla. *USAir Magazine* March, 1988;96,99,100.

[5] Kumar A, et al. The mystery of ingredients: sweeteners, flavorings, dyes, and preservatives in analgesic/antipyretic, antihistamine/decongestant, cough and cold, antidiarrheal, and liquid theophylline preparations. *Pediatrics* 1993;91:927-33

[5] Warwick ZS, et al. Taste and smell sensations enhance the satiating effect of both a high-carbohydrate and a high-fat meal in humans. *Physiol Behav* 1993;53:553-63.

Veratrum

SCIENTIFIC NAME(S): *Veratrum* species (Family: Liliaceae)

BOTANY: Included among its approximately 30 species are the following:

Scientific Name	Common Names	Distribution
V. album L.	White hellebore, langwort	Europe and Northern Asia
V. viride A.	Green hellebore, false hellebore, itchweed, Indian poke	Eastern US and Canada
V. californicum Dur	California false hellebore, Western hellebore	Western US
V. nigrum L.	Black false hellebore	Central Europe
V. fimbriatum	Fringed false hellebore	North America
V.frigidum[1,2]		Mexico

Veratrum album or white hellebore (WH) is a perennial that has a wide distribution throughout Europe, northern Asia, and North America. It grows to 5 feet and is characterized by a hairy stem. Its large, oval, yellow-green leaves alternate around the stem and have a slightly hairy undersurface. The lower leaves can reach a foot in length. Its greenish flowers bloom in June and July. The rhizome has an acrid taste and onion-like odor. The fruit is a capsule.[3]

Veratrum viride or green hellebore (GH) can grow to 8 feet in height and is found in damp areas such as marshes and swamps. It has oval to linear leaves, with green flowers on short stalks. Its habitat is northern North America, west of the Rockies.[4] The dried rhizome is the part of the plant used.[5] The plant's flowers are greenish yellow in color.[2]

WH resembles GH in structure and appearance (ie, similar leaves),[2] although its external color is much lighter.[5] The rhizomes of the 2 species are histologically, chemically, and toxicologically similar. WH may be more poisonous and contain more alkaloids than GH.[2]

HISTORY: *Veratrum* comes from the Latin *vere* meaning "truly," and *ater* meaning "black." In 1900, both species (*V. album* and *V. viride*) were recognized.[2]

The use of *V. album* centers around its toxic potential. It had been used as a poison during Roman times and an extract of the plant was used as an arrow tip poison. Small doses had been used to treat symptoms of cholera, often with less than desirable effects. White hellebore had been used in place of *Colchicum* for the treatment of gout, to aid in the treatment of hypertension, and externally to treat herpetic lesions, but its use has always been limited by its toxicity.

Green hellebore derives its name from the Latin *viride* meaning "green." This species was used by certain Indian tribes to treat congestion and arthritic pain. European settlers used the plant as a delousing agent. Like WH, GH is also highly toxic and rarely used in herbal medicines today except homeopathy in some cases.[4]

CHEMISTRY: Important alkaloids of both species in general include esters of highly hydroxylated parent alkanolamine bases, mainly cervine, germine, and protoverine. Other alkanolamines include jervine, rubijervine, pseudojervine, and isorubijervine. Alkaloids present in both species include veratrobasine and geralbine.[2] Veratrum alkaloids (cyclopamine, cycloposine, jervine, and veratramine) have been evaluated by carbon-13 and proton nuclear magnetic resonance spectra analyses.[6] Analysis of jervine from *Veratrum* species has also been performed using densitometry, thin layer, and liquid chromatography methods.[7] In addition, alkaloids from 17 species of veratrum have been identified and reviewed.[8,9]

White hellebore has been found to contain 2 related alkaloids, protoveratrine A and B. The rhizome contains about 1.5% total alkaloids, which also include germerine, jervine, pseudojervine, and veratrosine.[10] Minor and other alkaloids have been described.[11,12] Non-alkaloidal compounds have also been isolated from WH "above ground" parts and include cinnamic, isoferulic, caffeic, chlorogenic, fumaric, and succinic acids, and tectochrysin.[13] Organic acids veratric and vanillic are also present.[14] Other reports concerning WH-specific chemistry include: Phenolic compounds from aerial plant parts,[15] isolation of flavonoids chrysoeriol and apigenin,[16] determination of beta-adrenoceptor agonist, "o-acetyljervine,"[17] and identification of glycoside veratramarine.[18]

Three alkaloid groups are present in:
1.) Esters of steroidal bases (alkamines) with organic acids, including cevadine, germidine, germitrine, neogermitrine, neoprotoveratrine, protoveratrine, and veratridine;
2.) The glucosides of the alkamines pseudojervine and veratrosine;
3.) The alkamines themselves including germine, jervine, rabijervine, and veratramine.[5,19] Alkaloid mixtures alkavervir and cryptenamine are also specifically mentioned as being constituents in WH.[20]

Other *Veratrum* species chemistry is available, including vertaline B structure from *V. taliense*,[21] steroidal alkaloid isolation from *V. californicum*,[22] isolation of alkaloids verazine and angeloylzygadenine from *V. maacki*,[23] and isolation of a new indole alkaloid echinuline from *V. nigrum*.[24]

PHARMACOLOGY: The white and green varieties of veratrum have been used for their antihypertensive properties.[5,25,26,27] When administered intravenously, protoveratrine A and B cause a rapid reduction in blood pressure. Protoveratrine A is more active orally than B. Extracts of this plant have sometimes been combined with rauwolfia alkaloids in the treatment of hypertension.[28] Some alkaloids of *Veratrum* species exhibit a cardiotonic, digitalis-like effect.[9] Other sources report the ester alkaloids to reduce systolic and diastolic pressure, slow the heart rate, and stimulate peripheral blood flow.[2,19] (Large doses of plant extracts may cause respiratory depression.) Neurophysiological studies show certain alkaloids of GH work on the pacemaker area of the heart, and are of possible use in management of tachycardia or fibrillations.[2] In another report, protoveratrines caused prompt improvement of cardiac and respiratory functions in rats suffering from severe hypotension and respiratory depression, warranting further experimentation in the area of such crisis management as massive blood loss, etc. The mechanism could be attributable to an increase in total peripheral resistance and cardiac output.[29] However, the use of veratrum derivatives in the 1950s for hypertension therapy diminished with the discovery of more effective agents in the 1960s.[30]

Other actions of veratrum include stimulation of cardiac receptors, inhibiting ADH secretion in dogs,[31] and possible serotonin-agonist actions of constituent veratramine.[32]

Certain veratrum alkaloids exhibit in vitro cytotoxic effects on leukemia cells.[33] A later report discusses the demonstration of hemolytic and cytotoxic effects of the alkaloids.[34]

At least 1 report is available discussing a synthetic veratrum derivative and how it may be of use in myasthenia gravis treatment.[35]

Veratrum species have also been used as insecticides.[5,19] One report on *V. album* discusses its insecticidal activity against *Drosophila*, *Tribolium*, and *Aedes* species.[36]

Other uses for veratrum include treatments for cancers, respiratory problems, convulsions, mania, neuralgia, headaches, analgesia, inflammations, fluid retention, vomiting, toothache, amenorrhea, hiccoughs, measles, and sunstroke.[19]

Other *Veratrum* species literature is available concerning antiplatelet principles of *V. formosanum*,[37] absorption studies of *V. nigrum*,[38] and hemodynamic effects of *V. nigrum*.[39]

TOXICOLOGY: All *Veratrum* species are irritating;[19] however, *V. album*-specific poisonings have been the most often observed. For example, 7 cases have been reported to the Austrian Poison Information Center from 1977 to 1981.[40] Usual symptoms include hypotension, bradycardia, and gastrointestinal distress.[19,20,41] One source suggests ingestion of the alkaloids causes a burning sensation in the upper abdominal area followed by salivation, vomiting, and gastric erosion. Symptoms have been described as "having a heart attack." However, symptoms often disappear within 24 hours.[42]

Stereochemical configuration of veratrum alkaloids offer reason for the plant's teratogenicity.[43] Parasympathetic stimulation and increase in the permeability of sodium channels also contribute to its toxic mechanisms.[3]

Inhalation of the powdered rhizome induces a runny nose and violent sneezing.[44] Seven cases of intoxications have been reported from *V. album* alkaloids present in sneezing powder.[45] The fatal human dose of powdered rhizome is 1 to 2 g.[18]

Five cases of *V. album* poisoning have been reported, all having occurred shortly after ingestion of what was believed to be gentian wine (homemade; *V. album* was mistaken for *Gentiana lutea* when harvested because of similarities in appearance and habitat). Clinical effects included nausea, vomiting, abdominal pain, hypotension, and bradycardia. Therapy with atropine led to recovery within a few hours.[46] Another case of "mistaken identity" of *V. album* with *G. lutea* describes similar gastrointestinal and cardiac symptoms.[47]

Two additional *V. album* poisonings have occurred within 30 minutes of ingestion. Symptoms included vomiting, decrease in blood pressure, and bradycardia. Both cases had favorable outcomes.[48]

Six cases of *V. viride* poisonings have been reported, the symptoms being similar to those of *V. album* toxicity.[49]

Congenital tracheal stenosis occurred in 7 of 9 lambs born to 6 ewes who ingested the related species *V. californicum*. All 7 died from asphyxia within 5 minutes after birth.[50] Poisoning by this species is a veterinary problem in the US.

SUMMARY: Veratrum includes many species, most notably *V. album* and *V. viride*, which are similar. Their chemistry includes numerous alkaloids, some of which are toxic. Both species have been used for their antihypertensive properties. Different constituents may cause bradycardia, respiratory depression, or stimulation of peripheral blood flow. Other actions of veratrum include use as an insecticide and as a cytotoxic agent. *V. album* is considered toxic, with many reports of hypotension, bradycardia, and gastrointestinal distress. The toxicity of veratrum is so high that its use is not recommended.

PATIENT INFORMATION – Veratrum

Uses: Veratrum has been used to treat high blood pressure.

Side Effects: Veratrum is irritating and ingestion can result in a burning sensation in the upper abdominal area followed by salivation, vomiting, gastric erosion, hypotension, and bradycardia. There have been several poisonings reported in humans with the different species, but all had favorable outcomes.

---

[1] Hocking G. *A Dictionary of Natural Products.* Medford, NJ: Plexus Publishing, Inc., 1997;841-42.
[2] Osol A, et al. *The Dispensatory of the United States of America,* 25th ed. Philadelphia, PA: J.B. Lippincott Co., 1955;1486-92.
[3] Bruneton J. *Pharmacognosy, Phytochemistry, Medicinal Plants.* Paris, France: Lavoisier Publishing, 1995;872-75.
[4] Chevallier A. *Encyclopedia of Medicinal Plants.* New York, NY: DK Publishing, 1996;279.
[5] Tyler VE, et al. *Pharmacognosy,* 9th ed. Philadelphia, PA: Lea & Febiger, 1988;238-39.
[6] Gaffield W, et al. *J Nat Prod* 1986(Mar-Apr);49:286-92.
[7] Sarsunova M, et al. *Farmaceuticky Obzor* 1986;55(11):495-500.
[8] Grancai D, et al. *Ceska A Slovenska Farmacie* 1994(Apr);43:147-54.
[9] Grancai D, et al. *Ceska A Slovenska Farmacie* 1994(May);43:200-8.
[10] Schaeunberg P, Paris F. *Guide to Medicinal Plants.* New Canaan, CT: Keats Publishing, 1977.
[11] Foldesiova V, et al. *Farmaceuticky Obzor* 1995(Jul-Aug);64:193-96.
[12] Tomko J, et al. *Farmaceuticky Obzor* 1981;50(2):115-22.
[13] Grancai D, et al. *Farmaceuticky Obzor* 1991(Oct);60:473-77.
[14] Grancai D, et al. *Farmaceuticky Obzor* 1981;50(12):617-20.
[15] Foldesiova V, et al. *Farmaceuticky Obzor* 1996(Feb);65:31-33.
[16] Grancai D, et al. *Farmaceuticky Obzor* 1981;50(11):563-67.
[17] Gilani A, et al. *Archives of Pharmacal Research* 1995;18(2):129-32.
[18] Morton JF. *Major Medicinal Plants.* Springfield, IL: Charles C. Thomas Co., 1977.
[19] Duke J. *CRC Handbook of Medicinal Herbs.* Boca Raton, FL: CRC Press Inc., 1989;506-7.
[20] Reynolds E, ed. *Martindale, The Extra Pharmacopoeia,* 31st ed. London, England: Royal Pharmaceutical Society, 1996;964-65.
[21] Min Z, et al. *Yao Hsueh Hsueh Pau* 1988;23(8):584-87.
[22] Browne C, et al. *J Chromatogr* 1984;336(1):211-20.
[23] Zhao W, et al. *Chung Yao Tung Pao Bull Chin Materia Medica* 1986(May);11:294-95.
[24] Zhao W, et al. *Chung-Kuo Chung Yao Tsa Chih — China Journal of Chinese Materia Medica* 1991;16(7):425-26.
[25] Page L, et al. *N Eng J Med* 1972(Nov 23);287:1074-81.
[26] Petkov V. *Am J Chin Med* 1979;7(3):197-236.
[27] Atta-Ur-Rahman, et al. *Planta Med* 1993;59(6):569-71.
[28] Kupchan SM. *J Pharm Sci* 1961;50:273.
[29] Bertolini A, et al. *Experientia* 1990;46(7):704-8.
[30] Moser M. *Am J Med* 1986;80(5B):1-11.
[31] Thames M, et al. *Am J Physiol* 1980;239(6):H784-78.
[32] Izumi K, et al. *Brain Res Bull* 1978;3(3):237-240.
[33] Fuska J, et al. *Nemoplasma* 1981;28(6):709-14.
[34] Badria F, et al. *Pharmazie* 1995(Jun);50:421-23.
[35] Flacke W. *N Eng J Med* 1973(Jan 4);288:27-31.
[36] Sener B, et al. *Gazi Universitesi Eczacilik Fakultesi Dergisi* 1991;8(1):31-40.
[37] Chung M, et al. *Planta Med* 1992;58(3):274-76.
[38] Lin N, et al. *Chung Kuo Chung Yao Tsa Chih* 1992;17(1):43-45.
[39] Li S, et al. *Chinese Pharmaceutical Journal* 1997(Jul);32:407-9.
[40] Hruby K, et al. *Wien Klin Wochenschr* 1981;93(16):517-19.
[41] DeSmet P, et al, eds. *Adverse Effects of Herbal Drugs 1.* Berlin, Germany: Springer-Verlag, 1992;4.
[42] Lampe KF, McCann MA. *AMA Handbook of Poisonous and Injurious Plants.* Chicago: Am. Medical Assn., 1985.
[43] Gaffield W, et al. *Adv Exp Med Biol* 1984;177:241-51.
[44] Kinghorn DA, ed. *Toxic Plants.* New York: Columbia University Press, 1979.
[45] Fogh A, et al. *Journal of Toxicology — Clinical Toxicology* 1983;20(2):175-79.
[46] Garnier R, et al. *Ann Med Interne* 1985;136(2):125-28.
[47] Festa M, et al. *Minerva Anestesiol* 1996;62(5):195-96.
[48] Quatrehomme G, et al. *Hum Exp Toxicol* 1993;12(2):111-15.
[49] Jaffe A, et al. *J Emerg Med* 1990;8(2):161-67.
[50] Keeler R, et al. *Teratology* 1985;31(1):83-88.

White Cohosh

SCIENTIFIC NAME(S): *Actaea alba* (L.) Mill. (also known as *A. pachypoda* Ell.) and *A. rubra* (Ait.) Willd. Family: Ranunculaceae

COMMON NAME(S): White Cohosh, baneberry, snakeberry, coralberry, doll's eye

BOTANY: White cohosh is a bushy, herbaceous perennial, that can grow to 3 feet tall. Its wide leaves have 6 or more sharp leaflets. The small flowers are white and grow in clusters. The berries of the plant can be red or white.[1] The plant is found from Alaska to California and east to the mid-United States.[1] Anatomical structure has been investigated.[2]

HISTORY: The plant has been used in a manner similar to that of black and blue cohosh to stimulate menstruation and to treat other "female disorders." Certain tribes, such as Cherokee and Cheyenne, used the root to cure itching, colds and cough, urogenital disorders, stomach disorders and to revive those near death. It has also been used as a purgative and in childbirth.[3]

CHEMISTRY: The chemistry of the plant is poorly defined. A compound called protoanemonin is believed to be responsible for the irritant effect. In addition, the plant contains an essential oil. Fruits and seeds contain trans-aconitic acid.[3]

PHARMACOLOGY: Little is known about its pharmacologic effects. There are no studies confirming its effects in the treatment of women's disorders. Homeopaths have used the roots for arthritis and rheumatism.[3]

TOXICOLOGY: All parts of the plant are toxic, especially the roots and berries, which contain the toxic glycosides and an essential oil. Ingestion of these parts results in acute stomach cramping, headache, increased pulse rate, vomiting, delirium, and circulatory failure. As few as 6 berries can cause severe symptoms, persisting for hours.[4] The protoanemonin-like compound can inflame and blister the skin.[3] Gastric lavage, emesis, and supportive treatment are recommended if ingested.[1,3]

SUMMARY: There is no evidence that white cohosh is of any therapeutic value. Its ingestion can lead to toxicity. Its use should be discouraged. Few reports are available on this topic.

PATIENT INFORMATION – White Cohosh

Uses: White cohosh has been used historically to treat women's disorders. Homeopaths have used white cohosh to treat arthritis and rheumatism.

Side Effects: Ingestion of white cohosh results in stomach cramping, headache, increased pulse rate, vomiting, delirium, and circulatory failure.

---

[1] Turner N, et al. *Common Poisonous Plants and Mushrooms.* Portland, OR: Timber Press. 1991;99–100.
[2] Bukowiecki H, et al. *Acta Poloniae Pharmaceutica* 1972;29(4):425–30.
[3] Duke J. *CRC Handbook of Medicinal Herbs.* Boca Raton, FL: CRC Press, Inc. 1985;16.
[4] Hardin JW, Arena JM. *Human Poisoning from Native and Cultivated Plants.* Durham, NC: Duke University Press. 1974.

Wild Yam

SCIENTIFIC NAME(S): *Dioscorea villosa* L. Dioscoreaceae (Yams)

COMMON NAME(S): Wild yam root, colic root, yuma, devil's bones, rheumatism root, China root

BOTANY: *Dioscorea villosa* is a twining vine native to the central southeastern US and found less frequently in the Appalachian region. It is a dioecious plant with inconspicuous white to greenish yellow female flowers and smooth heart-shaped leaves. A Chinese species, *Dioscorea opposita* Thunb., is also occasionally found in herbal commerce. There are more than 500 species of *Dioscorea* worldwide.

HISTORY: Wild yam was popularized by the Eclectic medical movement in the 19th century for its supposed antispasmodic properties and prescribed for biliary colic and spasm of the bowel. More recently, it has been promoted for the relief of nausea in pregnancy, and for amenorrhoea and dysmenorrhea.[1] Further indications have been reported for urinary tract infections, rheumatoid arthritis, cholera, nervous excitement, and gas expulsion.

CHEMISTRY: While substantial amounts of chemical investigation have been made on other species of *Dioscorea*, there is little current work on *D. villosa*. As with many species of *Dioscorea*, *D. villosa* is a source of diosgenin.[2,3,4] It is not as prolific a producer of diosgenin as *D. zingiberensis*, *D. floribunda*, or other species. Diosgenin is not typically found in the free state in plants but commonly occurs as the saponins dioscin and gracillin. The saponins of *D. villosa* have not been elucidated, nor have other constituents of the species been investigated. A high performance liquid chromatography (HPLC) method for separation of dioscin, gracillin, and other *Dioscorea* saponins has been reported.[5]

PHARMACOLOGY: The root of *D. villosa* is reported to be diaphoretic and expectorant in a dose of 4 g.[6] Much of the current herbal use of wild yam is predicated on the misconception that the diosgenin contained in the product can be converted by the human body into steroid hormones, particularly progesterone, through the intermediate dehydroepiandrosterone (DHEA). This notion appears to be based on diosgenin's use as a synthetic precursor of cortisone[7] and of the steroids found in birth control pills. There is no scientific evidence to support the notion that diosgenin or dioscin can be converted by the body into human hormones. In a pilot study of women using wild yam products (*D. villosa*), it was found that progesterone synthesis appeared to be suppressed compared with controls.[8] No direct effect of wild yam extract on the estrogen or progesterone receptors was found.

Work with ginseng saponins has shown that metabolism by specific microbes in the gut can substantially enhance uptake of the metabolites into the body.[9,10] Thus, one may postulate a similar mechanism of uptake with other, otherwise poorly absorbed plant saponins such as dioscin. Research needs to be done to understand the pharmacodynamics of saponin-containing plants in humans.

Topical formulations of *Dioscorea* are also poorly understood, though it is unlikely that they can serve as "progesterone replacement" vehicles. The sale of supplemental DHEA as an "anti-aging" product has carried over to *Dioscorea* by analogy. In fact, several products containing *Dioscorea* and DHEA are available.

TOXICOLOGY: In large doses, *D. villosa* root may cause nausea, vomiting, and diarrhea.

SUMMARY: Wild yam root is currently recommended for the treatment of menstrual dysfunction; however, little scientific evidence supports its use in medicine. The potential for toxicity is modest; however, in the absence of evidence of benefit, it cannot be recommended. A monograph of wild yam can be found in the *British Herbal Pharmacopoeia*, vol. 2.[11]

PATIENT INFORMATION – Wild Yam

Uses: *Dioscorea* has been promoted for the treatment of menstrual dysfunction, nausea in pregnancy, urinary tract infections, rheumatoid arthritis, cholera, nervous excitement, and gas expulsion.

Side Effects: In large doses, *D. villosa* root may cause nausea, vomiting, and diarrhea.

[1] Brinker F. A comparative review of eclectic female regulators. *J Naturopathic Med* 1996;7:11.

[2] Marker R, et al. Sterols. CIV. Diosgenin from certain American plants. *J Am Chem Soc* 1940;62:2542.

[3] Wall M, et al. Steroidal sapogenins. XII. Survey of plants for steroidal sapogenins and other constituents. *J Am Pharm Assoc Sci Ed* 1954;43:503.

[4] Sauvaire Y, et al. Diosgenin, (25R)-spirost-5-en-3b-ol; problems of the acid hydrolysis of saponins. *Lloydia* 1978;41:247.

[5] Xu C, et al. Comparison of silica-C18-and NH2-HPLC columns for the separation of neutral steroid saponins from Dioscorea plants. *J Liq Chromatogr* 1985;8:361.

[6] Claus E. *Textbook of Pharmacognosy*, 5th ed. Philadelphia, PA: Lea & Febiger, 1956:151-52.

[7] Cornell D, et al. The search for plant precursors of cortisone. *Econ Bot* 1955;9:307.

[8] Zava D, et al. Estrogen and progestin bioactivity of foods, herbs, and spices. *Proc Soc Exp Biol Med* 1998;217:369.

[9] Akao T, et al. Appearance of compound K, a major metabolite of ginsenoside Rb1 by intestinal bacteria, in rat plasma after oral administration-measurement of compound K by enzyme immunoassay. *Biol Pharm Bull* 1998;21:245.

[10] Hasegawa H, et al. Main ginseng saponin metabolites formed by intestinal bacteria. *Planta Med* 1996;62:453.

[11] *British Herbal Pharmacopoeia*, vol 2. Great Britain: British Herbal Medicine Association, 1996.

Willard Water

COMMON NAME(S): Willard's water, catalyst altered water, CAW, carbonaceous activated water, Biowater

HISTORY: Willard water is a product with a history that dates to the early twentieth century. This product was developed by John Wesley Willard, PhD, a professor of chemistry at the South Dakota School of Mines and Technology. During the 1930s, Willard patented an industrial cleanser used to degrease and clean train parts. The liquid was named "carbonaceous activated water" or "catalyst activated water." However, over the years, the product became legendary among townfolks who used "Willard's water" to treat practically every recognized animal and human disease. In the early 1970s, Willard distributed a product called "Dr. Willard's Water XXX" with lignite, which was advertised as a plant growth stimulator. In 1980, the CBS network program "60 Minutes" featured Dr. Willard and the water, showing fruits and plants that had grown to many times their normal size, allegedly because of treatment with Willard water. Thereafter, a national sales system developed, with some distributors suggesting exaggerated indications for the product, including the treatment of arthritis, acne, anxiety, nervous stomach, hypertension, ulcers, hair growth, and food preservation, in addition to serving as a laundry aid and a treatment for bovine and feline leukemia.

The Willard family has ackowledged that the product does not have the capability to cure disease. The FDA does not recognize Willard water as an approved drug and does not recognize claims of medical benefits for the product.

CHEMISTRY: The formula of Willard water appears to have changed over the decades. Analysis of Willard water products by the FDA found that they contain various combinations of rock salt, lignite, sodium metasilicate, sulfated castor oil, calcium chloride, and magnesium sulfate.

PHARMACOLOGY: There are no valid data describing the botanical, animal, or human effects of Willard water. One advertisement indicates that the product is a "powerful free radical scavenger [and] antioxidant and enables any organism - plant or animal - to tolerate stressful conditions better, assimilate nutrients more efficiently, and recover from injuries faster."

TOXICOLOGY: No reports of toxicity had been reported to the FDA as of 1982, and the product has not been generally associated with significant toxicity problems.

SUMMARY: Willard water is a solution of electrolytes and other compounds, and had originally been developed as an industrial cleanser. Over the past 60 years, exaggerated claims have been made for the product, including its use for the treatment of various diseases. There are no data to suggest that the product is of any significant therapeutic value.

PATIENT INFORMATION – Willard Water

Uses: There are no proven pharmacological effects of willard water, but in the past it has been used as an industrial cleanser.

Side Effects: There are no reported side effects.

---

[1] No references.

Willow Bark

SCIENTIFIC NAME(S): *Salix alba* L., *Salix purpurea* L., *Salix fragilis* L., and other species. Family: Salicaceae (willow family)

COMMON NAME(S): Willow, weidenrinde, white willow (*S. alba*), purple osier willow/basket willow (*S. purpurea*), crack willow (*S. fragilis*)

BOTANY: Willows are small trees or shrubs, many of which grow in moist places or along riverbanks in temperate and cold climates. Most of the several hundred species are dioecious, with male and female catkins (flowers) on separate plants. Largely insect pollinated, different species of willow hybridize freely. Medicinal willow bark is collected in the early spring from young branches (2 to 3 years of age) of the species listed above. Other species of *Salix* have similar chemistry and pharmacology.

HISTORY: For centuries, the bark of European willows has been used to treat fevers, headache and other pain, and arthritis. North American willows have also been used in folk medicine. Most of the European medicinal willows have been introduced to the Americas and have escaped cultivation. In the late 19th century, salicylic acid was widely used in place of willow bark, and its derivative aspirin was discovered to be less irritating to the mouth and stomach.[1,2]

CHEMISTRY: Salicylate derivatives are the primary medicinal constituents of willow bark. While small amounts of salicylic acid can be detected in most species, the principle salicylates of *S. alba* are the phenolic ester glycoside salicortin[3,4] and glycoside salicin, its acid hydrolysis product. Salicin is hydrolyzed in the intestine to saligenin (o-hydroxybenzyl alcohol), which is absorbed and then oxidized to salicylic acid.[5] Salicortin and other related salicylates are chemically unstable (for example, to the boiling water in teas)[6] and avoidance of loss of these compounds requires careful drying of the bark.[6,7,8] Extraction protocols that avoid decomposition of the native glycosides have been developed. Most standards for medicinal willow bark require salicylates to be greater than 1% of dry weight; however, this standard is difficult to achieve with many source species. This has stimulated surveys of the salicylate content of many other species of *Salix*[9,10] as well as aspen (*Populus*), which also contains salicylates.[11] While the leaves generally contain lower concentrations of salicylates than the bark, several species contain medicinally useful quantities of salicylates in their leaves.[12] Salicylates have been quantified in willows by spectrophotometry,[13] by thin-layer chromatography (TLC),[14] by high-performance liquid chromatography (HPLC) after enzymatic deglycosylation,[15] and by capillary electrophoresis.[16] A method using gas chromatography of silyl derivatives of salicylates gave comparable results to HPLC.[17] An HPLC method was used to compare the salicylate content of different cultivated clones of *Salix myrsinifolia* grown in a single location.[18] NMR spectra of the principle salicylates of willows have been reported and assigned.[19] The ecological role of salicylates has also been investigated.[20] Naringenin glycosides,[21] oligomeric procyanidins,[22] and condensed tannins presumably derived from the simpler flavonols have been obtained from commercial willow barks.

PHARMACOLOGY: The ester glycosides salicortin, tremulacin, and fragilin can be considered to be pro-drugs of salicylic acid, that deliver this compound into the systemic circulation without irritating the GI tract.[23] The pharmacokinetics of salicylic acid delivered from willow bark have been studied, and the plasma half-life is determined as approximately 2.5 hours.[24] The mechanism of action of salicylic acid is inhibition of cyclooxygenase enzymes, which are involved in prostaglandin synthesis. The anti-inflammatory efficacy of tremulacin (a derivative of salicin) has recently been studied.[25] A clinical trial of a willow bark preparation found mild efficacy in arthritis.[26]

TOXICOLOGY: There are no reports of adverse effects due to the use of willow bark; although, additive effects with synthetic salicylates must be considered. Use with caution in patients with peptic ulcers and other medical conditions in which aspirin is contraindicated.

SUMMARY: Willow bark was approved by the German Commission E for diseases accompanied by fever, rheumatic ailments, and headaches. It is monographed by ESCOP, the British Herbal Pharmacopeia, and is official in the German Pharmacopeia. An American Herbal Pharmacopeia monograph is due to be published shortly.

Willow bark can be an effective analgesic if the content of salicylates is adequate. Adverse effects are those of salicylates in general. Use with caution in patients with peptic ulcers and other medical conditions in which aspirin is contraindicated.

PATIENT INFORMATION – Willow Bark

Uses: Willow bark can be an effective analgesic if the content of salicylates is adequate.

Side Effects: Adverse effects are those of salicylates in general. Use with caution in patients with peptic ulcers and other medical conditions in which aspirin is contraindicated.

[1] Weissmann G. Aspirin. *Sci Am* 1991;264(1):84-90.

[2] Jourdier S. A miracle drug. *Chem Ber* 1999;35:33.

[3] Thieme H. Die phenolglykoside der Salicaceen. *Planta Med* 1965;13:431.

[4] Pearl I, et al. The structures of salicortin and tremulacin. *Phytochem* 1971;10:3161.

[5] Meier B, et al. Pharmaceutical aspects of the use of willow in herbal remedies. *Planta Med* 1988;54:559.

[6] Steele J, et al. Phytochemistry of the Salicaceae. VI. The use of a gas-liquid chromatographic screening test for the chemotaxonomy of *Populus* species. *J Chromatogr* 1973;84(2):315-18.

[7] Julkunen-Tiitto R, et al. The effect of the sample preparation method of extractable phenolics of Salicaceae species. *Planta Med* 1989;55:55.

[8] Julkunen-Tiitto R, et al. Further studies on drying willow (*Salix*) twigs: the effect of low drying temperature on labile phenolics. *Planta Med* 1992;58:385.

[9] Julkunen-Tiitto R. Chemotaxonomical screening of phenolic glycosides in northern willow twigs by capillary gas chromatography. *J Chromatogr* 1985;324:129.

[10] Meier B, et al. A chemotaxonomic survey of phenolic compounds in Swiss willow species. *Planta Med* 1992;58:A698.

[11] Clausen T, et al. A simple method for the isolation of salicortin, tremulacin, and tremuloiden from quaking aspen (*Populus tremuloides*). *J Nat Prod* 1989;52:207.

[12] Julkunen-Tiitto R. A chemotaxonomic survey of phenolics in leaves of northern Salicaceae species. *Phytochem* 1986;25:663.

[13] Afsharypour S, et al. Estimation of salicin in barks and leaves of *Salix* species by a TLC-spectrophotometric method. *J Sch Pharm* 1995;4:8.

[14] Vanhaelen M, et al. Quantitative determination of biologically active constituents in medicinal plant crude extracts by thin-layer chromatography-densitometry. *J Chromatogr* 1983;281:263.

[15] Luo W, et al. Determination of salicin and related compounds in botanical dietary supplements by liquid chromatography with fluorescence detection. *J AOAC Int* 1998;81(4):757-62.

[16] Zaugg S, et al. Capillary electrophoretic analysis of salicin in *Salix* spp. *J Chromatogr A* 1997;781:487.

[17] Meier B, et al. Comparative high-performance liquid and gas-liquid chromatographic determination of phenolic glucosides in Salicaceae species. *J Chromatogr* 1988;442:175.

[18] Julkunen-Tiitto R, et al. Variation in growth and secondary phenolics among field-cultivated clones of *Salix myrsinifolia*. *Planta Med* 1992;58:77.

[19] Dommisse R, et al. Structural analysis of phenolic glycosides from Salicaceae by NMR spectroscopy. *Phytochem* 1986;25:1201.

[20] Roininen H, et al. Oviposition stimulant for a gall-inducing sawfly, *Euura lasiolepis*, on willow is a phenolic glucoside. *J Chem Ecol* 1999;25:943.

[21] Pearl I, et al. Phenolic extractives of *Salix purpurea* bark. *Phytochem* 1970;9:1277.

[22] Kolodziej H. Olimeric flavan-3-ols from medicinal willow bark. *Phytochem* 1990;29:955.

[23] Kaul R, et al. Willow bark. Renaissance of a phyto-analgesic. *Deutsche Apoth Ztg* 1999;139:3439.

[24] Pentz R. Bioverfügbarkeit von salicylsäure und coffein aus einem phytoanalgetischen kominationspräparat. *Deutsche Apoth Ztg* 1989;92.

[25] Cheng G, et al. Anti-inflammatory effects of tremulacin, a salicin-related substance isolated from *Populus tomentosum* Carr leaves. *Phytomed* 1994;1:209.

[26] Mills S, et al. Effect of a propietary herbal medicine on the relief of chronic arthritis pain: a double-blind study. *Br J Rheumatol* 1996;35(9):874-78.

Wine

SOURCE: Wine is an agricultural product created by the natural fermentation of sun-ripened grape juice. Yeast-induced fermentation converts endogenous sugars to alcohol, and the flavors associated with each wine depend on the grape variety, harvest, and fermentation conditions. While most wines are derived from grapes, fermentation of other fruits and vegetables has yielded alcoholic wine-like beverages. Wine production includes a series of steps including extraction of juice, fermentation, clarification, and aging.[1,2]

HISTORY: Wine has played an important role in societal development for thousands of years. The first cultivated grapes were grown in Asia Minor around 6000 BC. Archaeologists have uncovered the remains of a 2600-year-old winery in Israel.[1] Egyptian accounts of wine-making date back to 2500 BC. The Bible mentions raising grapes to make wine.[2] Hippocrates (450 to 370 BC) was said to be the first physician to realize the healing value of wine.[3] The Romans disseminated the science and art of wine-making throughout much of the world, and Europe subsequently became the center of wine-growing expertise. Wine-making techniques were kept alive during the Dark Ages by the clergy. Early fermentation procedures produced heavy wines that often were exceedingly sweet. Refinement of the fermentation process resulted in the development of numerous varieties of wines, each with unique flavors and typical alcohol contents. Wine has had a role in societal interactions and many religious ceremonies. The growth of the American wine industry during the 20th century was halted by prohibition (1919 to 1933) but has risen steadily since. Today, almost every state in the US produces wines, with boutique wineries accounting for a growing proportion of the production.[1,2] Several historical articles discussing the history of wine and wine in the practice of medicine are available.[4,5,6,7,8,9,10,11,12,13]

CHEMISTRY: The chemical composition of wine is varied and complex. A typical wine contains more than 300 components other than alcohol, often containing minerals and vitamins not found in other fermented beverages.[1] Alcohol concentrations may vary from 10% to 14% for table wines and up to 20% for certain aperitifs. While the prevalent alcohol is ethanol, glycerol plus more than a dozen alcohols have been isolated from wines.[14] The polyphenols in wine have desirable biological properties, including phenolic acids (p-coumaric, cinnamic, caffeic, gentisic, ferulic, and vanillic) and trihydroxy stilbenes (polydatin, resveratrol).[12,15] One Japanese report ana-lyzes resveratrol and piceid (and their isomers) content in 42 different wines. The average stilbene content was 4.37 mg/L in red wines and 0.68 mg/L in white.[16] Wine flavonoids are also present (1 to 3 g/L in red wines, 0.2 g/L in white) and include flavonols, anthocyanins, flavanols (catechins, quercetin), oligomers (procyanidins), and polymers (tannins) of the catechins.[12,17] Champagnes and sparkling wines contain ≈ 1.5% carbon dioxide. Other wine components include carbonyl compounds, organic acids, tannins, carbohydrates, and esters.[1,14]

PHARMACOLOGY: The correlation between wine consumption and reduced heart disease and mortality has been widely reported. World Health Organization data show that fat consumption is associated with coronary heart disease (CHD) mortality. However, certain populations where daily consumption of wine is highest (eg, Italy, Switzerland, France) had high-fat intake but low CHD mortality rates. This was termed the "French paradox."[18] Researchers previously had seen that there was a population-based association between CHD mortality and increased wine consumption.[19] Subsequent reports confirm that moderate intake of wine lowers CHD mortality.[20,21,22] In one study, the rate of CHD mortality per 1000 men decreased from ≈ 22 among those who did not drink alcohol to ≈ 8 for those who had 2 drinks per day.[23] The Copenhagen City Heart Study (CCHS) (Copenhagen, Denmark), initiated in 1976, analyzed 13,329 patients 45 to 84 years of age for 16 years to determine risk of first stroke. Although this report did not address factors such as genetic diversity, existing risk factors, or type (red or white) or amount of wine consumed, it confirmed that wine has beneficial effects. It was concluded that compounds other than ethanol in wine are responsible for the protective effect on risk of stroke.[24] The National Stroke Association (NSA) states that heavy drinking increases stroke risk. They agree that modest consumption, such as a 4 oz glass of wine per day, may lower stroke risk, provided that there is no other medical reason to avoid alcohol.[25]

Recent reports confirm the relationship between alcohol consumption and decrease in cardiovascular (CV) risk. A review of 30 population studies suggests this correlation but also emphasizes that the effect of alcohol and CV risk is highly dependent on other risk factors. Alcohol as a "heart medicine" was deemed insufficient in this report.[26] A later study agrees that alcoholic intake is associated with lower CHD risks but also comments that mortality can be influenced by lifestyle characteristics (eg, smoking, obesity).[27]

Red wine phenolic compound has positive effects on plasma antioxidant capacity.[28] Antioxidants prevent the oxidation of LDL cholesterol into plaque, which is known to clog arteries, leading to cardiovascular disease (CVD).[29] The most potent antioxidants for LDL (in descending order) are the phenolics (epicatechin, catechin, and resveratrol).[30]

Several mechanisms have been suggested as to the beneficial CV effects of wine polyphenols. Nitric oxide production by vascular endothelium, modulation of lipoproteins by decreasing total cholesterol and increasing HDL levels, and carcinogenesis inhibition have all been reported.[12,31] Red wine polyphenols are thought to inhibit several pathways leading to CHD. A range of 300 to 500 mg of extract appears to protect against CVD. Its vasorelaxing activity and inhibition of platelet aggregation can be beneficial for disease prevention.[15]

Wine flavonoids and phenolics inhibit clotting by platelet aggregation inhibition.[17] This is apparently done by inhibition of either oxygenase enzymes[32] or thromboxane synthesis.[12]

Purple grape juice may have the same effects as red wine in reducing heart disease risk.[33] Fruit consumption has also correlated highly with reduced CHD mortality.[22]

Aside from cardiovascular disease, a large body of evidence has accumulated regarding the benefits of moderate wine intake in the management of other afflictions. These include emotional tension, anxiety, and inability to relax. The pharmacology of ethanol has been well characterized (including its effects on the CNS and smooth and skeletal muscles).[2,14] Also included are achlorhydria and related gastric disorders and malabsorption syndromes.[14,19] Certain substances in wine promote better absorption of minerals such as calcium, magnesium, phosphorus, and zinc. The aroma and taste of wine stimulate the appetite, especially in elderly and debilitated patients.[2,14] White wine also significantly shortens gastric emptying time.[34] Wine also may be of benefit topically to stimulate wound healing and to improve rheumatoid skin ulcerations.[35]

TOXICOLOGY: Alcohol consumption has detrimental physical, medical, social, and economic ramifications.

This monograph will not address these well-known facets of alcohol (and wine) consumption. The danger of drinking too much wine is available in a concise summary.[2] In addition, a recent report on the management of heavy drinkers is referenced as well.[36]

Typically, adverse reactions to pure wine are rare. The vast majority of commercially prepared wines now contain sulfites as preservatives, and those sensitive to these chemicals may develop severe allergic reactions, including wheezing and tachycardia. Those sensitive to yeasts may experience allergies to some wines. While a glass of wine before bedtime has long been an accepted treatment for temporary insomnia, a larger amount may be counterproductive because it depresses respiration resulting in sleep apnea.[37]

Headaches following the ingestion of some wines (particularly chianti) have been associated with histamine or tyramine content although the relationship has not been firmly established. Tyramine may result in a severe drug interaction (eg, hypertensive crisis) in patients taking MAO inhibitors.[38]

Patients with gastroesophageal reflux should ingest wine cautiously because wine worsens reflux.[39,40]

A direct association has been made between increasing wine consumption and the rate of ovarian cancer in women in Italy.[41] Excessive wine consumption has been associated with a reversible rise in systolic blood pressure levels.[42]

Women should not drink alcoholic beverages during pregnancy because of the risk of birth defects. Alcohol consumption is contraindicated in people with viral hepatitis such as hepatitis B and C.

SUMMARY: Wine has been a part of civilization for thousands of years. Wines are complex mixtures of flavors and fragrances. They have been used as beverages and as the basis for traditional medicines. The correlation between wine consumption and reduced heart disease has been shown in many reports. Other factors do play a role, including amount consumed, smoking, and certain lifestyle habits. Wine has antioxidant activity and inhibits clotting by altering platelet aggregation. Other benefits include reduction in anxiety and better absorption of certain nutrients. Adverse reactions to pure wine are rare. Some people may be sensitive to other ingredients in wine.

PATIENT INFORMATION – Wine

Uses: Studies suggest that wine may lower the incidence of cardiovascular disease.

Drug Interactions: Tyramine in certain wines (particularly chianti) may cause life-threatening hypertensive crisis in patients receiving MAO inhibitors concurrently or for at least 4 weeks after MAO inhibitor therapy is discontinued.[43]

Side Effects: Adverse reactions to pure wine are rare. Headaches following the ingestion of some wines have been associated with histamine or tyramine content. Patients with gastroesophageal reflux should ingest wine cautiously because it may worsen reflux. Alcohol consumption is contraindicated in people with viral hepatitis such as hepatitis B and C.

[1] *Wine and America*. Emeryville, CA: Wine Growers of California, 1986.

[2] Ensminger A, et al. *Foods and Nutrition Encyclopedia*, 2nd ed. vol. 2. Boca Raton FL: CRC Press, Inc. 1994;2336-44.

[3] Van Laere J. Nonnius, 'dietetics' and oenology. *Verh K Acad Geneeskd Belg* 1996;58(3):301-17.

[4] Berland T. Wine as a medicine. *West Med Med J West* 1966 Apr;7(4):80-83.

[5] Leake C, et al. The clinical use of wine in geriatrics. *Geriatrics* 1967;22(2):175-80.

[6] Cambon K. Wine and otolaryngology. *Trans Pac Coast Otoophthalmol Soc Annu Meet* 1968;52:69-80.

[7] Favazza A. Wine in medicine. *Mich Med* 1968;67(21):1355-56.

[8] Anon. Wine in the practice of medicine. *Pa Med* 1969;72(1):20.

[9] Lucia S. Wine: A food throughout the ages. *Am J Clin Nutr* 1972 Apr;25(4):361-62.

[10] Spring J, et al. Three centuries of alcohol in the British diet. *Nature* 1977;270(5638):567-72.

[11] Van Laere J. Hieronymus Fracastorius, from syphilographist to oenologist. *Verh K Acad Geneeskd Belg* 1993;55(4):305-17.

[12] Soleas G, et al. Wine as a biological fluid: History, production, and role in disease prevention. *J Clin Lab Anal* 1997;11(5):287-313.

[13] Haas C. Barley, the olive and wine, dietary and therapeutic triad of ancient Mediterranean people. *Ann Med Interne* 1998;149(5):275-79.

[14] *Uses of Wine in Medical Practice*. San Francisco, CA: Wine Advisory Board, 1975.

[15] Halpern M, et al. Red-wine polyphenols and inhibition of platelet aggregation: Possible mechanisms, and potential use in health promotion and disease prevention. *J Int Med Res* 1998;26(4):171-80.

[16] Sato M, et al. Contents of resveratrol, piceid, and their isomers in commercially available wines made from grapes cultivated in Japan. *Biosci Biotechnol Biochem* 1997;61(11):1800-5.

[17] Anon. *Chemistry and Industry*. 1995 May 1:338-41.

[18] Renaud S, et al. Wine, alcohol, platelets, and the French paradox for coronary heart disease. *Lancet* 1992;339(8808):1523-26.

[19] St. Leger A, et al. Factors associated with cardiac motility in developed countries with particular reference to the consumption of wine. *Lancet* 1979;i:1017-20.

[20] Marmot M, et al. Alcohol and mortality: A U-shaped curve. *Lancet* 1981;i:580.

[21] Klatsky A, et al. Alcoholic beverage choice and risk of coronary artery disease mortality: Do red wine drinkers fare best? *Am J Cardiol* 1993;71;467-69.

[22] Criqui M, et al. Does diet or alcohol explain the French paradox? *Lancet* 1994;344:1719-23.

[23] Blackwelder W, et al. Alcohol and mortality: The Honolulu Heart Study. *Am J Med* 1980;68:164.

[24] Truelsen T, et al. Intake of beer, wine, and spirits and risk of stroke: The Copenhagen City Heart Study. *Stroke* 1998;29:2467-72.

[25] National Stroke Association Web site. (www.stroke.org)

[26] Gronbaek M. Positive effects of alcohol drinking? *Nord Med* 1997;112(10):367-69.

[27] Wannamethee S, et al. Type of alcoholic drink and risk of major coronary heart disease events and all-cause mortality. *Am J Public Health* 1999;89(5):685-90.

[28] Carbonneau M, et al. Supplementation with wine phenolic compounds increases the antioxidant capacity of plasma and vitamin E of low-density lipoprotein without changing the lipoprotein Cu(2+)-oxidizability: Possible explanation by phenolic location. *Eur J Clin Nutr* 1997;51(10):682-90.

[29] Esterbauer H, et al. *Free Radical Communication* 1992;13:341-90.

[30] Frankel E, et al. Inhibition of human LDL oxidation by resveratrol. *Lancet* 1993;341:1103-4.

[31] Harada K, et al. Alcohol consumption, serum lipids and severity of angiographically determined coronary artery disease. *Am J Cardiol* 1990;65:287-89.

[32] Mower R, et al. *Biochem Pharmacol* 1994;36:317-22.

[33] American Heart Association's 71st Scientific Session.

[34] Pfeiffer A, et al. Effect of ethanol and commonly ingested alcoholic beverages on gastric emptying and gastrointestinal transit. *Clin Investig* 1992;70(6):487.

[35] Alterescu V, et al. Wine treatment of rheumatoid skin ulcerations. *Arthritis Rheum* 1983;26(7):934.

[36] Haines A, et al. Management of heavy drinkers. *Occas Pap R Coll Gen Pract* 1992;53:39-43.

[37] Block A, et al. Alcohol increases sleep apnea and oxygen desaturation in asymptomatic men. *Am J Med* 1981;71:240.

[38] Kalish G. *Lancet* 1981;i:1263.

[39] Rubinstein E, et al. Oesophageal and gastric potential difference and pH in healthy volunteers following intake of coca-cola, red wine, and alcohol. *Pharmacol Toxicol* 1993;72(1):61.

[40] Pehl C, et al. Low-proof alcoholic beverages and gastroesophageal reflux. *Dig Dis Sci* 1993;38(1):93.

[41] La Vecchia C, et al. Alcohol and epithelial ovarian cancer. *J Clin Epidemiol* 1992;45(9):1025.

[42] Periti M, et al. Alcohol consumption and blood pressure. An Italian study. *Eur J Epidemiol* 1988;4(4):477-81.

[43] Tatro D, et al. *Drug Interaction Facts*. St. Louis, MO: Facts and Comparisons. 1999.

Wintergreen

SCIENTIFIC NAME(S): *Gaultheria procumbens* L. and other related species. Family: Ericaceae

COMMON NAME(S): Wintergreen, teaberry, checkerberry, gaultheria oil, boxberry, deerberry, mountain tea, Canada tea, partridgeberry

BOTANY: The wintergreen is a perennial evergreen shrub with thin creeping stems from which arise leathery leaves with toothed, bristly margins. It is a low-growing plant native to North America. Its white flowers bloom in late summer, developing a scarlet fruit.[1]

HISTORY: Wintergreen oil is obtained by steam distillation of the warmed, water-macerated leaves. Wintergreen oil is used interchangeably with sweet birch oil or methyl salicylate for flavoring foods and candies. The berries have been used to make pies.[2] The plant and its oil have been used in traditional medicine as an anodyne and analgesic, carminative, astringent, and topical rubefacient. Teas of the plant have been used to relieve cold symptoms and muscle aches.[3]

CHEMISTRY: Wintergreen oil contains approximately 98% methyl salicylate. The plant has little odor or flavor until the methyl salicylate is freed. During steam distillation, gaultherin (also described as primeveroside or monotropitoside) present in the leaves is enzymatically hydrolyzed to methyl salicylate, which is subsequently obtained through the distillation process.[1,4] In addition, D-glucose and D-xylose are obtained. The yield of oil from the leaves is in the range of 0.5% to 0.8%.[5]

PHARMACOLOGY: Small oral doses of wintergreen oil stimulate digestion and gastric secretion.[2] Topically, the oil is a counterirritant and may offer some analgesic effect due to the structural similarity of methyl salicylate to aspirin.

TOXICOLOGY: Large doses of wintergreen oil, as with other volatile oils, can induce vomiting, and deaths have been reported following the ingestion of large amounts of the oil.[2] The oil may be particularly toxic to children. As little as 4 to 10 ml of the oil has been reported to cause death.[6,7] Because of this toxicity, official labeling requirements were changed so that no drug product may contain more than 5% methyl salicylate or else it would be regarded as misbranded.[8] No deaths have been reported from the ingestion of the plant itself.[1]

The compound lectine, has been shown to have mutagenic properties[2] and the extract is used in some insecticides.[1]

The essential oil and its component can be absorbed through the skin. Because of the structural similarity between methyl salicylate and acetylsalicylic acid (aspirin) (methyl salicylate is a methyl ester of aspirin), a toxic syndrome similar to that seen in salicylism has been observed in persons who have ingested wintergreen for prolonged periods of time. This syndrome has been characterized by tinnitus, nausea, and vomiting.[2]

The highest amount of methyl salicylate typically used in candy flavoring is 0.04%.

SUMMARY: Wintergreen and its oil are used commonly in topical analgesic and rubefacient preparations for the treatment of muscular and rheumatic pains. The oil is widely used as a flavor. As with other volatile oils, ingestion of large amounts may be toxic, and smaller amounts may pose a danger to young children.

PATIENT INFORMATION – Wintergreen

Uses: In addition to being used as a flavoring, wintergreen and its oil have been used in topical analgesic and rubefacient preparations for the treatment of muscular and rheumatic pains.

Side Effects: Large doses of wintergreen oil can induce vomiting and in some cases death. Children should not take wintergreen or its oil.

[1] Simon JE. *Herbs: an indexed bibliography, 1971-1980.* Hamden, CT: Shoe String Press, 1984.

[2] Duke JA. *Handbook of Medicinal Herbs.* Boca Raton, FL: CRC Press, 1985.

[3] Dobelis IN, ed. *Magic and Medicine of Plants.* Pleasantville, NY: Reader's Digest Association, Inc., 1986.

[4] Spoerke DG, Jr. *Herbal Medications.* Santa Barbara, CA: Woodbridge Press, 1980.

[5] Leung AY. *Encyclopedia of Common Natural Ingredients Used in Food, Drugs, and Cosmetics.* New York, NY: J. Wiley and Sons, 1980.

[6] Tyler VE, et al. *Pharmacognosy,* ed. 9. Philadelphia, PA: Lea and Febiger, 1988.

[7] Dreisbach RH, Robertson WO. *Handbook of Poisoning,* ed. 12. Norwalk, CT: Appleton and Lange, 1987.

[8] Fink JL, et al, eds. *Pharmacy Law Digest.* St. Louis, MO: Facts and Comparisons, 1992.

Witch Hazel

SCIENTIFIC NAME(S): *Hamamelis viginiana* L. Family: Hamamelidaceae

COMMON NAME(S): Witch hazel, hamamelis, snapping hazel, winter bloom, spotted alder, tobacco wood, hamamelis water.

BOTANY: Witch hazel grows as a deciduous bush or small tree, often reaching about 20 feet in height. The plant is found throughout most of North America. Its broad, toothed leaves are ovate, and the golden yellow flowers bloom in the fall. Brown fruit capsules appear after the flowers, then when ripe, eject its two seeds away from the tree. The dried leaves, bark and twigs are used medicinally.[1,2]

HISTORY: Witch hazel is a widely known plant with a long history of use in the Americas. One source lists more than 30 traditional uses for witch hazel including the treatment of hemorrhoids, burns, cancers, tuberculosis, colds, and fever. Preparations have been used topically for symptomatic treatment of itching and other skin inflammations and in ophthalmic preparations for ocular irritations.[3]

The plant is used in a variety of forms including the crude leaf and bark, fluid extracts, a poultice, and commonly as witch hazel water. The latter, also known as hamamelis water or distilled witch hazel extract, is obtained from the recently cut and partially dormant twigs of the plant. This plant material is soaked in warm water followed by distillation and the addition of alcohol to the distillate. Witch hazel water is the most commonly found commercial preparation, usually kept in most homes as a topical cooling agent or astringent.[2,3]

Traditionally, witch hazel was known to native North American people as a treatment for tumors and eye inflammations. Its internal use was for hemorrhaging. Eighteenth century European settlers came to value the plant for its astringency, and it is still used today for this and other purposes.[2]

CHEMISTRY: Witch hazel leaves contain about 7% to 10% of tannins. There is some dispute as to the actual composition of the tannin with hamamelitannin, digally-hamamelose and various gallotannins having been identified.[4] It is not clear whether hamamelitannin is found in the leaves.[5] Recent sources list from 8%[3,6] to no hamamelitanin in leaves.[1] The bark contains from 1% to 7%

hamamelitannin and smaller amounts of condensed tannins.[7,8] Other components include flavonoids (eg, kaempferol, quercetin), gallic acid, saponins, a fixed oil, and a volatile oil. The volatile oil contains small amounts of safrole and eugenol and numerous other minor components, such as resin, wax, and choline. Because witch hazel water is a steam distillate of the extract, it does not contain any tannins.[2,6]

PHARMACOLOGY: Witch hazel leaves, bark, and its extracts have been reported to have astringent and hemostatic properties. These effects have been ascribed to the presence of a relatively high concentration of tannins in the leaf, bark, and extract. Tannins are protein precipitants in appropriate concentrations.[9]

Witch hazel water is absent of tannins but still retains its astringency. This suggests other constituents may possess astringent-like qualities.[2]

The mechanism of witch hazel astringency involves the tightening of skin proteins, which come together to form a protective covering that promotes skin healing.[2] This quality is desirable in treatment of hemorrhoids (including preventive measures for recurring hemorroids).[10] A preparation of tea has been used in cases of diarrhea, dysentery, and colitis.[1,2,3,6]

Skin problems are also treated with witch hazel. Its drying and astringent effects help treat skin inflammations such as eczema. Witch hazel's action on skin lesions also protects against infection.[2] Skin lotions may also contain witch hazel for these purposes.[1] Inflammation of mucous membranes including mouth, throat and gums may also be treated with witch hazel in the form of a gargle.[1]

Witch hazel is also used to treat damaged veins. Its ability to tighten distended veins and restore vessel tone is employed in varicose vein treatment and is also valuable for bruises and sprains.[1,2] This hemostatic property of witch hazel is said to stop bleeding instantly, and if used as an enema, offers a rapid cure for "inwardly bleeding piles."[3] In Europe, an alcoholic fluid extract is taken internally to treat varicose veins and fluid extracts administered parenterally to rabbits have been found to be vasoconstrictive.[11]

TOXICOLOGY: Although the volatile oil contains the carcinogen safrole, this is found in much smaller quantities than in plants such as sassafras.[3] Although extracts of witch hazel are available commercially, it is not recommended that these extracts be taken internally because the toxicity of the tannins has not been well defined.[6] Although tannins are not usually absorbed following oral administration, doses of 1 g of witch hazel will cause nausea, vomiting, or constipation, possibly leading to impactions; hepatic damage may occur if the tannins are absorbed to an appreciable extent.[1,12] Witch hazel water is not intended for internal use. Teas can be brewed from

leaves and twigs available commercially in some health-food stores, but their safety is undefined.

At least one report is available discussing contact allergy to witch hazel.[13]

SUMMARY: Witch hazel leaves, bark, and extracts are high in tannins and have been used as topical astringents. Witch hazel water, most commonly found in the home, is a product of the steam distillation of the leaves and twigs; it contains no tannins, but is still used for its astringency. This "skin-tightening" effect of witch hazel is of value in treating hemorrhoids, other GI problems, skin afflictions and vein damage. It has anti-inflammatory and hemostatic properties as well. Witch hazel has a low toxicity profile, but internal use is not recommended.

PATIENT INFORMATION – Witch Hazel

Uses: Witch hazel has astringent and hemostatic properties, making it useful as a skin astringent to promote healing in hemorrhoid treatment, diarrhea, dysentery, and colitis, as well as other skin inflammations such as eczema. It can also be gargled to treat mucous membrane inflammations of the mouth, throat, and gums. Witch hazel has been used to treat damaged veins, bruises, and sprains; it rapidly stops bleeding making it useful as an enema.

Side Effects: Internal use is not recommended. Doses of 1 g of witch hazel will cause nausea, vomiting, or constipation, possibly leading to impactions. Hepatic damage may occur if the tannins are absorbed to an appreciable extent.

---

[1] Bisset N. *Herbal Drugs and Phytopharmaceuticals.* Stuttgart, Germany: CRC Press, 1994.

[2] Chevallier A. *Encyclopedia of Medicinal Plants.* New York, NY: DK Publishing Inc., 1996.

[3] Duke JA. *Handbook of Medicinal Herbs,* Boca Raton, FL: CRC Press, 1985.

[4] Bernard P, et al. *J Pharm Belg* 1971;26:661.

[5] Friedrich VH, Kruger N. *Planta Medica* 1974;26:327.

[6] Newall C, et al. *Herbal Medicine.* London: Pharmaceutical Press, 1996.

[7] Leung AY, et al. *Encyclopedia of Common Natural Ingredients Used in Food, Drugs and Cosmetics,* 2nd ed. New York, NY: Wiley and Sons, 1996.

[8] Vennat B, et al. *Planta Medica* 1988;54:454.

[9] Bate-Smith EC. *Phytochemistry* 1973;12:907.

[10] Weiner B, et al. *Nat Assoc Retail Drug J* 1983;105(Apr):45–9.

[11] *J Pharm Belg* 1972;27:505.

[12] Spoerke DG. *Herbal Medications.* Santa Barbara, CA: Woodbridge Press, 1980.

[13] Granlund H. *Contact Dermatitis* 1994;31(3):195.

Withania

SCIENTIFIC NAME(S): *Withania somnifera* (L.) Dunal, also *W. coagulans* Dunal Family: Solanaceae (nightshade family)

COMMON NAME(S): Withania, Ashwagandha, Aswaganda, Winter Cherry, Indian ginseng, Ajagandha, Kanaje Hindi, Samm Al Ferakh, Asgand (Hindi), Amukkirag (Tamil), Amangura (Kannada), Asvagandha (Bengali), Ashvagandha (Sanskrit), Asundha (Gujarati), Kuthmithi, Clustered Wintercherry

BOTANY: *W. somnifera* is an erect, greyish, slightly hairy evergreen shrub with fairly long tuberous roots. It is widely cultivated in India and throughout the Middle East, and is found in eastern Africa. The flowers are small and greenish, single or in small clusters in the leaf axils. The fruit is smooth, round, fleshy, and has many seeds, orange-red when ripe, enclosed in a membranous covering.

HISTORY: The root of *W. somnifera* is used to make the Ayurvedic sedative and diuretic "Ashwagandha," which is also considered an adaptogen. Other parts of the plant (eg, seeds, leaves) are used as a pain reliever, to kill lice, and to make soap. The fresh berries have been used as an emetic.

CHEMISTRY: The principal bioactive compounds of *W. somnifera* are withanolides, highly oxygenated C-28 steroid derivatives. Over 40 withanolides have been isolated and identified from *W. somnifera*. Three chemotypes of the plant have been defined[1]: Indian (I), which contains withanone[2] and withaferin A[3,4] as major constituents; Israeli (II), whose major withanolides are withanolide D[5] and 27-hydroxywithanolide D;[1] and Israeli (III), containing principally withanolide E.[6] The biosynthesis of withanolides from the cholesterol pathway has been studied,[7] and the C-13 NMR spectra of withanolides have been assigned.[8] An HPLC separation of withanolides has been reported.[9]

W. somnifera roots also contain nicotine and assorted piperidine and pyrrolidine alkaloids.[10] The leaves have been found to contain flavonol glycosides and phenolic acids.[11]

PHARMACOLOGY: The majority of studies of *W. somnifera* pharmacology have not related bioactivity to specific chemical constitutents present. Given the noted variation in withanolides, it is obvious that this has limited reproducibility of results.

Adaptogenic effects: Pretreatment with the alcoholic extract of defatted seeds increased swimming endurance in mice, and significantly reduced cold-, stress-, restraint-, and aspirin-induced ulcers in rats.[12] A combination of withaferin A and two sterol glucosides from roots of *W. somnifera* showed antistress activity in a panel of tests.[13] Aqueous suspensions from the roots of Ashwagandha and ginseng were compared in a mouse swimming model and for anabolic activity (weight gain) in rats and both were found to possess oral activity when animals were treated for 7 days.[14] Ashwagandha extract given orally to rabbits and mice prevented stress-induced increases in lipid peroxidation.[15] Stress-induced increases in plasma corticosterone, phagocytic index, and avidity index were blocked by administration of *W. somnifera* to rats, while swimming time was increased.[16] Another study in rats and frogs found the extract to be adaptogenic when given as a pretreatment for up to 3 months, as measured by swimming tests, glycogen content of various tissues, coagulation time, and catecholamine content, among others.[17] The effect of *W. somnifera* extract on thyroid hormone levels[18] and corticosterone levels[19] in animals has been studied. A review of adaptogenic effects of *W. somnifera* and other Ayurvedic adaptogens has been published.[20]

Immunomodulatory and anti-inflammatory effects: *W. somnifera* extracts given IP suppressed rat paw edema induced by carrageenan,[21] as well as in a granuloma pouch assay.[22] Orally administered proprietary extracts of *W. somnifera* were found to have modest activity in an active paw anaphylaxis model and to suppress cyclophosphamide-induced delayed-type hypersensitivity.[23] Withanolides inhibit murine spleen cell proliferation,[24] and an extract of *W. somnifera* reversed ochratoxin's suppressive effect on murine macrophage chemotaxis.[25] Withanolide glycosides activated murine macrophages, phagocytosis, and increased lysosomal enzymatic activity secreted by the macrophages, while also displaying anti-stress activity and positive effects on learning and memory in rats.[26] Alpha-2 macroglobulin synthesis stimulated by inflammation was reduced by *W. somnifera* extract.[27] Similarly, the extract prevented myelosuppression caused by cyclophosphamide, azathioprine, or prednisolone in mice.[28]

The stimulation of macrophages was invoked to explain activity versus experimental aspergillosis in mice.[29] Similar activity in other experimental infections was observed in rats.[30]

Cancer: Withaferin A was first isolated as a cytotoxic agent,[3] and a considerable amount of investigation followed. The compound produced mitotic arrest in Ehrlich ascites carcinoma cells in vitro[31] while in vivo effects were mediated by macrophage activation.[26,32] Further investigations on peripheral blood lymphocytes determined that withaferin A destroyed spindle microtubules of cells in metaphase.[33] Mouse sarcoma cells showed similar effects, with additional effects on nuclear membranes of cells.[34] A structure-activity comparison of withaferin A analogues in P388 cells attributed reaction of its lactone and epoxide moieties with cysteine as important to its cytotoxicity.[35] Withaferin was synergistic with radiation treatment in a mouse Ehrlich ascites carcinoma model.[36] Recently, several withanolides were identified as inducers of differentiation of myeloid leukemia cells.[37]

CNS: Withania extract protected against pentylenetetrazol-induced seizures in a mouse anticonvulsant model when administered over a 9-week period.[38] The same research group found the extract active in a rat status epilepticus model.[39] A further study of the extract found that it inhibited the development of tolerance to morphine in mice, while suppressing withdrawal symptoms precipitated by naloxone.[40] A withanolide-containing fraction reversed morphine-induced reduction in intestinal motility and confirmed the previous finding of inhibition of development of tolerance to morphine.[41] A depressant effect on the CNS was indicated by potentiation of pentobarbital effects on the righting reflex in mice.[42] Effects on learning and memory attributed to the plant in Ayurvedic medicine were supported by an experiment in which ibotenic acid-induced lesions in intact rat brain which led to cognitive deficit, as measured by performance in a learning task, were found to be reversed by treatment with a withanolide mixture.[43]

Miscellaneous: *W. somnifera* seed extract was found to protect against carbon tetrachloride-induced liver damage in rats.[44] The leaf extract also showed a modest protective effect in a subacute model of liver damage, as well as an anti-inflammatory effect.[45] Damage to the bladder by cyclophosphamide was ameliorated by *W. somnifera* extract given IP,[46] as was leukopenia induced by cyclophosphamide.[47] The extract decreased arterial and diastolic blood pressure in normotensive dogs, while preventing the hypotensive effect of acetylcholine and increasing the hypertensive effects of adrenaline.[48]

TOXICOLOGY: Acute toxicity of *W. somnifera* is modest. In mice an LD-50 was determined to be 1750 mg/kg PO[12] in one study and 1260 mg/kg by the intraperitoneal route.[49] Subacute IP toxicity studies at 100 mg/kg/day for 30 days led to decreased spleen, thymus, and adrenal weights, but no mortality or hematological changes.[49] A longer-term study (180 days) in rats at a dose of 100 mg/kg PO found no lethality but unfavorable increases in catecholamine content of the heart and decreases in the adrenal glands.[17]

SUMMARY: Withania appears in the *WHO Monographs on Selected Medicinal Plants* (vol. 2). An American Herbal Pharmacopoeia monograph is forthcoming. A book-length review was published.[50] Ashwagandha is a well-known Ayurvedic drug with a multitude of observed pharmacologic effects. It is generally thought to be non-toxic. The withanolides are considered to be the principal bioactive compounds in the root; however, their complexity and variation have made correlation of the complex pharmacology with chemistry difficult.

PATIENT INFORMATION – Withania

Uses: Withania has adaptogenic, immunomodulatory, and anti-inflammatory effects in animals; it also has been studied in animals as a cytotoxic agent and has different CNS applications.

Side Effects: Acute toxicity of *W. somnifera* is modest. A 180-day study involving rats found unfavorable increases in catecholamine content of the heart and decreases in the adrenal glands.

[1] Nittala S, et al. Chemistry and genetics of withanolides in *Withania somnifera* hybrids. *Phytochemistry* 1981;20:2741.

[2] Kirson I, et al. Constituents of *Withania somnifera* Dun. Part XII. The withanolides of an Indian chemotype. *J Chem Soc* (C) 1971;2032.

[3] Kupchan S, et al. The isolation and structural elucidation of a novel steroidal tumor inhibitor from *Acnistus arborescens*. *J Am Chem Soc* 1965;37:5805.

[4] Lavie D, et al. Constituents of *Withania somnifera* Dun. Part IV. The structure of withaferin A. *J Chem Soc* 1965;7517.

[5] Lavie D, et al. Constituents of *Withania somnifera*. X. The structure of withanolide D. *Isr J Chem* 1968;6:671.

[6] Lavie D, et al. Crystal and molecular structure of withanolide E, a new natural steroidal lactone with a 17-alpha-side-chain. *Chem Comm* 1972;877.

[7] Lockley J, et al. Biosynthesis of steroidal withanolides in *Withania somnifera*. *Phytochem* 1976;15:937.

[8] Gottlieb H, et al. 13C NMR spectroscopy of the withanolides and other highly oxygenated C28 steroids. *Org Magn Res* 1981;16:20.

[9] Hunter I, et al. Separation of withanolides by high-pressure liquid chromatography with coiled columns. *J Chromatogr* 1979;170:437.

[10] Schwarting A, et al. The alkaloids of *Withania somnifera*. *Lloydia* 1963;26:258.

[11] Kandil F, et al. Flavonol glycosides and phenolics from *Withania somnifera*. *Phytochem* 1994;37:1215.

[12] Singh N, et al. *Withania somnifera* (Ashwagandha), a rejuvenating herbal drug which enhances survival during stress (an adaptogen). *Int J Crude Drug Res* 1982;20:29.

[13] Bhattacharya S, et al. Anti-stress activity of sitoindosides VII and VIII, new acylsterylglucosides from *Withania somnifera*. *Phytother Res* 1987;1:32.

[14] Grandhi A, et al. A comparative pharmacclogical investigation of ashwagandha and ginseng. *J Ethnopharmacol* 1994;44:131.

[15] Dhuley J. Effect of ashwagandha on lipid peroxidation in stress-induced animals. *J Ethnopharmacol* 1998;60:173.

[16] Archana R, et al. Antistressor effect of *Withania somnifera*. *J Ethnopharmacol* 1999;64:91.

[17] Dhuley J. Adaptogenic and cardioprotective action of ashwagandha in rats and frogs. *J Ethnopharmacol* 2000;70:57.

[18] Panda S, et al. *Withania somnifera* and *Bauhinia purpurea* in the regulation of circulating thyroid hormone concentrations in female mice. *J Ethnopharmacol* 1999;67:233.

[19] Singh A, et al. Adrenocorticosterone alterations in male, albino mice treated with *Trichopus zeylanicus*, *Withania somnifera*, and *Panax ginseng* preparations. *Phytother Res* 2000;14:122.

[20] Rege N, et al. Adaptogenic properties of six rasayana herbs used in Ayurvedic medicine. *Phytother Res* 1999;13:275.

[21] al Hindawi M, et al. Anti-inflammatory activity of some Iraqi plants using intact rats. *J Ethnopharmacol* 1989;26:163.

[22] al Hindawi M, et al. Anti-granuloma activity of Iraqi *Withania somnifera*. *J Ethnopharmacol* 1992;37:113.

[23] Agarwal R, et al. Studies on immunomodulatory activity of *Withania somnifera* (Ashwagandha) extracts in experimental immune inflammation. *J Ethnopharmacol* 1999;67:27.

[24] Bähr V, et al. Immunomodulating properties of 5,20-alpha(R)-dihydroxy-6-alpha-7-alpha-epoxy-1-oxo-(5-alpha)-witha-2,24-dieno lide and solasodine. *Planta Med* 1982;44:32.

[25] Dhuley J. Effect of some Indian herbs on macrophage functions in ochratoxin A treated mice. *J Ethnopharmacol* 1997;58:15.

[26] Ghosal S, et al. Immunomodulatory and CNS effects of sitoindosides IX and X, two new glycowithanolides from *Withania somnifera*. *Phytother Res* 1989;3:201.

[27] Anbalagan K, et al. *Withania somnifera* (Ashwagandha), a rejuvenating herbal drug which controls a-2 macroglobulin synthesis during inflammation. *Int J Crude Drug Res* 1985;23:177.

[28] Ziauddin M, et al. Studies on the immunomodulatory effects of Ashwagandha. *J Ethnopharmacol* 1996;50:69.

[29] Dhuley J. Therapeutic efficacy of Ashwagandha against experimental aspergillosis in mice. *Immunopharmacol Immunotoxicol* 1998;20:191.

[30] Thatte U, et al. Immunotherapeutic modification of experimental infections by Indian medicinal plants. *Phytother Res* 1989;3:43.

[31] Shohat B, et al. Effect of withaferin A on Ehrlich ascites tumor cells–cytological observations. *Int J Cancer* 1970;5:244.

[32] Shohat B, et al. Effect of withaferin A on Ehrlich ascites tumor cells. II. Target tumor cell destruction in vivo by immune activation. *Int J Cancer* 1971;8:487.

[33] Shohat B, et al. The effect of withaferin A on human peripheral blood lymphocytes. An electron-microscope study. *Cancer Lett* 1976;2:63.

[34] Shohat B, et al. The effect of withaferin A, a natural steroidal lactone, on the fine structure of S-180 tumor cells. *Cancer Lett* 1976;2:71.

[35] Fuska J, et al. Novel cytotoxic and antitumor agents. IV. Withaferin A: Relation of its structure to the in vitro cytotoxic effects on P388 cells. *Neoplasma* 1984;31:31.

[36] Devi P, et al. In vivo growth inhibitory and radiosensitizing effects of withaferin A on mouse Ehrlich ascites carcinoma. *Cancer Lett* 1995;95:189.

[37] Kuroyanagi M, et al. Cell differentiation inducing steroids from *Withania somnifera* L. (Dun.). *Chem Pharm Bull* 1999;47:1646.

[38] Kulkarni S, et al. Anticonvulsant action of *Withania somnifera* (Ashwaganda) root extract against pentylenetetrazol-induced kindling in mice. *Phytother Res* 1996;10:447.

[39] Kulkarni S, et al. Protective effect of *Withania somnifera* root extract on electrographic activity in a lithium-pilocarpine model of status epilepticus. *Phytother Res* 1998;12:451.

[40] Kulkarni S, et al. Inhibition of morphine tolerance and dependence by *Withania somnifera* in mice. *J Ethnopharmacol* 1997;57:213.

[41] Ramarao P, et al. Bioactive phytosterol conjugates. 8. Effects of glycowithanolides from *Withania somnifera* on morphine-induced inhibition of intestinal motility and tolerance to analgesia in mice. *Phytother Res* 1995;9:66.

[42] Ahumada F, et al. Effect of certain adaptogenic plant extracts on drug-induced narcosis in female and male mice. *Phytother Res* 1991;5:29.

[43] Bhattacharya S, et al. Bioactive phytosterol conjugates. 9. Effects of glycowithanolides from *Withania somnifera* on an animal model of Alzheimer's disease and perturbed central cholinergic markers of cognition in rats. *Phytother Res* 1995;9:110.

[44] Singh N, et al. An experimental evaluation of protective effects of some indigenous drugs on carbon tetrachloride-induced hepatotoxicity in mice and rats. *Quart J Crude Drug Res* 1978;16:8.

[45] Sudhir S, et al. Pharmacological studies on leaves of *Withania somnifera*. *Planta Med* 1986;36:61.

[46] Davis L, et al. Effect of *Withania somnifera* on cyclophosphamide-induced urotoxicity. *Cancer Lett* 2000;148:9.

[47] Davis L, et al. Suppressive effect of cyclophosphamide-induced toxicity by *Withania somnifera* extract in mice. *J Ethnopharmacol* 1998;62:209.

[48] Ahumada F, et al. *Withania somnifera* extract. Its effect on arterial blood pressure in anaesthetized dogs. *Phytother Res* 1991;5:111.

[49] Sharada A, et al. Toxicity of *Withania somnifera* root extract in rats and mice. *Int J Pharmacognosy* 1993;31:205.

[50] Singh S, et al. *Withania somnifera*: The Indian ginseng ashwagandha. New Dehli: Vedams Books Intl.,1998.

Woodruff, Sweet

SCIENTIFIC NAME(S): *Galium odoratum* (L.) Scop. also known as *Asperula odorata* L. Family: Rubiaceae

COMMON NAME(S): Woodruff, sweet woodruff, master of the wood, woodward

BOTANY: Sweet woodruff is a small perennial that grows to about a foot in height. It has creeping rhizomes and lance-shaped leaves. It is native to Eurasia and North Africa and now grows throughout North America. The small white flowers appear from April to June. The dried whole plant is used in traditional medicine. When cut, the plant develops a characteristic smell of fresh-cut hay.

HISTORY: Sweet woodruff has been used as a sedative, antispasmodic, diuretic, and sweat inducer. In homeopathy, the plant extract is used as an antispasmodic and to treat liver impairment. The bruised leaves have been applied topically to reduce swelling and improve wound healing. Extracts and teas have been administered as expectorants. Woodruff is usually taken as a tea. The dried herb is used in sachets, and the extract is used in perfumes and other fragrances. It is a flavoring component in May wines (woodruff soaked in sweet white wine), vermouth, and some bitters and is used in food and candy flavorings.

CHEMISTRY: It is widely described that woodruff contains coumarin in a glycosidic form that is freed by enzymatic action during the drying process. However, at least one study did not detect any coumarins in woodruff.[1]

The plant contains a number of minor components including asperuloside (0.05%), monotropein,[2] tannins, a fixed oil, and a bitter principle. The root contains a red dye.

PHARMACOLOGY: Asperuloside has been reported to have anti-inflammatory activity.[1] When evaluated in vivo in rats, an extract of *G. odoratum* administered orally inhibited carrageenan-induced rat paw edema by 25% this compared favorably with the 45% inhibition observed following indomethacin administration.[3] The whole herb has been said to have antibacterial activity.[4]

TOXICOLOGY: The plant is generally recognized as safe for use in foods as a flavoring. Some concern has been raised over the toxic potential of the coumarin content of the plant. Dietary feeding of coumarin to animals has been associated with liver damage, growth retardation, testicular atrophy,[4] and impaired blood clotting. However, it is highly unlikely that these events would occur with normal dietary intake of the plant or its extracts.

SUMMARY: Woodruff is a common herb that is used as a fragrance and flavoring in foods. Although the plant has been used medicinally for a variety of purposes, there is only scant evidence to support these uses.

PATIENT INFORMATION – Woodruff, Sweet

Uses: Sweet woodruff is reported to have anti-inflammatory and antibacterial activities but is commonly used as a fragrance and flavoring in foods.

Side Effects: The plant is generally recognized as safe for use in foods. There is some concern over the toxic potential of the plant's coumarin content.

---

[1] Leung AY. *Encyclopedia of Common Natural Ingredients Used in Food, Drugs, and Cosmetics*. New York, NY: J. Wiley and Sons, 1980.
[2] Sticher O. *Pharm Acta Helv* 1971;46:121.
[3] Mascolo N, et al. *Phytotherapy Research* 1987;1:28.
[4] Duke JA. *Handbook of Medicinal Herbs*. Boca Raton, FL: CRC Press, 1985.

Wormwood

SCIENTIFIC NAME(S): *Artemisia absinthium* L. Family: Compositae

COMMON NAME(S): Wormwood, absinthium, armoise, wermut, absinthe, absinthites, ajenjo.

BOTANY: The wormwood is an odorous perennial shrub native to Europe. Today the plant is naturalized in the United States where it grows widely throughout the Northeast and North Central regions. The leaves and stems are covered with fine silky hairs and the plant grows to a height of about 3 feet.[1] The small flowers are green-yellow and the indented leaves have a silver-gray color.

HISTORY: The name wormwood is derived from the ancient use of the plant and its extracts as an intestinal anthelmintic. The leaves and flowering tops were used as a bitter aromatic tonic, sedative,[2] and flavoring. A tea of the plant was used traditionally as a diaphoretic. Wormwood extract was the main ingredient in absinthe, a toxic liqueur that induces absinthism, characterized by intellectual enfeeblement, hallucinations,[3] psychosis, and possible brain damage. The drink is now outlawed but had been popular until the early part of the 20th century. The emerald green color of absinthe liqueur came from chlorophyll; however, there had been reports of copper and antimony salts being added as colorants to inferior batches, with toxic consequences. Thujone-free wormwood extract is currently used as a flavoring, primarily in alcoholic beverages such as vermouth.

CHEMISTRY: The bitter taste of wormwood is due to the glucosides absinthin and anabsinthin and several related compounds.[4] The plant contains a pleasant-smelling volatile oil (about 1% to 2% by weight); up to 12% of the oil is a mixture of alpha- and beta-thujone with smaller amounts of phellandrene, pinene, azulene and more than a half-dozen other minor components.[5] Flowers may contain oil composed of up to 35% thujones. Cis- and trans-epoxyocimenes account for up to 57% of the volatile oil derived from Italian absinthium.[1]

PHARMACOLOGY: The anthelmintic activity of the plant is probably due to lactones related to santonin, found in wormseed and other species of Artemisia.[1] In addition, thujone can stun roundworms, which can then be expelled by normal intestinal peristalsis.[3]

TOXICOLOGY: In rats, injection of thujone in concentrations as low as 40 mg/kg induces convulsions, with a dose of 120 mg/kg being fatal.[4] The subcutaneous LD_{50} of thujone in mice is 134 mg/kg.[6]

Ingestion of absinthe may lead to a constellation of neurologic symptoms described as "absinthism." The syndrome is characterized by digestive disorders, thirst, restlessness, vertigo, trembling of the limbs, numbness of the extremities, loss of intellect, delirium, paralysis and death.[5] One commonly cited report indicates that 15 g of the volatile oil can cause convulsions and unconsciousness in humans.[5]

Thujone bears a superficial structural resemblance to camphor, pinene, anethole, and citral, and it has been postulated that Vincent van Gogh's demented craving for not only absinthe but also other terpenes, including turpentine, certain paints, and camphor, may have represented a type of pica.[7]

Although some of the nervous system effects of thujone are similar to those observed with camphor, comprehensive structural dimensional analyses suggest that thujone more likely conforms to the same receptor as tetrahydrocannabinol (THC).[8] Both compounds appear to have an affinity for a common receptor binding site and for similar oxidative metabolic pathways.

The FDA has classified wormwood as an unsafe herb, although thujone-free derivatives have been approved for use in foods.

The oil is used as an ingredient in rubifacient preparations; flowers may induce topical eruptions in sensitized persons.[5]

SUMMARY: Wormwood and its extracts have been used traditionally in the treatment of worm infections and as flavoring agents. Wormwood extract was the most important component of the liqueur absinthe, a toxic drink that was banned early in the 20th century. Wormwood toxicity is caused by thujone, which may exert its central effect by interacting with receptors for tetrahydrocannabinol.

PATIENT INFORMATION – Wormwood

Uses: Wormwood was traditionally used in the treatment of worm infections and as flavoring agents.

Side Effects: The FDA classified wormwood as an unsafe herb. Ingestion of wormwood may result in neurologic symptoms described as "absinthism." The syndrome is characterized by digestive disorders, thirst, restlessness, vertigo, trembling of the limbs, delirium, paralysis, and death.

[1] Leung AY. *Encyclopedia of Common Natural Ingredients Used In Food, Drugs, and Cosmetics.* New York, NY: J. Wiley and Sons, 1980.

[2] Spoerke DG. *Herbal Medications.* Santa Barbara, CA: Woodbridge Press, 1980.

[3] Arnold WN. *Sci Am* 1989;260:112.

[4] Tyler VE. *The New Honest Herbal.* Philadelphia, PA: G.F. Stickley Co., 1987.

[5] Duke JA. *Handbook of Medicinal Herbs.* Boca Raton, FL: CRC Press, 1985.

[6] Windholz M, ed. *The Merck Index*, 10th ed. Rahway, NJ: Merck and Co., 1983.

[7] Arnold WN. *JAMA* 1988;260:3042.

[8] del Castillo J, et al. *Nature* 1975;253:365.

Yarrow

SCIENTIFIC NAME(S): *Achillea millefolium* L.; Family: Compositae

COMMON NAME(S): Yarrow, thousand-leaf, mil foil, green arrow, wound wort, nosebleed plant

BOTANY: The name yarrow applies to any of roughly 80 species of daisy plants native to the north temperate zone. *A. millefolium* L. has finely divided leaves and whitish, pink, or reddish flowers. It can grow up to 3 feet in height. This hardy perennial weed blooms from June to November. Golden yarrow is *Eriophyllum confertiflorum*.[1,2]

HISTORY: Yarrow is native to Europe and Asia and has been naturalized in North America. Its use in food and medicine is ancient, dating back to the Trojan War, around 1200 BC.[3] In legend, Achilles used it on the Centaur's advice, hence the name. In classical times, yarrow was referred to as "herba militaris" because it stopped wound bleeding caused by war.[2] Yarrow leaves have been used for tea, and young leaves and flowers have been used in salads. Infusions of yarrow have served as cosmetic cleansers and medicines. Sneezewort leaves (*A. ptarmica*) have been used in sneezing powder, while those of *A. millefolium* have been used for snuff.[1] Yarrow has been used therapeutically as a "strengthening bitter tonic" and astringent. Chewing fresh leaves has been suggested to relieve toothaches.[3,4] Yarrow oil has been used in shampoos for a topical "healing" effect.

CHEMISTRY: As many as 82 constituents have been identified in the essential oil (of which yarrow yields 1%).[5] Some of these components include linalool, sabinene, allo-ocimene, azulene, eugenol, menthol, alpha-pinene, borneol, cineole (less than 10%), limonene (less than 11%), camphor (18% to 21%) and chamazulene (up to 50%).[2,3,5,6,7,8] Quantitative determination of chamazulene and prochamazulene has been performed.[9-10] Tetraploid species contain azulene, while hexaploid and octaploid species do not.[5,11] The precursors of azulene in the tetraploid species *A. millefolium* sp collina Becker are prochamazulenes that confirm the genera *Matricaria, Artemisia* and *Achillea* are closely related.[12]

Sesquiterpene lactones, including alpha-peroxyachifolid and others, have been determined.[13,14] Sesquiterpenoids, achimillic acids A, B, and C, and alpha-methylene sesquiterpene lactones have also been isolated from yarrow.[15] Two guaianolide-peroxides from the plant's blossoms have been found.[16] Other triterpenes and sterols identified in yarrow include beta-sitosterol, alpha-amyrin, stigmasterol, campesterol, cholesterol, beta-amyrin, taraxasterol, and pseudotaraxasterol.[17]

Flavonoids present in yarrow include apigenin, artemetin, casticin, luteolin, and rutin.[5,8] The alkaloids achiceine, achilletin, betaine, betonicine, choline, moschatine, stachydrine, and trigonelline have been found in yarrow.[3,8] Among the amino acids are alanine, histodine, aspartic acid, glutamic acid, and lysine.[3,8] Fatty acid constituents include linoleic, myristic, oleic, and palmitic. Other acids found are salicylic, ascorbic, caffeic, folic, and succinic.[8]

Other components found in yarrow include polyacetylenes, coumarins (± 0.35%), tannins (3% to 4%), and sugars (dextrose, glucose, mannitol, sucrose).[5,8] The constituents of yarrow have been reviewed in detail.[18]

PHARMACOLOGY: Yarrow is used as a **sudorific** (to induce sweating). It is also classified as a **wound-healing** herb because it stops wound bleeding.[4] It has been used for this purpose for centuries and is a component in some healing ointments, lotions, and percolates or extracts.[2,5] Its healing and regenerating effects have been reported when used as a constituent in medicated baths to remove perspiration and remedy inflammation of skin and mucous membranes.[5,19,20] One study reports wound-healing properties of yarrow oil in napalm burns.[21]

Chamazulene, a constituent in yarrow essential oil, has **anti-inflammatory** and **anti-allergenic** properties. In animal studies, this anti-inflammatory activity has been demonstrated using mouse and rat paw edema models.[8]

The yarrow component achilleine arrests internal and external bleeding.[2] IV injection (0.5 g/kg) in rabbits has decreased blood clotting time by 32%. Hemostasis persisted for 45 minutes with no toxic effect.[2] Achilletin has also reduced coagulation time in canines.[3]

Yarrow helps **regulate the menstrual cycle** and reduces heavy bleeding and pain.[2,8] It has been used as an herbal remedy for **cerebral and coronary thromboses**.[8] Yarrow has also been used to lower **high blood pressure, improve circulation,** and **tone varicose veins**.[2,3]

Antispasmodic activity of yarrow has also been documented, probably caused by the plant's flavonoid fractions[2,8] or azulene.[8] Yarrow has relieved **GI ailments** such as diarrhea, flatulence, and cramping.[5] Yarrow's **antimicrobial** actions have also been documented. In vitro fungistatic effect from the oil has been proven.[22] The oil has also exhibited marked activity against *S. aureus* and *C. albicans*.[23] Another report discusses **antistaphylococcal** activity from yarrow grass extract.[24] Antibacterial actions have also been demonstrated against *B. subtillus*, *E. coli*, *Shigella sonnei*, and *flexneri*.[8] One report found yarrow's sesquiterpenoids, achimillic acids, to be active against mouse leukemia cells in vivo.[15] Other actions of yarrow include: **Growth inhibiting effects on seed germination** caused by constituents phenylcarbonic acids, coumarins, herniarin, and umbelliferone,[25] marked **hypoglycemic** and **glycogen-sparing properties**[26] and **CNS-depressant activity** and sedative actions in mice.[8] Yarrow is a natural source for food flavoring and is used in alcoholic beverages and bitters.[8] Thujone-free yarrow extract is generally recognized as safe (GRAS) for use in beverages.

TOXICOLOGY: Contact dermatitis is the most commonly reported adverse reaction from yarrow. Guaianolide peroxides from yarrow have caused this reaction,[16] as have alpha-peroxyachifolid,[14] 10 sesquiterpene lactones, and 3 polyines.[13] A Danish report evaluates routine patch testing in 686 patients to determine sensitivity to compositae plants and their sesquiterpene lactones. Terpinen-4-ol, a yarrow oil component, has irritant properties and may contribute to its diuretic actions.[8] Thujone, a known toxin and minor component in the oil, is in too low a concentration to cause any health risk.[8] Yarrow is not generally considered toxic.[3,8]

SUMMARY: Yarrow is the name for many plant species used for teas, herbal infusions, and other remedies. Yarrow contains many diverse compounds (acids, alkaloids, flavonoids, and volatile oils), several of which have pharmacologic activity. It is used as a healing agent and for its anti-inflammatory properties. It has also been used for circulatory disorders and thromboses. The plant has choleretic, antispasmodic, antimicrobial, and other actions. Yarrow is contraindicated in individuals with an existing hypersensitivity to any member of the composite (asteraceae) family. The yarrow's volatile oil is not recommended during pregnancy or in epileptic patients.

PATIENT INFORMATION – Yarrow

Uses: Yarrow has been used to induce sweating and to stop wound bleeding. It can also reduce heavy menstrual bleeding and pain. It has been used to relieve GI ailments, for cerebral and coronary thromboses, to lower high blood pressure, to improve circulation, and to tone varicose veins. It has antimicrobial actions, is a natural source for food flavoring, and is used in alcoholic beverages and bitters.

Side Effects: Contact dermatitis is the most commonly reported side effect. It is generally not considered toxic.

---

[1] Seymour ELD. *The Garden Encyclopedia*. Wise, 1936.
[2] Chevallier A. *Encyclopedia of Medicinal Plants*. New York, NY:DK Publishing 1996;54.
[3] Duke J. *CRC Handbook of Medicinal Herbs*. Boca Raton, FL: CRC Press Inc. 1989;9-10.
[4] Loewenfeld C and Back P. *The Complete Book of Herbs and Spices*. London: David E Charles 1979.
[5] Bisset N. *Herbal Drugs and Phytopharmaceuticals*. Stuttgart, Germany: CRC Press 1994;342-44.
[6] Merck Index, 10th edition. Rahway: Merck and Co. 1983.
[7] Verzar-Petri, et al. *Herba Hun* 1979;18:83.
[8] Newall C, et al. *Herbal Medicines*. London, England: Pharmaceutical Press 1996;271-73.
[9] Verzar-Petri G, et al. *Sci Pharm* 1977 Sep 30;45:220-34.
[10] Falk AJ, et al. *Lloydia* 1974;37:598.
[11] Verzar-Petri G, et al. *Planta Med* 1979;36:273.
[12] Hausen B, et al. *Contact Dermatitis* 1991;24(4):274-80.
[13] Rucker G, et al. *Pharmazie* 1994;49(2-3):167-69.
[14] Tozyo T, et al. *Chem Pharm Bull* 1994;42(5):1096-100.
[15] Rucker G, et al. *Archiv Der Pharmazie* 1991;324(12):979-81.
[16] Chandler R, et al. *J Pharm Sci* 1982 Jun 71:690-93.
[17] Chandler R. *Can Pharm J* 1989 Jan;122:41-43.
[18] Koerber G. *Seifen, Oele, Fette, Wachse* 1969 Dec;95:951-54.
[19] Gafitanu E, et al. *Revista Medico-Chirurgicala A Societatii de Medici Si Naturalisti Din Iasi* 1988;92(1):121-2.
[20] Taran D, et al. *Voenno-Meditsinskii Zhurnal* 1989;(8):50-52.
[21] Popovici A, et al. *Rev Med* 1970;16(3-4):384-89.
[22] Kedzia B, et al. *Herba Polonica* 1990;36(3):117-25.
[23] Molochko V, et al. *Vestnik Dermatologii I Venerologii* 1990;(8):54-56.
[24] Detter A. *Pharmazeutische Zeitung* 1981 Jun 4;126:1140-42.
[25] Molokovskii D, et al. *Problemy Endokrinologii* 1989;35(6):82-87.
[26] Paulsen E, et al. *Contact Dermatitis* 1993;29(1):6-10.

Yellow Dock

SCIENTIFIC NAME(S): *Rumex crispus* L. Family: Polygonaceae

COMMON NAME(S): Yellow dock, curly dock, curled dock, narrow dock, sour dock, rumex

BOTANY: A perennial herb that grows to 3 to 4 feet, yellow dock has narrow, slender light green leaves with undulated margins. It flowers in June and July.[1] Although native to Europe, it grows throughout the United States. The yellow roots (deep, spindle-shaped) and rhizomes are used medicinally.

HISTORY: The spring leaf stalks of this plant have been used as a potherb in salads but is disagreeable to some because of its tart sour-sweet taste. The plant must be boiled and rinsed thoroughly before being eaten. Due to its astringent properties, the plant has been used (generally unsuccessfully) in the treatment of venereal diseases and skin conditions. The powdered root has been used as a natural dentifrice. Larger amounts have been given as a laxative and tonic.

CHEMISTRY: The plant contains oxalate, most probably in the form of potassium oxalate crystals.[2] Anthroquinones (emodin, chrysophanic acid, physcion) have been identified, and the total anthroquinone content of the root (approximately 2%) exceeds that of medicinal rhubarb (Rheum rhaponticum, 1.4%), also a member of the family Polygonaceae.[3]

PHARMACOLOGY: Little is known about the pharmacology of yellow dock. The anthroquinone content most likely contributes to the laxative effect of the plant. The tannin component, however, may cause constipation. The related plant R. hymenosepalus (dock) contains a tannin that, upon hydrolysis, yields leucodelphinidin and leucopelargonidin, 2 compounds with potential antineoplastic activity.[4]

TOXICOLOGY: The oxalate crystals damage mucosal tissue resulting in severe irritation and possible tissue damage. The ingestion of large amounts of oxalates may result in gastrointestinal symptoms; systemic absorption of oxalates may result in kidney damage. Ingestion of the plant by livestock has resulted in death. The stewed leaf stalks can be eaten as a potherb, but mature and uncooked leaves should be avoided. Overdoses of the root extract may cause diarrhea, nausea, and polyuria in humans.

One traditional remedy for dermatitis and rashes suggest applying the juice of Rumex spp. However, sensitive people may develop dermatitis after contact with yellow dock.

SUMMARY: The roots of yellow dock and related Rumex species exert a laxative effect. The oxalate content of the leaf is significant enough to warrant boiling young leaves eaten as salads; older and uncooked leaves should not be eaten.

PATIENT INFORMATION – Yellow Dock

Uses: The roots of yellow dock exert a laxative effect.

Side Effects: The oxalate content of the leaves may result in GI symptoms or kidney damage. The stewed leaf stalks can be eaten as a potherb, but mature and uncooked leaves should be avoided. Overdose of the root may cause diarrhea, nausea, and polyuria.

---

[1] Meyer JE. *The Herbalist*. Hammond, IN: Hammond Book Co., 1934.
[2] Spoerke DG. *Herbal Medications*. Santa Barbara, CA: Woodbridge Press, 1980.
[3] Tyler VE. *The Honest Herbal*. Philadelphia, PA: G.F. Stickley Co., 1981.
[4] Lewis WH, Lewis MPF. *Medical Botany*. New York, NY: J. Wiley & Sons, 1977.

Yellow Root

SCIENTIFIC NAME(S): *Xanthorhiza simplicissima* Marsh. synon. with *Zanthorhiza apiifolia*. Family: Ranunculaceae.

COMMON NAME(S): Yellow root, parsley-leaved yellow root, yellow wart, shrub yellow root. Not to be confused with "yellow root," also referring to goldenseal (*Hydrastis canadensis* L.).

BOTANY: A shrub-like plant indigenous to the east coast of North America that grows from New York to Florida, yellow root is commonly found growing near stream banks and shady areas. It flowers in April and derives its names from the bright yellow color of the rhizome.[1]

HISTORY: Yellow root had been used by people living in the southern United States for the treatment of hypertension and diabetes.[1] It was popular in folk medicine and has been used for mouth infections and sore throat, diabetes, and childbirth.[2]

CHEMISTRY: Berberine is the major alkaloid in yellow root with the minor alkaloids jatrorhizine and mognoflorine also having been identified.[3] In addition, 2 cytotoxic isoquinoline alkaloids, liriodenine and palmatine have been isolated in a later report.[4] The major alkaloid berberine is present in 23 genera, spanning 7 plant families.[5] Berberine content in yellow root ranges between 1.2% to 1.3%[2] puntarenine, an isohomoprotoberberine alkaloid has recently been isolated as well.[6]

PHARMACOLOGY: Yellow root has been used as a source for yellow dye.[2] Various pharmacokinetic information of yellow root constituent berberine in animals is available.[5]

Berberine-containing plants have been used for thousands of years in China and India, mostly for treatment of diarrhea. Berberine is reportedly effective against diarrhea caused by such enterotoxins as *Vibrio cholerae* and *E. coli*. In several clinical trials, diarrhea treatment from berberine has proven successful.[7] However, some contraversy exists on the validity of this type of treatment in children, not only caused by underlying pathophysiological processes, but to the fact that berberine salts were often given as part of a mixture of agents (ie, with anticholinergic compounds).[5]

Yellow root constituent berberine has been used not only in folk medicine, but as an **antibiotic, immunostimulant, anticonvulsant, sedative, hypotensive, uterotonic,** and **choleretic**.[7]

Berberine produces a transient drop in blood pressure and appears to antagonize the pharmacologic effects of acetylcholine and histamine.[8] Its hypotensive effects have been studied in animals.[7]

Berberine decreases anticoagulant actions of heparin in dog and human blood. It exhibits antipyretic activity in rats.[7]

Yellow root has been used as a bitter tonic for mouth and gum sores, especially in denture care.[2]

A broad spectrum of antimicrobial action has been found for berberine, including activity against bacteria, fungi, and protozoa.[7] Yellow root extracts were found to exhibit antimicrobial activity against *Candida albicans*, *Cryptococcus neoformans*, and *Mycobacterium intracellularae*.[6] Extract of yellow root has also been shown to inhibit RNA and DNA synthesis in leukemia cells.[9]

Yellow root has also been reported to be used as an adulterant for the more expensive goldenseal.[10]

TOXICOLOGY: A case of a man who developed chronic arsenic poisoning after drinking yellow root tea for 2 years has been reported. Yellow root is not a natural concentrator of arsenic and the contamination was thought to be secondary to pollution in the plant's habitat.[11]

Yellow root constituent berberine is generally considered non-toxic (as other berberine plants). Coagulant activity opposing heparin's actions and cardiac stimulation have been reported from the plant, which may be of concern. In addition, berberine has been known to stimulate uterine activity; its use during pregnancy should be avoided.[7]

The oral LD-50 of berberine in mice is 3.29 mg/10 g. Experimentation with other laboratory animals being administered berberine in various amounts has produced GI irritation, tremors, emesis, and sedation.[5]

SUMMARY: Yellow root derives its name from the yellow color of the rhizome. It was a popular plant in folk medicine, with its major alkaloid being berberine. Berberine's activities include antibiotic, immunostimulant, anticonvulsant, sedative, hypotensive, utertonic, choleretic, and carminative. It is generally considered non-toxic, with exceptions being anticoagulation interactions, cardiostimulation, and uterine stimulatory.

PATIENT INFORMATION – Yellow Root

Uses: Yellow root has been used in folk medicine for mouth infections and sore throat, diabetes, and childbirth, and as an antibiotic, immunostimulant, anticonvulsant, sedative, hypotensive, utertonic, and choleretic.

Side Effects: It is generally considered non-toxic, exceptions being anticoagulation interactions, cardiostimulation, and uterine stimulatory. Berberine can stimulate uterine activity; use during pregnancy should be avoided.

---

[1] Der Marderosian A. *Natural Product Medicine*. Philadelphia, PA: George F. Stickley Co., 1988;369-70.
[2] Hocking G. *A Dictionary of Natural Products*. Medford, NJ: Plexus Publishing, Inc., 1977;872.
[3] Hussein F, et al. *Lloydia* 1963;26:254.
[4] Wu Y, et al. *Kao Hsiung I Hsueh Ko Hsueh Tsa Chih* 1989;5(7):409-11.
[5] DeSmet P, ed. *Adverse Effects Of Herbal Drugs 1*. NY: Springer-Verlag, 1992;97-104.
[6] Okunade A, et al. *J Pharm Sci* 1994;83(3):404-6.
[7] Newall C. *Herbal Medicines*. London, Eng: Pharmaceutical Press, 1996;151-52.
[8] Kulkarni S, et al. *Jpn J Pharmacol* 1972;22:11.
[9] Baker V. *Am J Med Sci* 1989;298(5):283-88.
[10] Osol, ed., et al. *The Dispensatory of the United States of America,* 25th ed. Philadelphia, PA: J.B. Lippincott Co.,1955;660-1.
[11] Parsons J. *NC Med J* 1981;42:38.

Yerba Santa

SCIENTIFIC NAME(S): *Eriodictyon californicum* (Hook. & Arn.) Torrey. Also known as *E. glutinosum* Benth. and *Wigandia californicum* Hook. & Arn. Family: Hydrophyllaceae

COMMON NAME(S): Yerba santa, eriodictyon, tarweed, consumptive's weed, bear's weed, mountain balm, gum plant[1]

BOTANY: The plant is an evergreen aromatic shrub with woody rhizomes. The hairy, lance-shaped leaves are glutinous.[2] Native to the southwestern regions of North America, yerba santa is often cultivated as an ornamental shrub. The plant grows to more than 2 meters in height at elevations exceeding 3500 feet and has white to lavender flowers.

HISTORY: The name yerba santa ("holy weed") was given by the Spanish priests who learned early from the native American Indians of the medicinal value of the shrub. The plant has a long tradition of use in the United States. The thick sticky leaves, used either fresh or dried, were boiled to make a tea or taken as treatment for coughs, colds, asthma, and tuberculosis. The leaves have been powdered and used as a stimulating expectorant.[3] A liniment was applied topically to reduce fever. A poultice of fresh leaves was used to treat bruises and young leaves were applied to relieve rheumatisms.[4,5] The plant is contained in a number of over-the-counter herbal preparations. Yerba santa has been used as a pharmaceutical flavoring, particularly to mask the flavor of bitter drugs.[6] The fluid extract is used in foods and beverages.

CHEMISTRY: Yerba santa contains a volatile oil, up to 6% eriodictyonine, about 0.5% eriodictyol (the aglycone of eriodictin) and several related alcoholic compounds, ericolin and a resin.[2]

PHARMACOLOGY: Eriodictyol is reported to exert an expectorant action.[1] Little other animal or human experience with the plant has been published.

TOXICOLOGY: There are no reports of significant toxicity associated with the topical or systemic use of yerba santa.

SUMMARY: Yerba santa is a traditional American plant used widely by Native Americans for the preparation of a tea and medicinally for the management of bruises, inflammations and rheumatic pain. The plant is also used as an expectorant and in the treatment of respiratory diseases. There are no good studies to evaluate these effects.

PATIENT INFORMATION – Yerba Santa

Uses: Yerba santa has been used in tea, and medicinally for the management of bruises and rheumatic pain. The plant is also used as an expectorant and in the treatment of respiratory diseases.

Side Effects: There are no reports of significant toxicity associated with the topical or systemic use of yerba santa.

---

[1] Windholz M, et al, eds. *The Merck Index,* tenth edition. Rahway, NJ: Merck & Co., 1983.

[2] Leung AY. *Encyclopedia of Common Natural Ingredients Used in Food, Drugs, and Cosmetics.* New York, NY: J. Wiley and Sons, 1980.

[3] Lewis WH, Elvin-Lewis MPF. *Medical Botany.* New York, NY: J. Wiley and Sons, 1977.

[4] Balls EK. *Early Uses of California Plants.* Berkeley, CA: University of California Press, 1962.

[5] Sweet M. *Common Edible and Useful Plants of the West.* Healdsburg, CA: Naturegraph Publishers, 1976.

[6] Morton JF. *Major Medicinal Plants.* Springfield, IL: C.C. Thomas, 1977.

Yew

SCIENTIFIC NAME(S): Taxus bacatta L. and *T. cuspidata* Sieb. and Zucc. The native species of the US, *T. canadensis* Marsh. is found throughout the eastern United States; other species found in North America include *T. floridana* Nutt. and the western or California yew, *T. brevifolia* Nutt. Family: Taxaceae

COMMON NAME(S): Yew, ground hemlock

BOTANY: This common evergreen is found throughout woods and forests and is often used as an ornamental hedge bush. The trunk supports a crown of spreading branches with long, narrow, dark green shiny leaves. It is dioecious, with male and female flowers being produced on different trees. The ovoid seed is black and is surrounded by a red, fleshy covering called the aril. Yews flower in March and April.

HISTORY: The Celts coated their arrows with yew sap as a nerve toxicant. The alkaloid taxine has been used as an antispasmodic. A tincture of the leaves had been used to treat rheumatisms and liver and urinary tract conditions.[1]

CHEMISTRY: The entire plant, with the exception of the red, fleshy aril, contains approximately 19 taxane alkaloids, of which the best known is taxine.[2] Other alkaloids (milossine, ephedrine), the glycoside taxicatin, paclitaxel and its derivatives,[3] and pigments are found throughout the plant. Bristol-Myers Squibb recently received FDA approval to market paclitaxel (*Taxol*)[4] as an antineoplastic agent for ovarian cancer, and concern has been raised regarding the environmental impact of debarking Pacific yew trees to harvest the drug. Consequently, methods have been developed to produce paclitaxel from precursors found in the leaves, twigs and needles of yews common in Europe and Asia, and others are attempting to synthesize paclitaxel from pinene, a common compound found in pine trees. Paclitaxel content varies from 0.00003% to 0.069% of the plant.[5] The approved generic name, paclitaxel, was previously referred to as "taxol." *Taxol* is now the trademarked brand name for paclitaxel.

PHARMACOLOGY: The compound paclitaxel is an anticancer agent that is available commercially in the United States and a number of countries. It is derived from several species of yew but primarily from the western yew, *T. brevifolia*. It has a novel mechanism of action causing mitotic abnormalities and arrest, and promoting microtubule polymerization into aggregated structures resulting in the inhibition of cell replication.[6]

Paclitaxel has been widely tested in the United States and approval has been swift. Clinical response has ranged up to approximately 40% with response periods lasting up to two years. Myelosuppression has been the most common adverse event.[7] In other clinical trials, intravenous paclitaxel has resulted in a 12% response rate among patients with metastatic melanoma, with durable response lasting 6 to 17 months.[6] Dose-limiting myelosuppression was observed in early trials that used single or divided intravenous doses. The drug was generally well tolerated except for significant hypersensitivity reactions occurring as skin rashes, bronchospasms, and anaphylaxis. These reactions have been limited by administering the drug as a slow infusion over 6 to 24 hours.

Taxotere, a derivative of paclitaxel derived from the more common English yew, is being investigated for treatment of ovarian, breast, and lung cancer.

TOXICOLOGY: Excluding the red aril, most of the plant is poisonous. Following ingestion, symptoms of dizziness, dry mouth, mydriasis and abdominal cramping develop rapidly. A rash may appear, and the skin can become pale and cyanotic. Bradycardia, hypotension, and dyspnea may be accompanied by coma, leading to death caused by respiratory or cardiac failure. A number of deaths in humans have been reported following the ingestion of yew leaves or teas brewed from yew. The administration of digoxin-specific FAB antibody fragments has been associated with the improvement of cardiac conduction abnormalities following ingestion of yew leaves and berries.[2]

General supportive measures have also been suggested for the management of yew intoxication. The stomach should be emptied and a charcoal slurry administered. The patient should be treated symptomatically.[8]

SUMMARY: The yew has been used in herbal medicine for centuries. The plant is now considered to be of major medical importance, with one extract approved for its antineoplastic activity. Because it is one of the most common foundation plantings in North America, it is often associated with childhood and animal poisonings. All parts of the plant are toxic with the exception of the red fruit.

PATIENT INFORMATION – Yew

Uses: The yew plant has been used to treat rheumatisms, liver and urinary tract conditions, and most recently to treat cancer cells.

Side Effects: The ingestion of the plant results in dizziness, dry mouth, mydriasis, and abdominal cramping. Rash and pale cyanotic skin may develop. It may eventually result in death.

[1] Schauenberg P, Paris F. *Guide to Medicinal Plants.* New Canaan, CT: Keats Publishing, 1977.
[2] Cummins RO, et al. *Ann Emerg Med* 1990;19:38.
[3] Senilh V, et al. *J Nat Prod* 1984;47:131.
[4] Olin BR, ed., et al. *Drug Facts and Comparisons.* St. Louis, MO: Facts and Comparisons, Inc., 1993.
[5] Vidensek N, et al. *J Nat Prod* 1990;53:1609.
[6] Legha SS. et al. *Cancer* 1990;65:2478.
[7] McGuire WP, et al. *Ann Intern Med* 1989;111:273.
[8] Lampe KF. *AMA Handbook of Poisonous and Injurious Plants.* Chicago, IL: Chicago Review Press, 1985.

Yogurt

SOURCE: Yogurt is the general term for a fermented, slightly acidic milk product that contains essentially no alcohol. Most commonly it is prepared by the addition of live cultures of *Streptococcus thermophilus* and *Lactobacillus bulgaricus* to heated whole or skimmed cow's milk. The mixture is incubated and homogenized to a semisolid. Condensed skimmed milk or dry milk solids are sometimes added to produce a custard-like texture. If cultures of *Lactobacillus acidophilus* are added, the product is called acidophilus milk. Bulgarian yogurt is yogurt that has been concentrated by a factor of about 1.5 and contains the highest amount of lactose.

PHARMACOLOGY:

Lactose Intolerance: Yogurt has been at the center of a controversy regarding milk products that can be tolerated by people with lactose-deficiency syndromes. Although a *Lancet* editorialist concluded that "yogurt, cheese, and double creams contain little lactose and can be freely used by most patients,"[1] numerous respondents suggested that the use of yogurt might be inadvisable.

Milk contains 4.6% lactose and yogurt about 3% (after fermentation). Bulgarian yogurt contains about 4.5% lactose, an amount almost equal to that in milk. High lactose levels in yogurt, however, seem to be better tolerated than similar levels in milk. This may be because of the microbial beta-galactosidase in yogurt, because pasteurized yogurt containing little of the enzyme produces more malabsorption of lactose than does active-culture yogurt. Nevertheless, yogurt tolerance by lactase-deficient individuals may be independent of malabsorption, because these individuals tolerate pasteurized yogurt well.[2]

Hydrogen breath tests of lactase-deficient persons have shown that hydrogen production is lower after ingestion of unflavored yogurt than after milk ingestion, with flavored yogurt producing intermediate levels. Neither yogurt type, however, produced symptoms of lactose intolerance. Subjects tolerated frozen yogurt to about the same extent as ice cream or ice milk.[3]

Patients with short-bowel syndrome have been found to better absorb lactose from yogurt than from milk; because a lactose dose of up to 20 g from yogurt was well-tolerated in this study, the investigators suggested that lactose in this form may not need to be excluded from the diets of these patients.[4]

Antimicrobial activity: Yogurt has been promoted to restore the GI flora after systemic antibiotic therapy and to alleviate anal pruritus, aphthous ulcers, and canker sores.

Ingestion of yogurt may also be effective in the prevention of recurrent vaginal yeast infections. The large number of bacteria in active yogurt (each ml of commercial brands contains about 125 million *L. bulgaricus* and 125 million *S. thermophilus*) may hasten the colonization of the colon, thereby removing the reservoir of yeast infection. More than a decade ago, bacterial replacement therapy with live cultures was found to have "no established value in the prevention or treatment of such disorders."[5]

There has been some interest in the direct vaginal instillation of yogurt for the treatment of candida infections. While some lay texts suggest using dilutions of yogurt in water as a douche, its use in full-strength also has been reported.[6] Whatever effect is obtained might be because of the lactic acid content (about 1%) or low pH (about 4) of the product. One study assessed the effects of the intravaginal application of commercial yogurt in 32 pregnant women with bacterial vaginosis. A continuous improvement in vaginal pH and *Lactobacillus* flora was noted; the therapy was well-tolerated.[7] However, the clinical effects of this therapy have not been defined in well-controlled studies and this practice cannot be widely recommended, particularly in pregnant women.

Yogurt possesses intrinsic antibacterial activity against *Salmonella typhimurium*, probably because of its lactic acid content; the low oxidation-reduction potential of the product may also contribute. The small amount of acetic acid present (about 0.2%) is not sufficient for antibacterial activity.[8] The compound bulgaricum is elaborated by some strains of *L. bulgaricus* and has inhibitory activity against gram-negative and gram-positive bacteria.[9] This bacterium also produces amounts of hydrogen peroxide that are inhibitory to *Staphylococcus aureus*.[10] In vitro tests have shown yogurt to kill all 11 tested strains of *Campylobacter jejuni* within 25 minutes. Lactic acid is quite bactericidal against these organisms, but it is probably not the only factor in eliminating the bacteria.[11]

In spite of yogurt's antibacterial properties, it has been speculated that the product offers a suitable medium for the proliferation of toxic fungi. Conditions during the production of yogurt or during cooling (from 45°C to 4°C) meet the requirements for fungal growth; this has been associated with the production of small amounts of aflatoxin. It is unclear, however, whether lactic acid levels affect fungal growth and aflatoxin production.[12]

Two studies have shown that yogurt consumption increases the ability of weanling Sprague-Dawly rats to withstand gastrointestinal challenge by *Salmonella enter-itidis* in comparison with milk. Although yogurt did not prevent disease, it reduced mortality and the deceleration of weight gain. The differences between yogurt and milk did not appear to be related to differences in vitamin and mineral content.[13,14] The clinical importance of these findings is poorly understood.

It should be noted, however, that particularly in the elderly, the live bacteria found in yogurt do not necessarily pass through the gut. In one study, only a mucosal-adhering strain of *Lactobacillus gasseri* passed through the intestinal tract after ingestion of yogurt, suggesting that some bacterial stains may have a greater ability to remain within the gut than others.[15] In another study, women given yogurt containing live *Lactobacillus* demonstrated significant changes in fecal enzymatic activity and also had significant increases in fecal bacterial counts, indicating that yogurt supplementation could modify the colonic bacterial environment.[16] However, recent evidence indicates that ingestion of yogurt supplemented with *Bifidobacterium longum* does not alter the normal fecal aerobic or anaerobic counts, suggesting that the bacterial composition of human fecal flora may not be readily influenced by dietary supplementation with active culture yogurt.[17]

Antineoplastic activity: Experiments with cells from murine Peyer's patches suggest that yogurt may boost host immunocompetence by potentiating cell-mediated immune responses. This involves increases in the percentage of B lymphocytes and PHA- and LPS-induced proliferation responses as shown in suspensions of Peyer's patch cells.[18]

Several Russian investigators have reported the isolation of compounds from the cell wall of *L. bulgaricus* capable of inhibiting the proliferation of tumors in laboratory animals, and others have isolated an antitumor compound produced by *L. bulgaricus* var. tumornecroticans. Yogurt has an inhibitory effect on Ehrlich ascites tumor cell proliferation.[19] In vivo antitumor activity was demonstrated in mice with similar tumors; the activity resides in the water-soluble fraction of yogurt and may be a component(s) with molecular weight of less than 14,000. This compound is active orally and parenterally.[20] A case-control study of nearly 3,000 subjects that analyzed consumption of alcohol and dairy products found that yogurt consumption was associated with a drop in the incidence of breast cancer.[21]

The results of a more recent study that followed 120,852 Dutch men for approximately 3 years found that the risk of colorectal cancer decreased slightly as the consumption of fermented dairy (ie, yogurt) increased; however, unlike the findings from some other studies, increases in the total dietary intake of calcium were not associated with decreases in the risk for colorectal cancer.[22]

Lipid-lowering effects: A study of the dietary habits of the Masai, a nomadic tribe inhabiting southern Kenya, found that the Masai had low serum cholesterol levels and a low incidence of ischemic heart disease. Their diet consisted mostly of fermented milk product similar to yogurt, and they rarely ate meat. When challenged with a "western" diet, their cholesterol levels increased, ruling out a protective genetic factor.[23]

The data suggest that Masai yogurt contained a component that influenced cholesterol levels in man. These findings have been disputed; on autopsy, many Masai were found to have significant atherosclerotic deposits in their aortas. However, because they are a robust nomadic people, their cardiac vessels were found to be significantly larger than in sedate persons, thereby providing relatively unobstructed blood flow even in the presence of atherosclerosis.

When western subjects had their normal diets supplemented with a daily intake of the yogurt from 2 or 4 L of whole milk, from 2 L of skimmed milk or simply 2 L of fresh milk, both the whole and skimmed milk yogurt produced significant reductions in cholesterol levels of up to 29% within 20 days. The ingestion of fresh milk generally did not affect serum cholesterol levels.[24]

Results of other metabolic studies suggest that yogurt contains a factor that inhibits the synthesis of cholesterol from acetate, resulting in lower levels even when dietary cholesterol intake is large; the compound is thought to be hydroxymethyl glutaryl G coenzyme-A cholesterol biosynthesis. This finding has been disputed because the levels of HMG in yogurt are variable, indicating that HMG may not be solely responsible for the cholesterol-lowering effect. Other data suggest that the levels of calcium present in yogurt (equivalent to an intake of about 850 mg/day) may contribute to serum cholesterol reduction.[25]

In one test, rabbits were fed either yogurt, milk, or calcium, along with a high-cholesterol diet. When the study groups were compared after 16 weeks, the yogurt group showed significantly lower cholesterol levels than the milk group, but these decreases were similar to those observed in the calcium group. Because milk can also reduce cholesterol levels (to a lesser extent, however, than yogurt) calcium alone or with other factors such as HMG is responsible for yogurt's hypocholesterolemic effects.[26] Research continues into the identification of a hypocholesterolemic factor in milk and other dietary products.[27]

TOXICOLOGY: Yogurt is not associated with any significant adverse events. As described above, people intolerant to lactose may not be able to digest yogurt. One report of 11 children who developed hemolytic uremic syndrome from a toxic strain of *Escherichia coli* that contaminated a batch of yogurt in North West England suggests that stringent bacterial control must be applied to the production of this food product.

SUMMARY: Yogurt is a widely enjoyed milk product. It is a good source of calcium and may be more readily digested than milk by some lactose-deficient people. It has some antibacterial and antitumor activity, although the clinical implications are unknown. Reports of its use in treatment of enteric and vaginal infections are preliminary. The daily ingestion of yogurt may confer some protection against hypercholesterolemia, although the minimum amount of dietary yogurt required for this effect has not been established.

PATIENT INFORMATION – Yogurt

Uses: Yogurt has been used as a substitute for those who are lactose-intolerant and to prevent recurring vaginal yeast infections. Yogurt also inhibits other antimicrobial activity, antineoplastic activity, and lipid-lowering effects.

Side Effects: Yogurt is not associated with any significant adverse events.

---

[1] Arneil GC, Chin KC. *Lancet* 1979;2:840.
[2] Savaiano DA, Levitt MD. *J Dairy Sci* 1987;70(2):397.
[3] Martini MC, et al. *Am J Clin Nutr* 1987;46(4):636.
[4] Arrigoni E, et al. *Am J Clin Nutr* 1994;60(6):926.
[5] Anon. *Med Lett Drugs Ther* 1972;14(16):59.
[6] Joseph ST. *Am J Nurs* 1983;4:524.
[7] Neri A, et al. *Acta Obstet Gynecol Scand* 1993;72(1):17.
[8] Rubin HE, Vaughan F. *J Dairy Sci* 1979;62(12):1873.
[9] Reddy GV, Shahani JM. *J Dairy Sci* 1971;54:748.
[10] Dahiya RS, Speck ML. *J Dairy Sci* 1968;51(10):1568.
[11] Cuk Z, et al. *J Appl Bacteriol* 1987;63(3):201.
[12] Blanco JL, et al. *Z Lebensm Unters Forsch* 1988;186(4):323.
[13] Hitchins AD, et al. *Am J Clin Nutr* 1985;41(1):92.
[14] Pedrosa MC, et al. *Am J Clin Nutr* 1995;61(2):353.

[15] Ling WH, et al. *J Nutr* 1994;124(1):18.
[16] Bartram HP, et al. *Am J Clin Nutr* 1994;59(2):428.
[17] DeSimone C, et al. *Immunopharmacol Immunotoxicol* 1987;9(1):87.
[18] Reddy GV, et al. *J Natl Cancer Inst* 1973;50(3):815.
[19] Ayebo AD, et al. *J Dairy Sci* 1981;64(12):2318.
[20] Le MG, et al. *J Natl Cancer Inst* 1986;77(3):633.
[21] Kampman E, et al. *Cancer Res* 1994;54(12):3186.
[22] Mann GV, et al. *J Atheros Res* 1964;4:289.
[23] Mann GV. *Atherosclerosis* 1977;26(3):335.
[24] Hepner G, et al. *Am J Clin Nutr* 1979;32(1):19.
[25] Thakur CP, Jha AN. *Atherosclerosis* 1981;39(2):211.
[26] Eichholzer M, Stahelin H. *Int J Vitam Nutr Res* 1993;63(3):159.
[27] Morgan D, et al. *Epidemiol Infect* 1993;111(2):181.

Yohimbe

SCIENTIFIC NAME(S): *Pausinystalia yohimbe* (K Schumann) Pierre. Synonymous with *Corynanthe johimbe*. Family: Rubiaceae. The alkaloid yohimbine also is obtained from *Aspidosperma quebracho blanco* and *Rauwolfia serpentina*.

COMMON NAME(S): Yohimbe, yohimbehe, yohimbine

BOTANY: This tree grows throughout the African nations of Cameroon, Gabon, and Zaire.

HISTORY: The bark of the West African yohimbe tree is rich in the alkaloid yohimbine, and both the crude bark and purified compound have long been hailed as aphrodisiacs. The bark has been smoked as a hallucinogen and has been used in traditional medicine to treat angina and hypertension. Today the drug is being investigated for the treatment of organic impotence.

CHEMISTRY: The bark contains approximately 6% yohimbine (also known as aphrodine, quebrachine or corynine). Yohimbine is an indole analog. Other minor alkaloids include corynantheidine and allo-yohimbine.

PHARMACOLOGY: Yohimbine is generally classified as an alpha-2-adrenergic blocking agent. Small doses have a stimulant action in humans resulting in autonomic and psychic changes commonly associated with the subjective experience of anxiety.[1] Yohimbine has been reported to be an inhibitor of monoamine oxidase[2] but more likely has a weak calcium channel blocking effect.[3]

Yohimbine dilates blood vessels, thereby lowering blood pressure; however, its use as an antihypertensive agent has long been abandoned. The drug causes a significant increase in blood pressure after an oral dose of 5 mg in patients with orthostatic hypotension secondary to pure autonomic failure or multisystem atrophy. This response is associated with an increased heart rate and increased plasma noradrenaline levels.

Because yohimbine can cause both the dilation of peripheral and mucous membrane blood vessels along with central nervous system stimulation, the drug has been investigated for the treatment of organic impotence. It should be noted that both the crude drug and yohimbine have a long history of use as aphrodisiacs.

Sexual-stimulant products available over-the-counter often contain yohimbine, sometimes combined with hormones such as methyltestosterone.

One older prescription product (*Afrodex,* Bentex Pharmaceuticals) combined 5 mg each of yohimbine HCl, methyltestosterone, and nux vomica in a capsule for the treatment of male climacteric and impotence. Although a number of clinical trials were conducted with this product,[4] the results were generally unimpressive leading the *Medical Letter* to conclude that "there is still no good evidence that *Afrodex* and similar drugs have more than placebo effects."[5]

More recent investigations now strongly suggest that higher doses of the drug (6 mg three times a day) may be effective in the treatment of organically impotent men.[6] One study found that 10 of 23 men treated with the drug derived a benefit from treatment. Eleven of the 23 men were diabetics.[7] One prescription product containing 5.4 mg yohimbine HCl (*Yocon,* Palisades Pharmaceuticals) is indicated as a sympathicolytic and mydriatic that also may have activity as an aphrodisiac. Yohimbine appears to be effective and may exert its activity by increasing the norepinephrine content of the corpus cavernosum.[8]

TOXICOLOGY: Yohimbine may be toxic if ingested in high doses. The drug causes severe hypotension, abdominal distress, and weakness. Larger doses may cause central nervous system stimulation and paralysis. This drug should not be used in the presence of renal or hepatic disease. It has been suggested that because of its monoamine oxidase inhibiting activity the usual precautions for concomitant drug use with this class of agents be followed.[2] Yohimbine may precipitate psychoses in predisposed individuals. The drug or crude product should never be self administered, but should only be taken under supervision of a physician.

SUMMARY: Yohimbine is an alkaloid derived from the African yohimbe tree. Both the crude drug and purified alkaloid have been used as an aphrodisiac and hallucinogen. Recent studies suggest that the drug may be effective in the treatment of male organic impotence, in particular that associated with diabetes.

PATIENT INFORMATION – Yohimbe

Uses: Yohimbe has been investigated for the treatment of organic impotence, in particular those with diabetes, and for the use as aphrodisiacs.

Side Effects: Yohimbe may be toxic if ingested in high amounts. It causes severe hypotension, abdominal distress, and weakness and may cause CNS stimulation and paralysis.

[1] Ingram CG. *Clin Pharm Ther* 1962;3:345.
[2] Tyler VE. *The New Honest Herbal.* Philadelphia, PA: G.F. Stickley Co., 1987.
[3] Watanabe K, et al. *J Pharm Pharmacol* 1987;39:439.
[4] Miller WW. *Curr Ther Res* 1968;10:354.

[5] Anon. *Med Lett Drugs Ther* 1968;10:97.
[6] Anon. *Medical World News* 1982;23:115.
[7] Morales A, et al. *J Urol* 1982;128:45.
[8] Morales A, et al. *N Engl J Med* 1981;305:1221.

Yucca

SCIENTIFIC NAME(S): *Yucca* spp. Family: Agavaceae

COMMON NAME(S): Yucca, Spanish bayonet, Our Lord's candle, Joshua tree, Adam's needle

BOTANY: The name yucca applies to as many as 40 species of trees and shrubs found mostly in arid portions of North America. The common names noted above can apply to different species. The Spanish bayonet s *Y. aloifolia* and Our Lord's candle is *Y. whipplei*.[1] Other common yuccas include *Y. schidigera* (Mohave yucca) and *Y. brevifolia* (Joshua tree), which grows to 60 feet in height and is commonly found at the bases of desert mountains.[2] Yucca plants are characterized by stiff, evergreen, sword-shaped leaves crowded on a stout trunk. There is a dense terminal flowerhead (panicle) faintly resembling a candle. The flowers are white or greenish. All yucca plants depend for pollination on nocturnal yucca moths (*Tegeticula*).[3] Each variety of moth is adapted to a single species of yucca.

HISTORY: Yucca plants have served American Indians for centuries for a variety of uses including fiber for rope, sandals and cloth; the roots have been used in soap. The Indians and early Californian settlers used the green pods for food. Indian uses included boiling and baking the fruits, eating the blossoms, chewing the raw leaves and fermenting the fruits to produce a beverage for high rituals. In modern times yucca has been used in soaps, shampoos and food supplements. Yuccas contain saponins that have a long-lasting soaping action. The plant has been purported to be beneficial for treating hypertension, arthritis, migraine headaches, colitis, and a variety of other disorders. A solid extract is derived from the leaves;[2] the Mohave yucca is the most common commercially used plant. Current commercial uses of yucca extracts include foaming agents in carbonated beverages, flavorings, and for use in drug synthesis research.

CHEMISTRY: The roots of the yucca contain saponin glycosides consisting of a sapogenin and a sugar.[4] Saponins are characterized by their bitter taste and their ability to foam when shaken with water.[1] Most species of Yucca contain sarsasapogenin and tigogenin.[2,5] Cortical cells in the roots of *Y. torreyi* have been found to contain microbodies containing crystalline nucleoid inclusions that have been identified as unspecialized peroxisomes.[6] *Y. aloifolia* leaves contain up to 1.4% tigogenin and this compound can be used as a starting point in the commercial synthesis of steroidal hormones.

PHARMACOLOGY: Aqueous alcoholic extracts of the flowers of *Y. glauca* have been shown to have antitumor activity against B16 melanoma in mice. Analysis of these extracts has identified two galactose-containing polysaccharides effective against B16 melanoma but ineffective against L1210 and P388 leukemias in mice.[7] Yucca leaf protein has been found to inhibit herpes simplex virus types 1 and 2 and human cytomegalovirus.[8] Some saponins have been shown to allow bacterial, plant and animal cells to thrive under harsh environmental conditions. However, yucca saponins do not enhance weight gain, food conversion, or digestive coefficients when fed to young turkeys.[9]

One report found that the oral administration of daily doses of a yucca saponin extract for up to 15 months was effective and well-tolerated for the treatment of various arthritic conditions.[1] However, the Arthritis Foundation found the study to be poorly controlled and designed, and the conclusions to have been based on inconsistent results.[1,10] Interestingly, the patients who received the extract for 6 months had significant reductions in blood pressure and serum cholesterol levels, and a reduction in the incidence of migraine headaches from baseline.

TOXICOLOGY: It is generally recognized that saponins are poisonous to lower forms of life, but are however, nearly nontoxic to humans when taken orally. However, their injection into the bloodstream causes hemolysis, dissolving red blood cells even if the saponins are present at extreme dilutions. This effect, however, is more pronounced in vitro than in vivo.[2] Little is known about the toxicity of yucca saponins. The effects of long-term ingestion of these saponins is not well defined. A 12-week feeding study in rats found Mohave yucca extract to be essentially nontoxic.[11]

SUMMARY: Yucca is a hardy plant native to arid areas of North America. It has long been used for a variety of purposes, including as a fiber, soap, and for consumable products. When taken orally, it appears to be relatively nontoxic. While some evidence suggests the extract may be effective in the management of arthritis, hypertension, and hypercholesterolemia, there is no published corroborative evidence. Extracts may have potential as antiviral agents.

PATIENT INFORMATION – Yucca

Uses: Yucca has been historically used as a fiber, soap, and for consumable products. Some evidence suggests the extract may be effective in the management of arthritis, hypertension, and hypercholesterolemia.

Side Effects: Little is known about the toxicity of yucca plants.

[1] Tyler V. *The Honest Herbal: a sensible guide to the use of herbs and related remedies.* Binghamton, NY: The Haworth Press, 1993.

[2] Leung AY. *Encyclopedia of Common Natural Ingredients Used in Food, Drugs and Cosmetics.* New York, NY: J. Wiley and Sons, 1980.

[3] Bull JJ, Rice WR. *J Theor Biol* 1991;149:63.

[4] Dewidar AM, el-Munajjed D. *Planta Med* 1970;19:87.

[5] Evans, WC. *Trease and Evans' Pharmacognosy.* 13th ed. London: Balliere Tindall, 1989.

[6] Kausch AP. *Eur J Cell Biol* 1984;34:239.

[7] Ali MS, et al. *Growth* 1978:42:213.

[8] Hayashi K, et al. *Antiviral Res* 1992;17:323.

[9] Dziuk HE, et al. *Poult Sci* 1985:64:1143.

[10] Bennett CC. *Public Information Memo.* New York: The Arthritis Foundation, Feb 22, 1977.

[11] Oser BL. *Food Cosmet Toxicol* 1966;4:57.

APPENDIX

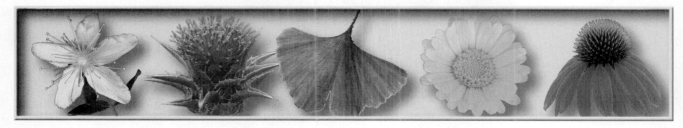

Potential Herb-Drug Interactions

There have been relatively few reports of interactions with the coadministration of herbs and conventional drug therapies. The table below profiles potential drug-herb interactions based on reported herbal constituents and known pharmacological actions. Many of the interactions are inconsequential. However, some could be serious depending on the herb quality, concentration, and sensitivity of the patient.

Monitoring is imperative. Always ask patients if unusual herbs or foods are being taken concomitantly with standard medications.

Report findings of interactions through FDA Medical Products Reporting Program (MedWatch) by phone at (301) 443-1240, or fax at 1-800-FDA-0178. Review MedWatch reports at www.fda.gov/medwatch.

Herb/Conventional Drug Interactions[1]		
Medications/ Therapeutic Class	Potential Herbal Interactions	Possible Adverse Effects
Central Nervous System		
Analgesics	Herbal-containing principles with diuretic activity (eg, corn silk, dandelion, juniper, uva ursi)	These may pose an increased risk of toxicity with the anti-inflammatory analgesic drugs.
	Herbs containing agents with corticosteroid activity (eg, licorice, bayberry)	These may induce reduction in plasma-salicylate concentration.
	Herbs containing agents with sedative properties (eg, calamus, nettle)	Possible enhancement of sedative side effects.
Anticonvulsants	Herbs with active principles which have sedative effects (eg, calamus, nettle, ground ivy, sage, borage)	Possible increase in sedative side effects. May increase risk of seizure.
	Herbs with salicylates (eg, poplar, willow)	May cause transient potentiation of phenytoin therapy.
	Ayurvedic Shankapushpi[2]	May shorten phenytoin's half-life and diminish its effectiveness.
Antidepressants	Herbs containing sympathomimetic amines (eg, agnus castus alkaloids, calamus amines, cola alkaloids, broom alkaloids, licorice)[2]	Increased risk of hypertensive crisis with MAO inhibitors. May potentiate sedative side effects.
	Ginkgo biloba	Use with tricyclic antidepressants or other medications known to decrease the seizure threshold is not advised.
Antiemetic and antivertigo drugs	Herbs containing sedative principles (eg, calamus, nettle, ground ivy, sage, borage)	May increase activity of sedative side effects.
	Herbs containing anticholinergic principles	May be antagonistic.
Antiparkinsonism agents	Herbs containing anticholinergic principles	Possible potentiation and increased risk of side effects.
	Herbs containing principles with cholinergic activity	Possible antagonism.

Herb/Conventional Drug Interactions[1]		
Medications/ Therapeutic Class	Potential Herbal Interactions	Possible Adverse Effects
Antipsychotics	Herbs containing diuretic principles (eg, corn silk, dandelion, juniper)	Possible potentation of lithium action; increased risk of toxicity.
	Herbs with anticholinergic principles (eg, corkwood tree)	May reduce plasma levels of phenothiazines; possible increased risk of seizures.
	Ginseng, yohimbine, and ephedra[2]	Concomitant use with phenelzine and other MAO inhibitors may result in insomnia, headache, and tremulousness.
Anxiolytics/hypnotics (eg, alprazolam)	Several herbs with claimed sedative properties (eg, calamus, kava, nettle, ground ivy, sage, borage)	Potentiation.
Phenobarbital[2]	Thujone-containing herbs (eg, wormwood, sage) and gamolenic acid-containing herbs (eg, evening primrose oil, borage)	May lower seizure threshold.
Nonsteroidal anti-inflammatory drugs (NSAIDs)[2]	Feverfew	NSAIDs may reduce the effectiveness of feverfew perhaps mediated by its prostaglandin inhibition effects.
	Herbs with antiplatelet activity (eg, ginkgo biloba, ginger, ginseng, garlic)	May increase the risk of bleeding due to gastric irritation.
Stimulants	Ginseng (Panax spp.)	Increased risk of side effects.
Cardiovascular System		
Antiarrhythmic	Herbs with cardioactive principles	Antagonize or affect efficiency of therapy.
	Herbs with diuretic properties (eg, corn silk, dandelion, juniper, uva ursi)	If hypokalemia occurs, may be antagonistic.
Anticoagulants	Herbs containing coagulant or anticoagulant principles (coumarins; eg, alfalfa, red clover, chamomile, ginkgo biloba)	Possible risk of antagonism or potentiation.
	Garlic[2]	May decrease platelet aggregation.
	Ginger[2]	Inhibits thromboxane synthetase, prolonging bleeding time.
	Herbs with high salicylate content (eg, meadowsweet, poplar)	Possible risk of potentiation.
Antihyperlipidemic drugs	Herbs containing hypolipidemic principles (eg, black cohosh, fenugreek, garlic, plantain)	Possible additive effects.

Herb/Conventional Drug Interactions[1]		
Medications/ Therapeutic Class	Potential Herbal Interactions	Possible Adverse Effects
Antihypertensives	Herbs containing hypertensive ingredients (eg, blue cohosh, cola, ginger)	May be antagonistic.
	Herbs containing principles with mineralo-corticoid action (eg, licorice, bayberry)	
	Herbs containing hypotensive principles (eg, black cohosh, devil's claw, hawthorn)	Possible potentiation.
	Herbs containing high levels of amine compounds or sympathomimetic action (eg, Agnus castus, black cohosh, cola, maté, St. John's wort)	May be antagonistic.
	Herbs containing diuretic ingredients (eg, corn silk, dandelion, juniper, uva ursi)	Possible risk of potentiation.
Beta-adrenergic blocking agents	Herbs containing cardioactive principles (cardiac glycosides)	Possible antagonism.
	Herbs with high levels of amines or sympathomimetic action (eg, Agnus castus, black cohosh, cola, maté, St. John's wort)	Possible risk of severe hypertension.
Cardenolides (cardiac glycosides)	Herbs with cardioactive constituents (eg, mistletoe [viscotoxin, negative inotropic properties], cola nut [caffeine], figwort [cardioactive glycosides])	Decreased effectiveness or potentiation; increased potential for side effects.
	Hawthorn, Siberian ginseng, Kyushin, and uzara root[2]	May increase the risk of bleeding.
Diuretics	Herbs containing diuretic properties (eg, corn silk, dandelion, gossypol, juniper, uva ursi)	Increased risk of hypokalemia.
	Herbals having hypotensive properties (eg, agrimony, black cohosh, devil's claw, mistletoe)	May cause difficulty in controlling diuresis.
Nitrates and calcium-channel blocking agents	Herbs with cardioactive constituents (eg, broom, squill)	Interferes with therapy (eg, broom may slow heart rate, cause arrhythmias).
	Herbs containing hypertensive principles (eg, bayberry, blue cohosh, cola)	Antagonistic effects.
	Herbs containing anticholinergic principles	Possible reduced buccal absorption of nitroglycerin.
Sympathomimetics	Herbs containing sympathomimetic amines (eg, aniseed, capsicum, parsley, vervain)	Possible increased risk of hypertension.
	Herb principles having hypertensive action (eg, bayberry, broom, blue cohosh, licorice)	
	Herb principles with hypotensive action (eg, agrimony, celery, ginger, hawthorn)	Antagonistic effects.

Herb/Conventional Drug Interactions[1]		
Medications/ Therapeutic Class	Potential Herbal Interactions	Possible Adverse Effects
Anti-infective agents		
Antifungals	Herbs containing anticholinergic agents (eg, corkwood tree)	Possible decreased absorption of ketoconazole.
Endocrine System		
Antidiabetic drugs	Herbs containing hypo- or hyperglycemic principles (eg, alfalfa, fenugreek, ginseng)	Possible antagonism or potentiation of action.
	Herbs containing diuretic principles (eg, broom, buchu, corn silk, juniper)	Antagonistic effects.
	Chromium, karela[2]	May affect blood glucose levels, complicating insulin and chlorpropamide requirements, respectively.
Corticosteroids	Herbs containing diuretic principles (eg, broom, buchu, corn silk, juniper)	Possible risk of increased potassium loss.
	Herbs containing corticosteroid principles or action (eg, bayberry)	Increased risk of side effects (eg, sodium retention).
	Herbs, vitamins, and minerals with immunostimulating effects (eg, echinacea, astragalus, licorice, alfalfa sprouts, vitamin E, zinc)	May offset the immunosuppressive effects of corticosteroids.
Sex hormones	Herbs containing hormonal principles (eg, alfalfa, bayberry, black cohosh, licorice)	Potential interactions with existing therapy (eg, black cohosh may decrease the response to estrogens).
Drugs used to treat hyper- and hypothroidism	Herbs containing high levels of iodine	Interferes with therapy.
	Horseradish (eg, goiterogenic myrrh) and kelp[2]	
Drugs Used in Obstetrics and Gynecology		
Estrogens[2]	Herbs containing phytoestrogens (eg, dong quai, red clover, alfalfa, licorice, black cohosh, soybeans)	Concomitant use may result in symptoms of estrogen excess such as nausea, bloating, hypotension, breast fullness or tenderness, migraine, or edema.
Oral contraceptives	Herbs containing principles with hormonal action (eg, black cohosh, licorice)	Possible interactions with exisitng drugs; may also reduce effectiveness of oral contraception.
Antineoplastics Drugs/Drugs with Immunosuppressive Activity		
Methotrexate	Herbs containing sufficient levels of salicylates (eg, willow, poplar, meadowsweet)	Possible increased risk of toxicity.
Immune-system affecting drugs	Herbs containing immunostimulant principles (eg, boneset, echinacea, mistletoe)	Possible antagonism or potentiation.
Drugs for Joint and Musculoskeletal Disorders		
Probenecid	Herbs containing sufficient levels of salicylates (eg, meadowsweet, poplar, willow)	Possible inhibition of uricosuric effect of probenecid.

Herb/Conventional Drug Interactions[1]		
Medications/ Therapeutic Class	Potential Herbal Interactions	Possible Adverse Effects
Diuretics		
Acetazolamide	Herbs containing sufficient levels of salicylates (eg, meadowsweet, poplar, willow)	Increased potential for toxicity.
Anesthetics		
General anesthetics	Herbs containing hypotensive principles (eg, black cohosh, goldenseal, hawthorn)	Potentiation of hypotensive action.
Muscle relaxants	Herbs containing diuretic principles (eg, broom, buchu, corn silk)	Possible potentiation if hypokalemia occurs.
Depolarizing muscle relaxants	Herbs containing cardioactive principles (eg, cola, figwort, hawthorn)	Possible risk of arrhythmias.

[1] Adapted from "*Herbal Medicines*" by C. Newall, et al. The Pharmaceutical Press, London, 1996.

[2] *Arch Intern Med* 1998;158:2200-211.

Specific Herb-Drug Interactions

Clinical Considerations for Specific Herb-Drug Interactions & Potential Adverse Effects of Herbs

	Adverse Effects	Interactions and Clinical Concerns
Aloe (Cape aloe, Barbados aloe, Curaçao aloe; *Aloe vera* L., *A. perryi* Baker)	*External:* May cause allergic contact dermatitis.	*External:* Do not use in deep vertical (surgical) wounds; may delay healing.
	Internal: Excessive consumption of juice may cause painful intestinal contractions.	*Internal:* Juice and exudate. Possible loss of intestinal K^+ leading to a decrease in serum K^+. This may potentiate effects of **cardiac glycosides** and **antiarrhythmics**. Concurrent use of **thiazides**, **licorice**, **steroids**, and other **K^+-wasting drugs** may be potentiated by aloe juice. Avoid juice if pregnant. The dried leaf exudate (not gel or juice) contains anthraquinone glycosides which are irritating laxatives. Avoid in children under 12 years of age and during menstruation, nursing, stomach or intestinal inflammation, ulcerative colitis, Crohn's disease, inflamed hemorrhoids, intestinal obstruction, and kidney disorders.
Bilberry fruit (*Vaccinium myrtillus*)	Excessive consumption of dried fruits (high in tannins) may lead to constipation.	Because of reported antiaggregation effect on platelets (anthocyanosides), monitor patients on **antiplatelet drugs** and **anticoagulants**. Myrtillin has hypoglycemic effects; monitor patients with diabetes.
Cayenne (hot pepper; *Capsicum frutescens* L., *C. annuum* L.)	*External:* Strong initial burning sensation, particularly in sensitive areas (eg, eyes, face).	Use oily (olive oil) or acidic (vinegar) solutions to wash away irritating capsaicin. Eat bananas or yogurt, or drink milk to diminish GI irritation. Because it stimulates GI secretions, it may help protect against **NSAID** damage (30 minutes before giving NSAIDs). Cayenne reduces platelet aggregation and increases fibrinolytic activity; therefore, monitor patients taking **antiplatelet drugs** or **anticoagulants**.
	Internal: Stomach upset and discomfort. Diarrhea with burning sensations. Contraindicated in asthmatics because of bronchoconstrictive effects of capsaicin. Avoid use on damaged skin and in the presence of gastric ulcers.	
Chamomile (*Matricaria chamomilla* L. = German Chamomile)	Pollen in flowers may cause hypersensitivity leading to sneezing, runny nose, anaphylaxis, dermatitis, and GI upset. The dried flowering heads can be emetogenic if ingested in large amounts.	Should be consumed regularly for desired effect. This may delay concomitant drug absorption from the gut. Avoid during pregnancy because of emmenagogue effect.
English Chamomile (*Anthemis nobilis*) Compositae family (Asteraceae)	Avoid chamomile in individuals with known sensitivity to any members of the Compositae family (Asteraceae).	Excessive doses may interfere with **anticoagulant** therapy because of the coumarin constituents. English chamomile is reported to be an abortifacient and to affect the menstrual cycle.

Clinical Considerations for Specific Herb-Drug Interactions & Potential Adverse Effects of Herbs

	Adverse Effects	Interactions and Clinical Concerns
Dong quai (*Angelica*) *polymorpha* Maxim. var. *sinensis*	Some species of *Angelica* are phototoxic or photosensitizing because of furanocoumarins. Lowers blood pressure. Possible CNS stimulation.	Contains vasodilatory and antispasmodic coumarin derivatives. Monitor warfarin patients. Possible synergism with calcium channel blockers. *Angelica Archangelica* L. is reported to be an abortifacient and to affect the menstrual cycle. *A. sinensis* has uterine-stimulant activity.
Echinacea spp. (*Echinacea angustifolia* DC., *E. purpurea* L. Moench and *E. pallida* Nutt. Britton) Compositae family	Cross-sensitivity in persons allergic to Compositae family pollen. Reported tingling and numbing sensation on tasting. Fever from freshly prepared juice.	Long-term use not recommended, particularly in people with autoimmune disorders (eg, lupus, rheumatoid arthritis). Also contraindicated in progressive disorders like multiple sclerosis, collagenosis, AIDS or HIV infection, and tuberculosis. Lack of toxicity data necessitates caution of excessive use, particularly during pregnancy.
Ephedra; Ma Huang (*Ephedra sinica*)	In large doses, ephedrine causes nervousness, headache, insomnia, dizziness, palpitations, skin flushing, tingling, vomiting, anxiety, and restlessness. Toxic psychosis could be induced by ephedrine. Skin reactions also have been observed in sensitive patients.	Contains the alkaloid ephedrine which is a CNS stimulant. Ephedrine stimulates the heart and increases heart rate. Dysrhythmias may occur when used in combination with **cardiac glycosides** or **anesthetics** (eg, halothane). Ephedrine constricts peripheral blood vessels and increases blood pressure; it has enhanced sympathomimetic effects when used with **guanethidine** and hypertensive crises are possible if used concomitantly with **MAOI antidepressants**. Avoid simultaneous use of **vasoconstrictor sympathomimetics**. Hypertension may occur when used with **oxytocin**, possibly severe with concomitant **beta blockers**. Bronchodilation, uterine contraction, and diuresis are other activities reported with ephedrine. Crude aerial parts have caused hyperglycemia as well as hypoglycemia. Patients with high blood pressure and diabetes should exercise caution when using these plants.
Feverfew (*Tanacetum parthenium*) Compositae family	Contact or chewing leaves may lead to aphthous ulcers. Dermatitis reported. Some abdominal pain, indigestion, diarrhea, flatulence, nausea, and vomiting reported.	May take several months (4 to 6) to see effects. Hence, it should not be discontinued abruptly. Can reduce platelet aggregation and increase fibrinolytic activity. Monitor patients on **anticoagulants** or **antiplatelet agents**. Has uterine-stimulant effects and should be avoided in pregnant women. Can modify menstrual flow. Avoid in children less than 2 years of age. Tachycardia has been reported. May prevent 5-HT (serotonin) release from platelets; possible potentiation of methysergide reported. A "post-feverfew" syndrome has been described with symptoms including nervousness, tension headaches, insomnia, stiffness/pain in joints, and tiredness. Some feel that feverfew should only be used for migraines when conventional drugs have failed. In ragweed family, cross-sensitivity possible.

Clinical Considerations for Specific Herb-Drug Interactions & Potential Adverse Effects of Herbs

	Adverse Effects	Interactions and Clinical Concerns
Garlic	Considered non-toxic, but can cause oral and GI irritation.	Because of inhibition of platelet aggregation and increased fibrinolytic properties, monitor patients on **antiplatelet drugs** or **anticoagulants**. Therapeutic doses of garlic are not recommended for those with blood that clots slowly. Use caution in patients on anticoagulant therapy. May increase serum **insulin** levels, decreasing blood glucose. Garlic may also lower cholesterol and lipid levels. High doses are reported to induce anemia because of both decreased hemoglobin synthesis and hemolysis. May potentiate the antithrombotic effects of **aspirin**. Also is likely to be synergistic with **eicosapentenoic acid** (EPA) in fish oils. Doses of garlic greatly exceeding amounts used in food should not be taken during pregnancy and lactation.
Ginger (*Zingiber officinale* Roscoe)	High doses may cause GI irritation and discomfort when taken on an empty stomach. Fresh ginger is considered more effective. A 1/4 inch slice of fresh equals ≈ 1 to 2 grams of powder.	Because ginger inhibits platelet aggregation, patients on **antiplatelet drugs** or **anticoagulants** should be monitored. Increased calcium uptake by heart muscle may alter **calcium channel blocker** effect. Contraindications include pregnancy (large amounts) and gallstones because of its cholagogue effect. Low doses are commonly used in the management of nausea of pregnancy (hyperemesis gravidarum). The German Commission E Monographs state that ginger should not be used for treatment of vomiting in pregnancy.
Ginkgo (*Ginkgo biloba* L.)	The extract may rarely cause GI discomfort and headache.	Therapeutic response may occur in 2 to 3 weeks and must be taken continuously. Inhibits platelet-activating factor (PAF); bleeding episodes reported. Use caution with patients on **antiplatelet drugs** and **warfarin**. No studies have been done on leaf extracts in pregnant and lactating women; it should be avoided in this population. Avoid the small oval fruits of the female tree because contact or ingestion of the fruit pulp has caused severe allergic reactions (eg, edema, erythema, blisters, itching). The bad smell is caused by butyric acid, but the toxin in the seed is 4-0-methylpyridoxine. Curiously, the boiled or cooked seeds are eaten and available canned in Asian food shops.

Clinical Considerations for Specific Herb-Drug Interactions & Potential Adverse Effects of Herbs		
	Adverse Effects	Interactions and Clinical Concerns
Ginseng (*Panax quinquefolium* L. = American ginseng; *P. ginseng* L. = Asian ginseng)	Generally low toxicity with high-quality standardized products. Breast tenderness in women, nervousness, and excitation have been reported, which diminish with lower doses or longer use. Women may experience estrogenic side effects.	Use in cyclic fashion (2 weeks on and 2 weeks off). Can cause diminished platelet adhesiveness, so monitor patients on **anticoagulants**. High doses may inhibit early stage of infection immune function. Ginseng may potentiate the action of MAOIs (inhibits uptake of various neurotransmitter substances), and at least 2 cases of suspected interaction with phenelzine have been reported. Generally ginseng is contraindicated in acute illness, any form of hemorrhage and during the acute phase of coronary thrombosis. Also avoidance is recommended in nervous, tense, hysteric, manic, and schizophrenic individuals. Do not use with **stimulants** (even **caffeine**), **antipsychotic drugs**, or while being treated with **hormones**. Use with caution in patients with diabetes, cardiac problems, hypo- and hypertensive disorders, and in patients receiving **steroid therapy**. If possible, avoid during pregnancy and lactation.
Eleutherococcus or Siberian Ginseng (not the same as Panax ginseng but in the same family) (Araliaceae); *Eleutherococcus senticosus* (Rupr. & Maxim.) Maxim; synonymous with *Acanthopanax senticosus*	High doses associated with irritability, insomnia, and anxiety. Other adverse effects include skin eruptions, headache, diarrhea, hypertension, and pericardial pain in rheumatic heart patients.	Possible estrogenic effect in females. Side effects, toxicity, contraindications, and warnings similar to those for *Panax* species (see ginseng). Russian experience suggests this product not be used for people under the age of 40 and that only low doses be taken on a daily basis. Patients are advised to abstain from alcohol, sexual activity, bitter substances, and spicy foods. Avoid during pregnancy and lactation. Possible assay interference with **digoxin**; concomitant therapy increased digoxin level to greater than 5 mg/ml without symptoms of toxicity (case report).

Clinical Considerations for Specific Herb-Drug Interactions & Potential Adverse Effects of Herbs		
	Adverse Effects	Interactions and Clinical Concerns
Goldenseal (*Hydrastis canadensis* L.)	Has CNS-stimulant properties. May interfere with the ability of the colon to manufacture the B vitamins or decrease their absorption.	Has been used in conjunction with standard antimicrobial therapy. Because of hypoglycemic properties, monitor diabetics. Has been used prophylactically for traveler's diarrhea (eg, 1 week before, during, and 1 week after travel). Do not use for greater than 2 months at a time. Contraindicated in patients with hypertension. Berberine has coagulant activity and can antagonize the action of **heparin**. It also has cardiac-stimulant properties. Do not use goldenseal as a douche because of its potential local ulcerative effects. Do not use locally for purulent ear discharge because of possibility of rupturing ear drum. Hydrostine, beberine, etc., alkaloids are potentially toxic, and thus excessive use should be avoided. Symptoms of alkaloid toxicity include stomach upset, nervous symptoms, depression, exaggerated reflexes, convulsions, paralysis, and death from respiratory failure. Alkaloids are also uterine stimulants and should be avoided during pregnancy. Avoid use during lactation.
Hawthorn (*Crataegus oxyacanthoides* Therill.; *C. monogyna* Jacq. Rosaceae family	High doses may lead to hypotension and sedation. Nausea, fatigue, sweating, and rash on the hands have been reported.	May take up to 2 weeks to see effects. Hawthorn's polymeric procyanidins may increase the activity of **cardiotonic drugs** like digitalis or they may reduce the toxicity of the cardiac glycosides via coronary vasodilating and antiarrhythmic effects. Because of cardioactive, hypotensive, and coronary vasodilatory properties of hawthorn, monitor other drugs with these actions (eg, **antihypertensives**) or avoid use. Hawthorn extracts have uteroactivity (reduction in tone and motility); avoid in pregnancy and lactation.
Kava-Kava (*Piper methysticum* Frost)	Masticated kava causes numbness of mouth (local anesthetic action). Monitor for excessive CNS depression.	Contraindicated in pregnancy because of loss of uterine tone. Avoid in lactation because of possible passage of pyrone compounds into milk. Also avoid in endogenous depression because of the sedative properties of the pyrones (kwain, methysticin, yangonin). Chronic ingestion of kava drink has led to "kawaism," characterized by dry, flaking, discolored skin, and reddened eyes. Because of euphoric effects, avoid other **CNS stimulants** or **depressants**. Heavy kava users are more likely to complain of poor health including low weight, reduced protein levels, "puffy faces," scaly rashes, increases in HDL and cholesterol counts, hematuria, blood cell abnormalities (eg, decreased platelets, lymphocytes), and pulmonary hypertension. Using kava along with **benzodiazepine** drugs (eg, alprazolam [*Xanax*]) may cause "semicomatose state" because of interaction. Avoid concomitant use.

Clinical Considerations for Specific Herb-Drug Interactions & Potential Adverse Effects of Herbs

	Adverse Effects	Interactions and Clinical Concerns
LaPacho (Pau d'arco, Tahubo, *Tabeluia ipe, T. avellanedae*)	Chronic administration may lead to moderate-to-severe anemia. Whole-bark decoction has no reports of human toxicity.	Purchase standardized products containing at least 2% to 4% lapachol. The various quinone derivatives (lapachol, 2-methylanthra-quinone, etc.) have proven antibacterial, antiviral, antiparasitic, anti-inflammatory, and anticancer activity. Concomitant use of similar-acting agents may have synergistic effects. Anti-vitamin K activity has been reported for lapachol, but the presence of several vitamin K-like substances in the whole bark suggests that this may not be a problem.
Licorice (*Glycyrrhiza glabra* L.)	Low doses are safe and widely used in true licorice candy products. Excessive or prolonged ingestion (over several ounces per day of candy) can result in symptoms known as pseudoaldosteronism (hypertension; sodium, chloride, and water retention; hypokalemia; weight gain). Low levels of plasma renin activity, aldosterone, and antidiuretic hormone also may be seen. Most "licorice" candy in the US is flavored with anise oil. Read the label carefully to determine if it has licorice mass. If so, this is real licorice. European licorice is real licorice, containing large amounts of the root extract. Deglycyrrhizenated licorice is available to avoid steroidal effects.	Aldosterone-like effects may be reversed using a high-potassium and low-sodium diet. Avoid licorice in hypertensive patients, in those with renal or liver failure, or cardiovascular disease. Also, avoid with **cardiac glycoside** therapy since licorice may potentiate its action. It may also increase levels of endogenous **corticosteroids** as well as those of systemically or topically administered steroids. Hypokalemia can aggravate glucose intolerance, and licorice may interfere with existing hypoglycemic therapy. Excessive consumption during pregnancy and lactation should be avoided. Licorice has uterine-stimulant action and may affect the menstrual cycle. Licorice is contraindicated in gall bladder disease, kidney disease, pheochromocytoma and other adrenal tumors, diseases which cause low serum potassium levels (eg, 1° and 2° aldosteronism and severe chronic alcoholism), diseases that may result from low potassium levels (eg, certain kinds of flaccid paralysis of limb disorders), fasting, anorexia, bulimia, and untreated hypothyroidism.
Milk thistle (*Silibum marianum* L. Gaertn.) Compositae family	Generally non-toxic. Possible loose stools related to increased bile flow. Some individuals may show mild allergic response.	Loose stools can be controlled with oat bran or psyllium. Phosphatidylcholine-bound silymarin is claimed to be more effective. Helps prevent liver damage from various hepatoxins and drugs (eg, **butyrophenones**, **phenothiazines**, **acetaminophen**, **halothane**, **phenytoin** and **ethanol**, due to liver membrane-stabilizing and antioxidant effects of the flavolignans [silybin, silydianin, silychristin]). Silybin reduces biliary cholesterol and increases bile secretion, cholate excretion, and bilirubin excretion. Be aware of related drugs and avoid milk thistle. Also keep in mind potential effects of milk stimulation and steroid secretory modulation. Widely used in Europe for Amanita mushroom poisoning.

Clinical Considerations for Specific Herb-Drug Interactions & Potential Adverse Effects of Herbs

	Adverse Effects	Interactions and Clinical Concerns
Peppermint (*Mentha X piperita* L.)	*External*: Possible contact dermatitis.	Use with caution in patients with hiatal hernia because peppermint relaxes the esophageal sphincter, thus potentiating esophageal reflux. Has wide range of effects causing concern about related drugs with similar or antagonistic action. Peppermint has carminative, antispasmodic, choleretic, and external analgesic action. Widely used as a tea (infusion) and as enteric-coated capsule for treating irritable bowel syndrome (1 to 2 capsules with 0.2 ml per capsule) 3 times daily with meals. Topical preparations of peppermint and menthol increase dermatitis potential when used in conjunction with heating pads. Contraindicated in pregnancy because of its emmenogogue effect and in gallstones because of its choleretic activity.
	Internal: Local mouth irritation and burning, skin rash, heartburn, and muscle tremor. Hypersensitivity reactions (skin rash) have been reported as well as heartburn, bradycardia, and muscle tremor.	
Herbs with phototoxic principles (eg, St. John's wort, celery, angelica)	Phototoxicity	Avoid UV or solarium light therapy or sun tanning because of potential photosensitizing effects.
St. John's wort (*Hypericum perforatum* L.) Hypericaceae family	Photosensitivity well documented with high doses because of hypericin. Pollen in flowers may cause severe allergic reaction and anaphylaxis.	Usually taken with food to prevent GI irritation or upset. The predominant mechanism of action is unclear but has been shown to be similar to **SSRIs** and **MAOIs**; therefore, concomitant use with these agents is not recommended. Also use caution with foods and drugs that interact with SSRIs and MAOIs. Contraindicated in pregnancy because of its emmenagogue and abortifacient effects and its uterine stimulant action. Avoid UV or solarium light therapy or sun tanning because of its potential photosensitizing effects. Also avoid in severe endogenous depression since it only has been shown to be effective in mild-to-moderate depression. St. John's wort enhances the sleeping time of **narcotics** and antagonizes the effects of **reserpine**. Avoid use in pregnancy and lactation.
Saw palmetto (*Serenoa repens* [Bartr.]) Small, Palmae family	Possible gastric side effects.	Because of well documented antiandrogen and antiestrogenic activity, avoid taking with any **hormone** therapy including oral contraceptive and hormone replacement therapy. Also has shown immunostimulant and anti-inflammatory activity; hence, watch for patients taking drugs that may increase or decrease these effects. For reproducible effects, it is recommended that the fat-soluble saw palmetto extracts standardized to contain 85% to 95% fatty acids and sterols be taken at the recommended dosage of 160 mg twice daily. Effects occur in 4 to 6 weeks. No demonstrated effect on serum prostate-specific antigen levels. Because of antiestrogenic effect, avoid during pregnancy and in patients with breast cancer.

Clinical Considerations for Specific Herb-Drug Interactions & Potential Adverse Effects of Herbs

	Adverse Effects	Interactions and Clinical Concerns
Systemic lupus erythematosus	Alfalfa	Contraindicated.
Valerian (*Valeriana officinalis* L.) Valerianacea family	Strong disagreeable odor, rare morning drowsiness, headache, excitability, uneasiness, and cardiac disturbances.	Can reduce morning sleepiness. Can potentiate effects of other **CNS depressants**. Reduction of caffeine consumption combined with exercise can increase effectiveness of this mild sedative. The volatile components of valerian can increase the sleeping time induced by **pentobarbital**. Acts on GABA receptor and is potentially additive to **benzodiazapines**. The depressant action of valerian is reported not to be synergistic with alcohol. Avoid in pregnancy and lactation. Related species (*V. wallichi*) have shown abortifacient properties and can affect the menstrual cycle. The valepotriate compounds are unstable and this may affect shelf life and efficacy of product.

[1] *The Review of Natural Products*. St. Louis, MO: Facts and Comparisons.

[2] Newall C, et al. *Herbal Medicines*. London: The Pharmaceutical Press, 1996.

[3] DeSmet P, et al. *Adverse Effects of Herbal Drugs*. NY: Springer-Verlag, 1992-1995:1-3.

[4] Murray, M. *The Healing Power of Herbs*. CA: Prima Publishing, 2nd ed., 1995.

[5] Brinker, F. *Herb Contraindications and Drug Interactions*. Oregon: Eclectic Institute, Inc., 1997.

[6] McDermott, J. Herbal Chart for Health Care Professionals. *Pharmacy Today*, 1997 Feb.

[7] Bergner, P. Herb-Drug Interactions in Medical Herbalism. *J for Herbal Practitioners*.

Herbal Diuretics

PHARMACOLOGY: Diuretics remain among the most frequently prescribed drugs in the United States. In addition to the widespread use of prescription diuretics, over-the-counter (OTC) and natural diuretics continue to play an important role in the self-treatment of menstrual distress, edema, and hypertension.

Numerous OTC menstrual distress preparations contain xanthine alkaloids such as caffeine and theobromine, which are most often derived from inexpensive natural sources. Of these compounds, only caffeine has been found to be both safe and effective for use as an OTC diuretic. In its review of these products, the FDA Advisory Review Panel on Menstrual Drug Products concluded that the frequently used dandelion root (*Taraxacum officinale* Wiggers), a preparation once thought to have strong diuretic properties, is safe but ineffective in the treatment of dysmenorrhea. Nor is there evidence that dandelion is an effective diuretic.

Teas and extracts of buchu (*Barosma betulina*) and quack grass (*Agropyron* spp.) are popular, but their diuretic activity is probably no greater than that of the xanthine alkaloids in coffee or ordinary tea. Significant toxicity from buchu and quack grass have not been reported.[1]

Diuretic teas that should be avoided include juniper berries (*Juniperus communis*), which contain a locally irritating volatile oil capable of causing renal damage, and shave grass or horsetail (*Equisetum* spp.) a weakly diuretic plant that contains several toxic compounds including aconitic acid, equisitine (a neurotoxin), and nicotine.[2] In grazing animals, the ingestion of horsetail has caused excitement, convulsions, and death. Thiamine deficiency has been reported in sheep after the experimental administration of shave grass.

Other teas, such as ephedra (ma huang), contain the mildly diuretic stimulant ephedrine. These teas should be used with caution by hypertensive patients.

All plants and herbal extracts included in OTC products for use as diuretics are not toxic; however, the majority are either clinically ineffective or no more effective than caffeine. The following table lists plants that have been reported to possess diuretic activity. This list has been compiled from old materia medica, herbals, and when documentation is available, the scientific literature. There is generally little scientific evidence to justify the use of most of these plants as diuretics. Some are toxic even in very low doses. The fact that some have been used for centuries in herbal medicine does not necessarily attest to their effectiveness; rather it suggests that such plants have a relatively broad margin of safety and their use does not usually result in toxicity.

HERBAL DIURETICS		
Scientific Name	*Common Name*	*Part Used*
Abutilon indicum	—	Bark
Acalypha evrardii	—	Flower, leaf
Acanthus spinosus	—	Entire plant
Acorus calamus*	**Calamus**	**Rhizome**
Adonis vernalis	Pheasant's eye herb	Above ground
Agave americana	Agave	Roots
Agrimonia eupatoria	**Agrimony**	**Entire plant**
Agropyron	**Couch grass**	**Rhizomes, roots, stems**
Alchemilla arvensis	**Lady's mantle**	**Entire plant**
Alisma plantago	—	Entire plant
Allium cepa	Onion	Bulb
Ammi visnaga	—	**Fruit**
Anemone spp.*	Windflower	Entire plant
Apium graveolens*	**Celery**	**Stalk, oil**
Apocynum cannabinum*	—	Entire plant

HERBAL DIURETICS

Scientific Name	Common Name	Part Used
Arctostaphylos uva-ursi*	**Uva ursi**	**Leaves**
Arctium lappa	**Burdock**	**Root**
Asparagus officinale	**Asparagus**	**Roots**
Bacopa monnieri	—	Entire plant
Barosma spp.	**Buchu**	**Leaves**
Begonia cucullata	Begonia	Entire plant
Betula alba*	Betula	Leaves, twigs
Blumea lacera	—	Entire plant
Boerhaavia diffusa	—	Entire plant
Borago officinalis	**Borage**	**Leaves, tops**
Buddleja americana	—	Bark, leaf, root
Callistris arborea	—	Gum
Calystegia soldanella	—	Entire plant
Camellia sinensis	Common tea	Leaves
Capsella bursa-pastoris	Shepherd's purse	Above ground
Carex arenaria	—	Entire plant
Chamaelirium luteum	—	Root
Chelidomium majus	Celandine	Root, leaves, latex
Chicorium intybus	**Chicory**	**Root**
Chimaphilia umbellata	Pipsissewa	Above ground
Claytonia sibirica	—	Entire plant
Clematis spp*	—	**Entire plant**
Coffea arabica	Coffee	Fruit
Collinsonia canadensis	Stoneroot	Root
Convallaria majalis*	Lily of the valley	Flowering tops
Costus spicatus	—	Sap
Curanga fel-terrae	—	Leaf
Cynanchium vincetoxi-cum	—	Entire plant
Cytisus scoparius*	**Broom**	**Flowering tops**
Daucus carota	**Carrot**	**Root**
Digitalis purpurea*	**Foxglove**	**Leaves**
Drosera rotundifolia	Drosera	Entire plant
Ephedra spp.	**Ephedra**	**Stems**
Equisetum spp.	**Horsetail**	**Above ground**
Eryngium yuccifolium	—	Entire plant
Fumaria officinalis	**Fumitory**	**Flowering tops**
Gaillardia pinnatifida	—	Entire plant
Galega officinalis	Goat's rue	All but root
Galium aparine	Cleavers	Above ground
Glycyrrhiza glabra	**Licorice**	**Rhizome, root**
Helianthus annus	Sunflower	Seeds
Hemidesmus indicus	—	Entire plant
Herniaria glabra	Rupturewort	Above ground
Hibiscus spp.	**Hibiscus**	**Flowers**

HERBAL DIURETICS		
Scientific Name	*Common Name*	*Part Used*
Hydrangea arborescens*	Hydrangea	Roots
Hypericum perforatum	**St. John's Wort**	**Entire plant**
Hypochoeris scarzonerae	—	Entire plant
Ilex paraguayensis*	**Maté**	**Leaves**
Iris florentina	Orris	Peeled rhizome
Juniperus communis*	**Juniper**	**Berries**
Laportea meyeniana	—	Leaf, root
Levisticum officinale	**Lovage**	**Roots**
Paullinia cupana	**Guarana**	**Seeds**
Petroselinum crispum*	**Parsley**	**Leaves, seeds**
Peumus boldus	**Boldo**	**Leaves**
Pinus silvestris	Pine	Cones
Psoralae corylifolia	—	Seeds
Rafnia perfoliata	—	Leaf
Rehmannia lutea	—	Entire plant
Sambucus nigra	**Elderberry**	**Flowers**
Santalum album	**Sandalwood**	**Oil**
Sassafras albidum	**Sassafras**	**Root**
Senecionis herba	Senecio herb	Above ground
Serenoa repens	**Saw palmetto**	**Ripe fruits**
Smilax spp.	Sarsaparilla	Roots
Solanum dulcamara*	**Bittersweet**	**Twigs, branches**
Spiranthes diuretica	—	Entire plant
Tagetes multifida	—	Entire plant
Taraxacum officinale	**Dandelion**	**Leaves**
Theobroma cacao	**Cocoa**	**Seeds**
Trianthema portulacastrum	—	Leaves
Tribulus terrestris	—	Fruit
Urginea maritima*	**Squill**	**Bulb**
Urtica dioica*	**Nettle**	**Leaves**
Viola odorata	Violet	Leaves, flowers
Withania somnifera*	**Withania**	**Root**

* Noted as toxic in reference; all others should not be considered safe for general use in the absence of valid safety.

Plants in **bold** are described in their own monograph in this system.

[1] *Med Let* 1979;21:29. [2] DerMarderosian AH. *Am Druggist* 1980 Aug:35.

Mushroom Poisoning Decision Chart

Mushroom poisoning represents an important aspect of plant toxicology. The toxic events caused by mushrooms are not limited to any group by age, race, or sex. Infants and children readily eat wild mushrooms because of their unique texture and often mild flavor. Adults experimenting with freshly collected, but misidentified, mushrooms often fall victim to intoxication.

Despite the many varieties of mushrooms that grow throughout North America, only a few types are responsible for the majority of mushroom intoxications. Therefore, determining the general type of mushroom intoxication is not always an impossible task.

While it is important to obtain a sample of the mushroom suspected in the poisoning, this is not always practical or possible. Consultation with a local mycologist and poison control center should always be considered when establishing the cause of a mushroom poisoning event (see monograph "Mushroom Societies"). If a mushroom intoxication is suspected, asking 6 simple questions will usually provide sufficient information to make a tentative determination of the causative agent. These are:

1.) When were the mushrooms eaten and how long after this did the symptoms first occur?
2.) What were the initial symptoms?
3.) Was more than 1 kind of mushroom eaten?
4.) Did anyone who did not eat mushrooms become sick?
5.) Did everyone who ate the mushrooms become sick?
6.) Was an alcoholic beverage consumed within 72 hours after the mushroom meal?

These questions, formulated by Lampe and McCann,[1] are useful in establishing a causative association between the mushroom and the intoxication.

The flow chart on the reverse of this page is designed to aid in determining the possible causative genus in a suspected mushroom intoxication. This chart should be used as a guide in determining which mushroom was most likely involved in the intoxication. The clinician should recognize that factors such as the amount of mushroom ingested, the season, individual sensitivities, and the possibility that toxic materials other than the mushroom may have been ingested, can confuse the diagnostic picture.

[1] *AMA Handbook of Poisonous and Injurious Plants*, AMA, Chicago Review Press, 1985.

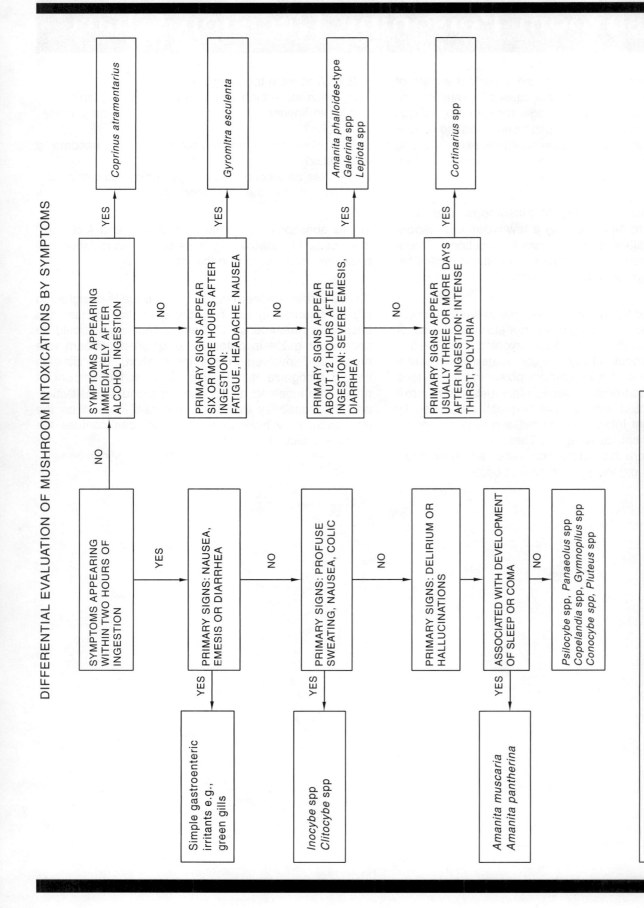

DIFFERENTIAL EVALUATION OF MUSHROOM INTOXICATIONS BY SYMPTOMS

SYMPTOMS APPEARING WITHIN TWO HOURS OF INGESTION

NO → SYMPTOMS APPEARING IMMEDIATELY AFTER ALCOHOL INGESTION — YES → *Coprinus atramentarius*

NO ↓

PRIMARY SIGNS APPEAR SIX OR MORE HOURS AFTER INGESTION: FATIGUE, HEADACHE, NAUSEA — YES → *Gyromltra esculenta*

NO ↓

PRIMARY SIGNS APPEAR ABOUT 12 HOURS AFTER INGESTION: SEVERE EMESIS, DIARRHEA — YES → *Amanita phalloides*-type Galerina spp Lepiota spp

NO ↓

PRIMARY SIGNS APPEAR USUALLY THREE OR MORE DAYS AFTER INGESTION: INTENSE THIRST, POLYURIA — YES → *Cortinarius spp*

YES ↓

PRIMARY SIGNS: NAUSEA, EMESIS OR DIARRHEA

YES → Simple gastroenteric irritants e.g., green gills

NO ↓

PRIMARY SIGNS: PROFUSE SWEATING, NAUSEA, COLIC

YES → *Inocybe spp* *Clitocybe spp*

NO ↓

PRIMARY SIGNS: DELIRIUM OR HALLUCINATIONS

↓

ASSOCIATED WITH DEVELOPMENT OF SLEEP OR COMA

YES → *Amanita muscaria* *Amanita pantherina*

NO ↓

Psilocybe spp, *Panaeolus* spp *Copelandia* spp, *Gymnopilus* spp *Conocybe spp, Pluteus spp*

Use this chart as a guide to aid in determining possible causes of mushroom intoxications. Other mushrooms may be involved. Factors such as the amount ingested, the season, individual sensitivity and possibility that toxic materials other than the mushrooms may have been ingested can confuse the diagnosis.

Mushroom Societies

Mushroom poisonings remain one of the most important causes of plant toxicities. The management of these poisonings varies depending on the type of mushroom ingested. Therefore, proper identification of the mushroom suspected to have caused the toxicity is of primary importance.

In order to facilitate the identification of a mushroom, it is important to obtain a fresh, undamaged specimen. It is not uncommon for several species of mushroom to grow close together. Therefore, the identification of a single mushroom from a collected batch may mislead the clinician in the treatment of the poisoning. Ideally, several mushrooms will be available for use in identification. The mushrooms should be placed in a paper bag (not plastic) and refrigerated.

Identification of cooked mushrooms is much more difficult. However, material from the meal should be obtained for physical and chemical analysis.

The Infectious Disease Section of the Centers for Disease Control in Atlanta, GA (USA), offers assistance in cases of suspected mushroom poisoning. Information is also available from local mycological societies, botany departments of local universities, and poison control centers. The following list provides the addresses of organizations that may be helpful in offering assistance in the identification of edible and toxic mushrooms:

Botanical Society of America
Business Office
1735 Neil Ave.
Columbus, OH 43210–1293
614/292–3519
www.botany.org/

National Center for Infectious Diseases
Centers for Disease Control and Prevention
1600 Clifton Rd. NE
Atlanta, GA 30333
404/639–3311
www.cdc.gov/ncidod/ncid.htm

International Society for Human and Animal Mycology
c/o Prof. W. Loeffler
Gellerstrasse 11 A
CH-4052 Basel, Switzerland

International Society for Mushroom Science
c/o Dr. K.S. Burton, Executive Secretary
Horticultural Research Institute
Wellesbourne, Warwick CV35 9EF United Kingdom

Medical Mycological Society of the Americas
c/o Dr. Jim Harris
2501 Timberline Dr.
Austin, TX 78746
410/955–5077

Mycological Society of America
c/o David H. Griffin, *Mycologia* Editor-in-Chief
Environmental and Forest Biology Faculty
State University, College of Environmental Science and
    Forestry
1 Forestry Dr.
Syracuse, NY 13210–2788
315/470–6794 (phone/fax)

c/o Marin Klich, Secretary, USDA, ARS, SRRC
1100 Robert E. Lee Blvd.
New Orleans, LA 70124
www.erin.utoronto.ca/%7Ew3msa/index.html

American Association of Poison Control Centers
3201 New Mexico Ave. NW, Ste. 310
Washington, DC 20016
202/362–7217 (phone)
202/362–8377 (fax)
www.aapcc.org/frrbotto.htm

International Mycological Association
Meredith Blackwell, Secretary-General
Department of Plant Biology
LA State University
Baton Rouge, LA 70803
lsb380.plbio.lsu.edu/ima/index.html

American Society for Microbiology Division F
    Medical Mycology
www.asmusa.org/division/f/divf_main.htm

North American Mycological Association
www.namyco.org/

Boston Mycological Club
6 Oak Ridge Dr. #4
Maynard, MA 01754–2470
www.ultranet.com/griner/BMC/

Poison Control Centers

Alabama

Alabama Poison Center, Tuscaloosa
2503 Phoenix Dr.
Tuscaloosa, AL 35405
800/462–0800 (AL only)
205/345–0600

Regional Poison Control Center
The Children's Hospital of Alabama
1600 7th Ave. S.
Birmingham, AL 35233–1711
205/939–9201
205/933–4050
800/292–6678 (AL only)

Alaska

Anchorage Poison Control Center
Providence Hospital Pharmacy
P.O. Box 196604
Anchorage, AK 99519–6604
907/261–3193
800/478–3193 (AK only)

Arizona

Samaritan Regional Poison Center
Good Samaritan Regional Medical Center Ancillary-1
1111 E. McDowell Rd.
Phoenix, AZ 85006
602/253–3334
800/362–0101 (AZ only)

Arizona Poison and Drug Information Center
Arizona Health Sciences Center
1501 N. Campbell Ave., Rm. 1156
Tucson, AZ 85724
800/362–0101 (AZ only)
520/626–6016

Arkansas

Arkansas Poison and Drug Information Center
University of Arkansas for Medical Sciences
4301 W. Markham St. - 552
Little Rock, AR 72205
800/376–4766

Southern Poison Center, Inc.
875 Monroe Ave., Ste. 104
Memphis, TN 38163
901/528–6048
800/288–9999 (TN only)

California

California Poison Control System—Fresno
Valley Children's Hospital
3151 N. Millbrook, IN31
Fresno, CA 93703
800/876–4766 (CA only)

California Poison Control System—San Diego Division
UCSD Medical Center
200 W. Arbor Dr.
San Diego, CA 92103–8925
800/876–4766 (CA only)

California Poison Control System—Sacramento Division
UCDMC — HSF Rm. 1024
2315 Stockton Blvd.
Sacramento, CA 95817
800/876–4766 (CA only)

Colorado

Rocky Mountain Poison and Drug Center
8802 E. 9th Ave.
Denver, CO 80220–6800
800/332–3073 (outside metro-CO only)
800/446–6179 (Las Vegas, NV only)
303/739–1123 (Denver metro)

Connecticut

Connecticut Regional Poison Center
University of Connecticut Health Center
263 Farmington Ave.
Farmington, CT 06030
800/343–2722 (CT only)

Delaware

The Poison Control Center
3600 Sciences Center, Ste. 220
Philadelphia, PA 19104–2641
800/722–7112 (PA only)
215/386–2100

District of Columbia

National Capital Poison Center
3201 New Mexico Ave., NW, Ste. 310
Washington, DC 20016
202/625–3333
202/362–8563 (TTY)

Florida

Florida Poison Information Center—Jacksonville
University of Florida Health Science Center—Jacksonville
655 W. 8th St.
Jacksonville, FL 32209
904/549–4480
800/282–3171 (FL only)

Florida Poison Information Center—Miami
University of Miami, School of Medicine
Department of Pediatrics
P.O. Box 016960 (r-131)
Miami, FL 33101
305/585–5253
800/282–3171 (FL only)

Florida Poison Information Center—Tampa
Tampa General Hospital
P.O. Box 1289
Tampa, FL 33601
813/253–4444 (Tampa)
800/282–3171 (FL only)

Georgia

Georgia Poison Center
Hughes Spalding Children's Hospital
Grady Health System
80 Butler St. SE, P.O. Box 26066
Atlanta, GA 30335–3801
800/282–5846 (GA only)
404/616–9000

Hawaii

Hawaii Poison Center
Kapiolani Medical Center for Women and Children
Honolulu, HI 96826
800/362–3585 (outer islands of HI only)
800/362–3586
808/941–4411

Idaho

Rocky Mountain Poison and Drug Center
8802 E. 9th Ave.
Denver, CO 80220–6800
800/860–0620 (ID only)
303/739–1123

Illinois

BroMenn Poison Control Center
BroMenn Regional Medical Center
Franklin at Virginia
Normal, IL 61761
309/454–6666

Interstate Center-Cardinal Glennon Children's Hospital
Regional Poison Center
1465 S. Grand Blvd.
St. Louis, MO 63104
800/366–8888 (Western IL only)

Indiana

Indiana Poison Center
Methodist Hospital of Indiana
1–65 at 21st St., P. O. Box 1367
Indianapolis, IN 46206–1367
800/382–9097 (IN only)
317/929–2323

Interstate Center-Kentucky Regional Poison Center of Kosair Children's Hospital
P.O. Box 35070
Louisville, KY 40232–5070
502/589–8222 (southern IN only)

Iowa

Iowa Poison Center
St. Luke's Regional Medical Center
2720 Stone Park Blvd.
Sioux City, IA 51104
712/277–2222
800/352–2222

Interstate Center-The Poison Center
Children's Memorial Hospital
8301 Dodge St.
Omaha, NE 68114
800/955–9119

Kansas

Mid-America Poison Control Center
University of Kansas Medical Center
3901 Rainbow Blvd., Room B-400
Kansas City, KS 66160–7231
913/588–6633
800/332–6633 (KS only and Kansas City metro area)

Interstate Center-Cardinal Glennon Children's Hospital
Regional Poison Center
1465 S. Grand Blvd.
St. Louis, MO 63104
800/366–8888 (Topeka, KS only)

Kentucky

Kentucky Regional Poison Center of Kosair Children's Hospital
P.O. Box 35070
Louisville, KY 40232–5070
502/629–7275
800/722–5725 (KY only)

Kentucky Regional Poison Center
Medical Towers S., Ste. 572
234 E. Gray St.
Louisville, KY 40202
502/589–8222

Louisiana

Louisiana Drug and Poison Information Center
School of Pharmacy
Northeast Louisiana University
Monroe, LA 71209–6430
800/256–9822 (LA only)
318/362–5393

Maine

Maine Poison Control Center
Maine Medical Center
Department of Emergency Medicine
22 Bramhall St.
Portland, ME 04102
207/871–2950
800/442–6305 (ME only)

Maryland

Maryland Poison Center
20 N. Pine St.
Baltimore, MD 21201
410/528–7701
800/492–2414 (MD only)

National Capital Poison Center (D.C. suburbs only)
3201 New Mexico Avenue, NW, Ste. 310
Washington, DC 20016
202/625–3333
202/362–8563 (TTY)

Massachusetts

Massachusetts Poison Control System
300 Longwood Ave.
Boston, MA 02115
617/232–2120
800/682–9211 (MA only)

Michigan

Blodgett Regional Poison Center
1840 Wealthy, SE
Grand Rapids, MI 49506
800/POISON-1 (800/746–7661)
800/356–3232 (TTY only)

Children's Hospital of Michigan Poison Control Center
4160 John R. Harper Office Bldg., Ste. 616
Detroit, MI 48201
800/764–7661 (MI only)
313/745–5711

Marquette General Hospital Poison Center
420 W. Magnetic St.
Marquette, MI 49855
906/225–3497
800/562–9781

Minnesota

Hennepin Regional Poison Center
Hennepin County Medical Center
701 Park Ave.
Minneapolis, MN 55415
612/347–3141
800/764–7661 (MN only)
612/337–7387 (petline)

Minnesota Regional Poison Center
8100 34th Ave. S.
P.O. Box 1309
Minneapolis, MN 55440–1309
800/222–1222 (MN only)
612/221–2113
800/764–7661

North Dakota Poison Information Center
MeritCare Medical Center
720 4th St. N.
Fargo, ND 58122
701/234–5575
800/732–2200 (ND, MN, SD only)

Mississippi

Mississippi Regional Poison Control Center
University of Mississippi Medical Center
2500 N. State St.
Jackson, MS 39216
601/354–7660

Southern Poison Center, Inc.
875 Monroe Ave., Ste. 104
Memphis, TN 38163
901/528–6048
800/288–9999 (TN only)

Missouri

Cardinal Glennon Children's Hospital Regional Poison Center
1465 S. Grand Blvd.
St. Louis, MO 63104
314/772–5200
800/366–8888 (MO, Western IL, and Topeka, KS only)
800/392–9111 (MO only)

Children's Mercy Hospital Poison Control Center
2401 Gillham Rd.
Kansas City, MO 64108
816/234–3430

Interstate Center-The Poison Center
8301 Dodge St.
Omaha, NE 68114
800/955–9119

Montana

Rocky Mountain Poison and Drug Center
8802 E. 9th Ave.
Denver, CO 80220–6800
800/525–5042 (MT only)
303/739–1123

Nebraska

The Poison Center
8301 Dodge St.
Omaha, NE 68114
402/354–5555 (Omaha only)
800/955–9119 (NE and WY only)

Nevada

Rocky Mountain Poison and Drug Center
8802 E. 9th Ave.
Denver, CO 80220–6800
800/446–6179 (Las Vegas, NV only)
303/739–1123

Washoe Poison Center
Washoe Medical Center
77 Pringle Way
Reno, NV 89520–0109
702/328–4129

New Hampshire

New Hampshire Poison Information Center
Dartmouth-Hitchcock Medical Center
1 Medical Center Dr.
Lebanon, NH 03756
603/650–8000
603/650–5000 (between 11 p.m. and 8 a.m.)
800/562–8236 (NH only)

New Jersey

New Jersey Poison Information and Education System
201 Lyons Ave.
Newark, NJ 07112
800/764–7661 (NJ only)

New Mexico

New Mexico Poison and Drug Information Center
University of New Mexico
Health Sciences Library, Room 125
Albuquerque, NM 87131–1076
505/272–2222
505/843–2551
800/432–6866 (NM only)

New York

Central New York Poison Control Center
SUNY Health Science Center
750 E. Adams St.
Syracuse , NY 13210
315/476–4766
800/252–5655 (NY only)

Finger Lakes Regional Poison Center
University of Rochester Medical Center
601 Elmwood Ave., Box 321
Rochester, NY 14642
800/333–0542 (NY only)
716/275–3232
716/273–4155

Hudson Valley Regional Poison Center
Phelps Memorial Hospital Center
701 N. Broadway
Sleepy Hollow, NY 10591
800/336–6997 (NY only)
914/366–3030

Long Island Regional Poison Control Center
Winthrop University Hospital
259 First St.
Mineola, NY 11501
516/542–2323

New York City Poison Control Center
NYC Department of Health
455 First Ave., Rm. 123
New York, NY 10016
212/340–4494
212/POISONS
212/447–2205
212/689–9014

Western New York Regional Poison Control Center
Children's Hospital of Buffalo
219 Bryant St.
Buffalo, NY 14222
800/888–7655 (NY Western regions only)
716/878–7654

North Carolina

Carolinas Poison Center
Carolinas Medical Center
5000 Airport Center Parkway, Ste. B
P.O. Box 32861
Charlotte, NC 28232–2861
704/355–4000
800/848–6946 (NC only)

North Dakota

North Dakota Poison Information Center
MeritCare Medical Center
720 4th St. N.
Fargo, ND 58122
701/234–5575
800/732–2200 (ND, MN, SD only)

Ohio

Central Ohio Poison Center
700 Children's Dr.
Columbus, OH 43205–2696
614/228–1323
800/682–7625 (OH only)
614/228–2272 (TTY)

Cincinnati Drug and Poison Information Center
Regional Poison Control Center
2368 Victory Parkway, Ste. 300
Cincinnati, OH 45206
513/558–5111
800/872–5111 (OH only)
330/379–8562

Greater Cleveland Poison Control Center
11100 Euclid Ave.
Cleveland, OH 44106
216/231–4455

Oklahoma

Oklahoma Poison Control Center
Children's Hospital
940 NE 13th St.
Oklahoma City, OK 73104
405/271–5454
800/POISON–1

Oregon

Oregon Poison Center
Oregon Health Sciences University
3181 SW Sam Jackson Park Rd., CB 550
Portland, OR 97201
503/494–8968
800/452–7165 (OR only)

Pennsylvania

Central Pennsylvania Poison Center
Penn State University Hospital
Milton S. Hershey Medical Center
Hershey, PA 17033
800/521–6110
717/531–6111

The Poison Control Center
3600 Sciences Center, Ste. 220
Philadelphia, PA 19104
800/722–7112 (PA only)
215/386–2100

Pittsburgh Poison Center
3705 Fifth Ave.
Pittsburgh, PA 15213
412/681–6669

Rhode Island

Lifespan Poison Center
593 Eddy St.
Providence, RI 02903
401/444–5727

South Dakota

Iowa Poison Center
St. Luke's Regional Medical Center
2720 Stone Park Blvd.
Sioux City, IA 51104
712/277–2222
800/352–2222

Tennessee

Middle Tennessee Poison Center
The Center for Clinical Toxicology
Vanderbilt University Medical Center
1161 21st Ave. S.
501 Oxford House
Nashville, TN 37232–4632
615/322–6435 (local)
800/288–9999 (TN only)
800/936–2034

Southern Poison Center, Inc.
875 Monroe Ave., Ste. 104
Memphis, TN 38163
901/528–6048
800/288–9999 (TN only)

Texas

Central Texas Poison Center
Scott and White Memorial Hospital
2401 S. 31st St.
Temple, TX 76508
800/764–7661 (TX only)
254/724–7401

North Texas Poison Center
5201 Harry Hines Blvd.
P.O. Box 35926
Dallas, TX 75235
800/764–7661 (TX only)

South Texas Poison Center
University of Texas Health Science Center
Forensic Science Bldg., Rm. 146
7703 Floyd Curl Dr.
San Antonio, TX 78284–7849
800/764–7661 (TX only)

Southeast Texas Poison Center
The University of Texas Medical Branch
301 University Ave.
Galveston, TX 77555–1175
409/765–1420
800/764–7661 (TX only)

Texas Poison Center Network at Amarillo
P.O. Box 1110
1501 S. Coulter
Amarillo, TX 79175
800/764–7661

West Texas Regional Poison Center
4815 Alameda Ave.
El Paso, TX 79905
800/764–7661

Utah

Utah Poison Control Center
410 Chipeta Way, Ste. 230
Salt Lake City, UT 84108
801/581–2151
800/456–7707 (UT only)

Vermont

Vermont Poison Center
Fletcher Allen Health Care
111 Colchester Ave.
Burlington, VT 05401
802/658–3456

Virginia

Blue Ridge Poison Center
University of Virginia Health System
P.O. Box 437
Charlottesville, VA 22908
804/924–5543
800/451–1428 (VA only)

National Capital Poison Center (Northern VA only)
3201 New Mexico Ave., NW, Ste. 310
Washington, DC 20016
202/625–3333
202/362–8563 (TTY)

Virginia Poison Center
Virginia Commonwealth University
P.O. Box 980522
Richmond, VA 23298–0522
800/552–6337 (VA only)
804/828–9123

Washington

Washington Poison Center
155 NE 100th St., Ste. 400
Seattle, WA 98125
206/526–2121
800/732–6985 (WA only)
206/517–2394 (TDD)
800/572–0638 (TDD)

West Virginia

West Virginia Poison Center
3110 MacCorkle Ave. SE
Charleston, WV 25304
800/642–3625 (WV only)
304/348–4211

Wisconsin

Poison Center of Eastern Wisconsin
P.O. Box 1997
Milwaukee, WI 53201
414/266–2222
800/815–8855 (WI only)

Wyoming

The Poison Center
8301 Dodge St.
Omaha, NE 68114
402/354–5555 (Omaha)
800/955–9119 (WY and NE only)

Scientific and Trade Organizations

The following list provides the names and addresses of organizations that can be helpful in providing information in specific areas of natural product research, evaluation, and education.

American Association of Oriental Medicine
433 Front St.
Catasauqua, PA 18032
610/266-1433
FAX: 610/264-2768
www.aaom.org

American Botanical Council
P.O. Box 144345
Austin, TX 78714-4345
512/926-4900
FAX: 512/926-2345
www.herbalgram.org

American Herbal Products Association
8484 Georgia Ave., Ste. 370
Silver Spring, MD 20910
301/588-1171
FAX: 301/588-1174
www.ahpa.org

American Foundation of Traditional Chinese Medicine
505 Beech St.
San Francisco, CA 94133
415/776-0502
FAX: 415/776-9053

American Nutraceutical Association
4647T Highway 280 East #133
Birmingham, AL 35242
205/980-5710
FAX: 205/991-9302
ana@mericanutra.com

American Society of Pharmacognosy
Attn: R. J. Krueger, Ph.D., Treasurer
College of Pharmacy
901 S. State St.
Big Rapids, MI 59307
616/592-2236
FAX: 616/592-3829
www.phcog.org

Association of Delegates of the Professional Organizations of Producers and Collectors of Medicinal and Aromatic Plants of the Environmental Export Council
6 bd Marechal-Joffre
F-91490 Milly-la-Foret, France

Association of Natural Medicine Pharmacists
P.O. Box 150727
San Rafael, CA 94915-0727
415/453-3534
FAX: 415/453-4963
www.anmp.org

Botanical Society of America
Office of Publications
1735 Neil Avenue
Columbus, OH 43210-1293
614/292–3519
www.botany.org

Centers for Disease Control and Prevention
Department of Health and Human Services
1600 Clifton Rd. NE
Atlanta, GA 30333
404/639–3311
www.cdc.gov

European Confederation of Distributors, Producers, and Importers of Medicinal Plants
23 Rue du Peintre Lebrun
F-78000 Versailles, France

Ginseng Research Institute of America
Attn: Bob Romang, President
16 H Menard Plaza
Wausau, WI 54401-4119
715/845-7300
FAX: 714/845-8006

Herb Research Foundation
1007 Pearl St., Ste. 200
Boulder, CO 80302
303/449–2265
800/748-2617
FAX: 303/449-7849
www.herbs.org

Inter-African Committee on African Medicinal Plants
c/o OAU/STRC — PM Bag 2359
Lagos, Nigeria
(01) 633430, 633289

International Herb Association
P.O. Box 317
Mundelein, IL 60060-0317
847/949-4372
FAX: 847/949-5896
www.herb-pros.com

Medical Mycological Society of the Americas
Attn: Dr. Jim Harris, Secretary
2501 Timberline Dr.
Austin, TX 78746
410/955-5077
FAX: 410/955-0767

Mycological Society of America
Attn: David H. Griffin, *MYCOLOGIA* Editor-in-Chief
Environmental and Forest Biology Faculty
State University, College of Environmental Science &
    Forestry
1 Forestry Dr.
Syracuse, NY 13210-2788
315/470-6794
www.erin.utoronto.ca

Attn: Marin Klich, Secretary, USDA, ARS, SRRC
1100 Robert E. Lee Blvd.
New Orleans, LA 70124
(For additional mycological organizations, see
    monograph entitled "Mushroom Societies.")

National Council Against Health Fraud
P.O. Box 1276
Loma Linda, CA 92354
909/824–4690
FAX: 909/824-4838
www.ncahf.org

National Nutritional Foods Association
3931 MacArthur Blvd., Ste. 101
Newport Beach, CA 92660
949/622-6272
FAX: 949/622-6266
www.nnfa.org

Natural Products Research Institute
Seoul National University
28 Yeongeon-dong, Chongro-Ku
Seoul 110–460, Korea Republic

Society for Economic Botany
Dr. Brian Boom
New York Botanical Garden
Bronx, NY 10458-5126
718/817-8632
FAX: 718/220-6783
www.econbot.org

World Association of Natural Medicine
Ave. Becquerel BP 37
F-16701 Pierrelatte CEDAX, France

Sources of Natural Product Information

NATURAL PRODUCT INFORMATION – WHERE ELSE TO LOOK

The burgeoning field of biomedical science has created an information glut that often makes finding useful facts a problem. There are more than 900 biomedical journals and newsletters published in the United States alone (Kruzas AT, Medical Health Information Directory, Gale Research Co, Detroit, 1980). Of these, only a few address the study of natural products.

A full appreciation of natural products requires an understanding of their origin, history, nomenclature, chemistry, pharmacology, toxicology, availability, and therapeutic uses. Little more than a dozen journals deal specifically with these topics. Many of the remaining scientific and medical journals represent excellent secondary sources of information about natural products.

Table 1 presents a selected list of American and foreign periodicals devoted to the study of natural products.

Books continue to be valuable sources of data about natural products. Many original works, no longer in publication, continue to set the standards in their fields (eg, Ernest Guenther's, The Essential Oils, Vols. 1–5 D, Van Nostrand Co, NY, 1948–1952). Table 2 is not an all-inclusive book list; rather, it offers suggestions for a well-rounded library on natural products.

With the increasing use of computer-accessible data bases, on-line indexing systems have become critical in the retrieval of references describing natural products. The biomedical field has at its disposal a variety of computer-based abstracting/indexing services. Of these, few specialty indexing services are available for the field of natural products (Table 3). Several excellent broac-based services do, however, provide quite adequate access to information about natural products.

It is hoped that this review of information sources will make the task of data retrieval and evaluation somewhat less overwhelming.

TABLE 1: Periodicals

Acta Botanica Indica, Society for Advancement of Botany, Meerut, India

American Journal of Natural Medicine – Impakt Communications, Green Bay, WI

Botanical Review – The New York Botanical Gardens, Bronx, NY

Bulletin on Narcotics – United Nations, New York, NY

Canadian Journal of Botany, NRC Research Press, Ottawa, Canada

Canadian Journal of Herbalism, Ontario Herbalists' Association, Ontario, Canada

Economic Botany, The Society for Economic Botany, The New York Botanical Garden, Bronx, NY

European Journal of Herbal Medicine: Phytotherapy, The National Institute of Medical Herbalists, Exeter, Devon, UK

Herb Companion, Interweave Press, Loveland, CO

Herb Quarterly, San Anselmo, CA

HerbalGram, The Journal of the American Botanical Council and the Herb Research Foundation, Austin, TX

International Herb Association Newsletter, International Herb Association, Mundelein, IL

International Journal of Aromatherapy, The American Alliance of Aromatherapy, Depoe Bay, OR

Journal of Economic and Taxonomic Botany, The Society for Economic and Taxonomic Botany, Scientific Publishers, India

Journal of Ethnopharmacology, The Journal of The International Society of Ethnopharmacology, Elsevier Science, Philadelphia, PA

Journal of Natural Products, The American Chemical Society and the American Society of Pharmacognosy, Columbus, OH

Medical Anthropology: Cross-Cultural Studies in Health and Illness, Gordon and Breach Science Publishers, International Publishers Distributor, Newark, NJ

Medical Herbalism: A Journal for the Clinical Practitioner, Bergner Communications, Boulder, CO

Natural Health, Natural Health Limited Partnership, Brookline Village, MA

Natural Product Letters, Harwood Academic Publishers, International Publishers Distributor, Newark, NJ

Natural Product Reports, The Royal Society of Chemistry, Cambridge, UK

NCAHF Newsletters, The National Council Against Health Fraud, Inc., Loma Linda, CA

Pharmaceutical Biology (formerly *International Journal of Pharmacognosy*), Swets & Zeitlinger Publishers, Royersford, PA

Phytochemistry: The International Journal of Plant Biochemistry and Molecular Biology, The Journal of the Phytochemical Society of Europe and the Phytochemical Society of North America, Pergamon Press, Elsevier Science, New York, NY

Phytomedicine: International Journal of Phytotherapy and Phytopharmacology, Gustav Fischer Verlag, Jena, Germany

Phytotherapy Research, John Wiley & Sons, Inc., New York, NY

Plant Foods for Human Nutrition (formerly *Qualitas Plantarum*), Kluwer Academic Publishers, Hingham, MA

Planta Medica: Natural Products and Medicinal Plant Research, Thieme, New York, NY

Toxicon: An Interdisciplinary Journal on the Toxins Derived from Animals, Plants and Microorganisms, Elsevier Science, New York, NY

Veterinary and Human Toxicology, American College of Veterinary Toxicologists, Manhattan, KS

Z. Naturforsch. Verlag der Zeitschrift fur Naturforshung, Tubingen, Germany

TABLE 2: Books

Aikman L. *Nature's Healing Arts: From Folk Medicine to Modern Drugs*. Washington, DC: National Geographic Society; 1977.

Baslow H. *Marine Pharmacology: A Study of Toxins and Other Biologically Active Substances of Marine Origin*. Baltimore: Williams & Wilkins Co; 1969.

Beal JL, Reinhard E, eds. *Natural Products as Medicinal Agents: Plenary Lectures of the International Research Congress on Medicinal Plant Research, Strasbourg, July 1980*. Stuttgart: Hippokrates Verlag; c1981.

Blackwell WH. *Poisonous and Medicinal Plants*. Englewood Cliffs, NJ: Prentice Hall; 1990.

Bricklin M. *The Practical Encyclopedia of Natural Healing*. New rev ed. Emmaus, PA: Rodale Press; 1983.

British Herbal Pharmacopoeia. Great Britain: British Herbal Medicine Association; 1996.

Bucherl W, Buckley EE, Deulofeu V, eds. *Venomous Animals and Their Venoms*. 3 vols. New York: Academic Press; 1968-71.

Castleman M. *The Healing Herbs: The Ultimate Guide to the Curative Power of Nature's Medicines*. Emmaus, PA: Rodale Press; 1991.

Densmore F. *How Indians Use Wild Plants for Food, Medicine, and Crafts*. Washington, DC: Government Printing Office; 1928. Reprint, New York: Dover; 1974.

Der Marderosian AH, Liberti LE. *Natural Product Medicine: A Scientific Guide to Foods, Drugs, Cosmetics*. Philadelphia: G.F. Stickley; 1988.

Duke JA. *CRC Handbook of Medicinal Herbs*. Boca Raton, FL: CRC Press; 1985.

Evans WC. *Trease and Evans' Pharmacognosy*. 14th ed. London: WB Saunders; 1996.

Facciola S. *Cornucopia: A Source Book of Edible Plants*. Vista, CA: Kampong Publications; 1990.

Foster S. *Tyler's Honest Herbal: A Sensible Guide to the Use of Herbs and Related Remedies*. 4th ed. New York: Haworth Herbal Press; 1998.

Halstead BW. *Poisonous and Venomous Marine Animals of the World.* 2d rev. ed. Princeton, NJ: Darwin Press; 1988.

Henslow G. *The Plants of the Bible: Their Ancient and Mediaeval History Popularly Described.* London: Masters; 1906.

Hoffmann D. *The Herbal Handbook: A User's Guide to Medical Herbalism.* Rochester, VT: Healing Arts Press; 1998.

Hoffmann D, ed. *The Information Sourcebook of Herbal Medicine.* Freedom, CA: Crossing Press; 1994.

Kerr RW. *Herbalism through the Ages.* 7th ed. San Jose, CA: Supreme Grand Lodge of AMORC; 1980.

Kingsbury JM. *Deadly Harvest: A Guide to Common Poisonous Plants.* New York: Holt, Rinehart and Winston; 1965.

Kingsbury JM. *Poisonous Plants of the United States and Canada.* Englewood Cliffs, NJ: Prentice-Hall; 1964.

Krogsgaard-Larsen P, Christensen SB, Kofod, H, eds. *Natural Products and Drug Development: Proceedings of the Alfred Benzon Symposium 20 Held at the Premises of the Royal Danish Academy of Sciences and Letters, Copenhagen, 7-11 August 1983.* Copenhagen: Munksgaard; 1984.

Lampe KF, McCann MA. *AMA Handbook of Poisonous and Injurious Plants.* Chicago: American Medical Association; 1985.

Leung AY. *Encyclopedia of Common Natural Ingredients Used in Food, Drugs, and Cosmetics.* 2d ed. New York: Wiley; 1996.

Lewis WH, Elvin-Lewis MPF. *Medical Botany: Plants Affecting Man's Health.* New York: Wiley; 1977.

Liener IE, ed. *Toxic Constituents of Plant Foodstuffs.* 2d ed. New York: Academic Press; 1980.

Mabberly DJ. *The Plant-book: A Portable Dictionary of the Vascular Plants Utilizing Kubitzki's....* 2d ed. Cambridge: Cambridge University Press; 1997.

Meyer JE. *The Herbalist.* Rev ed. Glenwood, IL: Meyerbooks; 1986.

Morton JF. *Atlas of Medicinal Plants of Middle America: Bahamas to Yucaton.* Springfield, IL: C.C. Thomas; 1981.

Morton JF. *Major Medicinal Plants: Botany, Culture, and Uses.* Springfield, IL: Thomas; 1977.

Ody P. *The Complete Medicinal Herbal.* New York: Dorling Kindersley; 1993.

Osol A, Pratt R, eds. *The United States Dispensatory.* 27th ed. Philadelphia: Lippincott; 1973.

Penso G. *Inventory of Medicinal Plants Used in the Different Countries.* Geneva: World Health Organization; 1980.

Reader's Digest Magic and Medicine of Plants. Sydney: Reader's Digest; 1994.

Robinson T. *The Organic Constituents of Higher Plants: Their Chemistry and Interrelationships.* 6th ed. North Amherst, MA: Cordus Press; 1991.

Rosengarten F. *The Book of Spices.* Wynnewood, PA: Livingston Pub. Co; 1969.

Schauenberg P. *Guide to Medicinal Plants.* New Canaan, CT: Keats; 1977.

Simon JE. *Herbs, An Indexed Bibliography, 1971-1980: The Scientific Literature on Selected Herbs, and Aromatic and Medicinal Plants of the Temperate Zone.* Hamden, CT: Shoe String Press; 1984.

Spoerke DG. *Herbal Medications.* Santa Barbara, CA: Woodbridge Press; 1990.

Steiner RP, ed. *Folk Medicine: The Art and the Science.* Washington, DC: American Chemical Society; 1986.

Swain T, ed. *Plants in the Development of Modern Medicine.* Cambridge, MA: Harvard University Press; 1972.

Sweet M. *Common Edible and Useful Plants of the East and Midwest.* Healdsburg, CA: Naturegraph Publishers; 1975.

Sweet M. *Common Edible and Useful Plants of the West.* Healdsburg, CA: Naturegraph Publishers; 1976.

Tyler VE, Brady LR, Robbers, JE. *Pharmacognosy.* 9th ed. Philadelphia: Lea and Febiger; 1988.

Youngken HW, Karas JS. *Common Poisonous Plants of New England*. U.S. Public Health Service pub. no. 1220. Washington, DC: Government Printing Office; 1964.

Zohary M. *Plants of the Bible: A Complete Handbook... with 200 Full-color Plates Taken in the Natural Habitat*. New York: Cambridge University Press; 1982.

TABLE 3: Abstracting, Indexing, and Retrieval Services

BIOSIS, the world's largest collection of abstracts and bibliographic references to worldwide biological and medical literature. Available in several formats, including *Biological Abstracts* in print and CD-ROM. BIOSIS, 2100 Arch Street, Philadelphia, PA 19103-1399, 1-800-523-4806, http://www.biosis.org/home.html

Chemical Abstracts Service, producer of the world's largest and most comprehensive databases of chemical information. CAS, 2540 Olentangy River Road, Columbus, OH 43202, 1-800-753-4227, http://www.cas.org/

Current Contents and *Science Citation Index*, published by the Institute for Scientific Information (ISI), producer of databases of scholarly research information. ISI, 3501 Market Street, Philadelphia, PA 19104, 1-800-336-4474, http://www.isinet.com/

Excerpta Botanica. Sectio A, Taxonomica et Chorologica, an annotated bibliography of periodical literature. International Association for Plant Taxonomy. G. Fischer Verlag, Stuttgart, New York.

GlobalHerb Software, Natural Medicine Computer Software, http://www.chiron-h.com/globalherb/

The Herb Research Foundation, a nonprofit research and educational organization focusing on herbs and medicinal plants. Library includes 150,000 scientific articles, up-to-date information on thousands of herbs, thorough files on traditional use of herbs and historical information. Herb Research Foundation, 1007 Pearl St., Suite 200, Boulder, CO 80302, 1-800-748-2617, http://www.herbs.org/

MEDLINE, MEDLARS, National Library of Medicine, index system of medical bibliographies. For access and information about these and other NLM databases, visit http://www.nlm.nih.gov/

IPA (International Pharmaceutical Abstracts), the American Society of Health-System Pharmacists, 7272 Wisconsin Ave., Bethesda, MD 20814, 301-657-3000, http://info.cas.org/ONLINE/DBSS/ipass.html. Database contains international coverage of pharmacy and health-related literature.

Herbal newsgroup: http://metalab.unc.edu/herbmed/

NAPRALERT (Natural PRoducts ALERT) file contains bibliographic and factual data on natural products from 1650 to the present. Updated monthly. Scientific and Technical Information Network (STN), c/o Chemical Abstracts Service, P.O. Box 3012, Columbus, OH 43210, 614-447-3600, http://stneasy.cas.org.

NAPRONET, an electronic scientific forum to discuss the chemistry and biology of natural products. For more information: http://chemistry.gsu.edu/post_docs/koenwnaprone.html

Lynn Index, a bibliography of phytochemistry, Massachusetts College of Pharmacy.

Medicinal and Aromatic Plants Abstracts, Publications and Information Directorate, Council of Scientific and Industrial Research (CSIR), New Delhi, India.

Poisindex System, identifies ingredients for hundreds of thousands of commercial, pharmaceutical, and biological substances. For information, MICROINDEX, 800-525-9038, info@mdx.com or http://www.microdex.com/po-pdx.htm.

Toxicology Information Response Center (TIRC), an information center offering direct access to virtually all of the world's scientific and technical databases. Toxicology and Risk Assessment (TARA) section of the Life Sciences Division (LSD) of the Oak Ridge National Laboratory (ORNL), 1060 Commerce Park, MS 6480, Oak Ridge, TN 37830, 423-576-1746, http://www.ornl.gov/TechResources/tirc/hmepg.html.

TOXLINE, the National Library of Medicine's extensive collection of online bibliographic information covering the biochemical, pharmacological, physiological, and toxicological effects of drugs and other chemicals. Available free of charge at: http://igm.nlm.nih.gov.

THERAPEUTIC INDEX

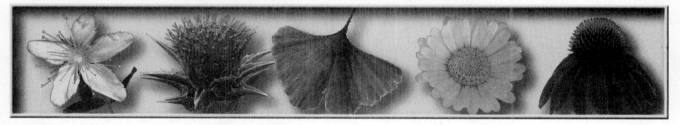

Therapeutic Uses Index

The Therapeutic Uses Index cross references the multiple applications noted within *The Review of Natural Products* monographs, which are presented alphabetically. The information contained in this index is intended to be a starting point when seeking information about natural products. It is imperative to read the entire monograph before advising patients on taking any phytomedicinal or herb. Urge patients to consult a qualified medical professional for serious or long-term problems.

The Therapeutic Uses Index entries are presented alphabetically. Boldface entries refer to the condition, followed by the monograph name in which the condition is discussed. The distinction between current and folkloric uses is designated by the following key:

> C – Clinical (Physiologic effects in humans and animals. Includes data from clinical studies. Information will be found within the pharmacology section of each monograph.)
>
> V – In vivo/In vitro (Preliminary studies show in vivo or in vitro action. Information will be found within the pharmacology section of each monograph.)
>
> H – Historic/Folkloric (Reviews the historical and folk uses of the topic. Information will be found within the history section of each monograph.)
>
> M – Multiple (Application of topic noted in more than one category within the monograph. Example: In the Echinacea monograph, the immunostimulant properties of echinacea are cited as a folkloric application, a clinical use, and in studies in vivo/in vitro.)

Please remember the uses cited in this index are not FDA-approved uses. In addition, listing of potential uses are not endorsements or recommendations of Facts and Comparisons®. As a health care professional, use your own judgment when dispensing advice.

Abdominal pain, see
Allspice, H
Betony, H
Chaparral, H
Lemongrass, H
Pennyroyal, H
Peppermint, C
Poppy, C
Rue, H
Abdominal tumors, see
Devil's Dung, H
Abdominal wounds, after Caesarean section, see
Honey, C
Abortifacient, see
Chinese Cucumber, M
Dong Quai, C
Laminaria, C
Nutmeg, H
Parsley, H
Pennyroyal, H
Poinsettia, H
Precatory Bean, H
Quinine, H
Rosemary, H
Rue, H
Slippery Elm, M
Abscesses, see
Gotu Kola, H
Chinese Cucumber, H
Maggots, H
Nigella Sativa, H
Slippery Elm, M
Acetylcholinesterase inhibitor,
see Calabar Bean, C
Achlorhydria, see
Wine, C
Acid-peptic disease, see
Acidophilus, V

Acne, see
Arnica, H
Asparagus, H
Fruit Acids, H
Jojoba, C
Labrador Tea, H
Lavender, H
Lemon, M
Onion, H
Soapwort, H
Tea Tree Oil, C
Willard Water, H
Acrocyanosis, see
Ginkgo, C
Adaptogenic effects, see
Eleutherococcus, C
Ginseng, H
Jiaogulan, C
Maca, C
Sarsaparilla, M
Schisandra, C
Withania, M
Adhesive, see
Karaya Gum, C
Adrenoleukodystrophy, see
Lorenzo's Oil, H
Adrenomyeloneuropathy, see
Lorenzo's Oil, H
Adsorbent, bind gastrointestinal toxins, see Kaolin, M
Afterbirth, expelling, see
Chaste Tree, H
Horseradish, H
Aging, see Ginseng
KH-3, C
Kinetin, M
Melatonin, C
Morinda, H
Nettles, H
Red Bush Tea, C
SAMe, M
Sour Cherry, C
Ubiquinone, H
Wild Yam, M

Ague, see Aletris, H
AIDS/HIV, see
Astragalus, M
Bitter Melon, M
Burdock, V
Cat's Claw, C
Chinese Cucumber, C
Gossypol, C
Hyssop, C
Nettles, V
SAMe, C
St. John's Wort, C
Albuminuria, see
Artichoke, H
Alcoholism, see
Evening Primrose Oil, C
Kudzu, H
Allergies, see
Bee Venom, C
Devil's Claw, H
Dong Quai, M
Eyebright, H
Methylsulfonylmethane, M
Milk Thistle, C
Nettles, C
Nigella Sativa, C
Perilla, C
Uva Ursi, C
Alzheimer's disease, see
SAMe, C
Amebicide, see Ipecac, C
AMP intracellular concentrations, see
Hawthorn, C
Amyloidosis, adjunctive treatment, see
Autumn Crocus, H
Amyotropic lateral sclerosis,
see Octacosanol, C
Anabolic effects, see
Bovine Colostrum, C
Anal fissures, see
Plantain, C
Analeptic, see Maté, H

Analgesic, see
Angelica, C
Arnica, H
Bitter Melon, C
Brahmi, C
Butterbur, M
Castor, C
Clove, H
Dong Quai, M
Gelsemium, H
Ginseng, C
Green Tea, M
Lemongrass, H
Lettuce Opium, H
Meadowsweet, M
Muira Puama, C
Passion Flower, H
Poppy, C
Precatory Bean, C
Quinine, C
Rosemary, V
Sour Cherry, M
Turmeric, H
Veratrum, M
Willow Bark, M
Wintergreen, M
Anemia, see
Anise, C
Artichoke, H
Bee Pollen, C
Fo-Ti, C
Parsley, H
Taheebo, H
Anesthetic, see
Allspice, C
Barberry, C
Cat's Claw, C
Corn Cockle, H
Kava, C
KH-3, H
Propolis, H

Angina, see
Ammi, C
Hawthorn, H
Musk, C
Yohimbe, H
Anorexia, see
Ginger, C
Quassia, H
Anthelmintic, see
Alpinia, C
Aspidium, M
Boldo, M
Brahmi, C
Carrot Oil, H
Catnip, H
Cat's Claw, H
Chamomile, H
Citronella Oil, H
Clove, C
Corn Cockle, H
Cucurbita, M
False Unicorn, H
Horehound, H
Horseradish, H
Indigo, H
Levant Berry, H
Morinda, V
Neem, H
Nigella Sativa, H
Papaya, H
Peru Balsam, H
Pineapple, C
Podophyllum, H
Quassia, H
Rue, H
Sarsaparilla, M
Storax, H
Tansy, H
Terminalia, C
Wormwood, H
Antiandrogenic, see
Saw Palmetto, C
Antiaphrodisiac, male, see
Maca, H
Savory, H
Antibacterial, see
Aconite, C
Aloe, C
Althea, C
Apple, V
Barberry, C
Boron, C
Buchu, C
Calendula, V
Chamomile, H
Citronella Oil, V
Clove, C
Coltsfoot, M
Cranberry, C
Cumin, V
Feverfew, V
Garlic, M
Ginger, M
Hibiscus, V
Honey, C
Lemon, M
Lemon Verbena, C
Lemongrass, C
Linden, V

Mace, H
Mastic, C
Musk, C
Neem, V
Parsley, V
Passion Flower, C
Peppermint, V
Propolis, M
Quassia, M
Quinine, V
Rue, V
Savory, C
Schisandra, C
Scullcap, V
Shark Derivatives, C
St. John's Wort, V
Stevia, M
Storax, C
Tansy, V
Tea Tree Oil, C
Turmeric, C
Turpentine, V
Woodruff, Sweet, C
Yellow Root, C
Yogurt, M
Antibiotic, see
Goldenseal, C
Lemon Verbena, V
Propolis, V
Sarsaparilla, M
Yarrow, C
Anticholinergic, see
Corkwood Tree, C
Anticoagulant, see
Dong Quai, C
Laminaria, C
Antidermatophytic, see
Clove, C
Antidiuretic, see Savory, C
Antidote, emergency, see
Charcoal, C
Antidote, poisonous herbs,
mushrooms, snakebites,
see Fennel, H
Senega Root, H
Antifungal, see
Aconite, C
Allspice, V
Alpinia, C
Angelica, C
Boron, C
Carrot Oil, C
Celery, V
Cinnamon, H
Clove, C
Garlic, V
Ginger, C
Lemon, M
Lemongrass, C
Mace, H
Mastic, C
Methylsulfonylmethane, M
Onion, C
Parsley, V
Propolis, M
Quassia, M
Rue, V
Sassafras, V
Savory, C

Scullcap, V
Shark Derivatives, C
Terminalia, C
Antigonadotropic, see
Comfrey, C
Antihepatotoxic, see
Elderberry, C
Turmeric, C
Antihistamine, see
Clove, C
Eleutherococcus, C
Musk, C
Anti-infective, see
Echinacea, H
Anti-inflammatory, see
Alchemilla, H
Aloe, C
Althea, C
Angelica, C
Astragalus, C
Bitter Melon, C
Bupleurum, C
Butcher's Broom, M
Butterbur, M
Calendula, H
Cat's Claw, H
Chamomile, H
Chestnut, C
Chicory, C
Clematis, C
Coltsfoot, M
Comfrey, C
Devil's Claw, C
Dong Quai, C
Emblica, C
Eyebright, H
Evening Primrose Oil, C
Ginger, C
Guggul, V
Indigo, H
Juniper, C
Larch, C
Lemon Balm, M
Mace, H
Marijuana, H
Meadowsweet, M
Milk Thistle, C
Musk, C
Neem, C
New Zealand Green-Lipped
Mussel, H
Nigella Sativa, M
Onion, H
Passion Flower, H
Pineapple, M
Plantain, H
Prickly Pear, C
Propolis, M
Pycnogenol, M
Sarsaparilla, M
Saw Palmetto, C
Scullcap, C
SOD, C
Sour Cherry, C
St. John's Wort, M
Veratrum, M
Willow Bark, C
Withania, M
Woodruff, Sweet, C

Antilactogen, see Celery, C
Antimicrobial, see
Agropyron, C
Aloe, C
Ammi, C
Anise, C
Australian Tea Tree, C
Bitter Melon, M
Black Cohosh, V
Blue Cohosh, C
Burdock, C
Cinnamon, H
Eleutherococcus, C
Emblica, C
Green Tea, M
Hops, C
Lemon, M
Lemongrass, C
Lentinan, C
Mace, H
Methylsulfonylmethane, M
Myrrh, V
Neem, C
Nigella Sativa, M
Olive Leaf, M
Olive Oil, C
Onion, C
Parsley, H
Passion Flower, C
Pawpaw, M
Propolis, C
Royal Jelly, C
Rue, C
Sage, C
Sassafras, V
Taheebo, C
Tea Tree Oil, C
Terminalia, C
Uva Ursi, M
Yogurt, C
Antimutagenic, see
Ammi, C
Chicory, V
Ginger, C
Green Tea, M
Lemongrass, C
Sarsaparilla, M
Antineoplastic, see
Autumn Crocus, V
Boneset, C
Boron, C
Chaparral, H
Goldenseal, C
Mistletoe, V
Periwinkle, C
Saffron, C
Sassafras, C
Tanning Tablets, C
Yarrow, C
Yellow Dock, C
Yew, C
Yogurt, C

Antioxidant, see
Alchemilla, C
Allspice, C
Artichoke, C
Astragalus, C
Bilberry Fruit, C
Chaparral, C
Cocoa, C
Cumin, C
Garlic, C
Ginger, C
Green Tea, M
Jiaogulan, C
Jojoba, C
Lemon, M
Lemongrass, C
Lycopene, M
Mastic, C
Melatonin, C
Milk Thistle, C
Olive Leaf, M
Onion, C
Propolis, M
Red Bush Tea, V
Rosemary, C
Sage, C
Sour Cherry, M
Turmeric, C
Ubiquinone, C
Willard Water, H
Wine, C

Antiprotozoal, see
Shark Derivatives, C
Taheebo, C

Antipsychotic, see Ginseng, C

Antipyretic, see
Ackee, H
Aconite, H
Arnica, H
Apple, H
Barberry, H
Bayberry, C
Boneset, H
Bupleurum, H
Burdock, C
Butterbur, M
Calamus, H
Calendula, H
Catnip, C
Chamomile, H
Chinese Cucumber, H
Clematis, H
Clove, C
Cranberry, H
Devil's Club, H
Ephedras, H
Feverfew, H
Fo-Ti, C
Gotu Kola, H
Holly, H
Indigo, H
Lemon, M
Lemon Balm, H
Lemon Verbena, H
Lemongrass, H
Lettuce Opium, H
Marijuana, H
Meadowsweet, M
Poinsettia, H

Quassia, H
Quinine, H
Safflower, H
Sarsaparilla, M
Vanilla, H
Witch Hazel, H
Yellow Root, C
Yerba Santa, H

Antiradical properties, see
Lemongrass, C

Antisecretory, see
Althea, C
Sage, C

Antiseptic, see
Agrimony, C
Allspice, C
Buchu, H
Clove, H
Garlic, C
Goldenseal, C
Honey, H
Larch, M
Lemongrass, H
Lettuce Opium, H
Meadowsweet, M
Myrrh, H
Peppermint, H
Peru Balsam, C
Sage, H
Sandalwood, M
Storax, C
Tea Tree Oil, M
Tolu Balsam, C

Antispasmodic, see
Alchemilla, H
Aletris, H
Althea, C
Anise, C
Blue Cohosh, H
Butterbur, M
Calamus, M
Chamomile, M
Citronella Oil, H
Clove, C
Dong Quai, M
Ginger, C
Hawthorn, H
Hops, C
Lavender, H
Lemon Balm, M
Lemon Verbena, H
Lemongrass, H
Musk, C
Myrrh, H
Nettles, H
Olive Leaf, C
Peppermint, H
Perilla, H
Quinine, C
Rosemary, H
Rue, V
Sage, M
Savory, C
Tansy, M
Valerian, C
Veratrum, M
Wild Yam, H
Woodruff, Sweet, H
Yew, H

Antithrombotic activity, see
Clove, C
Garlic, C
Ginger, C
Leeches, V
Onion, C

Antitrypanosome, see
Shark Derivatives, C
Taheebo, C

Antiviral, see
Agrimony, C
Asparagus, V
Bitter Melon, M
Calendula, V
Cat's Claw, V
Cranberry, V
Lemon, M
Lemon Balm, M
Lentinan, C
Prickly Pear, C
Propolis, M
Quassia, M
Reishi Mushroom, C
St. John's Wort, C
Terminalia, C
Yucca, C

Anxiety, see
Betony, H
Ginseng, C
Kava, C
Maca, C
Passion Flower, M
Schisandra, C
St. John's Wort, H
Valerian, M
Willard Water, H
Wine, C

Aphrodisiac, see
Avocado, H
Burdock, H
Carrot Oil, H
Celery, C
Damiana, H
Devil's Dung, H
Eleutherococcus, H
Fennel, H
Gotu Kola, H
Guarana, H
Iboga, H
Maca, C
Muira Puama, H
Nutmeg, H
Parsley, H
Saffron, H
Sarsaparilla, M
Savory, H
Terminalia, H
Tonka Bean, H
Vanilla, H
Wine, C
Yohimbe, H

Aphthous ulcers, see
Yogurt, C

Appetite stimulant, see
Calamus, C
Capsicum Peppers, H
Chicory, C
Dandelion, H
False Unicorn, H
Gentian, M
Ginger, C
Hyssop, H
Lemon Verbena, H
Marijuana, H
Mustard, H
Onion, H
Quassia, H
Sarsaparilla, M
Wine, C
Yellow Root, C

Appetite suppressant, see
Fennel, H
Guarana, C
Guar Gum, C
Khat, H

Aromatherapy, see
Bayberry, M
Lavender, M
Peppermint, H
Rosemary, M
Tea Tree Oil , C

Arrhythmias, see
Betony, H
Broom, M
Chicory, C
Dichroa Root, C
Hawthorn, H
KH-3, H
Licorice, C
Passion Flower, M
Quinine, C
Ubiquinone, H

Arteriosclerosis, see
Lemon, M

Arthritis, see
Alfalfa, H
Angelica, H
Bee Venom, C
Cat's Claw, H
Catnip, C
Celery, H
Chestnut, H
Devil's Claw, H
Devil's Club, H
Ephedras, H
Feverfew, H
Gentian, H
Glucosamine, C
Guggul, H
Juniper, H
KH-3, H
Lemon, M
Meadowsweet, M
Methylsulfonylmethane, M
Morinda, M
Mustard, H
Oats, H
Parsley, H
Pokeweed, H
Potato, H
SAMe, M
Sarsaparilla, M

Sour Cherry, H
Tea Tree Oil, H
Uva Ursi, C
White Cohosh, H
Willard Water, H
Willow Bark, M
Yucca, H
Asthma, see
Agrimony, H
Alfalfa, H
Ammi, C
Anise, C
Apricot, H
Bitter Melon, H
Brahmi, H
Butterbur, M
Coltsfoot, M
Devil's Dung, H
Digitalis, H
Ephedras, H
Feverfew, H
Gelsemium, H
Ginkgo, H
Honey, C
Hyssop, H
Labrador Tea, H
Lettuce Opium, H
Marijuana, H
Mullein, H
Nettles, H
Nigella Sativa, C
Oleander, H
Onion, C
Passion Flower, M
Perilla, H
Prickly Pear, H
Reishi Mushroom, H
Sage, H
Senega Root, H
Tung Seed, H
Yerba Santa, H
Astringent, see
Agrimony, M
Alchemilla, M
Alkanna Root, H
Apricot, H
Barberry, H
Bayberry, H
Betony, H
Boron, H
Canaigre, C
Cat's Claw, H
Chamomile, H
Elderberry, H
Green Tea, M
Holly, H
Horsetail, H
Karaya Gum, H
Labrador Tea, H
Larch, M
Lemon, H
Lemongrass, H
Meadowsweet, M
Mullein, C
Myrrh, M
Neem, H
Prickly Pear, H
Raspberry, M
Rosemary, H

Sage, H
Sandalwood, H
Savory, H
Slippery Elm, M
St. John's Wort, C
Terminalia, C
Uva Ursi, C
Wintergreen, H
Witch Hazel, M
Yarrow, H
Atherosclerosis, see
Butcher's Broom, H
Eleutherococcus, H
Flax, C
Fo-Ti, C
Garlic, C
Ginseng, H
Hawthorn, H
Oats, H
Onion, C
Terminalia, C
Athlete's foot, see
Lemon, M
Tea Tree Oil, C
Attention disorders, see
Evening Primrose Oil, C
Passion Flower, H
Back pain, see
Butterbur, M
**Bacterial flora, replenishment
of normal, see**
Acidophilus, C
Baldness, see
Aloe, H
Asparagus, H
Avocado, H
Evening Primrose Oil, C
Jojoba, C
KH-3, H
Nettles, H
Parsley, H
Quinine, H
Rosemary, H
Royal Jelly, H
Saffron, C
Willard Water, H
Bed-wetting, see Damiana, H
Uva Ursi, C
Bedsores, see Beta Glycans, C
Maggots, C
Tolu Balsam, C
Bell's palsy, see
Lysine, C
Rue, C
Benget's disease, see
Autumn Crocus, H
Beriberi, see
Muira Puama, M
Bile disorders, see
Alfalfa, V
Artichoke, M
Black Culver's Root, H
Boldo, H
Butterbur, M
Dandelion, H
Fumitory, C
Ginger, C
Nettles, C
Uva Ursi, C

Bladder cancer, see
Shark Liver Oil, C
Bladder disorders, see
Acidophilus, C
Agropyron, H
Alfalfa, H
Ammi, H
Celery, H
Gotu Kola, C
Hops, H
Horsetail, H
Nettles, C
SOD, C
Tea Tree Oil, C
Uva Ursi, H
Withania, C
Bleeding, see
Agrimony, H
Ginseng, H
Peru Balsam, H
Trillium, H
Bleeding, postpartum, see
Trillium, H
Blistering agent, see
Clematis, H
Blood disorders, see
Alfalfa, M
Brahmi, C
Ginseng, H
Wine, C
Blood flow, postoperative, see
Leeches, C
Blood purifier, see
Black Culver's Root, H
Echinacea, H
Fo-Ti, C
Gymnema, C
Karaya Gum, C
Milk Thistle, M
Periwinkle, C
Sarsaparilla, M
Blood vessels, dilate see
Cat's Claw, C
Hawthorn, C
Blood volume determination,
see Chromium, C
Boils, see
Barley, H
Bitter Melon, M
Fenugreek, H
Lovage, H
Potato, H
Slippery Elm, M
Soapwort, H
Taheebo, H
Tea Tree Oil, H
**Bone destruction during sur-
gery, see**
Maggots, C
Bone formation,
see Propolis, V
Bone healing, see
Maca, C
Rose Hips, C
Bone pain, see
Cat's Claw, H
Ephedras, H
Bradykininase activity, see
Aloe, V

Brain cancer, see
Maitake, C
Brain disorders, see
Bupleurum, C
Breast cancer, see
Bloodroot, H
Green Tea, M
Maitake, C
Melatonin, M
Methylsulfonylmethane, C
Onion, C
Pawpaw, C
Soy, C
Yew, C
Breast pain, see
Evening Primrose Oil, C
Breast size, increase, see
Saw Palmetto, H
Breath sweetener, see
Mastic, H
Bronchial conditions, see
Agropyron, H
Alpinia, H
Comfrey, H
Ephedras, H
Eyebright, H
Ginkgo, C
Labrador Tea, H
Mastic, C
Passion Flower, H
Bronchitis, see
Anise, C
Barley, C
Borage, H
Chaparral, H
Coltsfoot, M
Dichroa Root, C
Ginger, C
Juniper, H
Lettuce Opium, H
Milk Thistle, H
Nigella Sativa, C
Onion, H
Quillaia, H
Slippery Elm, M
Bronchodilator, see
Barley, C
Ephedras, C
Bruising, see
Alchemilla, H
Arnica, H
Comfrey, H
Lemon, M
Mullein, H
Parsley, H
Prickly Pear, H
Slippery Elm, H
Witch Hazel, C
Yerba Santa, H
Burns, see
Aloe, C
Australian Tea Tree, H
Bitter Melon, M
Chaparral, H
Comfrey, H
Devil's Club, H
Digitalis, H
Honey, C
Maggots, H

Safflower, C
Terminalia, C
Wine, C
Yogurt, C
Cholesterol levels, increase, see
Alfalfa, M
Cholesterol synthesis, inhibit, see Oats, C
Cholinesterase inhibitor, see
Iboga, C
Choriocarcinomata, see
Chinese Cucumber, C
Chronobiotic, see
Melatonin, C
Circulation, see
Arnica, H
Barley, C
Broom, H
Butcher's Broom, H
Ginger, C
Lettuce Opium, H
Mastic, C
Monascus, H
Olive Leaf, C
Pycnogenol, H
Cirrhosis, see
Autumn Crocus, M
Milk Thistle, C
SAMe, C
SOD, C
Climacteric complaints, see
Fennel, H
CNS depressant, see
Ginseng, C
Lavender, C
Musk, C
Nettles, C
CNS stimulant, see
Clematis, C
Cocoa, C
Corkwood Tree, H
Ephedras, C
Ginseng, C
Holly, H
Levant Berry, C
Maté, C
Musk, C
Schisandra, C
Yohimbe, C
CNS toxicity, anticholinergic drugs,
see Calabar Bean, C
Coagulant, see Agrimony, H
Boneset, C
Colds, see
Ackee, H
Althea, C
Anise, C
Beta Glycans, C
Betony, H
Boldo, H
Borage, M
Bupleurum, M
Burdock, H
Catnip, H
Chaparral, H
Devil's Club, H
Echinacea, C

Ephedras, H
Eyebright, H
Flax, H
Horehound, M
Hyssop, H
Labrador Tea, H
Lavender, H
Lemon, M
Life Root, H
Meadowsweet, M
Mullein, H
Peppermint, M
Turpentine, H
White Cohosh, H
Wintergreen, H
Witch Hazel, H
Yerba Santa, H
Colic, see
Butterbur, M
Calamus, H
Catnip, M
Chamomile, H
Devil's Dung, H
Ginger, C
Horseradish, H
Hyssop, H
Melatonin, C
Nigella Sativa, C
Parsley, H
Wild Yam, H
Colitis, see
Bee Pollen, C
Cat's Claw, H
Dandelion, C
Ginseng, H
Lemongrass, H
Prickly Pear, M
Witch Hazel, C
Yucca, H
Collagen degradation, see
Pycnogenol, M
Colon cancer, see
Chicory, C
Green Tea, M
Methylsulfonylmethane, C
Pawpaw, C
Pectin, C
Colorectal cancer, see
Echinacea, C
Green Tea, M
Condylomata, see
Podophyllum, H
Congenital defects, prevent, see Eleutherococcus, C
Congestion, see
Betony, C
Broom, H
Chestnut, H
Ephedras, M
Lovage, C
Onion, H
Congestive heart failure, see
Digitalis, C
Ubiquinone, M
Conjunctive tissue protectant, see Alchemilla, C

Conjunctivitis, see
Andrachne, H
Apricot, H
Eyebright, H
Nigella Sativa, H
Peppermint, H
Periwinkle, H
Precatory Bean, H
Sassafras, C
Witch Hazel, H
Connective tissue, protectant, see
Alchemilla, C
Constipation, see
Agrimony, H
Aletris, H
Allspice, H
Aloe, M
Apple, C
Apricot, M
Asparagus, H
Bee Pollen, C
Betony, C
Bitter Melon, M
Black Culver's Root, C
Boldo, H
Boneset, C
Broom, H
Burdock, H
Butcher's Broom, H
Cascara, M
Castor, H
Chicory, C
Clematis, H
Dandelion, H
Devil's Club, H
Elderberry, H
Fenugreek, C
Flax, H
Fo-Ti, C
Fumitory, H
Glucomannan, C
Hibiscus, C
Holly, H
Karaya Gum, C
Mate, H
Nigella Sativa, C
Oats, C
Olive Oil, M
Ostrich Fern, H
Parsley, H
Pineapple, M
Plantain, M
Podophyllum, M
Pokeweed, H
Rose Hips, M
Safflower, C
Senega Root, H
Senna, M
Slippery Elm, M
Soapwort, H
Tung Seed, H
Uva Ursi, H
White Cohosh, H
Yellow Dock, H

Contraceptive, see
Asparagus, H
Bitter Melon, M
Cat's Claw, M
Chicory, C
Gossypol, M
Gotu Kola, V
Melatonin, M
Neem, C
Nigella Sativa, C
Precatory Bean, H
Quassia, C
Contraceptive, Male see
Gossypol, C
Convulsions, see
Barberry, C
Betony, H
Devil's Dung, H
Ginseng, C
Lemongrass, C
Veratrum, M
Withania, C
Cornea, post-herpetic opacities, see
Honey, C
Corns, see
Agrimony, H
Devil's Dung, H
Oleander, H
Tea Tree Oil, C
Cough, see
Acacia Gum, C
Agropyron, H
Althea, M
Apricot, H
Anise, C
Barberry, H
Betel Nut, C
Bloodroot, H
Butterbur, M
Chinese Cucumber, H
Coltsfoot, M
Devil's Club, H
Ephedras, H
Eyebright, H
Flax, H
Ginger, M
Honey, M
Horehound, M
Hyssop, H
Ipecac, H
Labrador Tea, H
Lemon Verbena, H
Lemongrass, H
Lettuce Opium, H
Marijuana, H
Meadowsweet, M
Mullein, H
Nigella Sativa, C
Peppermint, C
Poppy, V
Quillaia, H
Reishi Mushroom, H
Schisandra, H
Senega Root, M
Slippery Elm, M
Tea Tree Oil, C
Terminalia, C
Turpentine, H

White Cohosh, H
Yerba Santa, H
Counterirritant, topical, see
Arnica, M
Betel Nut, C
Clove, H
Mustard, H
Turpentine, M
Wintergreen, C
Crohn's disease, see
Evening Primrose Oil, C
Croup, see
Devil's Dung, H
Mullein, H
Cystitis, see
Acidophilus, C
Chamomile, H
Hops, H
Larch, M
Olive Leaf, M
Slippery Elm, M
Tea Tree Oil, C
Uva Ursi, H
Cytomegalovirus inhibitor, see
Nettles, V
Cytoprotective effects, see
Mastic, C
Dandruff, see
Burdock, C
Marijuana, H
Quillaia, H
Squill, H
Deafness, see Garlic, H
Dementia, see
Calabar Bean, C
Ginseng, H
Jiaogulan, C
KH-3, H
SAMe, C
Demulcent, see
Acacia Gum, C
Althea, C
Chickweed, H
Flax, H
Hyssop, C
Mullein, C
Olive Oil, M
Slippery Elm, H
Tragacanth, C
Dengue fever, see
Boneset, H
Dental analgesic, see
Bloodroot, M
Dental caries prevention, see
Grape Seed, C
Green Tea, M
Vanilla, H
Dental disorders, see
Anise, H
Asparagus, H
Betony, H
Clove, C
Nigella Sativa, H
Peppermint, H
Peru Balsam, C
Propolis, C
Turpentine, H
Yarrow, H

Dentifrice, see
Apple, H
Neem, H
Tea Tree Oil, H
Yellow Dock, H
Deodorant, see
Chamomile, H
Depilatory, see Poinsettia, H
Depression, see
Borage, H
Juniper, C
KH-3, C
Khat, H
Melatonin, C
Milk Thistle, H
SAMe, M
Schisandra, H
St. John's Wort, M
Valerian, M
Dermatitis, see
Aloe, C
Althea, C
Ammi, C
Autumn Crocus, H
Evening Primrose Oil, C
Feverfew, H
Uva Ursi, C
Diabetes, see
Alfalfa, H
Ammi, H
Apple, H
Astragalus, H
Barley, C
Bitter Melon, M
Buchu, H
Carrot Oil, H
Chicory, C
Chinese Cucumber, H
Dandelion, H
Eleutherococcus, H
Emblica, H
Evening Primrose Oil, C
Fenugreek, H
Ginseng, H
Guar Gum, C
Gymnema, M
Karaya Gum, C
Lavender, H
Maitake, C
Milk Thistle, C
Morinda, H
Neem, H
Nettles, H
Onion, H
Periwinkle, M
Prickly Pear, C
Savory, C
Senega Root, M
Stevia, M
Taheebo, H
Tragacanth, C
Ubiquinone, C
Uva Ursi, C
Yellow Root, H
Diabetic retinopathy, see
Bilberry Fruit, H
Bitter Melon, C

Diaphoretic, see
Angelica, H
Bupleurum, H
Burdock, M
Catnip, M
Ephedras, H
Horehound, H
Lemon, H
Lemon Balm, H
Rosemary, H
Saffron, H
Senega Root, H
Wormwood, H
Diarrhea, see
Acidophilus, M
Agropyron, C
Alchemilla, M
Aletris, H
Allspice, H
Apple, C
Avocado, H
Barberry, C
Bayberry, H
Betony, M
Bilberry Fruit, M
Black Culver's Root, C
Bovine Colostrum, C
Cat's Claw, H
Chamomile, C
Chicory, C
Emblica, C
Fenugreek, C
Gentian, H
Honey, C
Kaolin, M
Labrador Tea, H
Lemon, M
Linden, H
Mace, H
Meadowsweet, M
Nigella Sativa, C
Nutmeg, C
Pectin, H
Poppy, C
Prickly Pear, M
Quassia, H
Raspberry, H
Sage, H
Savory, M
Schisandra, H
Storax, H
Tragacanth, C
Witch Hazel, C
Digestive aid, see
Alchemilla, H
Artichoke, M
Bitter Melon, M
Betel Nut, C
Betony, C
Black Culver's Root, C
Boldo, H
Calamus, M
Capsicum Peppers, H
Catnip, M
Chamomile, H
Gentian, H
Ginkgo, H
Green Tea, M
Lemon Verbena, H

Meadowsweet, M
Morinda, C
Nigella Sativa, M
Onion, H
Papaya, M
Sage, H
Sarsaparilla, H
Terminalia, H
Yellow Root, C
Wintergreen, C
Diphtheria, see Broom, H
Disease resistance, in salmon, see Beta Glycans, H
Disinfectant, see
Boron, C
Soapwort, H
Diuretic, see
Agrimony, H
Agropyron, H
Alchemilla, H
Alpinia, C
Ammi, H
Angelica, H
Anise, H
Artichoke, M
Asparagus, H
Astragalus, C
Bittersweet Nightshade, H
Boldo, H
Boneset, C
Borage, M
Brahmi, H
Broom, M
Buchu, H
Burdock, M
Butcher's Broom, H
Calamus, H
Carrot Oil, H
Catnip, M
Cat's Claw, C
Celery, H
Citronella Oil, H
Clematis, H
Cocoa, C
Corn Cockle, H
Dandelion, M
Devil's Dung, H
Digitalis, H
Elderberry, H
Ephedras, M
False Unicorn, H
Fumitory, H
Ginger, M
Goldenseal, H
Green Tea, M
Herbal Diuretics
Hibiscus, H
Holly, H
Hops, H
Horehound, H
Horseradish, H
Horsetail, M
Juniper, M
Larch, M
Lavender, H
Lemon, H
Licorice, H
Lovage, H

Gingivitis, see
Lemon, M
Neem, C
Glaucoma, see
Betel Nut, C
Calabar Bean, C
Marijuana, C
Glycolysis, accelerate, see
Ginseng, C
Gonorrhea, see
Ambrette, H
Autumn Crocus, H
Boldo, H
Cat's Claw, M
Gout, see
Agropyron, H
Autumn Crocus, M
Boldo, H
Burdock, H
Carrot Oil, H
Goldenseal, H
Labrador Tea, H
Larch, C
Lemon, M
Mullein, H
Sarsaparilla, M
Sassafras, C
Senega Root, H
Slippery Elm, M
Sour Cherry, H
Veratrum, H
White Hellebore, H
Graves' disease, see
Lemon Balm, M
Gum inflammation, see
Lemon, M
Neem, C
Witch Hazel, C
Gums, gargle for, see
Betony, C
Lemon, H
Terminalia, C
Gynecologic disorders, see
Bupleurum, M
Dong Quai, H
Gotu Kola, C
Life Root, H
Hair preparations, see
Squill, H
Nettles, H
Hallucinogen, see
Catnip, H
Iboga, H
Nutmeg, H
Yohimbe, H
Hand cleanser, see
Grape Seed, C
Hand pain, see
Labrador Tea, H
Headache, see
Betony, M
Butterbur, M
Celery, H
Damiana, H
Devil's Claw, H
Ephedras, H
Evening Primrose Oil, C
Eyebright, H
Feverfew, M

Green Tea, M
Labrador Tea, H
Lavender, H
Lemongrass, H
Linden, H
Melatonin, C
Morinda, C
Nigella Sativa, M
Rue, H
SAMe, M
Sandalwood, H
Veratrum, M
Willow Bark, M
Yucca, H
Healing agent, see
Honey, H
Morinda, H
St. John's Wort, H
Yarrow, M
Heart disease, see
Apple, H
Carrot Oil, H
Cocoa, C
Digitalis, C
Eleutherococcus, C
Emblica, C
Evening Primrose Oil, C
Green Tea, M
Guggul, V
Hawthorn, M
Holly, H
Jiaogulan, C
Lemon, M
Lycopene, M
Morinda, C
Olive Oil, M
Onion, C
Rue, C
SOD, C
Sour Cherry, C
Terminalia, H
Ubiquinone, H
Wine, C
Heart rate, lower, see
Cat's Claw, C
Hemorrhage, see
Apricot, H
Chaste tree, H
Life Root, H
Milk Thistle, H
Periwinkle, H
Turmeric, H
Witch Hazel, C
Hemorrhoids, see
Aloe, H
Bitter Melon, M
Black Culver's Root, C
Bupleurum, C
Catnip, C
Cat's Claw, H
Chestnut, H
Comfrey, H
Corn Cockle, H
Indigo, H
Marijuana, H
Mullein, H
Nigella Sativa, C
Passion Flower, H
Peru Balsam, C

Plantain, C
Prickly Pear, H
Quinine, M
Slippery Elm, M
St. John's Wort, H
Storax, H
Witch Hazel, M
Hepatic damage caused by psychotropic drugs, see
Milk Thistle, C
Hepatitis, see
Aloe, C
Autumn Crocus, C
Danshen, C
Green Tea, M
Ipecac, C
Larch, C
Milk Thistle, C
Reishi Mushroom, C
SAMe, C
Sarsaparilla, M
St. John's Wort, C
Turmeric, H
Herbicide, see
Lemongrass, C
Herniated lumbar interverte-bral disc, see
Papaya, C
Heroin detoxification, see
Lysine, C
Herpes simplex, see
Bitter Melon, M
Capsicum Peppers, C
Lemon, M
Lemon Balm, M
Mace, H
Nutmeg, C
Octacosanol, C
Peppermint, C
Reishi Mushroom, C
Slippery Elm, M
St. John's Wort, C
Tea Tree Oil, H
White Hellebore, H
Yogurt, C
High blood pressure, see
Barberry, H
Bitter Melon, M
Cat's Claw, C
Celery, C
Eleutherococcus, H
Evening Primrose Oil, C
Garlic, C
Gotu Kola, M
Hawthorn, H
Herbal Diuretics, C
Holly, H
Jiaogulan, C
KH-3, H
Lemongrass, H
Morinda, H
Nigella Sativa, C
Olive Leaf, C
Olive Oil, C
Passion Flower, M
Periwinkle, C
Reishi Mushroom, C
Saffron, C
Stevia, M

Ubiquinone, M
Veratrum, M
White Hellebore, M
Willard Water, H
Withania, C
Yellow Root, H
Yohimbe, C
Yucca, H
HIV/AIDS, see
Astragalus, M
Beta Glycans, C
Bitter Melon, M
Burdock, V
Calanolide A, M
Cat's Claw, C
Chinese Cucumber, V
Gossypol, C
Hyssop, C
Nettles, V
SAMe, C
St. John's Wort, C
Hives, see Catnip, H
Hodgkin's disease, see
Periwinkle, C
Human polymorphonuclear leukocyte (PMN), see
Milk Thistle, V
Hyperactivity, see
Evening Primrose Oil, C
Passion Flower, H
Hyperglycemia, see
Alfalfa, H
Ammi, H
Apple, H
Barley, C
Buchu, H
Carrot Oil, H
Chinese Cucumber, H
Dandelion, H
Eleutherococcus, C
Evening Primrose Oil, C
Fenugreek, H
Ginseng, H
Guar Gum, C
Gymnema, M
Karaya Gum, C
Lavender, H
Milk Thistle, C
Morinda, H
Neem, H
Nettles, H
Periwinkle, M
Senega Root, M
Stevia, M
Taheebo, H
Tragacanth, C
Ubiquinone, C
Uva Ursi, C
Yellow Root, H
Hyperkeratotic conditions, see
Fruit Acids, H
Hyperlipemia, see
Eleutherococcus, C
Guar Gum, C
Monascus, C
Hyperlipoproteinemia, see
Plantain, C
Hyperprolactinemia, see
Chaste Tree, C

Poison ivy, see
Jewelweed, H
Plantain, C
Soapwort, H
Poison ivy, prophylactic, see
Jewelweed, H
Poliovirus, see
Bitter Melon, M
Porphyrias, see
Tanning Tablets, C
Potassium channel blocker,
see Rue, C
Poultice, see
Devil's Club, H
Fenugreek, C
Slippery Elm, M
Turmeric, H
Premenstrual syndrome, see
Bupleurum, M
Evening Primrose Oil, C
Ginkgo, C
Kombucha, H
Preservative, see
Mastic, H
Prickly heat, see
Labrador Tea, H
Prostaglandin inhibitor, see
Alpinia, C
Feverfew, V
Juniper, V
Nutmeg, C
Prostate cancer, see
Maitake, C
Soy, C
Prostate disorders, see
Alfalfa, H
Autumn Crocus, H
Cucurbita, M
Lycopene, M
Nettles, C
Parsley, H
Saw Palmetto, M
Protein source, see
Spirulina, H
Pruritus, see
Aloe, C
Clematis, H
Labrador Tea, H
Sarsaparilla, M
White Cohosh, H
Witch Hazel, H
Yogurt, C
Pseudogout, see
Autumn Crocus, H
Psoriasis, see
Aloe, C
Ammi, C
Anise, C
Autumn Crocus, H
Bergamot Oil, C
Bitter Melon, M
Chickweed, H
Gotu Kola, C
Jojoba, C
Juniper, C
Olive Oil, M
Sarsaparilla, M
Soapwort, H

Psychoactive effects, see
Marijuana, H
Nutmeg, H
Puberty, see
Melatonin, C
Pulmonary disorders, see
Arnica, H
Labrador Tea, H
Schisandra, H
Pupil, contraction,
see Calabar Bean, C
Purgative, see
Agrimony, H
Aletris, H
Allspice, H
Aloe, M
Apple, C
Apricot, H
Asparagus, H
Bee Pollen, C
Betony, C
Boldo, H
Boneset, C
Broom, H
Burdock, H
Butcher's Broom, H
Cascara, M
Castor, H
Clematis, H
Dandelion, H
Devil's Club, H
Elderberry, H
Fenugreek, C
Flax, H
Fo-Ti, C
Fumitory, H
Glucomannan, C
Hibiscus, C
Holly, H
Karaya Gum, C
Mate, H
Oats, C
Ostrich Fern, H
Parsley, H
Pineapple, H
Plantain, M
Podophyllum, M
Pokeweed, H
Rose Hips, M
Safflower, C
Senega Root, H
Senna, M
Soapwort, H
Tung Seed, H
Uva Ursi, H
White Cohosh, H
Yellow Dock, H
Rabies, see
Lemon, M
Scullcap, H
Radiation exposure, see
Ginseng, H
Laminaria, C
Pectin, C
Shark Liver Oil, C

Radioprotective, see
Echinacea, C
Eleutherococcus, C
Reishi Mushroom, C
Shark Liver Oil, C
Rash, see
Agrimony, C
Chickweed, H
Labrador Tea, H
Prickly Pear, H
Sarsaparilla, M
Schisandra, H
Raynaud's disease,
see Ginkgo, C
Reflex responses, increase,
see Schisandra, C
Rejuvenating effect, see
Black Cohosh, C
KH-3, H
Hops, H
Respiratory disorders, see
Agropyron, C
Alpinia, H
Ambrette, H
Ammi, H
Angelica, H
Catnip, M
Chicken Soup, H
Coltsfoot, M
Comfrey, H
Echinacea, C
Ephedras, H
Eyebright, H
Gelsemium, H
Ginkgo, C
Labrador Tea, H
Larch, M
Meadowsweet, M
Mullein, H
Nigella Sativa, M
Passion Flower, H
Rose Hips, H
Schisandra, C
Slippery Elm, M
Terminalia, C
Veratrum, M
Yerba Santa, C
Respiratory function, improve,
see Ephedras, H
Restorative, see [ ]
Chicken Soup, H
Schisandra, C
Retinitis pigmentosa, see
Bilberry Fruit, H
Rheumatic disorders, see
Agropyron, H
Alpinia, H
Angelica, H
Cat's Claw, H
Chamomile, H
Ginger, C
Lemongrass, H
Scullcap, C
Turpentine, H
Willow Bark, M

Rheumatic pain, see
Chaparral, H
Chickweed, H
Lavender, H
Lemongrass, H
Rheumatism, see
Aletris, H
Alfalfa, H
Allspice, H
Asparagus, H
Autumn Crocus, H
Bittersweet Nightshade, H
Black Cohosh, H
Bloodroot, H
Blue Cohosh, H
Boldo, H
Boneset, H
Borage, H
Burdock, H
Cat's Claw, C
Celery, H
Chestnut, H
Devil's Claw, H
Dong Quai, H
Gotu Kola, H
Holly, H
Labrador Tea, H
Lemon, M
Lemongrass, H
Mace, H
Meadowsweet, M
Muira Puama, H
Mustard, H
Nettles, H
Nigella Sativa, C
Nutmeg, H
Pokeweed, H
Sarsaparilla, M
Sassafras, C
Senega Root, H
Slippery Elm, M
White Cohosh, H
Yerba Santa, H
Yew, H
Rheumatoid arthritis, see
Evening Primrose Oil, C
Lysine, C
New Zealand Green-Lipped
Mussel, H
Podophyllum, C
SOD, C
Wild Yam, H
Ringworm, see
Clove, C
Lemon, M
Pokeweed, H
Turmeric, H
Rubefacient, see
Aconite, H
Calamus, C
Capers, H
Capsicum Peppers, H
Clematis, H
Mustard, C
Pennyroyal, H
Turpentine, C
Wintergreen, H
Salivary gland atrophy, see
Evening Primrose Oil, C

Horsetail, H
Labrador Tea, H
Mullein, H
Propolis, C
Witch Hazel, H
Yerba Santa, H
Tuberculosis of the lymph glands, see Fo-Ti, C
Tumors, see
Aconite, V
Agrimony, H
Alpinia, C
Aspidium, H
Beta Glycans, C
Betony, H
Bitter Melon, M
Burdock, C
Canaigre, C
Cat's Claw, M
Chinese Cucumber, H
Clematis, H
Corn Cockle, H
Cucurbita, C
Digitalis, C
Echinacea, C
Eleutherococcus, H
Larch, C
Lemongrass, C
Lentinan, M
Maté, C
Meadowsweet, M
Nigella Sativa, C
Parsley, H
Pawpaw, M
Propolis, C
Pycnogenol, C
Quassia, C
Reishi Mushroom, V
Saffron, V
Sour Cherry, C
St. John's Wort, C
Tung Seed, H
Witch Hazel, H
Yogurt, C
Ulcerative colitis, see
Bovine Colostrum, V
Evening Primrose Oil, C
Ulcers, see
Alpinia, C
Bilberry Fruit, C
Bitter Melon, M
Black Culver's Root, C
Calendula, C
Cat's Claw, H
Clematis, H
Clove, C
Goldenseal, H
Gotu Kola, H
Honey, C
Licorice, C
Maggots, M
Mastic, C
Meadowsweet, M
Neem, H
Peru Balsam, C
Propolis, H
Raspberry, H
Slippery Elm, M
Taheebo, C

Willard Water, H
Withania, C
Yogurt, C
Ulcers, aphthous, see Yogurt, C
Ulcers, foot, see Maggots, C
Ulcers, pressure, see Maggots, C
Ulcers, venous stasis, see Maggots, C
Urethritis, see Uva Ursi, H
Uric acid levels, lower, see Oats, H
SOD, C
Urinary acidifier, see Cranberry, H
Urinary deodorant, see Cranberry, C
Urinary incontinence, see Damiana, H
Uva Ursi, C
Urinary tract antiseptic, see Kava, H
Uva Ursi, M
Urinary tract cancers, in women, see Cat's Claw, M
Urinary tract disorders, see Acidophilus, C
Agropyron, C
Ammi, H
Butterbur, M
Cranberry, C
Flax, H
Goldenseal, H
Hyssop, H
Juniper, C
Kava, H
Lettuce Opium, H
Marijuana, H
Onion, H
Slippery Elm, M
Uva Ursi, H
Wild Yam, H
Yew, H
Urination, excessive, see Chinese Cucumber, H
Urogenital disorders, see Boldo, H
Sandalwood, H
White Cohosh, H
Urolithiasis, see Burdock, C
Uterine bleeding, see Gossypol, C
Trillium, H
Uterine myoma, see Gossypol, C
Uterine pain, see Carrot Oil, H
Uterine stimulant, see Barberry, C
Blue Cohosh, H
Broom, H
Dong Quai, C
Ephedras, C
False Unicorn, H
Rue, C
Schisandra, H
Uterus, hard swellings, see Corn Cockle, H

Uterus, therapeutic radium, see Laminaria, C
UV/UVB Photodamage, see Echinacea, C
Vaccinia, see Peppermint, C
Vaginal infection, see
Acidophilus, H
Apricot, C
Australian Tea Tree, C
Terminalia, C
Yogurt, C
Varicella, see
Chaparral, H
Labrador Tea, H
Varicose veins, see
Chestnut, H
Gotu Kola, C
Lemon, M
Milk Thistle, H
Quinine, M
Witch Hazel, C
Vascular disorders, see
Arnica, H
Bilberry Fruit, C
Butcher's Broom, C
Chestnut, C
Ginkgo, C
Gotu Kola, C
Larch, C
Leeches, C
Pycnogenol, C
Witch Hazel, C
Vasodilator, see
Ammi, C
Ginkgo, C
Horehound, C
Olive Leaf, C
Vasoprotectant, see
Bilberry Fruit, C
Venereal disease, see
Clematis, H
Ephedras, H
Yellow Dock, H
Venous stasis ulcers, see
Maggots, C
Vertigo, see
Echinacea, H
Ginger, C
Gingko, C
Holly, H
Rue, H
Vesicant, see Clematis, H
Vision improvement, see
Bilberry Fruit, H
Fennel, H
Rue, H
Vitamin C source, see
Acerola, M
Rose Hips, H
Vitiligo, see
Ammi, C
Bergamot Oil, C
St. John's Wort, C
Tanning Tablets, C

Vomiting, see
Chamomile, H
Clove, H
Dichroa Root, C
Gentian, H
Ginger, M
Lemon, M
Lemongrass, H
Marijuana, C
Raspberry, H
Veratrum, M
Vomiting, induce, see
Alfalfa, C
Avocado, H
Betony, C
Black Culver's Root, H
Bloodroot, H
Blue Cohosh, H
Broom, H
Carrot Oil, H
Celery, H
Corn Cockle, H
Devil's Club, H
False Unicorn, H
Fennel, H
Holly, M
Indigo, H
Ipecac, M
Lavender, H
Mustard, H
Myrrh, H
Nutmeg, H
Pennyroyal, H
Pokeweed, H
Rosemary, H
Rue, M
Senega Root, H
Squill, H
Tansy, H
White Cohosh, H
Withania, H
Warts, see
Agrimony, H
Apple, H
Bloodroot, H
Corn Cockle, H
Lemon, M
Onion, H
Podophyllum, M
Rue, C
Weakness, see
Bee Pollen, C
Ginseng, H
Pennyroyal, H
Weight loss, see
Bee Pollen, C
Chaparral, H
Glucomannan, C
Green Tea, M
Guar Gum, C
Guarana, C
Guggul, H
Wheezing, see
Coltsfoot, H
Ephedras, H
Meadowsweet, M
Schisandra, C
Whooping cough, see
Onion, H

PRIMARY INDEX

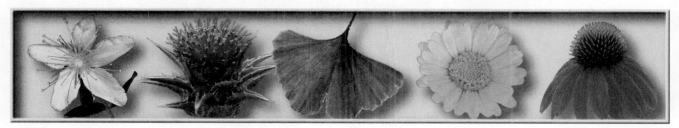

Larch, 343
Large fennel, see Fennel
Larix, see Larch
Larix dahurica, see Larch
Larix decidua, see Larch
Larix eurolepsis, see Larch
Larix gmelinii, see Larch
Larix kaempferi, see Larch
Larix laricina, see Larch
Larix leptolepsis, see Larch
Larix occidentalis, see Larch
Larix sibirica, see Larch
Larrea divaricata, see Chaparral
Larrea glutinosa, see Chaparral
Larrea tridentata, see Chaparral
Latherwort, see Soapwort
Lathyrus, 345
Lathyrus cicera, see Lathyrus
Lathyrus clymenum, see Lathyrus
Lathyrus hirsutus, see Lathyrus
Lathyrus incanus, see Lathyrus
Lathyrus odoratus, see Lathyrus
Lathyrus pusillus, see Lathyrus
Lathyrus sativus, see Lathyrus
Lathyrus sylvestris, see Lathyrus
Laurier rose, see Oleander
Laurus persea, see Avocado
Lavandin, see Lavender
Lavandula angustifolia, see Lavender
Lavendula dentata, see Lavender
Lavandula latifolia, see Lavender
Lavandula officinalis, see Lavender
Lavandula pubescens, see Lavender
Lavandula spica, see Lavender
Lavandula stoechas, see Lavender
Lavender, 347
Lavender angustifolia, see Lavender
Lavender dentata, see Lavender
Lavender latifolia, see Lavender
Lavender officinalis, see Lavender
Lavender pubescens, see Lavender
Lavender spica, see Lavender
Lavender stoechas, see Lavender
Lawn chamomile, see Chamomile
Lecithin, 350
Lecithol, see Lecithin
Ledum groenlandicum, see Labrador
  Tea
Ledum latifolium, see Labrador Tea
Ledum palustre, see Labrador Tea
Leeches, 352
Lei gong teng, see Thunder God Vine
Lei-kung t'eng, see Thunder God Vine
Lemon, 354
Lemon Balm, 356
Lemon Verbena, 358
Lemongrass, 359
Lentinan, 363
Lentinula edodes, see Lentinan
Lentinus edodes, see Lentinan

Lentisk, see Mastic
Leontodon taraxacum, see Dandelion
Leopard's bane, see Arnica
Lepidium meyenii, see Maca
Leptandra, see Black Culver's Root
Leptandra virginica, see Black Culver's
  Root
Leptandra-Wurzel, see Black Culver's
  Root
Lettuce Opium, 366
Leucanthemum parthenium, see
  Feverfew
Levant Berry, 368
Levisticum officinale, see Lovage; see
  also Herbal Diuretics
Licorice, 369; see also Herbal Diuretics
Life-giving vine of Peru, see Cat's Claw
Life Root, 371
Light kaolin, see Kaolin
Lily of the valley, see Herbal Diuretics
Lime flower, see Linden
Lime tree, see Linden
Linden, 373
Ling chih, see Reishi Mushroom
Ling zhi, see Reishi Mushroom
Linoleic acid, see Safflower
Linseed, see Flax
Lint bells, see Flax
Linum, see Flax
Linum usitatissimum, see Flax
Lion's mouth, see Digitalis
Lion's tooth, see Dandelion
Lipoic Acid, see Alpha Lipoic Acid
Lipoicin, see Alpha Lipoic Acid
Lippia citriodora, see Lemon Verbena
Liquidamber orientalis, see Storax
Liquidamber styraciflua, see Storax
Liverwort, see Agrimony
"Living antiseptic," see Maggots
Lobster flower plant, see Poinsettia
Lochnera rosea, see Periwinkle
Longwort, see Mullein
Lorenzo's Oil, 375
Louisa, see Lemon Verbena
Louisiana long pepper, see Capsicum
  Peppers
Louisiana sport pepper, see Capsicum
  Peppers
Louseberry, see Levant Berry
Lovage, 377; see also Herbal
  Diuretics
Love bean, see Precatory Bean
"Love in the mist," see Nigella Sativa
Lowbush cranberry, see Cranberry
Lucilia caesar, see Maggots
Lupanine, see Broom
Lupulin, see Hops
Lupulone, see Hops
Lycopene, 379
Lysine, 381

Ma-huang, see Ephedras
Maca, 383
Mace, 385; see also Nutmeg
Machona, see Marijuana
Macrotys actaeoides, see Black
  Cohosh
Mad-dog weed, see Scullcap
Madagascar lemongrass, see Lemon-
  grass
Madagascar periwinkle, see Periwinkle
Magdalena, see Periwinkle
Maggi plant, see Lovage
Maggots, 387
Magnesium carbonate, see Dolomite
Mahonia aquifolium, see Barberry
Maidenhair tree, see Ginkgo
Maino, see Maca
Maitake, 389
Malaleuca alternafolia, see Australian
  Tea Tree
Male fern, see Aspidium
Malic acid, see Fruit Acids
Malpighia glabra, see Acerola
Malpighia punicifolia, see Acerola
Maltose, see Barley
Malus sylvestris, see Apple
Malvaceae, see Gossypol
Manchurian "fungus," see Kombucha
Manchurian tea, see Kombucha
Mandrake, see Podophyllum
Manzanita, see Uva Ursi
Mao, see Ephedras
Mao-kon, see Ephedras
Marapuama, see Muira Puama
Margosa, see Neem
Margosan-O, see Neem
Marian thistle, see Milk Thistle
Marigold, see Calendula
Marihuana, see Marijuana
Marijuana, 391
Markweed, see Poison Ivy
Marrubiin, see Horehound
Marrubium alysson, see Horehound
Marrubium vulgare, see Horehound
Marsh tea, see Labrador Tea
Marshmallow, see Althea
Mary thistle, see Milk Thistle
Marybud, see Calendula
Marygold, see Calendula
Maspiron, see Gamma Oryzanol
Master of the Wood, see Woodruff,
  Sweet
Mastic, 394
Mastich, see Mastic
Mastick (tree), see Mastic
Mastix, see Mastic
Maté, 396; see also Herbal
  Diuretics
Matricaria, see Feverfew
Matricaria chamomilla, see Chamomile